Functional and Occupational Performance in Older Adults

FIFTH EDITION

Functional and Occupational Performance in Older Adults

FIFTH EDITION

Bette Bonder, PhD, OTR/L, FAOTA

Professor Emerita, School of Health Sciences
Cleveland State University
Cleveland, OH

Noralyn D. Pickens, PhD, OT, FAOTA

Associate Dean for Interprofessional Education and Strategic Initiatives
College of Health Sciences and College of Nursing
Professor, Occupational Therapy
Texas Woman's University
Denton, TX

Vanina Dal Bello-Haas, PhD, Med, BSc(PT)

Associate Professor
School of Rehabilitation Science
Assistant Dean, Physiotherapy
McMaster University
Hamilton University, Ontario, Canada

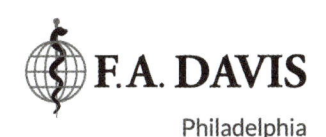

F.A. DAVIS

Philadelphia

F. A. Davis Company
1915 Arch Street
Philadelphia, PA 19103
www.fadavis.com

Copyright © 2024 by F. A. Davis Company

Copyright © 2024 by F. A. Davis Company. All rights reserved. This product is protected by copyright. No part of it may be reproduced, stored in a retrieval system, or transmitted in any form or by any means, electronic, mechanical, photocopying, recording, or otherwise, without written permission from the publisher.

Printed in the United States of America

Last digit indicates print number: 10 9 8 7 6 5 4 3 2 1

Editor-in-Chief: Margaret M. Biblis
Publisher: Christa A. Fratantoro
Director of Content Development: George W. Lang
Developmental Editor: Patricia Gillivan
Content Project Manager: Elizabeth Stepchin
Art and Design Manager: Carolyn O'Brien

As new scientific information becomes available through basic and clinical research, recommended treatments and drug therapies undergo changes. The author(s) and publisher have done everything possible to make this book accurate, up to date, and in accord with accepted standards at the time of publication. The author(s), editors, and publisher are not responsible for errors or omissions or for consequences from application of the book, and make no warranty, expressed or implied, in regard to the contents of the book. Any practice described in this book should be applied by the reader in accordance with professional standards of care used in regard to the unique circumstances that may apply in each situation. The reader is advised always to check product information (package inserts) for changes and new information regarding dose and contraindications before administering any drug. Caution is especially urged when using new or infrequently ordered drugs.

Library of Congress Cataloging-in-Publication Data

Names: Pickens, Noralyn D., editor. | Bonder, Bette, editor. | Dal Bello-Haas, Vanina, editor.
Title: Functional and occupational performance in older adults / [edited by] Noralyn D. Pickens, Bette Bonder, Vanina Dal Bello-Haas.
Other titles: Functional performance in older adults.
Description: Fifth edition. | Philadelphia : F. A. Davis Company, [2024] | Preceded by Functional performance in older adults / [edited by] Bette R. Bonder, Vanina Dal Bello-Haas. Fourth edition. [2018]. | Includes bibliographical references and index.
Identifiers: LCCN 2023045463 (print) | LCCN 2023045464 (ebook) | ISBN 9781719647908 (hardback) | ISBN 9781719651530 (epub) | ISBN 9781719651547 (pdf)
Subjects: MESH: Aging—physiology | Health Services for the Aged | Occupational Therapy | Healthy Aging | Activities of Daily Living | Aged
Classification: LCC QP86 (print) | LCC QP86 (ebook) | NLM WT 104 | DDC 612.6/7—dc23/eng/20231108
LC record available at https://lccn.loc.gov/2023045463
LC ebook record available at https://lccn.loc.gov/2023045464

Authorization to photocopy items for internal or personal use, or the internal or personal use of specific clients, is granted by F. A. Davis Company for users registered with the Copyright Clearance Center (CCC) Transactional Reporting Service, provided that the fee of $.25 per copy is paid directly to CCC, 222 Rosewood Drive, Danvers, MA 01923. For those organizations that have been granted a photocopy license by CCC, a separate system of payment has been arranged. The fee code for users of the Transactional Reporting Service is: 978-1-7196-4790-8/24 0 + $.25.

For our older family, friends, and clients, who are models of living occupationally rich lives.

—*NP and BRB*

PREFACE

It is hard to believe that 30 years have passed since the first edition of this volume was published in 1994. It has been a fascinating process analyzing the situation in 2023 and comparing it to years past, and it is heartening to see the many ways in which older adults around the world have seen improvements in their circumstances. It has also been sobering to consider the ongoing challenges for older adults, including the vast impact of the COVID-19 pandemic.

Updating and expanding the text has taken on personal immediacy over the years as some of us ourselves are reaching old age. We have taken care of—and in some instances lost—older loved ones. We have adjusted to changes in our physical capacities, activities, social networks, and living situations. As is true for all older adults, these changes have tested our adaptive capacities and required flexibility and, often, courage. Thus, the material in this book has increasing salience in our own lives. This has encouraged us to be ever more mindful of reflecting not only the facts associated with aging but also the emotional realities of the experience.

One bit of evidence about the realities of the aging experience is the changing of the guard as a new editor takes the helm. The teamwork required to ensure a smooth transition is itself a demonstration of ways in which adaptation is required as we age.

Those of you who have read previous editions will note that the content has been dramatically reconfigured. We have tried to ensure a comprehensive picture of aging. We are well aware that this is not really possible in a single volume; even if we could do so, it would be a snapshot in time. Writing and publishing a text of this scope takes time, and science and reality march on in the meantime. We hope readers will check the literature regularly to see what has happened since this book was written and will actively use the online resources. We made a concerted effort to address interprofessional practice as this edition has limited its main focus to occupational therapy. Interprofessional collaboration is more vital than ever and in the best interests of clients.

We hope you will find the new content and features of this book helpful and engaging, and that the updated material is worthy of your time and helpful in your professional and personal lives.

ACKNOWLEDGMENTS

This edition is a reconceptualization of Functional Performance in Older Adults. It has been a labor of love for many people who have been instrumental in making it the best book it could possibly be. Dr. Bonder is particularly appreciative of the excellent new editor and section editors who have made the process a smooth one and ensured a high quality outcome. She has been actively involved in the project, and grateful to know that this and subsequent editions are in good hands.

Dr. Pickens thanks Dr. Marsha Neville and Dr. Jenny Martinez, section editors, for their thoughtful work, and our many excellent authors for their important contributions. We also thank our reviewers, who offered helpful observations that have greatly improved the final product. We appreciate the input from our students over the years, and we are deeply grateful to the many clients who have enabled us to learn from their experiences. We are deeply grateful to Katie Shepard, OTD, OTR, and Christine Haines, PhD, OTR, who as graduate assistants provided editorial assistance to Dr. Pickens throughout this project. Their insights and organizational skills were essential this project.

We thank F. A. Davis for its continuing support and confidence in this project. In particular, Christa Fratantoro, Pat Gillivan, George Lang, Elizabeth Stepchin, Michael Kern, and Paul Marino. Our sincere apologies if we left anyone off this list; many F. A. Davis staff work hard and effectively behind the scenes.

As always, we thank our families. The process of bringing this edition to completion has been a long term, and at times intensive, effort, and they have not only provided helpful input, but have handled household chores and soloed countless weekends during the process.

CONTRIBUTORS

Samantha M. Barefoot, OTD, MOT, OTR/L, BCPR
Assistant Clinical Professor and Curriculum Coordinator
Bowling Green State University
Bowling Green, OH

Leslie E. Bennett, OTD, OTR/L
Associate Professor-Academic Fieldwork Coordinator
Russell Sage College
Troy, NY

Megan Bewernitz, PhD, OTR/L, ECHM
Associate Professor
Jacksonville University
Jacksonville, FL

Sarah E. Blaylock, PhD, OTR/L
Assistant Professor
Hawai'i Pacific University
Honolulu, HI

Patricia Bowyer, EdD, MS, OTR, FAOTA, SFHEA
Professor
Dr. Sophie Lin Rydin School of Occupational Therapy
Texas Woman's University
Houston, TX

Carly Braun, MS, OTR/L
Occupational Therapist
Cardinal Hill Rehabilitation Hospital
Lexington, KY

Brent Braveman, PhD, OTR, FAOTA
Director
Rehabilitation Services
M. D. Anderson Cancer Center
Houston, TX

Cara L. Brown, PhD, OTReg(MB)
Assistant Professor
Department of Occupational Therapy
Rady Faculty of Health Sciences
Winnipeg, Manitoba, Canada

Suzanne Perea Burns, PhD, OTR/L
Associate Professor
Division of Occupational Therapy
University of New Mexico
Albuquerque, NM

Marianne Capps, OTD, OTR/L
Occupational Therapist
University of Virginia Health System
Charlottesville, VA

Kelly Casey, OTD, OTR/L, BCPR, ATP, CPAM
Rehabilitation Therapy Manager
Department of Physical Medicine and Rehabilitation
Johns Hopkins Hospital
Baltimore, MD

Monique Chabot, OTD, OTR/L, SCEM, CLIPP, CAPS
Associate Professor
Occupational Therapy
Widener University
Chester, PA

Pei-Fen Chang, PhD, OTR
Professor
Dr. Sophie Lin Rydin School of Occupational Therapy
Texas Woman's University
Houston, TX

Janice Kishi Chow, PhD, DOT, OTR/L
Occupational Therapist
VA Palo Alto Health Care System
Palo Alto, CA

Brenda Fagan, MSDA, OTR/L
Program Manager
University of California San Francisco Division of Geriatrics

Beth Fields, PhD, OTR/L, BCG
Assistant Professor
Department of Kinesiology
University of Wisconsin
Madison, WI

Carol Getz Rice, PhD, OTR/L
Adjunct Professor
School of Occupational Therapy
Texas Woman's University
Denton, TX

Kristine Haertl, PhD, OTR/L, FAOTA, ACE
Professor
Department of Occupational Science and Therapy
Saint Catherine University
St. Paul, MN

Christine E. Haines, MBA, PhD, OTR/L
Occupational Therapist
Michael E. DeBakey Veterans Administration Hospital
Houston, TX

Kendra Heatwole Shank, PhD, OTR/L, CAPS
Associate Professor
Towson University
Towson, MD

Kimberly Hiroto, PhD
Clinical Psychologist
VA Palo Alto Health Care System
Palo Alto, CA

Brenda S. Howard, DHSc, OTR, FAOTA
Associate Professor
Occupational Therapy
University of Indianapolis
Indianapolis, IN

Elizabeth G. Hunter, PhD, MS, OTR/L
Affiliate Associate Professor
University of Kentucky
Lexington, KY

Vanessa D. Jewell, PhD, OTR/L, FAOTA
Associate Professor
Division of Occupational Science and Occupational Therapy
Chapel Hill, NC

Kristin Bray Jones, MS, OTD, OTR/L
Assistant Professor
Occupational Therapy Department
Dominican University of California
San Rafael, CA

Camille Ko, OTD, OTR, CBIS
Assistant Clinical Professor
Texas Woman's University
Denton, TX

Emily A. Kringle, PhD, OTR/L
Assistant Professor
School of Kinesiology
University of Minnesota
Minneapolis, MN

Christine Kroll, OTD, MS, OTR, FAOTA
Assistant Professor
University of Indianapolis
Indianapolis, IN

Karen la Cour, MSc, PhD, OT
Associate Professor
Head of Research, Occupational Science, Research Unit for User Perspectives & Community-Based Interventions, Department of Public Health
University of Southern Denmark
Odense, Denmark

Isabelle Laposha, OTD, OTR/L
Occupational Therapist
St. Louis Children's Hospital
St. Louis, MO

Line Lindahl-Jacobsen, PhD, MPH
Associate Professor
University College Absalon
Naestved, Denmark

Jennifer L. Martin, OTD, OTR, CHT, CLT
Assistant Clinical Professor
School of Occupational Therapy
Texas Woman's University
Dallas, TX

Jenny Martínez, OTD, OTR/L, BCG, FAOTA
Associate Professor
Associate Director, Clinical Research
ECOG-ACRIN Cancer Research Group
Philadelphia, PA

Michele L. McCarroll, PhD, FAACVPR, ACSM-CCEP, CCRP
Associate Professor
College of Graduate Studies
Northeast Ohio Medical University
Rootstown, OH

Keegan McKay, OTD, MOT, OTR
Assistant Professor
College of Health Sciences
University of St. Augustine for Health Sciences
Irving, TX

Chloe Muntefering, MS, OTR
Research Assistant
University of Wisconsin
Madison, WI

Katelyn Mwangi, OTD, MSOT, OTR/L
Assistant Teaching Professor
Department of Occupational Therapy
University of Missouri
Columbia, MO

Marsha Neville, PhD, OT
Professor Emeritus
Texas Woman's University School of Occupational Therapy
Dallas, TX

An T. Nguyen, OTD, OTR/L
Project Scientist
Cedars-Sinai Medical Center
Los Angeles, CA

Marc Sampedro Pilegaard, OT, MSc, PhD
Associate Professor and Senior Researcher
Department of Social Medicine and Rehabilitation, Gødstrup Hospital; DEFACTUM, Central Denmark Region and; Department of Clinical Medicine
Aarhus University
Aarhus, Denmark

Elizabeth K. Rhodus, PhD, MS, OTR/L
Assistant Professor
Department of Behavioral Science
University of Kentucky
Lexington, KY

Hillary Richardson, MOT, OTR/L, DipACLM
Practice Manager
American Occupational Therapy Association
North Bethesda, MD

Lydia Royeen, PhD, OTR/L
Assistant Professor
Midwestern University
Downers Grove, IL

Jessica Salazar Sedillo, MSW, MOT, OTR
Lecturer II
University of New Mexico
Albuquerque, NM

Stacy Smallfield, DrOT, OTR/L, BCG, FAOTA
Associate Program Director, Associate Professor, Doctoral Capstone Coordinator
Occupational Therapy Program
University of Nebraska Medical Center
Omaha, NE

Jeanine M. Stancanelli, OTD, MPH, OTR/L
Associate Professor
Department of Occupational Therapy
Mercy College
Dobbs Ferry, NY

Madison Tate, OTD, OTR/L
Occupational Therapist
Autumn Care of Mechanicsville
Richmond, VA

Patricia J. Watford, OTD, MS, OTR/L
Assistant Professor
Augusta University
Augusta, GA

REVIEWERS

Kayla Curtis Abraham, MA, OTR/L
Assistant Professor
School of Health Related Professions
University of Mississippi Medical Center
Jackson, Mississippi

Jessica Alden, OTD, OTR/L
Assistant Professor
Occupational Therapy
Howard University
Washington, District of Columbia

Sandra J. Allen, OTR, CHT, MHSc
Assistant Professor & Academic Fieldwork Coordinator
Department of Rehabilitation Sciences
Master of Occupational Therapy
Shawnee State University
Portsmouth, Ohio

Susan Coppola, OTD, OT/L, FAOTA
Clinical Professor
Division of Occupational Science and Occupational Therapy
University of North Carolina at Chapel Hill
Chapel Hill, North Carolina

Ellie Cusic, OTD, OTR/L
Assistant Professor of Occupational Therapy
Department of Occupational Therapy
College of St. Mary
Omaha, Nebraska

Sharon Glover, OTD, OTR/L
Assistant Professor
Department of Occupational Therapy
University of St. Augustine for Health Sciences
St. Augustine, Florida

Cara Lekovitch, CScD, MOT, OTR/L, BCG
Assistant Professor
Department of Occupational Therapy
University of Pittsburgh
Pittsburgh, Pennsylvania

Whitney Lucas Molitor, PhD, OTD, OTR/L, BCG
Assistant Professor, Doctoral Capstone Coordinator
Department of Occupational Therapy
University of South Dakota
Vermillion, South Dakota

Debora Oliveira, PhD, OTR/L
Professor/Program Director
Department of Occupational Therapy
Florida A&M University
Tallahassee, Florida

Christine Raber, PhD, OTR/L
Professor/Provost Fellow
Department of Rehabilitation Sciences
Shawnee State University
Portsmouth, Ohio

Nancy Schneider Smith, PT, DPT, PhD
Associate Professor
Department of Physical Therapy
Winston Salem State University
Winston Salem, North Carolina

Tonia Taylor, PhD
Professor
Department of Occupational Therapy
University of Mississippi Medical Center
Jackson, Mississippi

Jayne Marie Yatczak, PhD, OTRL
Associate Professor
Department of Occupational Therapy
Eastern Michigan University
Ypsilanti, Michigan

CONTENTS

PREFACE   vii
ACKNOWLEDGMENTS   ix
CONTRIBUTORS   xi
REVIEWERS   xv
INTRODUCTION TO THE FIFTH EDITION   xxxiii

PART I   The Context of Aging   1

1   Aging in Context   3
Noralyn D. Pickens, PhD, OT, FAOTA
Bette Bonder, PhD, OTR, FAOTA

  Context of Aging   4
    Life Expectancy   4
    Historical Roles of Older Adults   5
    Cohort Effects   5
  Factors Affecting the Experience of Aging   7
    Social Determinants of Health   7
    Physical Environment   8
    Sociocultural Factors   9
    Personal Factors   11
    Socioeconomic and Gender Factors   11
  Positive Aging   12
  Social and Occupational Justice and Aging   12
  Who ICF: A Framework for Health and Participation   13

2   Meaningful Occupations in Later Life   19
Bette Bonder, PhD, OTR, FAOTA
Noralyn D. Pickens, PhD, OT, FAOTA

  The Search for Meaning   19
  Occupation, Co-Occupation, and Meaning   21
    Themes of Meaning   21
    Spirituality and Religion as Contributors to Meaning   24
    Meaning and Identity   24
  Supporting Meaning Through the Occupational Therapy Process   25
    Theoretical Considerations in Assessment and Intervention   25
    Evaluation   26
    Intervention   26
    Individual and Cultural Considerations   28
  Occupation, Home, and Place   29

3 Theories of Aging   35
Elizabeth K. Rhodus, PhD, MS, OTR/L
Elizabeth G. Hunter, PhD, MS, OTR/L

Gerontology   36
What Do Gerontologists Want to Explain?   36
Biological Theories   36
Programmed Theories   36
Error Theories   37
Genetic Theories   37
Psychological Theories of Aging   37
Life Span Development Theory   38
Selective Optimization With Compensation Theory   38
Socioemotional Selectivity Theory   38
Personality and Aging Theories   38
Cognition and Aging Theories   38
Environmental Theories   39
Foundational Theories   39
Contemporary Theories   40
Sociological Theories of Aging   41
The Life Course Perspective   41
Social Exchange Theory   41
Social Constructionist Perspectives   41
Political Economy of Aging Perspective   41
Critical Perspectives of Aging Theories   41
Classifications and Taxonomies That Guide Practice   42
Occupation-Based Theories and Models   43
Population Health   44

4 Aging and Culture   49
Janice Kishi Chow, PhD, DOT, OTR/L
Pei-Fen Chang, PhD, OTR
Kimberly Hiroto, PhD

Defining Culture   50
Effects of Cultural Perceptions of Aging on Participation   52
Ageism   52
Intersectionality With Aging   53
Effect of Environmental Systems on Older Adult Health Outcomes   53
Access to Resources   53
Effect of Long-Term Stress Within Environmental Systems   56
Clinical Implications: Using Cultural Humility to Promote Participation   57

5 Identity, Sexuality, and Relationships   63
Jennifer L. Martin, OTD, OTR, CHT, CLT
Michele L. McCarroll, PhD, FAACVPR, ACSM-CCEP, CCRP

Social Relationships and Networks   64
Social Network Types   64
Family Constellations   65
Grandparenting   66
Widowhood   67
Gender Identity   67
Aging Concerns of LGBTQIA+ Adults   68

Isolation and Touch   69
   Isolation   69
   Touch   69
Sexuality   70
   Age Related Changes   70
Living Environment Considerations   72
Implications for Occupational Therapy Practitioners   72

6 Legal and Ethical Issues   79
Brenda Howard DHSc, OTR, FAOTA
Leslie E. Bennett, OTD, OTR/L
Christine Kroll, OTD, OTR

Introduction   79
Ethical Principles   80
Laws and Policy Affecting Older Adults   80
   Ageism and Healthcare   81
   Ethics of Billing and Productivity   82
Ethical Considerations in Advance Care Planning & End-of-Life Care   83
   What are Advance Directives?   83
   Ethical Considerations at End-of-Life   84
   What can Occupational Therapy Practitioners do?   85
Elder Abuse and Neglect   85
   Laws and Reporting   86
   Forms of Abuse and Neglect   86
   Addressing Elder Abuse   88
Unique Ethical Considerations in Later Life   89
Guide to Ethical Decision Making   90
Interprofessional Practice   91

PART II Aging: Body Structures and Body Functions   97

7 Special Concerns in Care and Prevention   99
Carol Getz Rice, PhD, OTR/L
Janice Kishi Chow, PhD, DOT, OTR/L

Introduction   99
Frailty With Aging   99
   Influencers of Frailty With Aging   100
   Assessment of Older Adult Frailty   100
   Implications for the Older Adult in Treatment: Frailty   100
Medication Management With Aging   102
   Influencers of Medication Effectiveness and Adherence With Aging   102
   Assessment of Older Adult Medication Management   103
   Implications for the Older Adult in Treatment: Medication Management   103
Oral Health With Aging   104
   Influencers of Oral Health With Aging   104
   Assessment of Older Adult Oral Health   105
   Implications for the Older Adult in Treatment: Oral Health   105
Nutrition and Hydration With Aging   105
   Influencers of Nutrition and Hydration With Aging   106
   Assessment of Older Adult Nutrition   108

Assessment of Older Adult Hydration   108

Implications for the Older Adult in Treatment: Malnutrition and Dehydration   109

Urinary Management With Aging: Urinary Tract Infection & Urinary Incontinence   109

Urinary Tract Infection   109

Urinary Incontinence   110

Falls With Aging   112

Influencers of Falls With Aging   112

Assessment of Older Adult Falls   113

Implications for the Older Adult in Treatment: Falls   116

8 Metabolic Conditions   123
Suzanne Perea Burns, PhD, OTR/L
Emily Kringle, PhD, OTR/L
Jessica Salazar Sedillo, MSW, MOT, OTR

Noncommunicable Diseases   123

Understanding the Metabolic System   125

CVD and Aging   125

Cancer and Aging   128

Pulmonary Diseases and Aging   129

Diabetes and Aging   129

Gastrointestinal Disorders and Aging   130

Theories and Practice Frameworks   130

Examples of Nonoccupation-Based Theories and Models   131

Examples of Occupation-Based Theories and Models   131

Implications for the Older Adult in Treatment   132

Nutritious Diet   132

Physical Activity and Sedentary Behavior   134

Sleep   135

Mental Health   136

Energy-Balance Behaviors: Implications for the Older Adult   136

Medication Management   137

Interprofessional Colleagues   138

Collaboration and Referrals   138

9 Cardiopulmonary and Cardiovascular Conditions   145
Samantha M. Barefoot, OTD, MOT, OTR/L, BCPR

Introduction   145

Theoretical Frameworks   146

Cardiovascular Function and Age-Related Changes   146

Electrical Behavior   146

Mechanical Behavior   146

Blood Vessels   147

Blood   147

Net Effects of Age-Related Cardiovascular Changes   147

Cardiopulmonary Function and Age-Related Changes   148

Airways   148

Lung Parenchyma   148

Alveolar Capillary Membrane   149

Chest Wall   149

Respiratory Muscles   149

Net Effect of Age-Related Cardiopulmonary Changes 149
Heart Disease 150
Major Cardiac Conditions 150
Functional Impairment Associated With Cardiovascular Conditions 152
Pulmonary Disease 153
Major Pulmonary Conditions 153
Nonsurgical Intervention 154
Surgical Intervention 154
Functional Impairment Associated With Cardiopulmonary Conditions 155
Practice Frameworks 155
Implications for the Older Adult in Treatment 156
Interprofessional Colleagues 161

10 Sensory Function and Health Conditions 165
Sarah E. Blaylock, PhD, OTR/L
Megan Bewernitz, PhD, OTR/L, ECHM

Visual System 167
Age-Related Visual System Changes 167
Major Conditions: Pathological Changes of the Visual System 169
Treatment Implications for the Older Adult With Vision Changes 171

Auditory System 173
Age-Related Auditory System and Hearing Changes 173
Major Conditions: Pathological Changes of the Auditory System 175
Auditory Implications for the Older Adult in Treatment 175
Social Consequences of Hearing Loss 175

Chemosensory System 176
Age-Related Taste and Olfactory Changes 176
Olfactory and Taste Implications for the Older Adult in Treatment 177

Somesthesis and Integumentary System 179
Age-Related Somesthesis and Integumentary System Changes 179
Temperature 179
Somesthesis and Integumentary Implications for the Older Adult in Treatment 180

Pain 180
Aging and Pain 180
Pain Implications for the Older Adult in Treatment 181
Pain Assessment 181
Pain Interventions 182

Interprofessional Practice 182

11 Musculoskeletal Function and Health Conditions 187
An T. Nguyen, OTD, OTR/L
Marianne Capps, OTD, OTR/L
Madison Tate, OTD, OTR/L

Typical Age-Related Changes in the Musculoskeletal System 188
Typical Age-Related Changes in Muscle Strength and Power 189
Typical Age-Related Changes in Muscle Structure 190
Typical Age-Related Muscle Changes and Occupational Performance 192
Typical Age-Related Changes in the Skeletal System 192
Typical Age-Related Changes in Cartilage, Joints, and Tendons 193

Atypical Age-Related Changes in the Musculoskeletal System   195
- Osteoarthritis   195
- Osteoporosis, Falls, and Fractures   197
- Amputation in Older Adults   199

Implications for Occupational Therapy Practice With Older Adults: Assessment of the Musculoskeletal System   201
- ROM and Flexibility Assessment   201
- Muscle Strength and Power Assessment   201
- Management of Musculoskeletal Impairments in Older Adults   202

12 Neuromuscular and Neuromotor Conditions   211
Cara L. Brown, PhD, OTReg(MB)
Vanina Dal Bello-Haas, PhD, Med, BSc(PT)

Typical Age-Related Changes in the Neuromotor System and Related Functions   212
- Proprioception   213
- Balance   213
- Coordination   214
- Upper Extremity Movement   215

Neuromotor Health Conditions Common in Older Adults   216
- Stroke   216
- Traumatic Brain Injury   220
- Parkinson's Disease   220

Theories and Practice Frameworks   221
- Motor Control Frame of Neurodevelopmental Theory   222
- Motor Learning Frames: Contemporary Task-Oriented Approaches   222
- Restoration Versus Adaptation   224
- Integrating Frameworks   224

Occupational Therapy Assessment and Intervention With the Older Adult With a Neuromotor Condition   224
- Assessment of Body Structures and Functions for Neuromotor Conditions   225
- Interventions for Neuromotor Conditions   227
- Assessing and Promoting Task Performance, Occupational Participation   230

Interprofessional Colleagues   231
- Physical Therapy Collaboration   232
- Speech–Language Therapy Collaboration   232
- Vision and Hearing Experts   232
- Medical Staff – Physicians and Nurses   232
- Social Worker Collaboration   232

13 Neurobehavioral Function and Health Conditions   237
Marsha Neville, PhD, OT

A Perspective on Cognition and Aging   238

Cognitive Processes and Implications for Older Adults   238
- Attention   238
- Memory   240
- Executive Functioning   240
- Intellectual Abilities   240
- Wisdom   241
- Implicit and Explicit Processing   241
- Functional Cognition   241

Cognitive Theories of Aging   243
- Speed of Processing   243
- Sensory Deficit Theory   243

Memory Deficit and Dual-Process　243
　　Structural Changes in Aging　243
　Summary of Typical Cognitive Functioning in Older Adults　243
　Neuropathologies and Impact on Cognitive Functioning in Older Adults　244
　　Delirium　244
　　Mild Cognitive Impairment　245
　　Dementia　245
　　Factors Impacting Functioning for Persons Living With Dementia　247
　　Occupational Therapy Interventions for Persons With Dementia　247
　Stroke　249
　　Occupational Therapy Assessment and Practice With Older Adults With Stroke　249
　　Interprofessional Practice With Older Adults With Stroke　250
　Mental Health Conditions　250
　　Depression　251
　　Anxiety Disorders　251
　　Schizophrenia　251
　　Bipolar Disorder　252
　　Substance Use Disorders　252
　Optimizing Cognitive Functioning in Older Adults　252
　　Cognitive and Mental Stimulation　252
　　Physical Activity and Exercise　253
　　Socialization　253
　　Occupational Therapy Interventions for Mental Health　253
　Summary of Cognitive Functioning in Persons with Neuropathologies　254
　Interprofessional Practice　254

PART III　Active Aging　261

14　Self-Care　263
Kristine Haertl, PhD, OTR/L, FAOTA, ACE

　Defining Self-Care　264
　Significance of Self-Care　265
　　Practical Importance of Self-Care: Health and Safety　266
　　Importance of Self-Care for Self-Identity and Socialization　266
　　Importance of Self-Care for Psychological Well-Being　266
　　Prevalence and Type of Limitations of ADLs Among Older Adults　266
　Impact of Health Conditions on Self-Care Performance　267
　　Stroke　267
　　Cardiovascular Disease　267
　　Neurocognitive Disorders and Cognitive Decline　267
　　Joint Inflammation and Disease　268
　　Sensory Problems　268
　Theoretical Approaches　269
　　Competence, Value, and Meaning in Self-Care　269
　Interprofessional Practice　270
　Assessments for Self-Care　270
　　Special Considerations in Evaluation of Self-Care　271
　　ADL Assessments　271
　　Assessing Environmental Factors　272

Intervention for Self-Care Activities of Daily Living 272
- Skill Training 272
- Environmental Modifications 273
- Assistive Technology Devices for Self-Care 274
- Task Modifications 274

15 Home Management 279
Elizabeth G. Hunter, PhD, MS, OTR/L
Hillary Richardson, MOT, OTR/L, DipACLM
Elizabeth K. Rhodus, PhD, MS, OTR/L
Carly Braun, MS, OTR/L

Defining Home Management 280
Impact of Health Conditions on Performance of Home Management Activities and Related IADLs 280
- Complexities of Aging: Physical, Environmental, and Social Factors 281
- Common Physical Changes Influencing Home Management and IADL Performance 282

Theoretical Approaches 282
- Environmental Press Theory 282
- Person-Environment-Occupation-Performance (PEOP) Model 283
- Task-Oriented Approach 283

Assessments for Home Management and IADLs 284
- Special Considerations in Assessment 284
- The Occupational Profile and the Canadian Occupational Performance Measure (COPM) 284
- Home Management and IADL Assessments 284
- Home Safety Assessments 284

Intervention for Home Management and IADLs 284
- Task Adaptation 286
- Energy Conservation 286
- Task-Specific Skill Training 286
- Assistive Technology 287
- Home Environmental Modification 287
- Disaster Preparedness 288
- Care Partner Training 288

16 Health Management and Sleep 293
Stacy Smallfield, DrOT, OTR/L, BCG, FAOTA
Katelyn Mwangi, OTD, MSOT, OTR/L
Isabelle Laposha, OTD, OTR/L

Defining Health 294
Health Management 294
- Social Determinants of Health 295
- Accessing and Using Health Care Services 295
- Impact of Health Conditions on Health Management 296

Sleep and Restoration 298
- Sleep in Older Adults 298

Theoretical Approaches to Successful Health Management in Older Adulthood 299
Occupational Therapy Assessment of Health Management and Sleep 299
Occupational Therapy Interventions to Address Health Management and Sleep 299
- Social and Emotional Health Promotion and Maintenance 301
- Symptom and Condition Management 302
- Communication With the Health Care System 302

Medication Management 303
Physical Activity and Fall Prevention 303
Nutrition Management 303
Personal Device Management 304
Sleep and Rest 304

17 Leisure 311
Jenny Martínez, OTD, OTR/L, BCG, FAOTA
Monique Chabot, OTD, OTR/L, SCEM, CLIPP, CAPS
Brenda Fagan, MSDA, OTR/L

Defining Leisure 311
Engagement and Leisure 312

Theoretical Approaches 313
Multi-Level Leisure Mechanisms Framework 313
Socioemotional Selectivity Theory 313
Selective Optimization With Compensation Model 313
Activity Theory 313
Continuity Theory 314
Life Course Theory 314

Impact of Environments and Health Conditions on Leisure Performance 314
The Role of Environments and Contexts on Leisure Participation 314
The Role of Disability on Leisure Participation 315
The Impact of Isolation on Leisure Participation 315

Lifelong Learning as Leisure 315
Learning Opportunities for Older Adults Internationally 316

Assessments 316
Applied Scenario 317

Exemplar Interventions 317
Skills2Care 317
Community Aging in Place—Advancing Better Living for Elders (CAPABLE) 317
Lifestyle Redesign® 317
Use of Assistive Technology to Support Leisure 318

Interprofessional Collaboration in Evaluation and Intervention 318

18 Work and Retirement 323
Brent Braveman, PhD, OTR, FAOTA
Patricia Bowyer, EdD, MS, OTR, FAOTA, SFHEA

Defining Older Workers and Retirement 324
Culture and Demographics 324
Impact of Health Conditions on Work and Retirement 325

Models of Retirement and Transition to Retirement 326
Theoretical Approaches to the Retirement Process 327
Barriers to Successful Continued Employment Faced by Older Workers 327

A Global Lens 328
Generational and Cultural Perspectives on Work and Retirement 329
Legislative and Policy Issues Around the World 329

Assessments 330
Special Considerations in Assessment 330

Exemplar Interventions 330
Ergonomic and Assistive Technologies 331
Technology and the Environment 331

19 Community Mobility and Driving   337
Kendra Heatwole Shank, PhD, OTR/L, CAPS

    Interprofessional Colleagues   331

    Volunteerism and Leisure   332

Defining Community Mobility Including Driving as an Occupation   338
- Community Mobility Options   338

Driving as an Occupation   338
- Driving and Client Factors   339
- Driving and Technology   340

Impact of Health Conditions on Community Mobility and Driving   341
- Visual Functions and Driving Performance and Safety   341
- Cognitive Functions and Driving Performance and Safety   341
- Other Medical Conditions Affecting Driving Performance and Safety   342

Occupational Therapy, Driving, and the Continuum of Care   342

Specialized Practice and the Interprofessional Team   342
- Driving Rehabilitation Specialists   343
- Certificate in Driving and Community Mobility   343
- Occupational Therapy Process and Collaboration   343

Assessment of Driving   343
- Medical and Driving History and Performance Patterns   343
- Types of Assessment and Screening   344
- Special Considerations in Assessment   345

Exemplar Interventions to Support Driving   346
- Interventions for Functional Mobility and Pain   346
- Interventions for Cognition and Perception   346
- Vehicle Modification and Technology Interventions   346
- On-Road Driving Rehabilitation Interventions   346

Driving Cessation   346
- Implications of Driving Cessation   347
- Initiating the Decision to Alter or Stop Driving   347
- Family Involvement in Driving Decisions   348

Mobility Alternatives to Driving   348
- Mobility Options Beyond Driving   348
- Envisioning Community Mobility Services and Solutions   349
- Advocacy and Education   349

20 Caregiving   355
Beth Fields, PhD, OTR/L, BCG
Chloe Muntefering, MS, OTR

Prevalence and Trends Affecting Family Caregiving   355
- Demographics and Contextual Characteristics of Family Caregivers   356
- Family Caregiving Responsibilities   356

Impact of Family Caregiving: A Public Health Issue   358

Levels of Prevention in Caregiving   359
- Example   359

Policies to Support Family Caregivers   359

Occupational Therapy's Role in Integrating Caregivers in Care   361

Exemplar Interventions   362

PART IV The Context of Service Delivery 367

21 Special Concerns Around Evaluation of the Older Adult 369
Camille Ko, OTD, OTR, CBIS
Christine E. Haines, MBA, PhD, OTR/L

Evaluating Functional and Occupational Performance 369
Defining Functional and Occupational Performance 370
Importance of Evaluating Functional and Occupational Performance 370
Purposes and Types of Assessment and Evaluation 370
Special Considerations for Choosing Assessment Tools 371
Ethical Considerations for Evaluating Older Adults 372

Models Underpinning Assessment 373

What to Assess When Focusing on Function in Older Adults 374
ADLs and IADLs 374
Functional Mobility 374
Upper-Extremity Function 375
Cognition 375
Social Participation and Leisure 376

Specific Issues Related to Evaluation of Functional Performance 376
Sensory Changes With Aging 376
Fatigue 377
Education 377
Caregiver Support 377

22 Wellness and Community-Based Services 383
Kristin Bray Jones, MS, OTD, OTR/L
Jeanine Stancanelli, OTD, OTR/L, MPH
Noralyn D. Pickens, PhD, OT, FAOTA

Community-Based Wellness Services 384
Wellness in Older Adults 384
Community-Based Wellness Services 384
Contexts of Community-Based Wellness Services 386
Service Utilization 387
Connecting Older Adults With Services 387

Role of Occupational Therapy and Interprofessional Partners 388
Occupational Therapy as Direct Care 388
Occupational Therapy as Indirect Care 389
Interprofessional Partners 389

Specific Issues for Promoting Wellness of Older Adults in Community-Based Settings 389
Social Determinants of Health 390
Health Factors 390
Psychosocial Factors 391

Intervention 391
Models to Guide Interventions 391
Program Development 392
Health Promotion, Management, and Maintenance Interventions 392
Chronic Condition Management 393
Health Education, Health Coaching, and Health Promotion 393
Lifestyle Redesign 393
Cognitive Activities 394

Social Activities 394

Physical Activity 394

Nutritional Intervention 395

Documentation, Payment Systems, and Reimbursement 396

Advocacy for Community-Based Wellness Services 396

23 Primary Care Services 401
Lydia Royeen, PhD, OTR/L

Primary Care and Primary Health Care 402

Integrating Rehabilitation Professionals and Services in Primary Care 402

Theoretical Frameworks and Approaches 403

A Conceptual Framework for Access to Healthcare 404

Conceptual Framework in Clinical Practice 404

Occupational Therapy Approach and Primary Healthcare 405

The Expanded Chronic Care Model 405

Roles for Interprofessional Partners 406

Role of Occupational Therapy 406

Interprofessional Partners 407

Integration of Occupational Therapy Within the Primary Care Team 408

Specific Issues for Working With Older Adults 408

Patient-Centeredness in Primary Care 408

Assessment and Intervention Exemplars 409

Functional Assessment 409

Cognition 409

Lifestyle Interventions 410

Health Coaching and Motivational Interviewing 410

Behavioral Health Intervention Approach 411

Chronic Disease Self-Care Management 411

Documentation, Payment Systems, and Reimbursement 412

International Reimbursement and Models 412

Advocacy for Patients and Services 412

24 Acute Care Services 419
Kelly S. Casey, OTD, OTR/L, BCPR, ATP, CPAM

The Acute Care and ICU Setting 420

Role of the Occupational Therapist and Interprofessional Partners 420

Role of Occupational Therapy in Acute Care 420

Interprofessional Integrated Care 420

Communication in the Hospital Setting 421

Occupational Therapy Evaluation in the Acute Care Hospital Setting 422

Assess Common Comorbidities Often Seen in Hospitalized Older Adults 423

Intervention Exemplars 424

Discharge Planning as Intervention 424

Early Mobility and Early Activity 424

Fall Prevention in the Hospital 425

Pain Management 425

Skin and Joint Protection 426

Addressing Visual Impairment 427

Addressing Cognitive Impairment 427

Assistive Technology: Considerations for the Older Adult in the Hospital 429

Addressing Spirituality in the Hospitalized Older Adult 429

Acute Care Documentation 429

Payment Systems and Reimbursement for Acute Care Services (US) 430

Advocacy for Patients and Occupational Therapy Services 431

25 Rehabilitation Services 435
Cara L. Brown, PhD, OTReg(MB)
Vanina Dal Bello-Haas, PhD, Med, BSc(PT)

Rehabilitation and Service Contexts 436

Rehabilitation Settings and Services 437

Role of Occupational Therapy and Interprofessional Partners 441

Interprofessional Partners 441

Specific Issues for Working With Older Adults 441

Personal Factors 441

Environmental Factors That May Influence Rehabilitation 443

Intervention Exemplars 443

Comprehensive Geriatric Assessment 443

Case Management 444

Integrated Care Models 445

Documentation, Payment Systems, and Reimbursement 445

Documentation 445

Payment Systems and Reimbursement 446

Advocacy for Older Adults and Rehabilitation Service 446

26 Home Health Services 451
Keegan McKay, OTR, MOT, OTD

Defining Home Health Services 452

The Context of Home Health 452

The Role of Occupational Therapy in Home Health 453

Interprofessional Partners 453

Physical Therapy 453

Speech Therapy 454

Skilled Nursing 454

Social Services and Home Health Aides 454

Administrative Staff 455

Home Health Agencies and Medicare 455

Criteria for Medicare Reimbursement to Home Health Agencies 456

Criteria for Coverage of Home Health Services for Medicare Beneficiaries 456

Home Health Assessment 457

Outcome and Assessment Information Set and Section GG 458

The Initial Visit and Comprehensive Assessment 458

Intervention in the Context of Home 459

Documentation and Reimbursement 460

Initial Evaluation 461

Reassessment 461

Payment Systems 461

International Home Health and Domiciliary Care 462

Advocacy in Home Health 462

27 Long-Term Care Services 467
Patricia J. Watford, OTD, MS, OTR/L
Vanessa Jewell, PhD, OTR/L, FAOTA

  Define Long-Term Care Services Context 467
    Profile of Nursing Home Residents 468
  Role of Occupational Therapy and Interprofessional Partners 469
    Interprofessional Partners 469
  Specific Issues for Working With Older Adults in Long-Term Care 471
    Intensity of Rehabilitation After Hospitalization 471
    The Value of Restorative Care 471
    Addressing Oral Hygiene 472
    Depression 472
    Dementia 472
  Occupational Therapy Evaluation and Intervention Exemplars 472
    Evaluation 472
    Intervention Exemplars 473
    Outcomes of Occupational Therapy Services in Long-Term Care 476
  Documentation, Payment Systems, and Reimbursment 477
    Payment Systems and Reimbursement 477
    State Regulations 478
    International Reimbursement and Models 478
  Advocacy for Clients and Service 478

28 Hospice and Palliative Care 483
Karen la Cour, MSc, PhD, OT
Line Lindahl-Jacobsen, PhD, MPH
Marc Sampedro Pilegaard, OT, MSc, PhD

  Hospice and Palliative Care 484
  The Role of Occupational Therapy 487
    Assessment 487
    Intervention 487
    Evaluation of Outcomes 488
  Interprofessional Partners 488
  Specific Issues for Working With Older Adults 489
  Grief and Bereavement 490
  Intervention Exemplars 491
    Hospice Day-Care Intervention 492
    Cancer Home-Life Intervention 492
    Resource-Oriented Intervention 494
  Documentation, Payment Systems, and Reimbursement 495
  Advocacy for Clients and Service 498

29 The Future of Aging 503
Noralyn D. Pickens, PhD, OT, FAOTA
Bette Bonder, PhD, OTR, FAOTA

  Demographic and Societal Trends 504
    Healthy Aging 504
    Living Arrangements 504
    Reemergence of Ageism 505
    Climate Change and Aging 505
    Aging in the Future 505

Trends in Healthcare   506
   Telehealth and Virtual Care   506
   Facilitating Transitions and Interprofessional Practices   507
   Acute Care at Home   508
   Creative Response to Staff Shortage and Funding Issues   508

Technology in Healthcare and Social Environments   509
   Health Monitoring   509
   Smart Homes   510
   Transportation   511
   Robotics   511

Caregiving in the Future   511

Implications for Occupational Therapy   512

APPENDIX A ANSWERS TO CRITICAL THINKING QUESTIONS   517

APPENDIX B INDEX OF ASSESSMENTS   527

GLOSSARY   535

INDEX   541

INTRODUCTION TO THE FIFTH EDITION

Three decades have passed since the first edition of this book was published in 1994. Since then, occupational therapy practice with older adults has grown significantly as the global population of older adults has surged. Health care systems have changed, society has changed, but occupational therapy's commitment to supporting occupationally enriched lives for older adults remains steadfast.

In western societies, health care for older adults provides an array of services for those who can afford care. In these same societies and across the globe, older adults may not have adequate health care, or even safe and stable living environments. Many continue to be marginalized and devalued. Good health is not a certainty, particularly in economically developing nations and among lower socioeconomic groups. Ensuring adequate financial and instrumental resources can be a struggle for many. There is much work for occupational therapists to do to support older adults' physical, social, emotional, and spiritual wellbeing. Part of the occupational therapist's role is to affirm the many ways in which older adults live meaningful lives and make important contributions to their families, communities, and societies.

Many readers will recognize a subtle, but important change in the title of this textbook – Functional and *Occupational* Performance in Older Adults. This edition is written solely for occupational therapy students and clinicians. There is an increased emphasis on meaning and occupation and occupational performance in context. The holistic lens of occupation is paramount.

The major organizing framework continues to be the International Classification of Function (ICF; World Health Organization, n.d.). The ICF provides structure to health care services globally as is reflected in international occupational therapy practice and it emphasizes the importance of wholistic care that integrates disciplines in tending to the needs of their clients. Beyond the title, this edition has other significant changes.

- Part I has new and reorganized chapters on culture, identity, relationships, and ethics. It puts meaning and occupation at the forefront, threaded through every chapter.
- Part II, with a focus on body structures and body functions, has the most significant change as it provides a continuum perspective on health conditions – from typical aging to illness and/or dysfunction that may emerge in later life. New to this section is a chapter on special issues, including comorbidities and falls; and a chapter on metabolic conditions. Other material has been reorganized into a chapter on neuromotor conditions and a chapter on neurocognitive conditions, both reflecting up to date understandings of neuroscience.
- Part III provides a deep dive into a range of occupations with new chapters on homemaking, sleep and self-management, and caregiving. Community mobility and driving are one chapter, also in recognition of the continuum of transportation needs and options. Rather than a separate chapter on technology, environmental modifications and assistive technologies are embedded in each chapter's exemplar interventions.
- Lastly, Part IV offers a continuum of care review, starting with an important chapter focused on evaluation with older adults, and adding a new chapter on acute care. Each chapter has an emphasis on interprofessional partners and advocating for both clients and services. The future of aging chapter bookends the early chapters in forecasting advances in healthcare, social changes, and technology.

Our intention in these changes is to address the complexity of the aging experience in the current environment and enhance occupational therapy services for older adults.

Using this Book

The changes in this fifth edition are designed to help students and instructors engage fully with the book as a whole. There are intentional areas where content is introduced and later addressed in a different context. To help readers follow these overlapping concepts, content is referenced to other chapters. The content has been significantly updated with best evidence for practice.

Each chapter begins with a mini-case study and questions intended to provoke thought while reading the materials. These same questions can be used to guide students' professional reasoning. Threaded case studies are incorporated within the chapters to encourage in-the-moment reflections on the content being read. Students and faculty are encouraged to think beyond the answers provided to additional responses to the question prompts. The reader will find that Part II case studies continue into Part IV – with the intention of helping students appreciate how occupational therapists provide services to older adults with conditions (as introduced in Part II) in different care contexts (found in Part IV).

Embedded in the chapters are boxes, figures, tables, and promoting best practice resources, designed to offer helpful strategies and insights on specific topics. Each chapter ends with critical thinking questions to help readers explore their new understandings. The author's responses to these questions are in Appendix A, thus providing the students and instructors ample space to create their own answers before considering the author's perspectives. Appendix B is an assessment table, organized by ICF factors. While the textbook chapters reference literally hundreds of assessments, the table provides information about those most relevant to older adult practice, occupation, and psychometrically best practice. This same attention is paid to the glossary terms, where terms specific to understanding the chapter content are highlighted. Additional terms are clearly defined in the chapters themselves.

For the instructors, online resources include chapter PowerPoint presentations, learning activities, a test bank, and instructor's guide. We hope that the online materials will serve as strong resources for practice and instruction.

Understanding later life and focusing on enhancing positive aging benefits not just older adults but their families, friends, communities, and society. We hope that as you read and as you move from learning to application, you will consider the ways in which this material can help you make a difference in your communities, your work, and in your own lives.

Reference

World Health Organization, (n.d.) *International classification of functioning, disability, and health (ICF)*. https://icd.who.int/dev11/l-icf/en

PART I

The Context of Aging

The number of older adults across the globe continues to grow dramatically, while the number of births, especially in northern hemisphere countries, declines (World Health Organization [WHO], 2023). This inversion has important implications for aging, society, and healthcare. The context of aging takes into consideration social policy, medical and social service access, and housing and transportation options. In addition, social shifts in embracing diversity in identity, ethnicity, family constellations, and culture influence how older adults engage in life's meaningful occupations. Recognizing these intersections of person and society, occupational therapists help older adults, their families, and communities adapt and find meaning in change.

The vast majority of older adults, even those with physical or cognitive limitations, live in the community and adapt well to the changes that are an inevitable part of aging. Many continue to participate in meaningful occupations that contribute to quality of life. Individuals find ways to manage the typical decrements in physical and cognitive skills that often occur in later life. These differences are not all negative. Individuals may have to adjust to reduced vision or hearing, but they also have life experience and knowledge that can help them cope. For example, as can be seen in this text, although older adults may learn differently from how younger people do, they are still quite capable of acquiring new skills and abilities, and through wisdom, may offer valuable insights and observations to younger people as well. It is essential to understand both the universal aspects of aging and the individual experience and how these experiences are shaped by current sociocultural and historical contexts.

Part I of this book provides an overview of the aging experience, the meanings of occupation in later life, and the social and cultural environment in which aging occurs. In addition, the section offers an introduction to biological and psychosocial theories of aging and legal and ethical considerations around aging. These chapters offer a framework in which the experience of growing old in contemporary society can be understood. To ensure the best care, providers must understand the individual, including their identity, relationships, history, needs, and wishes. It is also essential to think of the individual in context, not as separate from life experiences and community. Context includes those in the older adult's immediate surroundings: the built environment, social networks, neighborhood characteristics, and local and national policies. But they also include the more global contexts: societal attitudes toward aging, cultural values in the society, public policy affecting later life, and many other factors. This section of the book is designed to provide an understanding of the context in which aging occurs and the experiences of individuals and populations as they age.

– Noralyn Pickens, PhD, OT, FAOTA and Bette Bonder, PhD, OTR, FAOTA Part 1 Section Editors

World Health Organization. (2023). Ageing. https://www.who.int/health-topics/ageing#tab=tab_1

CHAPTER 1

Aging in Context

Noralyn D. Pickens, PhD, OT, FAOTA ■ Bette Bonder, PhD, OTR, FAOTA

> *"People tell me I look good these days. I look good because I feel good. I know people who are older than I am who are twenty-five... It's all about attitude. To me, age is just a number."*
>
> —Rita Moreno

LEARNING OUTCOMES

By the end of this chapter, readers will be able to:

1-1. Analyze demographic characteristics of older adults and their influence on global aging.
1-2. Explain how social determinants of health and public policy affect older adults.
1-3. Compare how different physical contexts influence the aging experience.
1-4. Analyze the impact of socio-cultural factors, including attitudes on the experience of aging.
1-5. Create interventions that support positive aging.
1-6. Describe social and occupational justice efforts to support the health and wellbeing of older adults.
1-7. Explain the WHO ICF model as foundational to occupational therapy practice with older adults.

Mini Case Study

Ms. Brown is a 72-year-old woman who had many jobs as an adult, from motel housekeeper to grocery clerk to school cafeteria cook. She retired from the school cafeteria at age 70, when being on her feet all day was too fatiguing. She has limited income from Social Security. She quit school at age 16 when she ran away from her abusive family home. She has always rented homes and currently lives in a home with her daughter, a granddaughter, and two great grandchildren who are in high school. Her daughter has mental health issues and receives Supplemental Security Income (SSI). Her granddaughter works in a local meat packing plant in their semirural community. Ms. Brown has diabetes, peripheral neuropathy, high blood pressure, degenerative joint disease affecting her back, and grade 1+ cataracts. She has difficulty getting to medical appointments in the larger community 40 minutes away. She reports stumbling in and around her home and has started limiting some community activities. She enjoys watching television, visiting with neighbors, and going to church services when feeling strong enough to do so.

Provocative Questions
1. What are the social determinants of health factors that influence Ms. Brown's health and wellbeing?
2. How would an occupational therapist address International Classification of Functioning, Disability, and Health (ICF) aspects of body functions and structure, activity, and participation?
3. How could Ms. Brown's environmental factors and personal factors influence the therapist's intervention plan?

This chapter provides an overview of many influences on individuals' experiences of later life. The first section explores definitions of aging and relevant demographic data followed by historical perspectives on aging. Factors that influence aging are discussed, including social determinants of health (SDOH); health literacy; and personal, environmental, and socioeconomic factors. The interrelationships among these elements and the experience of aging are examined, as are concepts of positive and successful aging. Social and occupational justice are explored, followed by an examination of the World Health Organization (WHO) International Classification of Functioning, Disability and Health (ICF) as a framework for practice.

Occupational therapists support older adults' health and participation through enabling occupations "that bring meaning, provide economic benefit and add to the cultural fabric of their communities" (World Federation of Occupational Therapists [WFOT], 2021). Throughout this book, evidence is presented with regard to the importance of various occupations in the lives of older adults and the outcomes of interventions focused on enabling occupational performance and supporting occupational justice. Therapists interested in fostering positive aging can look to this literature for guidance about how best to proceed. They can also use these findings to support efforts to improve the context in which aging occurs through interventions focused on policy change and on access to care for older adults.

Context of Aging

The world is growing older. In the United States, the population of people over age 65 is projected to increase from 54.1 million in 2019 to 94.7 million in 2060 (Administration on Aging [AOA], 2021). There will be more older people in the next several decades, both in absolute numbers and as a percentage of the population. This demographic trend is, in part, the result of improved wellness practices and improved healthcare. However, in the United States, 40% of individuals over the age of 65 have at least one disability (Centers for Disease Control and Prevention [CDC], 2020a). By age 75, over 50% report having one or more disabilities (ADA National Network, 2018).

Though adults experience positive aging well into their 90s, adults are still globally categorized as "older adult" at age 65. This is further subdivided into youngest-old (65 to 74 years), middle-old (75 to 84 years), and oldest-old (85+ years) (Lee et al, 2018).

Simply defining what is meant by the term "old" can be complicated. Some of the youngest-old may have more in common with individuals who are very old than with their age peers. Chronological definitions may be of limited value because extreme individual variability characterizes later life. Self-perceptions of aging relate more to function than to chronological age. Escourrou and colleagues (2022) found the shift to very-old age occurred when people experienced the "irreversibility of aging and its effects" leading to living more day-to-day. Importantly, for the purposes of occupational therapy intervention, the study found that this perceptual shift was preceded by reduced social participation, losses of health and close friends and family, and a disconnect from younger adults. Supporting social participation is a critical area for older adult health, advocacy, and justice. For the purposes of this book, old age is considered in the context of function rather than absolute chronological age. To evaluate the context of aging, one should examine current trends in life expectancy, understand historical roles and how they have evolved, and recognize shared cohort experiences.

Life Expectancy

Life expectancy is a mathematical construct capturing the estimate of the average age at which a person from a particular population category will die; it is influenced by such realities as war, poverty, and disease. (This is not to be confused with the human **life span,** the maximum years a human can live. The human life span is around 120 years, although modern science is pushing that forward.) In the premodern world, the average life expectancy was roughly 30 years (Roser et al, 2019). Even into the beginning of the 19th century, the average life expectancy globally was no more than 40 years of age. Starting during the European Renaissance and early emergence of modern medicine, life expectancies began to increase. Further improvements occurred with the introduction of public health measures in the early 20th century, and life expectancy in wealthy countries doubled by 2019. There continue to be great disparities in life expectancy globally and regionally. For example, people in Canada and Sweden have a life expectancy of 82, whereas those in Sierra Leone and Central Africa Republic have a life expectancy of 52 (Roser et al, 2019).

Life expectancy overall is influenced by premature mortality. The United States stood out among other wealthy countries for a drop in life expectancy due to opioid overdoses, suicides, and obesity-related organ system failures among younger people beginning in the mid-2010s (Arias et al, 2022; Raleigh, 2019). Life expectancy was negatively impacted globally by the 2019 coronavirus (COVID-19) pandemic and related excess deaths. See Figure 1-1 Life expectancy at birth, by sex, United States 2000 to 2021.

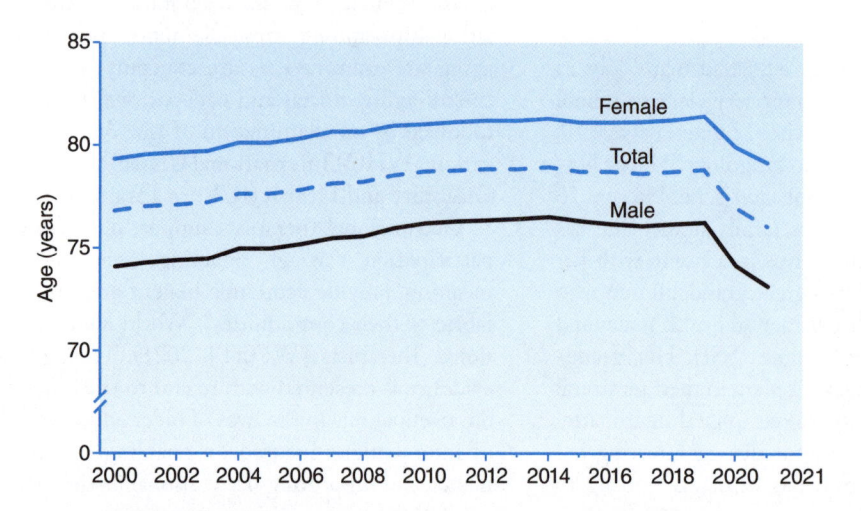

Notes: Estimates are based on provisional data for 2021. Provisional data are subject to change as additional data are received.
Estimates for 2000–2020 are based on final data.
Source: National Center for Health Statistics, National Vital Statistics System, Mortality.

FIGURE 1-1 Life expectancy at birth, by sex, United States 2000 to 2021. *(Adapted from: National Center for Health Statistics, National Vital Statistics System, Mortality.)*

During the late 20th century, the proportion of older adults to younger adults in the United States and much of the world increased dramatically due to innovations in medicine and public health, allowing for greater life expectancy, while at the same time society saw lowered birth rates. The aging of the global population has political, economic, and social impacts as people remain healthy and live longer (Sciubba, 2020). However, there are racial and ethnic differences. For babies born in the United States in 2019, life expectancy was 81 years for white women, 83 years for Hispanic women, 76 years for non-Hispanic black women, 76 years for white men, 77 years for Hispanic men, and 68 years for non-Hispanic black men. Pre-COVID-19 pandemic data suggests that white men and women who were 65 years of age in 2019 could expect to live an average of another 19 years, Hispanic men and women another 21 years on average, and non-Hispanic black men and women another 17 years (Arias et al, 2021).

Causes of Death

The leading causes of death in the United States in 2020, excluding COVID-19 (which ranked third that year), included heart disease, cancer, stroke, Alzheimer disease, diabetes, chronic lower respiratory diseases, and influenza and pneumonia. Although the rankings differ, these conditions are consistently the leading causes across all genders, races, and ethnicities (CDC, 2020b; Murphy et al, 2021) and across other high-income countries. Older adults in lower-income countries have higher death rates from communicable diseases such as lower respiratory conditions and diarrheal conditions (WHO, 2020). Knowing causes of death assists healthcare providers and policy makers direct funds for treatment and research. Changes in life expectancy have altered expectations and perceptions about the place of older individuals in society, their communities, and in families.

Historical Roles of Older Adults

Expectations about appropriate or expected functions for older people have varied over time (Cossar, 2012). In ancient and medieval society, contemplation was considered the central purpose of old age, and older adults were both cared for and revered (Troy, 2022). Other activities, including work, sex, and the military, were not thought to be appropriate. For years, conventional wisdom suggested that older adults did well in agrarian societies, where their supportive efforts were a vital part of the culture (Achenbaum & Sterns, 1978). In poor urban areas, however, those without family were sent to poorhouses as were people with mental illnesses and physical disabilities (Troy, 2022). Certainly in Native American groups, older adults were central to the well-being of the community (Eden & Eden, 2010). Even in agrarian cultures, individuals who did not live on farms or with extended families were denied clear roles (Hagestad, 1986), and older adults in industrial settings were denigrated because they could not contribute to their families' economic well-being (Achenbaum & Sterns, 1978). However, in some specific areas, including politics, religion, and academia, older adults—specifically, older white men—were valued for their experience and wisdom (Cossar, 2012).

Cohort Effects

Individuals age in particular clusters or cohorts that experience a set of historical events that influence personal behavior and the experience of aging. For example, today's cohort of the very old in the United States, those born before 1945, often called the silent generation or "maturists" may have lived through both the Great Depression that began in 1929 and World War II in the 1940s. These experiences led to a strong value placed on frugality as well as great patriotism that may have contributed to their tendency to vote in large numbers throughout their lives. They are less likely to use complex technologies and more likely to trust in medicine and the value of vaccines, including the COVID-19 vaccine due to their and their children's historical experience with polio and other potentially deadly diseases (Wang et al, 2022). People born between 1945 and 1964, commonly referred to as baby boomers, experienced more independence in healthcare decisions than prior generations. They access healthcare information on the internet, are more assertive with care providers, and expect to live longer, healthier lives (Kahana & Kahana, 2014).

Baby boomers lived through significant social, political, technological, and economic changes. These changes impact attitudes toward family values and religious beliefs (Vera-Toscano & Meroni, 2021). The baby boomer generational cohort is large, and there are differences among those born early in this cohort (the mid-1940s through early 1950s) and those born toward the end of the cohort (the early 1960s). Similar to former generational cohorts, earlier born baby boomers have a high value on religion and more traditional family values, whereas later born baby boomers are more accepting of divorce and nonmarried couples and place lower importance on religion but continue to hold traditional views on gender roles (Vera-Toscano & Meroni, 2021).

At the same time, within a given cohort, experiences and environment can lead to considerable variability among older adults. Education, gender, and socioeconomic status (SES) influence individuals' traits. Table 1-1 shows the characteristics attributed to some of the generations currently alive in the United States. Groups in other countries will have different experiences that affect cohort values and behaviors, although individuals within a given cohort may vary significantly from these stereotypes.

CASE STUDY

Occupational Profile

Mr. Bearheart is a 68-year-old of Ojibwe descent. He and four siblings live in the Lac du Flambeau tribal community. His wife died a year ago, and his only daughter lives with her husband and children in a midsized city 140 miles

TABLE 1-1 Generational Characteristics in the Western Countries

GENERATION	BORN	FORMATIVE EXPERIENCES	CORE LIFE VALUES	WORK-RELATED ETHIC AND VALUES
Maturists (aka Silent, Traditionalists)	1922–1945	Wartime rationing, rock n' roll, nuclear families, defined roles	Respect for authority Conformity Discipline	Sacrifice Hard work Duty before pleasure
Baby Boomers	1946–1964	Cold War, Woodstock, moon landings, family-oriented	Optimism Involvement Personal gratification/growth	Driven Personal fulfillment Questioning authority
Generation X	1965–1980	Fall of Berlin Wall, Live Aid, early mobile technology, increasing divorce rates	Fun Balance Informality	Risk takers Skeptical Self-reliance
Generation Y	1981–1995	9/11 terrorist attacks, social media, Middle and Far East conflicts, reality TV	Confidence Realism Social	Flexibility Collectivistic Entrepreneurial
Generation Z	Born after 1995	Economic downturn, global warming, mobile devices, cybersecurity concerns	Truth Dialogue Network	Multitaskers Seamless job shifts Apprenticeship

Developed from McKinsey & Company, n.d.; Tolbize, 2008.

away. His son died in a motor vehicle accident 25 years earlier. The loss of his son contributed to his alcoholism and difficulty holding a job. He and his wife lived in a small one-bedroom home. His wife worked at a local food market part-time early in their marriage but was otherwise a homemaker. Mr. Bearheart has arthritis, migraines, and diabetes, with beginning stages of peripheral neuropathy. When his wife was diagnosed with terminal cancer, he found support to end his drinking and help his wife navigate her end of life. As part of their time together, they worked with tribal youth on projects around sharing language, verbal traditions and knowledge, and traditional games and activities and became part of a canoe repatriation project. His immediate tribal community has limited access to healthcare; he drove his wife to her medical appointments in the town his daughter lives in. Since his wife's death, he has found purpose in mentoring youth with opioid and methamphetamine addictions. His diabetes continues to be poorly controlled, and he has had more problems with tripping and falling. He sees a nurse practitioner at the tribal health clinic supported by the Indian Health Service one town away.

Identified Problem Areas Related to Aging in Context

The occupational therapist working with Mr. Bearheart recognizes that access to regular diabetic care is important for his personal health management. The occupational therapist assessed Mr. Braveheart's instrumental activities of daily living performance, including health management and food preparation, balance and fall risk, his home and close community environment for safety barriers and supports, and his social participation. The assessment findings suggest that Mr. Bearheart would benefit from health and diabetes education, including medication management, nutrition, and simple food preparation skills and safety and fall prevention through balance activities and home and community safety modifications. Mr. Bearheart noted he wanted to continue to develop his role as an elder in the community and support his tribal youth.

Goals for OT
Mr. Bearheart will:
1. Explore and begin participation in a strengthening and balance program, such as WELL Balanced (Wise Elders Living Longer). (https://www.nrcnaa.org/well-balanced)
2. Demonstrate competence in diabetic medication and care management.
3. Demonstrate meal planning and food preparation in medically tailored meals after consulting with a registered dietitian (RDN).
4. Complete home modifications with assistance of family and community.
5. Advocate with the tribal council to address shared community space accessibility assessment and intervention when possible.

Intervention Plan

The occupational therapy provider and Mr. Bearheart will consult with an RDN for medically tailored meals from which to use recipes in meal planning and preparation. The occupational therapist and Mr. Bearheart will develop a routine for diabetic checks and medications. The occupational therapist will enroll Mr. Bearheart in WELL Balanced, which she helps facilitate at the community center, and provide an introduction to the recreation center fitness director for equipment orientation. The occupational therapist will work with Mr. Bearheart, family members, neighbors, and community leaders to make modifications to his home and potential community locations.

Factors Affecting the Experience of Aging

Many factors that affect aging are discussed in the following section. Using an ecological approach facilitates an examination of societal factors, including SDOH and public policy, and community factors, such as physical and social environments, that influence how an older adult experiences aging.

Social Determinants of Health

There has been growing attention to SDOH (U.S. Department of Health and Human Services [USDHHS], 2020), which can be linked directly to the experience of aging (Rudolph, 2021). The WHO defines **social determinants of health** as "the nonmedical factors that influence health outcomes. They are conditions in which people are born, grow, live, and age, and the wider set of forces shaping the conditions of daily life" (WHO, 2022b). SDOH are social, economic, and environmental conditions that can help or hinder older adults' ability to maintain their health and well-being (Jurkowski & Guest, 2021). These factors include: (a) education – access and quality, (b) healthcare – access and quality, (c) neighborhood and built environments (including safe housing), (d) economic stability (including income and access to nutritious food), and (e) social and community context (including social opportunity). Negative SDOH can significantly impact an older adult's health and aging experience, especially their ability to live independently and potentially age in place (Pooler & Srinivasan, 2018). The effects of SDOH can be exacerbated for older adults, particularly if they have had poor resources across their life span (Hunter & Guest, 2021). Loneliness and social isolation have a significant impact on overall health of older adults (CDC, 2020a). For those who grow up poor, the disadvantages of that poverty such as poor housing and nutrition and lack of access to healthcare can continue to accumulate across the life span, resulting in increasing health disparities (Dannefer, 2020; Ferraro & Morton, 2018). In the United States, older adults living in rural communities have even greater health disparities compared with their urban and suburban counterparts. Geographic location, along with lower social economic status and lower rates of comprehensive insurance, creates limited access to adequate and quality healthcare general providers and specialists (Coughlin et al, 2019; see also Rural Health Information Hub, 2022). Internationally, the rural – urban comparisons often differ. For example, in Taiwan, while older adults' education level was related to urban dwellers' social participation, independent living, and healthcare access, those living in rural communities were still likely to perform physical activities, feel physically safe, have better mental well-being, and have higher social respect and integration than those in urban areas (Hsu et al, 2019).

Differences in SDOH contribute to health status, including the risk for frailty (Hoogendijk et al, 2019), mental health concerns (Wang et al, 2018), oral health issues (Peres et al, 2019), and vascular disease and cognitive impairment (Zlokovic et al, 2020). Consider the role of occupational therapy as you examine Figure 1-2 – Social Determinants of Health Model. Occupational therapists should screen their clients for SDOH factors. See Promoting Best Practice 1-1 for an example of an SDOH screening tool.

Health Literacy

An important aspect of health equality is **personal health literacy,** "the degree to which individuals have the ability to find, understand, and use information and services to inform health-related decisions and actions for themselves and others" (USDHHS, Office of Disease Prevention and Health Promotion, 2022). As part of the Healthy People 2030 initiative, the definition emphasizes the ability to *use* information and to make *well-informed* decisions. Second, Healthy People 2030 acknowledges that organizations, staff, and direct care providers have a responsibility to address health literacy.

Occupational therapists play an important role in ensuring their clients can find, access, and take action on health

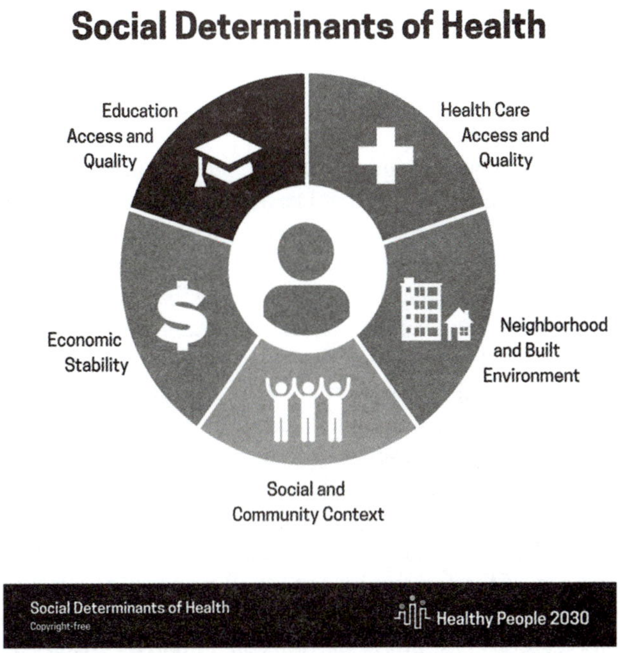

FIGURE 1-2 Social Determinants of Health model. *(From: https: health.gov/healthypeople)*

information. Providing written handouts with exercises with one successful demonstration during therapy does not ensure a client is well informed. Considering that many clients have chronic health conditions, educating them on how to find and verify health information is critical, especially because many people (or their family members) go to the internet as a primary resource. Armstrong-Heimsoth and colleagues (2019) developed an educational course to assist individuals and caregivers in finding and evaluating online health information. The participants reported improvements in understanding and retrieving future materials. Many studies demonstrate a relationship between poor health literacy and poor health outcomes. For occupational therapists, the second part of the personal health literacy definition should generate action to help clients "use information and services to inform health-related decisions and actions." Whether through helping clients develop self-management routines or gain self-advocacy skills, health literacy interventions are critical to support older adults' health. For more information about Healthy People 2030 initiatives and tools for action, visit https://health.gov/healthypeople

PROMOTING BEST PRACTICE 1-1
Screening for Social Determinants of Health Factors

Occupational therapists may want to screen clients for factors addressing social determinants of health. The Centers for Medicare & Medicaid Services developed the Health-Related Social Needs Screening Tool, available in English and Spanish. The 10-item tool can be used as a self-screen or in partnership with a health professional. The tool addresses housing instability, food insecurity, transportation needs, utility needs, and interpersonal safety. https://innovation.cms.gov/files/worksheets/ahcm-screeningtool.pdf

Physical Environment

Place of Residence

The geographic location in which an older adult resides and the quality of housing in that location are among the characteristics of the physical environment that influence late life. There are strong links between housing, health, and function (Swope & Hernandez, 2019). Stable neighborhoods provide social interaction, familiar access, and meaning. Beyond the home, considerations include the nature of the immediate physical environment—for example, whether there is access to safe outdoor space for physical activity (keeping in mind that one aspect of such safety is good air quality); the location—urban, suburban, or rural; and the familiarity of the individual to the location.

In rural environments, older adults are likely to be an integral part of the community and are often involved in volunteer activities and social networks (Carver et al, 2018). The grocery store, post office, and bank are important sources of socialization and support, and informal networks are effective for both maintaining health and providing care for those who are ill. These supports are essential to positive quality of life, whether they are provided by family or by others (Keating et al, 2011).

Although there is often good social support in small towns, older adults who live a distance from town may have limited social opportunities and more difficulty obtaining needed assistance in part because of distance and transportation difficulties. This can result in poor access to care or age-friendly programming and lower satisfaction (Colibaba et al, 2020). In contrast, Carver and colleagues (2018) found that the lack of formal services, including healthcare, was less important than attachment to place and social connections.

For suburban elders, transportation historically was a problem for healthcare access. This is changing with telehealth options, ride-share growth, and older adults driving in later life (Golant, 2019). Still, the need remains for automobile transportation for basic services, groceries, and social gatherings. Many older adults are first-generation suburban dwellers; they also share an attachment to the place where they raised their families and established roots.

In high-density urban cities, older adults may have the greatest access to transportation and services, resulting in greater access to healthcare and social activities than low-density urban dwellers have (Adorno et al, 2018). However, in disadvantaged urban communities, older adults have less access to transportation options and technology (Mitra et al, 2019). The built environment, the constructed aspects of the community, can be perilous in urban settings. Walking is an important mode of transportation, yet it can be dangerous due to poor infrastructure. Pedestrian collisions involving older adults often result in serious injury or death (Kim, 2019).

Aging in Place

Many older adults want to age in place, that is, to remain living in their home and/or community safely and independently. The CDC defines aging in place as the ability to live in one's own home and community safely, independently, and comfortably, regardless of age, income, or ability level (CDC, 2013). Aging in place is supported by adequate housing, transportation, social participation, respect and inclusion, civic participation and employment, communication and information, and outdoor spaces and buildings (Colibaba et al, 2020). Occupational therapists can play a major role in helping older adults remain in place through home modifications and advocating for walkable, accessible transportation, and accessible neighborhood services (see Chapter 15 for more information about home modifications and Chapter 19 for driving and community mobility options).

For some older adults, aging in place is not a choice but a reality. In some economic environments, they may not have the financial resources or options to move. Those "stuck in place" may be disabled and have limited social and financial resources to make necessary safety modifications (Granbom et al, 2021). When older adults choose not to age in place or cannot do so for reasons of health, economics, or other factors, careful consideration must be given to supporting successful transitions. Such transitions can be disruptive and unsettling. The decision to move seems to be most positive when it is made by the individual when they are still capable of the cognitive, physical, and emotional adjustment to a new environment. As the number of older adults has increased, a range of options has emerged. Options created by circumstance—for example, naturally occurring retirement communities (NORCs) in some condominium settings—and independent care facilities are among the many possibilities (see Chapter 2 for more information about home as a place of meaning).

Institutionalization

Few older adults are institutionalized. In 2019, roughly 1.2 million people aged 65 or older lived in nursing homes. The percentage increases from 1% of people who are young-old (age 65 to 74) to 2% middle-old (75 to 84) to 8% old-old (over age 84 years) (AOA, 2021). Often a "last address," occupational therapists have an important role serving older adults in nursing care facilities to help improve or maintain residents' quality of life. Older adults are frequently institutionalized due to high-level care needs, often related to cognitive impairments (e.g., dementia), neurological impacts (e.g., stroke), and frailty. Occupation-based interventions and maintenance programs can focus on improving mental health (e.g., depression, anxiety), physical health (e.g., self-care, mobility), and socialization. From their meta-analysis, de Medeiros and colleagues (2020) found three areas that are important to quality of life. These areas are relevant to occupational therapy practice and resident advocacy: (a) engaging in "past-present-future" activities (e.g., through reminiscence); (b) addressing intimacy, the need for companionship and social participation; and (c) providing sensory opportunities through normal everyday activities in an occupationally rich environment. Refer to Chapter 27 for more information on long-term care. While living in a nursing home may not be the life plan for most people, they can provide a caring and supportive community.

Domestic Migration

Domestic migration—the pattern of moving from one geographic region to another—has consequences for older adults. People move for reasons of economy, access to healthcare, proximity to family, climate, and amenities (Zhang et al, 2021). More than three million older adults in the United States move each year. The most popular destinations include southern and western states (Mateyka & He, 2022). Some individuals develop a pattern called "snowbirding," in which they maintain two households—one in their community of long-standing residence and one in a warmer climate where they live during the winter. In a "boomerang effect," older adults have been known to return "home" to have that proximity to family and familiar neighborhoods (Henderson, 2016). Many northern states in the United States have more robust Medicare payments for older adults than do southern states, allowing for care when financial resources are limited.

International Migration

People who migrate to another country later in life often experience challenges accessing healthcare. Internationally the proportion of migrants 65 and older is about 12% of 281 million migrants in 2020. Europe, North America, and Oceania received the greatest number of older adult migrants (United Nations, 2020). This population is not often considered in healthcare services or costs. Additionally, many international families host their older relatives part time in their homes for periods of time. Occupational therapists need to appreciate family and community culture while addressing mental health and psychosocial adaptation and health literacy, among other migrant needs (Hawkins et al, 2022).

Homelessness

Economic challenges have driven many older adults to become homeless. Homeless adults have a significantly lower life span (age 55) than the average adult, along with more health conditions (e.g., urinary incontinence and cognitive, sensory, and physical impairments) and a higher number of falls (Abbs et al, 2020). For individuals who are homeless, the environment is challenging to navigate, healthcare systems are inconsistent, and food access is uncertain. Survival is, of necessity, a primary focus of activity, leaving little time for concern about positive aging. Occupational therapists who work in hospitals and other care facilities that serve individuals who are homeless need to be aware of limited discharge options for rehabilitative physical or mental healthcare. Community-based practice therapists may have a growing role in sustaining older adults who live "rough," outside, or "surf" from one family or acquaintance's home to another. Addressing basic needs, including adequate shelter, food, and physical and psychological safety by working with social services, is a primary concern.

Sociocultural Factors

Attitudes

Attitudes have the potential to affect the experience of growing old in several ways. Positive attitudes toward aging can enhance the experience, increasing the potential for good quality of life in later life (Reich et al, 2020). Older adults with positive beliefs about aging were more likely to fully recover from a disabling condition than those with negative beliefs. In contrast, those with negative stereotypes of aging have more and earlier-life cardiovascular events.

Ageism is the process of systematic stereotyping or discrimination against people because of their age (Levy et al, 2020). Stereotypes of aging compete with the various realities. Although there are positive media portrayals of active and healthy older adults (e.g., *Grace and Frankie, Black-ish, The Kominsky Method*), too often older adult characters are portrayed as foolish or inept (e.g., Grandpa on *The Simpsons*, the Woody Grant character in the movie *Nebraska*, just about every Disney older adult). Negative social media messaging, especially during the COVID-19 pandemic, played a role in devaluing older adults, their healthcare, and their lives, negatively affecting older adults' mental health (Levy et al, 2022). Finding a nonageist birthday card can be a challenge.

Stereotypes of aging contribute to relatively pervasive if increasingly subtle ageism. There is a strong relationship between ageism and ableism, the discrimination in favor of able-bodied people (Oxford, n.d.). In their study of occupational therapy students, Friedman and VanPuymbrouck (2021) found that 70% of their student sample was ageist, with ableism being a strong covariate. Interventions to address community-based ageism include education and increasing positive interactions with older adults. The Positive Education about Aging and Contact Experiences (PEACE) model demonstrates that basic information about older adult health and life experiences, coupled with structured intergenerational interactions, improved relations in communities (Levy, 2018). Intergenerational service learning (Ramamonjiarivelo et al, 2021) and reverse mentoring (Leedahl et al, 2020) demonstrate improved attitudes toward older adults by healthcare students.

Cultural Factors

Historical and demographic trends are important, but they are not the same for all cultures. To understand the experience of aging, cultural factors must also be examined. "Age is a social construction and the experience of growing old is culturally mitigated" (Fry, 1996, p. 123).

Culture may affect individuals' expectations about what old age will be like, their plans and goals for this period of their lives, their values and attitudes about being older and about healthcare, and their motivations for engaging in or withdrawing from activity. Cultural realities also affect community acceptance and support for older adults, the extent to which they have meaningful roles in those communities, and the availability of meaningful roles in their families and the broader society. In the United States, one reason for increasing interest in cultural factors is the growing recognition of significant health disparities and the racial and ethnic differences associated with rates of disease, views on healthcare, access to care, and outcomes of care. Culture as it affects aging is discussed in greater detail in Chapter 4.

Public Policy and Aging

Public policies emerge from cultural values and beliefs in particular societies and have a substantial impact on individuals' lives. For example, retirement income and healthcare coverage are among the issues closely tied to legislation. Policies about pensions, investments, and healthcare can greatly influence the extent to which older adults are sufficiently secure financially in later life. Policy can also support or impede positive aging as it supports or impedes individual health and function (WHO, 2018). Let us consider one example: financial support for older adults.

Until relatively recently, in most societies, older adults undertook various instrumental tasks, such as farming, gathering, and child care, until they were too infirm to continue. At that point, they were tended to by families, or they managed as best they could on their own until they died, usually soon thereafter. The industrial revolution led to the gradual implementation of pensions over several decades beginning in the late 1800s in Germany (Hawthorne, 2013). In the United States, Social Security was instituted in the 1930s as a response to the Great Depression (Hawthorne, 2013). The system encouraged older adults to retire to open jobs for younger individuals. Other forms of pension became more common after World War II at a time when wages were federally controlled to minimize the threat of massive inflation.

Social Security has reduced poverty among older adults (Romig, 2022). Recent concern about Social Security focuses on the fact that the population of the United States has an increasing proportion of older adults relative to the population of working-age individuals (typically defined as 22 to 65 years of age) due to increasing longevity and decreasing fertility (Huston, 2019). Policy analysts suggest this dependency ratio—the ratio of those in the workforce to children and older adults depending on workers to provide their financial support through taxes—is projected to increase to 35% by 2025 (and 40% by 2065), meaning that for every 100 working age people, there are 35 people collecting benefits (Huston, 2019). This has contributed to the reduced number of pension plans, as concerns increase about the financial burden on younger individuals.

Now, however, employer funded pensions are rapidly disappearing in the United States and being replaced by employee driven investment schemes (Butrica et al, 2009). Employers now offer 401(k) plans with required employee investment. Whereas pensions provided stability for the worker, it put the investment risk on the employer; the 401(k) plans put the investment planning in the hands of employees (Forbes, 2018). For those older adults who had the benefit of investing, the Great Recession in 2008 and 2009 and the pandemic-related economic downturn in 2022 have affected long-term savings toward a planned retirement. One result of these various factors coming together at this point in time is substantial economic uncertainty for older adults. This is particularly problematic, because they do not have the luxury of a long time frame to recoup investment losses or to earn additional income. Social security benefits are not fully available to retirees until age 67 for those born after 1960 (Huston, 2019). As a result, many older adults find it necessary to remain in the workforce longer than initially planned. (See Chapter 18 on work and retirement.)

Personal Factors

The experience of aging is unique to each individual, even in the context of the broader society. Individual genetic traits, personality characteristics, and personal experience throughout the life span are central to a person's later life circumstances, behaviors, and attitudes. Genetic factors, age, health experiences, gender, and gender expression all play a role in the experience of aging. (See also Chapter 5, Identity, Sexuality, and Relationships.)

Genetic factors vary among individuals and have a significant impact on aging. As human genetic structure is better understood, it is clear that differences in DNA among individuals (and among species) are small, but those differences can have profound implications for development of each person (Sutphin & Kaeberlein, 2011). Genetic explanations have been proposed for a variety of disorders commonly seen in later life, including relationships between Alzheimer disease and depression, diabetes, and heart disease (Santiago & Potashkin, 2021). However, there is also compelling evidence that a variety of environmental and social factors can mediate the expression of genes (Belsky et al, 2018).

Personal experience includes the cumulative advantage or disadvantage that results from differences in SES and education that can influence health status and outlook in later life. Stress has a significant influence on well-being in later life, as experienced in the COVID-19 pandemic, when many older adults experienced loss of partners, loss of social opportunities, and loneliness. Among older adults with positive perception of their health, healthy family functioning, resilience, gratitude, and acceptance fared well, suggesting a focus on building personal resources is a means to combat stress in older adults (Lopez et al, 2020).

Socioeconomic and Gender Factors

As can be seen from the discussion to this point, SES factors play a significant role in aging. Education, occupation, and income level influence the experience of aging, along with morbidity and mortality. Public policies that encourage or discourage social and economic mobility (sociocultural environment) and the availability of effective schools (physical environment) also play a role in SES.

Globally, the consequences of long-standing socioeconomic disadvantage have received particular attention, especially in how early-life SES affects health later in life. For example, SES is associated with cognitive function in later life (Greenfield & Moorman, 2019), cardiovascular health (Hossin et al, 2021), and epigenetic (cellular) aging (Austin et al, 2018). Middle-life low SES is associated with poor oral health (Ramsay et al, 2018) and psychiatric disorders and substance abuse, which later associate with renal diseases, cardiopulmonary diseases, and dementias (Kivimaki et al, 2020).

For a variety of reasons, the financial circumstances of older adults tend to deteriorate as they live longer, and it seems likely that the extent of poverty in retirement is undercounted (Butrica et al, 2009). These findings are less true for individuals who have more education and financial resources. Some disadvantaged older adults have protective resources that ameliorate the negative consequences of low SES (Dupree & George, 2011). Among the protective factors are a stable marriage, the presence of adult children, and expecting to live to age 85. It seems possible that this last is a marker of optimism and resilience. One potential explanation, which is considered in Chapter 2, is the differential occupational patterns in which older adults engage—that is, the extent to which the individual finds life meaningful.

Impact of Economics and Gender

Historically, the wealthy have always lived the longest. The elements that contributed to this reality are similar to those that persist to this day: access to adequate diet, healthcare, and information. Wealth also affected general perceptions about older adults. Men of wealth were more likely than poor men to be thought of as wise. In medieval Italy, older clergy and men of means took on positions of increased authority later in life. Those who were impoverished, however, worked until they could no longer do so and were then perceived as burdensome (Cossar, 2012).

Gender has also influenced the experience of aging throughout history. As discussed earlier, women's life expectancy is longer than men's. However, their quality of life and specific circumstances of later life depend in part on their wealth. Historically, in societies where widows could not keep their late husbands' resources, older women lived in poverty. But even in societies in which they were able to retain resources, they were generally treated with suspicion (Haber, 1997). When pensions were introduced as a benefit of employment in the middle of the 20th century, these often stopped at the husband's death (or even earlier). To this day, older women are far more likely than older men to live in poverty, regardless of race, educational background, or marital status (Morrissey, 2016). The expectation that women will stay home to raise children, lack of availability of child care, and lower pay for female employees have all impacted women's earnings (Steinmayr et al, 2020) and thus available income and stability in retirement.

Women's higher rates of late-life disability present significant challenges, as they are more likely to develop Alzheimer disease, experience bone fractures, and have other compromising health conditions. This means that they are more likely to require assistance, because they are also more likely to be widowed, with less access to informal care and fewer financial resources (Morrissey, 2016). Men also face unique challenges. Although older men have fewer financial difficulties, men who are alone experience greater social isolation and loneliness (Neville et al, 2018). Greater loneliness is experienced by older men who are unpartnered and have low SES, limited social networks, and poor mental health. The suicide rate for men over the age of 85 is higher than any other group. Financial troubles, loss of partner or health, chronic pain, and cognitive impairment are frequently associated with suicide (National Council on Aging, 2021). Despite these challenges, most older adults are generally more satisfied and optimistic as they age.

Positive Aging

While most older adults want to live and age well, there are cultural differences in how people experience aging, their expectations, and their concerns. In their systematic review of multiethnic, cross-cultural literature on older adult perspectives on aging, Reich et al (2020) found that maintaining a positive attitude was most important to coping with aging. Other themes from their review included social engagement, independence, physical health, cognitive health, and spirituality. In the reviewed articles, representing people from North American, Western Europe, the Middle East, Asian, and Oceanic regions, *how* the older adults expressed the themes varied. For example, the social importance of giving back to communities and families demonstrated successful aging for the people of Middle East, Asia, and Oceanic regions. An important finding is that older adults viewed successful aging through psychological and social factors, not biomedical factors. Poor health was overcome with a positive attitude in a variety of circumstances (Reich et al, 2020).

Physical and psychosocial change is inevitable with age; however, such change does not define an individual's affective experience of aging. Older adults' attitudes and behaviors differ in ways that can dramatically affect their quality of life and life satisfaction. Theories of positive aging, stemming from positive psychology, focus on psychological well-being, de-emphasizing dysfunction and impairment to focus on psychologically healthy transitions across the life span. Positive aging is an adaptive process in which biological, lifestyle, and environmental factors interact to promote positive views on health. It also considers the benefits of aging to the individual, community, and society (Killen & Macaskill, 2020). In their study of positive well-being through life events, Killen and Macaskill (2020) found a positive attitude and approach to life can be facilitated through:

- Social interaction
- Participation in enjoyable activities
- Interaction with the physical environment
- Being of value
- Feeling capable
- Having a future orientation
- Taking time for contemplation, including religious and spiritual experiences
- Personal health and wellbeing
- Celebrating good outcomes for others

It is not difficult to see the role occupational therapists can play in supporting positive aging through enabling occupation. Whether occupations are the *means* of therapy (e.g., learning to use virtual technologies to visit with family or regaining strength to garden) or the *ends* of therapy (e.g., resilience and positive life view), keeping a focus on positive aging will promote best practice.

Social and Occupational Justice and Aging

The Occupational Justice Framework (OJF) (Stadnyk et al, 2010) provides a means to address fairness, equity, and empowerment in supporting occupational participation. The framework can be applied to individuals, groups, and populations and has direct relevance to the realities of aging. Social participation can be enabled by addressing institutional and contextual factors. Using the OJF as their theoretical foundation, Lewis and Lemieux (2021) found that enablers to social participation in Canada included providing community support staff, accessible physical environments, and programs tailored to older adults. Barriers to participation included cultural values and ageist attitudes. This is notably an international issue. In a study of older adults in India, older adults valued independence in community mobility, yet they experienced the same physical, social, and attitudinal barriers (Ramachandran & Dsouza, 2018). Lack of community mobility options for urban dwellers limited occupational opportunities, with older adults reporting being underoccupied, although concerns about health and safety also affected participation (Fritz & Cutchin, 2017). To address these issues, occupational therapists need to address home and community access, social skills, and crafting manageable routines for daily activities. They also need to provide interventions focused on changing unjust and discriminatory policies that impede positive aging. These interventions include advocating for older adults via political action, informing agencies and communities about the needs of older adults, and helping clients find resources to advocate for themselves.

For institutionalized older adults with dementia, a focus on client-centered, meaningful occupations and recognition of the individual as a person with a past, present, and future were empowering to occupational therapists and other staff (Du Toit et al, 2019). With this lens, Du Toit and colleagues created occupational opportunities for the older adult participants in their effort. Acquiring basic necessities is an occupational justice issue. For people with disabilities living in rural South Africa, water and sanitation are not a guarantee. Community politics and power, coupled with poverty and negative attitudes toward people with disabilities, led to discrimination and lack of community participation (Wrisdale et al, 2017).

As demonstrated, justice for older adults is a major concern internationally, one that was highlighted during the height of the COVID-19 pandemic as older individuals were simply advised to stay at home (CDC, 2021). See Box 1-1 describing the United Nations' initiatives for its Decade of Healthy Ageing (2021 to 2030).

CHAPTER 1 ■ Aging in Context 13

| BOX 1-1 | United Nations Decade of Healthy Ageing 2021–2030 |

Further addressing aging worldwide, the United Nations has declared 2021–2030 the Decade of Healthy Ageing, with four initiatives, including (WHO, n.d.):

1. **Age-friendly environments:** Removing physical and social barriers and implementing policies, systems, services, products, and technologies that enable participation.
2. **Combatting ageism:** Challenging negative stereotypes, prejudice, and discrimination to support health and well-being.
3. **Integrated care:** Providing access to services for prevention, promotion, curative, rehabilitative, palliative, and end-of-life care that is safe, affordable, and effective through essential medicine, dental care, and assistive technology.
4. **Long-term care:** Providing access to quality long-term care environments where clients maintain function, enjoy basic human rights, and live with dignity.

Who ICF: A Framework for Health and Participation

The WHO is the United Nations agency with a mission to promote health, keep the world safe, and serve the vulnerable (WHO, 2022a). The ICF is a taxonomy categorizing functions and factors that affect a person's health and participation as a member of society (WHO, n.d.). The ICF model demonstrates the interrelationships between health condition, environmental factors, and personal factors. Functioning and disability are on a continuum and are described in terms of body structures and body functions – impairments, activities – activity limitations, and participation – participation restrictions. Environmental factors include barriers and facilitators to support function (WHO-FIC Collaborating Centre for the Africa Region, n.d.). See Figure 1-3 – The ICF Framework for the model.

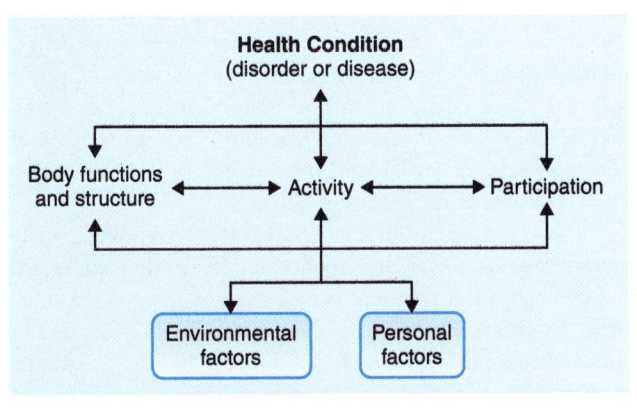

FIGURE 1-3 The WHO-ICF Framework. (*Adapted from https://www.who.int/standards/classifications/international-classification-of-functioning-disabilityand-Health*)

The ICF addresses health and disability as critical to active participation at personal, community, and societal levels. Recognizing that disability is on a continuum encourages participation of all people, regardless of their body functions and structure functioning, and takes into account societal factors, such as attitudes, that affect access. The World Health Organization Disability Assessment Schedule 2.0 (WHO-DAS 2.0; WHO, 2012) is an efficient and psychometrically sound measure of health and disability from an ICF lens. (See Promoting Best Practice 1.2 for more information about WHODAS 2.0.)

Occupational therapists will recognize the influence of the ICF on professional domains and taxonomies, for example, the American Occupational Therapy Association's Occupational Therapy Practice Framework (OTPF). Assessment and interventions can be organized around addressing the different aspects of the ICF. Some occupational therapy assessments and interventions focus on body structure and body function impairments, others on activity limitations, still others on participation restrictions. Some assessments and interventions address environmental and social factors. Maritz and colleagues (2018) completed a detailed analysis of three assessments to demonstrate how aspects of the ICF domains and codes are linked to occupational therapy concepts, models, and their related assessment tools. The Assessment of Motor and Process Skills (AMPS; Fisher & Bray Jones, 2014), Canadian Occupational Performance Measure (COPM; Law et al, 2014), and Model of Human Occupation Screening Tool (MOHOST; Parkinson et al, 2006) demonstrated linking to ICF codes that can assist occupational therapists in documentation and alignment to global practice. Refer to the assessment table in this text for a list of assessments discussed by chapter authors and as categorized by ICF domain by textbook editors.

PROMOTING BEST PRACTICE 1-2
WHODAS 2.0

To measure health and disability from an ICF lens, the WHODAS 2.0, a psychometrically sound, short, 5- to 20-minute assessment can be used across diseases and health disorders to measure and address change over time for individuals. It is applicable across cultures for adult populations. It directly links to the ICF domains, specifically integrating activity and participation. The six domains of the tool are cognition (understanding and communicating), getting around (mobility), self-care, getting along (social and interpersonal functioning), life activities (home, academic, and occupational functioning), and participation (in family, social, and community activities). The manual and its 12- and 36-item versions are available online, along with population norms. Review and download at: https://www.who.int/standards/classifications/international-classification-of-functioning-disability-and-health/who-disability-assessment-schedule

CASE STUDY (CONTINUED)

Discharge Status

Mr. Bearheart has managed his diabetes with minimal diabetic incidents. He cooks at home 2 to 3 days a week, following recipes provided by his registered dietitian. He regularly attends the WELL-Balanced program and goes to the community center fitness gym to work out twice a week. He reports he has not tripped or fallen in the home, and he continues to be careful in the community. Mr. Bearheart is integral to the fabric of his community, supporting youth programs, tribal language, and tradition sharing.

Questions

1. What do you see in this description of Mr. Bearheart that contributes to positive aging?
2. How do SDOH affect Mr. Bearheart?
3. In what ways does Mr. Bearheart's culture influence his experience of aging?
4. What elements of Mr. Bearheart's occupational profile suggest occupations that give his life meaning? What might he need as his capacity to pursue these occupations alters?

Answers

1. Mr. Bearheart and his wife addressed her health condition with a positive approach by focusing on others, being of value, and participating in activities together. These foci helped Mr. Bearheart after his wife's death and with his continued health concerns.
2. Mr. Bearheart has limited access to healthcare, especially specialized care. His community is open to modification, but it needs work to make the community more accessible to all people. He does not live in a community that has many economic opportunities for young people, but it is rich with cultural opportunities, including social and educational.
3. Mr. Bearheart's Native American culture has provided opportunities for him and his wife to engage with other generations in their community. The history and language projects provide temporal continuity for him to his tribe. While his personal history was difficult because of his addiction, he was able to refocus his life by embracing culturally rich, generational activities.
4. Mr. Bearheart clearly derives satisfaction and meaning from his activities with youth in his community, which are focused on maintaining traditional activities, language, and history. Over time, he may find it difficult to get to meetings and need transportation help. He may also find his dexterity diminished, requiring him to provide greater verbal description as he becomes less able to demonstrate skills. It is possible his memory—especially for recent events—may diminish, at which point recording stories of his youth and history might become the focus of his interaction with the young people with whom he works.

SUMMARY

Clearly there is no unitary description of old age that adequately conveys the roles and circumstances of all older adults. Individual and cultural differences are great. Furthermore, roles and circumstances change over time. What is true today may not be true tomorrow, and predictions based on current situations may or may not turn out to be accurate. Changes in cognitive, physical, sensory, and psychosocial performance occur in all older adults. Individual differences exist within the broad parameters of these predictable changes. Social and environmental events are also at least somewhat predictable. For example, whether they are married, single, or divorced and whether they are from large or small families, older individuals experience loss of significant others. Functional limitations increase with age; however, statistics reflect averages and do not provide definitive information about a given individual. The challenge for occupational therapists and other healthcare providers is to understand not only general patterns but also the factors that mold individual experience of growing older. Every client, no matter the age, must be regarded as a unique individual with special interests, abilities, and needs. However, the common realities of the aging process must be addressed to help the individual prepare for probable changes.

Circumstances that influence the performance of older adults are highly complex, including all the factors described in this chapter and the normal biological, social, and psychological changes that accompany aging. All healthcare providers must be sensitive to myriad interacting considerations that affect function. Interventions risk being irrelevant to the client if they are planned without attention to the nature of the culture, family structure, and place and types of residence; demographic factors; the demands of life in terms of physical and social environment and cultural institutions; work and leisure roles and the value placed on each; the degree of choice of activity available to the individual; and the unique characteristics of the individual.

When reading the chapters in this textbook, consider the environmental, social, and economic factors that undergird the description of different experiences of aging. Reflect on how the continuum of health and disability is described in the health conditions chapters. Consider how occupational performance is facilitated through addressing barriers and applying a strengths-based approach to participation. Lastly, engage curiosity for how older adults engage in occupation individually and with others and how they thrive.

Critical Thinking Questions

1. How could ageism and health literacy interact to negatively affect the healthcare being provided to older adults?
2. What can an occupational therapist do to address the four initiatives of the UN Decade of Healthy Ageing?

REFERENCES

Abbs, E., Brown, R., Guzman, D., Kaplan, L., & Kushel, M. (2020). Risk factors for falls in older adults experiencing homelessness: Results from the HOPE HOME cohort study. *Journal of General Internal Medicine, 35,* 1813–1820. https://doi.org/10.1007/s11606-020-05637-0

Achenbaum, W. A., & Sterns, P. N. (1978). Essay: Old age and modernization. *Gerontologist, 18,* 307–312. https://doi.org/10.1093/geront/18.3.307

ADA National Network. (2018). *Aging and the ADA* [Fact sheet]. https://adata.org/factsheet/aging-and-ada

Administration on Aging (AOA). (2021). *The 2020 profile of older Americans.* Administration for Community Living (ACL). https://acl.gov/sites/default/files/aging%20and%20Disability%20In%20America/2020 Profileolderamericans.final_.pdf

Adorno, G., Fields, N., Cronley, C., Parekh, R., & Magruder, K. (2018). Ageing in a low-density urban city: Transportation mobility as a social equity issue. *Ageing and Society, 38*(2), 296–320. https://doi.org/10.1017/S0144686X16000994

Arias, E., Tejada-Vera, B., & Ahmad, F. (2021). Provisional life expectancy estimates for January through June, 2020. *Vital Statistics Rapid Release* (010), 1–8. https://www.cdc.gov/nchs/data/vsrr/VSRR10-508.pdf

Arias, E., Tejada-Vera, B., Kochanek, K. D., & Ahmad, F. B. (2022). Provisional life expectancy estimates for 2021. https://www.cdc.gov/nchs/data/vsrr/vsrr023.pdf

Armstrong-Heimsoth, A., Johnson, M. L., Carpenter, M., Thomas, T., & Sinnappan, A. (2019). Health management: Occupational therapy's key role in educating clients about reliable online health information. *The Open Journal of Occupational Therapy, 7*(4), 1–12. https://doi.org/10.15453/2168-6408.1595

Austin, M. K., Chen, E., Ross, K. M., McEwen, L. M., Maclsaac, J. L., Kobor, M. S., & Miller, G. E. (2018). Early-life socioeconomic disadvantage, not current, predicts accelerated epigenetic aging of monocytes. *Psychoneuroendocrinology, 97,* 131–134. https://doi.org/10.1016/j.psyneuen.2018.07.007

Belsky, D. W., Domingue, B. W., Wedow, R., & Harris, K. M. (2018). Genetic analysis of social-class mobility in five longitudinal studies. *PNAS, 115*(31). E7275–E7284. https://doi.org/10.1073/pnas.180123811

Butrica, B. A., Iams, H. M., Smith, K. E., & Toder, E. J. (2009). The disappearing defined benefit pension and its potential impact on the retirement income of baby boomers. *Social Security Bulletin, 69,* 3. https://www.ssa.gov/policy/docs/ssb/v69n3/v69n3p1.html

Butrica, B. A., Murphy, D. P., & Zedlewski, S. R. (2009). How many struggle to get by in retirement? *Gerontologist, 50,* 482–494. http://dx.doi.org/10.1093/geront/gnp158

Carver L. F., Beamish, R., Phillips, S.P., & Villeneuve, M. A. (2018). Scoping review: Social participation as a cornerstone of successful aging in place among rural older adults. *Geriatrics, 3*(4), 75. https://doi.org/10.3390/geriatrics3040075

Centers for Disease Control and Prevention. (2013). *The state of aging and health in America 2013.* Atlanta, GA. https://www.cdc.gov/aging/pdf/state-aging-health-in-america-2013.pdf

Centers for Disease Control and Prevention. (2020a). *Disability impacts all of us infographic.* https://www.cdc.gov/ncbddd/disabilityandhealth/infographic-disability-impacts-all.html

Centers for Disease Control and Prevention. (2020b, December 31). *Social determinants of health and Alzheimer's disease and related dementias.* https://www.cdc.gov/aging/disparities/social-determinants-alzheimers.html

Centers for Disease Control and Prevention. (2021, August 4). *COVID-19 recommendations for older adults.* https://www.cdc.gov/aging/covid19-guidance.html

Colibaba, A., McCrillis, W., & Skinner, M. W. (2020). Exploring rural older adult perspectives on the scope, reach and sustainability of age-friendly programs. *Journal of Aging Studies, 55,* 100898. https://doi.org/10.1016/j.jaging.2020.100898

Cossar, R. (2012). Portraits of aging men in late medieval Italy. *Gerontologist, 52,* 553–560. https://doi.org/10.1093/geront/gnr149

Coughlin, S. S., Clary, C., Johnson, J. A., Berman, A., Heboyan, V., Benevides, T., Moore, J., & George, V. (2019). Continuing challenges in rural health in the United States. *Journal of Environment and Health Sciences, 5*(2), 90–92. https://www.ncbi.nlm.nih.gov/pmc/articles/PMC7043306/

Dannefer, D. (2020). Systemic and reflexive: Foundations of cumulative dis/advantage and life-course processes. *The Journals of Gerontology: Series B, 75*(6), 1249–1263. https://doi.org/10.1093/geronb/gby118

de Medeiros, M. M. D., Carletti, T. M., Magno, M. B., Maia, L. C., Cavalcanti, Y. W., & Rodrigues-Garcia, R. C. M. (2020). Does the institutionalization influence elderly's quality of life? A systematic review and meta-analysis. *BMC Geriatrics, 20*(1), 44. https://doi.org/10.1186/s12877-020-1452-0

Dupree, M. E., & George, L. K. (2011). Exceptions to the rule: Exceptional health among the disadvantaged. *Research on Aging, 33,* 115–144. http://dx.doi.org/10.1177/0164027510391988

Du Toit, S. H. J., Shen, X., & McGrath, M. (2019). Meaningful engagement and person-centered residential dementia care: A critical interpretive synthesis. *Scandinavian Journal of Occupational Therapy, 26*(5), 343–355. https://doi-org/10.1080/11038128.2018.1441323

Eden, J., & Eden, N. (2010). Views of older Native American adults in colonial New England. *Journal of Cross Cultural Gerontology, 25,* 285–298. http://dx.doi.org/10.1007/s10823-010-9125-7

Escourrou, E., Laurent, S., Leroux, J., Oustric, S., & Gardette, V. (2022). The shift from old age to very old age: An analysis of the perception of aging among older people. *BMC Primary Care, 23,* 3. https://doi.org/10.1186/s12875-021-01616-4

Ferraro, K. F., & Morton, P. M. (2018). What do we mean by accumulation? Advancing conceptual precision for a core idea in gerontology. *The Journals of Gerontology: Series B, 73*(2), 269–278. https://doi.org/10.1093/geronb/gbv094

Fisher, A. G., & Bray Jones, K. (2014). *Assessment of motor and process skills: Vol. 2. User manual.* Fort Collins, CO: Three Star Press.

Forbes. (2018, Feb 9). *Where did all the pensions go?* https://www.forbes.com/sites/impactpartners/2018/02/09/where-did-all-the-pensions-go/?sh=71c3eca43aab

Friedman, C., & VanPuymbrouck, L. (2021). Ageism and ableism: Unrecognized biases in occupational therapy students. *Physical & Occupational Therapy in Geriatrics, 39*(4), 354–369. https://doi.org/10.1080/02703181.2021.1880531

Fritz, H., & Cutchin, M. P. (2017). Changing neighborhoods and occupations: Experiences of older African-Americans in Detroit. *Journal of Occupational Science, 24*(2), 140–151. https://doi-org/10.1080/14427591.2016.1269296

Fry, C. (1996). Age, aging, and culture. In R. H. Binstock & L. K. George (Eds.), *Handbook of aging and the social sciences* (4th ed., pp. 117–136). San Diego: Academic Press.

Golant, S. M. (2019). Stop bashing the suburbs: Mobility limitations of older residents are less relevant as connectivity options expand. *Journal of Aging Studies, 50,* 100793. https://doi.org/10.1016/j.jaging.2019.100793

Granbom, M., Nkimbeng, M., Roberts, L. C., Gitlin, L. N., Taylor, J. L., & Szanton, S. L. (2021). "So I am stuck, but it's OK": Residential reasoning and housing decision-making of low-income older adults with disabilities in Baltimore, Maryland. *Housing and Society, 48*(1), 43–59. https://doi.org/10.1080/08882746.2020.1816782

Greenfield, E. A., & Moorman, S. M. (2019). Childhood socioeconomic status and later life cognition: Evidence from the Wisconsin longitudinal study. *Journal of Aging and Health*, *31*(9), 1589–1615. https://doi.org/10.1177/0898264318783489

Haber, C. (1997). Witches, widows, wives, and workers: The historiography of elderly women in America. In J. M. Coyle (Ed.), *Handbook on women and aging* (pp. 29–51). Westport, CT: Greenwood Press.

Hagestad, G. O. (1986). The aging society as a context for family life. *Daedalus*, *115*, 119–139. http://dx.doi.org/10.1007/978-1-4612-0423-7_5

Hawkins, M. M., Holliday, D. D., Weinhardt, L. S., Florsheim, P., Ngui, E., & AbuZahra, T. (2022). Barriers and facilitators of health among older adult immigrants in the United States: An integrative review of 20 years of literature. *BMC Public Health*, *22*(1), 755. https://doi.org/10.1186/s12889-022-13042-x

Hawthorne, F. (2013). *A brief history of American pensions—The origins of U.S. retirement plans*. Stamford, CT: Asset International.

Henderson, T. (2016). *Can you go home again? Some older retirees say yes*. Pew Charitable Trust. https://www.pewtrusts.org/en/research-and-analysis/blogs/stateline/2016/10/06/can-you-go-home-again-some-older-retirees-say-yes

Hoogendijk, E. O., Afilalo, J., Ensrud, K. E., Kowal, P., Onder, G., & Fried, L. P. (2019). Frailty: Implications for clinical practice and public health. *The Lancet*, *394*(10206), 1365–1375. https://doi.org/10.1016/S0140-6736(19)31786-6

Hossin, M. Z., Koupil, I., & Falkstedt, D. (2021). Early life socioeconomic position and mortality from cardiovascular diseases: An application of causal mediation analysis in the Stockholm Public Health Cohort. *BMJ Open*, *9*(26), e026258. https://doi.org/10.1136/bmjopen-2018-026258

Hsu, H. C., Liang, J., Luh, D. L., Chen, C. F., & Wang, Y. W. (2019). Social determinants and disparities in active aging among older Taiwanese. *International Journal of Environmental Research and Public Health*, *16*(16), 3005. https://doi.org/10.3390/ijerph16163005

Hunter, E. G., & Guest, M. A. (2021). Identifying barriers to care and support: Aging in Central Kentucky. *Local Development & Society*, *3*(2), 153–165. https://doi.org/10.1080/26883597.2021.1928534

Huston, B. F. (2019*). Social security: Demographic trends and the funding shortfall*. Congressional Research Service, R45990. https://sgp.fas.org/crs/misc/R45990.pdf

Jurkowski, E. T., & Guest, M. A. (2021). *Healthy aging through social determinants of health*. Alpha Press.

Kahana, E., & Kahana, B. (2014). Baby boomers' expectations of health and medicine. *American Medical Association Journal of Ethics: Virtual Mentor*, *16*(5), 380–384. https://doi.org/10.1001/virtualmentor.2014.16.5.msoc2-1405

Keating, N., Swindle, J., & Fletcher, S. (2011). Aging in rural Canada: A retrospective and review. *Canadian Journal on Aging*, *30*, 323–338. http://dx.doi.org/10.1017/S0714980811000250

Killen, A., & Macaskill, A. (2020). Positive ageing: To what extent can current models of wellbeing categorise the life events perceived as positive by older adults? *International Journal of Applied Positive Psychology*, *5*, 99–119. https://doi.org/10.1007/s41042-020-00028-6

Kim, D. (2019). The transportation safety of elderly pedestrians: Modeling contributing factors to elderly pedestrian collisions. *Accident Analysis & Prevention*, *131*, 268–274. https://doi.org/10.1016/j.aap.2019.07.009

Kivimäki, M., Batty, G. D., Pentti, J., Shipley, M. J., Sipilä, P. N., Nyberg, S. T., Suominen, S. B., Oksanen, T., Stenholm, S., Virtanen, M., Marmot, M. G., Singh-Manoux, A., Brunner, E. J., Lindbohm, J. V., Ferrie, J. E., & Vahtera, J. (2020). Association between socioeconomic status and the development of mental and physical health conditions in adulthood: A multi-cohort study. *The Lancet Public Health*, *5*(3), e140–e149. https://doi.org/10.1016/S2468-2667(19)30248-8

Law, M., Baptiste, S., Carswell, A., McColl, M., Polatajko, H., & Pollock, N. (2014). *Canadian Occupational Performance Measure (5th ed.)*. Ottawa, ON: CAOT Publications ACE.

Lee, S. B., Oh, J. H., Park, J. H., Choi, S. P., & Wee, J. H. (2018). Differences in youngest-old, middle-old, and oldest-old patients who visit the emergency department. *Clinical & Experimental Emergency Medicine*, *5*(4), 249–255. https://doi.org/10.15441/ceem.17.261

Leedahl, S. N., Brasher M. S., LoBuono, D. L., Wood, B. M., & Estus, E. L. (2020). Reducing ageism: Changes in students' attitudes after participation in an intergenerational reverse mentoring program. *Sustainability*, *12*(17), 6870. https://doi.org/10.3390/su12176870

Levy B. R., Chang, E-S., Lowe, S. R., Provolo, N., & Slade, M. D. (2022). Impact of media-based negative and positive age stereotypes on older individuals' mental health. *The Journals of Gerontology: Series B*, *77*(4), e70–e75. https://doi.org/10.1093/geronb/gbab085

Levy, B. R., Slade, M. D., Chang, E. S., Kannoth, S., & Wang, S. Y. (2020). Ageism amplifies cost and prevalence of health conditions. *The Gerontologist*, *60*(1), 174–181. https://doi.org/10.1093/geront/gny131

Levy, S. R. (2018). Toward reducing ageism: PEACE (Positive Education about Aging and Contact Experiences) model. *The Gerontologist*, *58*(2), 226–232. https://doi.org/10.1093/geront/gnw116

Lewis, E., & Lemieux, V. (2021). Social participation of seniors: Applying the framework of occupational justice for healthy ageing and a new approach to policymaking. *Journal of Occupational Science*, *28*(3), 332–348. https://doi.org/10.1080/14427591.2020.1843069

Lopez, J., Perez-Rojo, G., Noriega, C., Carretero, I., Velasco, C., Martinez-Huertas, J. A., Lopen-Frutos, P., & Galarraga, L. (2020). Psychological well-being among older adults during the COVID-19 outbreak: A comparative study of the young-old and old-old adults. *International Psychogeriatrics*, *32*(11), 1365–1370. https://doi.org/10.1017/S1041610220000964

Maritz R, Baptiste S, Darzins SW, Magasi S, Weleschuk C., & Prodinger B. (2018). Linking occupational therapy models and assessments to the ICF to enable standardized documentation of functioning. *Canadian Journal of Occupational Therapy*, *85*(4):330–341. doi:10.1177/0008417418797146

Mateyka, P. J., & He, W. (2022). *Domestic migration of older Americans: 2015–2019*. U.S. Census Bureau. https://www.census.gov/content/dam/Census/library/publications/2022/demo/p23-218.pdf

McKinsey & Company. (n.d.) *Generation Z*. https://www.mckinsey.com/featured-insights/generation-z

Mitra, S. K., Bae, Y., & Ritchie, S. G. (2019). Use of ride-hailing services among older adults in the United States. *Transportation Research Record*, *2673*(3), 700–710. https://doi.org/10.1177/0361198119835511

Morrissey, M. (2016). *Women over 65 are more likely to be poor than men, regardless of race, educational background, and marital status*. Economic Policy Institute. https://www.epi.org/publication/women-over-65-are-more-likely-to-in-poverty-than-men/

Murphy, S. L., Kochanek, K. D., Xu, J., & Arias, E. (2021). Mortality in the United States, 2020: NCHS Data Brief No. 427, December 2021. CDC.gov. https://www.cdc.gov/nchs/data/databriefs/db427.pdf

National Council on Aging. (2021). *Suicide and older adults: What you should know*. https://ncoa.org/article/suicide-and-older-adults-what-you-should-know

Neville, S., Adams, J., Montayre, J., Larmer, P., Garrett, N., Stephens, C., & Alpass, F. (2018). Loneliness in men 60 years and over: The association with purpose in life. *American Journal of Men's Health*, *12*(4), 730–739. https://doi.org/10.1177/1557988318758807

Oxford. (n.d.). Ableism. In *oed.com dictionary*. Retrieved December 5, 2022, from https://www.oed.com/

Parkinson, S., Forsyth, K, & Kielhofner, G. (2006). *The model of human occupation screening tool (MOHOST) version 2.0*. MOHO Clearinghouse.

Peres, M. A., Macpherson, L. M., Weyant, R. J., Daly, B., Venturelli, R., Mathur, M. R., Listel, S., Celeste, R K., Cuarnizo-Herreno, C., Kearns, C., Benzian, H., Allison, P., & Watt, R. G. (2019). Oral diseases: A global public health challenge. *The Lancet*, *394*(10194), 249–260. https://doi.org/10.1016/S0140-6736(19)31146-8

Pooler, J. A., & Srinivasan, M. (2018). Cost-related medication nonadherence for older adults participating in SNAP, 2013–2015. *American Public Health Association*, *108*(2), 224–230. https://doi.org/10.2105/AJPH.2017.304176

Raleigh, V. S. (2019). OECD Health working paper No. 108. Trends in life expectancy in EU and other OECD Countries: Why are improvements slowing? https://www.oecd.org/officialdocuments/publicdisplaydocumentpdf/?cote=DELSA/HEA/WD/HWP(2019)1&docLanguage=En

Ramachandran, M., & Dsouza, S. A. (2018). Older adults' experiences of community mobility in an indian metropolis: A qualitative study. *Physical & Occupational Therapy in Geriatrics, 38*(2/3), 315–329. https://doi.org/10.1080/02703181.2018.1508170

Ramamonjiarivelo, Z., Renick, O., & Osborne, R. (2021). Intergenerational service learning: A way to increase cultural competency and decrease ageism. *The Journal of Health Administration Education, 38*(3), 785–808. https://www.proquest.com/openview/2ea51d7dcab979a7f454f4fd3adee387/1?pq-origsite=gscholar&cbl=105455

Ramsay, S., Papachristou, E., Watt, R. G., Lennon, L. T., Papacosta, A. O., Whincup, P. W., & Wannamethee, S. G., (2018). Socioeconomic disadvantage across the life-course and oral health in older age: Findings from a longitudinal study of older British men. *Journal of Public Health, 40*(4), e423–e430. https://doi.org/10.1093/pubmed/fdy068

Reich, A. J., Claunch, K. D., Verdeja, M. A., Dungan, M. T., Anderson, S., Clayton, C. K., Goates, M. C., & Thacker, E. L. (2020). What does "successful aging" mean to you? Systematic review and cross-cultural comparison of lay perspectives of older adults in 13 countries, 2010–2020. *Journal of Cross-Cultural Gerontology, 35*, 455–478. https://doi.org/10.1007.s10823-020-09416-6

Romig, K. (2022). *Social security lifts more people above the poverty line than any other program*. Center on Budget and Policy Priorities. https://www.cbpp.org/sites/default/files/atoms/files/10-25-13ss.pdf

Roser, M., Ortiz-Ospina, E., & Ritchie, H. (2019). *Life expectancy*. OurWorldInData.org. https://ourworldindata.org/life-expectancy

Rudolph, J. (2021). The intersection of aging and social determinants of health (SDoH). *Rhode Island Medical Journal*, 14–25. http://www.rimed.org/rimedicaljournal/2021/05/2021-05-14-sdoh-rudolph.pdf

Rural Health Information Hub. (2022). https://www.ruralhealthinfo.org/

Santiago, J. A., & Potashkin, J. A. (2021). The impact of disease comorbidities in Alzheimer's Disease. *Frontiers in Aging Neuroscience, 13*, 631770. https://doi.org/10.3389/fnagi.2021.631770

Sciubba, J. (2020, August 27). Population aging as a global issue. *Oxford Research Encyclopedia of International Studies*. https://oxfordre.com/internationalstudies/display/10.1093/acrefore/9780190846626.001.0001/acrefore-9780190846626-e-559

Stadnyk, R., Townsend, E., & Wilcock, A. (2010). Occupational justice. In C. H. Christiansen & E. A. Townsend (Eds.), *Introduction to occupation: The art and science of living* (2nd ed., pp. 329–358). Pearson Education.

Steinmayr, D., Weichselbaumer, D., & Winter-Ebmer, R. (2020). Gender differences in active ageing: Findings from a new individual-level index for European countries. *Social Indicators Research, 151*, 691–721. https://doi.org/10.1007/s11205-020-02380-1

Sutphin, G. L., & Kaeberlein, M. (2011). Comparative genetics of aging. In E. J. Masoro & S. N. Austad (Eds.), *Handbook of the biology of aging* (pp. 215–241). San Diego: Elsevier Academic Press.

Swope, C. B., & Hernandez, D., (2019). Housing as a determinant of health equity: A conceptual model. *Social Science & Medicine, 243*, 112571. https://www.ruralhealthinfo.org/

Tolbize, A. (2008). Generational differences in the workplace. Retrieved from http://rtc.umn.edu/docs/2_18_Gen_diff_workplace.pdf

Troy, D. (2022*). How did the elderly used to be looked after in the past? 18th Century History – The age of reason and change*. https://www.history1700s.com/index.php/articles/14-guest-authors/1631-how-did-the-elderly-used-to-be-looked-after-in-the-past.html

U.S. Department of Health and Human Services. (2020). *Social determinants of health*. Social Determinants of Health - Healthy People 2030. https://health.gov/healthypeople/objectives-and-data/social-determinants-health

U.S. Department of Health and Human Services, Office of Disease Prevention and Health Promotion, (2022). *Healthy people 2030*. https://health.gov/healthypeople

United Nations Department of Economic and Social Affairs, Population Division. (2020). *International migrant stock*. United Nations. https://www.un.org/development/desa/pd/content/international-migrant-stock

Vera-Toscano, E. & Meroni, E. C. (2021). An age-period-cohort approach to disentangling generational differences in family values and religious beliefs: Understanding the modern Australian family. *Demographic Research. 45*, 653–692. https://doi.org/10.4054/DemRes.2021.45.20

Wang, J., Mann, F., Lloyd-Evans, B., Ma, R., & Johnson, S. (2018). Associations between loneliness and perceived social support and outcomes of mental health problems: A systematic review. *BMC Psychiatry, 18*(1), 1–16. https://doi.org/10.1186/s12888-01801736-5

Wang, V. H-C., Silver, D., & Pagán, J. A. (2022). Generational differences in beliefs about COVID-19 vaccines. *Preventive Medicine, 157*. https://doi.org/10.1016/j.ypmed.2022.107005

World Health Organization. (n. d.). *International classification of functioning, disability, and health (ICF)*. https://icd.who.int/dev11/l-icf/en

World Health Organization. (2012). *Measuring health and disability: Manual for WHO Disability Assessment Schedule (WHO–DAS 2.0)*. https://www.who.int/publications/i/item/measuring-health-and-disability-manual-for-who-disability-assessment-schedule-(-whodas-2.0)

World Health Organization. (2018). *Public spending on health: A closer look at global trends*. Geneva: World Health Organization. https://www.who.int/publications/i/item/WHO-HIS-HGF-HFWorkingPaper-18.3

World Health Organization. (2020). *Leading causes of death*. https://www.who.int/news-room/fact-sheets/detail/the-top-10-causes-of-death

World Health Organization. (2022a). *About WHO*. https://www.who.int/about

World Health Organization. (2022b). *Social determinants of health*. https://www.who.int/health-topics/social-determinants-of-health

World Health Organization. (2023). *Ageing*. https://www.who.int/health-topics/ageing

WHO-FIC Collaborating Centre for the Africa Region. (n.d.) *What is ICF?* ICF Education. https://icfeducation.org/what-is-icf

World Federation of Occupational Therapists (WFOT). (2021). *Position statement: Occupational therapy and ageing across the life course*. https://wfot.org/resources/occupational-therapy-and-ageing-across-the-life-course

Wrisdale, L., Mokoena, M. M., Mudau, L. S., & Geere, J. (2017). Factors that impact on access to water and sanitation for older adults and people with disability in rural South Africa: An occupational justice perspective, *Journal of Occupational Science, (24)*3, 259–279. https://doi.org/10.1080/14427591.2017.1338190

Zhang, X., Mu, K., & Shannon, J. (2021). The relationship between older adult migration and destination characteristics in Georgia. *Applied Geography, 132*, 102464. https://doi.org/10.1016/j.apgeog.2021.102464

Zlokovic, B. V., Gottesman, R. F., Bernstein, K. E., Seshadri, S., McKee, A., Snyder, H., Greenberg, S., Yaffe, K., Schaffer, C., Yuan, C., & Chen, J. (2020). Vascular contributions to cognitive impairment and dementia (VCID): A report from the 2018 National Heart, Lung, and Blood Institute and National Institute of Neurological Disorders and Stroke Workshop. *Alzheimer's & Dementia, 16*(12), 1714–1733. https://doi.org/10.1002/alz.12157

CHAPTER 2

Meaningful Occupations in Later Life

Bette Bonder, PhD, OTR, FAOTA ■ Noralyn D. Pickens, PhD, OT, FAOTA

"None are so old as those who have outlived enthusiasm."

—Henry David Thoreau

LEARNING OUTCOMES

By the end of this chapter, readers will be able to:

2-1. Explain the importance of meaning in the lives of older adults.
2-2. Discuss the role of occupation and co-occupation in supporting meaning in the lives of older adults.
2-3. Identify and describe four primary categories of meaningful occupation.
2-4. Define spirituality and religion and discuss their relevance in later life.
2-5. Create occupational therapy interventions to promote and support meaningful occupation and co-occupation for older adults.
2-6. Discuss theories regarding meaningful occupation and well-being, emphasizing occupational impact on health, subjective well-being, self-efficacy, and life satisfaction.
2-7. Debate the importance of home and place as integral to meaning in later life.

Mini Case Study

Claudette Odon is a 71-year-old African American woman who resides in a large West Coast city where she has lived her entire life. She is widowed, having lost her husband 6 years ago after 48 years of a marriage she describes as happy. She has two adult daughters who live in the same city and six grandchildren, most of whom are currently at universities around the United States. She had a son, but he was killed in a drive-by shooting when he was 16, a loss that remains central to her awareness.

Ms. Odon worked for many years in a nonprofit organization that promoted the arts, especially theater, in her city and retired 3 years ago. She continues to be very involved in the arts community, serving on the boards of several organizations and attending frequent performances. She has a large circle of friends, mostly related to the arts, and she is very involved in her Baptist church.

Ms. Odon reports having arthritis that interferes with her ability to move comfortably. The discomfort has led her to give up gardening, and she reports having difficulty preparing her meals because standing and handling food preparation tools are uncomfortable as well.

Provocative Questions

1. Do you think that Ms. Odon has a satisfying occupational profile? Are there areas of occupation that are missing from her profile? If there are, what might be some explanations for their absence?
2. How might the loss of her son and her husband affect her occupational profile and her satisfaction with the associated activities?
3. How might an occupational therapist help Ms. Odon prepare for adaptations she may need for future occupational participation in valued occupations?

Later life is characterized by significant change—change in physical capacity, change in roles, change in family constellations, change in living arrangements. All these changes can present daunting challenges in the absence of a sense of purpose and meaning. Occupational therapy can make important contributions in helping older adults find purpose and thereby enhance quality of life. This chapter considers the ways in which older adults construct meaningful lives, the centrality of occupations to life, and strategies that occupational therapists can employ to help older adults find meaning.

Throughout this book, evidence is presented regarding the importance of various occupations in the lives of older adults and the outcomes of interventions focused on enabling occupational performance. Therapists interested in fostering positive aging can look to this literature for guidance about how best to proceed. They can also use these findings to support efforts to improve the context in which aging occurs through interventions focused on policy change and on access to care for older adults.

The Search for Meaning

Everyone needs a reason to get up in the morning, and these reasons relate to making sense of one's life—feeling that what one does is valuable and matters to the world. In this sense, meaning is typically expressed both by one's actions and by the interpretation of those actions. Meaning can be thought of as "what we create for ourselves in our mind that explains experiences and, in turn, motivates us and spurs us on to create new experiences" (Polatajko et al, 2013, p. 61).

George and Park (2016) suggest that meaning in life is multidimensional, consisting of three factors: **comprehension** (feeling as though one's life makes sense), **purpose** (feeling directed and motivated by valued goals), and **mattering** (feeling one's existence is significant). These characteristics are often expressed through what we do. In this sense, meaning is typically expressed both by our actions and by our interpretation of those actions.

Csikszentmihalyi (1990) offers a three-part definition: Meaning includes achieving purpose, expressing intentionality, and creating internal harmony. Meaningful occupation is a multifaceted, richly interconnected system of positive subjective experiences associated with occupation. Such a system is sensitive to an individual's history and unique constellation of occupations and is influenced by the sociocultural contexts within which occupations arise (Eakman et al, 2018).

Meaning in life is associated with positive psychological health and function, good physical health, reduced morbidity—including lower incidence of cardiac events and Alzheimer disease, and overall reduced morbidity (Hooker et al, 2017). Meaning in life reduces stress, improves coping, and encourages healthy behaviors (Hooker et al, 2017). Meaningful engagement reduces loneliness (Tam & Chan, 2019). Meaning is associated with resilience (Mohseni et al, 2019), well-being, and overall quality of life (Eakman, 2014; Steptoe & Fancourt, 2019). These factors are particularly salient in later life. Steptoe and Fancourt have noted that "maintaining a sense that life is worthwhile may be particularly important at older ages when social and emotional ties often fragment, social engagement is reduced, and health problems may limit personal options" (2019, p. 1207).

All individuals strive to find meaning in their lives (Hasselkus & Dickie, 2021; Hill & Turiano, 2014). They ascribe meaning to the objects around them, to their social relationships, and to what they do with their time. Aristotle noted that "all human happiness or misery takes the form of action, the end for which we live is a certain kind of activity, not a quality" (cited in Lind, 1957, p. XXVIII). This view is consistent with the fundamental principles of occupational science (Pierce, 2014). Occupational therapy focuses on enabling individuals to maintain function in support of those occupations they need or want to do and helping individuals determine what occupations matter most and how to sustain them. In doing so, occupational therapy supports the ability to live a meaningful life.

Western societies often fail to provide meaningful roles for older adults, such that they must construct meaning themselves (Achenbaum, 2020; Steptoe & Fancourt, 2019). The notion of retirement commonly found in developed countries allows—even encourages—withdrawal from paid employment. Children have been raised and are creating their own lives. Thus older adults may lose both work and childrearing as sources of meaning. Hypothetically, this offers a greater degree of personal choice, although for some, retirement is not voluntary, and childrearing may be reintroduced if they assume responsibility for raising grandchildren. Perhaps because of the diversity introduced by greater choice and less predictable life course, there is little clarity about occupational patterns among older adults or the personal meanings of the occupations that they undertake. For older adults, the search for meaning is highly individual and begins with few reference points.

The importance of meaningful occupation in later life has been the subject of considerable discussion (Hooker et al, 2017; Steptoe & Fancourt, 2019). In addition to occupational scientists, psychologists explore "positive psychology" focused on understanding what makes life worth living (Seligman & Csikszentmihalyi, 2000). Csikszentmihalyi (1990) described optimal experience as "flow," the intense and consuming engagement in occupations that promotes a sense of well-being and happiness. Optimal experiences, as he describes them, are characterized by concentration, attention, and creative use of personal skills. Occupational therapy emphasizes the value of such engagement (AOTA], 2020a), but other disciplines like nursing have also recognized that meaning in life is an important outcome of care for older adults (Hupkens et al, 2018) and that meaning is intertwined with occupation.

The relationship between occupation and meaning is central to quality of life for older adults. However, the creation of personal meaning is not a one-time event, but a process (Raanas et al, 2019; Webster et al, 2014). In later life, "searching for meaning entails a motivated process to find and engage with sources of meaning" (Morgan & Robinson, 2013, p. 999). In this chapter, some types of meaning that have particular relevance in the lives of older adults and the interaction between meanings and occupations are discussed, as are some important therapeutic considerations in helping older adults create and maintain meaningful occupational lives.

CASE STUDY

Occupational Profile

Claire is an 83-year-old woman living in her own home in an urban community. She has five grown children—three in the same city, two living across the country from her—and 11 grandchildren. Her husband died 12 years earlier from heart disease. She wears glasses and hearing aids. She had been experiencing problems with some favored activities, which she attributed to arthritis in her hands and wrists, but otherwise is in good health. Claire drives, though limits her driving at night. She enjoys attending her grandchildren's school events and keeping in touch with them via a range of social media apps. She was a schoolteacher and continues to be involved in after-school reading programs for the children at her church's grade school 3 days a week. She participates in Bible studies and teaching Sunday school. She has vegetable and flower gardens, frequently trading plants with neighbors. Recently, one of her grandchildren was killed in a car accident while driving home from college.

Identified Problem Areas

Claire's hand and wrist pain worsened, and she was diagnosed with carpal tunnel syndrome in her right wrist (dominant) and was referred to an outpatient hand clinic. The occupational therapist completed an occupational profile, along with standard biomechanical and motor assessments. Claire reported her involvement in after-school and Sunday school programs has waned since the death of her grandchild. She has found it difficult, and at times painful, to use her garden and cooking tools. She has reduced her time on the computer in both school activities and social media.

Goals for Occupational Therapy

1. Reduce pain in bilateral U/E wrists
2. Improve R U/E function
3. Demonstrate successful use of assistive technology for computer use
4. Demonstrate successful use of ergonomic gardening tools
5. Demonstrate adapted cooking skills

Occupation, Co-Occupation, and Meaning

Occupational therapy holds that humans are occupational beings whose identities are strongly related to the occupations they pursue (AOTA, 2020a; Hooper & Wood, 2019). This perspective means that occupational therapy focuses on the ways in which engagement with occupations contributes to purpose and meaning in life (Bar et al, 2016).

Occupation is described as having four dimensions of doing, being, becoming, and belonging (Hitch et al, 2014) that are necessary for understanding older adult occupation and meaning. Doing reflects a sense of purpose and activity. Being is about presence and oneness with the self. Becoming is change, transition, and adaptation. Belonging encompasses both social and place aspects of occupation. Occupational therapists are interested in helping older adults *do* their occupations, so that they can have a sense of maintaining their *selves*. Occupations help people transform and *become*. Engaging with others helps create a sense of belonging. All four dimensions create meaning for the older adult.

Occupation is an essential component of meaning in later life (Jessen-Winge et al, 2018). Occupation plays a central role in identity throughout the life span, and factors that interfere with occupation, including life crises, can negatively affect both self-concept and well-being (Hooper & Wood, 2019); although aging is not a life crisis, it involves numerous changes and transitions that require adaptation and resourcefulness.

Humans are co-occupational beings in that much adaptation and meaning is dependent on and shared with others. **Co-occupations** are occupations that have aspects of shared physicality, shared emotionality, shared intentionality, and shared communication (Beckinger et al, 2016; Pizur-Barnekow & Pickens, 2019). Co-occupations are engaged in by dyads and small and large groups. Examples of co-occupations include washing dishes together, playing charades, and singing in a choir. Importantly for older adults, co-occupations create meanings through regular and even mundane shared activities. Consider the morning routine of a long-partnered couple, the weaving of their activities to prepare a shared morning meal of making coffee, breakfast, reading the paper, and planning their day. Although these activities could be completed alone, the shared aspects of emotion and intention create co-occupation. Consider now one of the partners experiencing a stroke that affects their physical and communication skills and how the morning routine may have heightened shared physicality and shared verbal communication to support both partners engaging in the morning routine. The amount and intensity of sharing is on a continuum depending on the partners' needs. For couples managing chronic health conditions, mutual caregiving and co-creating meaning was found to be important in their daily activities (Antonelli et al, 2020).

Although most researchers and care providers recognize that occupation and co-occupation are essential components of quality of life in later life, there is a lack of clarity about what factors are most salient in establishing meaningful occupations and co-occupations for older adults. As noted earlier, the inevitable change in performance skills, client factors, and environmental circumstances that characterize later life require adjustment in activity patterns.

Erlandsson, Eklund, and Persson (2011) describe meaning as central to understanding of occupations. As the individual makes choices, **occupational value**—the individual's assessment of the importance of the activity—informs meaning. The reasons for the choice and the outcomes from participation in the specific occupation reflect the meaning as perceived and enacted by the individual (Erlandsson et al, 2011). "The values of occupations, generated in the interaction between the person, the task performed, and the environment, constantly contribute to building an overarching experience of meaning in life" (p. 73). Although occupations have socially constructed meanings, those meanings are filtered through the screen of personal interpretation to create what we will call personal meaning.

Themes of Meaning

Many of the psychosocial theories described in Chapter 3 focus on understanding how older adults can live meaningful lives. Early developmental theories were written at a time when life expectancy and good health were more limited than today. For example, Erikson (1963) suggested that the major tasks of later life are generativity (productivity and creativity) versus stagnation and ego integrity versus despair. Neugarten (1975) identified acceptance of imminent death, coping with increasing infirmity, dealing with care decisions, and maintaining social ties as the important developmental tasks of later life. Levinson (1986) described two stages for older adults. The first is a transition stage, during which tasks involve coping with physical decline and moving from formal authority to a more informal life structure. The second, in late adulthood, is characterized by decreasing concern with formal authority, status, and formal rewards; forming a broader life perspective and greater inner resources; and contributing to the wisdom of others. In each of these theories, there is an implicit or explicit assumption that in accomplishing these tasks, older adults will find later life meaningful and satisfying.

It is clear that later life now extends substantially from when these scholars wrote. It is unlikely that Erikson anticipated in 1963 that later life might last two or more decades. Cohen (2005) proposed a life span theory based on human potential stages. He suggested that in middle age (35 to 65), individuals experience a midlife reevaluation followed by a liberation phase, a summing up, and, by age 75, an encore, an opportunity for reflection, continuation, and spirituality that lasts until death. He placed particular emphasis on the importance of creativity in later life, suggesting that creative capacity is maintained or enhanced with age. This and other more recent theories make it clear that meaning changes throughout the life course and that later life is characterized by gains as well as losses (Boudiny, 2013; Erlandsson et al, 2011).

Meaning is highly individual and subjective (Black et al, 2019; Eakman, 2014). However, there are some general considerations in understanding older adults' occupational choices in that context (Hooker et al, 2017). A qualitative exploration of older adults' perspectives found that older adults perceived activity as contributing to well-being, a means to express and manage identity, an organizer of time, and a connector to the past, present, and future. Occupational meaning is also influenced by individuals' cultural experiences and identity and the social environment in which they are situated (AOTA, 2020a; Black et al, 2019; George & Park, 2016). As an example, independence in instrumental occupations like self-care tend to be highly meaningful in Western societies but less important in other, more communal cultural groups (Black et al, 2019).

For purposes of this discussion, meanings will be clustered into four main themes: instrumental meanings, evaluative meanings, existential meanings, and self-identity. Even though there are undoubtedly many other ways to organize themes of meaning—Persson and colleagues (2001) have a conceptual model identifying concrete value, self-reward value, and symbolic value—the literature about aging seems to suggest that the four listed here are particularly salient in later life. These themes overlap to some extent, and the same occupation can have different meanings for specific individuals or in particular contexts (Persson et al, 2001). Instrumental meanings are not completely separate from self-identity or evaluative meanings. Because ability to complete instrumental activities may be more tenuous for older adults than younger individuals, it is an important theme to consider separately.

Some occupations, or the conditions in which those occupations occur, span all four of these meaning categories. Social engagement (Carstensen, 2021) is an example of this kind of occupation. Carstensen notes that in spite of the reality of loss of social connections as friends and family die or move away, older adults recognize the shortened time frame of their own lives and make use of their adaptive and cognitive resources to sustain social occupations to give their lives meaning.

Social interaction is well-established as essential to well-being in later life (Santini et al, 2020). Social interactions can certainly address instrumental meanings (e.g., providing shopping and home maintenance support may allow an older adult to age in place). They also support evaluative meanings as individuals experience the satisfaction of deep supportive relationships or the loneliness of their absence. They contribute to existential meanings through opportunities for life review and for leaving a legacy and are a source of identity exploration and understanding as interactions clarify personal characteristics and provide external validation.

Instrumental Meanings

Instrumental meanings are those typically associated with occupations that support daily life. For younger individuals, accomplishing daily tasks is habitual. As performance skills diminish with age, those habits may be disrupted. Older adults may need to focus much greater attention on bathing, dressing, and taking nourishment than do their younger counterparts. Other occupations that may have instrumental meanings, including work and caring for others, may likewise be affected by changes in physical and psychological abilities. These occupations become imbued with important meanings, particularly in terms of the individual's perceptions about independence and dependence (Barken, 2019). These instrumental occupations meet basic daily needs, but they are also foundational to other meaningful occupations (Eakman, 2014).

Instrumental tasks structure meaning in later life in that they provide everyday routines (Söderbacka et al, 2016). Older adults who can accomplish instrumental tasks experience less disability and greater satisfaction than peers who struggle with these tasks (Ferreira et al, 2012). Many occupations have outcomes that support function in important ways and thus can be categorized as instrumental. For example, reading supports cognition, emotional regulation, and other performance skills needed to accomplish an array of other occupations (cf. Candler et al, 2021).

Subjective usefulness and self-rated functional ability correlate with mortality; that is, older adults who perceive themselves as capable are likely to live longer than others (Okamata & Tanaka, 2004). A variety of functional activities, including work, hobbies (e.g., needlework, carpentry), and participation in social groups like clubs have all been identified as having instrumental meaning for older individuals (Beauchet et al, 2020; Söderbacka et al, 2016). Some of these occupations also address evaluative meanings and contribute to self-identity.

Aging is associated with some degree of decline in performance skills as well as change in contexts such as family and social networks. Ability to adapt and maintain routines can, in itself, be a meaningful attribute of instrumental occupations (Barken, 2019; Shank & Cutchin, 2010).

Evaluative Meanings

For most of us, occupations contribute to our evaluation of well-being and happiness (Steptoe & Fancourt, 2019). Life span theories suggest that this evaluation is a central concern of later life, and research confirms that for older adults, occupation has a central role in subjective assessments about satisfaction with life (Roberts & Bannigan, 2018). A number of interrelated constructs are used in the research examining this issue: **happiness, life satisfaction, subjective well-being,** and **quality of life.** There are subtle distinctions among these constructs. Happiness refers to a sense of pleasure or positive affect in the present, and life satisfaction refers to an overall life evaluation with which one is content. Well-being reflects a feeling that current circumstances are, in general, positive. Quality of life is perhaps the most inclusive of these evaluative terms, because it conveys satisfaction with circumstances and health and also reflects external, concrete markers of well-being, such as income, type of housing, and education.

Erlandsson and colleagues (2011) developed a direct theoretical connection between occupational value and meaning. Their Value and Meaning in Occupations (ValMO) model posits that there is a person-task-environment interrelationship. According to the ValMO model, this interrelationship generates three kinds of value assessment: **concrete value** (features that are concrete and visible in an occupation), **symbolic value** (what the occupation signifies to the individual), and **self-reward value** (the immediate reward resulting from participation in a particular occupation).

As noted earlier, there is overlap among the themes discussed here. For example, productive activities like paid employment and volunteering can support a sense of meaning and control (Söderbacka et al, 2016). Therefore, accomplishing an instrumental purpose can contribute to a positive evaluation of occupation and thus to well-being. This would reflect the concrete value of work, the symbolic value based on the importance of the role to the person's identity, and the self-reward value derived from feeling one has been effective in one's work.

A great deal of research literature suggests that positive evaluations of life are associated with occupation. Some of the literature examines specific performance areas such as leisure (Provencher et al, 2018), productive activities like volunteering (Huo et al, 2021), creativity (Carpenter et al, 2021), and social participation (Steptoe & Fancourt, 2019). Other literature examines more global aspects of the association between occupation and well-being (Söderbacka et al, 2016). Although there are differences among nations in reported subjective well-being, work and social occupations are associated with subjective well-being around the world. Research examining the opposite side of the same coin finds that decreased activity is associated with decreased happiness (Menec, 2003), and stressors such as retirement or loss of a spouse that affect highly valued roles erode meaning (Krause, 2004).

Older adults also evaluate specific occupations and occupational patterns. So not only do occupations help determine whether individuals feel their lives are well-lived, but they also evaluate their satisfaction with regard to the things they do (Bar et al, 2016). Individuals may consider the balance of those occupations (Eakman, 2016; Hovbrandt et al, 2019). For example, is enough time being spent in social occupations, productive occupations, or creative occupations? For some older adults, too much activity can feel oppressive (Nesteruk & Price, 2011). This, too, is an evaluative consideration as older individuals consider their occupational choices. There is some lack of clarity about optimal engagement, in large part as a result of the wide range of individual difference.

Occupational patterns in later life may contribute to a sense of fulfillment, restoration, and connection (Roberts & Bannigan, 2018). All these considerations reflect both evaluation of occupational engagement and the contributions of occupations to overall well-being and satisfaction with life.

Existential Meanings

Of course, the question about whether life is worth living defines the existential challenge of living, a challenge that certainly becomes more critical as death nears. One of the major ways in which older adults maintain ego integrity and avoid despair is through engagement in meaningful occupations. These are the occupations through which older adults address important philosophical questions about their lives: Has my life been worth living? Have I made a contribution to the world around me? Hicks and colleagues (2012) label this "eudaemonic well-being," a sense that one is living a life of meaning. Many older individuals are particularly focused on ensuring that they leave a legacy, reflecting a sense of concern about how they will be remembered and what they leave for the next generation (Newton et al, 2020). Older adults must draw on "human strengths that act as buffers against mental illness: courage, future mindedness, optimism, interpersonal skill, faith, work ethic, hope, honesty, perseverance, and the capacity for flow and insight" (Seligman & Csikszentmihalyi, 2000, p. 5). Meaningful occupations allow older adults to sustain these attributes in the face of the challenges of later life. Refer to Table 2-1 for further descriptions of these themes of meaning.

Spirituality and Religion as Contributors to Meaning

"A **religion** is a set of beliefs about life and the self, is usually associated with established rituals and is certainly spiritual" (Stevens, 2016, p. 156). **Spirituality** is harder to define but can be thought of as reflecting a sense of something transcendent or sacred in the universe, larger than the individual (Steinhauser et al, 2017). Religion is spiritual, but not all spiritual beliefs are religious in nature.

Spirituality, identified as a contextual factor in the American Occupational Therapy Association's Occupational Therapy Practice Framework (OTPF; 2020a), is a form of occupation whose central purpose is to address existential meanings. Gerontology and occupational therapy literature are replete with studies of participation in religious or spiritual occupations (cf. Pham et al, 2022). **Religious occupations** are those undertaken in association with formally constituted religious organizations, such as churches, mosques, or synagogues. **Spiritual occupations** are those that individuals identify as connecting them to a higher power (Amirav et al, 2021). These occupations may not have an obvious association with organized religion; for example, someone who enjoys hiking and canoeing might report that being close to the natural world has a spiritual component.

Both religion and spirituality are associated with positive outcomes in later life. Individuals who participate in religious activities report higher levels of life satisfaction, self-esteem, and optimism, a finding that is particularly pronounced among some minority groups in the United States (Hodge et al, 2012). Religious and spiritual activities are associated with lower levels of chronic illness, higher levels of activity, and lower mortality (Avelar-González et al, 2020). Spiritual occupations contribute to meaning and well-being for individuals in residential care, including those with dementia (Dewitte et al, 2021). Occupations that are perceived as having religious or spiritual significance foster hope (Amirav et al, 2021) and a sense of optimism and joy (Gabriel et al, 2020). They offer a sense of security and a belief in one's ability to cope (Söderbacka et al, 2016).

Spiritual experiences have also been found to reduce fear of death and dying (Renz et al, 2018). Anxiety is reduced, and a sense of calm may be profound, perhaps because spiritual occupations increase death acceptance by offering an explanation of the self in the world (Surall & Steppacher, 2020).

Meaning and Identity

To a great extent, we are what we do. Thus, a fourth meaning of occupations in later life is the maintenance of a sense of identity (Mulholland & Jackson, 2018). "Identities are shaped through daily occupations within a social context, and individuals seek to make sense of who they were, who they are and who they want to become through a coherent story of their activities" (p. 658). Especially during such life transitions as retirement, the occupations that allow for exploration and personal growth can be supportive and meaningful.

For older adults, later-life occupations allow a continued sense of mastery and control in the face of significant physical and social change (Tovel & Carmel, 2014). Barken (2019) notes that the ability to take care of oneself is highly valued in Western society; as a result, maintaining such ability may powerfully influence self-identity.

Self-efficacy, confidence in physical performance in specific contexts, is associated with reduced frailty and greater function in later life (Hladek et al, 2021). A strong sense of self-efficacy can mediate the effects of anxiety about loss during later life, reducing the incidence of depression (Dutt & Wahl, 2019).

As is true for self-efficacy, perceived control is an important factor in overall well-being and health in later life (Hülür et al, 2017), making a clear contribution to positive aging (Finkenzeller et al, 2019). Perceived control is related to better use of resources and improved ability to address challenges.

What, then, are the essential elements of occupations that provide for a sense of control? In particular, occupations that are productive, health-promoting, and family-related seem to contribute to a positive sense of identity (Križaj et al, 2019). Cultural relevance of occupation is also important in promoting a sense of control (Wang et al, 2019). Although predictable routines are important, adaptability and incorporating new occupations into identity also affect perceived control (Tatzer et al, 2012).

Consider the example of volunteering, an occupation many older adults participate in later in life (Jiang et al,

TABLE 2-1 ■ Themes of Meaning

THEME	DESCRIPTION	EXAMPLES
Instrumental	Occupations that support daily life	Dressing Cooking Financial management
Evaluative	Assessing current well-being, previous achievements	Life review Reminiscence Sharing life stories with family
Existential	Assessing overall meaning of one's life, whether life has been worth living	Spiritual and/or religious activity Immersion in nature
Identity	Occupations that support conceptions of the self	Creative occupations Interaction with loved ones

2021). Volunteering is a socially recognized contribution to others, one that enhances a sense of purpose and competence. It has thus been identified as an occupation that has major implications for older adults as a way to maintain identity (Greenfield & Marks, 2004). Note that it also can support evaluative meanings by promoting a sense of well-being and existential meanings by giving life a purpose beyond the self.

A particular challenge in maintaining identity in later life relates to the impact of transitions (Raanaas et al, 2019). Change in physical capacity, social networks, and occupational patterns is inevitable in later life, and these changes can disrupt sense of self. Adaptation to these new realities may well be linked to modifying or reestablishing meaningful occupational participation.

Creativity

Some special consideration should be given to the role of creative occupations in maintaining and expressing identity in later life. There is a considerable body of evidence suggesting that creative occupations such as drama, art, writing, and dance offer opportunities for self-expression and for processing emotion related to aging (Carpenter et al, 2021; Swinnen, 2018).

Although maintaining or reestablishing identity are key outcomes of creative occupations, they serve other values as well. Gallistl (2021) notes that individuals who participate in creative occupations maintain cognitive skill and social connections. Creative occupations also support processing of difficult emotions and life challenges. They have particular value in supporting clients at the end of life (Caserta, 2018). They allow for expression for older individuals who may not have strong verbal skills, but they also allow for reflection on life and opportunities to leave a legacy for others.

An arts-based action research project found that individual and group music composition supported a sense of wellbeing through control over materials, opportunities for creativity and identity making, and social engagement (Habron et al, 2013). There are many such examples reflecting the wide range of creative and nature-based occupations that contribute to self-identity in later life (Sia et al, 2020).

Supporting Meaning Through the Occupational Therapy Process

Throughout this textbook, there is information about particular aspects of function, the performance skills necessary to enable them, and the contexts in which older adults engage in occupations and receive services. It is important to remember that it is *meaningful* occupation that is critical later in life. Strategies for selecting the most salient occupations, optimizing the ability to engage in those occupations, and compensating for those that must be abandoned can greatly enhance life satisfaction and subjective well-being (George & Park, 2016; Taylor & Jones, 2017).

The *Occupational Therapy Practice Framework* (OTPF) (AOTA, 2020a) identifies the steps in occupational therapy intervention. These include evaluation, composed of completion of an occupational profile and an analysis of occupational performance; intervention, composed of establishing an intervention plan, implementing it, and reviewing its effectiveness; and outcomes defined in terms of engagement in an occupation to support participation (AOTA, 2020b). Such participation is also described in the International Classification of Function as involvement in life situations (World Health Organization, 2013). At every step in this process, having a model or framework that organizes the kinds of questions and forms of intervention can help ensure that the therapist works with the client to establish a helpful, comprehensive, and meaningful plan.

Theoretical Considerations in Assessment and Intervention

Numerous theories have attempted to explain the human need to engage in occupation. Although they differ in some details, identifying a theory of occupation can organize conceptualization of a client's needs and can improve intervention outcomes. Theories of aging are described more comprehensively in Chapter 3.

The need for purpose and drive for occupation has been known for over a century. In the 1920s and 1930s, Russian psychologists proposed a theory of human activity that holds that the need to meet a goal is the primary human motivation for activity (cf. Vygotsky, 1978). Occupation is also a fundamental biological need (Wilcock, 2007). This and other theories, including the Model of Human Occupation (MOHO; Kielhofner, 2008), emphasize not only doing activities but also what motivates that engagement. MOHO describes a volition subsystem that encompasses personal causation, values, and interests (Kielhofner, 2008). According to Kielhofner, an important early discovery in life is the connection between personal intention, action, and consequences. The individual must identify those actions that are important and that he or she wishes to pursue.

The desire to act is insufficient to ensure the ability to act, however. Roles must be identified and habits developed. These processes constitute the habituation subsystem. In many ways, roles dictate activity patterns. For example, the role of grandmother may involve such activities as playing with grandchildren, attending their sporting events, and advising their parents. Roles alone, however, are not sufficient to fully explain activity. Grandmothers differ greatly in the specific types of activities they undertake in that role, selecting from the many possible activities that can make up the role. One might take her grandchildren to see her office, whereas another might sew elaborate Halloween costumes.

Even when values, goals, and roles have been identified, the ability to accomplish them affects activity. Skills are required that enable the grandmother to talk with her grandchildren, bake cookies for them, and so on. Skills include the ability to perceive and respond, to process information, and to communicate. In determining what activity means to older adults in this framework, each of the subsystems must be considered (Kielhofner, 2008). A problem that becomes immediately obvious is the absence of prescribed roles for older adults, other than "retiree" (if indeed the person has retired) and grandparent (if indeed the person has grandchildren). In addition, older adults vary greatly with regard to values, habits, and skills.

Eakman (2013, 2014, 2016) has proposed the Meaningful Activity and Life Meaning model (MALM). This model posits a relationship among basic psychological needs, meaningful activity, and meaning in life. Research findings suggest that meaningful activity has both a direct impact on meaning in life and an indirect impact through its effect in addressing psychological needs. For example, engagement in a creative occupation like painting or writing poetry might reinforce a sense of mastery, supporting a positive evaluation of identity. A psychometrically sound assessment for measuring meaning is the Engagement in Meaningful Activities Survey (EMAS) (Eakman et al, 2010; Goldberg et al, 2002; Cheraghifard et al, 2022), which was also translated into Japanese (Kawakatsu et al, 2022) and Spanish (Fernández-Solano et al, 2022) and has been validated for Iranian people with chronic stroke (Cheraghifard et al, 2022). The EMAS (Eakman, 2012) can provide numerical scores that reflect subjective qualities of participation.

Evaluation

Evaluating meaningfulness in occupations and identifying strategies for enhancing participation in those occupations that matter the most can be challenging. Certainly, it is easier to determine whether a client can dress independently than it is to discern whether this occupation has meaning for the individual or whether he or she would rather get help with this and invest energy in other occupations. Together, the client and the occupational therapist must "find ways to reengage with the meaningfulness of occupations and life itself" (Taylor & Jones, 2017, pp. 440 to 441).

The OTPF (AOTA, 2020a) recommends that a first step is the completion of an occupational profile. This is typically done through interview, with a focus on understanding what the individual needs and wants to do. Questioning might include analyzing which of those occupations the person feels are going well and which are presenting problems. The Meaningful Activity Wants and Needs Assessment (MAWNA; Eakman, 2015) is an assessment tool that can be used to supplement this conversation with a more standardized approach.

In addition to this kind of qualitative assessment, a number of instruments can evaluate particular aspects of occupational meaning. The Spirituality Index of Well-Being (Frey et al, 2005) is one such instrument that explores self-efficacy and life scheme as related to spirituality. The Spiritual History Scale in Four Dimensions (Hays et al, 2001) measures factors labeled "God helped," "family history of religiousness," "lifetime religious social support," and "cost of religiousness." Other quantitative measures designed for older adults capture different elements of life satisfaction or well-being. These include the Life Satisfaction Index (Havighurst et al, 1968) and the Satisfaction With Life Scale (SWLS) (Pavot & Diener, 1993). The SWLS, in particular, is quick and easy to administer, can provide a global view of the older adult's well-being, and has been adequately tested for reliability and validity. The Life Satisfaction Inventory has questionable validity and is particularly problematic when used with individuals from cultures with different values. When this instrument was administered to Mayan older adults in Guatemala, it was clear that the constructs did not translate conceptually, despite the careful linguistic translation that had been done. Because it is based, to some extent, on comparing current circumstances with the past and with other individuals, it did not fit Mayan values, because the Maya view this kind of comparison as promoting jealousy or dissatisfaction (Bonder, 2001).

A strategy that can be used both as an assessment and an intervention is the creation of workbooks to explore the meaning of occupations (Taylor & Jones, 2017). The *What Now?* workbook allows for analysis of what various occupations mean to specific individuals, with an emphasis on consideration of location (society, time, place, mind), activity (the active self); and change (the changing self). This last element is particularly relevant to older adults whose capacities change regularly.

One instrument that incorporates both qualitative and quantitative methods is the Canadian Occupational Performance Measure (Law et al, 2005). This instrument asks the individual first to identify important occupations. These are then rated numerically in terms of satisfaction with ability to perform it and its importance in the individual's life. These numbers can be tracked throughout the intervention process to determine whether progress is being made toward enabling those important occupations.

Intervention

Occupational therapists have opportunities to intervene to support engagement in meaningful occupations and co-occupations through the many life and care transitions of the older adult.

Many late-life activities support well-being and meaning (Morgan & Robinson, 2013). Those that encourage expression and management of identity and those that connect the older adult to the past, present, and future can enhance the individual's sense of meaning and purpose in later life. A wide array of occupations can be considered in working with clients to refine their occupational profiles to better address important life meanings for them. Research has clearly established that occupational therapy interventions emphasizing wellness and meaningful occupation promote mental health, social functioning, functional status, and physical functioning (Clark et al, 2012). Clark and colleagues compared occupational therapy intervention to a nonintervention control group and a generalized group activity group. The occupational therapy intervention, perhaps because of its emphasis on meaningful occupation, was superior to the two other conditions in one of the few well-controlled studies of occupational therapy interventions with older adults. Numerous intervention programs now use this Lifestyle Redesign® approach for different conditions and populations.

Among other occupations, reminiscence and storytelling are particularly valued by older adults (Lee, 2016; Zuiderveen et al, 2016). These occupations relate directly both to leaving a legacy and to the importance of connections with the past, present, and future. Life review contributes to resilience in later life (Randall, 2012; Webster et al, 2014). There are other ways to leave a legacy. For example, the woman shown in Figure 2-1 derives great satisfaction by combining her love of music with her love of family. By teaching a grandchild to play, she might pass along some of her heritage, and by playing at family gatherings, she might provide her family with positive memories of her.

Likewise, creative occupations like writing offer opportunities for self-reflection, connection with others, and meaning-making generally (Edwards & Owen-Booth, 2021). Creative occupations may include painting, sketching, writing poetry, memoir, or fiction, dance, photography, and many other outlets for personal expression. "Creative occupations provide more or different types of meaningfulness, and thus therapeutic opportunities" (Roberts & Bannigan, 2018, p. 387). Figure 2-2 shows older individuals involved in a group activity at an art museum during which they are encouraged to explore the feelings they experience when viewing others' creations.

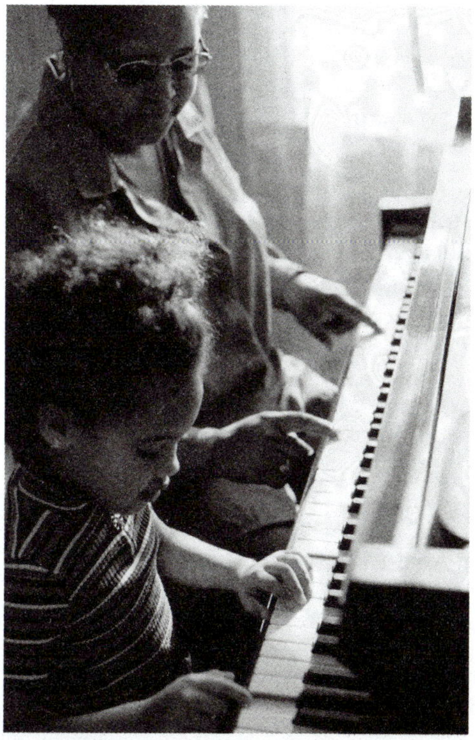

Spiritual interventions may be both direct and indirect (Box 2-1). They take many forms and often provide added meanings. For example, physical activity may occur in outdoor settings that provide spiritual benefits as well.

Physical activity has particular salience in later life (Amireault et al, 2018). It is meaningful in and of itself but also contributes to the ability to participate in other important activities, such as work and other productive occupations (Matz-Costa et al, 2012; Versey & Newton, 2013). Worldwide, physical activity is positively correlated with life satisfaction and happiness, increasing significance with increasing age (An et al, 2020; Patria, 2022).

Occupational Therapy Intervention Considering Co-Occupation

Occupational therapy often emphasizes independence over interdependent occupational performance. However, most people who live or interact with other people develop routines that require the other to act or perform a part of a task for occupations of meaning. If an older adult couple enjoyed

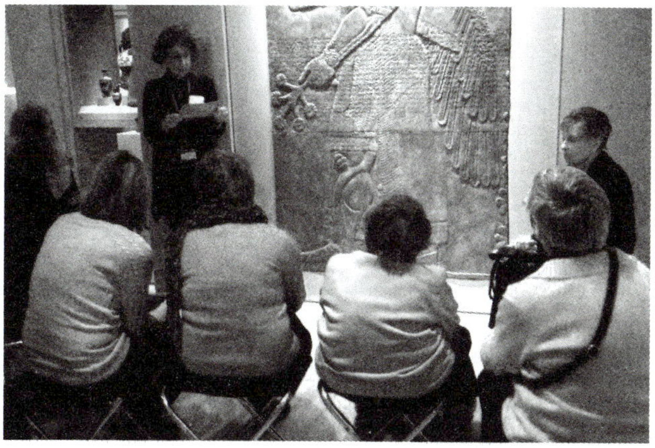

FIGURE 2-2 Art in the Afternoon is an engaging and meaningful activity. A group studies a massive wall relief depicting a winged genie at the Cleveland Museum of Art. *(Courtesy of Cleveland Museum of Art.)*

FIGURE 2-1 This grandmother shares her love of music with her granddaughter. *(Buccina Studios/Photodisc/Thinkstock.)*

BOX 2-1 Religious and Spiritual Interventions

Intervention type	Description
Direct	Occupations that support participation in specific religious rituals or exploration of religious tenets and beliefs
Indirect	Occupations that consider the relationship of a variety of occupations to a sense of greater purpose, without reference to specific religious rituals

a routine of year-round daily walks and porch-sitting, a focused co-occupation of donning warm coats would be a valuable therapy training for someone with hemiparesis. Likewise, for a woman with dementia and her adult son, family education could focus on grading favorite card games. For more examples and research on co-occupation with older adults and practice implications, see Promoting Best Practice 2-1.

PROMOTING BEST PRACTICE 2-1
Examples of Co-Occupations and Practice Implications

ARTICLE	CO-OCCUPATION	PRACTICE IMPLICATIONS
An Ethnographic Analysis of a Church Supper in New England (Crepeau, 2015)	Coordinated tasks, collaborative routines, and shared meaning create community co-occupation steeped in rich cultural, social, and temporal context	Understand the transactional nature of context for individuals' continued engagement in community co-occupations to support meaning and social participation.
Views on Co-Occupation Between Elderly Persons With Dementia and Family (Ono et al, 2014)	Difficult to perform, "troublesome" co-occupations were recognized as challenges for family caregivers of people with dementia, affecting shared quality of life and ability to provide care in the home.	Provide education, training, care coordination, and respite resources to caregivers. Create routines where shared occupations are positively experienced.
Exploring Co-Occupation Between University Students and Older Adults Living Together in a Retirement Home (Gorjup, 2020)	Informal co-occupations in a shared intergenerational living environment provided a means of connection between young and older adults.	Provide opportunities for older adults to engage in intergenerational co-occupations to develop shared understandings and shared meaning.
One Body, Three Hands and Two Minds: A Case Study of the Intertwined Occupations of an Older Couple After a Stroke (van Nes et al, 2009)	Weaving of time and space in two people with health conditions performing valued occupations alone and together	Emphasize value of co-occupations rather than "independence-focused" rehab to patients and families. Include partners in hands-on treatment sessions.

Occupational Therapy Interventions in Support of Spiritual and Religious Meanings

There has been a tremendous growth of attention to the importance of interventions that emphasize spirituality (Thompson et al, 2018). Recognition of the centrality of both spiritual needs and religious needs has increased attention in occupational therapy to addressing these needs effectively. The Practice Framework (AOTA, 2020a) specifically incorporates these as appropriate objectives for occupational therapy intervention.

It is important to recognize the purpose of spiritual and religious intervention in the occupational therapy process. The goal is not to encourage religious adherence or evaluate religious beliefs. Instead, the goal is to offer opportunities for the individual to identify the importance of religious and spiritual occupations and to find ways through therapy to support those occupations if the client wishes. This is an important distinction, as it is an area in which recognizing the domain of occupational therapy can be essential.

There are two primary strategies for addressing religious and spiritual needs of clients: direct and indirect. Direct strategies include such occupations as attending church, praying together, and otherwise engaging in religious rituals. These kinds of interventions are valuable when clients clearly identify religion as a central and meaningful part of their lives.

Other individuals might focus more on spiritual meanings that do not involve participation in organized religion and rituals. For such individuals, indirect intervention would be a more supportive approach. Indirect intervention strategies might emerge from discussion during the identification of an occupational profile about how individuals frame the existential questions in their lives.

As an example, consider the case of two women who described religion as being very important in their lives (Bonder & Martin, 2000). One went to church regularly, rarely missing a Sunday, and participated in a number of church committees and activities. The other never went to church services but instead choreographed intergenerational dance at the church. The first of these women might benefit from direct intervention in the event she began to struggle with her beliefs or with the skills required to participate in church services. The second woman might benefit from a more indirect form of intervention, focused on strategies for spiritual expression during her dance practices and performances.

Individual and Cultural Considerations

The two women described above (Bonder & Martin, 2000) were actively engaged in an array of other occupations as well. Within a given category, variability in the occupations that were undertaken and the meanings each woman assigned to them were so great as to make the occupation label almost meaningless. For example, one woman enacted grandparenting by having fun with her granddaughter through such activities as Halloween trick-or-treating. She enjoyed providing child care as a way to get to know her granddaughter. The other enacted grandparenting through child care provided on days when school was closed and during the summer. She experienced these activities as somewhat burdensome but expected. Reducing occupational patterns through simple categorization on a single dimension may mask issues of vital importance to the individual—in particular, the unique contribution of each occupation to meaning and quality of life. This is but one example of the individual variability that is typical in occupational choice and enactment.

A major factor that influences individual choice is the cultural background of the individual. Every individual has multiple cultures, so it is essential for the therapist to have a clear understanding of the person's cultural identification and the associated occupational choices (Bonder, 2001; Bonder & Martin, 2013). Having a general sense of cultural values is helpful and necessary as well. Understanding historical realities and social contexts contributes essential information about occupational choices of individuals and groups (Gerlach et al, 2018).

An Example of Evaluation and Intervention to Support Meaning

How does this process translate into an individual life? Mrs. Anthony was a 72-year-old widow who had been working full time for the past 30 years. However, her hearing had worsened, and her hearing aid was not effective in addressing this loss, making it difficult to continue her job as a social worker. Her daughter was recently divorced and was a single parent with two young children. An occupational therapist and Mrs. Anthony reviewed her occupational profile, occupational performance, and performance patterns, skills, contexts, and client factors. Applying the selection, optimization, and compensation (SOC) model (see Ch. 3), Mrs. Anthony and the therapist considered a careful selection of meaningful occupations and strategies for optimizing her performance and satisfaction in those occupations. In addition, they considered ways to substitute new occupations for those she could no longer perform. On the basis of this evaluation, Mrs. Anthony decided to retire and assume a substantial role in the care of her grandchildren. The specific constellation of activities that constituted the roles of "retiree" and "grandparent," in Mrs. Anthony's view, included spending days with her grandchildren, arriving early enough that her daughter could get to work on time, taking them to school, or, on days when they had no school, helping them with homework and baking cookies.

Unfortunately, as much as she loved her grandchildren, Mrs. Anthony did not like baking cookies and felt personally unfulfilled in the new roles she had identified. She was frustrated by what she perceived as a lack of productivity. She was also concerned at what she perceived as a loss of mobility and endurance as a result of diminished physical activity during retirement. Thus, the outcomes of this first plan were unsatisfactory, so the therapist and Mrs. Anthony revisited her occupational profile and reconsidered her decisions. This led to a new set of choices. One possibility was to redefine "retiree" and "grandparent" to reflect more adequately her personal values and beliefs. This included substituting some activities that Mrs. Anthony perceived as productive because this is an important value for her. She decided to volunteer at a hospital while her grandchildren were in school and to give guest lectures at the local school of social work. She optimized her involvement with her grandchildren by engaging with them in more "productive" kinds of activities as well, including homework and visits to museums to enhance their education. She also considered whether her volunteer and grandparenting roles compensated for the worker role she had relinquished, along with the possibility of returning to work and alternatives such as part-time employment. If she decided to do so and felt that she was abandoning her daughter, providing financial assistance might resolve the dilemma. She also visited with a physical therapist for a comprehensive evaluation and began to implement an exercise program to regain some of the endurance and mobility she had lost. Concerns about her decreasing ability to work effectively could be assuaged by a visit to an audiologist to determine whether newer hearing aid technology might improve her hearing to the point that it did not interfere with her work performance or by identifying a job in which she could function despite any decline in abilities.

Occupation, Home, and Place

Home is a place of identity, continuity, relationship, refuge, and meaning. Home can also be a place of isolation, burden, and oppression (Barry et al, 2018). How a person experiences home changes over time and as the person ages. Home includes objects of meaning. These objects have pragmatic purposes that are used by the older adult in their doing of daily activities. Objects also have symbolic purposes connecting people and time through photographs and family keepsakes. Sixsmith and colleagues (2014) undertook a qualitative study to explore the ways older adults in five European countries understood healthy aging in the context of the home. They discovered five primary themes, of which three related to activities. Those three reflected keeping active, managing lifestyles, and balancing social life. These occupations, in the context of the home, contribute to meaningful and positive aging.

Seamon describes the phenomenological perspective of place as "any environmental locus that gathers human experiences, action, and meaning, spatially and temporally" (p. 2, 2018). People become attached to places, such as their home, experiencing security. Home, as place, fosters space–time routines that provide comfort and familiar rhythms for older adults. A person becomes *one-with* their environment often providing the best context for aging-in-place. It is when the body and place are no longer congruent—for example mobility problems coupled with stairs to sleeping quarters—that the home no longer supports a place of safety and security.

The decision to move from one's home to a "safer" environment, whether the home of an adult child, a senior living community, or a care home, disrupts place-attachment and can be distressing not only to the older adult(s) moving but also to family members who may have experienced a sense of place in that same home.

Around the world, older adults prefer to age in place, which is the concept of living out one's life in their own home and community (Ailshire et al, 2018; Nakagawa et al, 2022). However, not everyone is able to—or chooses to—age in their primary residence. Alternatives to aging in place include aging in community in a shared home or cohousing environment. Pfaff and Trentham (2022) describe a Swedish cohousing community where individual apartments with communal kitchens and living spaces created shared occupations of meal making, cleaning, choir, and coffee groups. Younger residents took on more challenging tasks that older residents may have done years earlier in the same community. This form of housing also eased the minds of residents' children about caring for their parents.

Moving to a care home is an opportunity to support older adults' ability to maintain meaningful occupations. An exemplary care concept in the Netherlands provides care facilities with the look and feel of homes in a village. Each home has six to seven residents and a care provider. The homes have different lifestyle experiences, from traditional home to more cosmopolitan. The care community supports the individual's interests and needs. The village has a market, gardens, theatre events, and even a pub (more information can be found at https://hogeweyk.dementiavillage.com/).

CASE STUDY (CONTINUED)

Intervention Plan

Engage Claire in standard carpal tunnel syndrome exercises. Explore assistive technology options for computer use. Explore ergonomic gardening and cooking tools, along with activity analysis of gardening and cooking activities to make recommendations about body mechanics and routines. Invite Claire's children and grandchildren to participate in therapy sessions to support the implementation of new routines.

Discharge Status

Claire was discharged from outpatient therapy with reduced pain, improved strength, and a plan to manage her activities. She reports her children and grandchildren have taught her a new social media app where she has also joined an online writing collective called Reflections of Faith. She has returned to her church and school volunteering activities.

Questions

1. What themes of meaning did the therapist engage in addressing Claire's problems?
2. What occupations and co-occupations are important to Claire, as demonstrated in her profile and subsequent experiences during therapy? How are these important to her continued successful aging?

Answers

1. Instrumental meaning was addressed through supporting cooking tasks. Existential meaning and identity were addressed through focusing on gardening, computer, and cooking activities and engaging Claire's family in therapy. (Found in Section on occupation, co-occupation, and meaning.)
2. Claire's occupations include gardening, cooking, and driving to attend her grandchildren's events. She has a new co-occupation of a shared writing collective. She demonstrates continued engagement in meaningful activities along with the desire and ability to learn new technologies that support participation.

SUMMARY

The ultimate goal of occupational therapy is client well-being, a status that goes beyond physical health. This presents dilemmas for care providers who design programming or individual interventions for older adults. Public policy too often emphasizes self-care as the sole desired outcome of care and provides reimbursement according to guidelines that reflect this emphasis. Although this focus is understandable, given the lack of clarity about what occupations contribute to life satisfaction in later life, it may well be misguided because it is clear that "there is more to life than putting on your pants" (Radomski, 1995, p. 487). As will be seen in subsequent chapters, occupational therapists must consider strategies other than direct care in hospital settings. Community-based and population-based care has grown considerably and may offer greater latitude in addressing client needs that are vital to positive aging.

Pursuing an evaluation that incorporates all aspects of occupational performance is challenging, as is designing meaningful intervention plans. Further, intervention is not complete until reevaluation has occurred and outcomes are carefully examined. Simply developing a list of occupations is inadequate, because the nature of the occupation, the context in which it occurs, and individual skills, performance, and patterns are essential considerations. Occupations can be expressed in many ways, and thus occupational therapists must examine not only clients' occupations but also their essential meanings. They must then pursue a process through which they support individuals' meaningful occupational performance patterns and help remediate ongoing or new challenges to participation. A number of methods for accomplishing these goals are presented in the chapters that follow. It is clearly crucial that both evaluation and intervention must be undertaken with recognition of meanings that are important to the client.

Positive aging has become the focus of considerable research interest. Comprehensive review supports the idea that individuals who have lives with purpose are most likely to be among successful—as opposed to usual or even unsuccessful—agers. As Swensen (1983) noted, "People live as long as they have something to do that needs to be done" (p. 331). Healthcare providers, policy planners, and older adults must develop a clear understanding of what it means, both to the individual and to society, to have something that needs to be done. Specific developmental realities of later life are examined in detail throughout this book. It is vital to keep in mind that as these later-life changes occur, a central and vital goal of occupational therapy is to help clients maintain meaning in their lives.

Critical Thinking Questions

1. An older man is admitted to an assisted living community from a single-family home where he lived independently for 54 years until a recent fall resulted in a complex leg fracture and need for mobility aids. What routine occupations could the therapist promote continued participation in for this new resident?

2. In what ways can occupations related to spirituality and religion support clients' search for meaning?

3. In what way might the ability to carry out self-care activities contribute to meaning and satisfaction for an older individual? Does it seem likely that all older adults would value such activities, or might there be some for whom this is not an important element for creating meaning?

4. Occupations can be described as related to: doing, being, becoming, and belonging (Hitch et al, 2014). Consider the various occupational categories in the OTPF (AOTA, 2020a). Choose a category and describe some occupations in that category that might fulfill those four purposes.

REFERENCES

Achenbaum, W. A. (2020). *Old age in the new land: The American experience since 1790.* JHU Press.

Ailshire, J., Frochen, S., & Rodnyansky, S. (2018). Moving preference and determinants among U.S. older adults. *Innovations in Aging*, 11; 2(Suppl 1), 873. doi: 10.1093/geroni/igy023.3261

American Occupational Therapy Association. (2020a). Occupational therapy practice framework: Domain and process (4th ed.). *American Journal of Occupational Therapy*, 74(Suppl_2), 7412410010p1-7412410010p87. doi:10.5014/ajot.2020.74S2001. Retrieved from https://www.aota.org/practice/practice-essentials/documentation/improve-your-documentation-with-aotas-updated-occupational-profile-template

American Occupational Therapy Association. (2020b). *AOTA's occupational profile template.* https://www.aota.org/practice/practice-essentials/documentation/improve-your-documentation-with-aotas-updated-occupational-profile-template

Amirav, D. R., Larsen, D., & Taylor, E. (2021). Imbuing occupations with spiritual significance fosters experiences of hope. *OTJR: Occupation, Participation and Health*, 41(3), 163–168. doi:10.1177/1539449220985903

Amireault, S., Baier, J. M., & Spencer, J. R. (2018). Physical activity preferences among older adults: A systematic review. *Journal of Aging and Physical Activity*, 27(1), 128–139.

An, H. Y., Chen, W., Wang, C. W., Yang, H. F., Huang, W. T., & Fan, S. Y. (2020). The relationships between physical activity and life satisfaction and happiness among young, middle-aged, and older adults. *International Journal of Environmental Research and Public Health*, 17(13), 4817. https://doi.org/10.3390/ijerph17134817

Antonelli, M. T., Grace, P. J., & Boltz, M. (2020). Mutual caregiving: Living meaningfully as an older couple. *International Journal of Older People Nursing*, 15, e12340. https://doi.10.1111/opn.12340

Avelar-González, A. K., Bureau-Chávez, M., Durón-Reyes, D., Móndragón-Cervantes, M. I., Jiménez-Acosta, Y. del C., Leal-Mora, D., & Díaz-Ramos, J. A. (2020). Spirituality and religious practices and its association with geriatric syndromes in older adults attending to a geriatric's clinic in a university hospital. *Journal of Religion & Health*, 59(6), 2794-2806. doi: 10.1007/s10943-020-00990-0

Bar, M. A., Forwell, S., & Backman, C. L. (2016). Ascribing meaning to occupation: An example from healthy, working mothers. *OTJR: Occupation, Participation and Health*, 36(3), 148–158. doi:10.1177/1539449216652622

Barken, R. (2019). 'Independence' among older people receiving support at home: The meaning of daily care practices. *Ageing & Society*, 39(3), 518–540. doi: 10.1017/S0144686X17001039

Barry A., Heale R., Pilon R., & Lavoie A. M. (2018). The meaning of home for ageing women living alone: An evolutionary concept analysis. *Health and Social Care in the Community*, 26, e337–e344. https://doi.org/10.1111/hsc.12470

Beauchet, O., Bastien, T., Mittelman, M. Hayashi, Y., & Ho, A. H. Y. (2020). Participatory art-based activity, community-dwelling older adults and changes in health condition: Results from a pre–post intervention, single-arm, prospective and longitudinal study. *Maturitas*, 134, 8–14. https://doi.org/10.1016/j.maturitas.2020.01.006

Beckinger, A., Overturf, A., & Pickens, N. (2016). *Reliability and validity of the complexities of co-occupation (CoCO) scale,* 70(4_Supplement_1), 7011500065p1. doi:10.5014/ajot.2016.70S1-PO6021

Black, M. H., Milbourn, B., Desjardins, K., Sylvester, V., Parrant, K., & Buchanan, A. (2019). Understanding the meaning and use of occupational engagement: Findings from a scoping review. *British Journal of Occupational Therapy*, 82(5), 272–287. doi: 10.1177/0308022618821580

Bonder, B. R. (2001). Culture and occupation: A comparison of weaving in two traditions. *Canadian Journal of Occupational Therapy*, 65, 310–319. http://dx.doi.org/10.1177/000841740106800507

Bonder, B. R., & Martin, L. (2000). Personal meanings of occupation for women in later life: Two women compared. *Women and Aging*, 12, 177–193. http://dx.doi.org/10.1300/J074v12n03_11

Bonder, B. R. & Martin, L. (2013). *Culture in clinical care: Strategies for competence (2nd ed.).* Thorofare, NJ: Slack, Inc.

Boudiny, K. (2013). "Active ageing": From empty rhetoric to effective policy tool. *Ageing & Society*, 33, 1077–1098. http://dx.doi.org/10.1017/S0144686X1200030X

Candler, C., Mikeska, R, Lacy, K., Elliott, N., & Huddleston, A. (2021). Autoethnographies of reading as an occupation. *Open Journal of Occupational Therapy*, 9(1), 1–12. doi.org/10.15453/2168-6408.1718

Carpenter, S. M., Chae, R., Sung, Y., & Yoon, C. (2021). The influence of creativity on objective and subjective well-being in older adulthood. In A. Drolet & C. Yoon (Eds.), *The aging consumer: Perspectives from psychology and marketing* (2nd ed., pp. 279–297). New York: Routledge/Taylor & Francis Group.

Carstensen, L. L. (2021). Socioemotional selectivity theory: The role of perceived endings in human motivation, *The Gerontologist*, 61(8), 1188–1196. https://doi.org/10.1093/geront/gnab116

Caserta, M. S. (2018). Sky above clouds: Finding our way through creativity, aging, and illness. *Omega: Journal of Death and Dying, 77*(2), 188–191. doi: 10.1177/0030222817717321

Cheraghifard, M., Akbarfahimi, M., Azad, A., Eakman, A. M., & Taghizadeh, G. (2022). Validation of the Persian version of the Engagement in Meaningful Activities Survey (EMAS) in an Iranian stroke population: Predictors of participation in meaningful activities. *American Journal of Occupational Therapy, 76*(4), 7604205130. doi: 10.5014/ajot.2022.046623

Clark, F., Jackson, J., Carlson, M., Chou, C. P., Cherry, B. J., Jordan-Marsh, M., Knight, B. G., Mandel, D., Blanchard, J., Granger, D. A., Wilcox, R. R., Lai, M. Y., White, B., Hay, J., Lam, C., Marterella, A., & Azen, S. P. (2012). Effectiveness of a lifestyle intervention in promoting the well-being of independently living older people: Results of the Well Elderly 2 randomised controlled trial, *Journal of Epidemiology & Community Health, 66*, 782–790.

Cohen, G. D. (2005). *The mature mind: The positive power of the aging brain.* New York: Basic Books.

Crepeau, E. B. (2015). An ethnographic analysis of a church supper in New England. *Journal of Occupational Science, 22*(1), 54–70. doi:10.1080/14427591.2014.908817

Csikszentmihalyi, M. (1990). *Flow: The psychology of optimal experience.* Grand Rapids, MI: Harper & Row.

Dewitte, L., Vandenbulcke, M., Shcellekens, T., & Dezutter, J. (2021). Sources of well-being for older adults with and without dementia in residential care: Relations to presence of meaning and life-satisfaction. *Aging & Mental Health, 25*(1), 170–178. doi: 10.1080/13607863.2019.1691144

Dutt, A. J., & Wahl, H. W. (2019). Future time perspective and general self-efficacy mediate the association between awareness of age-related losses and depressive symptoms. *European Journal of Ageing, 16*(2), 227–236. doi: 10.1007/s10433-018-0482-3

Eakman, A. M. (2012). Measurement characteristics of the engagement in meaningful activities survey in an age-diverse sample. *American Journal of Occupational Therapy, 66*, e20–e29. http://dx.doi.org/10.5014/ajot.2012.001867

Eakman, A. M. (2013). Relationships between meaningful activity, basic psychological needs, and meaning in life: Test of the meaningful activity and life meaning model. *OTJR: Occupation, Participation and Health, 33*, 100–109. doi: 10.3928/15394492-2013022-02

Eakman, A. M. (2014). The meaningful activity wants and needs assessment: A perspective on life balance. *Journal of Occupational Science, 22*(2), 210–227. doi:10.1080/14427591.2013.769405

Eakman, A. M. (2015). The meaningful activity wants and needs assessment: A perspective on life balance. *Journal of Occupational Science, 22*(2), 210–227. doi: 10.1080/14427591.2013.769405

Eakman, A. M. (2016). A subjectively-based definition of life balance using personal meaning in occupation. *Journal of Occupational Science, 23*(1), 108–127. doi: 10/1080/14427591.2014.955603

Eakman, A. M., Atler, K. E., Rumble, M., Gee, B. M, Romriell, B., & Hardy, N. (2018). A qualitative synthesis of positive subjective experiences in occupation from the Journal of Occupational Science (1993–2010). *Journal of Occupational Science, 25*(3), 346-367. doi:10.1080/14427591.2018.1492958

Eakman, A. M., Carlson, M. E., & Clark, F. A. (2010). Factor structure, reliability, and convergent validity of the engagement in meaningful activities survey for older adults. *OTJR, 30*(3), 111–121. doi: 10.3928/15394492-20090518-01

Edwards, L., & Owen-Booth, B. (2021). An exploration of engagement in community based creative activities as an occupation for older adults. *Irish Journal of Occupational Therapy, 49*(1), 51–57. doi: 10.1108/AJOT-05-2020-0009

Erikson, E. H. (1963). *Childhood and society.* New York: W. W. Norton.

Erlandsson, L. K., Eklund, M., & Persson, D. (2011). Occupational value and relationships to meaning and health: Elaborations of the ValMO-model. *Scandinavian Journal of Occupational Therapy, 18*(1), 72–80. doi: 10.3109/11038121003671619

Fernández-Solano, A. J., Merchán-Baeza, J. A., Rodríguez-Bailón, M., & Eakman, A. (2022). Translation and cultural adaptation into Spanish of the engagement in meaningful activities survey. *Occupational Therapy International*. 4492582. doi. 10.1155/2022/4492582

Ferreira, O. G. L., Maciel, S. C., Costa, S. M. G., Silva, A. O., & Moreira, M. A. S. P. (2012). Active aging and its relationship to functional independence. *Texto & Contexto Enfermagem, 21*, 513–518.

Finkenzeller, T., Pötzelsberger, B., Kösters, A., Würth, S., Amesberger, G., Müller, E., & Dela, F. (2019). Aging in high functioning older adultly persons: Study design and analyses of behavioral and psychological factors. *Scandinavian Journal of Medicine & Science in Sports, 29*, 7–16. doi: 10.1111/sms.13368

Frey, B. B., Daaleman, T. P., & Peyton, V. (2005). Measuring dimension of spirituality for health research: Validity of the Spirituality Index of Well-Being. *Research on Aging, 27,* 556–577. http://dx.doi.org/10.1177/0164027505277847

Gabriel, S., Naidu, E., Paravati, E., Morrison, C. D., & Gainey, K. (2020). Creating the sacred from the profane: Collective effervescence and everyday activities. *Journal of Positive Psychology, 15*(1), 129–154. doi: 10.1080/17439760.2019.1689412

Gallistl, V. (2021). What's it worth? Value and valuation of late-life creativity. *Aging & Society, 41*(11), 2599-2614. doi: 10.1017/S0144686X20000495

George, L. S., & Park, C. L. (2016). Meaning in life as comprehension, purpose, and mattering: Toward integration and new research questions. *Review of General Psychology 20,* 205–220. doi: 10.1037/gpr0000077

Gerlach, A. J., Teachman, G., Laliberte-Rudman, D., Aldrich, R. M., & Huot, S. (2018). Expanding beyond individualism: Engaging critical perspectives on occupation. *Scandinavian Journal of Occupational Therapy, 25*(1), 35–43.

Goldberg, B., Brintnell, E. S., & Goldberg, J. (2002). The relationship between engagement in meaningful activities and quality of life in persons disabled by mental illness. *Occupational Therapy in Mental Health, 18*(2), 17–44.

Gorjup, R. J. (2020). Exploring co-occupation between university students and older adults living together in a retirement home. (Publication no. 7239) [Thesis, The University of Western Ontario]. Electronic Thesis and Dissertation Repository, https://ir.lib.uwo.ca/etd/7239

Greenfield, E. A., & Marks, N. F. (2004). Formal volunteering as a protective factor for older adults' psychological well-being. *Journal of Gerontology Series B: Psychological Sciences and Social Sciences, 59,* S258–S264. http://dx.doi.org/10.1093/geronb/59.5.S258

Habron, J., Butterly, F., Gordon, I., & Roebuck, A. (2013). Being well, being musical: Music composition as a resource and occupation for older people. *British Journal of Occupational Therapy, 76,* 308-316. http://dx.doi.org/10.4276/030802213X13729279114933

Hasselkus, B. R. & Dickie, V. A. (2021). *The meaning of everyday occupation,* 3rd ed. Thorofare, NJ: Slack.

Havighurst, R. J., Neugarten, B. L., & Tobin, S. S. (1968). Life satisfaction index. In R. A. Kane & R. L. Kane (Eds.), *Assessing the older adult: A practical guide to measurement* (pp. 174–189). Lexington, MA: Lexington Books.

Hays, J. C., Meador, K. G., Branch, P. S., & George, L. K. (2001). The spiritual history scale in four dimensions (SHS-4): Validity and reliability. *The Gerontologist, 41,* 239–249. http://dx.doi.org/10.1093/geront/41.2.239

Hicks, J. A., Davis, W. E., Trent, J., & King, L. A. (2012). Positive affect, meaning in life, and future time perspective: An application of socioemotional selectivity theory. *Psychology and Aging, 27,* 181–189. http://dx.doi.org/10.1037/a0023965

Hill, P. L., & Turiano, N. A. (2014). Purpose in life as a predictor of mortality across adulthood. *Psychological Science, 25,* 1482–1486. doi: 10.1177/0956797614531799

Hitch, D., Pépin, G., & Stagnitti, K. (2014). In the footsteps of Wilcock, part one: The evolution of doing, being, becoming, and belonging. *Occupational Therapy in Health Care, 28*(3), 231–246. DOI: 10.3109/07380577.2014.898114

Hladek, M. D., Zhu, J., Buta, B. J., Szanton, S. L., Bandeen, R. K., Walston, J. D., & Xue, Q. (2021). Self-efficacy proxy predicts frailty incidence over time in non-institutionalized older adults. *Journal of the American Geriatrics Society, 69*(12), 3507-3518. doi: 10.1111/jgs.17417

Hodge, D. R., Horvath, V. E., Larkin, H., & Curl, A. L. (2012). Older adults' spiritual needs in health care settings: A qualitative meta-synthesis. *Research on Aging, 34,* 131–155. http://dx.doi.org/10.1177/0164027511411308

Hooker, S. A., Masters, K. S., & Park, C. L. (2017). A meaningful life is a healthy life: A conceptual model linking meaning and meaning salience to health. *Review of General Psychology, 27*(1), 11–24. doi: 10.1037/gpr0000115

Hooper, B., & Wood, W. (2019). The philosophy of occupational therapy: A framework for practice. In B.A.B. Schell & G. Gillman (Eds). *Willard and Spackman's occupational therapy* (13th ed., pp. 43–55). Philadelphia, PA: Wolders Kluwer.

Hovbrant, P., Darlsson, G., Nilsson, K., Albin, M., & Håkansson, C. (2019). Occupational balance as described by older workers over the age of 65. *Journal of Occupational Science, 26*(1), 40–52. doi: 10.1080/14427591.2018.1542616

Hülür, G., Heckhausen, J., Hoppmann, C. A., Infurna, F. J., Wagner, G. G., Ram, N., & Gerstorf, D. (2017). Levels of and changes in life satisfaction predict mortality hazards: Disentangling the role of physical health, perceived control, and social orientation. *Psychology & Aging, 32*(6), 507–520. doi: 10.1037/pag0000187

Huo, M., Miller, L. M. S., Kim, K., & Liu, S. (2021). Volunteering, self-perceptions of aging, and mental health in later life. *Gerontologist, 61*(7), 1131–1140. doi:10.1093/geront/gnaa164

Hupkens, S., Machieelse, A., Goumans, M., & Derkx, P. (2018). Meaning in life of older persons: An integrative literature review. *Nursing Ethics, 25*(8), 973–991. doi: 10.1177/0969733016680122

Jessen-Winge, C., Petersen, M. N., & Morville, A. L. (2018). The influence of occupation on wellbeing, as experienced by the older adultly: A systematic review. *JBI Database of Systematic Reviews and Implementation Reports, 16*(5), 1174–1189. doi: 10.11124/JBISRIR-2016-003123

Jiang, D., Warner, L. M., Chong, A. M. L., Li, T., Wolff, J. K., & Chou, K. L. (2021). Benefits of volunteering on psychological well-being in older adulthood: Evidence from a randomized controlled trial. *Aging & Mental Health, 25*(4), 641–649.

Kawakatsu, Y., Yokoi, K., Tanno, K., Eakman, E. A. & Hirayama, K. (2022). Development of the Japanese Version of the Engagement in Meaningful Activities Survey. *OTJR: Occupation, Participation and Health, 42*(3), 209–218.

Kielhofner, G. (2008). *Model of human occupation: Theory and application* (4th ed.). Philadelphia: Lippincott, Williams & Wilkins.

Krause, N. (2004). Stressors arising in highly valued roles, meaning in life, and the physical health status of older adults. *Journal of Gerontology Series B: Psychological Sciences and Social Sciences, 59,* S287–S297. http://dx.doi.org/10.1093/geronb/59.5.S287

Križaj, T., Roberts, A., Warren, A., & Slade, A. (2019). Early hour, golden hour: An exploration of Slovenian older people's meaningful occupations. *Journal of Cross-Cultural Gerontology, 34,* 201–221. doi: 10.1007/s10823-019-09369-5

Križaj, T., Warren, A., & Slade, A. (2018). "Holding on to what I do": Experiences of older Slovenians moving into a care home. *Gerontologist, 58*(3), 512–520. doi:10.1093/geront/gnw150

Law, M., Baptiste, S., Carswell, A., McColl, M. A., Polatajko, H., & Pollock, N. (2005). *Canadian occupational performance measure.* Toronto: Canadian Association for Occupational Therapy.

Lee, T. (2016). Skilled listening and writing for story: From reminiscence to story-work with older adults' stories. *Educational Gerontology, 42*(6), 423–430. doi: 10.1080/03601277.2016.1139978

Levinson, D. J. (1986). A conception of adult development. *American Psychologist, 49,* 3–13. http://dx.doi.org/10.1037/0003-066X.41.1.3

Lind, L. R. (1957). *Ten Greek plays in contemporary translations.* Boston: Houghton Mifflin.

Matz-Costa, C., Besen, E., James, J. B., & Pitt-Catsouphes, M. (2012). Differential impact of multiple levels of productive activity engagement on psychological well-being in middle and later life. *Gerontologist, 54,* 277–289. doi: 10.1093/geront/gns148

Menec, V. H. (2003). The relation between everyday activities and successful aging: A 6-year longitudinal study. *Journal of Gerontology Series B: Psychological Sciences and Social Sciences, 58,* S74–S82. http://dx.doi.org/10.1093/geronb/58.2.S74

Mohseni, M., Iranpour, A., Naghibzadeh-Tahami, A., Kazazi, L., & Borhaninejad, V. (2019). The relationship between meaning in life and resilience in older adults: A cross-sectional study. *Health Psychology Report, 7*(2), 133–138. doi: 10.5114/hpr.2019.85659

Morgan, J., & Robinson, O. (2013). Intrinsic aspirations and personal meaning across adulthood: Conceptual interrelations and age/sex differences. *Developmental Psychology, 49,* 999–1010. doi: 10.1037/a0029237

Mulholland, F., & Jackson, J. (2018). The experience of older adults with anxiety and depression living in the community. Aging, occupation and mental wellbeing. *British Journal of Occupational Therapy, 81*(11), 657–666. doi: 10.1177/0308022628777200

Nakagawa, T., Noguchi, T., Komatsu, A., Ishihara, M., & Saito, T. (2022). Aging-in-place preferences and institutionalization among Japanese older adults: A 7-year longitudinal study. *BMC Geriatrics, 22*:66. https://doi.org/10.1186/s12877-022-02766-5

Nesteruk, O., & Price, C. A. (2011). Retired women and volunteering: The good, the bad, and the unrecognized. *Journal of Woman & Aging, 23,* 99–112. http://dx.doi.org/10.1080/08952841.2011.561138

Neugarten, B. L. (1975). *Middle age and aging.* Chicago, IL: University of Chicago Press.

Newton, N. J., Chauhan, P. K., & Pates, J. L. (2020). Facing the future: Generativity, stagnation, intended legacies, and well-being in later life. *Journal of Adult Development, 27,* 70-80. doi: 10.1007/s10804-019-09330-3

Okamata, K., & Tanaka, Y. (2004). Subjective usefulness and 6-year mortality risks among older adultly persons in Japan. *Journal of Gerontology Series B: Psychological Sciences and Social Sciences, 59,* P246–P249. http://dx.doi.org/10.1093/geronb/59.5.P246

Ono, K., Kanayama, Y., Iwata, M., & Yabuwaki, K. (2014). Views on co-occupation between elderly persons with dementia and family. *Journal of Gerontology and Geriatric Research, 3*(5), 1000185. doi:10.4172/2167-7182.1000185

Patria, B. (2022). Modeling the effects of physical activity, education, health, and subjective wealth on happiness based on Indonesian national survey data. *BMC Public Health, 22,* 959. https://doi.org/10.1186/s12889-022-13371-x

Pavot, W., & Diener, E. (1993). Review of the satisfaction with life scale. *Psychological Assessment, 5,* 164–172. http://dx.doi.org/10.1037/1040-3590.5.2.164

Persson, D., Erlandsson, L., Eklund, M., & Iwarsson, S. (2001). Value dimensions, meaning, and complexity inhuman occupation—a tentative structure for analysis. *Scandinavian Journal of Occupational Therapy, 8,* 7–18. http://dx.doi.org/10.1080/110381201300078447

Pfaff, R., & Trentham, B. (2022). Rethinking home: Exploring older adults' occupational engagement in senior cohousing, *Journal of Occupational Science, 29*(4), 562-576. DOI: 10.1080/14427591.2020.1821755

Pham, L., Sarnicola, R., Villasenor, C., & Vu, T. (2022). Spirituality in occupational therapy practice: Where is our spirituality now? *OTJR: Occupation, Participation & Health, 42*(2), 91-98. doi:10.1177/15394492211068216

Pierce, D. (2014). *Occupational Science for Occupational Therapy.* Slack.

Pizur-Barnekow, K., & Pickens, N. D. (2019). Introduction to occupation and co-occupation. In C. Brown, V. Stoffel, & J. P. Munoz (Eds.), *Occupational therapy in mental health: A vision for participation,* 2nd ed. (pp. 759–772). F.A. Davis Company.

Polatajko, H. J., Backman, C., Baptiste, S. Davis, J., Eftckhar, P., Harvey, A., Jarman, J., Krupa, T., Lin, N., Pentland, W., Laliberte-Rudman, D., Shaw, L., Amoroso, B., & Connor-Schisler, A. (2013). Human occupation in context. In E. A. Townsend, & H. J. Polatajko, *Enabling occupation II: Advancing an occupational therapy vision for health, well-being, and justice through occupation* (2nd ed., pp. 37–61). Ottawa, ON: CAOT Publications ACE.

Provencher, V., Carbonneau, H., Levasseur, M., Poulin, V., Filatrault, J., Giroux, D., & Filion-Tredeau, M. (2018). Exploring the impact of a new intervention to increase participation of frail older adults in meaningful leisure activities. *Activities, Adaptation & Aging, 42*(1), 1–18. doi: 10.1080/01924788.2017.137176

Raanaas, R. K., Lund, A., Sveen, U., & Asbjornslett, M. (2019). Re-creating self-identity and meaning through occupations during expected and unexpected transitions in life. *Journal of Occupational Science, 26*(2), 211–218. doi:10.1080/14427591.2019.1592011

Radomski, M. V. (1995). There is more to life than putting on your pants. *American Journal of Occupational Therapy, 49,* 487–490. http://dx.doi.org/10.5014/ajot.49.6.487

Randall, W. (2012). Composing a good strong story: The advantages of a liberal arts environment for experiencing and exploring the narrative complexity of human life. *Journal of General Education, 61*(3), 277–293.

Renz, M., Reichmuth, O., Buche, D., Traichel, B., Mao, M. S., Cerny, T., & Strasser, F. (2018). Fear, pain, denial, and spiritual experiences in dying processes. *American Journal of Hospice & Palliative Medicine, 35*(3), 478–391. doi: 10.1177/1049909117725271

Roberts, A. E. K., & Bannigan, K. (2018). Dimensions of personal meaning from engagement in occupation: A metasynthesis. *Canadian Journal of Occupational Therapy, 85*(5), 386–396. doi: 10.1177/0008417418820358

Santini, Z. I., Jose, P. E., York Cornwell, E., Koyanagi, A., Nielsen, L., Hinrichsen, C., Meilstrup, C., Madsen, K. R., & Koushede, V. (2020). Social disconnectedness, perceived isolation, and symptoms of depression and anxiety among older Americans (NSHAP): A longitudinal mediation analysis. *The Lancet Public Health, 5*(1), e62–e70.

Seamon, D. (2018). *Life takes place: Phenomenology lifeworlds, and place making.* Routledge.

Seligman, M. E. P., & Csikszentmihalyi, M. (2000). Positive psychology: An introduction. *American Psychologist, 55,* 5–14. http://dx.doi.org/10.1037/0003-066X.55.1.5

Shank, K. H., & Cutchin, M. P. (2010). Transactional occupations of older women aging-in-place: Negotiating change and meaning. *Journal of Occupational Science, 17,* 4–13. http://dx.doi.org/10.1080/14427591.2010.9686666

Sia, A., Tam, W. W. S., Fogel, A., Kua, E. H., Khoo, K., & Ho, R. C. M. (2020). Nature-based activities improve the well-being of older adults. *Scientific Reports, 10,* 18178. https://doi.org/10.1038/s41598-020-74828-w

Sixsmith, J., Sixsmith, A., Malmgren-Fänge, A., Naumann, D., Kucsera, C., Tomsone, S., Haak, M., Dahlin-Ivanoff, S., & Woolrych, R. (2014). Healthy ageing and home: The perspectives of very old people in five European countries. *Social Science & Medicine, 106,* 1–9. doi: 10.1016/j.socscimed.2014.01.006

Söderbacka, T., Nystrom, L., & Fagerstrom, L. (2016). Older persons' experiences of what influences their vitality—a study of 65- and 75-year-olds in Finland and Sweden. *Scandinavian Journal of Caring Sciences, 31,* 378–387. doi: 10.1111/scs.12357

Steinhauser, K. E., Fitchett, G., Handzo, G. F., Johnson, K. S., Koenig, H. G., Pargament, K. I., Puchalski, C. M., Sinclair, S., Taylor, E. J., & Balboni, T. A. (2017). State of the science of spirituality and palliative care research part I: Definitions, measurement, and outcomes. *Journal of Pain & Symptom Management, 54*(3), 428–440. doi: 10.1016/j.jpainsymman.2017.07.028

Steptoe, A., & Fancourt, D. (2019). Leading a meaningful life at older ages and its relationship with social engagement, prosperity, health, biology, and time use. *PNAS, 116*(4), 1207-1212. doi: 10.1073/pnas.1814723116

Stevens, B. A. (2016). Mindfulness: A positive spirituality for ageing? *Australasian Journal on Aging, 35*(3), 156–158. https://doi.org/10.1111/ajag.12346

Surall, V., & Steppacher, I. (2020). How to deal with death: An empirical path analysis of a simplified model of death anxiety. *Omega: Journal of Death & Dying, 82*(2), 261–277. doi.10.1177/0030222818808145

Swensen, C. H. (1983). A respectable old age. *American Psychologist, 9,* 327–334. http://dx.doi.org/10.1037/0003-066X.38.3.327

Swinnen, A. (2018). 'Writing to make ageing new': Dutch poets understandings of late-life creativity. *Ageing & Society, 38*(3), 543–567 .doi: 10.1017/S0144686X16001197

Tam, K. Y. Y., & Chan, C. S. (2019). The effects of lack of meaning on trait and state loneliness: Correlational and experience-sampling evidence. *Personality and Individual Differences, 141,* 76–80. doi.org/10.1016/j.paid.2018.12.023

Tatzer, V. C., van Nes, F., & Jonsson, H. (2012). Understanding the role of occupation in ageing: Four life stories of older Viennese women. *Journal of Occupational Science: Special Issue: Occupational Science in Europe, 19,* 138–149. http://dx.doi.org/10.1080/14427591.2011.610774

Taylor, J., & Jones, V. (2017). The development of a workbook to explore meaningful occupations after life-changing events. *British Journal of Occupational Therapy, 80*(7), 440–447. doi: 10.1177/0308022617698168

Thompson, K., Gee, B. M., & Hartje, S. (2018). Use of religious observance as a meaningful occupation in occupational therapy. *The Open Journal of Occupational Therapy, 6*(1). doi: 10/15453/2168-6408.1296

Tovel, H., & Carmel. S. (2014). Maintaining successful aging: The role of coping patterns and resources. *Journal of Happiness Studies, 15,* 255–270. http://dx.doi.org/10.1007/s10902-013-9420-4

van Nes, F., Runge, U., & Jonsson, H. (2009) One body, three hands and two minds: A case study of the intertwined occupations of an older couple after a stroke, *Journal of Occupational Science, 16*(3), 194–202, doi:10.1080/14427591.2009.9686662

Versey, H. S., & Newton, N. J. (2013). Generativity and productive pursuits: Pathways to successful aging in late midlife African American and white women. *Journal of Adult Development, 30,* 185–196. doi: 10.1007/s10804-013-9170-x

Vygotsky, L. S. (1978). *Mind in society. The development of higher psychological processes.* Cambridge, MA: Harvard University Press.

Wang, W. P., Wu, L. H., Zhang, W., & Tsay, R. M. (2019). Culturally-specific productive engagement and self-rated health among Taiwanese older adults. *Social Science & Medicine, 229,* 89–86. doi: 10.1016/j.socscimed.2018.07.037

Webster, J. D., Westerhof, G. J., & Bohlmeijer, E. T. (2014). Wisdom and mental health across the lifespan. *Journals of Gerontology: Series B: Psychological Sciences and Social Sciences, 69,* 209–218. doi:10.1093/geronb/gbs.121

Wilcock, A. A. (2007). Occupation and health: Are they one and the same? *Journal of Occupational Science, 14*(1), 3–8.

World Health Organization. (2013). *How to use the ICF: A practical manual for using the International Classification of Functioning, Disability and Health (ICF).* Exposure draft for comment. Geneva: WHO.

Zuiderveen, A., Ivey, C., Dordan, S., & Leiras, C. (2016). Encouraging occupation: A systematic review of the use of life review and reminiscence therapy for the treatment of depressive symptoms in older adults. *Occupational Therapy in Mental Health, 32*(3), 281–298. doi: 10.1080/0164212X.2016.1145090

CHAPTER 3

Theories of Aging

Elizabeth K. Rhodus, PhD, MS, OTR/L ■
Elizabeth G. Hunter, PhD, MS, OTR/L

"It is better to know some of the questions than all of the answers."

—James Thurber

LEARNING OUTCOMES

By the end of this chapter, readers will be able to

3-1. Discuss the importance of understanding various theories of aging.
3-2. Compare and contrast biological theories of aging.
3-3. Differentiate among psychological theories of aging.
3-4. Apply environmental theories of aging to practice with older adults.
3-5. Evaluate sociological theories of aging in relation to older adults.
3-6. Create approaches using theory as guiding practice with older adults.
3-7. Apply principles of population health in practice with older adults.

Mini Case Study

Ms. Estelle Arthur is a 73-year-old widow. Because of her long history of arthritis and a fear of falling, she walks slowly with feet wide apart. She spends most of her time in her urban apartment alone. The local Meals on Wheels program brings her three meals per week, as she is no longer able to cook due to arthritis in her hands. Her children live a few states away and visit when they can.

Mr. Bernard Morris is an 83-year-old married Black man living in a midsized rural community. He is active in his church Sunday School programs, makes community meals for his church members, and is considered an elder to the community beyond his church. He and his eldest son run a small machine shop, where Mr. Brown spends most of his time transporting materials to customers via the company truck. He had some back problems in the past but has no current back pain.

Provocative Questions
1. What makes these two stories so different?
2. How is occupation relevant to these individuals' daily lives?
3. What factors influence aging in relation to functional performance in daily activities?

The questions posed in the mini-case study raise fundamental issues about the life course. Why do we age? What is the nature of senescence, and can its process be altered? How can quality of life and health be maintained throughout older adulthood? What characteristics influence why some people age in a positive way and others do not? How can we better address the needs of older adults through occupation to facilitate and maximize their potentialities? These are important questions, and scientific theory is required to answer them. Theory is an attempt to explain what we observe in empirical research or practice. To develop theories, scientists most often start with definitions of concepts and put forward ordered propositions about the relationships among concepts. Concepts are linked to empirical phenomena through operational definitions, from which hypotheses are derived and then tested against empirical observations. Theories may incorporate knowledge from multiple disciplines, and can, likewise, inform intervention as framed by many professions, including rehabilitation science and occupational therapy (Bukhave & Creek, 2021). Theoretical frameworks are considered essential for designing evidence-based occupational therapy interventions.

Theories of aging go beyond the *what* of experiences associated with aging in order to examine the *why* and *how* of changes related to age. At the societal level, the shifting demographics of the population toward increased numbers of older adults (as the baby boomer generation enters old age) presents researchers and policymakers with new and difficult questions. In fact, all countries of the world are facing population aging and the **effect** of altering dependency ratios due to the dramatically increasing number of older adults who will need care. This chapter will discuss aging through the lens of gerontology by describing several theoretical approaches including biological, psychological,

35

environmental, and sociological perspectives. Application of these theories is described as related to the *Occupational Therapy Practice Framework (OTPF)* and occupational therapy theories.

Gerontology

Gerontology is the scholarly and scientific exploration of aging and old age. Since its inception after World War II, gerontology has had broadly defined interests. To understand and explain the multifaceted phenomena and processes of aging required the scientific insights of biology, medicine, psychology, and social sciences. Over time, the field expanded beyond these core disciplines to include anthropology, demography, economics, epidemiology, history, arts and humanities, political science, and social work, among many other professions that serve older persons (Libertini et al, 2021).

What Do Gerontologists Want to Explain?

Gerontologists focus on the aged person, the process of aging, and psychosocial implications of age as they attempt to analyze and understand the phenomena of aging. The *aged person* is the individual who is categorized as an older adult in terms of the duration of life lived or expected life span. The *process of aging* relates to the biological development of maturation and senescence and includes the biological processes across the life course. *Social gerontology* is the study of psychosocial implications within the structure and behavior within species. Social gerontologists are interested in how social organizations are created and changed in response to age-related patterns of birth, socialization, role transitions, retirement, and death. Although these emphases are quite different in focus and inquiry, they are nonetheless interrelated in gerontological research and practice. No one theory adequately explains observed phenomena. It seems increasingly likely that aging is the result of complex phenomena that incorporate elements of many of the theories presented here and others yet to be identified (Wahl et al, 2021).

CASE STUDY

Occupational Profile

Mr. Morales is a 76-year-old married Puerto Rican man living in a large Midwestern city. He appears much younger than his age; his hair retains some of its original dark color, and his skin has a relatively youthful look. Mr. Morales lives with his wife, who is quite disabled as a consequence of long-standing rheumatoid arthritis. As a result of her disability, he does most of the housework, including preparing the evening meal, cleaning, and doing the laundry and small home maintenance tasks. Despite ongoing bilateral knee pain from overuse and old soccer injuries, he provides care for his wife. He enjoys the company of many friends and is busy much of the time playing pool, attending dominoes tournaments, and driving friends to the Latino Cultural Center for senior events. He enjoys the lunches there, which are typically traditional Puerto Rican meals. On days that the weather is too bad for him to feel comfortable driving, he gets to the center using the van they provide. He maintains social activity and seeks out supports in his environment that facilitate his occupational engagement. He enjoys dancing and expresses enthusiasm for life. He and his wife have a good relationship, although he regrets that she is not able to participate in activities at the senior center. He is committed to providing care for her and takes satisfaction in finding ways to enrich her quality of life. In particular, he notes that he likes finding creative solutions to the limitations imposed by her physical limitations. The couple's two sons live in town and see their parents frequently.

Identified Problem Areas

Although he has diabetes that he developed in his early 20s, he reports he was in generally good health until recently experiencing tingling in his feet. His knee pain has become increasingly troubling. He reports his wife wonders if his hearing is becoming a problem.

Goals for Occupational Therapy
- Reduce pain.
- Reduce risk and injuries.
- Modify home environment to support homemaking and caregiving tasks.

Biological Theories

Biological theories address aging processes at the organism, molecular, and cellular levels. There are a multitude of theories, reflecting the fact that there is no single cause, mechanism, or basis for **senescence.** Biological theories often fall within one of three primary views: programmed theories, error theories, and genetic theories. These theories focus on body systems and body function as classified in the International Classification of Functioning, Disability and Health (ICF) (World Health Organization [WHO], 2001) and as described in the *OTPF* (American Occupational Therapy Association [AOTA], 2020) as performance skills and client factors. Table 3-1 summarizes the biological theories of aging.

Programmed Theories

These theories illustrate aging as a programmed phenomenon tied to the temporal context (Goldsmith, 2017). Over time, the body degrades through specific mechanisms that fail due to programmatic deterioration throughout the life course. Programmed theories include programmed longevity, endocrine theory, and immunologic theory (Jin, 2010).

TABLE 3-1 ■ Biological Theories of Aging

THEORY NAME	MAIN CONSTRUCTS	CONSTRUCT DEFINITION
Programmed theories	Programmed longevity Immunologic Endocrine	Aging is genetically programmed. The immune system is programmed to decline. Functional decrements in neurons and hormones Functional decrements in immune system
Error and damage theories	Somatic mutation Free radical	Defect in protein synthesis mechanism leads to errors in proteins. Damage from highly chemically reactive agents
Genetic theories	Cell senescence Epigenetics	Genetic errors/accidents over time lead to aging. Accumulation of behavioral, social, and environmental insults influence aging.

Programmed longevity depicts aging as the expression of genes as "on" or "off," whereby senescence occurring with age-related decline becomes apparent. *Endocrine theory* proposes the involvement of hormones related to the aging process. For example, a study of changes on neurotransmitter synthesis, availability, and function showed that these changes are correlated with the behavioral and cognitive changes observed in delirium (Maldonado, 2013). Aging is hormonally regulated, and the evolutionarily conserved insulin/IGF-1 signaling (IIS) pathway plays a key role in the hormonal regulation of aging (Bartke & Darcy, 2017).

Immunologic theory (Walford, 1969) depicts a gradual decline in functioning of the immune responses, thereby increasing vulnerability and the risk of infections, viruses, and other pathological changes. This theory is based on the observation that the functional capacity and fidelity of the immune system declines with age, as indicated by the strong age-associated increase in autoimmune disease. It is well documented that the effectiveness of the immune system peaks at puberty and gradually declines thereafter with advanced age. Dysregulated immune response has been linked to cardiovascular disease, inflammation, Alzheimer disease (AD), and cancer. Although direct causal relationships have not been established for all of these detrimental outcomes, the immune system has been at least indirectly implicated.

Error Theories

Error theories explain aging as resulting from the accumulation of environmental insults, which eventually reach a level incompatible with life. *Somatic mutation theory* states that accumulation of mutations and other genetic damage produces cell functional failure, eventually resulting in death (Franco & Eriksson, 2022). DNA damage occurs continuously in cells of living organisms. Though most of DNA damage is repaired, some accumulates, as the DNA polymerases and other repair mechanisms cannot correct defects as fast as they are produced. Genetic mutations occur and accumulate with increasing age, causing cells to deteriorate and malfunction. *Free radical theory* suggests that most DNA damage and subsequent aging changes are due to the production of free radicals—highly chemically reactive agents generated in single electron reactions to metabolism—during cellular respiration (Harman, 1956). This theory proposes that superoxide and other free radicals cause damage to the macromolecular components of the cell, giving rise to accumulated damage, thereby causing cells, and eventually organs, to stop functioning. The macromolecules such as nucleic acids, lipids, sugars, and proteins are susceptible to free radical attack (Lobo et al, 2010).

Genetic Theories

Genetic theories associate aging and age-related morbidities with inherited genetics and acquired genetic mutations. Scientists explored removal of certain genes in mice and were able to extend the duration of life by as much as 35% (Baker et al, 2016). *Cell senescence theory* states that accumulation of aged cells creates age-related decline and deterioration of stem cells over time. Genes specific to longevity allow extended healthy life; yet, specific components of DNA, such as telomeres, eventually die. Telomeres are repeated nucleotide sequences on the end of chromosomes that are believed to protect DNA strands and prevent them from fusing with other strands. Telomeres lose a bit of their length during each cell division. Eventually telomeres become too short to replicate after a fixed number of cell divisions. This causes the cell to stop growing and enter cellular senescence.

Epigenetics is the scientific exploration of how behavioral, social, and environmental factors affect genetic expression. These changes indicate that biological aging cannot be divorced from social and behavioral characteristics throughout the life span (Roseboom, 2019). This field has seen increased investigation in the past several years, with increased recognition of social determinants of health as well as the cumulative disadvantage. The social and environmental factors one faces as a child create potential negative implications that accumulate across the life span and can result in poorer health and quality of life in old age.

Psychological Theories of Aging

The psychology of aging is a complex field with several subfields (cognitive development, personality development, and social development) and topic areas (memory, learning, sensation and perception, psycholinguistics, social psychology, motor skills, psychometrics, and developmental psychology). Theories in psychology of aging seek to explain the multiple changes in individual behavior across these domains in the middle and later years of the life span (Drewelies et al, 2019). Psychological theories of aging focus largely on activity as described in the ICF (WHO, 2001) and on client factors, performance skills, and performance patterns as discussed in the practice framework (AOTA, 2020). See Table 3-2 for a summary of psychological theories of aging.

Life Span Development Theory

One of the most widely cited explanatory frameworks in the psychology of aging, *life span development theory* conceptualizes ontogenetic development as biologically and socially constituted and as manifesting both developmental universals (homogeneity) and interindividual variability (for example, differences in genetics and in social class). Cohort effect illustrates how similarities among individuals born during the same time period or in the same region can influence behavior and life course experiences (Loures & Cairns, 2021). Focus is on how these dynamics contribute to the optimal expression of human development. This perspective also proposes that the second half of life is characterized by significant individual differentiation, multidirectionality, and intraindividual plasticity.

Selective Optimization With Compensation Theory

This theory identifies fundamental mechanisms or strategies as selection, optimization, and compensation (SOC) (Baltes & Carstensen, 1996, 1999). *Selection* refers to the increasing restriction of an individual's life to fewer domains of functioning because of age-related loss in the range of adaptive potential. *Optimization* reflects the idea that people engage in behaviors that augment or enrich their general reserves and maximize their chosen life course. Like selection, *compensation* results from restriction of the range of adaptive potential and becomes operative when specific behavioral capacities are lost or are reduced below the standard required for adequate functioning. This lifelong process of selective optimization with compensation enables people to age positively (Wahl, 2020).

Socioemotional Selectivity Theory

In this theory, Carstensen (1992) combines insights from developmental psychology, particularly the SOC model, with social exchange theory to explain why the social exchange and interaction networks of older persons are reduced over time (a phenomenon that disengagement theory tried to explain). Through mechanisms of socioemotional selectivity, individuals reduce interactions with some people as they age and increase emotional closeness with significant others, such as an adult child or an aging sibling, with a goal of focusing on the need for emotional closeness with a specific group of others.

Personality and Aging Theories

Theories of personality and aging focus on the extent and nature of personality stability and change over the life span. There are two categories of explanation of age-related changes in personality. First are the *developmental explanations* as represented by Erikson's (1950) stages of development (in adulthood and old age, the stages of generativity versus stagnation and integration versus despair), and D. J. Levinson's (1978) stage theory of personality development. "Stage" theories of personality have fallen out of favor in recent years. Second are the *personality trait explanations*, based on the "big five" factors of personality (neuroticism, extroversion, openness to experience, agreeableness, and conscientiousness). These personality theories postulate that people show a high degree of stability in basic dispositions and personality, particularly during the latter half of their life course. There is growing consensus that personality traits tend to be stable with age, whereas key aspects of self, such as goals, values, coping styles, and control beliefs, are more amenable to change (Atherton et al, 2021). Emphasis is on understanding the mechanisms that promote the maintenance of personal integrity and well-being in the face of social loss and health constraints (Milad & Bogg, 2020).

Cognition and Aging Theories

Researchers of cognition differentiate between three types of cognitive abilities: *fluid intelligence*, reflecting genetic-biological determinants; *crystallized abilities*, representing sociocultural influences on general world knowledge; and most recently, *functional cognition*, as the representation of cognitive abilities related to occupation. Fluid abilities have been shown to decline with age, but crystallized abilities are more stable across the life span and may even display some

TABLE 3-2 ■ Psychological Theories of Aging

THEORY	MAIN CONSTRUCTS
Life span	The second half of life is characterized by significant individual differentiation, multidirectionality, and intraindividual plasticity
Selective optimization with compensation	A model of psychological and behavior adaptation identifying three fundamental mechanisms (selection, optimization, and compensation) for managing adaptive development in later life
Socioemotional selectivity	Describes individual choices in interaction, based on self-interested need for emotional closeness that leads to selective interactions
Personality and aging	Proximal determinant: Specific individual differences are the cause of cognitive change Theories that focus on the extent and nature of personality stability and change over time
Cognition and aging	Distal determinant: Factors that affect cognition reside outside the individual, for example, in the social and cultural environment

growth with age. Functional cognition is an emerging construct that is oriented to an individual's capacity to integrate information from environmental surroundings for return of occupational performance (Baum et al, In press; Giles et al, 2023).

Drawing from the fields of neurology, physiology, and psychology, the neuropsychology of aging is a relatively new discipline that scientifically investigates, clinically assesses, and develops treatments for age-related and neurodegenerative changes in brain function and behavior. Contemporary theories of neuropsychology and aging differentiate between typical age-related changes in brain function and neurodegenerative changes. These theories bridge the biological and the psychological as they attempt to describe organismal factors that influence behavior.

As discussed in greater detail in Chapters 7 and 12, a number of normal cognitive changes, particularly changes to the prefrontal cortex and in the ability to form declarative memory, occur in later life. Even though memory resides in a constellation of interacting brain areas, the medial temporal lobe circuitry for declarative memory appears to be most affected by processes of both normal and neuropathological aging. A number of pathological changes can be seen in later life, most notably AD, but also Parkinson disease, Huntington disease, and many others. Theories of AD relate to its neuropathological mechanisms (amyloid plaques and tangles associated with neuronal death) and its genetic predisposition (presence of e4 allele within the *ApoE* genotypes and other factors modulating its expression) (Rahimi, 2021).

These theories hold that aging leads to a reduction in the quantity of one or more processing resources, such as attentional capacity, working memory capacity, or speed of processing. However, there are emerging theories, such as neuroplasticity, that indicate a reductionistic approach may be too pessimistic. Increasing evidence shows that older adults can engage in a variety of nonpharmacological approaches, including exercise; novel cognitive activities, such as learning a new skill or performing a routine task in a different position or with a different technique; socialization; and a healthy diet, such as the Mediterranean diet, offer cognitive health benefits (Kivipelto et al, 2020). Cognitive change in later life and theories explaining this process are discussed in greater detail in Chapters 7 and 12.

Neuroplasticity theories include manipulating the cholinergic system (acetylcholine), manipulating brain excitation or signaling (blocking glutamate's ability to activate *N*-methyl-D-aspartate [NMDA] receptors, controlling the effect of calcium on NMDA receptors), blocking the formation of beta-amyloid (secretase inhibitors), and reducing brain inflammation (NSAIDs, statins). Advances in understanding of neuroplasticity have demonstrated neuroplastic changes in older adults, including those with cognitively impairing conditions, such as AD (Mercerón-Martínez et al, 2021). Activity engagement, meaningfulness of occupations, and novel cognitive challenges are associated with greater neuroplasticity in older adults (Smith et al, 2021). Evidence supports *enriched environments* as a tool to encourage neurogenesis, including neuronal cell and dendritic growth (Farioli-Vecchioli et al, 2022). Characteristics of enriched environments include social interaction, physical exercise, novel cognitive challenges, and healthy nutrition (Kentner et al, 2019). These characteristics promote sensory stimulation to encourage neural firing, thereby activating established and new neural networks (Karoglu-Eravsar et al, 2021).

Environmental Theories

Environmental gerontologists have long explored aging within the context of elements in the surrounding environment. Occupational therapists consider, alter, or rely on environmental factors to support the performance of the older person. Numerous occupational therapy theories pull components from theories established by environmental gerontologists.

Foundational Theories

As early as 1936, Kurt Lewin postulated that behavior was a direct function of the person and their environment, as indicated in his equation (B) = f (P, E) (Lewin, 1936). Several decades later, additional foundational theories of environmental gerontology were added. Lawton & Nahemow (1973) defined the *Ecological Model of Aging* to illustrate the effects of environmental press related to individual adaptation. The press model posits that when demands (environmental press) and individual competency are aligned, maximum performance and adaptative behaviors occur, thereby allowing ideal occupational performance. A theory developed to explain the interaction of competence and environment for older adults, it suggests that aging is a process of adaptation to the external environment and internal capacity. Environmental press includes external physical and social demands that evoke responses from the individual. The individual's capacity includes cognitive abilities and physical and emotional health. Adaption (or maladaptation) is the response to environmental demands to which people either improve their competence or lower the environmental press.

This concept was expanded by Kahana and colleagues (1980) as they described the relationship between the aging person and the environment in terms of *fit;* a person's capacity is congruent with the demands and affordances of the environment. Person-environment fit is vital for well-being, quality of life, and usability of one's environment, as an appropriate fit can promote activity, engagement, and a sense of being in place (Iwarsson et al, 2013).

Around the same time, Bronfenbrenner (1979) developed *ecological systems theory,* which framed nested levels of environmental influence (microsystem, mesosystem, exosystem, macrosystem, and chronosystem) based on proximity to the person. The model depicts five concentric circles with the word "Individual" in the center circle, "Microsystem" in the next circle, "Mesosystem" in the next circle, "Exosystem" in the next circle, and "Macrosystem" in outer-most circle. The circles are connected with arrows that cross between them. Each level affects the aging person's resources and supports to promote functional activity performance at varying levels of influence. Social and cultural structures of the environments are recognized as areas for intervention. Lawton & Nahemow's (1973) ecological theory, along with Bronfenbrenner's ecological systems theory, informed many occupational therapy theories.

Contemporary Theories

Theoretical perspectives have advanced to include psychoemotional factors of environmental influence. Golant's (2020) model of *aging in the right place* describes the importance of aging in an environment that is supportive to the person's unique needs and characteristics. There is no "one-size-fits-all" environment for older adults. Wahl and colleagues conceptualized *agency and belonging* (Oswald & Wahl, 2013; Wahl & Gerstorf, 2018; Wahl et al, 2012) to include autonomy, self-efficacy, and a sense of belonging within the surrounding environment. Chaudhury and Oswald (2019) defined an integrative framework that captures nuances of the individual capacities, environmental features, and psychosocial aspects of the person. Cutchin expanded these concepts by embracing the lens of John Dewey's pragmatism with an idea of *place integration* (Cutchin, 2001). Cutchin described human/environment relationships not within a stimulus/response or cause-and-effect rubric but rather as a transactional process evolving within a constantly changing situation. Person and environment become inseparable as they continuously evolve through experience. Cutchin envisions each person nested within their surroundings and experiencing a greater or lesser degree of belonging and being in place as they constantly adjust to the moment, the instabilities of change, and negotiability as each situation evolves (Rowles, 2018). See Table 3-3.

Lastly, environmental theories blend biological and social theories. For example, familiar environments can preserve occupational performance despite the onset of neuropathology related to AD and related dementias (Snowden et al, 2003), and environmental enrichment (incorporation of social, physical, and cognitively stimulation) has been described as neuroprotective in aging adults (Gonçalves et al, 2018). These theories offer critical frameworks for occupational therapists working with older adults. Rhodus and Rowles (2022) have developed an ecological care model for older adults. See Promoting Best Practice 3-1 for more information.

PROMOTING BEST PRACTICE 3-1

Models that incorporate an array of factors associated with the aging experience from social, environmental, and biological lens guide occupational therapists in creating client-centered goals and treatment plans. As a therapist, not only looking at the specific goal or occupation in greatest need but using a holistic view of the situation can provide greatest uptake and follow through from patients and their care partners. Rhodus and Rowles (2022) describe a comprehensive theoretical model, *Situational Model of Care*, that is grounded in the lived experiences of older adults (Fig. 3-1). The model identifies "being in place" as an ideal for the person cared for, as well as the care partner, within the specific situational context. These elements require *doing* of occupations to facilitate *being in place*. A comprehensive understanding of the older adult, their support system, personal goals, and resources available create best practices in occupational therapy services.

TABLE 3-3 Environmental Theories

THEORY	MAIN CONSTRUCTS
Ecological Model of Aging	Demands (environmental press) and individual competency are aligned, maximum performance and adaptive behaviors occur.
Ecological Systems Theory	Environmental influences (microsystem, mesosystem, exosystem, macrosystem, and chronosystem) based on proximity to the person
Aging in the right place	Describes the importance of aging in an environment which is supportive to the person's unique needs and characteristics
Place integration	Human/environment relationships are a transactional process evolving within a constantly changing situation.
Person-Environment-Occupation	Interaction of the person, environment, and occupation facilitates participation.
Situational Model of Care	Situational context influences occupational, emotional, and social factors.

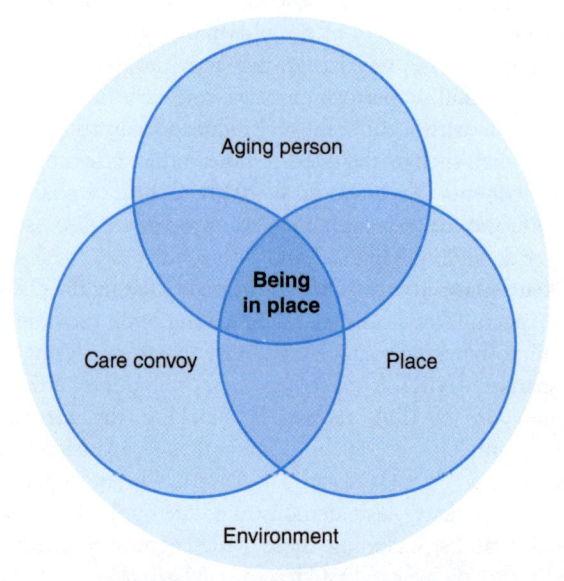

FIGURE 3-1 Situational Model of Care. (*From Elizabeth K Rhodus, PhD, OTR/L, Graham D Rowles, PhD, Being in Place: Toward a Situational Perspective on Care, The Gerontologist, Volume 63, Issue 1, February 2022, Pages 3–12, https://doi.org/10.1093/geront/gnac049, with permission.*)

Sociological Theories of Aging

Sociological theories of aging consider the social structure, culture, and context in which aging occurs; that is, they focus on social participation. These theories are summarized in Table 3-3. A predominate first-generation social gerontology theory, *disengagement theory* (Cumming & Henry, 1961), attempted to explain human aging as an inevitable process of individuals and social structures mutually disengaging and adaptively withdrawing from each other in anticipation of the person's inevitable death, but, when tested, its validity and generalizability claims could not be supported (Hochschild, 1975). In a second period of theoretical development, from approximately 1970 to 1985, several new theoretical perspectives emerged: *continuity theory* (Atchley, 1993), *social breakdown/competence theory* (Kuypers & Bengtson, 1973), *exchange theory* (Dowd, 1975), the *age stratification perspective* (Riley et al, 1972), and the *political economy of aging perspective* (Estes et al, 1984). Starting in the late 1980s, many of these theories have been refined and reformulated, and new theoretical perspectives have emerged. The following is an overview of contemporary theoretical perspectives in social gerontology.

The Life Course Perspective

The **life course perspective** is explicitly dynamic, focusing on the life cycle in its entirety while allowing for deviations in trajectories (Dannefer & Sell, 1988). This perspective is perhaps the most widely cited theoretical framework in social gerontology today. Its proponents argue that to understand the present circumstances of older people, we must take into account the major social and psychological forces that have operated throughout the course of their lives (Bernardi et al, 2019).

Researchers using this perspective are attempting to explain

- The dynamic, contextual, and processual (that is, process-driven) nature of aging,
- Age-related transitions and life trajectories,
- How aging is related to and shaped by social contexts, cultural meanings, and social structural location, and
- How time, period, and cohort shape the aging process for individuals as well as for social groups.

This approach is multidisciplinary, drawing content and methods from sociology, psychology, anthropology, and history, and emphasizes the social and cultural factors that might influence the experience of growing old for individuals from differing cultures.

Social Exchange Theory

Developed and extended by Dowd (1975), the social exchange theory as applied to aging attempts to account for exchange behavior between individuals of different ages as a result of the shift in roles, skills, and resources that accompany advancing age. A central assumption is that the various actors (such as parent and child or elder and youth) each bring resources to the interaction or exchange and that resources need not be material and will most likely be unequal. A second assumption is that the actors will only continue to engage in the exchanges for as long as the benefits are greater than the costs and as long as there are no better alternatives. This theoretical approach also assumes that exchanges are governed by norms of reciprocity: that when we give something, we trust that something of equal value will be reciprocated.

Social Constructionist Perspectives

Social constructivism focuses on individual agency and social behavior within larger structures of society, particularly on the subjective meanings of age and the aging experience. Examples include Gubrium's (1993) study of the subjective meanings of quality of care and quality of life for residents of nursing homes and how each resident constructs meanings from her or his own experiences. These meanings emerge from the qualitative analyses of life narratives but cannot be measured by predefined measurement scales, such as those used by most survey researchers.

Political Economy of Aging Perspective

These theories, which draw originally from Marxism (Marx, 1867/1967), conflict theory (Simmel, 1904/1966), and critical theory (Habermas, 1971), attempt to explain how the interaction of economic and political forces determines how social resources are allocated and how variations in the treatment and status of elderly individuals can be understood by examining public policies, economic trends, and social structural factors (Estes, 2020). Political economy perspectives applied to aging maintain that socioeconomic and political constraints shape the experience of aging, resulting in the loss of power, autonomy, and influence of older persons. Life experiences are seen as being patterned not only by age, but also by class, sex, race, and ethnicity. These structural factors, often institutionalized or reinforced by economic and public policy, constrain opportunities, choices, and experiences of later life.

Critical Perspectives of Aging Theories

In future theorizing, there may be greater emphasis placed on macrolevel phenomena and the structural contexts of aging. This is because there is increased awareness of social determinants of health as having effects on processes of aging independent of individual actions, and the recognition that structures and institutions are not socially constructed but based in fact (Wahl & Gerstorf, 2018).

Shifting the emphasis from theories *of* aging to theories *in* aging opens up a novel strategy for developing cross-disciplinary explanations and understanding in gerontology. Collective identification of the major issues in aging research by various disciplines and theoretical perspectives allows inquiry of discipline-specific theoretical knowledge to illuminate and resolve issues. Engaging in such a process holds the potential for forging a cross-disciplinary fertilization of ideas and possibly new and very practical approaches (Table 3-4).

Classifications and Taxonomies That Guide Practice

In addition to the many theories described here, several frameworks or organizing systems have been developed to structure the strategies by which healthcare professionals can conceptualize and approach the needs of their clients, whether individuals, groups, or communities. Two frameworks that are particularly relevant to occupational therapists are the ICF (WHO, 2001) and the *OTPF* (AOTA, 2020). The ICF was briefly introduced in Chapter 1 to set the framework for this textbook.

ICF

The ICF (WHO, 2001) serves diverse disciplines across mulitple countries and cultures to

- Provide a scientific basis for understanding and studying health and health-related states, issues, outcomes, and determinants,
- Establish a common, international language for describing health and health-related states to improve communication among professionals and with clients, and
- Allow for comparison of data across countries, healthcare disciplines, and health services.

The ICF framework (Fig. 3-2) is applicable to all people, regardless of their health condition, and emphasizes function rather than health conditions or diseases. Functioning and disability are viewed as a complex interaction between the health condition and personal factors of the individual and the contextual factors of the environment. Its three main domains—*body function, body structure*, and *activity and participation*—can be used to classify the effect of health on an individual (WHO, 2001). The body component includes classifications of body functions (e.g., functions of bones and joints, muscle functions) and body structures. Body functions are defined as the physiological functions of body systems and include psychological functions. Body structures are the anatomical parts of the body, such as organs, limbs, and their components. Abnormalities of function, as well as abnormalities of structure, are referred to as impairments. Impairments are defined as a significant loss or deviation (e.g., deformity) of structures (e.g., joints) or functions (e.g., decreased range of motion or muscle strength, pain, fatigue).

Activity and participation include all aspects of functioning from both the individual and societal perspectives. Activity is the execution of a task or action by an individual and represents the individual perspective of functioning. Participation refers to the involvement of an individual in a life situation and represents the societal perspective of functioning. Difficulties at an activity level are referred to as *activity limitations*, and problems an individual may experience in their involvement in life situations are denoted as *participation restrictions* (e.g., restrictions in community life, recreation, and leisure).

The ICF describes the health of an individual according to how he or she is functioning within his or her environment. Within this context, *functioning* is an umbrella term for body structures, body functions, activities, and participation and denotes the *positive* aspects of the interaction between an individual with a health condition and the contextual factors of the individual. *Disability* is an umbrella term for impairments, activity limitations, and participation restrictions, and denotes the *negative* aspects of the interaction between an individual with a health condition and the contextual factors of the individual.

TABLE 3-4 ■ Sociological Theories of Aging

THEORY	MAIN CONSTRUCTS
Life course	Focuses on expected and normal changes in life over its entire span
Social exchange	Individuals, including elders, make rational choices about interactions with others, based on their needs and on norms of reciprocity.
Social constructionist	Focuses on individual agency and social behavior within the larger structures of society and on subjective meanings of age and the aging experience
Political economy of aging	Focuses on the interaction of economic and political forces in explaining how the treatment and status of older adults can be understood
Critical perspectives of aging	Focuses either on humanistic dimensions of aging or on structural components in attempting to create positive models emphasizing strengths and diversity of age

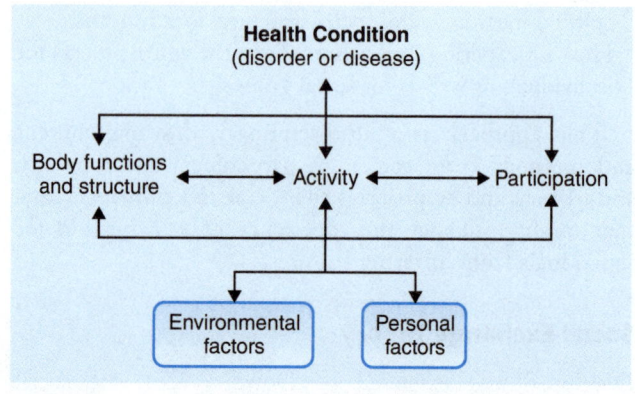

FIGURE 3-2 International Classification of Functioning, Disability, and Health. *(https://www.who.int/standards/classifications/international-classification-of-functioning-disabilityand-Health)*

The domains interact with each other but not necessarily in a linear manner, are influenced by contextual factors (*environmental and personal factors*), and produce a visual of *the person in his or her world* through the combination of factors and domains (WHO, 2001). The contextual factors represent the complete background of an individual's life and living situation: (1) the *environmental* factors that make up the physical, social, and attitudinal environment in which an individual lives and conducts his or her life are external to the individual and can be facilitators (positive) or barriers (negative) for an individual; (2) *personal* factors, such as sex, age, race, fitness levels, lifestyle, habits, and social background, are the particular background of an individual's life and living situation.

The Occupational Therapy Practice Framework, 4th edition

Individual disciplines often create their own systems for categorizing constructs relevant to their domains. For occupational therapists, that system is described in the *OTPF* (AOTA, 2020). The *OTPF* is a living document that is updated periodically to reflect best practices. The principles and characteristics closely align with the ICF, primarily focusing on "achieving health, well-being, and participation in life through engagement in occupation" (p. 5). It identifies the domain of occupational therapy as focused on occupation as reflecting interaction among client factors, performance skills, performance patterns, and contexts. For all healthcare professionals, practice should be grounded in conceptual practice models that derive from theory and are empirically supported. Doing so ensures that the needs of clients are carefully considered and addressed in the processes of assessment, intervention, and outcomes measurement.

Occupation-Based Theories and Models

The following brief descriptions highlight theories and models related to occupation applied to practice with older adults. Each model has greater depth and breadth beyond what is described here, as the purpose of this section is to provide an introduction rather than a full description of the models. This is not an exhaustive list, as numerous occupational therapy theories are applied while working with older adults in practice.

It is important to consider the emphasis on "function" in the theories previously discussed compared with theories specific to occupation. Some theories of aging emphasize the function of cells, neurotransmitters, biological systems (e.g., cardiovascular), whereas others emphasize the function of societal institutions. Occupational therapists emphasize function at the level of participation and performance. Therapists must be clear about the meaning of function as relevant to their areas of concern, so that the theories they emphasize can help guide their consideration of age and aging. Among the definitions relevant to therapy, function can be understood in the context of the ICF. "In ICF, the term functioning refers to all body functions, activities and participation" (WHO, 2001, p. 2). Occupational therapists emphasize the restoration, maintenance, and promotion of optimal "engagement in occupations" (AOTA, 2020, p. 4). Unless otherwise specified, function refers to the individual's ability to engage in the activities that support participation and in occupations that are necessary or meaningful, or both. This discussion of the meaning of function is necessary to explore theories that are specifically relevant to occupational therapy perspectives on aging. Understanding the various theories as well as the possible limitations of each is central to framing interventions for individuals and communities.

Person-Environment-Occupation

Foundational to occupational theories is the interaction of the person (P), environment (E), and occupation (O). Drawing from ecological and human development theories, Law and colleagues (1996) developed the PEO model, which demonstrates how performance and participation are facilitated through addressing the PEO factor's interaction and transaction. The person is viewed holistically; the environment is broadly conceptualized by place, culture, social, and socioeconomic aspects; and the occupation comprises those functional and meaningful tasks that a person does across their lifetime. By analyzing occupational performance, the occupational therapist can address any part of the PEO to create optimal *PEO fit*.

Person-Environment-Occupation-Performance

The PEO model was expanded to include the element of performance as described in the *Person-Environment-Occupation-Performance* model (PEOP; Bass et al, 2017; Christiansen, Baum, & Bass, 2015). This client-centered theory further explains the person's intrinsic factors interacting with the extrinsic environmental factors to create occupational performance. PEOP is a foundational theory within the practice of occupational therapy and used in a variety of settings and populations. The model offers an evidence-based approach to guide intervention development and improved functional outcomes for older adults (Rhodus et al, In press; Whyman, 2022).

Canadian Model of Occupational Performance and Engagement

The Canadian Model of Occupational Performance and Engagement (CMOP-E; Polatajko et al, 2007) is a holistic view of occupation to include three dimensions: person, occupation, and environment. Client-centered approaches foster interplay among these dimensions to allow for occupational performance and engagement within the surrounded contextual factors. This model is well established in guiding goal development and client-centered occupation outcomes across the life span. Evidence supports application of use with older adults to help improve performance and occupational engagement during the older adult years (Tuntland et al, 2020).

The Model of Human Occupation

The Model of Human Occupation (MOHO; Kielhofner, 2008) reflects a broader application of systems theory to understanding of client-centered behavior. MOHO was developed to provide insight into what motivates a client to engage in an occupation, how that occupation becomes habituated in terms of activity patterns and roles, and how the occupation is performed and supported by the client's social and physical environments. Strong evidence supports this model to be effective in guiding intervention for improved participation and function in adults living with disabilities (Jo & Kim, 2022).

Occupational Adaptation

Occupational adaptation is a normative process in which people adapt to press or changing abilities, conditions, needs, and demands across time (Schkade & Schultz, 1992). Central to occupational adaptation (OA) theory is a person's adaptive capacity to respond to these changes. Adaptative responses are hyperstable (no adaptive behavior), hypermobile (random behavior), or mature (the desired adaptive response of goal-directed behaviors). Relative mastery of adaptation is evaluated through efficiency, effectiveness, and satisfaction to the self and society. Evidence supports using OA theory in addressing the internal adaptive capacity and relative mastery of individuals after a hip fracture (Buddenberg & Schkade, 1998), in long-term care (Kirchen et al, 2017), and with dementia (McKay et al, 2021).

KAWA Model

The Kawa model of occupational therapy was developed by Japanese therapists through a lens of life course experiences (Iwama, 2006). The model uses metaphoric description of the life journey as a flowing river from high land to the ocean. As a professional reasoning tool, the Kawa model guides the occupational therapist and client to consider how environments, personal resources, and life circumstances might create or block life flow and create dysfunction, and thus indicate where to intervene. The model has been shown to increase therapeutic processes when working with older adults to foster aging in place and well-being (Newbury & Lape, 2021).

Population Health

Population health is defined as "a concept of health characterized by both objective and subjective determinants and health outcomes of a population" (Tkatch, et al, 2016, p. 1). Populations of adults and older adults consider their health as a whole in making social and health decisions for communities and groups of people.

Rapid population aging and higher dependency ratios, as described in Chapter 1, will create major changes for societies around the world over the next half century. Less obvious but equally important is the profound effect that population aging will have on social institutions, such as families. Who will care for the growing numbers of aging members of human societies? Will it be state governments? The older adults themselves? Their families? Private care providers? These challenges are the result of four remarkable sociodemographic changes that have occurred since the start of the 20th century but particularly during the past 3 decades.

1. Over this period, there has been a remarkable increase in life expectancy and an astonishing change in the typical, expected life course of individuals, especially in industrialized societies. The number of older individuals unable to live independently is expected to quadruple, with direct impact on healthcare institutions and social service agencies.

2. Increased longevity has added a generation to the social structure of societies. By 2050, the number of older adults over age 65 years is projected to outnumber the number of children under age 5 years (United Nations Department of Economic and Social Affairs, Population Division, 2021).

3. Changes in population proportions have added a whole generation to the structure of many families. High divorce rates, growing incidence of single parenting, and increased demands on the adult caretakers have placed a significant burden on families and contributed to changing expectations regarding the role of the state in the lives of individuals and families.

4. Governmental states in the industrialized world have slowed or reversed their assumption of responsibility for senior citizen well-being as states make efforts to reduce welfare expenditures.

It is important to demonstrate the interaction of occupational participation and health outcomes for groups and communities. Occupational therapists have an important role to play in addressing population health through population-based needs in the physical environment and social community, through addressing health disparities, and access to healthcare services (Braveman, 2017).

CASE STUDY (CONTINUED)

Intervention Plan
- Educate and train in pain management strategies.
- Evaluate home and caregiving routines for additional safety and task modifications.
- Provide and train in assistive technology for performance of caregiving tasks (e.g., safe lifting of wife via a hydraulic lift).
- Refer to physical therapist for mobility evaluation.
- Refer to audiologist for hearing evaluation.

Discharge Status

Mr. Morales and his wife demonstrated competence in using safe-patient-handling equipment in their home. He and their son are making needed modifications to the family home, including adding grab bars, a bath bench, toilet rails, and handrails at all stairs and rearranging furniture. Mr. Morales reports a slight reduction in knee pain when he performs his pain management routine, allowing him to continue dancing.

Questions

1. How might the various biological theories contribute to an understanding of the ways in which Mr. Morales has aged well?
2. Knowing Mr. Morales's interpersonal characteristics, what therapeutic modes might be effective when interacting with him? Justify your answer.
3. How would you use the PEOP model to inform a treatment plan for Mr. Morales? What aspects of the PEOP model would you emphasize and to what effect?

Answers

1. Several biological theories may be at play when considering Mr. Morales aging experience. For example, he may have genetics that support health in late adulthood, as well as lived a healthy lifestyle with exercise and good nutrition to reduce free radicals in his body. (LO 3.2)
2. A socioecological model could be beneficial when working with Mr. Morales. Incorporating his family, friends, and/or social routines into goal setting will allow increased buy in and follow through from him after completion of the occupational therapy plan of care. (LO 3.5)
3. The PEOP model provides a comprehensive approach to aligning a treatment plan with Mr. Morales's goals and life. Personal factors such as his strength, stamina, and preference for social interaction should be included. His environmental resources help determine the situational factors that will support treatment planning. Finally, occupational preferences and performance facilitation are end goals for occupational therapy. (LO 3.4)

SUMMARY

The goals of this chapter were to (1) examine the state of theory and knowledge building in the field of gerontology and gauge its prospects for future development and (2) present an overview of the major theories in its core disciplines: the biology of aging, the psychology of aging, environmental theory, and the sociology of aging. Theories relevant to occupational therapy were also considered.

In the quest to understand the diverse phenomena of aging, gerontologists focus on three sets of issues: older adults as individuals; the biological processes of aging, and age as a dimension of structure and social organization. Societal aging poses new problems for gerontologists. For example, developing knowledge that informs policies that can deal effectively with the challenges posed by growing numbers of older persons will be crucial in the coming decades.

Therapists and researchers need to make explicit their assumptions and theoretical orientations when engaging in client-centered care and presenting results and interpretations. There is a need to cross disciplinary boundaries and develop multidisciplinary and interdisciplinary causal explanations of broader theoretical scope. Explanation and understanding in the complex field of gerontology should draw from a range of theories and theoretical perspectives developed by its constitutive disciplines. Gerontology builds knowledge not only through the methods of formal theory development that characterize science but also from the understandings developed by interpretivists and critical theorists. This diversity of theoretical perspectives can offer complementary insights. But for these insights to occur, therapists and clinical researchers must pay more attention to the accumulated knowledge of the field and be explicit in their theoretical perspectives and insights.

Critical Thinking Questions

1. Of the theories presented here, which seem to best incorporate a comprehensive model that might explain the aging process? Might a combination of theories provide the best explanation of the phenomenon of aging?
2. Explain how occupational therapists use theory in practice when engaging with older adults.

REFERENCES

American Occupational Therapy Association. (2020). Occupational therapy practice framework: Domain and process (4th ed.). *American Journal of Occupational Therapy,* August 2020, 74(2 Suppl.), 1–87. https://doi.org/10.5014/ajot.2020.74S2001

Atchley, R. C. (1993). Critical perspectives on retirement. In T. R. Cole, W. A. Achenbaum, P. L. Jakobi, & R. Kastenbaum (Eds.), *Voices and visions: Toward a critical gerontology* (pp. 3–19). Springer.

Atherton, O. E., Grijalva, E., Roberts, B. W., & Robins, R. W. (2021). Stability and change in personality traits and major life goals from college to midlife. *Personality and Social Psychology Bulletin, 47*(5), 841–858. https://doi.org/10.1177/0146167220949362

Baker, D. J., Childs, B. G., Durik M, Wijer, M. E., Sieven, C. J., Zhong, J., Saltness, R. A., Jeganathan, K. B., Verzosa, G. C., Pezeshki, A., Khazaie, K., Miller, J. D., & van Deursen, J. A. (2016). Naturally occurring p16(Ink4a)-positive cells shorten healthy lifespan. *Nature, 530*(7589), 184-9. doi:10.1038/nature16932

Baltes, M. M., & Carstensen, L. L. (1996). The process of successful ageing. *Ageing and Society, 16,* 397–422. http://dx.doi.org/10.1017/S0144686X00003603

Baltes, M. M., & Carstensen, L. L. (1999). Social-psychological theories and their applications to aging: From individual to collective. In V. L. Bengtson & K. W. Schaie (Eds.), *Handbook of theories of aging* (pp. 209–226). Springer.

Bartke, A., & Darcy, J. (2017). GH and ageing: Pitfalls and new insights. *Best Practice & Research Clinical Endocrinology & Metabolism, 31*(1), 113–125. https://doi.org/10.1016/j.beem.2017.02.005

Bass, J. D., Baum, C. M., & Christiansen, C. H. (2015). Interventions and outcomes: The person-environment-occupational performance (PEOP) occupational therapy process. In C. Christiansen, C. Baum, J. Bass, (eds.), *Occupational therapy: Performance, participation, well-being.* (4th ed.). Thorofare, NJ: Slack

Bass, J. D., Baum, C. M., & Christiansen, C. H. (2017). Person-environment-occupation-performance (PEOP): An occupation-based framework for practice In P. Kramer, J. Hinojosa, & C. Royeen (Eds.), *Perspectives on human occupation: theories underlying practice* (2nd ed.). Philadelphia, PA: F.A. Davis

Baum, C. M., Lau, S. C. L., Heinemann, A. W., & Connor, L. T. (2023). Functional cognition: Distinct from fluid and crystallized cognition? *American Journal of Occupational Therapy, 77*(3), 770325020. https://doi.org/10.5014/ajot.2023.050010

Bernardi, L., Huinink, J., & Settersten, R. A. (2019). The life course cube: A tool for studying lives. *Advances in Life Course Research, 41,* 100258. https://doi.org/10.1016/j.alcr.2018.11.004

Braveman, B. (2017). Population health and occupational therapy. *American Journal of Occupational Therapy, 70*(1), 7001090010p1–7001090010p6. https://doi.org/10.5014/ajot.2016.701002

Bronfenbrenner, U. (1979). The ecology of human development: Experiments by nature and design. Harvard University Press.

Buddenberg, L. & Schkade, J. K. (1998). A comparison of occupational therapy intervention approaches for older patients after hip fracture. *Topics in Geriatric Rehabilitation, 13*(4), 52–68.

Bukhave, E. B., & Creek, J. (2021) Occupation through a practice theory lens. *Journal of Occupational Science, 28*(1), 95–101, http://dx.doi.org/10.1080/14427591.2020.1812105

Carstensen, L. (1992). Social and emotional patterns in adulthood: Support for socioemotional selectivity theory. *Psychology and Aging, 7,* 331–338. http://dx.doi.org/10.1037/0882-7974.7.3.331

Chaudhury, H., & Oswald, F. (2019). Advancing understanding of person-environment interaction in later life: One step further. *Journal of Aging Studies, 51,* 1–9. DOI: 10.1016/j.aging.2019.100821

Cumming, E., & Henry, W. (1961). *Growing old: The process of disengagement.* New York: Basic Books.

Cutchin, M. P. (2001). Deweyan integration: Moving beyond place attachment in elderly migration theory. *International Journal of Aging and Human Development, 52*(1), 29-44. DOI: 10.2190/AF2D-A0T4-Q14C-1RTW

Dannefer, W. D., & Sell, R. R. (1988). Age structure, the life course and aged heterogeneity: Prospects for research and theory. *Comprehensive Gerontology, 2,* 1–10.

Dowd, J. J. (1975). Aging as exchange: A preface to theory. *Journal of Gerontology, 30,* 584–594. http://dx.doi.org/10.1093/geronj/30.5.584

Drewelies, J., Huxhold, O., & Gerstorf, D. (2019). The role of historical change for adult development and aging: Towards a theoretical framework about the how and the why. *Psychology and Aging, 34*(8), 1021–1039. https://doi.org/10.1037/pag0000423

Erikson, E. H. (1950). *Childhood and society.* W. W. Norton.

Estes, C. L. (2020). The new political economy of aging: Introduction and critique. In M. Minkler & C. Estes (Eds.), *Critical perspectives on aging* (pp. 19–36). Routledge.

Estes, C. L., Gerard, L. E., Jones, J. S., & Swan, J. H. (1984). *Political economy, health, and aging* (pp. 1–22). Boston: Little, Brown.

Farioli-Vecchioli, S., Ricci, V., & Middei, S. (2022). Adult hippocampal neurogenesis in Alzheimer's disease: An overview of human and animal studies with implications for therapeutic perspectives aimed at memory recovery. *Neural Plasticity,* 9959044. DOI: 10.1155/2022/9959044

Franco, I., & Eriksson, M. (2022). Reverting to old theories of ageing with new evidence for the role of somatic mutations. *Nature Reviews Genetics, 23*(11), 645–646. https://doi.org/10.1038/s41576-022-00513-5

Giles, G. M., Edwards, D. F., Baum, C., Furniss, J., Skidmore, E., Wolf, T., & Leland, N. E. (2020). Making functional cognition a professional priority. *American Journal of Occupational Therapy, 74*(1), 11-16. doi:10.5014/ajot.2020.741002

Golant, S. M. (2020). The distance to death perceptions of older adults explain why they age in place: A theoretical examination. *Journal of Aging Studies, 54,* 1–9. https://doi.org/10.1016/j.jaging.2020.100863

Goldsmith, T. C. (2017). Externally regulated programmed aging and effects of population stress on mammal lifespan. *Biochemistry (Mosc), 82*(12), 1430-1434. doi:10.1134/S0006297917120033

Gonçalves, L. V., Herlinger, A. L., Ferreira, T. A. A., Coitinho, J. B., Pires, R. G. W., & Martins-Silva, C. (2018). Environmental enrichment cognitive neuroprotection in an experimental model of cerebral ischemia: Biochemical and molecular aspects. *Behavior Brain Research, 348,* 171–183. https://doi.org/10.1016/j.bbr.2018.04.023

Gubrium, J. F. (1993). *Speaking of life: Horizons of meaning for nursing home residents.* Aldine de Gruyter.

Habermas, J. (1971). *Knowledge and human interests.* Trans. J. J. Shapiro. Beacon Press.

Harman, D. (1956). Aging: A theory based on free radical and radiation chemistry. *Journal of Gerontology, 11,* 298–300. http://dx.doi.org/10.1093/geronj/11.3.298

Hochschild, A. R. (1975). Disengagement theory: A critique and a proposal. *American Sociological Review, 40,* 553–569. http://dx.doi.org/10.2307/2094195

Iwama, M. K. (2006). *The Kawa model: Culturally relevant occupational therapy.* Elsevier Health Sciences.

Iwarsson, S., Ståhl, A., & Löfqvist, C. (2013). Mobility in outdoor environments in old age. In G. Rowles, & M. Bernard (Eds.), *Environmental gerontology: Making meaningful places in old age.* New York: Springer Publishing Co.

Jin, K. (2010). Modern biological theories of aging. *Aging and Disability, 1,* 72–74.

Jo, Y. J., & Kim, H. (2022). Effects of the model of human occupation-based home modifications on the time use, occupational participation and activity limitation in people with disabilities: A pilot randomized controlled trial. *Disability and Rehabilitation: Assistive Technology, 17*(2), 127–133.

Karoglu-Eravsar, E. T., Tuz-Sasik, M. U., & Adams, M. M. (2021). Environmental enrichment applied with sensory components prevents age-related decline in synaptic dynamics: Evidence from the zebrafish model organism. *Experimental Gerontology, 149,* 1113–1146.

Kahana, E., Liang, J., & Felton, B. J. (1980). Alternative models of person-environment fit: Prediction of morale in three homes for the aged. *Journal of Gerontology, 35*(4), 584-595. https://doi.org/10.1093/geronj/35.4.584

Kentner, A. C., Lambert, K. G., Hannan, A. J., & Donaldson, S. T. (2019). Environmental enrichment: Enhancing neural plasticity, resilience, and repair. *Frontiers in Behavioral neuroscience, 13,* 75.

Kielhofner, G. (2008). *Model of human occupation: Theory and application* (4th ed.). Lippincott, Williams & Wilkins.

Kirchen, T., Ewing, K., Nguyen, J., & Peachey, A. (2017). Health benefits of group based cooking in a skilled nursing facility. *Journal of Aging and Geriatric Medicine, 1*(4), 1–6. doi: 10.4172/2576-3946.1000113

Kivipelto, M., Mangialasche, F., Snyder, H. M., Allegri, R., Andrieu, S., Arai, H., Baker, L., Belleville, S., Brodaty, H., Brucki, S. M., Calandri, I., Caramelli, P., Chen, C., Chertkow, H., Chew, E., Choi, S. H., Chowdhary, N. Crivelli, L., De La Torre, R., …Carrillo, M. C. (2020). World-wide FINGERS network: A global approach to risk reduction and prevention of dementia. *Alzheimer's & Dementia,* 16, 1078–1094. https://doi.org/10.1002/alz.12123

Kuypers, J. A., & Bengtson, V. L (1973). Social breakdown and competence: A model of normal aging. *Human Development, 16,* 181–201.

Law, M., Cooper, B., Strong, S., Stewart, D., Rigby, P., & Letts, L. (1996). The person-environment-occupation model: A transactive approach to occupational performance. *Canadian Journal of Occupational Therapy, 63*(1), 9–23.

Lawton, M. P., & Nahemow, L. (1973). Ecology and the aging process. In *The psychology of adult development and aging* (pp. 619–674). American Psychological Association.

Levinson, D. J. (1978). *The seasons of a man's life*. New York: Knopf.

Lewin, K. (1936). *Principles of topological psychology*. McGraw-Hill.

Libertini, G., Corbi, G., Conti, V., Shubernetskaya, O., & Ferrara, N. (2021). *Evolutionary gerontology and geriatrics: Why and how we age* (Vol. 2). Springer Nature.

Lobo, V., Patil, A., Phatak, A., & Chandra, N. (2010). Free radicals, antioxidants and functional foods: Impact on human health. *Pharmacognosy reviews*, *4*(8), 118–126. https://doi.org/10.4103/0973-7847.70902

Loures, C. R., & Cairns, A. J. (2021). Cause of death specific cohort effects in US mortality. *Insurance: Mathematics and Economics*, *99*, 190–199.

Maldonado, J. R. (2013). Neuropathogenesis of delirium: Review of current etiologic theories and common pathways. *American Journal of Geriatric Psychiatry*, *21*, 1190–1222. http://dx.doi.org/10.1016/j.jagp.2013.09.005

Marx, K. (1967). *Capital: A critique of political economy*. International Publishers. Original work published 1867–1895.

McKay, M. H., Pickens, N. D., Medley, A., & Evetts, C. L. (2021). Outcomes of team-centered, occupational adaptation-based versus traditional dementia workforce training. *Canadian Journal of Occupational Therapy*, *88*(4), 384–394. doi:10.1177/00084174211048017

Mercerón-Martínez, D., Ibaceta-González, C., Salazar, C., Almaguer-Melian, W., Bergado-Rosado, J. A., & Palacios, A. G. (2021). Alzheimer's disease, neural plasticity, and functional recovery. *Journal of Alzheimer's Disease*, *82*(1), S37–S50.

Milad, E., & Bogg, T. (2020). Personality traits, coping, health-related behaviors, and cumulative physiological health in a national sample: 10 year prospective effects of conscientiousness via perceptions of activity on allostatic load. *Annals of Behavioral Medicine: A Publication of the Society of Behavioral Medicine*, *54*(11), 880–892. https://doi.org/10.1093/abm/kaaa024

Newbury, R. S., & Lape, J. E. (2021). Well-being, aging in place, and use of the Kawa model: A pilot study. *Annals of International Occupational Therapy*, *4*(1), 15–25.

Oswald, F., & Wahl, H. W. (2013). Creating and sustaining homelike places in residential environments. *Environmental gerontology: Making meaningful places in old age*, 53–77.

Polatajko, H. J., Townsend, E. A. & Craik, J. (2007). Canadian model of occupational performance and engagement (CMOP-E). In E. A. Townsend & H. J. Polatajko (Eds), *Enabling occupation II: Advancing an occupational therapy vision of health, well-being, & justice through occupation* (pp. 22–36). CAOT Publications ACE.

Rahimi F. (2021). Alzheimer disease: Controversies in basic science research, different theories, and reasons for failed trials. *Biomedicines*. *9*(3), 254. https://doi.org/10.3390/biomedicines9030254

Rhodus, E. K., & Rowles, G. D. (2022). Being in place: Toward a situational perspective on care. *Gerontologist*, gnac049. https://doi.org/10.1093/geront/gnac049

Rhodus, E. K., Baum, C. M., Kryscio, R., Liu, C., George, R., Thompson, M. E., Lowry, K., Coy, B., Barber, J., Nichols, H., Curtis, A., Holloman, A., & Jicha, G. A. (2023). Feasibility of telehealth occupational therapy for behavioral symptoms of adults with dementia: Randomized controlled trial. *American Journal of Occupational Therapy*, *77*(4), 770405010. https://doi.org/10.5014/ajot.2023.050124

Riley, M. W., Johnson, M., & Foner, A. (1972). *Aging and society. Vol III: A sociology of age stratification*. Russell Sage Foundation.

Roseboom T. J. (2019). Epidemiological evidence for the developmental origins of health and disease: Effects of prenatal undernutrition in humans. *Journal of Endocrinology*, *242*(1), T135–T144. https://doi.org/10.1530/JOE-18-0683

Rowles, G. D. (2018). Being in place, identity and place attachment in late life. In M. Skinner, G. Andrews, & M. Cutchin (Eds.), *Geographical gerontology: Concepts and approaches* (pp. 203–2015). Routledge.

Schkade, J. K., & Schultz, S. (1992). Occupational adaptation: Toward a holistic approach for contemporary practice, Part 1. *The American Journal of Occupational Therapy*, *46*(9), 829–837. https://doi.org/10.5014/ajot.46.9.829

Simmel, G. (1966). *Conflict* (Trans. K. H. Wolff). Glencoe, IL: Free Press. Original work published 1904.

Smith, A. E., Dumuid, D., Goldsworthy, M. R., Graetz, L., Hodyl, N., Thornton, N. L., & Ridding, M. C. (2021). Daily activities are associated with non-invasive measures of neuroplasticity in older adults. *Clinical Neurophysiology*, *132*(4), 984–992.

Snowden, J. S., Gibbons, Z. C., Blackshaw, A., Doubleday, E., Thompson, J., Craufurd, D., Foster, J., Happé, F., & Neary, D.. (2003). Social cognition in frontotemporal dementia and Huntington's disease. *Neuropsychologia*, *41*(6), 688–701.

Tkatch, R., Musich, S., MacLeod, S., Alsgaard, K., Hawkins, K., & Yeh, C. S. (2016). Population health management for older adults: Review of interventions for promoting successful aging across the health continuum. *Gerontology & Geriatric Medicine*, *2*, 2333721416667877. https://doi.org/10.1177/2333721416667877

Tuntland, H., Kjeken, I., Folkestad, B., Førland, O., & Langeland, E. (2020). Everyday occupations prioritised by older adults participating in reablement: A cross-sectional study. *Scandinavian Journal of Occupational Therapy*, *27*(4), 248–258.

United Nations Department of Economic and Social Affairs, Population Division. (2021). *Global population growth and sustainable development*. UN DESA/POP/2021/TR/NO. 2.

Wahl, H. W. (2020). Aging successfully: Possible in principle? Possible for all? Desirable for all? *Integrative Psychological and Behavioral Science*, *54*(2), 251–268.

Wahl, H. W., & Gerstorf, D. (2018). A conceptual framework for studying context dynamics in aging (CODA). *Developmental Review*, *50*, 155-176. https://doi.org/10.1016/j.dr.2018.09.003

Wahl, H. W., Hoppmann, C. A., Ram, N., & Gerstorf, D. (2021). Healthy aging-relevant goals: The role of person–context co-construction. *The Journals of Gerontology: Series B* (2 Suppl.), S181–S190.

Wahl, H. W., Iwarsson, S., & Oswald, F. (2012). Aging well and the environment: Toward an integrative model and research agenda for the future. *The Gerontologist*, *52*(3), 306–316.

Walford, R. (1969). *The immunologic theory of aging*. Copenhagen, Denmark: Munksgaard.

Whyman, J. (2022). Geriatric occupational therapy: Achieving quality in daily living. *Pathy's Principles and Practice of Geriatric Medicine*, *2*, 1574–1584.

World Health Organization. (2001). *International classification of functioning, disability, and health (ICF)*. https://icd.who.int/dev11/l-icf/en

CHAPTER 4

Aging and Culture

Janice Kishi Chow, PhD, DOT, OTR/L ■ Pei-Fen Chang, PhD, OTR ■
Kimberly Hiroto, PhD

*Culture is the intersection of people and life itself. It's how
we deal with life, love, death, birth, disappointment…all of
that is expressed in culture.*

—Wendell Pierce

LEARNING OUTCOMES

By the end of this chapter, readers will be able to:

4-1. Describe culture and its importance in client-centered practice.
4-2. Identify factors that vary cultural perceptions within the same cultural group.
4-3. Articulate how cultural perceptions of aging affect older adult participation.
4-4. Articulate how environmental systems affect older adult health outcomes.
4-5. Discern whether one's own cultural biases hinder or facilitate client-centered practice.
4-6. Integrate cultural humility into client-centered interventions.

Mini Case Study

Ann is an 85-year-old woman who tripped on a raised portion of the sidewalk during her daily walk. She sustained a hip fracture and is now post-op day one after a total hip replacement. Ann is a retired registered nurse who values a thorough understanding of her medical care to make the best healthcare decisions for herself. Although a longtime healthcare provider at the community hospital, she also draws upon holistic medicine, including the use of homeopathic treatments and wellness interventions, such as massage therapy, yoga, acupuncture, and a vegetarian diet. A native urbanite raised by a self-reliant, single mother, Ann loves the vibrancy of the city and prides herself in being independent. Throughout her life, she has lived in different downtown areas and enjoys making new friends, learning about the latest trends, and trying different restaurants. As she has aged, it has become more difficult to negotiate public transportation (e.g., climbing the stairs to change subway platforms, walking distances between bus stops) to do her shopping, explore the city, or visit her friends across town. She now uses a rideshare application on her smartphone to get around. Ann lives alone and has a very supportive son who lives in the area and is willing to help her at home during her recovery. Yet, she sees her role as his mother to take care of him, not vice versa, and does not want to burden him.

Provocative Questions
- What are assumptions the occupation therapy practitioners may make based solely on Ann's age, sex, and/or work history? Could these assumptions hinder or support client-centered practice?
- How does the intersection of Ann's different experiences and life spheres shape her values, goals, and role expectations?
- How can the occupational therapy practitioners understand and integrate Ann's culture into their interventions to make occupational therapy meaningful for her?

In a fast-paced healthcare setting, occupational therapy practitioners may make assumptions based on the client's background and circumstances to quickly make clinical decisions. This, however, may lead to stereotyping, overgeneralization of the client's needs, and missed opportunities to provide personal and meaningful care (American Psychological Association [APA], 2017; Shepherd & Brochu, 2021). By understanding a client's culture, the practitioner may better understand how clients view themselves in relation to others, discover what the client finds valuable, and more thoughtfully develop client-centered, occupation-based interventions that promote quality of life. By understanding one's own culture, the practitioner can be aware of their own view of the world, assumptions, and biases which may hinder or facilitate the therapeutic process. This chapter discusses culture with regard to clinical practice with older adults and the ramifications on health outcomes. After defining *culture*, we will examine the effect of cultural perceptions of aging on participation and the effect of environmental systems on older adult health outcomes. The chapter ends by reflecting on the use of cultural humility to integrate culture into a client-centered practice and promote participation.

Defining Culture

Culture is defined by the shared languages, customs, beliefs, rules, arts, knowledge, and identities and memories of a group (Cole, 2019). These elements form a "collective agreement to the rules and norms that allow us to cooperate, function as a society, and live together..." (Cole, 2019, p. 1). Often people associate culture with an ethnic group, but cultures go well beyond ethnicity (Fig. 4-1). For example, a person of German descent may identify more strongly with other aspects of identity (e.g., sexuality, sex, their profession, hobbies) than with their German heritage. Meanwhile, another person without German heritage may identify strongly with this culture based on their time living in Germany (e.g., daily routines, rituals, foods, language).

Culture encompasses a shared way of engaging in life across a range of settings and environmental contexts. Environmental contexts as described by Spencer (2002) will be used to explore the complexities of the older adult client's culture. These environmental contexts are levels that start closest to the *individual* at the *immediate level* in their personal space, move outward to the *proximal level* where the individual interacts with others, further out to the *community level* within one's neighborhood, and most broadly to the *societal level*, encapsulating societal beliefs, attitudes, social institutions, and public policies. At the immediate level, the client may engage with their family through specific routines, traditions, foods, languages, and communication patterns. At the proximal level, the client's office may have a workplace culture with a particular mission that guides work duties, rules of engagement with coworkers and customers, and expectations of work performance. The client's community has its own culture, including a calendar of events (e.g., a new school year starts in August), holidays (e.g., Diwali, Super Bowl Sunday), social customs (e.g., saying hello to a stranger passing by on the street), terminology, (e.g., *soda* versus *pop*), and language. At the societal level, laws and policies reflect the values and priorities of the society. Table 4-1 provides more examples of cultural groups at different environmental levels.

An older adult's participation in a cultural activity may also vary at different environmental levels. Take, for example, celebrating the Lunar New Year (Figure 4-2). If a community does not recognize Lunar New Year, one may be limited to celebrate traditions only within their intermediate or proximal levels. The older adult may gather with just their family for a meal, eating foods representing cultural values such as dumplings for prosperity, a whole chicken for the reunion of family, and long noodles for longevity (Vincenty, 2020). They may give red envelopes filled with varying amounts of money to their younger, unmarried family members (Wirth, 2017). Family members may not be able to easily gather if their schools or workplaces do not recognize the holiday and allow time off to travel or visit. It may be difficult to acquire traditional foods at the local grocery store. Neighbors may not necessarily know about or celebrate the holiday. But if Lunar New Year is recognized at greater environmental levels, participation may widen with a greater sense of connection and belonging. The older adult may greet others in the community with holiday salutations, conveniently purchase traditional foods at their neighborhood grocery store, easily travel and gather with the whole family and friends during an observed holiday time-off, attend a parade, or view regional fireworks.

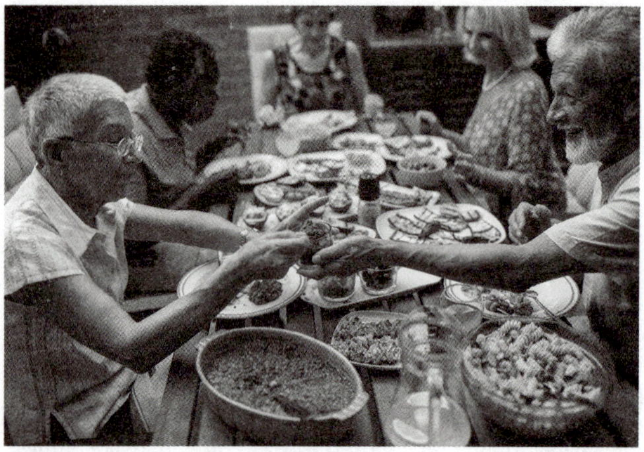

FIGURE 4-1 Often people associate culture with an ethnic group, but cultures go well beyond ethnicity. A culture is a collective agreement of how people engage together. It may be the routine of a group of when they meet, how they choose a restaurant, and what they do while together. *(vgajic/E+/Getty Images.)*

TABLE 4-1 ■ Examples of Cultural Groups by Environmental Levels

IMMEDIATE	PROXIMAL	COMMUNITY	SOCIETAL
Spouse	Workplace	Library Advisory Board	National Association of Stock Car Racing Fans
Partner	Lunch Group	Parkinson's Disease Support Group	National Organization for Women
Chosen Family	Bible Study	Community Walking Group	United States Tennis Association
Biological Family	Walking Group	Golf Club	
Roommates	Bridge Club	Faith Groups	

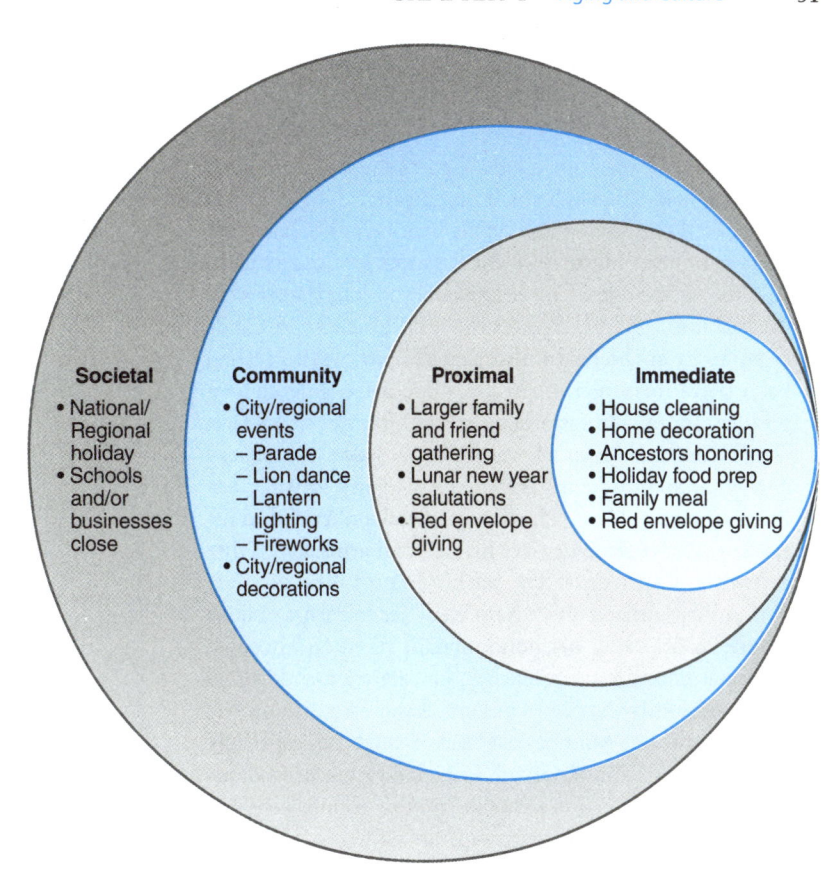

FIGURE 4-2 Example of Celebrating Lunar New Year Across Environmental Levels Note. Participation in Lunar New Year celebrations may vary depending on the cultural context at different environmental levels. Environmental levels are based on the definitions as described by Spencer (2002).

As with all people, the older adult is a simultaneous intersection of multiple spheres, all comprising an individual identity (APA, 2017). Identity encompasses a collective sense of self, based on emotional and cognitive experiences that may vary in different contexts and change over time (APA, 2017). An older adult's identity defines how they see themselves and how they relate to others, not just as adjectives describing themselves (e.g., outgoing, intelligent, athletic), but also how they see themselves in relationship to others as part of a group or community or perhaps in contrast to a community (e.g., member of a marginalized group). Examples of identity may include vocational roles (e.g., photographer, firefighter), class (e.g., low income), gender identity (e.g., cis-female, transgender), ethnic background (e.g., Pakistani American), indigenous heritage (e.g., Cherokee), and regional residency (e.g., Northern Californian).

Different identities reflect the different spheres of the older adult's life. The integration of these identities creates an intersection. **Intersectionality** "incorporates the vast array of cultural, structural, sociobiological, economic, and social contexts by which individuals are shaped and with which they identify" (APA, 2017, p. 19). The concept of intersectionality emerged from black feminist writings (Crenshaw, 1994) asserting that the experience of being a black female cannot be summed by considering race and sex: it is the accumulation and intersectionality of these identities that constitute the experiences faced by black women.

A person's intersection further underscores the unique point of view of each person and how people within the same cultural group may vary in cultural perceptions. In other words, two people can have similar cultural influences, yet the differences in personal and environmental factors can create a variance in experience.

Similarly, we cannot artificially separate aging processes from other aspects of the person's identity. For example, two U.S. military veterans may live in the same regional area, be of the same ethnic background, have combat experience, and thus share a camaraderie. However, with one being a 75-year-old male Vietnam War veteran and the other a 50-year-old female Persian Gulf War veteran, they may have very different values, perceptions of life circumstances, and reactions to these circumstances, based on generational differences, sex, and historical contexts. Furthermore, their relative proximity to social capital and power also determines their treatment and views by society (e.g., inequities in treatment based on age, sex, and other aspects of identity). Positionality is "the social and political context that creates identity in terms of race, class, sex, sexuality, and ability status" and describes "how your identity influences, and potentially biases, your understanding of and outlook on the world" (What does positionality mean?, 2018). Differences in positionality within society, influenced by one's intersecting identities, can also affect their access to resources and their consequent participation in society.

CASE STUDY

Occupational Profile

Sam was a 75-year-old, single, Caucasian man who grew up as an only child in a small beach town along the central coastal region of California where he enjoyed surfing and spending time with a small group of close friends. In 1966, at the age of 19 years, Sam and his friends were drafted into the U.S. Army. He found himself thousands of miles from home in Vietnam (Figure 4-3). He had been there for a year when he pulled a trip line and set off a landmine. He sustained shrapnel injuries to his face, skull, arms, and legs and was flown to Japan for surgery and rehabilitation. Sam regained his ability to walk, but he continued to live with pain, shrapnel embedded in his skull, extensive scarring over his face and arms, and right-sided partial paralysis. Two of his friends died in Vietnam; others drifted away. Sam went on to earn a college degree in art using his nondominant hand and become a special education art teacher; he related to nonverbal and profoundly disabled students. Like a soldier on the field, he did not want to leave anyone behind, especially his students. Sam observed special education students being treated like untouchables in the community. He felt the same as a Vietnam veteran with his facial and body scars. When he was diagnosed with colon cancer a few years ago, Sam assumed he would overcome cancer as well. After surgery and chemotherapy, Sam went into remission and was still able to live alone and volunteer at his local school, but within the past 3 months, he started to have abdominal pain, loss of appetite, and weakness. When Sam did not show up to school as expected, a friend checked in to find him collapsed on the floor of his home. After Sam was admitted to the local Veterans Affairs hospital, the doctors determined his cancer had extensively metastasized throughout his abdomen and recommended hospice.

Sam had continued pain that made self-care tasks and sleeping difficult. He felt a need to contribute to his students' education but was unsure how due to his progressive illness. His occupational therapist, Tamika, was intentional in asking Sam about his worldview of his experiences. He had a very complex view of life as a Vietnam veteran who had survived combat trauma, been marginalized for his war-related injuries, and become a special education art teacher to advocate for students similarly ostracized for their disabilities.

Goals

Tamika sat down with Sam and asked him more about his goals. He wanted to better manage his pain so he could "do the things that mattered." With some prompting from Tamika, Sam set a goal to compile a book of six different art lessons, write down the supply list and steps, create the projects, and take pictures of the finished projects to illustrate the lesson.

Effects of Cultural Perceptions of Aging on Participation

There are common American cultural perceptions of older adults. These perceptions may shape the older adult's membership in their communities and participation in older adulthood. Two concepts to consider are ageism and intersectionality with aging.

Ageism

Ageism is the act of stereotyping and discriminating against individuals or groups based on their age (Butler, 1969; World Health Organization [WHO], 2021). Ageist cultural perceptions continue to influence older adults' participation in activities. Consider the plethora of antiaging products inundating television and social media feeds. These industries rely on our collective desire to defer the aging process, if not rewind it completely (Thayer & Houghton, 2021). In Western societies, gray hair often symbolizes aging (Cecil et al, 2021). In a thematic analysis of survey responses among 81 women age 30 to 70 years, Cecil and colleagues (2021) noted that participants often dyed their gray hair for fear of looking old, incompetent, or unrelatable to younger people.

Consider the image of older adults in the media such as movies and television. Are there older adult characters?

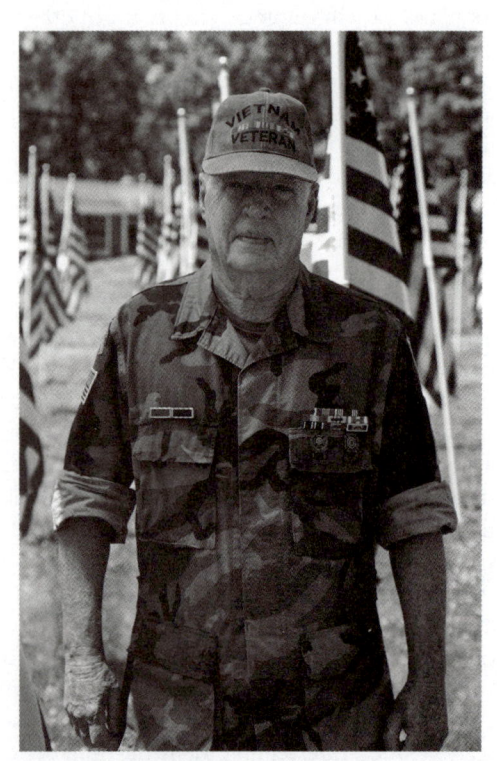

FIGURE 4-3 Image of Vietnam War veteran. *(Johnrob/E+/Getty Images Plus.)*

How are they portrayed? In an analysis of a 1.1-billion-word media database among genres in the United Kingdom and the United States, Ng (2021) noted six times more negative descriptors of older adults (e.g., frail, infirm) than neutral (e.g., society, group) or positive (e.g., acclaimed, valuable) descriptors. By internalizing ageist stereotypes, older adults may feel unattractive, see themselves as a burden on others, and limit their social engagement (WHO, 2021).

Like many other systemic oppressions, ageism is built into cultural perceptions within societal structures and systems of power. The commodification of the aging body maintains ageism by framing older adults as objects with decreasing returns on investment. North American fashion is typically marketed for younger people, ignoring the value of older adult consumers and narrowing clothing options for people older than 50 years and those with mature body types and postures (Veresiu & Parmentier, 2021). A workplace may not offer training to older employees nearing retirement, possibly affecting the employee's motivation to set developmental goals and reinforcing the idea that older adults need to make way for younger people (Rothermund et al, 2021).

The maintenance of society's aversion to aging also relies on our sense of exceptionalism: by distancing ourselves from older adults (even if we ourselves are considered old), we "other" and ostracize our future selves (Applewhite, 2020). Older adults may be geographically marginalized from communities that do not support aging-in-place with stairs, multilevel living spaces, and/or inaccessible transportation (WHO, 2021). As technology continues to expand, older adults are often labeled as inept digital immigrants, and younger adults are seen as proficient digital natives (Köttl et al, 2021; Figure 4-4). Köttl and colleagues (2021) observed that older adult, nontechnology user participants internalized these stereotypes, lacked self-efficacy, and further disengaged themselves from technology. Many older adults lack devices, internet access, and/or user-friendly computer interfaces that accommodate a range of abilities (Chu et al, 2022). As the digital divide widens, older adults are excluded from central social media discourse. Younger adults may be culturally conditioned as products of society to separate themselves from older adults, remaining complicit with ageist policies and systems rather than challenging them.

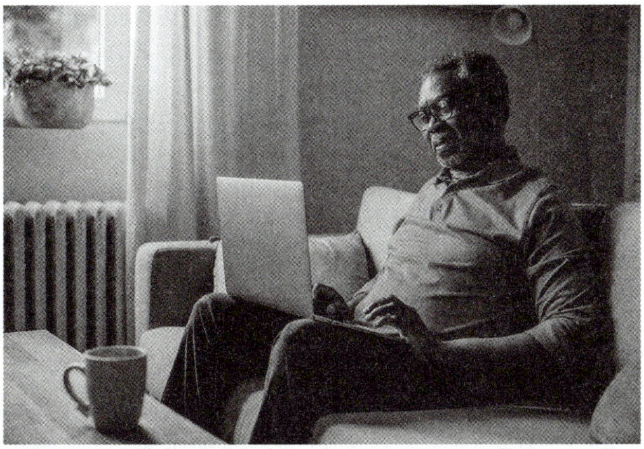

Intersectionality With Aging

To fully understand a client and their experiences in older adulthood, we need to examine the complex intersecting identities of individuals and communities whose experiences are shaped by cultural perceptions of aging within social structures and systems (Crenshaw, 1994). There is pervasive ageism at the workplace (WHO, 2021); however, Lössbroek & Radl (2019) found that older female employees were more often excluded from training opportunities than older male employees. Among transgender older adults with dementia, Baril and Silverman (2022) noted increased difficulty in older adulthood while negotiating ageism as well as the threat of violence for having a cognitive impairment and a transgender identity. It is important to consider the older adult's intersectional identities and the differential ways society may shape cultural perceptions of them.

Occupational therapy practitioners have an opportunity to address ageism and recognize a client's intersectionality in practice. By questioning society's (as well as one's own) assumptions about older adults, we may be able to identify discrimination, determine power imbalances, and counteract oppression with new and perhaps unconventional interventions that foster participation. By holistically seeing our client as the intersection of multiple spheres of their life, we may better perceive their potential rather than their limitations, develop interventions that better fit their abilities, and thus renew the client's motivation and interest in participation (American Occupational Therapy Association [AOTA], 2021b).

Effect of Environmental Systems on Older Adult Health Outcomes

Environmental systems as cultures in themselves at the societal, intermediate, and individual levels shape older adult participation and, consequently, health outcomes.

Access to Resources

Societal Level: Institutions

At a societal level, older adults may have limited healthcare access due to structural ageism at an institutional level. Structural ageism is any "explicit or implicit policies, practices, or procedures of societal institutions that discriminate against older persons" (Chang et al, 2020, p. 2). In a systematic review on the effect of ageism on older adult health

FIGURE 4-4 Older adults may internalize ageist stereotypes that older adults are inept digital immigrants. Occupational therapy practitioners have an opportunity to address ageism by challenging stereotypes and enabling participation in occupations that keep older adults active in society. *(svetikd/E +/Getty Images.)*

outcomes, Chang et al. (2020) found that in 84.6% of the reviewed studies, healthcare providers were more likely to determine treatment for older clients based on age rather than their needs despite potential benefit of the intervention. Remarkably, during the COVID-19 pandemic, healthcare providers rationed intensive care beds, ventilators, and other medical equipment for younger cohorts on the unfounded assumption that a greater life expectancy warranted a more generous resource use and without recognition that a healthier older adult might gain more than a younger adult with multiple comorbidities and poor health (Ayalon, 2020; Daniali et al, 2022; Inouye, 2021; Rueda, 2021). With routine dental care typically covered under employment insurance and excluded from Medicare benefits (U.S. federal health insurance for people 65 years or older), many older adults are uninsured or underinsured for dental needs in the United States, have limited access to oral healthcare, and are at higher risk of oral disease burden (Henshaw & Karpas, 2021). In a review of clinical trials, Chang et al. (2020) noted that 49% of the trials excluded older adults based on age alone, even among studies of diseases more prevalent in later life (e.g., Parkinson disease, Alzheimer disease). With less clinical evidence for older adults, there is limited understanding of a disease trajectory in older adulthood, increased risk of missed or delayed diagnoses, and less guidance for treatment recommendations and pharmaceutical dosing (Inouye, 2021). Lack of clinical data on older adults in artificial intelligence algorithms in healthcare proliferates *digital ageism* (age bias in technology) in healthcare predictive models (Chu et al, 2022).

Structural ageism may also affect health outcomes on an individual level. Antiaging messages and negative stereotypes of older adults precipitate feelings of low self-worth and inefficacy (Daniali et al, 2022). Compassionate ageism (or *benevolent ageism*) seems supportive with an underlying desire to help older adults but instead reinforces patronizing stereotypes of older adults as needy, declining, incompetent, and dependent on younger adults (Chu et al, 2022). Healthcare providers may use elder speak (Williams et al, 2009), infantilizing the older adult as "cute," referring to them "honey" or "sweetie" instead of by their preferred name, using simplified language or childish words, or speaking in a slower, singsong voice with the presumption that the older adult is cognitively impaired ("How do you talk to someone who has Alzheimer's?," 2018; Shaw et al, 2021). During the COVID-19 pandemic, older adults were frequently grouped as high-risk, fragile, and vulnerable, reinforcing learned helplessness (Vervaecke & Meisner, 2021). Studies on self-perceived ageism noted significant association with increased depressive symptoms, risky behaviors (e.g., medication nonadherence, smoking, drinking, unhealthy diet), and cognitive impairment (Chang et al, 2020). Older adults who reported experiencing higher levels of ageism were less likely to participate in health-promoting behaviors and consequently had decreased physical health and reduced longevity (Chang et al, 2020).

Healthcare providers may combat ageism at an institutional level by not using age as the sole determiner for treatment interventions (Ayalon, 2020; Rueda, 2021) but instead incorporating a more holistic review of a client's long-term prognosis, personal preferences, functional status, and outcomes to determine needs and interventions (Inouye, 2021). More attention needs to be given to the older adults' abilities and how their capacity may be further increased with support. Despite stereotypes that older adults are unable to utilize technology, older adults have demonstrated digital capability and proficiency. In a retrospective study of 17,103 older adults (mean age, 75.1 years) during the COVID-19 pandemic, 60.3% of patients accessed primary care via telemedicine (Ryskina et al, 2021).

Healthcare providers can build deeper therapeutic relationships by avoiding elder speak and instead professionally speaking as one would with a peer, in a normal tone with words typically used by adults and referring to the client by their preferred name ("How do you talk to someone who has Alzheimer's?," 2018). Training providers on **implicit biases** (Greenwald & Banaji, 1995) (unconscious attitudes and stereotypes), increasing utilization of preventive care with older adults (e.g., healthcare screening), developing healthcare digital capacity for older adult use, and building physical environments that accommodate visual, hearing, and cognitive impairment may more widely improve healthcare access to older adults (Inouye, 2021). Looking at the clinical practice area, how are older adults viewed or perceived? How do staff speak to older adults? Does this manner convey respect? Are older adults appropriately provided with a range of services as are other age groups? If clinical practice area culture does not support the autonomy of older adults, what could be done to advocate for older adults and shape the clinical culture?

Intermediate Level: Neighborhoods

Neighborhoods may be defined as "geographical places that can have social and cultural meaning to residents and nonresidents alike" (Duncan & Kawachi, 2018, p. 19). Neighborhood characteristics such as types of housing, personal and environmental safety, availability of food and other resources, transportation, and accessibility to affordable quality healthcare and community services in nearby surroundings can coalesce to form the culture and feel of a neighborhood. Moreover, these neighborhood characteristics may have larger consequences on health outcomes. Two significant neighborhood characteristics socioeconomic level and access to neighborhood resources—have been found to affect older adult health outcomes:

Research studies have found that a neighborhood's socioeconomic characteristic is strongly associated with health in older adults. In their seminal investigation, Browning and Cagney (2003) found that "neighborhood affluence" was a more significant predictor of health status in older adults than other individual factors (e.g., poverty, socioeconomic status, health behaviors, insurance coverage). Neighborhood affluence accounted for a substantial proportion of the racial gap in health status among older adults. Sequential studies reiterated these findings. Wight and colleagues (2008) found that adults age 70 years or older who live in a low-income neighborhood had poorer self-rated health than those who live in a wealthier neighborhood. Freedman et al. (2011) found that an economically disadvantaged neighborhood was significantly associated with increased mortality, heart disease, number of comorbidities, and poorly self-rated health. Lack of neighborhood affluence continues to lead to poor health status in older adulthood.

Another neighborhood factor that significantly affects health in older adults is access to resources and spaces. Limited access to nearby grocery stores may lead to poor nutrition and higher risk of medical conditions such as heart disease, diabetes, obesity, and substance abuse (Freedman et al, 2011). A shortfall and inaccessibility to parks and recreational facilities may lead to a decrease in physical activity or exercise, a decline in physical function, and an increase in emotional distress (Wight et al, 2008). McMaughan and colleagues (2020) noted globally the "wealth-health" gradient, in that wealthier older adults tended to have greater access to better healthcare (preventive to long-term care) and better healthcare status than older adults with a lower socioeconomic status.

One challenge many older adults experience today is living in rural areas, which often have fewer neighborhood resources. More than one in five older Americans live in rural areas (U.S. Census Bureau, 2021). In numerous states, including Maine, Vermont, Arkansas, Mississippi, Montana, South Dakota, and West Virginia, more than 50% of older adults live in rural areas, primarily in widely separated communities, and must often travel long distances to get to a store or access services. Compared with their urban counterparts, older adults living in rural areas were more disadvantaged with limited access to services and resources (Skoufalos et al, 2017). A study by Levasseur and colleagues (2020) assessed 139 participants from a rural regional county in Canada, revealing that social environment factors (availability of assistance or volunteers) and physical environment factors (distance to resources, recreational facilities, and social partners) created significant challenges that often prevented older adults from performing daily activities and socializing regularly. However, Suragarn and colleagues (2021) reported that older adults who have high social connections may change their cognitive interpretation of stress through emotional regulation, reinforcing the need for social connections as a protective health factor for older adults.

When working with older adults, the occupational therapy practitioner should be sensitive to the client's intermediate level environmental system. The practitioner must understand whether their interventions, prescribed assistive technologies, and recommendations are facilitated by the client's neighborhood social and physical characteristics to effectively support participation and in turn improve health outcomes. For example, the occupational therapist may prescribe use of a scooter to access a grocery store too far to walk to with a chronic condition; however, if the client does not have a place to safely store or charge the scooter, the individual will not be able to reap the benefits of power mobility. In this circumstance, the client may benefit more from practicing how to access available paratransit service within their community instead. Is the occupational therapist promoting the client's autonomy by enabling them to self-advocate, investigate their resources, build social connections, use available transportation, and so on? If not, how can they modify, adapt, or help locate other supports? Are there accessible resources? Is a referral to other disciplines, such as social work, indicated? By tailoring occupational therapy interventions to the client's neighborhood, the practitioner may enable the client to have a better fit with their physical and social neighborhood environment and draw upon environmental supports to improve health outcomes.

Individual Level: Influence of Culture on Personal Health Beliefs

Health beliefs are, "what people believe about their health, what they think constitutes their health, what they consider the cause of their illness, and ways to overcome an illness" (Misra & Kaster, 2012, "Health Beliefs" section). These health beliefs are strongly associated with each individual's cultures and may form a larger health belief system (Brega et al, 2015; Shahin et al, 2019). For example, health beliefs regarding the cause of disease may vary by cultural groups. While some cultures may consider disease a natural, scientific phenomena whose medical diagnosis and treatment should be based on evidence-based technologies, other cultures consider disease a result of supernatural phenomena whose treatment may require spiritual power (*How Culture Influences Health Beliefs*, n.d.). A culture may dictate how a family makes healthcare decisions. In some cultures, the oldest male in the family may determine healthcare decisions; in other cultures, the primary decision-maker may be the oldest female in the family (*How Culture Influences Health Beliefs*, n.d.). The client may also be more or less receptive to care and direction from a practitioner of a specific sex (Brega et al, 2015). A client's religious faith and spiritual beliefs may also influence the client's openness to accepting specific treatments and making behavioral changes (Brega et al, 2015). Culturally mediated health beliefs may shape the client's understanding of their illness, attitudes toward their medical care, expectations of healthcare delivery, personal coping mechanisms, and participation in their own care (Brega et al, 2015; Shahin et al, 2019).

Understanding the client's health beliefs can have a significant effect on the client's participation in their care and their health outcomes. In a systematic review of whether personal and cultural beliefs influence medication adherence in patients with chronic illness, Shahin and colleagues (2019) noted a statistically significant association between medication adherence and personal and cultural factors. It is therefore imperative that occupational therapy practitioners take time to understand their client's health beliefs to then work within their health belief systems and make interventions meaningful and beneficial. To develop interventions that are client-centered at this individual level, the practitioner needs to ask the client what their health beliefs are, if treatment recommendations are congruent with their belief system (or incongruent and thus unhelpful or impractical). The practitioner must also assess if they are working within the family's structure and communication style. By reflecting on whether interventions work within a client's health belief system, the practitioner may more effectively collaborate with the client, support their participation in their healthcare, and foster greater healthcare outcomes (Shahin et al, 2019).

Effect of Long-Term Stress Within Environmental Systems

When discussing cultural considerations, we must also consider disparities. Though cultural groups are often discussed in silos (e.g., black communities and lack of trust in healthcare institutions), we must consider systemic factors contributing to disparities. As mentioned before, cultures operate in various spheres of influence which contribute to the cultures that are deemed "dominant" and the ones that are minoritized. These larger spheres or systems can elevate some cultures and communities while denigrating others.

Sentinel events of 2020 in the United States (e.g., the murders of George Floyd and Breonna Taylor by law enforcement) elevated awareness of systemic injustice. These events highlighted what many have known for a long time: institutional and organizational systems prefer some groups and oppress others. The consequences of these systems date back centuries and affect intergenerational wealth and longevity. As a clear example, social systems in the United States (and other places in the world) legitimized slavery as a means of stigmatizing and dehumanizing black and brown individuals. After the abolition of slavery, the stigma and dehumanization manifested into Jim Crow laws. Once these laws were outlawed, the ongoing stigma evolved into the mass incarceration of largely black and brown individuals (for further reading, see Alexander, 2012). The stigmatization and dehumanization persisted even while the strategies used to carry out these views changed (Hatzenbuehler et al, 2013). As a result, black, brown, and indigenous communities remain disproportionately impoverished relative to other groups, resulting in poorer health, residence in less safe or unsafe neighborhoods, lower paying jobs, and less access to resources. The pandemic highlighted these disparities: once society recognized how COVID-19 spread, black, brown and indigenous communities became hardest hit because of limited access to privileges such as working from home, basic necessities (e.g., running water, electricity), or safe transportation (Clouston et al, 2021).

Centuries of systemic oppression lend themselves to reduced community trust. Too often this problem is identified as a community-based problem (e.g., black communities and lack of trust of healthcare systems. However, when examined more closely, the fault lies with healthcare systems not demonstrating their trustworthiness (e.g., historically using black individuals for medical experiments [Washington, 2006], inadequate pain management in black Americans [Aaron et al, 2021; Maly & Vallerand, 2018], higher maternal death rates among black women [Howell et al, 2016]). Such mistrust is not relegated to racial groups. Individuals identifying as sexually and gender diverse (e.g., lesbian, gay, bisexual, transgender, queer, intersex, asexual, plus; LGBTQIA+) note mistrust of healthcare settings to the point of avoiding care. (Chapter 5 provides an in-depth discussion on healthcare and LGBTQIA+ people). Religious groups may also not feel welcome to access local healthcare resources. Padela and Zaidi (2018) found that Islamic community members may avoid healthcare facilities due to the lack of cultural accommodation or awareness of religious values, widening health inequities within the Muslim community. The stress of being constantly subjected to bias—explicit or implicit—imposes a prolonged level of stress resulting in higher rates of chronic illness. For example, in a study examining whether stress, health behaviors, social isolation, and inflammation were associated with racial health disparities among 1,577 older adults (age 55 to 65 years, 32.7% black), black Americans were exposed to greater cumulative stress and had greater odds of stress- and age-related diseases compared with white Americans (McClendon et al, 2021). The onset of chronic diseases also reflects the systemic health effects of prolonged stress: Black Americans tend to acquire chronic diseases at a younger age and have a higher symptom burden and complication risk in older adulthood (Aaron et al, 2021). Similar studies demonstrate this pattern of higher chronic illness rates across historically oppressed racial groups (Ryskina et al, 2021).

The vulnerability imposed on communities by systems of power (governmental and housing policies; limited resources for education, health, and upward mobility) creates "stress proliferation," referring to the exponential effect of one stressor on an individual's life (Gee et al, 2012; Ong et al, 2009). Consider, for example, an older Latina lesbian ciswoman who recently lost her job. This one stressor creates ripple effects in her life: with limited income and difficulty finding other employment at her age, she may struggle to pay her bills and rent, resulting in food and housing insecurities. Due to increased stress and lack of income, she may be unable to afford insulin for her diabetes, resulting in poorer health and possibly higher risk of mortality. Many historically marginalized groups lacked the opportunity to accumulate intergenerational wealth, property, or other privileges that buffer the effects of acute and chronic stress. Their precarious social position, often created over generations of systemic oppression and marginalization, puts them at higher risk of experiencing precipitous declines in health due to the ripple effects of a single stressor (Gee et al, 2012).

Given this information, when working with clients, consider their age relative to their health and functional status. Consider how they came to this level of functioning at this age. What factors may have contributed to their current situation? How many of these factors were within their control, and how many were not? These aspects of the person's story are often invisible but are worthy of being seen. Keeping them hidden neglects aspects of the individual's personhood and risks overlooking their pain as well as their fortitude and resilience.

Clinical Implications: Using Cultural Humility to Promote Participation

For the past 20 years in the United States, public and private entities (e.g., medical schools, healthcare professionals, government services) have mandated **cultural competency** training to foster greater cultural understanding of various groups and to improve services (Lekas et al, 2020). These programs typically present attributes of these groups but lack standardized guidelines or define competency criteria (Lekas et al, 2020). Completion of a brief cultural competency training erroneously implies the trainee has mastered understanding the identified cultural groups and will thus provide better services (Hughes et al, 2020; Lekas et al, 2020). There is a paucity of evidence on whether cultural competency programs improve service provision (Lekas et al, 2020). Curricula based on group attributes increase the likelihood of stereotyping people, ignoring an individual's unique life experience, and reinforcing institutional power imbalances (Lekas et al, 2020). There is a need for a different approach to enrich client-centered practice to promote participation and improve health outcomes.

Cultural humility is "the ability to have a humble and other-oriented approach to others' cultures" (Rullo et al, 2022, p. 169). Rullo and colleagues (2022) explain further that cultural humility "recogniz[es] how one's values and beliefs are shaped by cultural identities and systemic structures of power and privilege in order to question stereotypes and learn from others" (p. 171). Instead of asserting mastery in understanding a client's culture, the practitioner recognizes the client as the expert of their own culture, commits to self-reflect on how personal biases may affect care provision, and acknowledges power imbalances (Bernstein & Gukasyan, 2019). Practitioners may more effectively promote occupational participation in older adulthood using cultural humility rather than cultural competency. In a cross-sectional study of whether cultural humility was associated with positive intergroup contact and reduced negative intergroup contact, participants with self-reported higher cultural humility were associated with more positive contact and less negative contact with an immigrant group of a different religious background (Rullo et al, 2022). In the International Classification of Functioning, Disability and Health model (WHO, n.d), personal factors of both the client's and practitioner's culture may affect occupational participation. The practitioner and the client come together in therapy and bring their unique cultural experiences and views. The quality of the therapeutic process may depend on dissonance or consonance of the practitioner and client exchanging their perceptions. Cultural humility may facilitate client-centered practice by looking to the client's expertise of their culture and shedding light on what the client finds meaningful and wants to prioritize in their treatment.

Everyone has implicit and explicit biases. **Implicit biases** are subconscious attitudes and beliefs that individuals have about people (Bernstein & Gukasyan, 2019). One way to recognize implicit biases is to take the Implicit Association Test through Project Implicit at https://www.projectimplicit.net/. Implicit biases can also be internalized and affect one's behavior. When subtly reminded of stereotypes of aging, which activate their own internalized ageism, older adults demonstrated changes in gait speeds: those who received positive stereotypes demonstrated increased gait speed compared with those who did not (Hausdorff et al, 1999). Similarly, when subtly reminded of cognitive decline with advanced age, older adults performed worse on tests of gross cognition than those who had not received this reminder (Levy, 2003). Practitioners must be mindful of their own implicit biases, often learned over a lifetime, to prevent unintentionally activating biases internalized by others. **Explicit biases** are conscious attitudes and beliefs we have about people ("Explicit Bias Explained," n.d.). Recognizing explicit biases involves self-reflection on messages received from the proximal and distal environments that influenced a person's development (e.g., neighborhood where they grew up, school cliques, portrayal of groups on television).

Cultural perceptions and societal expectations (or norms) shape biases. Biases influence treatment. Bernstein and Gukasyan (2019) suggest taking time to consider how these biases may affect how practitioners communicate with clients, their ability to have empathy and engage positively with them, and the types of interventions they provide. Practitioners may have biases about what older adults should or should not be doing that may limit the practitioner from what older adult clients want and feel they should be doing. For example, the practitioner may have a stereotype that an 80-year-old client should not be dating or be sexually active, but the 80-year-old client may feel otherwise. The practitioner may also make assumptions about an older adult based on their ethnicity with regard to language proficiency, social standing, financial means, and residency status and provide different treatment than for another older adult of another ethnicity. Conversely, the client may have biases that hinder participation. Perhaps the client perceives using a walker stigmatizes a person as "crippled," avoiding use and increasing risk of falling, instead of seeing the walker as holding possibilities for safety and empowerment. Biases may be shaped by historical and social contexts and continued throughout a person's life span. Older adult black Americans who lived under segregation and Jim Crow laws during their childhood to middle adulthood years may have different expectations of the medical care system today (e.g., provision of substandard care based on race) than those of people who have lived in integrated and progressive communities. It is important to consider both the practitioner's and the client's biases and how these biases may limit or support participation in a range of activities (e.g., work, leisure, self-care). For more information on implicit biases, see Box 4-1: Resources on Implicit Biases.

To further cultivate cultural humility in interacting with a client, Bernstein and Gukasyan (2019) suggested seeking first to understand the client's point of view, asking questions over offering advice, listening intently to both verbal and nonverbal communication, checking with the client's understanding, and asking if the client has any questions. When asking a question, consider whether the question is pertinent to providing quality client-centered care or is just to satisfy curiosity or fuel assumptions. Avoid pushing questions to check off a demographic checklist. Respect the client by refraining from answering or limiting their responses (e.g., finishing the sentence of someone with slowed speech). Allow the client to define their culture and identity and the amount of information they choose to provide. For suggestions on how to initiate a conversation about culture, see Promoting Best Practice 4-1. By taking the time to get to know the client and their preferences, practitioners can better collaborate with the client, provide better client-centered care, and offer interventions the client values and is motivated to pursue.

PROMOTING BEST PRACTICE 4-1
Starting a Conversation About a Client's Culture

Demonstration of cultural humility is a standard of occupational therapy practice (AOTA, 2021a). Conversations about culture involve a dialogue that "notices, recognizes, and responds to the [client's] different viewpoints on health wellness, family, and role expectations as they play out in individual lives" (Agner, 2020, p. 3). Yet, research has found that cultural humility does not translate well through standardized, didactic methods, as recited scripts contrive client interactions (Agner, 2020). Starting such cultural conversations can seem daunting.

The clinician can use therapeutic interactions (AOTA, 2020) and open-ended questions (Agner, 2020) to discover how the client defines themselves and avoid making assumptions. Simple prompts such as, "What is a typical day like for you?" or "What is the best part of the day?" allows the client to self-describe how they use time and what their valued occupations are. Asking them what music they like to listen to, foods they like to eat, or holiday they celebrate may identify their personal and cultural preferences that guide client-centered care. These conversations may take time before trust is built and cultivated between client and practitioner. Through a culturally humble lens, the clinician uses therapeutic use of self to tap into the client's expertise about themselves and to learn about their culture.

BOX 4-1 Resources on Implicit Biases

Agency for Healthcare Research and Quality

Health Literacy Universal Precautions Toolkit, 2nd Edition
https://www.ahrq.gov/health-literacy/improve/precautions/toolkit.html
This toolkit is a resource to help practitioners support various levels of health literacy. In particular, Tool #10 provides tips addressing a client's culture, customers, and beliefs.

Canadian Royal Arts College

10 Questions to Challenge Your Implicit Biases
https://ciracollege.com/2021/03/23/10-questions-to-challenge-your-implicit-bias/
This link provides the 10 questions to challenge your implicit biases and prompts further discussion.

Project Implicit

https://www.projectimplicit.net/
This nonprofit organization investigates implicit social cognition and offers a 10-minute test to help determine one's implicit biases.

University of California at Los Angeles, Office of Equity, Diversity, and Inclusion

https://equity.ucla.edu/know/implicit-bias/
This link offers a video series explaining more about implicit bias.

Upon finding out more about a client's culture, occupational therapy practitioners can integrate these elements into the client's treatment, as guided by the client (e.g., the practitioner refers to the client by their self-identified name and pronouns and recognize their chosen family). Activities of daily living can incorporate the client's clothing preferences (e.g., clothing that may be nonconforming to gender stereotypes) and personal grooming routines (e.g., application of makeup, choice of haircut). The client's schedule may be framed with personal rituals (e.g., starting the day with a particular routine, praying at certain times of day, engaging in holiday traditions), routines (e.g., having weekly taco Tuesday or fish Friday, exercising every morning), interests (e.g., watching World Cup soccer, working with children with disabilities), and values (e.g., spending time with family, being politically active). By bringing the client's culture into treatment as the client directs, the practitioner can build an inclusive, respectful, meaningful, and safe space to receive quality care.

CASE STUDY (CONTINUED)

Intervention Plan

The hospice team worked hard to help palliate Sam's pain. As a result, he started sleeping better and was able to eat. Interventions focused on basic mobility first, such as sitting up at the edge of the bed and then getting up to the wheelchair and grooming at the sink. He progressed to being able to complete a full routine each day with minimal assistance, adaptive equipment, and energy conservation principles.

Tamika engaged another veteran, a peer volunteer, to assist Sam with his art lessons project. Throughout each session and stage of the project, Tamika and his peer volunteer asked Sam for his input, direction, and preferences. While legacy projects were known to the hospice staff, Tamika advocated during an interdisciplinary team meeting for staff support to use "the commons," inviting other patients to drop in. Many began to do art projects themselves. Sam would beam in his role as art teacher, encouraging hesitant people to come in and engaging them in the art activity.

Discharge status

Sam worked on this project for a month but then grew weaker, slept more, and ate less. He insisted on completing one last art project, essentially directing his peer volunteer in completing the work. He held a faint smile as he oversaw the project. Tamika and the peer volunteer collected the lesson materials and photographed the products for a digital book. Sam died the following Monday morning. His art lesson book was presented to his school as a lasting legacy to his role and advocacy for his students.

Questions

1. How did Tamika incorporate Sam's culture and identity in treatment to help him develop new and valued occupational roles on the inpatient hospice unit?
2. How did Tamika check her biases and presumptions? Could she have done more to check her biases and presumptions?

Answers

1. Tamika took the time to find out more about Sam's culture and identity and utilized cultural humility to defer to him as the expert. Listening to Sam, she integrated the intersection of the different experiences and identities he shared (Vietnam veteran, survivor, rehabilitation graduate, and teacher) and suggested making an art lesson book. During treatment, she supported his development as an artist and teacher on the hospice unit, bringing his past roles into the present. See "Clinical Implications: Using Cultural Humility to Promote Occupational Participation."

2. Tamika asked questions instead of making assumptions, such as asking Sam what led him to become an art teacher. However, she could have done more to check her biases and presumptions by reflecting on how she was engaging with Sam and if there were any biases that were limiting their engagement. See "Clinical Implications: Using Cultural Humility to Promote Occupational Participation."

SUMMARY

Culture is a collective agreement of the rules and norms shared among a group. Each person within a cultural group has their own identity that encompasses a collective sense of self. The intersection of identities across multiple spheres of life underscores the unique point of view of each person and the variance of perceptions within the same cultural group. Cultural perceptions of aging, such as ageism and intersectionality with aging, can influence older adult participation in their community. Environmental systems at the societal, intermediate, and individual levels further shape older adult participation and, consequently, health outcomes. Occupational therapy practitioners are positioned within healthcare to challenge cultural biases and systems of power that limit participation. With cultural humility, the occupational therapy practitioner acknowledges the client as the expert in their own cultural experience and identity. Collaborating with the client and drawing upon the client's expertise of their culture, the occupational therapy practitioner can cultivate meaningful client-centered interventions that foster greater participation and health outcomes.

Critical Thinking Questions

1. How can a therapist integrate an older adult client's culture into their interventions?
2. If the context of care does not allow for a therapist to incorporate the client's culture into intervention, what steps can be taken to advocate for the client?

REFERENCES

Aaron, S. P., Gazaway, S. B., Harrell, E. R., & Elk, R. (2021). Disparities and racism experienced among older African Americans nearing end of life. *Current Geriatrics Reports, 10*(4), 157–166. https://doi.org/10.1007/s13670-021-00366-6

Agner, J. (2020). The issue is—moving from cultural competence to cultural humility in occupational therapy: A paradigm shift. *American Journal of Occupational Therapy, 74*, 7404347010. https://doi.org/10.5014/ajot.2020.038067

Alexander, M. (2012). *The new Jim Crow. Mass incarceration in the age of colorblindness*. The New Press.

American Occupational Therapy Association. (2020). Educator's guide for addressing cultural awareness, humility, and dexterity in occupational therapy curricula. *American Journal of Occupational Therapy,*

74(Suppl. 3), 7413420003p1–7413420003p19. https://doi.org/10.5014/ajot.2020.74S3005

American Occupational Therapy Association. (2021a). Standards of practice for occupational therapy. *American Journal of Occupational Therapy, 75*(Suppl. 3), 7513410030. https://doi.org/10.5014/ajot.2021.75S3004

American Occupational Therapy Association. (2021b, May 27). *AOTA's guide to addressing the impact of racial discrimination, stigma, and implicit bias on provision of services.* https://www.aota.org/-/media/corporate/files/aboutot/dei/guide-racial-discrimination.pdf

American Psychological Association. (2017). *Multicultural guidelines: An ecological approach to context, identity, and intersectionality.* https://www.apa.org/about/policy/multicultural-guidelines.pdf

Applewhite, A. (2020). *This chair rocks: A manifesto against ageism.* Celadon Books.

Ayalon, L. (2020). There is nothing new under the sun: Ageism and intergenerational tension in the age of the Covid-19 outbreak. *International Psychogeriatrics, 32*(10), 1221–1224. https://doi.org/10.1017/s1041610220000575

Baril, A., & Silverman, M. (2022). Forgotten lives: Trans older adults living with dementia at the intersection of cisgenderism, ableism/cogniticism and ageism. *Sexualities, 25*(1–2), 117–131. https://doi.org/10.1177/1363460719876835

Bernstein, C., & Gukasyan, S. (2019, February). *A tool box: Addressing patient needs through empathic inquiry.* https://ccalac.org/wordpress/wp-content/uploads/A-Tool-Box.pdf

Brega, A. G., Barnard, J., Mabachi, N. M., Weiss, B. D., DeWalt, D. A., Brach, C., Cifuentes, M., Albright, K., & West, D. R. (2015). *AHRQ health literacy universal precautions toolkit* (2nd ed.). https://www.ahrq.gov/health-literacy/improve/precautions/toolkit.html

Browning, C. R., & Cagney, K. A. (2003). Moving beyond poverty: Neighborhood structure, social processes, and health. *Journal of Health and Social Behavior, 44*(4), 552. https://doi.org/10.2307/1519799

Butler, R. N. (1969). Age-ism: Another form of bigotry. *Gerontologist, 9*(4), 243–246. https://doi.org/10.1093/geront/9.4_Part_1.243

Cecil, V., Pendry, L. F., Salvatore, J., Mycroft, H., & Kurz, T. (2021). Gendered ageism and gray hair: Must older women choose between feeling authentic and looking competent? *Journal of Women & Aging, 34*(2), 210–225. https://doi.org/10.1080/08952841.2021.1899744

Chang, E.-S., Kannoth, S., Levy, S., Wang, S.-Y., Lee, J. E., & Levy, B. R. (2020). Global reach of ageism on older persons' health: A systematic review. *PLoS One, 15*(1), e0220857. https://doi.org/10.1371/journal.pone.0220857

Chu, C. H., Nyrup, R., Leslie, K., Shi, J., Bianchi, A., Lyn, A., McNicholl, M., Khan, S., Rahimi, S., & Grenier, A. (2022). Digital ageism: Challenges and opportunities in artificial intelligence for older adults. *Gerontologist, 62*(7), 947–955. https://doi.org/10.1093/geront/gnab167

Clouston, S. A. P., Natale, G., & Link, B. G. (2021). Socioeconomic inequalities in the spread of coronavirus-19 in the United States: An examination of the emergence of social inequalities. *Social Science & Medicine, 268*(113554), 1–6. https://doi.org/10.1016/j.socscimed.2020.113554

Cole, N. L. (2019, August 2). *Defining culture and why it matters to sociologists.* https://www.thoughtco.com/culture-definition-4135409

Crenshaw, K. W. (1994). Mapping the margins: Intersectionality, identity, politics, and violence against women of color. In M. A. Fineman & R. Mykitiuk (Eds.), *The public nature of private violence: The discovery of domestic abuse* (pp. 93–118). Routledge.

Daniali, S. S., Rahimi, M., & Salarvand, S. (2022). Age discrimination in delivery of health services to old people during COVID-19 pandemic: A scoping review study. *Journal of Gerontology and Geriatrics, 70*(1), 68–82. https://doi.org/10.36150/2499-6564-n415

Duncan, D. T., & Kawachi, I. (2018, April). *Neighborhoods and health.* https://oxford.universitypressscholarship.com/view/10.1093/oso/9780190843496.001.0001/oso-9780190843496-chapter-1

Freedman, V. A., Grafova, I. B., & Rogowski, J. (2011). Neighborhoods and chronic disease onset in later life. *American Journal of Public Health, 101*(1), 79–86. https://doi.org/10.2105/ajph.2009.178640

Gee, G. C., Walsemann, K. M., & Brondolo, E. (2012). A life course perspective on how racism may be related to health inequities. *American Journal of Public Health, 102*(5), 967–974. https://doi.org/10.2105/ajph.2012.300666

Greenwald, A. G., & Banaji, M. R. (1995). Implicit social cognition: Attitudes, self-esteem, and stereotypes. *Psychological Review, 102*(1), 4–27. https://doi.org/10.1037/0033-295x.102.1.4

Hatzenbuehler, M. L., Phelan, J. C., & Link, B. G. (2013). Stigma as a fundamental cause of population health inequalities. *American Journal of Public Health, 103*(5), 813–821. https://doi.org/10.2105/AJPH.2012.301069

Hausdorff, J. M., Levy, B. R., & Wei, J. Y. (1999). The power of ageism on physical function of older persons: Reversibility of age-related gait changes. *Journal of the American Geriatrics Society, 47*(11), 1346–1349. https://doi.org/10.1111/j.1532-5415.1999.tb07437.x

Henshaw, M. M., & Karpas, S. (2021). Oral health disparities and inequities in older adults. *Dental Clinics of North America, 65*(2), 257–273. https://doi.org/10.1016/j.cden.2020.11.004

EuroMed Info. *How culture influences health beliefs.* (n.d.). https://www.euromedinfo.eu/how-culture-influences-health-beliefs.html/

Good Samaritan Society (2018). *How do you talk to someone who has Alzheimer's?* https://www.good-sam.com/resources/communicating-with-people-with-dementia

Howell, E. A., Egorova, N., Balbierz, A., Zeitlin, J., & Hebert, P. L. (2016). Black-white differences in severe maternal morbidity and site of care. *American Journal of Obstetrics and Gynecology, 214*(1), 122.e1–122.e7. https://doi.org/10.1016/j.ajog.2015.08.019

Hughes, V., Delva, S., Nkimbeng, M., Spaulding, E., Turkson-Ocran, R.-A., Cudjoe, J., Ford, A., Rushton, C., D'Aoust, R., & Han, H.-R. (2020). Not missing the opportunity: Strategies to promote cultural humility among future nursing faculty. *Journal of Professional Nursing, 36*(1), 28–33. https://doi.org/10.1016/j.profnurs.2019.06.005

Inouye, S. K. (2021). Creating an anti-ageist healthcare system to improve care for our current and future selves. *Nature Aging, 1*(2), 150–152. https://doi.org/10.1038/s43587-020-00004-4

Köttl, H., Gallistl, V., Rohner, R., & Ayalon, L. (2021). "But at the age of 85? Forget it!": Internalized ageism, a barrier to technology use. *Journal of Aging Studies, 59*(2021), 100971. https://doi.org/10.1016/j.jaging.2021.100971

Lekas, H. M., Pahl, K., & Fuller Lewis, C. (2020). Rethinking cultural competence: Shifting to cultural humility. *Health Services Insights, 13,* 117863292097058. https://doi.org/10.1177/1178632920970580

Levasseur, M., Routhier, S., Clapperton, I., Doré, C., & Gallagher, F. (2020). Social participation needs of older adults living in a rural regional county municipality: Toward reducing situations of isolation and vulnerability. *BMC Geriatrics, 20*(1), 456. https://doi.org/10.1186/s12877-020-01849-5

Levy, B. R. (2003). Mind matters: Cognitive and physical effects of aging self-stereotypes. *Journals of Gerontology: Series B, 58*(4), P203–P211. https://doi.org/10.1093/geronb/58.4.p203

Lössbroek, J., & Radl, J. (2019). Teaching older workers new tricks: Workplace practices and gender training differences in nine European countries. *Ageing and Society, 39*(10), 2170–2193. https://doi.org/10.1017/s0144686x1800079x

Maly, A., & Vallerand, A. H. (2018). Neighborhood, socioeconomic, and racial influence on chronic pain. *Pain Management Nursing, 19*(1), 14–22. https://doi.org/10.1016/j.pmn.2017.11.004

McClendon, J., Chang, K., J. Boudreaux, M., Oltmanns, T. F., & Bogdan, R. (2021). Black-white racial health disparities in inflammation and physical health: Cumulative stress, social isolation, and health behaviors. *Psychoneuroendocrinology, 131,* 105251. https://doi.org/10.1016/j.psyneuen.2021.105251

McMaughan, D. J., Oloruntoba, O., & Smith, M. L. (2020). Socioeconomic status and access to healthcare: Interrelated drivers for healthy aging. *Frontiers in Public Health, 8*(231). https://doi.org/10.3389/fpubh.2020.00231

Misra, R., & Kaster, E. C. (2012). Health beliefs. In S. Loue & M. Sajatovic (Eds.), *Encyclopedia of Immigrant Health.* Springer. https://link.springer.com/referenceworkentry/10.1007/978-1-4419-5659-0_332

Ng, R. (2021). Societal age stereotypes in the U.S. and U.K. from a media database of 1.1 billion words. *International Journal of Environmental Research and Public Health, 18*(16), 8822. https://doi.org/10.3390/ijerph18168822

Ong, A. D., Fuller-Rowell, T., & Burrow, A. L. (2009). Racial discrimination and the stress process. *Journal of Personality and Social Psychology, 96*(6), 1259–1271. https://doi.org/10.1037/a0015335

Padela, A. I., & Zaidi, D. (2018). The Islamic tradition and health inequities: A preliminary conceptual model based on a systematic literature review of Muslim health-care disparities. *Avicenna Journal of Medicine, 8,* 1–13, https://doi.org/10.4103/ajm.AJM_134_17

Perception Institute. *Explicit bias explained.* (n.d.). https://perception.org/research/explicit-bias/

Rothermund, K., Klusmann, V., & Zacher, H. (2021). Age discrimination in the context of motivation and healthy aging. *The Journals of Gerontology: Series B, 76*(Supplement_2), S167–S189. https://doi.org/10.1093/geronb/gbab081

Rueda, J. (2021). Ageism in the COVID-19 pandemic: Age-based discrimination in triage decisions and beyond. *History and Philosophy of the Life Sciences, 43*(3). https://doi.org/10.1007/s40656-021-00441-3

Rullo, M., Visintin, E. P., Milani, S., Romano, A., & Fabbri, L. (2022). Stay humble and enjoy diversity: The interplay between intergroup contact and cultural humility on prejudice. *International Journal of Intercultural Relations, 87,* 169–182. https://doi.org/10.1016/j.ijintrel.2022.02.003

Ryskina, K. L., Shultz, K., Zhou, Y., Lautenbach, G., & Brown, R. T. (2021). Older adults' access to primary care: Gender, racial, and ethnic disparities in telemedicine. *Journal of the American Geriatrics Society, 69*(10), 2732–2740. https://doi.org/10.1111/jgs.17354

Shahin, W., Kennedy, G. A., & Stupans, I. (2019). The impact of personal and cultural beliefs on medication adherence of patients with chronic illnesses: A systematic review. *Patient Preference and Adherence, 13,* 1019–1035. https://doi.org/10.2147/ppa.s212046

Shaw, C., Gordon, J., & Williams, K. (2021). Understanding elderspeak: An evolutionary concept analysis. *Innovation in Aging, 4*(Suppl_1), 451. https://doi.org/10.1093/geroni/igaa057.1459

Shepherd, B. F., & Brochu, P. M. (2021). How do stereotypes harm older adults? A theoretical explanation for the perpetration of elder abuse and its rise. *Aggression and Violent Behavior, 57,* 101435. https://doi.org/10.1016/j.avb.2020.101435

Skoufalos, A., Clarke, J. L., Ellis, D. R., Shepard, V. L., & Rula, E. Y. (2017). Rural aging in America: Proceedings of the 2017 connectivity summit. *Population Health Management, 20*(S2), S1–S10. https://doi.org/10.1089/pop.2017.0177

Spencer, J. C. (2002). Evaluation of performance contexts. In E. B. Crepeau, E. S. Cohn, & B. A. B. Schell (Eds.). *Willard & Spackman's occupational therapy* (10th ed., pp. 427–447). Lippincott, Wolters, Kluwer.

Suragarn, U., Hain, D., & Pfaff, G. (2021). Approaches to enhance social connection in older adults: An integrative review of literature. *Aging and Health Research, 1*(3), 100029. https://doi.org/10.1016/j.ahr.2021.100029

Thayer, C., & Houghton, A. (2021, April). *Women seek more authentic representation of aging in media and the marketplace.* https://www.aarp.org/research/topics/life/info-2019/womens-reflections-beauty-age-media.html

U.S. Census Bureau. (2021, October 8). *The older population in rural America: 2012–2016.* https://www.census.gov/library/publications/2019/acs/acs-41.html

U.S. Department of Veterans Affairs. (n.d.). Military health history pocket card: Vietnam. https://www.va.gov/oaa/docs/mhpcmobile.pdf

U.S. Department of Veterans Affairs. (2015, April 21). *Office of public and intergovernmental affairs: Federal benefits for veterans, dependents and survivors.* Veterans Affairs. https://www.va.gov/opa/publications/benefits_book/benefits_chap02.asp

Veresiu, E., & Parmentier, M.-A. (2021). Advanced style influencers: Confronting gendered ageism in fashion and beauty markets. *Journal of the Association for Consumer Research, 6*(2), 263–273. https://doi.org/10.1086/712609

Vervaecke, D., & Meisner, B. A. (2021). Caremongering and assumptions of need: The spread of compassionate ageism during COVID-19. *The Gerontologist, 61*(2), 159–165. https://doi.org/10.1093/geront/gnaa131

Vincenty, S. (2020, December 20). 11 traditional Lunar New Year foods to eat in 2021. *Oprah Daily.* https://www.oprahdaily.com/life/g34895835/traditional-lunar-new-year-foods/

Washington, H. (2006). *Medical apartheid the dark history of medical experimentation on black Americans from colonial times to the present.* Doubleday.

What does positionality mean? (2018). Dictionary.com. https://www.dictionary.com/e/gender-sexuality/positionality/

Wight, R. G., Cummings, J. R., Miller-Martinez, D., Karlamangla, A. S., Seeman, T. E., & Aneshensel, C. S. (2008). A multilevel analysis of urban neighborhood socioeconomic disadvantage and health in late life. *Social Science & Medicine, 66*(4), 862–872. https://doi.org/10.1016/j.socscimed.2007.11.002

Williams, K. N., Herman, R., Gajewski, B., & Wilson, K. (2009). Elderspeak communication: Impact on dementia care. *American Journal of Alzheimer's Disease & Other Dementias, 24*(1), 11–20. https://doi.org/10.1177/1533317508318472

Wirth, K. (2017, January 25). What's the significance of Lunar New Year red envelopes? https://www.seattletimes.com/life/whats-the-significance-of-lunar-new-year-red-envelope/

World Health Organization. (n. d.) *International classification of functioning, disability, and health (ICF).* https://icd.who.int/dev11/l-icf/en

World Health Organization, United Nations Office of the High Commissioner for Human Rights, United Nations Population Fund, & United Nations Department of Economic and Social Affairs (Eds.). (2021, March 18). *Global report on ageism.* World Health Organization. https://www.who.int/publications/i/item/9789240016866

Yeh, H. E., & McColl, M. A. (2019). A model for occupation-based palliative care. *Occupational Therapy in Health Care, 33*(1), 108–133. https://doi.org/10.1080/07380577.2018.1544428

CHAPTER 5

Identity, Sexuality, and Relationships

Jennifer L. Martin, OTD, OTR, CHT, CLT
Michele L. McCarroll, PhD, FAACVPR, ACSM-CCEP, CCRP

True belonging only happens when we present our authentic, imperfect selves to the world, our sense of belonging can never be greater than our level of self-acceptance.

—Brené Brown

LEARNING OUTCOMES

By the end of this chapter, readers will be able to:

5-1. Discuss the importance of social relationships, social networks, and social support in the lives of older adults.
5-2. Understand the impact of gender identity and gender-based attitudes and expectations on aging, relationships, and life satisfaction.
5-3. Examine the effects of social isolation, loneliness, and touch deprivation in older adulthood.
5-4. Identify how gender identity, sexuality, and relationships effect health status and healthcare delivery in older adults.
5-5. Examine the impact of the environment in which one lives on sexual expression.
5-6. Develop strategies for use in therapeutic interactions with older adults and families.

Mini Case Study

Esther Rose is a 74-year-old African American, cisgender woman who recently retired as a grocery store manager. Ms. Rose has a medical history that includes hypertension, high cholesterol, diabetes, diabetic retinopathy with vision loss, and osteoarthritis in her spine, hands, and knees. She currently lives in a senior apartment complex in a large Southern U.S. city and reports that she is having difficulty cooking and cleaning due to vision loss and pain in her hands and knees. Ms. Rose moved into the apartment complex after the death of her second husband, Marcus, approximately 1 year ago. Ms. Rose was married to her first husband, George, for 30 years and had three children with him. After his death, she married a friend from church. She and her second husband Marcus were married for 2 years before he suddenly died from complications due to COVID-19. Ms. Rose now spends most of her time watching television. She used to enjoy going to the library, Bible study, and church services but has recently stopped driving because of her vision loss. She served as a Sunday school teacher and helped at the church's food pantry in the past. She has not made many friends at the apartment complex yet but hopes to reach out to her neighbors soon. Of her three children, one lives in the same city but does not stop by to visit very often; the other two live across the country. She has four teenage grandchildren living with their parents 1,200 miles away. When asked by the occupational therapist to identify important activities that she is unable to do and would like to do in the future, she states that she would like to resume valued social activities such as going to church, teaching Sunday school, and working in the food pantry, all of which she is unable to because she can no longer drive.

Provocative Questions

1. What strengths do you see in Ms. Rose's social network? What weaknesses do you see in Ms. Rose's social network?
2. Who can Ms. Rose reach out to for social support? How can the occupational therapist facilitate this process?
3. How will Ms. Rose's social support needs change as she ages?

Healthy aging is the process of developing and maintaining the functional ability that enables well-being in older age (World Health Organization [WHO], 2015). Well-being is a combination of feeling good, functioning well, experiencing happiness, having a sense of purpose, and experiencing positive relationships (Ruggeri et al, 2020). Older adults report that maintaining these relationships is central to their well-being and that as they age, they may give increasing priority to this ability (WHO, 2015).

Occupational therapy practitioners help people achieve health, well-being, and participation in life through engagement in occupation (American Occupational Therapy Association [AOTA], 2020). All occupations occur within a person's context, which includes environmental and personal factors that act as facilitators or barriers that influence occupational engagement and participation. Environmental factors are the aspects of a person's physical, social, and attitudinal surroundings in which they live and conduct their lives. Support and relationships are considered part of a person's environment and such relationships provide not only support, but also nurturing, protection, assistance, and connections to other persons in the home and community, or in other aspects of their daily activities (AOTA, 2020).

A broad range of relationships is important to older people, including relationships with family members, intimate relationships, and informal relationships with friends, neighbors, and acquaintances, as well as more formal relationships with healthcare providers (Rook & Charles, 2017). The social networks of older adults can be diverse and complex, and occupational therapy practitioners should recognize these networks as an important resource for the promotion of healthy aging. This chapter will explore the variety and breadth of social relationships in the lives of older adults in a global population that is aging rapidly and becoming increasingly more diverse. This chapter will also explore the role of gender identity and sexuality in the social lives of older adults.

Social Relationships and Networks

The evidence is clear that positive social connections, the sense of having close relationships with others, are essential for health and well-being and for promoting healthy aging later in life. Older adults who are socially integrated and have access to social support have better physical health and reduced risks for cardiovascular disease, infections, and cognitive decline (Rook & Charles, 2017). Equitable relationships that provide reciprocal support affirm an older adult's self-esteem and identity. These relationships can reduce an older adult's risk for depression and helplessness and increase their ability to cope with chronic pain and functional limitations (Reynolds & Hean Lim, 2013).

All forms of social connections are important, including superficial interactions; therefore, it is important not to make assumptions about the types of social interactions or relationships that are most meaningful to an older person (Van Orden et al, 2020). Close social relationships are accumulated throughout one's life and often consist of a spouse or partner, children, family members, and friends (Rook & Charles, 2017). Older adults report greater satisfaction with their social relationships than do younger adults because they tend to retain relationships with their closest, most rewarding social connections and reduce their casual acquaintances and other peripheral social ties as they age (Rook & Charles, 2017).

Older adults report greater satisfaction with their relationships, most likely because they selectively engage with their most rewarding social ties and proactively avoid potential conflicts with others. Older adults who experience frequent negative interactions with their social networks may experience psychological distress and poor physical health outcomes (Rook & Charles, 2017). Some social ties that provide positive support and companionship may simultaneously serve as sources of strain or conflict; these relationships are considered **ambivalent** in nature (Rook et al, 2012). Older people may also find some relationships burdensome. Examples include providing long-term care for a spouse, which may affect the caregiver's mental health and their ability to take advantage of other opportunities, and raising grandchildren, which can place additional financial, emotional, and physical strains on grandparents (WHO, 2015).

Social connection is a multifactorial construct that includes structural, functional, and qualitative aspects that collectively contribute to various health-related risks and protections (Holt-Lunstad et al, 2017). The structural aspects of social connections include social network size, marital status, frequency of social contact, and living arrangements; functional and qualitative aspects include received and perceived social support, social isolation, loneliness, social inclusiveness, and relationship quality (Holt-Lunstad et al, 2017). It is important not to assume that older adults who live alone or are unmarried are socially disconnected or lonely. Measuring social *dis*connection can be difficult because of the multiple factors involved in defining this construct (Holt-Lunstad et al, 2017).

Social Network Types

Social networks are quantifiable relationships between individuals, families, and groups that are held together by a common interest, goal, or need (Siette et al, 2021). This network helps facilitate engagement in social activities and promotes access to social support. Social networks provide opportunities for social engagement and reinforce meaningful roles within the family and community, which in turn provides a sense of value, belonging, and attachment (WHO, 2015). Social networks can be further defined according to the type and frequency of interaction between members or the overall density of the network (Siette et al, 2021).

Li & Zhang (2015) described four types of social networks and their characteristics:

- Diverse social networks maintain a broad range of supportive relations with family, friends, and neighbors for social participation,
- Friend-focused social networks include frequent interactions with friends or neighbors but fewer interactions with family members,
- Family-focused social networks arrange social life around family and have few active relationships with other types, and
- Restricted social networks have limited engagement in all kinds of social relations.

Social Network Characteristics

The composition of social networks for older adults changes with age. Studies have found that older adults tend to transition from more diverse into less diverse types of social networks over time (Gouveia et al, 2016). This transition over time is due to death of close network members, health problems, children leaving home, and retirement. Network composition may also change as a result of natural disasters and pandemics. Older adults have been particularly susceptible to network loss during the COVID-19 pandemic. While digital media offer ways to connect to family, friends, and others, users must have access to technology and be technologically literate (Polizzi et al, 2020).

A larger, more diverse social network is positively associated with well-being, as older adults with larger networks demonstrate fewer depressive symptoms and higher life satisfaction than those with smaller networks (Gouveia et al, 2016). Diverse social networks might include relationships with a spouse or partner, family, friends, coworkers, or neighbors. Social network diversity is thought to enhance health and activity engagement by providing access to a broader range of support (Cohen, 2021); however, one study found that the diversity of ties is no more important than the number of ties at improving functional health (Brown & Rook, 2022). Smaller network sizes may be particularly damaging for the health and emotional well-being of older minority adults due to racial inequalities that limit social participation throughout the life course (Gauthier et al, 2020).

Social Support

Social support relates to how an individual perceives the availability of help or support from others in their social network (Siette et al, 2021):

- Instrumental support: help with activities of daily living (ADLs) and instrumental activities of daily living (IADLs) such as shopping, getting to appointments, household chores and paying bills
- Informational or appraisal support: advice, problem-solving, or information about particular needs
- Emotional support: love and friendship, understanding, caring, and recognition

Social networks tend to become more centered on close family members (kin) as individuals age, particularly among older women, African Americans, and Latinx (Verdery & Campbell, 2019). Among all racial and ethnic groups, kin ties provide more instrumental social support than do nonkin ties (Verdery & Campbell, 2019). Older people tend to prefer receiving practical, instrumental support from family than friends or neighbors; however, close friends offer welcome emotional support and companionship and have a large effect on morale (Reynolds & Hean Lim, 2013).

Emotional support offered by friends and close family plays an important role in helping older adults maintain their identity and self-esteem and offers an opportunity to share stressful experiences and receive advice (Reynolds & Hean Lim, 2013). Loss of friends can leave the older adult without support, especially those over the age of 80 years, leading to higher risk of depression. In western countries, declining rates of marriage and child-rearing may mean that older adults in the future will have fewer family members to provide social support (Rook & Charles, 2017). Nonkin ties are becoming more important sources of support than family relationships as the predominant family structures evolve in the United States and elsewhere.

Older women seem able to maintain their social support with age through joining community organizations, volunteer work, remaining active in religious communities, and making new friends (Reynolds & Hean Lim, 2013). Older cisgender, heterosexual men are particularly vulnerable to losing social support when they retire, and many depend on female relatives, especially spouses, for support. This may make older men more vulnerable to loneliness, especially if their spouse dies before them. Older adults value providing support to others in their social networks, such as to their adult children and grandchildren (Reynolds & Hean Lim, 2013).

Social Relationship Skills

Social participation is an occupation that involves social interaction with others and supports interdependence (AOTA, 2020). Maintaining social connection is an active process of cultivating social relationships, striving to belong to communities of importance, and connecting to a wider world (Löfgren et al, 2021). Maintaining social relationships might include making telephone calls, using the internet and social media, and having personal meetings. Social relationships change over time and may fade if not based on **reciprocity**. Reciprocity is mutual support rather than just one person caring for another (Löfgren et al, 2021). Active engagement is required to make commitments, take initiative, make plans, and invest time in others, and some older adults may need to accept that some relationships are not built on reciprocity.

Maintaining social connection over time is challenging, and there is a need to develop strategies and adapt to new circumstances, especially when a person's life is challenged in some way (Löfgren et al, 2021). Being able to build and maintain relationships and social networks is related to a range of competencies, such as the ability to form new relationships and behave in ways that are socially acceptable. How a person learns to engage with others is often shaped by their familial, cultural, and generational roots (Van Orden et al, 2020). When faced with declining capacity, older people may find it harder to maintain social networks, which consequently shrink over time (WHO, 2015).

Family Constellations

Family (chosen and/or genetic) is a socially complex concept that is variable, diverse, and dynamic as determined by marriage, birth, friendships, other relationships, death, and/or divorce. The family unit for today's older adult may include intimate relationships, nuclear families (adult children and grandchildren), extended families (nieces, cousins, aunts, siblings), and fictive kin (neighbors and friends who have both instrumental and emotional relationships with the individual) (Suanet et al, 2013). Older adult family members are an important primary resource for caregiving and social support, but these relationships are sometimes associated with ambivalence (Connidis, 2020). Family relationships seem to have protective effects for individuals by decreasing individual stress and positively affecting an individual's psychological and physical health; however, family support may not always promote well-being if the support is perceived as stressful, intrusive, or controlling. In families where conflict has been long-standing or interpersonal relationships have been strained, these difficulties will persist and characterize family relationships in later life as well unless active steps are taken by family members to resolve them.

Population-wide demographic changes create the need to recognize the wide range of different family structures compared with previous generations (Carr & Utz, 2020). Decreasing numbers of adults are growing old with their first and only spouse, while rising numbers are divorcing, remarrying, forming nonmarital romantic unions, or living single by choice (Brown & Wright, 2017). Remarriage and stepfamilies may pose new challenges to the family network as older adults negotiate complex decisions affecting their futures (Waite & Xu, 2015). Many factors shape roles and relationships within later-life families, including race and sex, childhood experiences, relationships with social networks, and factors such as public support for and cultural norms regarding families (Carr, 2019). Diminishing economic opportunities for young people have transformed intergenerational ties, with some grandparents acting as providers rather than recipients of care (Doley et al, 2015). This illustrates the interdependent, interconnected, and dynamic nature of older adults' family ties and shows how these ties are consequential for older adult well-being.

Future generational cohorts will be more ethnically and racially diverse which may influence how older adults interact with family members (Rook & Charles, 2017). Future cohorts will also be better educated than prior generations, and this is related to better health outcomes. These demographic changes in addition to declining rates of marriage and child rearing will impact family functioning (Rook & Charles, 2017). The reduced availability of adult children to provide care may well be counterbalanced by the increased physical health and reduced disability of the generation about to enter later life.

During the occupational therapy process, practitioners can help older adults identify those important family relationships that will help contribute positively to their participation in meaningful occupations. In some cases, practitioners may have to help the older adult redefine family to include those outside of the traditional definition, who can potentially provide much needed social, emotional, and instrumental support. Practitioners may also be in a position to help older adults define, identify, and communicate the types of support needed, and/or if necessary, advocate these needs on behalf of the older adult with family, other healthcare providers, and/or community resources.

Grandparenting

Older adults who are involved in caring for grandchildren report taking great pleasure in their roles and activities (Reynolds & Hean Lim, 2013). For many older adults, the grandparent–grandchild relationship is a source of joy and optimism with some describing the relationships as more enjoyable than raising their own children (Fig. 5-1; Mansson, 2016). Grandparents provide numerous benefits to their grandchildren and other family members including financial resources and instrumental and emotional support. Older adults with greater economic advantages tend to provide sporadic support, such as babysitting, transportation, and recreational activities (Carr & Utz, 2020).

Grandparent–grandchild relationships vary across demographic subgroups with racial and ethnic minorities, with those from lower socioeconomic status taking on more time and labor-intensive roles and often serving as custodial caregivers (Carr & Utz, 2020). Custodial grandparenting carries both costs and benefits (Laughlin, 2013), and although it can promote a sense of well-being, it can be problematic in families already struggling with dysfunction. There is little training for custodial grandparents; occupational therapy intervention may provide mechanisms for building skills.

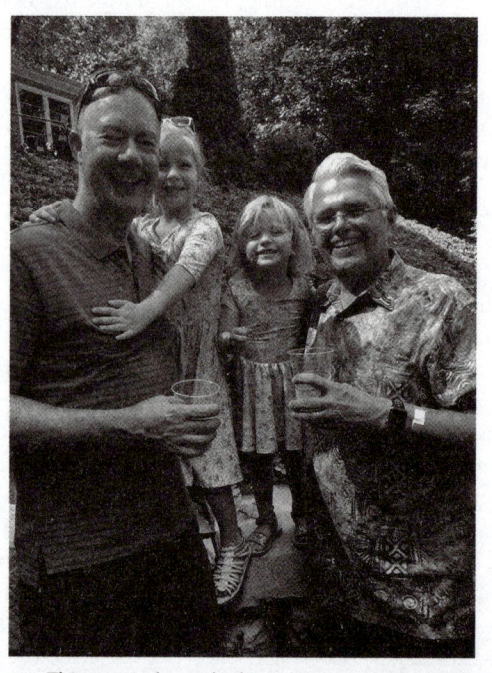

FIGURE 5-1 This married couple demonstrates joy and optimism in grandparent-grandchild relationships while participating in a community event.

Widowhood

One of the most important social relationships in later life is that with one's spouse. At least nine in 10 adults in the United States, age 60 years or older, have been married (Gurrentz & Mayol-Garcia, 2021). Widowhood is more common among older women compared with older men due to differences in life expectancy. Often the greatest challenge in an intimate relationship is the death of a spouse. By their mid 70s, nearly 60% of women and 22% of men are likely to be widowed (Rook & Charles, 2017). Older bereaved spouses are vulnerable to mental health symptoms such as depression, anxiety, grief, and loneliness, though most return to pre-loss levels of emotional well-being within 2 years of the spouse's death (Sasson & Umberson, 2014). The negative aspects of widowhood may be exacerbated by physical and psychological dysfunction (Carr & Utz, 2020). Healthcare providers can recognize that adaptation is the norm rather than the exception and therefore help the widow(er)s explore, grow, and re-engage interpersonally and socially (Carr & Utz, 2020).

CASE STUDY

Occupational Profile

Mr. Johnson is a 68-year-old Caucasian, cisgender man who has had a cerebrovascular accident that has left him with moderate right sided hemiplegia. Mr. Johnson spent 3 days in the hospital and 2 weeks in an inpatient rehabilitation facility and has been discharged home with home healthcare and assistance from his neighbor Sam. His physician has ordered home occupational therapy and physical therapy services for ADLs, home management, transfers, adaptive equipment, and therapeutic exercise. Mr. Johnson lives alone and lost his husband of 12 years unexpectedly about 6 months ago when he died from cancer. Before his stroke, Carter worked from home part-time as an accountant and volunteered weekly at a transitional living center teaching life-skills classes to program participants. Carter's social network includes his coworkers, other volunteers at the transitional living center, a small group of friends, and his neighbor, Sam. Carter does not have a relationship with his family because of their strong negative feelings about his sexual orientation. Carter lives in a small cottage in an urban neighborhood where he used to enjoy tending his vegetable and flower garden. Before his stroke, he was independent with his ADLs, IADLs, transfers, work, and leisure activities.

Identified Problem Areas

The occupational therapist evaluated Mr. Johnson in his home 3 weeks after his stroke. Mr. Johnson is right hand dominant and reports difficulty preparing his meals and cooking, driving, typing on his computer, doing his laundry, gardening, and grocery shopping. His neighbor Sam has been helping him with grocery shopping, laundry, and transportation to his medical appointments, but Mr. Johnson wants to do these activities on his own. He also hopes to return to his paid and volunteer work and leisure activities (gardening). Mr. Johnson appears quiet and tearful when talking about the loss of his husband and his lack of support.

Goals for OT

Mr. Johnson's occupational therapy goals include the following:

- Modified independence with simple meal preparation, cooking, and cleanup,
- Minimal assistance from neighbor, Sam, with carrying groceries into house and putting away in cupboards and refrigerator,
- Modified independence with doing small load of laundry,
- Explore current social network to determine support availability for higher level IADLs,
- Explore adaptive driving community resources,
- Explore adaptive gardening community resources,
- Explore opportunities for adapted work and volunteer activities.

Gender Identity

Gender, in the context of the older adult, typically refers to the characteristics of historical dichotomous categories of cisgender male and cisgender female, which are socially constructed from culture, religion, socioeconomic status, age, and geographic location (WHO, n.d.a.). **Gender identity** plays out in relationship roles and experiences, which are typically formulated from individuals, cultures, and society under a very limited contextual frame of reference. Today, Millennials and adults in Generation Z have a broader frame of reference of gender identity (Table 5-1) versus adults 60 years of age or older (United Nations, 1991).

Sexual and gender minority older adults face historic stigma, discrimination, and social exclusion which negatively impact their sexuality, relationships, health, healthcare access, and use of age-related social services globally (Flatt et al, 2022). It is estimated that 10% of older adults worldwide self-identify as LGBTQIA+ which includes, but is not limited to, lesbian, gay, bisexual, transgender, queer/questioning, intersex, asexual, plus (Fondationemergence, 2018). The 2015 U.S. Transgender Survey from the National Center for Transgender Equality found that the number of aging transgender individuals is increasing and there will be a need for gender-affirming care professionals in geriatric transgender communities specifically trained for their healthcare needs while addressing disparities often associated with this vulnerable population (Gamble et al, 2020; James et al, 2016). How an individual presents their gender identity (e.g., use of preferred **pronouns**) in parallel to masculine or feminine sociocultural gender roles in relationships,

TABLE 5-1 ■ Gender Identity

TERMINOLOGY	DESCRIPTION
Cisgender (cis)	A person whose gender identity is consistent in a traditional sense with their sex assigned at birth; for example, a person assigned female sex at birth whose gender identity is woman/female. The term cisgender comes from the Latin prefix cis, meaning "on the same side of."
Transgender	An umbrella term for people whose gender identity and/or expression is different from cultural expectations based on the sex they were assigned at birth. Being transgender does not imply any specific sexual orientation. Therefore, transgender people may identify as straight, gay, lesbian, bisexual, etc.
Sex	A person's biological status and is typically assigned at birth, usually on the basis of external anatomy. Sex is typically categorized as male, female, or intersex.
Nonbinary, gender nonconforming, or gender diverse	Terms that can be used by people who do not describe themselves or their genders as fitting into the categories of man or woman. A range of terms are used to refer to these experiences.
Intersex	An umbrella term used to describe people with differences in reproductive anatomy, chromosomes or hormones that don't fit typical definitions of male and female. Being intersex is not the same as being nonbinary or transgender, which are terms typically related to gender identity.
Gender	A social construct of norms, behaviours, and roles that varies between societies and over time. Gender is often categorized as male, female, or nonbinary.
Assigned female at birth/ assigned male at birth	Refers to the sex that is assigned to an infant, most often based on the infant's anatomical and other biological characteristics. Commonly abbreviated as AFAB (assigned female at birth) or AMAB (assigned male at birth).

Sources: Wamsley, 2021; The Trevor Project, 2021.

inequalities are present in society and manifest in different ways, thereby affecting those relationships, home life, familial attitudes, power, autonomy, self-esteem, workplace stressors, health outcomes, and mental health (Kerr et al, 2021).

Even though cisgender females tend to have a more positive perspective on the aging process compared with males, women in heterosexual relationships are often burdened with taking charge of healthy eating, meal planning, and healthcare for their male partners ensuring that their partners apply healthy lifestyle habits (Schladitz et al, 2022). These greater domestic responsibilities can negatively influence a woman's life satisfaction if they reduce time for other desired activities such as out-of-home mobility (e.g., walking, shopping, socializing), which are associated with more satisfaction in an older adult woman's life (Isaacson et al, 2020).

On the other hand, older cisgender, partnered heterosexual males fall into paternalistic sociocultural masculine role norms whereby occupation, a sense of duty to support the family, mental toughness, stoicism, self-sufficiency (outside of household tasks), and a spectrum of risky health behaviors take center stage (McCreary et al, 2020). These masculine gender scripts promote the "longevity gap" between cisgender men and women. Acting on perceived gender influences, cisgender men do not seek support services (including with family and friends) when they are experiencing health problems, which perpetuates negative health outcomes in the context of gender identity stigmas affecting treatment (e.g., failure to self-disclose symptoms, symptom minimization, or premature ending of treatment) (Milner et al, 2018). Males view doctor-seeking behavior as necessary only when severe illness or physical health severity is accompanied by significant pain (Novak et al, 2019). Essentially, traditional masculine role norms of cisgender men tend to ignore and downplay their aging symptoms as they choose to put family financial needs above their own health (Courtenay, 2011).

Aging Concerns of LGBTQIA+ Adults

For older, same-gendered partnered adults, sociocultural gender roles play less of a part in domestic household tasks, such as food roles and eating behaviors, as the roles tend to be carried out by the person designated for the task, such as the health or cooking expert (Peak et al, 2021). Evidence suggests that the stereotypical gender roles of performing household labor are shared whether the person in a relationship identifies as widow, transgender, intersex, nonbinary, gender non-conforming, or gender diverse (Peak et al, 2021).

Notably, older adults may shy away from explicitly discussing their gender identity due to a lack of familiarization of today's vocabulary or fear after a lifetime of oppression (Hurd et al, 2022). It is important to recognize their gender transformation experience as a sentinel life event related to adversity and resilience that has shaped their social networks, relationships, health, and well-being (Fredriksen-Goldsen et al, 2017). Though older gender diverse individuals may experience higher levels of anxiety and depression, they may be more adept at managing certain elements of aging given their resilience experience (Inventor et al, 2022). Throughout the literature, emphasis is placed on the importance of acknowledging diverse genders and empathizing with personal histories (Stinchcombe et al, 2021). Promoting Best

Practice 5-1 discusses occupational therapy interventions with LGBTQIA+ older adults.

PROMOTING BEST PRACTICE 5-1
Implications for Intervention with LGBTQIA+ Individuals

Occupational therapy students need to prepare to address the unique needs of older transgender, intersex, non-binary, gender non-conforming, or gender diverse individuals. Immersion clinicals, case studies, and didactic lectures encourage student self-exploration and reflection of implicit biases regarding sociocultural gender roles and gender identities (Simon et al, 2021). As both gender- and age-related discrimination are significantly associated with depression, occupational therapy practitioners can develop person-centered plans of care that foster community and social engagement. To do this, practitioners can help older LGBTQIA+ adults explore and develop multidimensional and multifunctional social support networks by facilitating access to creative social experiences such as activism or linking/pairing aging transgender adults with young transgender adults (e.g., "big" and "little" brothers or sisters) (August et al, 2022; White Hughto & Reisner, 2018).

Isolation and Touch

In the era of the COVID-19 pandemic, the world experienced deprivation in socialization and interpersonal touch correlating to declines in psychological wellbeing (von Mohr et al, 2021). The consequences of a lack of quality, supportive social connections, and nonsexual, affectionate touch for older adults can be social isolation and loneliness. Isolation and loneliness increase an older adult's risk for mortality, cardiovascular disease, stroke, diabetes, cognitive decline, depression, anxiety, suicide, and poor quality of life (Kuiper et al, 2015). Life transitions such as the loss of a spouse or friend, retirement, or loss of function put older adults at greater risk for isolation and loneliness and the COVID-19 pandemic and social distancing measures have exacerbated this problem (WHO, 2021).

Isolation

Social isolation is the objective lack or limited extent of social connections with others (Donovan & Blazer, 2020). An older adult who has a lack of social contact, participation in social activities, communication, or confidants may develop social isolation over time (Suragarn et al, 2021). Loneliness is a subjective experience, regardless of one's objective social network size. It is characterized by dissatisfaction with the quantity and quality of one's social life, feelings of social isolation, disconnectedness, and not belonging (Suragarn et al, 2021). Estimating the prevalence of social isolation and loneliness in a population can be difficult because there is no standard, internationally used valid measure (WHO, 2021).

Multiple factors can put people at risk of social isolation and loneliness, and healthcare providers are in a unique position to identify those most at risk and provide intervention (WHO, 2021).

According to the WHO (2021), the first step in combating social isolation and loneliness in the older adult population is identifying those affected and providing connection to community resources. Validated scales can be used to assess older adults at risk of social isolation and loneliness who might benefit from intervention. The Lubben Social Network Scale-6 (Lubben et al, 2006) and the Three-Item Loneliness Scale (Hughes et al, 2004) were developed for use in the older adult population and have been used extensively in research and clinical settings.

Individual level interventions include maintaining and improving social relationships as well as changing how one thinks and feels about their current relationships (WHO, 2021). Healthcare providers can facilitate older adults in developing new relationships by exploring opportunities to make more contributions to the community through leisure and volunteer occupations. Promising interventions are client-centered and may include social skills training, peer support, social activity groups, befriending services, cognitive behavioral techniques, mindfulness training, and the use of antidepressants (WHO, 2021). Occupational therapy practitioners can promote social participation with older adults by using health promotion strategies to maintain functional capability, create supportive environments, and adapt activities (Turcotte et al, 2018).

Digital technology (smart phones, internet, and social media) interventions are widely used and met social connection needs for some older adults during the COVID-19 pandemic. Digital interventions for older adults could include training in the use of the internet and computers, providing support for video communication, creating or joining online discussion groups, telephone befriending, participating in social networking sites, and providing virtual companions (WHO, 2021).

Touch

A consequence of social isolation, loneliness, and social distancing is touch deprivation, or skin hunger. Nonsexual and affectionate physical touch is a form of communication that is a universal and essential component of showing care, affection, and intimacy in social contexts. Touch deprivation is a longing to touch or be touched in a social way (Lee & Cichy, 2020). The amount of touch a person desires is personal, but people who are more likely to feel lonely are more likely to say they are deprived of touch (Lee & Cichy, 2020).

Physical touch may include hugging, being held, greeting with a pat on the back, or other close physical contact is linked to multiple physiological benefits such as lower blood pressure, lower heart rate, lower levels of inflammation, and higher oxytocin levels (Field, 2014). Moreover, a combination of high physical touch and high emotional/instrumental support can be protective against high blood pressure (Lee & Cichy, 2020). Physical touch from people who are not close family or friends also may be beneficial, as evidenced by the positive effect of physical touch from nurses on patients' improved sleep, blood pressure, respiratory rate, and pain (Papathanassoglou & Mpouzika, 2012). Occupational therapy practitioners could encourage positive physical touch among older adult household members to protect the older adult's health, stress levels, and well-being. Self-applied touch to one's palm of the hand has been linked to positive signals in the brain (Field, 2014), which may be helpful for older adults living alone who do not have access to physical touch from others.

Sexuality

Many myths, stereotypes, and misconceptions exist surrounding sexuality and aging. According to the WHO, adult sexuality contributes to the overall health and well-being of an individual and/or couple as long as the engagement is safe and free of coercion, discrimination, and violence (WHO, n.d.b). Although aging may bring about physiological changes (e.g., sexual dysfunction, body dysphoria, aging stigmas) and psychological complications (e.g., cognitive impairment, capacity to consent, inappropriate sexual behavior) due to varying differential diagnoses, sexuality remains an integral component to older adult quality of life (Srinivasan et al, 2019).

Humans are sexual beings, and most adults have a desire for some level of sexuality expression in late adulthood, whether it is partnered or solo (Forbes et al, 2017). Cismaru-Inescu et al (2022) reported that 79% of older adults were either sexually active or experienced physical tenderness in the past 12 months. It is important to have an open mind and a positive sexual attitude toward solo or partnered sexual experiences in later life (Fileborn et al, 2017). Solo sexual satisfaction is a common substitute for intercourse among contemporary older populations (Fileborn et al, 2017). Elderly partnered adults were more likely to resort to solo sexual satisfaction if the frequency of sexual events and orgasm satisfaction were not meeting their needs (Fileborn et al, 2017).

Though sexuality may ebb with age, a substantial number of cisgender women rate the desire for sexuality important, regardless of the old-age belief that all women lose interest in sex as they age (Thomas et al, 2019). According to Thomas et al, there are three distinct categories in a cisgender woman's feelings around sexuality as they get older: valued less, more important, or remained the same. For example, if a cisgender woman was having satisfying sex in her 40s, she is more likely to continue to highly value sex in her 50s and 60s (Thomas et al, 2019). Partnered older cisgender women are more likely to be sexually active than women without a partner, regardless of relationship history (e.g., divorced, separated, unmarried) or partner loss (Li et al, 2022). Older transgender women experience poorer sexual health (partnered or not) with aging due to genital and body dysphoria, less sexual desire, avoidance of sexual intercourse, and decreasing quality of life which negatively affect partner relations more than men (cisgender or transgender) (Holmberg et al, 2019).

For cisgender men (regardless of sexuality), 85% of those age 60 to 69 years, 60% of those age 70 to 79 years, and 32% of those over 80 years of age are sexually active (Smith et al, 2019). Among men, performance anxiety, erectile difficulties, or orgasm timing issues were the most highlighted difficulties showing a clear gradient with age (Richters et al, 2022). Older transgender men most likely have not undergone surgery to affirm their masculine identity but have received hormone replacement therapy (HRT) in the form of testosterone to suppress female secondary sex characteristics (Unger, 2016). Using implanted devices, an erection prosthesis, or artificial penis is believed to contribute to sexual satisfaction in transmasculine people, partnered or not, and should be considered when discussing ADLs (Morrison et al, 2016).

Older adults in same-gendered relationships reported high levels of relationship satisfaction whereby relationship satisfaction was positively correlated with sexual satisfaction (Fleishman et al, 2020). All things considered, multifactorial sexuality constructs exist with sexuality, aging, and gender; thus, occupational therapy practitioners can facilitate ameliorating barriers to healthy sexual expression, which can lead to an improved quality of life for all older adults and their loved ones (Srinivasan et al, 2019).

Age Related Changes

Perimenopause, menopause, chronic disease management, and health decline complicate sexuality for cisgender women entering middle and old age. Female sexual dysfunction (FSD) is a global term used to encompass a variety of issues including body alterations (dysphoria), intimacy avoidance (possibly due to a partner loss), depersonalization or lack of love with sex, lack of interest in sex (desire), and a reduced response to sexual activity (arousal) and/or reaching orgasm (American College of Obstetricians and Gynecologists [ACOG], 2020). According to ACOG, sexually active older people with a cervix experience hormonal changes (lowered levels of estrogen hormones), depression, anxiety, thyroid disorders, problems with their uterus, vaginal dryness, and pain with sex, which may affect sexual activities (ACOG, 2020). Many of the FSD issues and physiological changes can be addressed by using lubricants for vaginal dryness, conversing with a partner about aging changes that are occurring, exploring positions that are more pleasurable, trying non-sexual but sensual activities like massage, seeking cognitive behavioral therapy, and/or taking pain-relieving steps before sex (e.g., emptying the bladder, using over-the-counter pain reliever, taking a warm bath) (ACOG, 2020).

Cisgender male sexual dysfunction may include ejaculation disorders, erectile dysfunction, and hormone changes (lowered levels of testosterone). These, along with chronic health problems inhibit sexual desire and function (Cleveland Clinic, n.d.). Age-related erectile dysfunction (ARED) in cisgender men is the inability to achieve and/or maintain a penile erection during a sex act due to arterial insufficiency and high venous outflow (Antonio et al, 2022). The cause of ARED may be due to physiological (vascular problems affecting blood flow to the penis), hormonal, and psychogenic (anxiety and depression) factors, all of which are not fully understood (Antonio et al, 2022). Some cisgender men can seek to restore their sexual function by using phosphodiesterase inhibitors (sildenafil [Viagra, Pfizer], vardenafil [Levitra and Staxyn, Bayer/GlaxoSmithKline]), testosterone therapy, and cognitive behavioral therapy and discussing with their partner about mismatched sex drives. See Table 5-2 for a discussion of age-related changes in sexual response by gender identity.

Metabolic Changes

Atherosclerotic cardiovascular disease (ASCVD) remains the greatest reason for cognitive and physical impairment, making sexuality expression more difficult in older adults (Grundy et al, 2019). Lifestyle risk factors (e.g., smoking) in the older adult increase ASCVD risk as do chronic obstructive pulmonary disease) leading to hypoxemia, excessive stress or fatigue, limitation of sexual activity, and ARED (Turan et al, 2016). Sex hormones may also both negatively and positively affect aging and sexuality. The use of exogenous sex hormones (oral or transdermal) appears to have some positive effects on sexuality when an individual presents with hypogonadism (gonad deficiency), which helps with sexual function and libido; however, some long-term negative effects may occur in older age, such as increased risk of venous thromboembolism (VTE), thereby heightening adverse cardiovascular events (Slack & Safer, 2021). Prolonged HRT in aging transgender individuals may result in more negative effects, such as liver failure, ASCVD, VTE, and cognitive disorders, including dementia, causing further distress in an already vulnerable population (Gamble et al, 2020).

Musculoskeletal Changes

Older adults with arthritis or rheumatoid arthritis (RA) may experience joint pain, stiffness, fatigue, and limited mobility which interfere with sexual activity. Inflammatory arthritis negatively affects sexual function for all genders, causing stress in relationships (Restoux et al, 2020). Moreover, cisgender women with RA had significantly higher levels of sexual dysfunction versus cisgender men with RA (Zhao et al, 2018).

Neuromuscular Changes

Cerebrovascular diseases (e.g., stroke) may result in sexual dysfunction due to fundamental alterations (e.g., incontinence, paralysis, dysphagia) and can sometimes lead to a decrease in sexual activity. McGrath et al (2019) suggest that stroke survivors and their partners struggle to communicate about sexuality even though sexual intimacy remains important. It is important to address this topic during rehabilitation in order to support the patient and their partner on ways to adapt and modify sexual experiences to adjust to the survivor's changing body.

Neuromotor Changes

Non-motor and motor disease issues can affect sexual function for those diagnosed with Parkinson's disease (PD) across all stages and genders. Between 43% and 79% of men with PD report impaired sexual function due to erectile dysfunction, premature ejaculation, orgasm difficulties, and decreased libido, while 47% to 84% of women with PD report decreased libido and orgasm difficulties (Santa Rosa Malcher et al, 2021); motor symptoms, including tremor, rigidity, and immobility in bed, may cause difficulty during intimate activities such as touching and kissing. Depression affects up to 50% of patients with PD and is associated

TABLE 5-2 ■ Age-Related Changes in Sexual Response by Gender Identity

	CISGENDER FEMALE	CISGENDER MALE	TRANSGENDER/GENDER DIVERSE FEMALE	TRANSGENDER/GENDER DIVERSE MALE
Arousal	Delayed lubrication Decreased Bartholin gland secretion Reduced vaginal expansion Decreased elevation of the uterus	Delayed and less firm erection Longer interval to ejaculation Less testicular elevation	Gender dysphoria Genital and body dysphoria Avoidance of sexual intercourse (with gonads assigned male at birth and no vaginoplasty intervention) Biopsychosocial barriers	Gender dysphoria Genital and body dysphoria Vulvar pain (with gonads assigned female at birth and no phalloplasty) Dyspareunia Biopsychosocial barriers
Orgasm	Fewer orgasmic contractions	Shorter ejaculation time	Fewer orgasms	Fewer orgasms
Postorgasm	No dilation of cervix Longer refraction period	Rapid loss of erection	Longer refraction period	Longer refraction period

Sources: Abern et al, 2022; Schardein & Nikolavsky, 2021; and Pavanello Decaro et al, 2021.

with sexual dissatisfaction (Haktanir, 2022). Pain (including pelvic pain for men and women) and loss of sensation may also limit ability to enjoy sexual activities. Some medications prescribed to control PD symptoms cause sexual dysfunction and may need to be re-evaluated. Sex counseling or therapy would be beneficial in addition to managing pain, fatigue, depression, and medication monitoring (Bronner & Vodusek, 2011).

Cognitive Behavioral Changes

Psychiatric illnesses, especially major depression and dementia, are frequently associated with sexual dysfunction in late life. Age-specific depression, anxiety, and psychosocial stresses related to fear of self-injury or death because of a new medical condition (e.g., myocardial infarction, dementia), a newly acquired disability, the loss of a partner, or the death of loved ones may accelerate and negatively affect positive psychological factors and sexuality (Bell et al, 2022). When depression occurs, the loss of interest in personal appearance and hygiene may perpetuate a decreased libido, which could lead to the end of an individual's desire for sexual activity.

Alzheimer disease and related dementias (ADRD) can have a profound effect on sexuality in older adults. Sometimes sexual desire in people with ADRD increases and can result in unreasonable and exhausting demands, often at odd times, in inappropriate places, or with inappropriate people. Other individuals with ADRD may lose interest in a physical relationship and become withdrawn (Mahieu & Gastmans, 2015).

Medications

Sexual dysfunction in older adulthood is a common side effect of many classes of medication (Neel, n.d.). Over 500 prescription medicines are known to cause at least occasional problems with sexual desire and function for all sexualities and genders. Solomon et al. (2022) found a robust relationship between increasing medication use and decreasing physical function, including sexual function, across all racial and ethnic groups, in women more than men. Sometimes the problem is not with a single medication but may be a reaction to two or more medications taken in combination. Thus, pharmaceutical treatment approaches to combat disease layered with underlying physiological changes may prevent resumption or terminate sexual activity which negatively affects sexual relationships (Nowosielski, 2022).

Living Environment Considerations

Sexual expression in later life can be difficult from a lived environment perspective. Partner availability, cultural differences toward engagement in sexuality, housing arrangements, believing societal stereotypes and taboos surrounding older adult engagement in sexual or tender physical experiences impact sexual expression (Freak-Poli, 2020). After the death of a longtime spouse, partner, or companion, finding new relationships with expectations of sexual engagement can be challenging and intimidating (Sinković & Towler, 2019). The surviving partner may engage in a new relationship explicitly for sexual activity or have a more flexible definition of *relationship* (e.g., dating, living-apart-together, or cohabitation) than before the death of their partner (Sevcikova et al, 2021). Risky sexual behaviors are more prevalent in older adults who may feel that safe sex practices (e.g., condoms, dental dams) are unnecessary. These risky behaviors have caused a significant increase in sexually transmitted infections and HIV among all older adult groups, especially older cisgender men who have sex with men (Pilowsky & Wu, 2015).

The limited opportunities for sexual expression are even more pronounced in long term care (LTC) facilities (i.e., independent living facilities, assisted living communities, nursing homes, or continuing care retirement communities). LTC providers have cited concerns that patients might physically hurt themselves during sex or that staff do not see residents as sexually active beings and actively discourage sexual expression, especially for LGBTQIA+ adults (Dickson et al, 2022). Heteronormativity in LTCs is a concern of older LGBTQIA+ adults, as inherent biases exist among LTC staff who provide maltreatment, overtly express homophobic comments, or subtly create a toxic culture of care (Schwinn & Dinkel, 2015).

Consent is a critical component of a healthy sexual relationship, and it includes three legal criteria: sexual knowledge, intelligence, and voluntariness (Esmail & Concannon, 2022). Older adults with cognitive disability may not be able to give consent. Healthcare providers have to consider legal, clinical, and ethical issues to reduce the risk of unhealthy or harmful sexual behaviors. Healthcare providers should use a holistic, person-centered approach to determine an older adult's functional capacity when it comes to consenting to sexual activity. Healthcare providers can provide education on sexual knowledge, sexual consent, advanced directives, and recognizing abusive situations, which may facilitate an older adult's ability to participate in a healthy intimate relationship (Esmail & Concannon, 2022).

Implications for Occupational Therapy Practitioners

In a study that examined the beliefs, knowledge, and comfort levels of Canadian occupational therapists with respect to addressing clients' sexual health, a number of barriers and challenges were identified that affect a practitioner's ability to attend to a client's sexuality (Young et al, 2019). Respondents in this study believed that sexuality is a relevant occupation and an important part of a client's overall health, yet there was a gap between this belief and actual practice. Practitioners cited a lack of knowledge, skills, and competence that limited their ability to assess and treat their client's sexual health needs (Young et al, 2019).

Training that is specific to older adults in different practice settings may be necessary for practitioners to be prepared to address their client's needs in a meaningful way (Young et al, 2019). See Promoting Best Practice 5-2 for a communication model.

PROMOTING BEST PRACTICE 5-2
Plissit and Ex-Plissit Communication

The PLISSIT and Ex-PLISSIT models can be used by healthcare professionals to guide interventions related to client sexuality and sexual health needs (Taylor & Davis, 2006; Annon, 1976). The PLISSIT model is an acronym that signifies four levels of intervention: permission, limited information, specific suggestions, and intensive therapy (Annon, 1976; Taylor & Davis, 2006):

- **Permission:** providing affirmation to clients that their concerns with sexuality are appropriate and can be addressed by a healthcare professional. Permission can be provided as a handout on the role of occupational therapy and sexuality, an explicit question during the occupational therapy evaluation, or a mention of sexuality while explaining the role of occupational therapy.
- **Limited information:** information related to the effect of illness on sexuality and sexual function. Most clients will be curious about the changes to their bodies and when, if ever, they will be able to resume normal sexual activities.
- **Specific suggestions:** requires a problem-solving approach to address a particular issue. Specific suggestions need to be tailored to address specific needs and will require further assessment into the nature of the particular problem.
- **Intensive therapy:** most advanced stage of the PLISSIT model. Most occupational therapy practitioners will not have an adequate amount of training to provide intensive training so clients should be referred to other professionals when appropriate, such as neuropsychologists, sex therapists, or psychosexual counselors.

Occupational therapy sexuality interventions for older adults could include the following:

- Promote safe sex practices and use of condoms at an assisted living facility,
- Improve individual client factors that are required to engage in sexual activity or increase satisfaction, e.g., Increase endurance needed to maximize sexual participation,
- Suggest lubrication to reverse the adverse effects of vaginal dryness,
- Recommend positioning devices to maximize safety and promote independence with maintaining positions,
- Promote energy conservation techniques to compensate for fatigue,
- Provide information on using personal pleasure devices to engage in self-pleasure, and
- Recommend modified positions to compensate for activity limitations or restrictions and promoting intimacy in place of sexual intercourse,

- Sexuality is an ADL and very important to an older adult's quality of life. Occupational therapy practitioners can address sexuality issues and, through education and training, increase their comfort and confidence addressing this area in practice (Mohammed, 2017).

CASE STUDY (CONTINUED)
Intervention Plan

To explore social support available in Mr. Johnson's current social network, the occupational therapy practitioner will ask him to list his current close ties and the nature of their relationship. The occupational therapy practitioner will work with Mr. Johnson to identify support resources in his social network and ways that he can ask for assistance with higher level IADLS.

Discharge Status

Mr. Johnson was discharged from home health care to outpatient therapy to continue to work on motor function, work, volunteer, leisure, and driving activities.

Questions

1. How would you categorize Mr. Johnson's social relationships? Does Mr. Johnson have adequate social support to help him live independently in his community? How can an occupational therapist help Mr. Johnson foster current relationships and develop new relationships?
2. What factors in Mr. Johnson's case may contribute to his risk for developing loneliness, social isolation, and/or touch deprivation?

Answers

1. We could say that Mr. Johnson has a very limited set of family relationships due to his immediate and extended families' beliefs about his sexuality. Mr. Johnson does appear to have a close relationship with his neighbor, and we may be able to classify this family relationship as fictive kin. Mr. Johnson appears to have relationships with his coworkers and volunteer community, and the occupational therapist can help Mr. Johnson continue to participate in activities with these important sources of social support.
2. Mr. Johnson's recent change in physical functioning and the loss of his husband may contribute to his risk for loneliness and social isolation. Mr. Johnson would benefit from skilled occupational therapy to help him foster his current relationships and allow him to participate in valued activities.

SUMMARY

This chapter explored the diverse, complex, and varied forms of social networks, relationships, gender identity, and sexuality of older adults. Although maintaining functional capacity and performance are central to successful aging, these relational constructs affect an individual's ability to do so (WHO, 2015). The social lives of older adults are often misunderstood and tumultuous with changing environments, societal norms, and family units. Yet, the cornerstones of healthy aging are cemented in a sense of purpose, positive relationships, and participation in life through engagement in occupation (AOTA, 2020). Occupational therapy practitioners should derive an empathetic connection with how older adults may struggle with sexuality, intimacy, loneliness, and relationships and attempt to bridge the gap by recognizing each individual's relevant historical circumstances to foster thriving while aging.

Critical Thinking Questions

1. For older adults, what occupational and emotional needs are addressed through social and family interactions?
2. What are some ways that older adults who do not have blood relatives meet family-focused occupational needs?

REFERENCES

Abern, L., Maguire, K., Cook, J., & Carugno, J. (2022). Prevalence of vulvar pain and dyspareunia in trans masculine individuals. *LGBT Health, 9*(3), 194–198. https://doi.org/10.1089/lgbt.2020.0357

American College of Obstetrics and Gynecologists (ACOG). (2020, October). *Your sexual health.* https://www.acog.org/womens-health/faqs/your-sexual-health

American Occupational Therapy Association. (2020). Occupational therapy practice framework: Domain and process (4th ed.). *American Journal of Occupational Therapy, 74*(Suppl. 2), 7412410010. https://doi.org/10.5014/ajot.2020.74S2001

American Psychological Association. (n.d.a). *APA dictionary of psychology.* https://dictionary.apa.org/ambivalence

American Psychological Association. (n.d.b). *APA dictionary of psychology.* https://dictionary.apa.org/reciprocity

Annon, J. (1976). The PLISSIT model: A proposed conceptual scheme for the behavioral treatment of sexual problems, *Journal of Sex Education Therapy, 2*(1), 1–15.

Antonio, L., Wu, F. C. W., Moors, H., Matheï, C., Huhtaniemi, I. T., Rastrelli, G., Dejaeger, M., O'Neill, T. W., Pye, S. R., Forti, G., Maggi, M., Casanueva, F. F., Slowikowska-Hilczer, J., Punab, M., Tournoy, J., & Vanderschueren, D. (2022). Erectile dysfunction predicts mortality in middle-aged and older men independent of their sex steroid status. *Age and Ageing, 51*(4), afac094. https://doi.org/10.1093/ageing/afac094

August, K. J., Novak, J. R., Peak, T., Gast, J., & Miyairi, M. (2022). Examining foodwork and eating behaviors among heterosexual and gay male couples. *Appetite, 172,* 105953. https://doi.org/10.1016/j.appet.2022.105953

Bell, G., Singham, T., Saunders, R., John, A., & Stott, J. (2022). Positive psychological constructs and association with reduced risk of mild cognitive impairment and dementia in older adults: A systematic review and meta-analysis. *Ageing Research Reviews, 77,* 101594. https://doi.org/10.1016/j.arr.2022.101594

Bronner, G., Royter, V., Korczyn, A. D., & Giladi, N. (2004). Sexual dysfunction in Parkinson's disease. *Journal of Sex & Marital Therapy, 30*(2), 95–105. https://doi.org/10.1080/00926230490258893

Bronner, G., & Vodušek, D. B. (2011). Management of sexual dysfunction in Parkinson's disease. *Therapeutic Advances in Neurological Disorders, 4,* 375–383. DOI:10.1177/1756285611411504

Brown, C., & Rook, K. (2022). Does diversity of social ties really matter more for health and leisure activity than number of social ties? Evidence from later adulthood. *Journal of Aging and Health,* 8982643211066652. https://doi.org/10.1177/08982643211066652

Brown, S. L., & Wright, M. R. (2017). Marriage, cohabitation, and divorce in later life. *Innovation in Aging, 1*(2), 1–11. https://doi.org/10.1093/geroni/igx015

Carr, D. (2019). *Golden years? Social inequality in later life.* Russell Sage Foundation.

Carr, D. & Utz, R. L. (2020). Families in later life: A decade in review. *Journal of Marriage and Family, 82*(1), 346–363. https://doi.org/10.1111/jomf.12609

Cismaru-Inescu, A., Hahaut, B., Adam, S., Nobels, A., Beaulieu, M., Vandeviver, C., Keygnaert, I., & Nisen, L. (2022). Sexual activity and physical tenderness in older adults: Prevalence and associated characteristics from a Belgian study. *Journal of Sexual Medicine, 19*(4), 569–580. https://doi.org/10.1016/j.jsxm.2022.01.516

Cleveland Clinic. (n.d.). *Sexual dysfunction in males.* https://my.clevelandclinic.org/health/diseases/9122-sexual-dysfunction-in-males

Cohen, S. (2021). Psychosocial vulnerabilities to upper respiratory infectious illness: Implications for susceptibility to Coronavirus Disease 2019 (COVID-19). *Perspectives on Psychological Science, 16*(1), 161–174. https://doi.org/10.1177/1745691620942516

Connidis, I. (2020). Who counts as family later in life? Following theoretical leads. *Journal of Family Theory & Review, 12*(2), 164–179. https://doi.org/10.1111/jftr.12367

Courtenay, W. H. (2011). *Dying to be men: psychosocial, environmental, and biobehavioral directions in promoting the health of men and boys.* Routledge.

Dickson, L., Bunting S., Nanna A., Taylor M., Spencer M., & Hein L. (2022). Older lesbian, gay, bisexual, transgender, and queer adults' experiences with discrimination and impacts on expectations for long-term care: Results of a survey in the southern United States. *Journal of Applied Gerontology, 41*(3), 650–660. https://doi.org/10.1177/07334648211048189

Doley, R., Bell, R., Watt, B., & Simpson, H. (2015). Grandparents raising grandchildren: Investigating factors associated with distress among custodial grandparent. *Journal of Family Studies, 21*(2), 101–119. https://doi.org/10.1080/13229400.2015.1015215

Donovan, N. J. & Blazer, D. (2020) Social isolation and loneliness in older adults: Review and commentary of a National Academies report. *American Journal of Geriatric Psychiatry, 28*(12), 1233–1244. https://doi.org/10.1016/j.jagp.2020.08.005

Esmail, S. & Concannon, B. (2022). Approaches to determine and manage sexual consent abilities for people with cognitive disabilities: Systematic review. *Interactive Journal Of Medical Research, 11*(1), e28137. https://doi.org/10.2196/28137

Field, T. (2014). *Touch (2nd ed).* MIT Press.

Fileborn, B., Hinchliff, S., Lyons, A., Heywood, W., Minichiello, V., Brown, G., Malta, S., Barrett, C., & Crameri, P. (2017). The importance of sex and the meaning of sex and sexual pleasure for men aged 60 and older who engage in heterosexual relationships: Findings from a qualitative interview study. *Archives of Sexual Behavior, 46*(7), 2097–2110. https://doi.org/10.1007/s10508-016-0918-9

Flatt, J. D., Cicero, E. C., Kittle, K. R., Brennan-Ing, M., Anderson, J. G., Wharton, W., & Hughes, T. L. (2022). Advancing gerontological health research with sexual and gender minorities across the globe. *Journal of Gerontological Nursing, 48*(4), 13–20. https://doi.org/10.3928/00989134-20220304-03

Fleishman, J. M., Crane, B., & Koch, P. B. (2020). Correlates and predictors of sexual satisfaction for older adults in same-sex relationships. *Journal of Homosexuality, 67*(14), 1974–1998. https://doi.org/10.1080/00918369.2019.1618647

Fondationémergence. (2018). *Assurer la bientraitance des personnes aînées lesbiennes, gaies, bisexuelles et trans: Guide d'information* [Ensuring the well-treatment of lesbian, gay, bisexual and trans seniors: Information guide]. https://e06ef624-6c85-4f0d-961fa0bffcd58705.filesusr.com/ugd/cdd9d7_0b76e7afa1ed4bd4af60b0c947727f24.pdf

Forbes, M. K., Eaton, N. R., & Krueger, R. F. (2017). Sexual quality of life and aging: A prospective study of a nationally representative sample. *Journal of Sex Research, 54*, 137–148. https://doi.org/10.1080/00224499.2016.1233315

Freak-Poli, R. (2020). It's not age that prevents sexual activity later in life. *Australasian Journal on Ageing, 39 Suppl 1*(Suppl 1), 22–29. https://doi.org/10.1111/ajag.12774

Fredriksen-Goldsen, K. I., Bryan, A. E., Jen, S., Goldsen, J., Kim, H. J., & Muraco, A. (2017). The unfolding of LGBT lives: Key events associated with health and well-being in later life. *The Gerontologist, 57*(suppl 1), S15–S29. https://doi.org/10.1093/geront/gnw185

Gamble, R. M., Taylor, S. S., Huggins, A. D., & Ehrenfeld, J. M. (2020). Trans-specific Geriatric Health Assessment (TGHA): An inclusive clinical guideline for the geriatric transgender patient in a primary care setting. *Maturitas, 132*, 70–75. https://doi.org/10.1016/j.maturitas.2019.12.005

Gauthier, G. R., Smith, J. A., García, C., Garcia, M. A., & Thomas, P. A. (2020). Exacerbating inequalities: Social networks, racial/ethnic disparities, and the COVID-19 pandemic in the United States. *The Journals of Gerontology. Series B, Psychological Sciences and Social Sciences, 76*(3), e88–e92. https://doi.org/10.1093/geronb/gbaa117

Gouveia, O. M. R., Matos, A. D., & Schouten, M. J. (2016). Social networks and quality of life of elderly persons: A review and critical analysis of literature. *Revista Brasileira de Geriatria e Gerontologia, 19*(6), 1030–1040. https://doi.org/10.1590/1981-22562016019.160017

Grundy, S. M., Stone, N. J., Bailey, A. L., Beam, C., Birtcher, K. K., Blumenthal, R. S., Braun, L. T., de Ferranti, S., Faiella-Tommasino, J., Forman, D. E., Goldberg, R., Heidenreich, P. A., Hlatky, M. A., Jones, D. W., Lloyd-Jones, D., Lopez-Pajares, N., Ndumele, C. E., Orringer, C. E., Peralta, C. A., Saseen, J. J., ... Yeboah, J. (2019). 2018 AHA/ACC/AACVPR/AAPA/ABC/ACPM/ADA/AGS/APhA/ASPC/NLA/PCNA guideline on the management of blood cholesterol: A report of the American College of Cardiology/American Heart Association Task Force on Clinical Practice Guidelines. *Circulation, 139*(25), e1082–e1143. https://doi.org/10.1161/CIR.0000000000000625

Gurrentz, B., & Mayol-Garcia, Y. (2021, April 22). *Marriage, divorce, widowhood remain prevalent among older populations.* https://www.census.gov/content/dam/Census/library/publications/2021/demo/p70-167.pdf

Haktanır, D. (2022). Sexual dysfunction and related factors in patients with Parkinson's disease. *Journal of Psychosocial Nursing & Mental Health Services*, 1–11. https://doi.org/10.3928/02793695-20220907-02

Holmberg, M., Arver, S., & Dhejne, C. (2019). Supporting sexuality and improving sexual function in transgender persons. *Nature Reviews Urology, 16*(2), 121–139. https://doi.org/10.1038/s41585-018-0108-8

Holt-Lunstad, J., Robles, T., & Sbarra, D. A. (2017). Advancing social connection as a public health priority in the United States. *American Psychologist, 72*(6), 517–530. https://doi.org/10.1037/amp0000103

Hughes, M. E., Waite, L. J., Hawkley, L. C., & Cacioppo, J. T. (2004). A short scale for measuring loneliness in large surveys: Results from two population-based studies. *Research on Aging, 26*(6), 655–672. https://doi.org/10.1177/0164027504268574

Hurd, L., Mahal, R., Wardell, V., & Liang, J. (2022). "There were no words": Older LGBTQ+ persons' experiences of finding and claiming their gender and sexual identities. *Journal of Aging Studies, 60*, 100999. https://doi.org/10.1016/j.jaging.2022.100999

Inventor, B. R., Paun, O., & McIntosh, E. (2022). Mental health of LGBTQ older adults. *Journal of Psychosocial Nursing and Mental Health Services, 60*(4), 7–10. https://doi.org/10.3928/02793695-20220303-01

Isaacson, M., Tripathi, A., Samanta, T., D'Ambrosio, L., & Coughlin, J. (2020). Giving voice to the environment as the silent partner in aging: Examining the moderating roles of gender and family structure in older adult wellbeing. *International Journal of Environmental Research and Public Health, 17*(12), 4373. https://doi.org/10.3390/ijerph17124373

James, S., Herman, J., Rankin, S., Keisling, M., Mottet, L., & Anafi, M. (2016). *The report of the - National Center for Transgender Equality. The Report of the 2015 Transgender Survey.* https://transequality.org/sites/default/files/docs/usts/USTS-Full-Report-Dec17.pdf

Kerr, P., Barbosa Da Torre, M., Giguère, C. É., Lupien, S. J., & Juster, R. P. (2021). Occupational gender roles in relation to workplace stress, allostatic load, and mental health of psychiatric hospital workers. *Journal of Psychosomatic Research, 142*, 110352. https://doi.org/10.1016/j.jpsychores.2020.110352

Kuiper, J. S, Zuidersma, M. Oude Voshaar, R. C., Zuidema, S. U., van den Heuvel, E. R., Stolk, R. P., & Smidt, N. (2015). Social relationships and risk of dementia: A systematic review and meta-analysis of longitudinal cohort studies. *Ageing Research Reviews, 22*, 39–57. https://doi.org/10.1016/j.arr.2015.04.006

Laughlin, L. (2013). Who's minding the kids? Child care arrangements: Spring 2011. *Current Population Reports.* U.S. Census Bureau, 70e135.

Lee, J. E., & Cichy, K. E. (2020). Complex role of touch in social relationships for older adults' cardiovascular disease risk. *Research on Aging, 42*(7-8), 208–216. https://doi.org/10.1177/0164027520915793

Li, T., Luo, Y., Meng, Y., Yue, J., Nie, M., Fan, L., & Tong, C. (2022). Sexual activity and related factors of older women in Hunan, China: A cross-sectional study. *The Journal of Sexual Medicine, 19*(2), 302–310. https://doi.org/10.1016/j.jsxm.2021.11.020

Li, T. & Zhang, Y. (2015). Social network types and the health of older adults: Exploring reciprocal associations. *Social Science & Medicine, 130*, 59–68. https://doi.org/10.1016/j.socscimed.2015.02.007

Löfgren, M., Larsson, E., Isaksson, G., & Nyman, A. (2021). Older adults' experiences of maintaining social participation: Creating opportunities and striving to adapt to changing situations. *Scandinavian Journal of Occupational Therapy, 29*(7), 587–597. https://doi.org/10.1080/11038128.2021.1974550

Lubben, J., Blozik, E., Gillmann, G., Iliffe, S., von Renteln Kruse, W., Beck, J. C., & Stuck, A. E. (2006). Performance of an abbreviated version of the Lubben Social Network Scale among three European community-dwelling older adult populations. *The Gerontologist, 46*(4), 503–513. https://doi.org/10.1093/geront/46.4.503

Mahieu, L., & Gastmans, C. (2015). Older residents' perspectives on aged sexuality in institutionalized elderly care: A systematic literature review. *International Journal of Nursing Studies, 52*(12), 1891–1905. https://doi.org/10.1016/j.ijnurstu.2015.07.007

Mansson, D. H. (2016). The joy of grandparenting: A qualitative analysis of grandparents. *Journal of Intergenerational Relationships, 14*(2), 135–145. https://doi.org/10.1080/15350770.2016.1160738

McCreary, D. R., Oliffe, J. L., Black, N., Flannigan, R., Rachert, J., & Goldenberg, S. L. (2020). Canadian men's health stigma, masculine role norms and lifestyle behaviors. *Health Promotion International, 35*(3), 535–543. https://doi.org/10.1093/heapro/daz049

McGrath, M., Lever, S., McCluskey, A., & Power, E. (2019). How is sexuality after stroke experienced by stroke survivors and partners of stroke survivors? A systematic review of qualitative studies. *Clinical Rehabilitation, 33*(2), 293–303. https://doi.org/10.1177/0269215518793483

Milner, A., Kavanagh, A., King, T., & Currier, D. (2018). The influence of masculine norms and occupational factors on mental health: Evidence from the baseline of the Australian longitudinal study on male health. *American Journal of Men's Health, 12*(4), 696–705. https://doi.org/10.1177/1557988317752607

Mohammed, A. (2017). Addressing sexuality in occupational therapy. *OT Practice, 22*(9), CE-1–CE-7.

Morrison, S. D., Shakir, A., Vyas, K. S., Kirby, J., Crane, C. N., & Lee, G. K. (2016). Phalloplasty: A review of techniques and outcomes. *Plastic and Reconstructive Surgery, 138*(3), 594–615. https://doi.org/10.1097/PRS.0000000000002518

Neel, A. B. (n.d.). *7 meds that can wreck your sex life.* American Association of Retired Persons (AARP). https://www.aarp.org/health/drugs-supplements/info-04-2012/medications-that-can-cause-sexual-dysfunction.html

Novak, J. R., Peak, T., Gast, J., & Arnell, M. (2019). Associations between masculine norms and health-care utilization in highly religious, heterosexual men. *American Journal of Men's Health, 13*(3), 1557988319856739. https://doi.org/10.1177/1557988319856739

Nowosielski, K. (2022). Predictors of sexual function and performance in young- and middle-old women. *International Journal of Environmental Research and Public Health, 19*(7), 4207. https://doi.org/10.3390/ijerph19074207

Papathanassoglou, E. D., & Mpouzika, M. D. (2012). Interpersonal touch: Physiological effects in critical care. *Biological Research for Nursing, 14*(4), 431–443. https://doi.org/10.1177/1099800412451312

Pavanello Decaro, S., Van Gils, S., Van Hoorde, B., Baetens, K., Heylens, G., & Elaut, E. (2021). It might take time: A study on the evolution of quality of life in individuals with gender incongruence during gender-affirming care. *The Journal Of Sexual Medicine, 18*(12), 2045–2055. https://doi.org/10.1016/j.jsxm.2021.09.008

Peak, T., Gast, J., & Novak, J. R. (2021). Caregiving and caring with pride: Health behavior work among older gay married couples. *Journal of Gay & Lesbian Social Services, 33*:1, 123–136, https://doi.org/10.1080/10538720.2020.1850389

Pilowsky, D. J., & Wu, L. T. (2015). Sexual risk behaviors and HIV risk among Americans aged 50 years or older: A review. *Substance Abuse and Rehabilitation, 6*, 51–60. https://doi.org/10.2147/SAR.S78808

Polizzi, C., Lynn, S. J., & Perry, A. (2020). Stress and coping in the time of COVID-19: Pathways to resilience and recovery. *Clinical Neuropsychiatry, 17*(2), 59–62. https://doi.org/10.36131/CN20200204

Restoux, L. J., Dasariraju, S. R., Ackerman, I. N., Van Doornum, S., Romero, L., & Briggs, A. M. (2020). Systematic review of the impact of inflammatory arthritis on intimate relationships and sexual function. *Arthritis Care & Research, 72*(1), 41–62. https://doi.org/10.1002/acr.23857

Reynolds, F., & Hean Lim, K. (2013). The social context of older people. In A. Atwal & A. McIntyre (Eds.), *Occupational therapy and older people* (2nd ed., pp. 38–58). Chichester: Wiley-Blackwell.

Richters, J., Yeung, A., Rissel, C., McGeechan, K., Caruana, T., & de Visser, R. (2022). Sexual difficulties, problems, and help-seeking in a national representative sample: The second Australian study of health and relationships. *Archives of Sexual Behavior, 51*(3), 1435–1446. https://doi.org/10.1007/s10508-021-02244-w

Rook, K. S. & Charles, S. T. (2017). Close social ties and health in later life: Strengths and vulnerabilities. *American Psychologist, 72*(6), 567–577. http://dx.doi.org/10.1037/amp0000104

Rook, K. S., Luong, G., Sorkin, D. H., Newsom, J. T., & Krause, N. (2012). Ambivalent versus problematic social ties: Implications for psychological health, functional health, and interpersonal coping. *Psychology and Aging, 27*(4), 912–923. https://doi.org/10.1037/a0029246

Ruggeri, K., Garcia-Garzon, E., Maguire, A., Matz, S., & Huppert, F. A. (2020). Well-being is more than happiness and life satisfaction: A multidimensional analysis of 21 countries. *Health and Quality of Life Outcomes, 18*(192) https://doi.org/10.1186/s12955-020-01423-y

Santa Rosa Malcher C.M., Roberto da Silva Gonçalves Oliveira K., Fernandes Caldato M.C., Lopes Dos Santos Lobato B., da Silva Pedroso J., & de Tubino Scanavino M. (2021). Sexual disorders and quality of life in Parkinson's disease. *Sexual Medicine, 9*(1), 100280 https://doi.org/10.1016/j.esxm.2020.10.008

Sasson, I., & Umberson, D. J. (2014). Widowhood and depression: New light on gender differences, selection, and psychological adjustment. *The Journals of Gerontology Series B: Psychological Sciences and Social Sciences, 69B*(1), 135–145. https://doi.org/10.1093/geronb/gbt058

Schardein, J. N., & Nikolavsky, D. (2022). Sexual functioning of transgender females post-vaginoplasty: Evaluation, outcomes and treatment strategies for sexual dysfunction. *Sexual Medicine Reviews, 10*(1), 77–90. https://doi.org/10.1016/j.sxmr.2021.04.001

Schladitz, K., Förster, F., Wagner, M., Heser, K., König, H. H., Hajek, A., Wiese, B., Pabst, A., Riedel-Heller, S. G., & Löbner, M. (2022). Gender specifics of healthy ageing in older age as seen by women and men (70+): A focus group study. *International Journal Of Environmental Research and Public Health, 19*(5), 3137. https://doi.org/10.3390/ijerph19053137

Schwinn S. V. & Dinkel S. A. (2015). Changing the culture of long-term care: Combating heterosexism. *Online Journal of Issues in Nursing, 20*(2), 7. https://doi.org/10.3912/OJIN.Vol20No02PPT03

Ševčíková, A., Gottfried, J., & Blinka, L. (2021). Associations among sexual activity, relationship types, and health in mid and later life. *Archives of Sexual Behavior 50*, 2667–2677. https://doi.org/10.1007/s10508-021-02040-6

Siette, J., Pomare, C., Dodds, L., Jorgensen, M., Harrigan, N., & Georgiou, A. (2021). A comprehensive overview of social network measures for older adults: A systematic review. *Archives of Gerontology and Geriatrics, 97*, 104525. https://doi.org/10.1016/j.archger.2021.104525

Simon, P., Grajo, L., & Powers Dirette, D. (2021). The role of occupational therapy in supporting the needs of older adults who identify as lesbian, gay, bisexual, and/or transgender (LGBT). *The Open Journal of Occupational Therapy, 9*(4), 1–9. https://doi.org/10.15453/2168-6408.1742

Sinković, M., & Towler, L. (2019). Sexual aging: A systematic review of qualitative research on the sexuality and sexual health of older adults. *Qualitative Health Research, 29*(9), 1239–1254. https://doi.org/10.1177/1049732318819834

Slack, D. J., & Safer, J. D. (2021). Cardiovascular health maintenance in aging individuals: The implications for transgender men and women on hormone therapy. *Endocrine Practice: Official Journal of the American College of Endocrinology and the American Association of Clinical Endocrinologists, 27*(1), 63–70. https://doi.org/10.1016/j.eprac.2020.11.001

Smith, L., McDermott, D., & Jackson, S. (2019). Having sex in older age could make you happier and healthier: New research. Accessed on: April 26, 2022. Retrieved at: https://theconversation.com/having-sex-in-older-age-could-make-you-happier-and-healthier-new-research-122290

Solomon, D. H., Santacroce, L., Colvin, A., Lian, Y., Ruppert, K., & Yoshida, K. (2022). The relationship between 19-year trends in medication use and changes in physical function among women in the midlife: A study of women's health across the nation pharmacoepidemiology study. *Pharmacoepidemiology and Drug Safety, 31*(3), 283–293. https://doi.org/10.1002/pds.5355

Srinivasan, S., Glover, J., Tampi, R. R., Tampi, D. J., & Sewell, D. D. (2019). Sexuality and the older adult. *Current Psychiatry Reports, 21*(10), 97. https://doi.org/10.1007/s11920-019-1090-4

Stinchcombe, A., Kortes-Miller, K., & Wilson, K. (2021). "We are resilient, we made it to this point": A study of the lived experiences of older LGBTQ2S+ Canadians. *Journal of Applied Gerontology: the Official Journal of the Southern Gerontological Society, 40*(11), 1533–1541. https://doi.org/10.1177/0733464820984893

Suanet, B., van Tilburg, T. G., & Broese van Groenou, M. I. (2013). Nonkin in older adults' personal networks: More important among later cohorts?. *The Journals of Gerontology. Series B, Psychological sciences and social sciences, 68*(4), 633–643. https://doi.org/10.1093/geronb/gbt043

Suragarn, U., Hain, D., & Pfaff, G. (2021). Approaches to enhance social connection in older adults: An integrative review of literature. *Aging and Health Research, 1*(3), 100029. https://doi.org/10.1016/j.ahr.2021.100029

Taylor, B., & Davis, S. (2006). Using the Extended PLISSIT model to address sexual healthcare needs. *Nursing Standard, 21*(11), 35–40.

The Trevor Project. (2021, November 12). *Understanding gender identities.* https://www.thetrevorproject.org/resources/article/understanding-gender-identities/

Thomas, H. N., Hamm, M., Borrero, S., Hess, R., & Thurston, R. C. (2019). Body image, attractiveness, and sexual satisfaction among midlife women: A qualitative study. *Journal of Women's Health (2002), 28*(1), 100–106. https://doi.org/10.1089/jwh.2018.7107

Turan, O., Ure, I., & Turan, P. A. (2016). Erectile dysfunction in COPD patients. *Chronic Respiratory Disease, 13*(1), 5–12. https://doi.org/10.1177/1479972315619382

Turcotte, P. L., Carrier, A, Roy, V., & Levasseur, M. (2018). Occupational therapists' contributions to fostering older adults' social participation: A scoping review. *British Journal of Occupational Therapy, 81*(8), 427–449. https://doi.org/10.1177/0308022617752067

Unger C. A. (2016). Hormone therapy for transgender patients. *Translational Andrology and Urology, 5*(6), 877–884. https://doi.org/10.21037/tau.2016.09.04

United Nations. (1991). United Nations principles for older persons https://www.ohchr.org/en/instruments-mechanisms/instruments/united-nations-principles-older-persons

Van Orden, K. A., Bower, E., Lutz, J., Siva, C., Gallegos, A. M., Podgorski, C. A., Santos, M. D., & Conwell, Y. (2020). Strategies to promote social connections among older adults during "social distancing" restrictions. *American Journal of Geriatric Psychiatry, 29*(8), 816–827. https://doi.org/10.1016/j.jagp.2020.05.004

Verdery, A., & Campbell, C. (2019). Social support in America: Stratification and trends in access over two decades. *Social Forces, 98*(2), 725–752. https://doi.org/10.1093/sf/soz008

von Mohr, M., Kirsch, L. P., & Fotopoulou, A. (2021). Social touch deprivation during COVID-19: Effects on psychological wellbeing and craving interpersonal touch. *Royal Society Open Science, 8*(9), 210287. https://doi.org/10.1098/rsos.210287

Waite, L. J., & Xu, J. (2015). Aging policies for traditional and blended families. *Public Policy & Aging Report, 25*(3), 88–93. https://doi.org/10.1093/ppar/prv015

Wamsley, L. (2021, June 2). *A guide to gender identity terms.* https://www.npr.org/2021/06/02/996319297/gender-identity-pronouns-expression-guide-lgbtq

White Hughto, J. M., & Reisner, S. L. (2018). Social context of depressive distress in aging transgender adults. *Journal of Applied Gerontology: The Official Journal of the Southern Gerontological Society, 37*(12), 1517–1539. https://doi.org/10.1177/0733464816675819

World Health Organization. (2015). *World Report on Ageing and Health.* http://apps.who.int/iris/bitstream/handle/10665/186463/9789240694811_eng.pdf

World Health Organization. (2021). *Social isolation and loneliness among older people: Advocacy brief.* https://www.who.int/teams/social-determinants-of-health/demographic-change-and-healthy-ageing/social-isolation-and-loneliness

World Health Organization. (n.d.a.). *Gender and Health.* https://www.who.int/health-topics/gender#tab=tab_1

World Health Organization. (n.d.b.). *Sexual Health.* https://www.who.int/health-topics/sexual-health#tab=tab_1

Young, K., Dodington, A., Smith, C., & Heck, C. S. (2019). Addressing clients' sexual health in occupational therapy practice. *Canadian Journal of Occupational Therapy. Revue Canadienne D'ergotherapie, 87*(1), 52–62. https://doi.org/10.1177/0008417419855237

Zhao, S., Li, E., Wang, J., Luo, L., Luo, J., & Zhao, Z. (2018). Rheumatoid arthritis and risk of sexual dysfunction: A systematic review and metaanalysis. *The Journal of Rheumatology, 45*(10), 1375–1382. https://doi.org/10.3899/jrheum.170956

CHAPTER 6

Legal and Ethical Issues

Brenda Howard DHSc, OTR, FAOTA ■ Leslie E. Bennett, OTD, OTR/L ■ Christine Kroll, OTD, OTR

Ethics and equity and the principles of justice do not change with the calendar.

—D.H. Lawrence

LEARNING OUTCOMES

By the end of this chapter, readers will be able to:

6-1. Identify laws and policies that affect older adults, including policies on ageism and ethics of billing and productivity.
6-2. Determine the legal needs of older adults for advance care planning, end-of-life decision-making, and their ethical implications.
6-3. Analyze circumstances and factors that contribute to elder abuse and neglect.
6-4. Determine the responsibilities of occupational therapy practitioners in addressing elder abuse.
6-5. Critically reflect on key ethical issues relevant to the experience of older adults.
6-6. Apply ethical decision making to a case study regarding legal and ethical issues faced by older adults.
6-7. Explain the importance of multidisciplinary and interprofessional teams in ethical decision-making.

Mini Case Study

Ms. Parks is a 64-year-old female referred to outpatient occupational therapy for imbalance and frequent falls during activities of daily living (ADLs). During the history portion of the assessment, Ms. Parks reported she was essentially homeless and went back and forth between her ex-husband's home and her brother's home. She reported that her brother would yell at and berate her and sometimes take her money. However, when she was at her ex-husband's home, he would hit and shove her. She reported that sometimes her ex-husband would shove her so hard that "my head hits the wall." Ms. Parks quickly added, "But don't report me because then I won't have anywhere to live," and stated that she was afraid of what her brother or ex-husband would do if she reported them. The initial evaluation findings indicated the client's imbalance was caused by central nervous system impairment, likely from undiagnosed head trauma as a result of the abuse. The occupational therapy practitioner could not persuade the client to agree to report the abuse. Later, the occupational therapy practitioner recounted Ms. Parks' story to the outpatient facility's manager, who was also the social worker, asking for advice on how to proceed. The manager shrugged and stated, "If an adult of sound mind and in control of her own affairs requests to not report abuse, there is nothing I can do."

Provocative Questions

What are the legal and ethical issues at stake in this scenario?

1. Which ethical principles and standards from the American Occupational Therapy Association (AOTA) Code of Ethics (AOTA, 2020a) apply to Ms. Parks' case? Alternate: Which aspects of the World Federation of Occupational Therapists Code of Ethics apply? Which aspects of occupational therapy codes of ethics from around the world apply?
2. Is the social worker's assertion correct regarding reporting the abuse? Why or why not? What do the laws in your location say about mandatory reporting of abuse?

Introduction

Occupational therapy practitioners enter the profession as generally ethical people who want to do good in the world. However, the issues they will encounter are often more complex than just wanting to do good; sometimes, the "right" thing to do is not apparent. Occupational therapy practitioners often find themselves in circumstances where there are no good solutions; instead, there are choices between the lesser of evils and the necessity of uncovering the least objectionable option. For example, if the occupational therapy practitioner reports Ms. Parks' abuse, going against her expressed wishes, the occupational therapy practitioner violates her autonomy. But if the practitioner remains silent, the practitioner fails to keep Ms. Parks from harm, violating the ethical principle of beneficence. What would be the "good" and "right" thing to do?

This chapter explores legal and ethical considerations in working with older adults, including laws and policies, issues and practices affecting older adults, ageism and elder abuse, and the ethical issues that emerge in older adults' complex environments (see Chapter 4 for introduction to ageism). Readers will explore the occupational therapy practitioner's legal and ethical obligations to older adult clients. Finally, readers will apply an ethical problem-solving framework when working with older adults to manage legal and ethical problems. By preparing and practicing the ability to manage ethical and legal issues, the occupational therapy practitioner can manage these concerns and minimize *moral distress* and *moral injury* for their clients and themselves.

Ethical Principles

Managing ethical issues can be complicated, as Ms. Parks' story illustrates. However, understanding ethical principles can help the occupational therapy practitioner discern a path forward. Beauchamp and Childress (2019) have named six ethical principles commonly used in Western cultures, also used in the AOTA (2020a) Occupational Therapy Code of Ethics, that are useful for helping understand and categorize ethical problems: beneficence, nonmaleficence, autonomy, justice, veracity, and fidelity. Beneficence indicates a concern for the well-being and safety of service recipients, including the provision of competent, evidence-based care and removing persons from harm. Nonmaleficence means the care provider will refrain from actions that cause harm. Nonmaleficence includes providing due care and not having inappropriate relationships with service recipients. Autonomy requires that the service provider respects the right of the person to self-determination, privacy, confidentiality, and informed consent. Justice means that the occupational therapy practitioner will promote fairness and objectivity when providing services. Justice includes the timely response to a request for service, following laws and maintaining credentials, and addressing barriers to receiving occupational therapy services. Veracity indicates that the occupational therapy practitioner will be truthful in records, billing, marketing, and all other communication; will be comprehensive, objective, and accurate when representing the occupational therapy profession; will correct communication errors; and will not plagiarize. Fidelity requires that an occupational therapy practitioner treats service recipients and their families, colleagues, and other professionals with respect, fairness, discretion, and integrity. It includes safeguarding confidential information, being good stewards of resources, and avoiding harassment of all persons with whom they interact. An **ethical dilemma** occurs when two or more of these principles conflict, such as when Ms. Parks and the occupational therapy practitioner faced an issue concerning autonomy vs. beneficence. These ethical principles are not universal, however. In more communal cultures, autonomy may be much less important. Occupational therapy practitioners may need to consider other conceptualizations, including, for example, *narrative ethics,* which focuses on the person's lifeworld and experiences (Lo, 2010). Some ethical issues presented in late life may require different thinking about cultural, generational, and societal values (McArdle, 2012).

Laws and Policy Affecting Older Adults

The United States enacted the Social Security Act (SSA) in 1935. The SSA, written during the Great Depression, focused on providing a federal financial safety net for the elderly, unemployed, and disadvantaged. The SSA put in place a system to provide financial assistance to those over the age of 65 after a lifetime of payroll tax contributions. In 1965, the U.S. Congress enacted the Social Security Amendments Act, popularly known as the Medicare and Medicaid Act of 1965. The federally funded Medicare program provides health services to those who qualify for the program. The Medicaid program is funded through a combination of state and federal funds and provides services for those who meet the requirements, based primarily on low-income status. The SSA is a living document used to codify changes in policy over the decades, including the Medicare and Medicaid program, and continues to guide program implementation and policymaking.

Although the SSA initiated significant policy changes and provided financial assistance for those over age 65, issues of age discrimination led to nondiscrimination laws and resulted in policies to protect the rights of adults over certain ages. Allen and colleagues (2022) completed a survey of 2,035 adults aged 50 to 80 in 2021 and 2022. The survey found that 93% of the study participants regularly reported experiencing one or more forms of everyday ageism. Further, those 65 to 80 years reported significantly more occurrences of everyday ageism than persons aged 50 to 64. The survey used the Everyday Ageism Scale, which includes ageism items such as jokes or comments that place aging or older adults in a negative light and people assuming that older people have difficulty with technology or memory/cognition. Ageism is a significant everyday concern for older adults that may affect their physical and mental wellbeing.

Practitioners need to consider that the population of older adults is growing. By 2030, the United States will have more people over the age of 65 than younger than five (Fulmer et al, 2021), and globally, those of 60+ years will rise from 900 million to 2 billion by 2050 (WHO, 2022b, April 27). The issue of ageism applies to those in their 40s, with more than 30% of people experiencing some form of ageism in the workplace before they reach the age of 45 (Mistry, 2020). Ageism is persistent and continues to affect the workforce despite the aging of the U.S. workforce. Ageism can also affect social determinants of health, such as housing, healthcare, and other aspects of daily life. Ageism, based on young or old stereotypes, is harmful to society as a whole, as it affects how long people can or want to work, which takes a toll on both the financial health and well-being of our older population.

In response to the problem of ageism, national, state, and local governments and organizations/employers implemented various policies and laws. The laws addressed ageism in employment, financially assisted work programs, and housing. Table 6-1 lists three significant laws passed in the United States regarding ageism. The Age Discrimination in Employment Act (ADEA) of 1967 prohibits discrimination against people 40 years and older by labor organizations, employers with at least 20 employees, the federal government, and employment agencies. Legislation to address age discrimination in government programs prompted the passage of the Age Discrimination Act of 1975 (42 U.S.C. Sections 6101 to 6107). Although this act applied to all age groups and did not exclusively address ageism against older adults, it did allow for certain age distinctions. It is crucial to grasp that the issue of age discrimination had to reach a tipping point for legislative action.

State laws often imitate federal laws. One example is the Older Americans Act (OAA) of 1965. The OAA, reauthorized in 2020, established services for older adults through a national network of state agencies, Area Agencies on Aging (AoA), and other organizations and providers. The Administration on Aging, through the OAA, also developed the Long-Term Care (LTC) Ombudsman Program, which now exists in every state in the United States and acts as a third party to assist families and residents of LTC facilities in having their voices heard regarding their rights under federal and state laws (American Association of Retired Persons, 2022). The LTC Ombudsman program ensures that through each state's AoA, older adults receive representation, advocacy, and community-based services that assist them in participating in their communities, aging in place, and receiving protections when residing in LTC facilities (Administration for Community Living, 2022). State laws may also address ageism in the workplace, housing, or participation in programs. State regulations vary and may have a basis in federal laws such as the OAA, which charges the Administration on Aging to fund community programs, research, training, and services related to aging (Administration for Community Living, 2021).

Ageism is a global issue (Ageing Equal, n.d.). Older adults may face mandatory retirement requiring them to change jobs or careers to continue working after a certain age. Additionally, opportunities for education and lifelong learning are not always available for older adults. Further, housing may become an issue due to affordability, lack of access to loans to afford to adapt their home, or inability to receive the care they need in their home.

Ageism and Healthcare

Healthcare professionals are not immune to ageism. Inker (2018) found that there are fewer healthcare professionals seeking to specialize in the care of older adults due to ageist attitudes, lower pay, and lack of prestige related to geriatric care. Healthcare professionals also receive very little education on aging, some of which may be outdated and misleading (Inker, 2018). The focus of healthcare professions on the biomedical model of care also leads to ageist attitudes, as it provides a narrow lens through which aging is a pathological process that may be overtreated in an attempt to "fix" someone or undertreated due to the rationalization that the person cannot be cured (Inker, 2018). The persistence of ageism in healthcare professions is an ethical concern, because healthcare providers have authority and power regarding what treatments they offer to clients. Ageism is contrary to the ethical healthcare principle of nonmaleficence—not harming clients.

Kadıoğlu et al (2013) found that a sample of primary care providers in Turkey was sensitive to and recognized ethical issues surrounding geriatric care. However, the providers still reported incidents of a lack of respect for older adults related to assumptions about decision-making competency, ignoring the older adult's role in decision-making, ignoring complaints by older adults, and rejecting treatment without sharing it with the client due to their age. The implicit and explicit effects of ageism in healthcare workers may lead to worse outcomes and limited shared decision-making. It is a form of harmful discrimination.

During the COVID-19 pandemic and public health emergency, the popular press portrayed older adults as vulnerable and a burden to the economy and the younger generations. The Eurobarometer survey indicated that European older adults suffered the most from reforms and budget cuts (Ageing Equal, n.d.). In the United States, Fraser and colleagues (2020) noted a similar portrayal of the older adult as undervalued and the initial perception that the Coronavirus was an older adult problem. Fraser and colleagues (2020)

TABLE 6-1 United States Laws Addressing Ageism

FEDERAL LAWS	INTENT
The Age Discrimination in Employment Act of 1967 (ADEA)	Prohibits employers from discrimination against people who are 40+ years of age Applies to employers with at least 20 employees
The Age Discrimination Act of 1975	Prohibits age discrimination in programs receiving federal assistance and applies to all ages
Section 188 of the Workforce Investment Act of 1998 (WIA)	Prohibits age discrimination against applicants, employees, or participants in financially-assisted WIA programs; created the One-Stop delivery system

stated that policies meant to protect older adults might be patronizing and isolating, further communicating negative messages.

Older adults have internalized and exhibited attitudinal beliefs surrounding ageism, further adding to the deleterious effects of ageism. Ayalon & Cohn-Schwartz (2021) explored self-perceptions of aging and perceived age discrimination and found that both perceptions significantly predicted an increase in worries among older persons during the COVID-19 pandemic. Previtali and colleagues (2020) discussed the arbitrary use of chronological age to determine public policy during the pandemic and argued that this practice further spread ageist ideology. Previtali and colleagues (2020) also pointed out that policy based on chronological age led to the assumption that being "old" meant that one is automatically vulnerable, in poor health, and thus less valuable to society. Public policy based on arbitrary factors such as chronological age and healthcare providers' implementation of such policies led to more concern and isolation for older adults.

Models aimed at reducing ageism could benefit policymaking processes and advocacy. Levy et al (2020) studied the empirical application of the Positive Education about Aging and Contact Experiences (PEACE) model, which is focused on the reduction of ageism through education. They found knowledge about aging to be lacking at all levels, including the home environment through primary and secondary education, and professional programs. The PEACE model posits that through education and positive interactions with older adults, attitudes about aging, such as discrimination and stereotyping, can affect society policymaking and program development. Setting a foundation for education and coordinating positive interactions with older adults lead to changes in thinking and attitudes, reducing assumptions about aging.

The PEACE model supports the use of education and exposure to older adults through positive interactions, which may change perceptions and thus the focus of policy issues in governments and organizations. Occupational therapy practitioners could advocate for their clients to create positive experiences with older adults and legislators at the state and national levels. Table 6-1 lists several laws developed in response to issues on aging. As such, developing education through meetings and using evidence to support a need is a worthwhile advocacy effort. Policy guides actions through the creation of laws, regulations, and rules. Occupational therapy practitioners must become involved in policy to advocate for access to occupational therapy services and receive government consideration during policymaking. The AOTA, state occupational therapy associations, and other organizations actively advocate in a nonpartisan manner to work toward legislative actions that support clients, their families, and occupational therapy practitioners. Membership in professional organizations supports lobbying efforts and is one way to support policy development. Through professional organizations, occupational therapy practitioners can be active in volunteering their time and talent to support critical issues at the state and national levels.

The Strength and Vulnerability Integration (SAVI) model is another model developed to reduce ageism in policymaking. Marchiondo and colleagues (2019) empirically assessed the SAVI model to determine older adults' perceptions of age discrimination in the United States using longitudinal data. Using the Health and Retirement Study data from a group of Americans aged 51 and older and selecting those who worked full- or part-time, Marchiondo and colleagues (2019) found that as perceived age discrimination increased, so did depression, whereas job satisfaction and perceived overall health decreased. The SAVI model proposes that long-term age discrimination is deleterious to older adults over time, causing chronic stress, despite the higher emotional regulation skills as part of their coping strategies (Marchiondo et al, 2019). The study's findings support the need to expand legal support for older employees through the ADEA and to improve education about age stereotypes. Improving legal and educational support might improve the health of older workers and their ability to participate in the workforce longer, thereby benefiting organizations and employers by reducing age discrimination. The population is aging, and the need to work longer requires support for older adults to enable their participation.

Ethics of Billing and Productivity

Knowing laws, policies, and regulations relating to the elderly is critical for ethical treatment and advocacy for older adult clients. As practitioners working with older adults in the United States, healthcare workers must also be aware of and abide by laws, policies, and regulations that affect billing for services. Billing for the 65+ population in the United States means billing Medicare and Medicaid insurances for most services. Rules and regulations apply to these federal and state-run programs, and understanding those rules will assist in compliance and advocacy for access to care. The AOTA is a resource for occupational therapy practitioners regarding federal and state-specific changes to Medicare and Medicaid, as well as information on state-specific practice acts for occupational therapy practitioners (AOTA, 2022a).

Abiding by the AOTA Code of Ethics (2020a), the principles of justice and veracity apply to billing occupational therapy services. Referring to the Standards of Conduct (AOTA Code of Ethics, 2020a), section 3 on Documentation, Reimbursement, and Financial Matters specifies that compliance with laws, guidelines, and regulations and accurate reporting are ethical obligations of the occupational therapy practitioner. These legal and ethical obligations include billing equitably, documenting services adequate to requirements, and reporting/recording information accurately. These Standards of Conduct also apply to one's work and what one's employer may require in the workplace. Besides the ethical and professional standards, documentation and billing are part of medical records, and falsification or inaccurate medical records have legal implications that could affect a practitioner's professional license.

Productivity is a significant practice issue arising from changes in the healthcare system, especially in some settings where older adults are predominant, such as skilled nursing facilities and home health. As the cost of providing therapy has increased and reimbursement has decreased, employers have developed productivity requirements specific to their particular business. Occupational therapy practitioners have had ethical questions regarding productivity standards and their impact on practice. It is critical to identify how the employer is calculating productivity. However, if the productivity requirement does not allow the practitioner to maintain an evidence-based practice and provide the outcomes needed for the client, the AOTA Code of Ethics (2020a) principle of fidelity indicates that the practitioner needs to speak with management to maintain the employer-employee relationship and explore concerns. The Standards of Conduct further specify professional expectations in sections 4 and 5 on Services Delivery and Professional Competence, Education, Supervision, and Training (AOTA Code of Ethics, 2020a). These sections are worth considering regarding what practitioners are asked to do or not do in accordance with their workload to ensure they are acting in the best interest of the client and providing services congruent with their state practice act.

Ethical Considerations in Advance Care Planning & End-of-Life Care

Aging naturally puts persons at a higher risk for experiencing a medical crisis that could leave the person so ill or disabled that they are incapable of making healthcare decisions on their own. Even if a person is healthy and has never been sick, planning for their healthcare needs in the future, including treatment wishes, is essential. Advance care planning is "a process that supports understanding and sharing of personal values, life goals, and preferences regarding future medical care" (Casey, 2019, p. 17). It involves learning about the types of decisions that might need to be made during a medical crisis and allows a person to express their values and wishes regarding end-of-life care through formal written advance directives.

What are Advance Directives?

Advance directives are living documents that can speak for persons who can no longer do so for themselves (Table 6-2: Types of Advance Directives). Advance directives include information on a person's identified healthcare proxy or surrogate designated to make treatment decisions for the person if there is a time that person can no longer speak for themselves. These documents also include specific directives on treatment options that the person would or would not want to undergo, including cardiopulmonary resuscitation (CPR), mechanical ventilation, artificial nutrition and hydration, and comfort care measures, which include palliative and hospice care services (Table 6-3: End-of-Life Treatment Options).

TABLE 6-2 ■ Types of Advance Directives

TREATMENT	DEFINITION
POLST/MOLST forms	POLST: Physician Orders for Life-Sustaining Treatment MOLST: Medical Orders for Life-Sustaining Treatment ■ Generally instated when a person has a long-term chronic illness or terminal condition ■ Allows a person's treatment wishes to be carried over in emergency situations, such as a 911 call
Living will	Written document that details a person's treatment wishes when they are no longer able to speak for themselves; helps healthcare professionals and the person's family to make decisions on their behalf
Durable power of attorney	■ Legal document that identifies a person's healthcare proxy who can make decisions on their behalf when they no longer can speak for themselves

(NIH, 2022.)

Advance care planning can help to mitigate tough decisions later in life by family members. Resources are available to support individuals and their families as they negotiate this process. One such resource is the Five Wishes (2022) organization, the U.S.-only national advance care planning program. Additionally, there are several free resources that families can download to develop advance directives documents, which include healthcare proxy designation forms, a living will template, and an advance directive wallet card (American Hospital Association, 2022: Five Wishes, 2022). However, current statistics from the CDC indicate that only one in three Americans has any kind of advance directive in place or has done any advance care planning (Lendon, Caffrey, & Lau, 2018).

The failure to enact this planning is a consequence of sociocultural factors that influence perceptions of end-of-life and advance care planning, which includes a culture of avoidance of death. Magazines, commercials, and news stories emphasize staying young and healthy. People often avoid discussions about aging and end-of-life care. Moreover, a lack of preparation about how to handle these tough decisions regarding end-of-life has led to increased distrust in the medical system. Failure to adequately prepare professionals to facilitate these discussions may contribute to the overall problem.

Without advance care planning, people's family and friends face tough decisions regarding what treatments should be implemented, what treatments to avoid, and when to decide to withdraw treatments. Prognostic uncertainty, limited resources, and trying to weigh the risks of treatment interventions versus benefits have caused increased moral distress among family members and healthcare providers.

TABLE 6-3 ■ End-of-Life Treatment Options

TREATMENT	DEFINITION
CPR	Cardiopulmonary resuscitation: used to restore cardiac function during life-threatening events
DNR	Do not resuscitate order
Mechanical ventilation	Machine that assists persons to breathe
Artificial nutrition & hydration	If someone is unable to eat or take in fluids it may be necessary to use a feeding tube or initiate IV fluids to help them while they are recovering
Pain management	Interventions used to relieve pain: ■ Medicine ■ Massage ■ Meditation ■ Music ■ Acupuncture ■ Hot/cold packs
Palliative sedation	Generally used as a last resort; measure taken to sedate a person who is not getting sufficient pain relief from normal measures
Palliative care	Covers a broad population of persons with chronic or long-term conditions (life-limiting) ■ Team-oriented approach: addresses physical pain and impairments, disease symptoms, and emotional/social/spiritual pain ■ Focus is on increasing quality of life, comfort, and dignity ■ Examines body functions/structures, activities, and participation within the context of disease ■ Assesses environmental and personal factors
Hospice care	Provides quality and compassionate care for persons with a prognosis of 6 months or less to live

Ethical Considerations at End-of-Life

Expanding healthcare technology and treatment possibilities coupled with an increasingly complex health management system have created a culture focused on providing all measures to save someone's life. Increasing pressure to provide life-extending treatments past their ability to actually help has become common practice in many intensive care units. Without documentation of a person's treatment wishes, healthcare providers must develop a treatment plan that considers the client's and families'/proxies' values. Ultimately, the person is the only one who has the right to determine what will happen with and to their bodies. When they are unable to speak for themselves, and in the absence of documented advance directives, personal autonomy and self-determination are compromised. The decision-making then falls to the family or a designated proxy or surrogate who has the responsibility to speak for the client, ensuring that the rights of the person in a medical crisis are being addressed. The proxy also has rights that practitioners must respect. These include access to accurate, complete, and understandable information regarding the person's medical condition. It includes a right to be supported by the facility and healthcare providers while the proxy tries to make an informed decision, and they have a right to ultimately refuse treatments. It is important to remember that the proxy's purpose is to enact the client's wishes, not to substitute personal priorities.

Communication breakdowns between the client, family, and healthcare providers can result in ineffective symptom management or nonbeneficial care. More importantly, a lack of shared decision-making can affect timely treatment and lead to increased moral distress among all stakeholders. A reluctance of healthcare providers to address end-of-life needs results in ethical conflict. Barriers to proper care emerge from a simple lack of understanding of the options for treatment and misconceptions about end-of-life treatment choices. Additionally, with prognostic uncertainty, it can be difficult for healthcare providers to recognize when it is time to transition from curative treatment methods to more comfort care or palliative methods, which often results in delay in referring the person and the family to these services until very late in the course of treatment. This delay may contribute to additional suffering, violating the ethical principle of nonmaleficence (Beauchamp & Childress, 2019).

Ethical conflicts can occur when the cultural or religious beliefs of the person and their family conflict with recommended care. Healthcare providers have a moral and ethical duty to care for their clients and to do no harm. When clients and family members decline treatment based on their religious and cultural values, even if that treatment could benefit the person, practitioners have a difficult time making decisions regarding the best course of care. These tough decisions, which conflict with healthcare practitioners' duty to provide care, directly correlate with increased stress, anxiety, and burnout.

Lastly, what do healthcare practitioners do when there is no clear course of treatment? Providers must look to the client and their family to decide what is the best course for that person. Healthcare providers have a duty to provide the person with all available information on treatment options. If the person is unable to speak for themselves, then this discussion must include a healthcare proxy. It is essential that the healthcare team provides the person and proxy with all the necessary information to make the most informed decision regarding care and options at end-of-life. Transparency and honesty during the entire process must occur, and conversations about end-of-life care and death need to be more transparent.

What can Occupational Therapy Practitioners do?

Occupational therapy practitioners have a role in end-of-life care. Practitioners must function as advocates for their clients and help support the team in making decisions. Occupational therapy practitioners can also have a role in communicating with clients and their families to help them fully understand their medical conditions. Occupational therapy practitioners must use holistic treatment methods that focus on clients' values and beliefs to support treatment. It is beneficial to share knowledge of the person's values and belief systems with the entire healthcare team.

Additionally, practitioners need to address symptoms within their scope of practice and make sure they are communicating and coordinating with other team members. Educating other healthcare providers on occupational therapy's role at end-of-life is important. Ongoing education and engagement in policy development are critical. (See Chapter 28 for more information on occupational therapy in palliative and hospice care.)

Elder Abuse and Neglect

According to the World Health Organization (WHO, 2022a), one in six people age 60 years or older have experienced some form of abuse or neglect. Research indicates that these rates are much higher in institutions and LTC facilities. The National Council on Aging (2022) reports that 5 million elderly persons suffer abuse every year in the United States and that the financial cost of this abuse is upwards of $36.5 billion. The number of cases of abuse and neglect is predicted to continue to rise as the United States and the rest of the world experience a rapid increase in the aging population. In fact, the population of older adults in the world will more than double by the year 2050, exceeding 2 billion people (WHO, 2022a). Additionally, the rates of reported abuse and neglect significantly increased during the COVID-19 pandemic due to increased social and physical isolation, resulting in serious physical, psychological, and emotional harm in an already vulnerable population. It is essential that occupational therapy practitioners consider the overall impact on these persons and the role that they play in addressing abuse and neglect concerns.

Abusers are both male and female, and approximately 60% of abuse and neglect is perpetrated by a close family member or relative, two-thirds of whom are the elder's adult children or spouse (National Council on Aging, 2022). Research indicates that increased social isolation, cognitive decline, and other impairments put the elderly population at increased risk for experiencing abuse and neglect. Additionally, persons with disabilities are more vulnerable to abuse and neglect. The result is that those who are 60 years of age or older are at a 300% higher risk of death from abuse and neglect than the general population (National Council on Aging, 2022; WHO, 2022a).

In this section, readers will consider the different forms of elder abuse and neglect. Laws and policies regarding reporting abuse and neglect will be examined. The goal is to ensure understanding of the forms of abuse and neglect, the reasons and context in which this may occur, and strategies for recognizing and addressing abuse.

CASE STUDY

Occupational Profile

Mr. Thompson is a 68-year-old African American recently discharged from the local hospital after a stroke. The physician referred Mr. Thompson to outpatient occupational therapy services. At his initial evaluation, Mr. Thompson indicated that he lived alone but his son lived two doors down from him. Although Mr. Thompson is retired, he was working a part-time job to help with finances. Since returning home, he had not been able to return to work and was worried about being able to support himself.

Identified Problems

Mr. Thompson's deficits consisted of poor balance and safety, visual-perceptual deficits, and deficits in higher-level executive functioning. The occupational therapy practitioner initially observed poor hygiene management in Mr. Thompson, who often smelled of urine and had a very disheveled appearance. He seemed depressed and withdrawn, which the client indicated was not his normal baseline.

As the occupational therapy practitioner continued to work with Mr. Thompson, they started to worry about his safety and poor self-care habits. He reported that he had fallen at home a couple of times and was not eating because he could not afford groceries. The occupational therapy practitioner asked Mr. Thompson if his son was checking in on him at all, and he indicated that his son worked full-time and was busy with his children during the evenings and on weekends. Mr. Thompson was worried about being a burden to his son, so he had not asked for help.

Question

1. Evaluate Mr. Thompson's case and decide if he is experiencing elder abuse or neglect. Explain why or why not.

Answer

As the team has noted, Mr. Thompson certainly is experiencing endangerment to his physical and emotional well-being. He also displays signs of abuse and neglect consisting of appearing depressed and withdrawn and having poor hygiene and a disheveled appearance. However, the team cannot be certain that he is being abused and neglected until they investigate further. He may be experiencing elder abuse consisting of *abandonment,* as he has been left alone without assistance when he requires care. Determining whether the son is aware of the condition of Mr. Thompson's home and has made a commitment to be his caregiver would factor heavily into this conclusion. Further, Mr. Thompson may be committing *self-neglect* if he is choosing to not request assistance. If Mr. Thompson is fully capable of making his own decisions, then intervening in this neglectful situation could be a breach of client autonomy. Students can further discuss which ethical principle (autonomy or beneficence) is most important to uphold in this situation.

Laws and Reporting

The U.S. Congress passed the Elder Justice Act in 2006. This act was the first legislation of its kind to address elder abuse, neglect, and exploitation at the federal level. Under this new legislation, the U.S. federal government authorized a variety of new programs and initiatives to better coordinate responses to elder abuse and neglect. This act provided for grants focused on promoting elder justice research and additional funding for adult protective services systems. The legislation also provided additional protections for residents in LTC facilities.

All U.S. states and territories have enacted laws authorizing adult protective services in elder abuse situations (American Bar Association, 2022). Additionally, states have enacted mandated reporting laws for the reporting of potential abuse or neglect of the elderly population. These mandatory reporting acts identify certain professionals as mandatory reporters, and they commonly include physicians, nurses, mental health practitioners, and social workers. Occupational therapists and physical therapy practitioners are also responsible for reporting, although requirements vary from state to state, so it is important that occupational therapy practitioners know their state and local laws on mandatory reporting. Inpatient and LTC facilities are particularly susceptible to having quality of care issues and problems with the reporting of potential abuse or neglect (Office of the Inspector General, n.d.).

In 2019, Medicare revised its policies on Abuse and Neglect of Medicare Beneficiaries in these facilities to address these problems (Office of the Inspector General, n.d.). The Office of the Inspector General and the Centers for Medicare & Medicaid Services provide ongoing analysis, assessment, and revision of these policies. It is important from an ethical perspective that healthcare professionals monitor these updates and implement any changes that might affect their responses to cases regarding elder abuse. In locations where the government mandates abuse reporting, the occupational therapy practitioner may face legal jeopardy if they choose not to report abuse.

Forms of Abuse and Neglect

Abuse and neglect can take many different forms, and they can often be difficult to identify. Occupational therapy practitioners must have a basic understanding of the signs, risk factors, and forms of abuse and neglect so they can assist older adults in their care. Abuse can occur with anyone, regardless of the person's age, sex, gender, culture, religion, or ethnic background. It also can occur anywhere, including in the person's home, in assisted living facilities, and nursing homes. According to the National Institutes of Health (NIH): Institute on Aging (2022), types of abuse can include physical, emotional, sexual, and financial. For a full list of terms and definitions, please refer to Box 6-1. Additionally, neglect is prominent among older adults and can occur when the person or their caregiver(s) fail to meet the person's physical, psychological, social, or emotional needs. Abuse can include withholding food, medication, or access to needed medical care. In many cases, abuse and neglect can include abandonment of the person and exploitation of their resources - physical, emotional, or financial.

Signs and Risk Factors of Abuse & Neglect

Signs and risk factors associated with elder abuse and neglect are critical to decision-making and assistance in identifying, referring, and treating elder abuse. Common warning signs include the person seeming more depressed, confused, or

---

BOX 6-1 **Elder Abuse Definitions**

Elder abuse: Actions causing physical, psychological, emotional, or financial harm or neglect to an older adult. Elder abuse includes but is not limited to the following:

Abandonment: Leaving an older adult who requires care alone without any plans for assistance

Emotional abuse: Yelling, screaming, verbal threats, or ignoring an older adult in one's care; also referred to as psychological abuse

Exploitation: Misuse and/or mismanagement of property, belongings, and a person's assets without consent, under false pretenses, or through intimidation/manipulation tactics

Financial Abuse: Theft of money or belongings from a person; may include but is not limited to forging checks; taking someone's retirement/Social Security benefits; accessing and using someone's bank accounts without permission; stealing credit cards; changing names on a will, bank account, life insurance policy, or title to a house without permission

Neglect: Occurs when a caregiver stops responding to the needs of a vulnerable older adult in their care; may include but is not limited to physical, emotional, or social needs neglect or withholding food, medications, or access to medical care

Physical Abuse: Bodily harm that results from hitting, pushing, and/or slapping a person; may also include but is not limited to the use of restraints, being locked or confined to one's room, or being tied to furniture

Sexual Abuse: Being forced to watch or be part of sexual acts

withdrawn. Additionally, the practitioner should note if the person reports feeling isolated, specifically from family and friends. Are there unexplained bruises, burns, or scars? The occupational therapy practitioner should observe whether the person's appearance is altered, such as looking disheveled or unkempt. The appearance of new bed sores may suggest neglect. Lastly, the person may report a change in banking or spending patterns or indicate they cannot afford necessities. If any of these signs should occur, further investigation is warranted (Figure 6-1).

Screening or Assessment Instruments for Elder Abuse Detection

Screening or assessment instruments enhance the occupational therapy practitioner's ability to detect risk factors and signs of elder abuse and neglect. Such tools are important for ensuring practitioners do not miss clues to case identification. These instruments also assist with organizing the information collected about abuse victims and their circumstances and systematically documenting data for court proceedings or research purposes. The National Center on Elder Abuse (2016) indicates that currently, there is no gold standard tool for assessment. Additionally, most screening and assessment tools are designed to be used by healthcare providers and require additional training. Although these tools can identify cases of abuse and neglect, a positive screening does not ensure that actual abuse or neglect is occurring; further assessment is required. Moreover, asking the client, "do you feel safe at home?" is not sufficient, as some persons might interpret the question as if it is concerning accidental falls rather than abuse.

In 2020, the Task Force on Elder Abuse released a guide for screening cases of potential abuse and neglect,

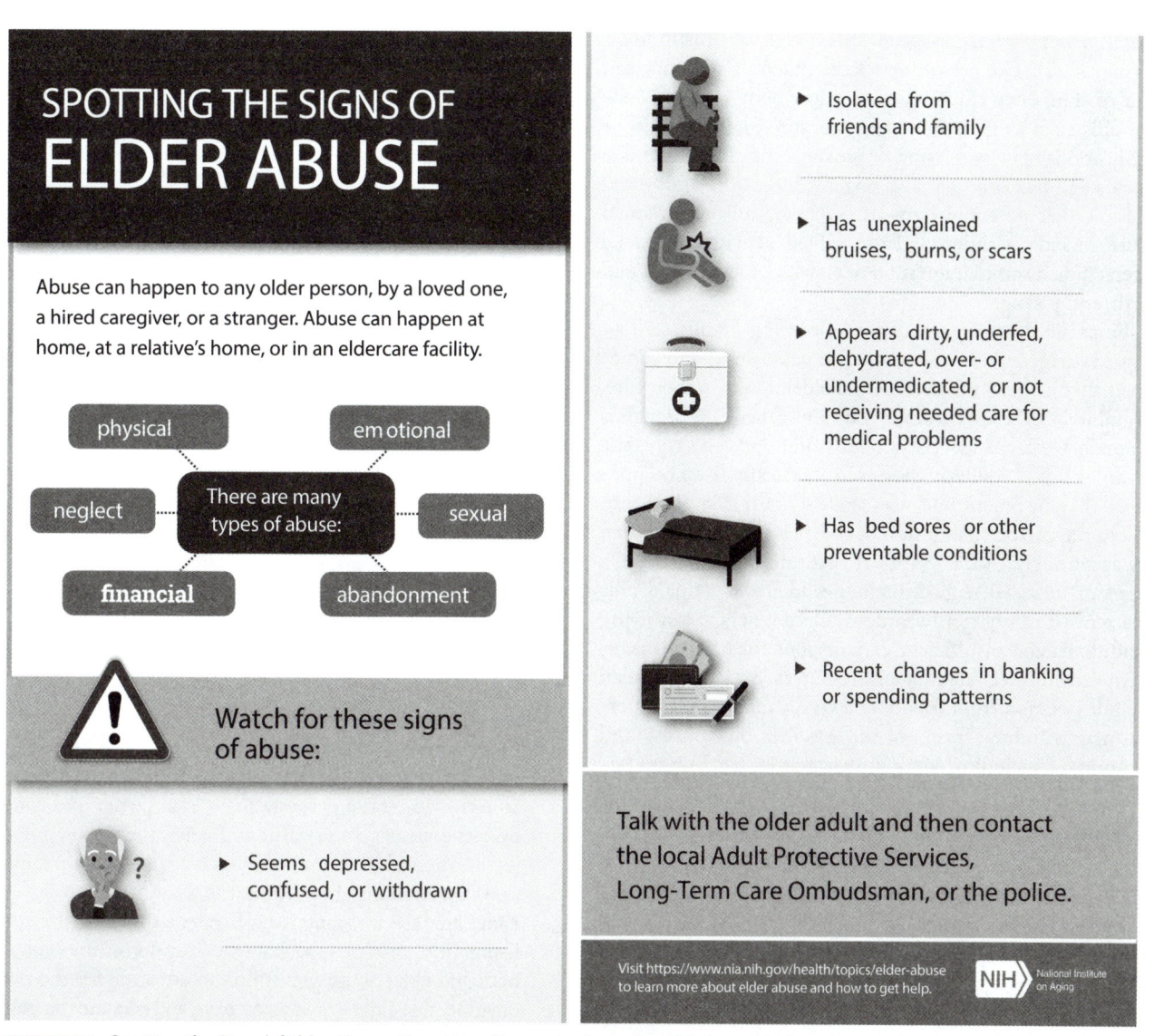

FIGURE 6-1 Spotting the Signs of Elder Abuse. *(From https://www.nia.nih.gov/health/infographics/spotting-signs-elder-abuse)*

including instructions for mediation. The pervasiveness of cases of elder abuse has called for better methods of screening, and many tools have been developed to address these needs. These new guidelines set forth by the Task Force on Elder Abuse assist healthcare professionals in identifying those at risk and offer strategies on how to move forward and deal with these cases. Among the most widely used instruments are the Hwalek-Sengstock Elder Abuse Screening Test Short, Elder Abuse Suspicion Index, Vulnerability to Abuse Screening Scale, Brief Abuse Screen for the Elderly, Caregiver Abuse Screen, and the Elder Assessment Instrument (National Center on Elder Abuse, 2016). Medicare developed the Elder Maltreatment Screen and Follow-up Plan (2019) that healthcare professionals have used widely with Medicare beneficiaries.

Signs

The signs of elder abuse and neglect can be physical, emotional, psychological, or social (NIH: National Institute on Aging, 2022). The person may look unkempt, with unclean hair or skin, dirty clothing, or very low body weight. Medical aids such as glasses, walkers, dentures, hearing aids, or medications may be missing or broken. Unexplained bruises or cuts and bed sores are also possible indicators of physical abuse. Other potential signs of psychological or emotional abuse include withdrawal from valued activities or social interaction, insomnia, agitation or violence, rocking back and forth, and pacing.

Financial abuse is particularly concerning. Family, staff, or unpaid caregivers have access to the possessions and sometimes the financial accounts of the older adults in their care. In home health, for example, staff and other care providers generally work unsupervised in the home and can easily take advantage of the elderly person in their care. If an occupational therapy practitioner sees these signs, it is important to talk to the person first to find out what is going on and then act accordingly (NIH: National Institute on Aging, 2022). Signs of financial neglect include evidence of unpaid bills like rent or mortgage; hazardous, unsafe, or unclean living conditions; and insufficient care or poor financial management despite adequate financial resources. Social neglect can include isolation from friends and family members. The person may withdraw from outside activities they once found meaningful, including community activities and events.

Risk Factors

Risk factors have greater power for predicting elder abuse when found in combination or with complex interaction; many risk factors have been proposed but can vary across nations, cultures, and religions. According to the WHO (2022b), risk factors occur at the individual level, the relationship level, and at the community level.

Multiple factors at the individual level can increase a person's risk for abuse and neglect. If the person is experiencing poor physical health or is functionally dependent for all self-care, home and food management, and other daily occupations, then healthcare professionals need to monitor the person closely. Second, the presence of a mental illness, poor mental health, or cognitive impairment can increase these risks. Low income and a history of substance abuse or dependency are also individual risk factors to consider (WHO, 2022a). Research indicates that most of these risk factors can lead to financial abuse and exploitation by the caregiver or partner. Close relationships can also place a person at a higher risk of abuse and neglect. The type of relationship and the person's marital status can be predictors. A spouse or partner or even a child or parent can be the perpetrator of abuse.

There are many sociocultural factors to consider when examining the community level. Ageism, which has been discussed in this chapter, is an indicator of abuse and neglect. Healthcare providers must be aware of how different cultural norms—such as in communities that have normalized violence—can place a person at a higher risk for abuse or neglect. Additional contextual factors include the absence or the presence of strong social support and living alone (WHO, 2022a).

Addressing Elder Abuse

Approaches

Seven major approaches have emerged over the past half century for understanding and responding to elder abuse (Anetzberger, 2018). Together they represent multiple distinct perceptions of elder abuse with different disciplines, systems, or programs leading each approach. No single approach dominates. There is broad consensus around the importance of multidisciplinary efforts to best address the issue. The approaches reflect the following:

- Elder abuse as a social problem. Key activities include receipt and investigation of reports, assessment of client status and service needs, arrangement or provision of services to treat harm or prevent its recurrence, and obtainment of legal interventions as indicated.
- Elder abuse as a geriatric syndrome. Definitive diagnosis (typically using screening tools to identify established signs and risk factors) and clinical management (employing intervention protocols) are essential methods for treating and improving the victim's presenting condition.
- Elder abuse as an aspect of family violence. The domestic violence approach defines the issue as one of the coercive tactics used by the perpetrator to gain power and control over the victim. Interventions focus on empowering the victim through information, support, and safety planning, as well as holding the perpetrator accountable.
- Elder abuse as an aging issue. Strategies include the establishment of programs such as the long-term care ombudsman and elder abuse prevention to advocate for the rights of vulnerable elders, raise awareness, and educate the public.
- Elder abuse as criminal action. The criminal justice approach focuses more on the perpetrator than the victim.

Activities seek to protect society, maintain order, enforce law, control crime, and punish perpetrators (while preserving their rights).

- Elder abuse as a human rights violation. This approach to elder abuse requires government action and social will to enact legislation for incidence reporting and interventions such as information centers and hotlines.
- Elder abuse as a public health concern. In this approach, the emphasis is on government initiatives to protect the public using problem-prevention strategies, such as public education, screening, social action, and surveillance (Anetzberger, 2018).

See Promoting Best Practice 6-1 for resources and information on who can help when a healthcare provider or family member suspects elder abuse.

PROMOTING BEST PRACTICE 6-1
Who Can Help? Resources when suspecting elder abuse.

Elder abuse and neglect will not go away. With rising numbers in the elderly population, it is essential that healthcare providers step up to assist their clients. The best way to start is just to talk with the person you suspect is experiencing abuse or neglect. Let them know that you are worried about them and feel as though there is something going on. Offer them help, resources, and contacts.

1. National Center on Elder Abuse
   855-500-3537
   https://ncea.acl.gov
2. Eldercare Locator
   800-677-1116 (open weekdays)
   eldercarelocator@n4a.org
   https://eldercare.acl.gov
3. National Adult Protective Services Association
   202-370-6292
   https://www.napsa-now.org
4. National Domestic Violence Hotline
   800-799-7233 (24/7)
   800-787-3224 (TTY)
   https://www.thehotline.org/get-help
5. Long-Term Care (LTC) Ombudsman Program
   U.S. Department of Health and Human Services,
   Administration for Community Living:
   https://acl.gov/programs/Protecting-Rights-and-Preventing-Abuse/Long-term-Care-Ombudsman-Program
   AARP webpage with links to U.S. State's LTC Ombudsman program:
   https://www.aarp.org/caregiving/health/info-2020/long-term-care-ombudsman.html
6. Call 911 for urgent needs
7. National Elder Fraud Hotline
   833-372-8311
   https://stopelderfraud.ovc.ojp.gov

Team Management of Elder Abuse

Multidisciplinary teams (MDT) assembled for the purpose of identifying elder abuse and developing recommendations have been the most effective in involving professional disciplines to address elder abuse (Galdamez et al, 2018). These specialized teams provide case analyses, program planning, education, and advocacy (Galdamez et al, 2018) and offer a more holistic perspective to the problem than is possible with a single system or discipline (Anetzberger, 2018). Challenges to MDT effectiveness can include lack of participation by key disciplines or systems, inadequate administrative support, and inability to sustain involvement over time (Anetzberger, 2011, 2018).

Occupational Therapy's Role

Occupational therapy practitioners have a key role in identifying persons at risk for abuse and noticing signs of abuse and neglect in their clients (Sanders, 2020). Because occupational therapy practitioners are often in the home, they may identify situations and physical markers that other team members do not see. Occupational therapy practitioners frequently include caregivers in their treatment plans. Being aware of dynamic family relationships is essential to identifying those families more at risk for abuse and neglect. Caregiver burnout is a key contributor to cases of elder abuse and neglect. Occupational therapy practitioners evaluate the person, environment, and occupations using a client-centered approach to ensure that the person and their caregivers are safe. Occupational therapy practitioners, therefore, are in a critical position to intervene and help these families (Waite, 2014). Practitioners can consult with the team to ascertain the best way in which to report problematic situations to protect the client and ameliorate the abuse. Occupational therapy practitioners may work with clients and caregivers to identify coping skills that reduce frustration and burnout that can lead to abuse, whereas other healthcare practitioners can encourage the use of physical activity as a stress relieving mechanism. Education is critical to identifying elder abuse and neglect, and it is important that occupational therapy practitioners know the signs and risk factors associated with it. The ethical principles of autonomy, beneficence, and nonmaleficence are often in conflict with one another in cases of abuse and neglect. Practitioners must be able to assess each situation objectively and identify when the risks of a potentially abusive situation outweigh personal autonomy and confidentiality (Waite, 2014). Understanding the complex nature of elder abuse and neglect will go a long way toward supporting and identifying persons who need help (Sanders, 2020).

Unique Ethical Considerations in Later Life

Working with older clients can raise a variety of ethical issues, some similar to those in any therapeutic encounter, others more unique to this particular area of practice. For example, the ethical principles of autonomy and beneficence (Beauchamp & Childress, 2019) may be in conflict when an older adult is making decisions about where to live. Whereas the older adult may wish to be independent, family members may want to balance this need with concerns for the person's safety (Gawande, 2014). Occupational therapy practitioners may face unique challenges in making intervention decisions. For example, decisions about whether an older adult should continue to drive have a profound impact on the person's quality of life but also on their safety and the safety of the community. Such a decision becomes an ethical question rather than a straightforward treatment decision.

Table 6-4 contains common ethical issues occupational therapy practitioners face when working with older adults. Client autonomy is an ethical principle of particular concern. Older adults may have their ability to make treatment decisions taken away from them when high-cost intervention disbursement is based solely on the person's age and a cost-benefit analysis that says the benefit would not be worth the cost (Craig, 2010; Jecker, 2013). For example, an organ transplant may not be an option for older adults based solely on their age. Conversely, families and healthcare providers may encourage and pressure older adults to accept a treatment intervention that may prolong their life but at a reduced quality of life (Gawande, 2014). For example, an older adult with a cancer diagnosis may choose to forgo chemotherapy in order to spend quality time with their family while they feel well, but their choice may mean they will not live as long. Although these examples of undertreatment and overtreatment occur frequently, a more insidious violation of autonomy may be more pervasive. Older adults' reports of pain and other symptoms often go ignored (Denny & Guido, 2012; Lehti et al, 2021). Healthcare workers likewise will often disregard depression and other mental health conditions in older adults (Lamoureux-Lamarche et al, 2021). Vulnerable older adults with diagnoses such as dementia are especially at risk for undertreatment (Denny & Guido, 2012). When an occupational therapy practitioner encounters such disregard for the needs and concerns of an older adult, it is important to speak up and advocate for their needs.

When a healthcare practitioner encounters an ethical problem and does not know what to do, the practitioner may experience moral distress. Jameton (1984) first defined moral distress as the distress and discomfort one feels when one knows the right thing to do but is prevented from doing it. Morley et al (2021) updated the definition to state, "Moral distress is the psychological distress that is causally related to a moral event" (p. 2). A newer concept, moral injury, refers to the cumulative impact of experiencing moral distress over and over with little time to process, leading to reduced ability to manage subsequent occurrences of moral distress (Roycroft et al, 2020). Moral distress and moral injury have come to the forefront in occupational therapy practice, especially during the COVID-19 pandemic (Smallwood et al, 2021). Occupational therapy practitioners have confronted ethical issues during the pandemic of changing policies and rules regarding precautions and personal protective equipment, the duty to self and family vs. duty to clients, HIPAA issues with telehealth, and finding themselves working closely with clients who were actively dying of COVID (Howard et al, 2020).

Guide to Ethical Decision Making

When faced with ethical problems of any kind, occupational therapy practitioners need not address these challenges unassisted. Occupational therapy practitioners should consider who they might have as resources within their practice setting. These resources may include an ethics committee, supervisor, senior colleague, or trusted mentor within the profession. Other sources, such as AOTA's Ethics Program (AOTA, 2022b), can point the occupational therapy practitioner to helpful resources.

The AOTA Occupational Therapy Code of Ethics (2020a) provides guidance on principles and standards of behavior for occupational therapy practitioners. An occupational therapy practitioner can use a code of ethics to defend one's choice of actions. In the United States, Occupational Therapy State Practice Acts also provide guidance. The AOTA *Occupational Therapy Practice Framework* (AOTA, 2020b) provides guidance on what is within the scope of

TABLE 6-4 ■ Common Ethical Issues When Working With Older Adults

ETHICAL ISSUE	EXAMPLE
Client autonomy	Client refuses to participate in occupational therapy services
	Client chooses to act against medical advice
	Client chooses unsafe living conditions
	Client's priorities differ from those of healthcare team
Medical mismanagement	Undertreatment
	Overtreatment
	Misdiagnosis
End-of-life care issues	Disagreement over advance care directives
Elder abuse, neglect, discrimination	Self-neglect of a person living alone
Clinical decision-making conflicts	Generational and cultural differences
	Differences of opinion on care choices between clients, families, and the healthcare team
Financial matters and ethical practice	Medicare billing and coding
	Medicare fraud

practice for an occupational therapy practitioner. Practitioners can make use of the laws, standards, and policies of their government, professional organizations, and employers to defend and justify their ethical decision-making process.

An ethical decision-making framework (Fig. 6-2) can assist the occupational therapy practitioner in taking the ethical problem out of the realm of emotional anguish and moral distress and provide a way to step back and consider all the options. Promoting Best Practice 6-2 demonstrates how to apply an ethical problem-solving framework using Ms. Parks' case. As a practitioner follows these steps, it is important to note that one will need to gather outside information and resources. Bringing an ethical issue to a satisfactory conclusion requires being able to consider the issue from multiple points of view, listening to others, and approaching potential outcomes with humility.

PROMOTING BEST PRACTICE 6-2
Ethical Problem-Solving: Applying the Ethical Decision-Making Framework to Ms. Parks' Case

1. **Identify** - Ms. Parks' case represents a true *ethical dilemma* - a conflict between two (or more) ethical principles. In this case, Ms. Parks' occupational therapy practitioner is concerned about beneficence - removing Ms. Parks from harm and providing due care. However, Ms. Parks is concerned about autonomy - being able to make her own decisions about her life.
2. **Gather** - The occupational therapy practitioner will need to gather information from their state laws to determine whether they are required to report abuse. They should also gather information from their organization regarding policies, ethics committees, and assistance available for managing ethical issues like this one.
3. **Resources** - The occupational therapy practitioner will need to determine what resources are available. Is there a social worker available to step into the case? Are there community resources, such as organizations or shelters that support victims of domestic violence? Does Ms. Parks have untapped resources such as other relatives or a religious organization?
4. **Options** - Examples of what the occupational therapy practitioner can do include: (1) do nothing; (2) provide the client with information about a domestic violence prevention and victim support organization in the local community; or (3) report what Ms. Parks said about her living situation to her doctor and to the organization's ethics committee to gain assistance to make a legal complaint against Ms. Parks' abusive family members.
5. **Prioritize** - The occupational therapy practitioner determines that option 1, doing nothing, would not fulfill the requirements of the code of ethics to provide beneficence to clients but that option 3 would violate Ms. Parks' autonomy. The occupational therapy practitioner opts to protect Ms. Parks' autonomy and discuss the situation further with Ms. Parks at her next visit, providing Ms. Parks with information on the local domestic violence prevention and victim support organization.
6. **Act & Reflect** - Ms. Parks is receptive to the information provided by the occupational therapy practitioner and states that she knows she needs to "do something" to change her circumstances. However, Ms. Parks does not return to occupational therapy services after this encounter, and the occupational therapy practitioner does not know if Ms. Parks ever resolved her living situation. The occupational therapy practitioner reflects that, although not content with this outcome, the occupational therapy practitioner can live with the results knowing they did everything they could to respect Ms. Parks' autonomy while assisting her to find options in her abusive situation.

Interprofessional Practice

Ethical issues are complex and require input and discussion from multiple perspectives (Pleschberger et al, 2011). In addition to the person who is the primary client (when they are able to participate) and their family members, team members from multiple professions provide insights into

Identify
- What ethics are in conflict? What is the concern?

Gather
- What information is known and what additional information is needed?

Resources
- What are available supports?

Options
- What are the consequences of each option?

Prioritize
- Values?
- Principles?

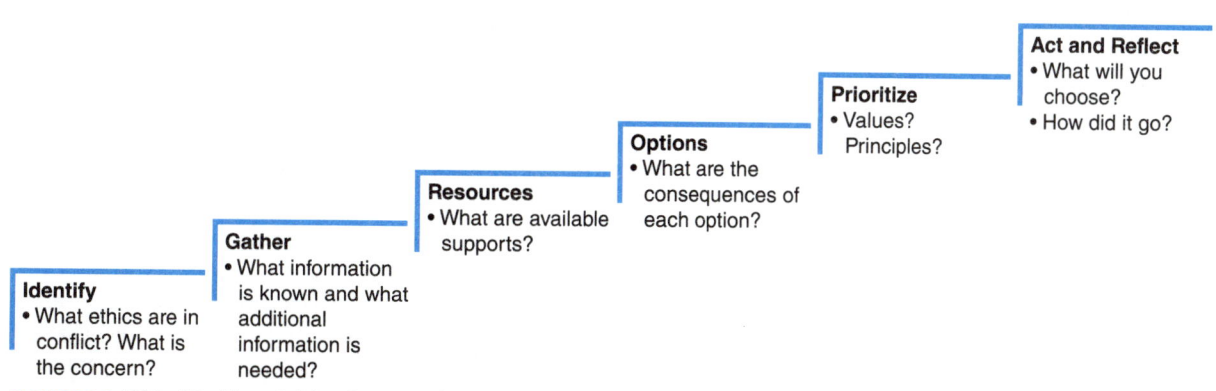

Act and Reflect
- What will you choose?
- How did it go?

FIGURE 6-2 Ethical Problem-Solving Framework. *(Yarett Slater, 2019; Doherty & Purtilo, 2016; graphic courtesy of Howard & Erler, 2021.)*

ethical decisions from many angles. Occupational therapy practitioners can contribute to the interprofessional team by assessing the older adult's occupational participation, activity performance, and quality of life, as well as considering how well the person's environment enables occupational performance. The interprofessional team helps the occupational therapy practitioner understand and address other considerations to understand the needs of the whole person within their context. Thus, the interprofessional team serves as a tremendous resource so the occupational therapy practitioner can make decisions on ethical issues in collaboration with others. Promoting Best Practice 6-3 contains a partial list of some interprofessional team members and their roles in aiding ethical decision making.

PROMOTING BEST PRACTICE 6-3
Interprofessional Team Members and Their Roles for Aiding in Ethical Decision Making

Interprofessional Team Member	Role	Ethical Decision Making
Physician	Coordinates the care team, diagnosis and prognosis determination	Listens to client's wishes; seeks help from ethics board or other entities when needed
Nurse	Provides information regarding the person's body structures and functions	Contributes to team discussion of an ethical issue regarding the person's physical and cognitive ability to manage their own medical care
Social worker	Provides information regarding the person's social context and resources	Shares abuse reporting systems and other community assistance resources with the team
Neuropsychologist	Assesses the person's capacity for executive function and decision making	Contributes to team's understanding of the person's cognitive capabilities for caring for their own safety and decision making
Occupational therapist	Determines the person's capacity for activity performance and occupational participation (physical, cognitive, psychosocial, occupational demands, and environmental considerations)	Contributes to team's ethical decision making by explaining the person's physical and cognitive abilities for safe ADL and instrumental ADL performance, including decision making, and environmental issues providing supports or barriers to occupational performance
Physical therapist	Determines the person's mobility needs and impairments	Contributes to team's ethical decision making by explaining the person's physical capabilities for safe home and community mobility
Clinical ethicist	Assists the interprofessional team in understanding the issues and possible paths to resolving those issues	Helps the team recognize the ethical principles in conflict and the values to consider when determining which ethical principle is most important in resolving the ethical issue
Pharmacist	Provides information regarding the impact of medication on the person, including intended effects and side effects	Contributes to team's ethical decision making by explaining the impact of prescribed medications, and in some cases, withholding medications or the person choosing to stop medications against medical advice

Interprofessional Team Member	Role	Ethical Decision Making
Dietitian	Provides information regarding the person's nutrition needs and how these needs may affect the person or their context	Contributes to team's ethical decision making by explaining options for providing or withholding nutrition, especially in end-of-life care

Ensuring that older adults have access to care and to a full range of occupations can present significant issues. Specific questions include whether to treat, what kinds of treatment to provide, when to terminate treatment, and whose wishes should be primary in framing occupational therapy assessment and intervention. By definition, ethical issues have no single "right" answer but require careful consideration based on appropriate ethical values. The interprofessional team affords the occupational therapy practitioner a variety of perspectives to aid in the ethical problem-solving process. Box 6-2 includes resource links for ethical decision making and legal supports for older adults.

> **BOX 6-2 Resource Links**
>
> **A)** For Ethical Issues and Problem-Solving
> National Association of Social Workers Essential Steps for Ethical Problem Solving: https://www.naswma.org/page/100/Essential-Steps-for-Ethical-Problem-Solving.htm
> World Federation of Occupational Therapists Code of Ethics: https://www.wfot.org/resources/code-of-ethics
> American Occupational Therapy Association Code of Ethics: https://www.aota.org/practice/practice-essentials/ethics
> Canadian Association of Occupational Therapists Code of Ethics: https://caot.in1touch.org/site/pt/codeofethics?nav=sidebar
> Occupational Therapy Australia Code of Ethics: chrome-extension://efaidnbmnnnibpcajpcglclefindmkaj/https://otaus.com.au/publicassets/73509493-3865-ed11-9475-005056be13b5/OTA%20Code%20of%20Ethics.pdf
> Royal College of Occupational Therapists Professional Standards for Occupational Therapy Practice, Conduct, and Ethics: https://www.rcot.co.uk/publications/professional-standards-occupational-therapy-practice-conduct-and-ethics
> National Board for Certification in Occupational Therapy (NBCOT) Code of Conduct: https://www.nbcot.org/-/media/NBCOT/PDFs/Code_of_Conduct.ashx?la=en
> Kennedy Institute of Ethics at Georgetown University: https://kennedyinstitute.georgetown.edu/
>
> **B)** For Older Adults for Legal Issues
> https://www.americanbar.org/content/dam/aba/administrative/law_aging/aba-elder-abuse-desk-guide.pdf

CASE STUDY (CONTINUED)

Intervention Plan and Status

The occupational therapy practitioner decided to reach out to Mr. Thompson's physical therapist and team social worker with their concerns, as they are concerned about the possibility of neglect. The social worker decided to meet with Mr. Thompson to assess his needs. Mr. Thompson indicated once again that he did not want to be a burden to his son because of his son's commitments. He stated he relied on Social Security for living expenses and did not identify any additional resources available to him at the time.

The team decided to complete a home visit to assess Mr. Thompson's home and make recommendations for modifications. When the team arrived at his house, it was clear that the house was in poor condition. The entrance was not accessible, and the inside was cluttered. There was evidence of rodents in the home, there were bags of garbage in the kitchen, Mr. Thompson had little food, and it was clear that he was not cleaning the home.

The team was worried about Mr. Thompson's living conditions and wanted to reach out to adult protective services to intervene, as they believed the home was not safe for him. They were also concerned about neglect, as Mr. Thompson was clearly unable to care for himself adequately, and it appeared the son was not checking in on him regularly. He appeared to be an endangered adult, so the social worker advised the team to consider the legal and ethical implication of their actions.

Questions

1. What further information do you need to gather to make decisions regarding Mr. Thompson's needs? Consider the legal and ethical issues that arose in this chapter (see especially the Laws and Policy Affecting Older Adults section).

2. Determine what the best course of action would be in this case if you were the occupational therapy practitioner working with Mr. Thompson. What actions would you take to resolve the ethical issue? (Guide to Ethical Decision Making)

Answers

1. Consider the legal and ethical issues that arose in this chapter. The occupational therapy practitioner must work with the healthcare team to find out more information before making decisions regarding Mr. Thompson. According to the Ethical Problem-Solving Framework (see Fig. 6.2), the team must first consider the ethical issues that are in conflict. The ethical principle of autonomy affords a person the

right to self-determination, privacy, confidentiality, and informed consent. The principle of beneficence indicates that a person's well-being and safety are paramount, and that the person should be removed from harm. Second, the team must consider how they might gather further information. The team might consider using a screening tool that could help identify abuse and neglect and provide guidance for mediation. The team should explore what resources the Area Agency on Aging may have available for Mr. Thompson. State and local programs may also be in place to assist older adults at risk for abuse and neglect. The Elder Justice Act of 2006 provided for grants and additional funding for adult protective services; the team should explore these resources as well. The team also needs to find out if their state requires mandatory reporting of Mr. Thompson's situation regardless of his wishes. To gather more information, the team can make use of resources listed in Promoting Best Practice Box 6.1: Who Can Help? These resources include the National Center on Elder Abuse, Eldercare Locator, and National Adult Protective Services Association.

2. According to the Ethical Problem Solving Framework, the team has now completed steps (1) identify, (2) gather, and (3) resources. The team now needs to (4) decide what their options are and the possible consequences for each option, (5) prioritize their choices based on ethical values and principles, and then (6) carry out the action and reflect on the outcome. The team knows that although they cannot arrive at a decision that all will be happy about, they can work with all parties to come to an agreement that all can live with. For example, the team may decide to prioritize Mr. Thompson's safety and well-being over his autonomy and may need to report his living situation to adult protective services. They may then work with Mr. Thompson and his son to negotiate bringing in more services, such as meals provided through the local Area Agency on Aging and companion and cleaning services through the Eldercare Locator. They may even find through mediation that Mr. Thompson's son did not know how dire his situation had become and would be more than willing to be more active in his care. In a best-case scenario, Mr. Thompson may not like having more people come into his home, but he may be willing to have these services to be able to continue living in his home.

SUMMARY

Ethical and legal issues are vital components of the context of care for older adults. This chapter has discussed laws and policies pertaining to older adults, end-of-life care, elder abuse and neglect, common ethical issues that arise when caring for older adults, an ethical problem-solving guide, and the role of the interprofessional team in managing ethical issues. Occupational therapy practitioners must be attentive to these factors as they plan and implement interventions to support function and quality of life. By staying aware of legal and ethical issues, occupational therapy practitioners work with the interprofessional team to ensure an environment of care that promotes the best outcomes for older adults.

Critical Thinking Questions

1. Analyze the role of the occupational therapy practitioner in preventing and mediating ageism.

2. Evaluate the outcome of Ms. Parks' case (see Promoting Best Practice 6-2). What ethical principles were at stake? Which ethical principle do you think was most important in this case? Did the outcome of the case uphold that principle?

REFERENCES

Administration for Community Living. (2021, July 8). *Older Americans Act | ACL Administration for Community Living.* https://acl.gov/about-acl/authorizing-statutes/older-americans-act

Age Discrimination Act of 1975, 42 U.S.C. § 6101–6107 (1975).

Age Discrimination in Employment Act, 29 U.S.C. § 621 to 29 U.S.C. § 634 (1968).

Administration for Community Living. (2022). Long-term care ombudsman program. https://acl.gov/programs/Protecting-Rights-and-Preventing-Abuse/Long-term-Care-Ombudsman-Program

Ageing Equal. (n.d.). Ageism and social rights. Retrieved April 13, 2022, from https://ageing-equal.org/ageism-and-social-rights/

Allen, J. O., Solway, E., Kirch, M., Kullgren, J. T., Moise, V., & Malani, P. N. (2022). Experiences of everyday ageism and the health of older US adults. *JAMA Network Open Geriatrics, 5*(6), e2217240. https://doi.org/doi:10.1001/jamanetworkopen.2022.17240

American Association of Retired Persons. (2022, April 15). How to find the long-term care ombudsman in every state. Retrieved August 5, 2022, from https://www.aarp.org/caregiving/health/info-2020/long-term-care-ombudsman.html

American Bar Association. (2022). Introduction to ABA section on Dispute Resolution Task Force: Elder Abuse and Neglect Screening Guidelines for Mediators. Retrieved from: https://www.americanbar.org/content/dam/aba/administrative/law_aging/2020-elder-abuse-screening-tool-abadr-section.pdf

American Hospital Association. (2022). Put it in writing. Retrieved from: https://www.aha.org/2017-12-11-put-it-writing

American Medical Association. (2019). Elder maltreatment screen and follow-up plan. https://qpp.cms.gov/docs/QPP_quality_measure_specifications/CQM-Measures/2020_Measure_181_MIPSCQM.pdf

American Occupational Therapy Association. (2020a). AOTA 2020 occupational therapy code of ethics. *American Journal of Occupational Therapy, 74*(Suppl. 3), 7413410005. https://doi.org/10.5014/ajot.2020.74S3006

American Occupational Therapy Association. (2020b). Occupational therapy practice framework: Domain and process (4th ed.). *American Journal of Occupational Therapy, 74*(Suppl. 2), 7412410010. https://doi.org/10.5014/ajot.2020.74S2001

American Occupational Therapy Association. (2022a). *Advocacy issues: Scope of practice.* Retrieved from https://www.aota.org/advocacy/issues/scope-of-practice-advocacy

American Occupational Therapy Association. (2022b). *Practice essentials: Ethics.* Retrieved from https://www.aota.org/practice/practice-essentials/ethics

Anetzberger, G. J. (2011). The evolution of a multidisciplinary response to elder abuse. *Marquette Elder's Advisor, 13,* 107–128.

Anetzberger, G. J. (2018). The intersection of public health and nontraditional partners and approaches to address elder abuse. In P. B. Teaster & J. Hall (Eds.), *Elder abuse and the public's health* (pp. 125–152). Springer Publishing Company.

Ayalon, L., & Cohn-Schwartz, E. (2021). Measures of self- and other-directed ageism and worries concerning COVID-19 health consequences: Results from a nationally representative sample of Israelis over the age of 50. *PLoS One, 16*(5), e0251577.

Beauchamp, T., & Childress, J. (2019). *Principles of biomedical ethics* (8th ed.). New York: Oxford University Press.

Casey, D. (2019). Hospice and palliative care: What's the difference? *MEDSURG Nursing, 28*(3), 196–197. https://www.proquest.com/docview/2242625554?pq-origsite=gscholar&fromopenview=true

Craig, H. D. (2010). Caring enough to provide healthcare: An organizational framework for the ethical delivery of healthcare among aging patients. *International Journal for Human Caring, 14,* 27–30.

Denny, D., & Guido, G. (2012). Undertreatment of pain in older adults: An application of beneficence. *Nursing Ethics, 19*(6), 800–809. doi: 10.1177/0969733012447015

Doherty, R., & Purtilo, R. (2016). *Ethical dimensions in the health professions* (6th Ed.). St. Louis, MO: Elsevier Saunders.

Elder Justice Act, S.2010, 109th Cong. (2006): https://www.congress.gov/congressional-report/109th-congress/senate-report/337

Five Wishes. (2022, July 31). Five wishes. Retrieved from: https://www.fivewishes.org/

Fraser, S., Lagacé, M., Bongué, B., Ndeye, N., Guyot, J., Bechard, L., Garcia, L., Taler, V., CCNA Social Inclusion and Stigma Working Group, Adam, S., Beaulieu, M., Bergeron, C. D., Boudjemadi, V., Desmette, D., Donizzetti, A. R., Éthier, S., Garon, S., Gillis, M., Levasseur, M., ... Tougas, F. (2020). Ageism and COVID-19: What does our society's response say about us? *Age Ageing, 49*(5), 692–695. https://doi.org/10.1093/ageing/afaa097

Fulmer, T., Reuben, D. B., Auerbach, J., Fick, D. M., Galambos, C., & Johnson, K. S. (2021c). Actualizing better health and health care for older adults. *Health Aff (Millwood), 40*(2), 219–225. https://doi.org/10.1377/hlthaff.2020.01470

Galdamez, G., Avent, E., Rowan, J., Wilbur, K. H., Mosqueda, L., Olsen, B., & Gassoumis, Z. D. (2018). Elder abuse multidisciplinary teams and networks: Understanding national intervention approaches. *Innov Aging, 2*(Suppl 1), 763. doi: 10.1093/geroni/igy023.2823

Gawande, A. (2014). *Being mortal: Medicine and what matters in the end.* New York: Metropolitan Books.

Howard, B., Argabrite-Grove, R., Bennett, L., Erler, K., Keith, J., Ritvo, R., Kennell, B., & Ewy, D. (2020). An ethical response to the COVID-19 pandemic: An AOTA Ethics Advisory Opinion. *OT Practice, 25*(6), 30–35. https://www.aota.org/~/media/Corporate/Files/Practice/Ethics/Advisory/Ethical-Response-to-COVID-19.pdf

Howard, B., & Erler, K. (2021, April 6). Moral distress in occupational therapy: Practicing in a post pandemic world. [Short Course]. AOTA 2021 Inspire Conference.

Inker, J. L. K. (2018). *Ageism among healthcare professionals: The influence of personal aging anxiety, job role, and work setting on attitudes toward older patients* [Virginia Commonwealth University]. https://doi.org/10.25772/F1VX-WY69

Jameton, A. (1984). *Nursing practice: The ethical issues.* Englewood Cliffs, N.J.: Prentice Hall.

Jecker, N. S. (2013). Justice between age groups: An objection to the Prudential lifespan approach. *Am J Bioeth, 13*(8), 3–15.10.1080/15265161.2013.802061

Kadıoğlu, F. G., Can, R., Nazik, S., & Kadıoğlu, S. (2013). Ethical problems in geriatrics: Views of Turkish primary healthcare professionals. *Geriatr Gerontol Int, 13*(4), 1059–1068.

Lamoureux-Lamarche, C., Berbiche, D., & Vasiliadis, H. M. (2021, September 15). Treatment adequacy and remission of depression and anxiety disorders and quality of life in primary care older adults. *Health Qual Life Outcomes, 19,* 218. https://doi.org/10.1186/s12955-021-01851-4

Lehti, T. E., Rinkinen, M. O., Aalto, U., Roitto, H. M., Knuutila, M., Öhman, H., Kautiainen, H., Karppinen, H., Tilvis, R., Strandberg, T., & Pitkälä, K. H. (2021). Prevalence of musculoskeletal pain and analgesic treatment among community-dwelling older adults: Changes from 1999 to 2019. *Drugs Aging, 38*(10), 931–937. https://doi.org/10.1007/s40266-021-00888-w

Lendon, J. P., Caffrey, C., & Lau D. T. (2018, September 12). Advance directive documentation among adult day services centers and use among participants, by region and center characteristics: National study of long-term care providers, 2016. *Natl Health Stat Report,* (117), 1–6. Retrieved from https://stacks.cdc.gov/view/cdc/58975

Levy, S., Lytle, A., Macdonald, J., & Apriceno, M. (2020). Reducing ageism: PEACE (Positive Education about Aging and Contact Experiences) model. *Innovation in Aging, 4,* 647–647. https://doi.org/10.1093/geroni/igaa057.2226

Lo, M. M. (2010). Cultural brokerage: Creating linkages between voices of lifeworld and medicine in cross-cultural clinical settings. *Health, 14,* 484–504. doi: 10.1177/1363459309360795

Marchiondo, L. A., Gonzales, E., & Williams, L. J. (2019). Trajectories of perceived workplace age discrimination and long-term associations with mental, self-rated, and occupational health. *J Gerontol B Psychol Sci Soc Sci, 74*(4), 655–663.

McArdle, P. (2012). Ageing: The new ethical frontier. *Journal of Religion, Spirituality & Aging, 24,* 20–29. doi: 10.1080/15528030.2012.633042

Medicare and Medicaid Act of 1965, 79 Stat. 286 (1965). https://www.govinfo.gov/features/medicare-law

Mistry, P. (2020, March 11). Ageism in the workplace: Laws and resources for employees. *The HR Digest.* https://www.thehrdigest.com/ageism-in-the-workplace-laws-and-resources-for-employees/

Morley, G., Bradbury-Jones, C., & Ives, J. (2021). The moral distress model: An empirically informed guide for moral distress interventions. *J Clin Nurs, 31*(9–10), 1309–1326. https://doi.org/10.1111/jocn.15988

National Center on Elder Abuse. (2016). Elder abuse screening tools for healthcare professionals. Retrieved from: http://eldermistreatment.usc.edu/wp-content/uploads/2016/10/Elder-Abuse-Screening-Tools-for-Healthcare-Professionals.pdf

National Council on Aging. (2022). *Issues for advocates: Get the facts on elder abuse.* Retrieved from https://www.ncoa.org/article/get-the-facts-on-elder-abuse

National Institute of Health. (2022, July 31). *Elder abuse.* Retrieved from: https://www.nia.nih.gov/health/elder-abuse#types

NIH: National Institute on Aging from U.S. Department of Health & Human Services. (2022). *Advanced care planning: Health directives.* Retrieved April 4, 2022, from nia.nih.gov/health/advance-care-planning-health-care-directives

Office of the Inspector General. (n.d.). *Advocating for the nation's elder population.* Retrieved from https://oig.hhs.gov/fraud/care/

Older Americans Act of 1965, 42 USC §3001 as amended (2020). Washington, D.C.: Administration on Aging, Office of Human Development Services, U.S. Department of Health, Education, and Welfare. https://acl.gov/sites/default/files/about-acl/2020-04/Older%20Americans%20Act%20Of%201965%20as%20amended%20by%20Public%20Law%20116-131%20on%203-25-2020.pdf

Pleschberger, S., Seymour, J. E., Payne, S., Deschepper, R., Onwuteaka-Philipsen, B. D., & Rurup, M. L. (2011). Interviews on end-of-life care with older people: Reflections on six European studies. *Qual Health Res, 21,* 1588–1600. doi: 10.1177/1049732311415286

Previtali, F., Allen, L. D., & Varlamova, M. (2020). Not only virus spread: The diffusion of ageism during the outbreak of COVID-19. *J Aging Soc Policy, 32*(4–5), 506–514. https://doi.org/10.1080/08959420.2020.1772002

Roycroft, M., Wilkes, D., Pattani, S., Fleming, S., & Olsson-Brown, A. (2020). Limiting moral injury in healthcare professionals during the

COVID-19 pandemic. *Occup Med (Lond), 70*(5), 312–314. https://doi.org/10.1093/occmed/kqaa087

Sanders, M. (2020). *What is elder abuse, and how can you address it in fieldwork?* Retrieved from: https://www.aota.org/publications/student-articles/career-advice/elder-abuse

Smallwood, N., Pascoe, A., Karimi, L., & Willis, K. (2021). Moral distress and perceived community views are associated with mental health symptoms in frontline health workers during the COVID-19 pandemic. *Int J Environ Res Public Health, 18*(16), 8723. https://doi.org/10.3390/ijerph18168723

Social Security Act of 1965, 42 USC Ch. 7 (1935). https://www.ssa.gov/history/35act.html

Waite, A. (2014). Elder abuse: Knowing when, why, and how to intercede. *OT Practice 19*, 9–12. http://dx.doi.org/10.7138/otp.2014.193f1

Workforce Investment Act of 1998, 20 USC § 9201 (1998).

World Health Organization. (2022a, July 31). *Abuse of older people.* Retrieved from https://www.who.int/news-room/fact-sheets/detail/abuse-of-older-people

World Health Organization. (2022b). *Ageing.* Retrieved April 27, 2022, from https://www.who.int/health-topics/ageing

Yarett Slater, D. (2019). Organizational ethics. In K. Jacobs & G. L. McCormack (Eds.), *The occupational therapy manager* (6th ed., pp. 539–545). Bethesda, MD: AOTA Press.

PART II

Aging: Body Structures and Body Functions

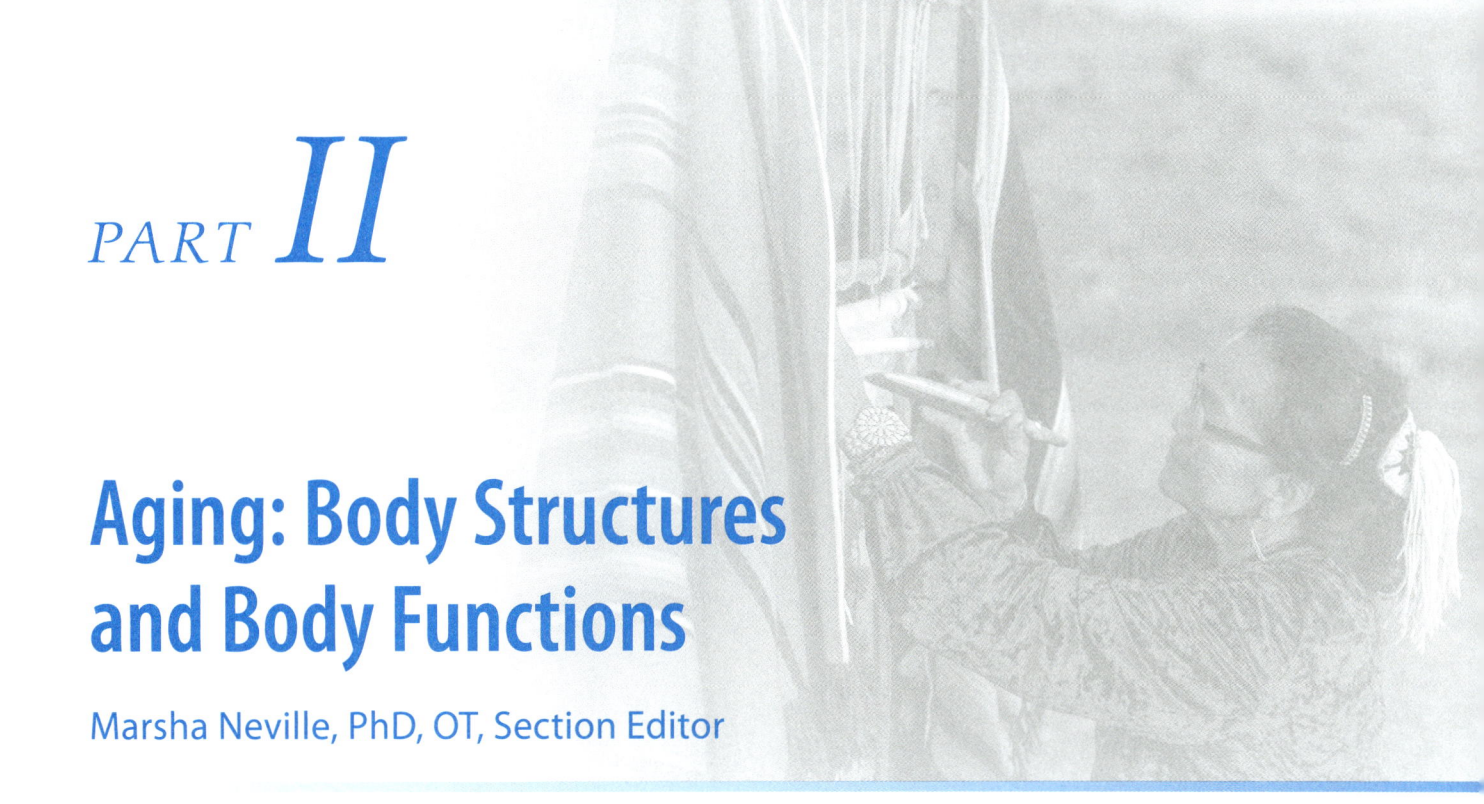

Marsha Neville, PhD, OT, Section Editor

Section I reviewed the sociocultural factors affecting persons later in life, as well as theoretical considerations. The focus now turns to individuals and to factors affecting healthy aging. Section II will delve into the effects of normal aging on body structures and body function, along with pathologies known to affect the healthy aging process.

The International Classification of Function (World Health Organization, 2020), the Occupational Therapy Practice Framework (American Occupational Therapy Association, 2020), and the Profile of Practice (Canadian Association of Occupational Therapists, 2012) all acknowledge that an individual's ability to participate fully in life is dependent to some extent on his or her biological and psychological function. A clear understanding of normal and pathological aging is one essential factor in a therapist's ability to frame effective interventions to support participation in meaningful occupations.

The next seven chapters provide an in-depth review of major body systems, the effect of normal aging on the systems, and pathologies affecting the systems. In addition, assessments and interventions for best practice in occupational therapy will be discussed, along with the role of the multidisciplinary team in addressing the occupational performance of older adults.

Look for the following when reading chapters:

- Changes in the body systems occur in the context of the sociocultural factors described in Chapters 1 through 6.
- Normal aging affects body structures and function. The various systems change to varying degrees for individuals. The reader will analyze factors contributing to changes, including environment, culture, lifestyle, education, genetics, and other factors contributing to changes due to aging.
- While the systems undergo changes due to normal aging, body systems can also be affected by pathologies. The reader will come to understand the differences between normal and pathological aging.
- There are interactions among the systems. Although they are presented here as if these systems function independently, the reality is far more complex. The reader will come to understand how systems are interrelated and the collective impact of these systems on occupational performance.
- And perhaps most important, changes in body systems, whether normal or pathological, alter a person's ability to participate in meaningful and rewarding occupations. Some individuals are able to find ways to manage change so that valued activities can be continued into very old age. Others struggle to cope with very minor differences in physical, cognitive, or sensory capacity. The reader will learn to assess client and environmental factors contributing to successful modifications and factors that deter adjustment to changes in body systems.

American Occupational Therapy Association. (2020). Occupational therapy practice framework: Domain and process (4th ed.). *American Journal of Occupational Therapy,* August 2020, 74(2 Suppl.), 1–87. https://doi.org/10.5014/ajot.2020.74S2001

Canadian Association of Occupational Therapists. (2012). *Profile of Practice of Occupational Therapists in Canada.* https://caot.ca/document/3653/2012otprofile.pdf

World Health Organization. (2020). Healthy ageing and functional ability. https://www.who.int/news-room/questions-and-answers/item/healthy-ageing-and-functional-ability

CHAPTER 7

Special Concerns in Care and Prevention

Carol Getz Rice, PhD, OTR/L ■ Janice Kishi Chow, PhD, DOT, OTR/L

"Old age ain't no place for sissies."
—Bette Davis

LEARNING OUTCOMES

By the end of this chapter, readers will be able to:

7-1. Identify preventative strategies to manage special concerns common among older adults.
7-2. Evaluate older adult frailty treatment options for best evidence-based, client-centered interventions.
7-3. Evaluate older adult medication management options for best evidence-based, client-centered interventions.
7-4. Evaluate older adult oral health and nutrition treatment options for best evidence-based, client-centered interventions.
7-5. Evaluate older adult hydration treatment options for the best evidence-based, client-centered interventions.
7-6. Evaluate older adult urinary management options for the best evidence-based, client-centered interventions regarding urinary tract infections and urinary incontinence.
7-7. Evaluate older adult fall prevention options for the best evidence-based, client-centered interventions.
7-8. Determine the implications for daily participation and health for older adults with these special concerns.
7-9. Generate strategies that foster interprofessional collaboration to manage special concerns common among older adults.

Mini Case Study

Peter is a 78-year-old male admitted to the emergency department today with dehydration, diarrhea, shortness of breath, and weakness. He has a history of hypertension, chronic obstructive pulmonary disease, and congestive heart failure. Peter retired 10 years ago and lost his dental insurance at that time. Paying for dental care out of pocket and living on a fixed income, he defers regular dental checkups to save on expenses. Peter now has a number of cavities, bleeding gums, and pain with chewing. Peter says he is having difficulty eating and has lost a significant amount of weight in the last 6 months. Peter also lives in an area of the city with contaminated water. Along with difficulty eating, he does not have access to clean drinking water, which has resulted in repeated bouts of diarrhea with concomitant dehydration.

Provocative Questions
1. What are Peter's various health issues?
2. How are these health issues linked or related?
3. How could occupational therapy practitioners help Peter manage these health issues to foster better quality of life and wellness?

Introduction

This chapter will discuss common health issues leading to special concerns for older adults. These health issues frequently co-occur in later life and include frailty, medication use, oral health, malnutrition, dehydration, urinary issues, and fall risk. At first glance, this chapter seems to introduce random health issues with no relationship to one another that perhaps do not fit elsewhere in this textbook. Yet these topics underscore the complexity of aging body structures and functions and the interdependence of multiple body functions, resulting in decreased participation, limitations in function, and occupational deprivation. The older adult's capacity for resiliency, adaptability, and healing diminishes with age because of inefficient body structures and body functions. Extra cognitive attention and effort are needed to participate in tasks because of the bodily inefficiencies caused by the aging process. Awareness is needed to understand the intersection of these common health issues, the physical and psychosocial effects on occupational participation, the consequent development of special concerns, and the role occupational therapy practitioners may play to support productive aging. The chapter is written with the lens of the Person-Environment-Occupation (PEO) model (Law et al, 1996) while using the constructs of the International Classification of Functioning, Disability, and Health (World Health Organization [WHO], 2001).

Frailty With Aging

Frailty is a geriatric syndrome characterized by multisystem dysregulation, decreased physiological reserve, and general decline. Weakness and fatigue can lead older adults to reduce their occupational participation and socialization, resulting in occupational deprivation. That is, the older adult's world narrows with fewer contexts, persons, and activities for engagement due to impaired occupational performance. As occupational participation lessens, occupational performance further declines as part of a vicious cycle.

Influencers of Frailty With Aging

Medication use, nutrition, hydration, oral health, and urinary management may support and maintain health in frailty or exacerbate it. But the aging process may cause inefficiencies in body functions and structures, leading to further debility and heightened risk for falls. Systemic chronic inflammation, obesity, and some diseases (e.g., cardiovascular disease and cancer) may exacerbate impairment. Thus, frailty increases an individual's vulnerability for dependency, disability, falls, institutionalization, hospitalization, and death (Bongue et al, 2017).

Assessment of Older Adult Frailty

Frailty is identified through a screen commonly based upon physical frailty as a biological state (Fried et al, 2001; Op het Veld et al, 2015) or deficit accumulation (Rockwood & Mitnitski, 2007), and can be measured with the Edmonton Frail Scale (Rolfson et al, 2006). The time-consuming Comprehensive Geriatric Assessment is considered the most evidenced-based process for identifying and grading the severity of frailty; however, the Vulnerable Elders-13 Survey for community dwellers has stronger prediction for falls (Bongue et al, 2017). Using Fried's criteria, a person with frailty has at least three of five outcomes: diminished strength, slowness, low physical activity, self-reported exhaustion, and unintentional weight loss (Travers et al, 2019). Each frailty assessment tool measures a different combination of domains, so results cannot be interpreted interchangeably (Bongue et al, 2017). Evaluation of the client's physiological response to activity (e.g., respiration rate, peripheral oxygen saturation [SpO_2], heart rate, blood pressure, rate of perceived exertion) is needed as the frail older adult decompensates more quickly than a well older adult.

Implications for the Older Adult in Treatment: Frailty

It is vital for occupational therapy practitioners to address frailty to mitigate declining occupational performance and participation. In an international systematic review, Travers et al (2019) identified clinically feasible, evidence-based interventions as strength training, mixed exercise, health education (e.g., nutrition, medication management, fall risk, supports, social supports), and nutritional supplementation (most notably protein supplementation). The studies identified efficacy for either one or a combination of strategies, with the combination of strength training and protein supplementation being the most effective and easiest to implement. Fritz et al's 2019 scoping review identified effective occupational therapy interventions for frailty in community dwellers such as providing recommendations and training for assistive devices and assistive technology, conducting self-care training, and conducting home hazard evaluation with recommendations for home modifications. See Promoting Best Practice 7-1.

PROMOTING BEST PRACTICE 7-1
Interdisciplinary Teams in Assessment and Treatment of Frailty Syndrome

Assessment and intervention for frailty syndrome are addressed best by an interdisciplinary team (e.g., geriatrician, nurse, social worker, pharmacist, dietitian, and occupational and physical therapists) so that frailty may be reversed or attenuated (Travers et al, 2019). Per Bray and Bonder (2018), "Goals are to improve function, reduce hospitalization and adverse events, improve quality of life, and decrease early mortality" (p. 270). It is in the scope of practice for occupational therapy practitioners to provide these evidence-based interventions: health education, home hazard evaluation with recommendations and training, assistive device and technology training, basic and instrumental activities of daily living (IADLs) training, and strength or exercise training (Fritz et al, 2019; Travers et al, 2019).

Addressing frailty and other special concerns for older adults can lead to ethical dilemmas. For example, the client's preferred food and beverage choice may yield best consumption but conflict with dysphagia precautions (e.g., preferring a regular diet over pureed foods). Volkert et al (2018) noted that participants tended to drink less when limited to thickened liquids and ate less when restricted to a texture-modified diet (e.g., pureed), increasing the risk of dehydration and malnutrition respectively. Occupational therapists are key team members for identifying the client's preferred food and beverage choices, optimizing the person fit with tableware/cutlery/drinking ware, plus enabling the most desirable context for eating and drinking beverages (Rice, 2017). Risk assessment is needed to identify, weigh, and balance the client's benefits and risks so that choice for activity participation may be enabled. Tancock and Roberts (2019) provide a free online guide regarding risk enablement plans in the authors' *Living Well Through Activity in Care Homes: the toolkit* for care home staff (see Box 7-1 at the end of the chapter for more information). Within a risk enablement plan, the health-care team, including an occupational therapist, should consider the:

- Risks and benefits
- Risk likelihood
- Risk seriousness/severity
- Preventive measures to minimize risks
- Actions if risks occur (Tancock & Roberts, 2019)

BOX 7-1 Resources

Frailty

United Kingdom College of Occupational Therapist's Living Well in Care Homes-Tool Kit
http://www.COT.org.uk/living-well-care-homes
(For the risk enablement plan, on the first website page go to "Finding the right resources for you," select "care home staff," then select "Balancing risk and choice.")

Medication Management

Agency for Healthcare Research and Quality: Medication Management Strategy: Intervention
https://www.ahrq.gov/patient-safety/reports/engage/interventions/medmanage.html
Centers for Disease Control and Prevention: Medication Safety Program
https://www.cdc.gov/medicationsafety/index.html

Oral Health

American Dental Association: Oral Health Topics
https://www.ada.org/resources/research/science-and-research-institute/oral-health-topics
Centers for Disease Control and Prevention: Oral Health
https://www.cdc.gov/oralhealth/index.html

Nutrition and Hydration

Mini Nutritional Assessment Forms and Scoring
https://www.mna-elderly.com/mna-forms
https://www.mna-elderly.com/sites/default/files/2021-10/mna-guide-english.pdf
CDC Global Health & Nutrition Resources (for older adults and caregivers)
https://www.cdc.gov/nutrition/micronutrient-malnutrition/resources/index.html
Modified Food Guide Pyramid for 70+ Adults
https://www.semanticscholar.org/paper/Modified-Food-Guide-Pyramid-for-people-overseventy-Russell-Rasmussen/c5997248a1003b87aa06c9f5cd47f3e252301715
MyPlate for Older Adults
https://hnrc.tufts.edu/myplate/about/download-myplate
https://hnrca.tufts.edu/resources/my-plate-older-adults
United Kingdom DRIE Study (it provides assessment and tracking tools, best practice toolkits, activities, etc.)
http://driestudy.appspot.com/links.html
USDA Dietary Guidelines for Americans, 2020–2025
https://www.dietaryguidelines.gov/

Urinary Management

Office on Women's Health: Urinary Incontinence
https://www.womenshealth.gov/a-z-topics/urinary-incontinence
Urology Care Foundation: Urinary Incontinence
https://www.urologyhealth.org/urology-a-z/u/urinary-incontinence

Falls Assessment and Intervention

AOTA Quality Toolkit: Standardized Assessment and Screening Tools
https://www.aota.org/practice/practice-essentials/quality/quality-toolkit
New Jersey Division of Aging Services: A Matter of Balance
https://www.nj.gov/humanservices/doas/services/balance/
STEADI Resources for Falls (material for older adults and caregivers)
https://www.cdc.gov/steadi/materials.html
https://www.cdc.gov/steadi/pdf/STEADI-PocketGuide-508.pdf
https://www.cdc.gov/steadi/pdf/Steadi-Coordinated-Care-Plan.pdf
CDC: Injury Prevention & Control
https://www.cdc.gov/injury/features/older-adult-falls/index.html

CASE STUDY

Presenting Situation

Solveig is an 88-year-old woman. Recently her daughter, Mariane, has been concerned about her mother's health. Her daughter reports that Solveig typically eats a well-balanced diet and drinks copious amounts of water but has had a diminished appetite and thirst lately. In the past couple of weeks, she became fatigued easily and was exhausted, limiting her ability to do the things she enjoys. To have people over for lunch, Solveig would need several days to prepare.

Mariane always visits Solveig on Wednesday afternoons. On this day, as Mariane entered her mother's apartment and her mom staggered toward the door yelling, "Who are you? What are you doing in my house?!" Solveig then lost her balance and fell. Mariane called 911.

After arrival at the emergency department, Solveig was admitted to the hospital with delirium (see Chapter 13 for more information about delirium), fever (101.2°F, 38.4°C), hypotension (90/60 mm Hg), weight loss (12 pounds over 30 days), fatigue, and a fall. Solveig currently weighs 115 pounds, is 5´9˝, and has a body mass index (BMI) of 17.

After a number of tests and intravenous (IV) fluids, the emergency doctor diagnosed her with orthostatic hypotension (blood pressure 100/90 mm Hg seated and 90/52 mm Hg standing), dehydration (>300 mOsm/kg H_2O), a urinary tract infection including colony forming units (CFUs)/mL: 100,000 with fever and confusion, syncope, and frailty. Her Mini Nutritional Assessment® (MNA) score was 5/14 (reduced intake = 1, weight loss = 0, mobility = 0, stress/disease = 2, neuropsychological problems = 2, and BMI <19 = 0). Peripheral oxygen saturation (SpO_2) levels on room air when seated was 97% and when standing was 91%. Solveig has new-onset confusion, fever, and debilitation, but she has a supportive family and a number of meaningful life roles. IV antibiotics were started, and Solveig was transferred to acute care.

Occupational Profile

Solveig is a recent widow of Norwegian descent. She is very active in the lives of her four adult children, two of whom live nearby. She resides in a two-bedroom disability-accessible apartment in an independent living complex geared for aging in place. At the complex, she socializes during meals in the dining room, participates in various classes, and uses the exercise room and swimming pool. She enjoys cooking for her family and friends, attending her grandchildren's events, crafting, baking, swimming with her grandchildren, participating in book club, and attending church and a women's Bible study. Solveig seems more hesitant to participate in community outings now for fear of not making it to the bathroom on time, tiring too easily, or falling in public. Mariane tries to talk with her mom about being reluctant to participate in social activities in public due to urinary incontinence, weakness, and her fear of falling along with tooth pain, managing medications, eating, and beverage consumption. Solveig says that she is an adult and able to manage herself.

Medical History

She has a history of urge incontinence, noninsulin-dependent diabetes, hypertension, mild bilateral cataracts, and a fall at the senior center a month ago. Solveig complains of difficulty chewing her favorite snacks like celery sticks with peanut butter due to tooth pain and has lost 12 pounds over the past month.

List of Problems

Low vision
Medication management
Nutrition and fluid intake
Dental problems

List of Strengths

Strong support system
Access to social participation, cognitive stimulation, and exercise/activities
Mental health
Safe living environment

Questions

1. What assessments will you choose to evaluate special aging concerns regarding Solveig? Why?
2. What more do you need to know about Solveig that would be assessed by other team members? Which team member? What assessment?

Answers

1. Refer to the Assessment section for each special concern. Assessment selection should be based on the client's priorities, functional status, setting, available assessment time, and discharge placement. For example, assessments may include the Edmonton Frail Scale to assess frailty, the Geriatric Oral Health Assessment Index to assess oral health, and identification of daily food and beverage preferences along with consumption tracking at various times of day and in different settings to assess nutrition and hydration statuses.
2. Please refer to the Assessment section for each special concern, focusing on the input provided by other interdisciplinary team members. For example, one of the frailty or balance screens, medication management assessment tools, serum water osmolality test, or urine analysis may be conducted by other team members.

Medication Management With Aging

Many older adults have more than one chronic illness and frequently take multiple medications to manage these conditions (American Geriatrics Society Beers Criteria® Update Expert Panel [AGS], 2019; Ruscin & Linnebur, 2021a). There are benefits of medication use, such as symptom relief (e.g., pain relief), improved function (e.g., mobility due to pain relief), prevention of infectious disease (e.g., antibiotics for an infection), and management of chronic disease (e.g., insulin for diabetes) (Ruscin & Linnebur, 2021a). Older adult medication management can be complicated and highly risky due to adverse or counteractive drug interactions commingled with the aging process and because few pharmacological studies with older adult participants establish appropriate prescriptive guidelines (AGS, 2019; Ruscin & Linnebur, 2021a). Occupational therapy practitioners do not prescribe medications but can play an integral role in helping older adults develop safe medication management skills (Schwartz & Smith, 2017).

Influencers of Medication Effectiveness and Adherence With Aging

Aging body functions and structures may affect how the body processes a drug (**pharmacokinetics**) (Ruscin & Linnebur, 2022).

Some examples of this include:

- Slowed gastric motility can delay drug absorption, reduce peak drug concentrations, and lessen pharmacological effects.
- Increased body fat and decreased body water can cause fat-soluble drugs to accumulate in the body and water-soluble drugs to remain at higher concentrations.
- Hepatic metabolism decreases 30% to 40% with age, decreasing overall drug metabolism.

- After age 40, kidney filtration (glomerular filtration rate) may decrease an average of 8 mL/min/1.73 m per decade, affecting systemic elimination of drugs.
- Drug elimination may be further impeded if the older adult is ill or dehydrated (Ruscin & Linnebur, 2022).

Such factors may lead to reduced therapeutic effects, drug buildup in the body, negative side effects (e.g., impaired cognition, dizziness), hospital admission, toxicity, and possible death (Murphy et al, 2017).

Aging body functions and structures may alter how a drug affects the body (**pharmacodynamics**) (Ruscin & Linnebur, 2021b). Age-related changes to neuroreceptors may alter drug-receptor binding, postreceptor effects, chemical interactions, and drug concentration (Ruscin & Linnebur, 2021b). Common drug side effects include muscle cramps or confusion with statins and dizziness, shakiness, or nausea with benzodiazepines. Such side effects can increase the risk for falls and injury (Bray & Bonder, 2018, p. 270).

In addition to aging body functions, diet and a client's medication nonadherence can affect drug use. Foods and beverages can enhance or reduce the effect of a medication. For example, grapefruit juice enhances the effect of statins, whereas increased eating of vitamin K–laden foods such as broccoli lessens the effect of warfarin or coumadin. Common factors for medication nonadherence include multimorbidity, cognitive and functional impairments, miscommunication, health literacy, complex medication regimens, negative attitudes or beliefs toward medication, poor patient–prescriber relationships, cost, and lack of transportation and/or social support (Adila & Walpola, 2021; Murphy et al, 2017; Smaje et al, 2018). Nonadherence can also be based on personal decision. In a study on medication problem-solving among adults 65 years or older with heart failure, participants intentionally deviated from prescribed instructions upon weighing medication advantages and disadvantages against personal priorities and lifestyle (e.g., diuretic medications may manage cardiovascular fluid overload but cause frequent urination) (Meraz, 2019). In all, it is important for the clinical team to holistically consider the client and their support, develop interventions that are client-centered, pay close attention to cognitive impairments, simplify medication regimens, educate on diet, continually monitor medication effectiveness and side effects, and provide easily accessible resources promoting medication adherence (Meraz, 2019; Smaje et al, 2018). Over time, side effects could develop that require cessation of medication use.

Assessment of Older Adult Medication Management

Occupational therapy practitioners may play a vital role in supporting medication adherence as a part of an interdisciplinary team, thus helping the client and caregivers develop self-care skills to safely manage medications (American Occupational Therapy Association [AOTA], 2017). Following the PEO model, the occupational therapist may evaluate the person by obtaining an occupational profile, asking questions to determine the client's understanding of medications and management routines, and assessing body functions to perform medication management tasks (e.g., vision, dexterity, reading level, problem-solving skills) (AOTA, 2017). For the environment, the occupational therapist considers environmental factors and the context of medication management, such as whether the client has the resources and means to obtain medication (e.g., transportation, financial resources), safe and dependable access to the medication within their living environment (e.g., client is homeless or has their own apartment), a place to store medications per instructions (e.g., refrigeration of unopened insulin), and social support (e.g., caregiver, family, friends) (Murphy et al, 2017). For occupation, activity analysis may involve how the client engages with the prescriber, fills the prescription, understands health information, takes the medication, refills the prescription, monitors for changes (e.g., adverse reactions), and knows when to get medical attention (Schwartz & Smith, 2017).

Three standardized performance-based assessments for older adults include the Hopkins Medication Schedule (Carlson et al, 2005), the Pillbox Test (Zartman et al, 2013), and the In-Home Medication Management Performance Evaluation (Home-Rx) (Murphy et al, 2017). The Hopkins Medication Schedule consists of completing a schedule indicating when to take medication(s), drink water, and eat any snacks and filling a pillbox. The patient is given a schedule with directions, a pillbox, and a bottle labeled with instructions and filled with capsules with an inert powder (cornstarch). The Hopkins Medication Schedule has concurrent validity for participant-reported difficulty with IADLs and may identify clients at risk for poor medication adherence (Carlson et al, 2005). The Pillbox Test consists of five labeled pill bottles filled with colored beads and a pillbox. The client is asked to read the directions on the bottles and then fill the pillbox for one week's worth of medications. The Pillbox Test has good criterion-related validity and convergent validity and may be effective in assessing levels of executive dysfunction (Carlson et al, 2005). The Home-Rx is specifically designed for older adults in the community, assesses ability to manage medication routines, and identifies at-risk behaviors (Murphy et al, 2017). There are three sections: (1) an interview to assess knowledge of medication management routine, (2) a medication list compiling drug names and prescribing instructions, and (3) a performance-based assessment of medication management tasks. The Home-Rx had established content validity (Murphy et al, 2017) and good reliability and validity (Somerville et al, 2019).

Implications for the Older Adult in Treatment: Medication Management

Upon identification of barriers and supports, the occupational therapy practitioner helps the client develop medication management skills (see Promoting Best Practice 7-2). Intervention may include the client remediating or compensating for body function impairments (AOTA, 2017). Environmental modifications (e.g., a medication organizer or built-up grip bottle top; Fig. 7-1) may create a good fit with the client's abilities (AOTA, 2017). Practitioners may help clients build routines and integrate caregivers' support to improve medication adherence (Schwartz & Smith, 2017). When a client is taking medications, the practitioner may evaluate the client's status (e.g., appears sleepy) while engaging in occupation and report observations to the team to help make modifications to the medication regimen (AOTA, 2017). The occupational therapist can also collaborate with the prescriber on types of medications, schedules, and precautions to then provide practice and reinforcement of the client's specific medication management program in occupational therapy treatment sessions.

PROMOTING BEST PRACTICE 7-2
Key Intervention Points With Medication Management

According to AOTA (2017), key occupational therapy interventions for medication management include:

- Helping the client establish habits and routines congruent with medication adherence
- Remediating impairments as able to maximize success with medication management
- Identifying strategies to adapt the environment to fit the client's capabilities
- Alerting the interdisciplinary team of how negative medication effects may affect occupational performance and safety (e.g., hypotension increasing fall risk)
- Communicating with the interdisciplinary team any changes in response to medication(s) (e.g., dizziness, confusion, agitation)

Oral Health With Aging

It is important for occupational therapists to consider how oral body structures (e.g., teeth) and functions (e.g., oral motor skills) change with aging, be aware of influencers of oral health diseases, understand how to assess oral health, and provide indicated interventions. For body structures and their functions, aging-related histological changes of salivary glands—along with outcomes of radiation due to cancer and the influence of some medications—may decrease saliva volume and flow rate, resulting in **xerostomia** (dry mouth) (Xu et al, 2018). Saliva is essential for lubrication and cleansing of the mouth; decreased saliva production can not only affect taste and perception of food texture but also increase risk for plaque and cavities (Xu et al, 2018). For health conditions, poor oral health is highly associated with chronic illness. People with fair or poor general health, rheumatoid arthritis, asthma, diabetes, emphysema, heart disease, liver condition, or stroke were over twice as likely to have severe tooth loss than those without such health conditions (Parker et al, 2020). For participation, poor health behaviors and routines may also contribute to poor oral health. Smoking, alcohol, lack of brushing twice a day, diets high in sugar and starches, and low prevalence of dental visits are associated with increased prevalence of tooth decay, periodontal disease, and tooth loss (Parker et al, 2020). For environmental factors, inaccessible and unaffordable dental care may impede oral health. Many low-income older adults lack public dental insurance and are unable to afford out-of-pocket expenses for dental care (Centers for Disease Control and Prevention [CDC], 2021a). Others may not live in a community that offers healthy food choices and/or public transportation to dental care (CDC, 2021a). Dental facilities may be inaccessible for people with disabilities due to chronic illness (Parker et al, 2020). By considering these constructs, occupational therapy practitioners can more holistically understand the client's oral health status.

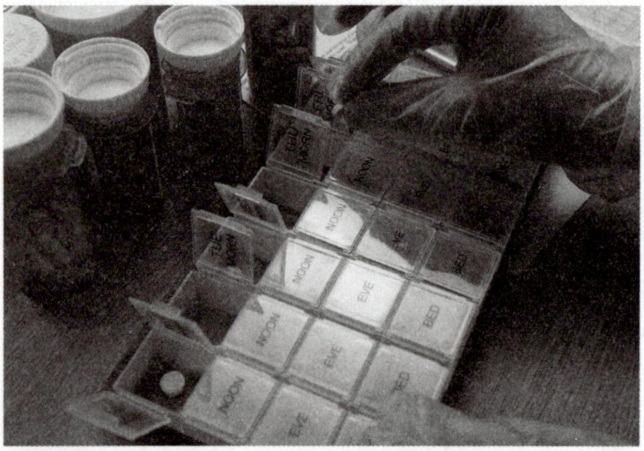

Influencers of Oral Health With Aging

Three major diseases that affect oral health are cavities, periodontal disease (gum disease), and oral cancer (CDC, 2022). Cavities, or tooth decay, may arise when sugars and starches interact with bacteria in the mouth and form a biofilm (plaque) that adheres to the teeth (Mayo Clinic, 2020). The acid from the bacteria erodes through the outer coating of the tooth (enamel) and into the root surface (CDC, 2022). Periodontal disease results from plaque on the tooth and gum line, causing irritation, swelling, and bleeding (Mayo Clinic, 2020). Left untreated, tooth decay and periodontal disease can lead to tooth loss, cause infection (abscess) under the gums, and spread disease to other parts of the body (CDC, 2022). Periodontal disease also precipitates an oral bacterial reservoir. Older adults who sleep with their dentures had greater amounts of oral candidiasis, tongue and denture plaque, and a 2.3-fold higher risk of developing pneumonia (Iinuma et al, 2015). Bacteria introduced into the bloodstream through bleeding gums may cause systemic inflammation of the cardiovascular system and atheroma formation (Sanchez et al, 2017). In addition to cavities and periodontal disease, oral cancers most often affect people over the age

FIGURE 7-1 An example of assistive technology for medication management: A weekly pill box organized by day of the week and three times a day. *(BanksPhotos/E+/Getty Images.)*

of 40 and affect twice as many men than women (National Institute of Dental and Craniofacial Research [NIDCR], 2018). Causes include smoking, alcohol use, and infection with human papillomavirus (NIDCR, 2018). Symptoms may include irritation, a lump, a white or red patch, swelling, and numbness in the oral cavity and may also include ear pain or difficulty moving the jaw or tongue, chewing, and swallowing (NIDCR, 2018). These three diseases may affect quality of life by limiting the ability to eat a range of food choices, impeding speech, changing facial appearance, hindering social interaction, causing systemic, chronic disease, and/or resulting in fatal conditions (Parker et al, 2020).

Assessment of Older Adult Oral Health

Beginning with an assessment, occupational therapists can screen for oral health status using tools such as the Geriatric Oral Health Assessment Index (GOHAI) (Atchison & Dolan, 1990). The GOHAI is a self-reported measure for assessing older adult oral health with a high level of internal consistency and reliability (Atchison & Dolan, 1990). Older adults answer 12 close-ended questions (on a four-point scale with 1 indicating good oral conditions and 4 indicating poor oral conditions) regarding oral pain, discomfort, and psychosocial impact (Venkatesan et al, 2020). Looking further into the client's ability to manage their oral health, occupational therapists may assess (1) self-care skills to perform oral hygiene, (2) daily routines supporting consistent oral care (e.g., brushing teeth twice a day or cleaning dentures daily), (3) healthy diet choices (e.g., diets low in sugar and starches), and (4) healthcare management (e.g., biannual dental checkup and cleaning) (Parker et al, 2020). The practitioner also assesses that the living environment allows for access to oral care supplies and enables performance of oral care. On the community level, the practitioner may consider whether the client has access to dental benefits, dental care, transportation, and nutritious food. If there are concerns outside occupational therapy's scope of practice, the practitioner needs to know how and when to refer to other disciplines (e.g., a dentist or a social worker).

Implications for the Older Adult in Treatment: Oral Health

Based on the assessment, the therapist may use the PEO model to help frame occupation-based interventions. For the person, the occupational therapist provides education to instill the value of oral health care, reinforcing the need to brush teeth twice a day or clean dentures daily, maintain a diet low in sugar and starches, avoid smoking, drink alcohol responsibly, and have dental checkups and teeth cleanings (CDC, 2021b). Edentulous clients also need regular dental checkups to check denture fit for effective dentition and to screen for oral cancer (Salinas, 2017). For the environment, the practitioner may prescribe indicated assistive technology to enable the client to perform good oral care (e.g., one-handed flosser), modify the home environment to make oral care easily accessible, and/or offer practice negotiating transportation systems to access dental care. The occupational therapist may collaborate with the social worker to help identify community resources and then work with the client to practice using transportation to access and negotiate the clinic environment. For the occupation, the practitioner helps the client establish healthy daily routines and offers opportunities to practice these routines and skills. It is important for practitioners to determine whether it is more advantageous to introduce more novel assistive technologies or draw on familiar patterns. In a study of tooth brushing ability after a left cerebrovascular accident, participants demonstrated more effective brushing with a familiar manual toothbrush using a nondominant hand than when provided an electric toothbrush with no instruction (Wu et al, 2016). The occupational therapy practitioner may collaborate with the dentist to reinforce specific dental hygiene techniques (e.g., using a prescribed mouthwash or toothpaste to prevent caries) or equipment (e.g., electric toothbrush, interdental brushes) during the self-care routine. Looking at the person, environment, and occupation, the occupational therapist provides client-centered, occupation-based interventions in collaboration with the team that enable the client to maintain their oral health (see Box 7-1 Resources).

Nutrition and Hydration With Aging

Not only does oral health affect nutritional status, but the aging process also places older adults at greater risk for malnutrition and dehydration than younger adults. The WHO classifies poor nutritional status as: (1) undernutrition; (2) micronutrient-related malnutrition; or (3) overweight, obesity, and diet-related noncommunicable diseases (2021). Undernutrition, defined as not having adequate intake of energy and nutrients, involves wasting where a person has low weight for their height (Maleta, 2006). **Micronutrient-related malnutrition** includes either deficiencies or excesses of vitamins and minerals that can occur because the aging process impedes their breakdown, absorption, and excretion (e.g., low vitamin B_{12} due to diminished stomach acid breaking it down for absorption). Globally, the most important micronutrients for any age are iodine, vitamin A, and iron (WHO, 2021), with iron deficiency being the most common form of malnutrition internationally (CDC, 2021c). Micronutrients in turn influence production of enzymes, hormones, and other necessary matter for bodily function. Being overweight or obese results from consuming more calories than are expended through activity. People may consume many calories and be overweight but consume few vitamins and minerals or have episodes of emesis and thus be malnourished despite being overweight. Diet also influences health status by leading to noncommunicable diseases such as diabetes, cardiovascular disease, high blood pressure, and some cancers (WHO, 2021). Malnutrition is evidenced in older adult Americans but disproportionately for those who are non-Hispanic black or have low incomes (Institute of Medicine [IOM], 2010), and malnutrition is pervasive in older adults from the United Kingdom (Clegg & Williams, 2018). Water is an essential nutrient for bodily processes such as nerve conduction, cardiac and renal function, muscle function, and postural balance. Yet the body's ability to retain and use water becomes impaired with aging. Water is lost through renal processes, respiration, and the skin and added through food and beverage ingestion. An overall fluid deficit leads to **dehydration**—a person using or losing more fluids than are ingested so there is not enough water for bodily needs. Malnutrition and dehydration are worldwide phenomena.

Starting around the age of 50, body functions change. A 5% to 25% reduction in one's basal or resting metabolic rate leads to subsequent body structure changes of weight gain (e.g., adipose redistributes around the abdomen and viscera) along with fluid, bone, and muscle losses of 20% to 40% by age 70 years, despite healthy dietary and exercise habits (Jafarinasabian et al, 2017). Declining bone density occurs disproportionately in women. Sarcopenia (muscle wasting), osteoporosis (bone tissue loss), fracture, and frailty risk increase with age as a result. Thus, older adults need a nutrient-dense diet with fewer calories and plenty of beverages, micronutrient supplementation, and physical activity. The Modified Food Guide Pyramid for 70+ Adults is an educational tool regarding food, beverages, and micronutrients (e.g., calcium, vitamins B_{12} and D_3) for the older adult (IOM, 2010) that may be familiar for older adults, although there are newer tools (see Resources). Note that a nutrient-dense diet includes minerals, vitamins, protein, and complex carbohydrates with few calories from sugar and saturated fat. For older adults, the needed nutrients include:

- Water
- Calcium
- Potassium
- Vitamin B_{12}
- Vitamin D_3
- Protein
- Dietary fiber (U.S. Department of Agriculture & U.S. Department of Health and Human Services [USDA & USHHS], 2020)

A review study by Clegg and Williams (2018) identified nutrient roles and recommendations for older adults. For example, protein ingestion supports maintaining muscle mass and promotes wound healing, skin integrity, immune response, and recovery from illness. The protein recommendations vary for older adults (e.g., same as or more than adult requirements), but Clegg and Williams recommend higher amounts for both healthy older adults (1.0 to 1.2 g protein/kg body weight/day) and for those at risk of malnutrition or those who are malnourished (1.2 to 1.5 g/kg body weight/day). To facilitate bone health, older adults should consume dark fish, calcium, vitamin D (Jafarinasabian et al, 2017), protein, magnesium, and potassium (IOM, 2010) in addition to participation in strength and balance activities (USDA & USHHS, 2020). Female older adults tend to ingest insufficient amounts of calcium, magnesium, and potassium and inadequate amounts of vitamins B_6, C, D_3, E, and K, where not only the amount but the ratio of these micronutrients is vital for body function (Jafarinasabian et al, 2017). The 2009 Institute of Medicine Food Forum workshop reported on various other vitamin and nutrient needs of older adults (IOM, 2010). Vitamin B_6 is involved in metabolism and immune and cognitive function, and low levels can lead to depression. Vitamin B_{12} is protective for bone and heart health plus nerve function, and vitamin D deficiency occurs with neurological and chronic conditions including reduced cognition—but not impaired memory. Vitamin E is important for antioxidant and immune function. On the other hand, folate and sodium tend to be overconsumed. It was also reported that omega-3 fatty acids and dietary fiber support heart health and metabolism, but it is not clear if supplementation is as effective as a food source.

Human fluid requirements are met mostly by beverage consumption (80%) and by food ingestion (20%). Water consumption is an issue for older adults because many do not consume enough fluids for bodily function needs. There is much debate about what constitutes adequate beverage intake for older adults, but experts, including the European Food Safety Authority, agree that at least 1,600 mL (females) to 2,000 mL (males) is needed (Jimoh et al, 2019). Community-dwelling older adults have a low prevalence of dehydration in Japan, the United States, and Sweden (Volkert et al, 2018). This prevalence increases up to 38% for those who are frail or live in long-term and residential care in the United States and United Kingdom and up to 58% for hospitalized patients in the United States and Sweden (Volkert et al, 2018).

Influencers of Nutrition and Hydration With Aging

There are a variety of causes for malnutrition involving the person, environment, and activity or occupation. In general, person factors include reduced cardiac, respiratory, gastrointestinal, and pancreatic exocrine function (e.g., digestive enzyme secretion); impaired fluid absorption and retention abilities (kidney function); and diminished intestinal flow and permeability and changes in villous architecture that occur with aging and with malnutrition. For example, stomach acid diminishes with age, limiting a person's ability to metabolize medications, break down food, and absorb needed substances. Consequently, the form of food (e.g., cooked vs. raw), vitamins (e.g., food or tablets or gel pills), and medications (e.g., coated or noncoated; liquid or solid) is important to consider for the older adult. At the 2009 Institute of Medicine Food Forum, functional foods were identified as those that support health for older adults "beyond their traditional nutrients" (IOM, 2010). That is, the nutritional benefits of functional foods extend to promoting optimal health and reducing the risk of disease. This may also include being in the correct form for absorption to counteract the aging effects of inefficient metabolism, low stomach acid, and poor absorption. Changes in dietary habits often occur with aging because of diminished appetite due to reduced physical activity (occupational participation), chronic medical conditions and medication effects, poor oral health, diminished taste, smell and vision, impaired swallowing, and food insecurity (IOM, 2010). In addition, unsafe storage of food by older home dwellers occurs because of either a too-warm refrigerator or expired foods, some of which are unopened but contain bacteria (Clegg & Williams, 2018). The unsafe food storage and consumption are likely due to diminished sensory perception (e.g., vision, smell, and taste).

Inadequate fluid intake for older adults occurs because of aging effects such as a lack of thirst sensation despite bodily functions requiring more fluids and premature satiation that occurs before adequate fluid consumption happens (Volkert et al, 2018). An impaired renal system also plays a role in dehydration. Person and environmental factors regarding mobility can support or impede hydration (e.g., easy access to fluids). Participation in daily routines also influences hydration status. An older adult may be sedentary versus regularly performing physical activity, or an adult may regularly self-limit beverage intake due to urinary incontinence issues. When poor fluid or electrolyte consumption are coupled with impaired absorption, then **homeostatic hydration** (balanced hydration) is at risk, leading to dehydration. All of these cumulative effects of aging (e.g., poor nutritional absorption, diminished muscle and bone, and dehydration) lead to increased risk of falls for older adults. See Table 7-1 for causes and examples of malnutrition and dehydration classified by PEO factors.

TABLE 7-1 Causes and Examples of Malnutrition and Dehydration Classified by PEO Factors

PEO FACTOR	CAUSE	EXAMPLE
Person factors (Body structures and function [physiology]; routines/habits)	Substance abuse	Alcohol is prioritized rather than food (water).
	Disease-related metabolic and absorption inefficiencies	Diabetes and Crohn disease lead to malnutrition.
	Age-related malabsorption	Inefficient gastrointestinal system fails to absorb nutrients.
	Surgery-related malabsorption	Intestinal resection results in less surface area for absorption.
	Impaired mobility and body function/capacity	Reduced mobility or reduced body function and capacity limit one's ability to shop and prepare nutritious meals.
	Poor oral health	The inability to chew or bite precludes selecting nutrient-dense fresh fruit or vegetables (malnutrition).
	Dysphagia	Difficulty swallowing results in self-limiting of nutrient-rich fresh vegetables and beverages.
	Aging-related loss of appetite and decreased taste and olfactory perception	Intake is reduced and consumption is limited because of poor appetite; food and beverages are unappetizing due to lack of taste and smell.
	Aging-related decreased saliva production	Food is difficult to chew, manipulate, and swallow due to reduced saliva.
	Depression	Depression can lead to over- or undereating (and/or drinking), where few needed nutrients are consumed in place of empty calories.
Environmental factors (Built environment; social environment)	Poverty	Poverty often involves a lack of access to or inability to afford nutrient-rich food or beverages (IOM, 2010).
	Social isolation	Social isolation can lead to eating less when alone eating processed foods (with poor nutritional quality) because they can be prepared quickly (Clegg & Williams, 2018), failure to prioritize, or forgetting to eat or drink when alone.
	Medications	Impaired medication metabolism may cause nutrient wasting for B vitamins (malnutrition) (IOM, 2010).
Occupation and participation	Physical activity level determines nutritional needs	A person who is bedfast requires fewer calories and less protein and water than a person who is physically active.
	Meaningfulness of food and beverage activity	A beverage occupation (client-directed drinking of a desired beverage in a meaningful setting using a "just right" container) improves fluid intake and hydration status (Rice, 2018).

Note. PEO = Person, environment, and occupation. The examples include both malnutrition and dehydration unless otherwise specified.

The outcome of these aging changes includes:

- Decreased reabsorption of water and electrolytes
- Diminished nutrient absorption
- Altered ion concentrations
- Reduced fluid for neural tissue function
- Reduced secretion of ions and fluids into the small and large bowel, which in turn may cause diarrhea

Diarrhea is associated with high risk for mortality in the malnourished. Muscle mass wasting from limited food consumption and poor absorption of protein and water result in impeded muscle function and diminished physical capacity. In addition, malnutrition results in poor immune response and wound healing as well as negative psychosocial effects (e.g., depression, apathy, anxiety, and self-neglect) (Saunders et al, 2011). Although older adults may be less active as they age, requiring fewer calories, they actually need to consume more nutrients due to poor absorption and utilization of such. It is important to note that there is a point of no return, where both malnutrition and dehydration become irreversible and lead to death.

Assessment of Older Adult Nutrition

Occupational therapists, nurses, and dietitians can use the revised MNA Short-Form to screen the nutritional status of clients aged 65 years and older in 3 to 5 minutes (see Box 7-1 Resources). The one-page gold standard tool has been validated in a variety of settings and has six questions regarding the past 3 months pertaining to the older adult client's food intake, weight loss, mobility, psychological status, and BMI, calf circumference, or both (Kaiser et al, 2009). A score ≥12 out of 14 possible points is normal nutrition status, 8 to 11 points indicates being at risk of malnutrition, and 0 to 7 points is malnourished. If the score is less than 12 points, then the MNA Long-Form is recommended to identify potential causes of malnutrition. The Interactive MNA Short-Form is available in a variety of languages. The MNA is included in the Comprehensive Geriatric Assessment. Occupational therapists should investigate the dietary habits and routines of the client, food and vessel preferences, body structures and functions, and the fit of the person with the setting. It is advisable to collaborate with nursing and dietary personnel regarding client habits and routines related to nutrition.

Assessment of Older Adult Hydration

The gold standard for assessment of hydration status is the blood test for serum plasma water osmolality (Lacey et al, 2019). Hooper et al (2015a) identified older adult serum osmolality values for being well hydrated as 275 to <295 mOsm/kg along with impending dehydration values (295 to 300 mOsm/kg) and current dehydration values (>300 mOsm/kg). Typical signs and symptoms of dehydration become unreliable indicators for older adults due to multiple other possible etiologies. For example, thirst, skin turgor, heart rate, urine color, urine volume, and dry mouth or tongue are not reliable indicators of dehydration in the older adult because the aging process, medications, and medical conditions can cause these signs and symptoms (Hooper et al, 2015b). Indicators that have some value as stand-alone tests for identifying older adult dehydration include fatigue, missed between-meal drinks, and bioeletrical impedance analysis resistance at 50 kHz, whereas beverage intake, urine osmolality and axilla moisture show some limited diagnostic accuracy (Hooper et al, 2015b). The combination of fatigue and missing some drinks between meals was sensitive at 0.71 (95% CI 0.29 to 0.96) and specific at 0.92 (95% CI 0.83 to 0.97) for identifying older adult dehydration (Hooper et al, 2015b). However, a combination of multiple factors is best to identify dehydration in any aged adult (Lacey et al, 2019).

Nutrition and hydration assessment in occupational therapy involves investigating the PEO factors that influence hydration in multiple contexts. To start, the occupational therapist interviews the older adult to identify client habits, routines, and preferences related to the eating and drinking experience and to toileting. Identification of desired food and beverages should include their temperature and form, preferred utensils and vessels, favored dining setting for each meal and between-meal ingestion, and timing for ingestion of food and fluids (e.g., length of the dining/drinking session, time of day, seasonal preference changes) (Rice, 2017). Body structures and functions are also assessed, such as sensory systems (e.g., vision, smell, taste, touch), range of motion, strength, postural balance, reach, mobility, and fatigue. Comorbidities are identified, as are their potential influences on hydration, such as incontinence. Observation of a meal in multiple contexts across a day is needed to identify the fit of the client with the demands of the physical built environment for lighting, room temperature, accessibility, and space for maneuvering along with the social environment for expectations and their availability and willingness to assist (Rice, 2017). For example, both dim lighting and glare require extra effort to see food and drink, small spaces require skilled precise movements for either arm reaching or for wheelchair maneuvering to access food and drink, and expectations from family or staff that the older adult will request a drink when thirsty do not match an impaired thirst mechanism or having dementia. The objects of the occupation are also examined for their client fit in terms of color contrast, weight, and shape and for the fit with the setting's features (Rice, 2017). For example, poor color contrast involving a clear glass containing water placed on a white table (or mashed potatoes and a chicken breast on a white plate) is difficult for aging eyes to discriminate. Heavy, wide drinking vessels without open handles impede independent drinking for someone with arthritis. An excessively hot or cold room or a vent blowing on the person during a meal may hasten the time spent dining, leading to poor intake. The occupational therapist should collaborate with nursing and dietary personnel regarding the client's nutrition and fluid requirements along with the client's habits, routines, and preferences related to hydration. In addition, the therapist should examine the medical chart for serum plasma water levels, nutrition, and fluid intake monitoring and possibly the MNA values.

Implications for the Older Adult in Treatment: Malnutrition and Dehydration

After the occupational therapist identifies the PEO fit for eating food and drinking beverages, then education on factors that influence aging is taught and recommendations given for optimizing the PEO fit. Intervention should view nutrition and hydration in terms of occupation—not just activity, where the eating and drinking experience is client-directed and meaningful and has purpose (Rice, 2017).

Questions for consideration include:

- What are the person's attitudes toward various foods and beverages?
- What are the client's motor, cognitive, postural, and sensory skills and performance?
- Does the client have any medical conditions that act as a support or barrier?
- Is the physical and social environment accessible, accommodating, and supportive to drinking and eating nutritious foods?
- What is the routine, frequency, method, timing (e.g., time of day; timing within a task), task (including its tools, equipment, and objects), culture, and meaning of the dining occupation for the client?
- Can the environment or occupation be adapted or modified to support performance and participation?

Intervention addresses the many PEO factors that were examined. The client's mobility status and ability to reach should align with the environment and occupation to enable easy access to food and beverages. The older adult's swallowing performance should match the form of food and drink. Preference should be considered and encompass not only the food and beverage but also the occupation and environment in terms of the dining setting (e.g., lighting, space, room temperature), utensils and dining vessels (e.g., color, size, weight, and shape), and portion size (Rice, 2017). Alignment of the dining objects with the person factors promotes food and beverage intake.

For example, a color contrast of vessels (e.g., red containers) with the food and with the table supports visibility of food and drink and thus enhances intake (Volkert et al, 2018). Often older adults, especially at the end of life, prefer smaller portions consumed frequently from smaller vessels. The weight and shape of containers can enable a person with arthritis to be independent in feeding or conversely can impede function. The environmental contexts may vary with time of day; thus intervention needs to include each context and its features (e.g., lighting, table height).

An occupation-based dining occupation experience should include:

- Favored edibles in person-centered vessels
- Beverage variety
- Just-right temperature
- Frequent accessibility
- Social setting

Flavor enhancers are known to increase food intake for hospitalized older adults in Hong Kong, and presenting a variety of food (Clegg & Williams, 2018) and a variety of preferred beverages (Rice, 2018) also facilitates intake for older adults. Preference needs to be incorporated at each food and drink offering—not assumed but re-asked, because the client may change their mind daily or seasonally. Participating in meal preparation and eating with other persons, where the focus is on a social experience rather than oral intake, facilitates more food and fluid consumption (Clegg & Williams, 2018). Beverages should be offered frequently (start, middle, end of session) during therapy sessions along with opportunities for toileting.

For those with frailty, home-cooked meals cannot only improve food variety and nutrition but also enable consumption of safe, edible food. Their declining body structures and functions result in fatigue and difficulty with package opening, and the older adult may select easily prepared, less nutritious meals that are stored incorrectly or kept too long due to the person's diminished sensory systems that fail to detect spoiled food (Clegg & Williams, 2018). Occupational therapy should collaborate with dietary staff regarding nutritional needs and client preferences in addition to educating nursing staff regarding the client's best dining PEO fit (see Box 7-1 Resources).

In mild or worse cases of malnutrition and dehydration, supplementation may be needed. Nutrition shakes with high calorie and protein or iron content are often advisable, and the dietitian determines which shake and micronutrients are needed. Nursing can offer the shake with medications. Occupational therapy ensures a good PEO fit for drinking the shake. To promote hydration, the following may be sufficient for rehydration: fluid tracking, plenty of fluids with medications, and frequent beverage offers. IV fluids are an alternative intervention that nursing uses for more severe cases of fluid depletion.

Urinary Management With Aging: Urinary Tract Infection & Urinary Incontinence

Urinary Tract Infection

A **urinary tract infection** (UTI) is an infection of any part of the urinary system—the kidneys, ureters, bladder, and urethra (Mayo Clinic, 2021a). The most common place of infection is the bladder (cystitis) and the urethra (urethritis)

(Mayo Clinic, 2021a). Women have UTIs more often than men, as a woman's urethra is shorter than a man's, decreasing the distance bacteria needs to travel to the bladder (Mayo Clinic, 2021a). Sexual activity, using a diaphragm, applying spermicidal agents, menopause (due to decreased estrogen), and toilet hygiene wiping from back to front (anus to vaginal/urethra areas) increases susceptibility to infection (Mayo Clinic, 2021a). UTIs are common and often treated with antibiotics; however, untreated UTIs may result in permanent kidney damage, urethral narrowing in men, and sepsis (Mayo Clinic, 2021a).

Assessment of Older Adult Urinary Tract Infection

Occupational therapy practitioners do not diagnose UTIs but can note the symptoms and alert the client and care team. Symptoms among older adults may include:

- Persistent urge to urinate
- Burning with urination
- Foul-smelling, cloudy, and/or bloody (red, bright-pink, or brownish color) urine
- Fever
- Nausea
- Vomiting
- Pain in the back, side, lower abdomen, and/or pelvic area (Mayo Clinic, 2021a)

Confusion in older adults may be a symptom but needs to be within the context of the described symptoms, as confusion alone does not necessarily allude to a UTI (Mayne et al, 2019). Either nursing or the primary care provider will order a urinalysis (test of urine for red blood cells, white blood cells, and bacteria) or urine culture (test of urine to determine what type of bacteria is in the urine) to diagnose a UTI (Cleveland Clinic, 2020). A laboratory result of 100,000 CFUs or greater of bacteria per mL of urine is indicative of a UTI (Kwon et al, 2012).

Implications for the Older Adult in Treatment: Urinary Tract Infection

Occupational therapy practitioners help older adults cope with UTIs primarily by being aware of the symptoms, alerting the client to get medical attention, or notifying the care team for further medical workup. Using the PEO model, occupational therapists can assess the person's understanding of a UTI and ability to provide self-care and educate the client on the signs and symptoms. For the environment, the practitioner can evaluate the person's access to regular and ample fluid intake, toileting areas, and healthcare services. For the occupation, a practitioner can teach the person preventive strategies such as: (1) drinking fluids to dilute urine and flush bacteria out of the urinary tract, (2) wiping from front to back to prevent bacteria from spreading from the anal area to the vagina and urethra, (3) emptying the bladder after intercourse to flush out bacteria, and (4) avoiding feminine products (e.g., deodorant sprays, scented pads, douches or powders, spermicidal agents) that may irritate the urethra (Mayo Clinic, 2021a).

Urinary Incontinence

Urinary incontinence is involuntary loss of urine in varying amounts and frequency (Mayo Clinic, 2021b). Impaired body structures that may cause incontinence include weakness of the muscles in the lower urinary tract, damage to the urinary tract or innervating nerves, or overactive bladder muscles that overtake the sphincter muscles (Stanford University Health Care, 2021).

There are six types of urinary incontinence (Mayo Clinic, 2021b):

- *Urge incontinence:* Frequent, sudden urge to urinate due to an overactive detrusor muscle, followed by involuntary urination loss (Lasak et al, 2018)
- *Overactive bladder:* Urgent urination with or without incontinence (Rogowski et al, 2021)
- *Stress incontinence:* Leaking urine with activity (e.g., jumping and sneezing); thought to stem from urethral or bladder neck hypermobility and intrinsic sphincter deficiency (Lasak et al, 2018)
- *Mixed incontinence:* Combination of urge and stress incontinence (Mayo Clinic, 2021b)
- *Overflow incontinence:* Frequent leakage with or without sensation and feelings of incomplete bladder emptying caused by weakness of the detrusor muscle or a blocked urethra (Lasak et al, 2018)
- *Functional or disability-associated urinary incontinence:* Incontinence related to physical, mental, or cognitive impairment (Mayo Clinic, 2021b)

Incontinence may be temporarily due to diuretic (causing increased urine excretion) foods, drinks, and medications such as alcohol, caffeine, carbonated drinks, artificial sweeteners, chocolate, foods high in spice, sugar, or acid, heart and blood pressure medications, and large doses of vitamin C (Mayo Clinic, 2021b). Short-term conditions that may cause incontinence include constipation, UTIs, and pregnancy (enlarging uterus pressing on bladder and/or weakening pelvic floor structures) (Mayo Clinic, 2021b). More chronic conditions include pelvic floor disorders, diabetes (due to increased urine production and/or peripheral neuropathy), menopause (due to hormonal changes and/or pelvic floor weakness), some neurological diseases that affect bladder control (e.g., multiple sclerosis, Parkinson disease, stroke, brain tumor, or spinal injury), and an enlarged prostate (Mayo Clinic, 2021b). The physical and social environment may also pose a barrier to bladder management, such as unsafe or inaccessible toilet areas or lack of caregiver support if needed (WHO, 2017). Although urinary incontinence affects many older adults, it is not a normal part of the aging process and warrants further workup to determine causes, barriers, and possible treatment options (Molitor & Nadeau, 2020).

There are varying associated risks for urinary incontinence. Women are two times more likely than men to have urinary incontinence. Patel et al (2022) calculated over 60% of community-dwelling women in the United States or 78,297,094 women have some level of urinary incontinence, of which 28,545,778 adult women have moderate to more severe incontinence. Other risks include age greater than 70 years, obesity (BMI >40), prior vaginal birth, smoking, family history of incontinence, anxiety, depression, functional dependence, and non-Hispanic white ethnicity and race (Patel et al, 2022).

Urinary incontinence is associated with reduced quality of life due to self-limiting occupational participation. In a study of 1,412 community-dwelling older adult women, participants with urinary incontinence were three times more likely to report feeling isolated, as a result of limiting social activities to avoid risk of urge incontinence (Yip et al, 2013). Urinary incontinence may precipitate embarrassment and poor self-perception, limit social interaction and physical activity, and impair sexual function (Dumoulin et al, 2018). In a study of 127 female patients with overactive bladder, there was a significant association of increased severity of overactive bladder symptoms with a history of psychiatric disorders and current use of at least two psychotropic medications (Rogowski et al, 2021). More specifically, there was an association of increased severity of stress urinary incontinence with history of depression and current treatment with serotonin reuptake inhibitor antidepressants (Rogowski et al, 2021). There is an increased risk for falls associated with incontinence. In a retrospective study of 348 women (mean age: 58.7 ± 15.8 years), Fisher et al (2022) found an increased fall risk of 40% among women with pelvic floor disorder. The number of urinary symptoms was a stronger risk predictor than the participants' primary diagnosis, with three or more urinary symptoms strongly correlating with a positive fall risk screening. Specific to urge incontinence, there was an increased fall risk with urgency or frequency. Based on a systematic review, Moon et al (2021) noted men and women ≥65 years old with urinary incontinence were 59% more likely to have a fall. The reasons for increased fall risk were unclear, but with urge incontinence, researchers speculated that velocity and gait stride change while rushing to the toilet may contribute to falling.

Assessment of Older Adult Urinary Incontinence

Assessments such as the Incontinence Impact Questionnaire (IIQ) (Shumaker et al, 1994) and International Consultation on Incontinence Questionnaire Short Form (ICIQ-SF) may help determine the effect incontinence has on quality of life. The IIQ is a 30-item self-report that is a measure of quality of life in women with stress urinary incontinence (Shumaker et al, 1994) with significant concurrent, predictive, and convergent validity and moderate to weak reliability (Kappa statistic ranging from 0.732 to 0.381) (Cobey, 2022). Developed by the WHO-sponsored International Consultation on Incontinence, the ICIQ-SF is a self-report, four-item questionnaire with three scored items and one unscored item on the prevalence, frequency, and self-perceived cause of incontinence and its impact on daily life (Avery et al, 2004; Sirls, 2008). This free assessment has good construct validity, acceptable convergent validity, and good reliability (Avery et al, 2004). Occupational therapists may specifically evaluate the client's ability to access the toilet, transfer on and off the toilet, and perform toileting tasks (e.g., dressing and hygiene).

Implications for the Older Adult in Treatment: Urinary Incontinence

Following the PEO model, the occupational therapist can work with the person to evaluate body structures and functions that enable and/or limit continence as well as feelings and thoughts about urinary incontinence. For the person, the practitioner can provide supportive listening and offer education on bladder function and continence, foods and medications that may cause excessive urination, and medical conditions that may cause incontinence and require further medical evaluation. For the environment, the occupational therapist may evaluate the physical and social environments—helping to make a clear, well-lit pathway to the toilet to decrease fall risk (especially at night) or providing modifications (e.g., grab bars, raised toilet seat, bedside commode) to increase accessibility and safety and involving family and caregivers as indicated to support toileting habits. For occupation, the practitioner can assess routines, habits, and toileting skills. The occupational therapist can help the client establish regular toileting habits, set phone reminders, schedule fluid intake, recommend assistive technologies (e.g., elastic waist pants, Velcro closures, incontinence products), and support development of toileting skills. By looking at the person, environment, and occupation, the occupational therapy practitioner can incorporate the client's preferences and individualize intervention to maximize continence management.

Occupational and physical therapy practitioners, nurses and nurses' aides, and primary care providers may all play a role in treating urinary incontinence. Nonpharmacological interventions for incontinence include prompted voiding, timed voiding, habit training, bladder training, and pelvic floor muscle training (PFMT) (WHO, 2017). Prompted voiding involves the person (with or without a cognitive impairment) initiating their own toileting by requesting that caregivers assist them with voiding. Timed voiding is voiding fixed by time or events and is not individualized but caregiver led. There is very low evidence that prompted and timed voiding improves incontinence (WHO, 2017). Habit training is a voiding schedule based on the person's natural pattern of urination and may not necessarily involve the individual in the process. There is low evidence that habit training improves incontinence (WHO, 2017). Bladder training involves the person actively working to increase the time between emptying the bladder to 3- to 4-hour intervals and the amount of fluid the bladder holds. Bladder training involves patient education about the bladder and how continence is maintained, scheduled voiding, positive reinforcement, and voiding schedule (WHO, 2017). It is recommended to provide bladder training for a minimum of 6 weeks, follow a strict schedule starting with bathroom visits every 2 hours, and gradually increase time between toileting (WHO, 2017). PFMT incorporates exercises for pelvic floor muscle contractions and is considered the first line of treatment for stress incontinence to help maintain continence and establish normal voiding (Lasak et al, 2018). Evidence from a systematic review demonstrated that women with stress incontinence who underwent PFMT were eight times more likely to report being cured, and women with any type of urinary incontinence were five times more likely to report being cured than those without treatment (Dumoulin et al, 2018). There is moderate evidence that PFMT with bladder training helps improve continence, and it is strongly recommended for urge, stress, or mixed incontinence for both men and women (WHO, 2017).

Other interventions include functional incidental training, Pilates, and yoga. Functional incidental training integrates endurance and strengthening exercises with focus on ambulating to the toilet, transferring on and off the toilet, and managing toileting tasks (e.g., hygiene, dressing tasks) (WHO, 2017). After an 8-week functional incidental training program using an individualized, function-based exercise program and prompted voiding with 528 Veterans Affairs nursing home patients, there were significantly improved outcomes in endurance, strength, and urinary incontinence but not for locomotion or toileting (Ouslander et al, 2005).

Pilates and yoga also offer an alternative for PFMT but are not shown to be as effective as PFMT. In a study comparing PFMT, yoga, and Pilates with 60 women 60 years old and older, each group participated once a week for 4 weeks and then had an audio-guided home exercise program for 8 weeks (Kannan et al, 2022). All groups had significant improvement on the ICIQ-SF at the 4-week and 12-week mark. The yoga and Pilates groups did not have a significant improvement compared with PFMT, but the yoga group had a significantly greater improvement than the Pilates group. In a study with 48 perimenopausal women comparing PFMT with yoga (Purba, 2021), participants received interventions three times a week for 8 weeks. The PFMT group scored significantly higher on the Incontinence Impact Questionnaire (IIQ-7) than the yoga group. PFMT has strong evidence of improving continence. Although not as effective as PFMT, yoga and Pilates are alternative means that offer significant benefits.

Specialized training is needed to address urinary incontinence. A primary care physician, urogynecologist, or urologist can assist with determining medical needs, prescribe medications, perform surgery, or recommend exercises (Molitor & Nadeau, 2020). Nursing can assist with developing bladder training programs. Pelvic floor physical therapists and yoga and Pilates instructors can provide a pelvic floor program. In addition to referring a client to these specialists, a generalist occupational therapist may collaborate with the nurse to develop a bladder program and practice strategies (e.g., integrating relaxation techniques for urge incontinence) within the context of the client's daily schedule to increase times between voiding while increasing social participation. The occupational therapy practitioner may also work with the pelvic floor training instructor to reinforce education (e.g., reminder to do Kegel exercises) and integrate the program within the client's daily routine (e.g., suggest doing Kegel exercises while stopped at red light). In all, the occupational therapy practitioners may play a vital role within the team to help older adults manage urinary incontinence and remain active in daily living (see Box 7-1 Resources).

Falls With Aging

The previous special concerns topics are all influencers of falling. A **fall** is defined as an unintentional landing of oneself on a lower surface with or without injury. Worldwide, 15% to 34% of community older adults fall annually, often with adverse outcomes (Montero-Odasso et al, 2022). Although both research and society find old age is associated with falling, it is not necessarily a normal part of aging.

Influencers of Falls With Aging

Falls may be classified as "mechanical" when external forces or objects from the environment precipitate the fall (Timsina et al, 2017). For example, clutter, throw rugs, toys, and obstacles may cause a fall. "Nonmechanical" falls are due to person factors involving aging body structures, aging body functions, behavior, and cognition. In healthy adults, falls rarely occur in the aforementioned circumstances due to postural resilience and occupational adaptation. The healthy, well-hydrated adult can adapt to walking on uneven sidewalks by harnessing muscle capacity and quick protective reactive-control reflexes to recover from tripping as noted by rapid stepping and outstretched arms to maintain balance. The adult may also use occupational adaptation by recruiting memories to select an action plan that accommodates a potential perturbation (external force).

Older adults most at risk of falling include women (Timsina et al, 2017), residents in long-term care, and hospitalized patients (Dal Bello-Haas & MacIntyre, 2018). Person factors such as vitamin D deficiency can lead to osteoporosis, muscle weakness, obesity, and fatigue, thereby heightening one's fall risk. The recommended daily adequate vitamin D intake for older adults of 600 to 800 IU is likely insufficient, whereas 4000 IU is deemed safe to promote bone health and attenuate frailty and falls for older adults (NIH, 2022).

Medical conditions involving chronic disease (e.g., diabetes and peripheral neuropathy) and acute illness can impair sensory feedback systems and functional capacity, leading to a fall. Sensory changes with aging for visual, auditory, tactile, proprioceptive, and vestibular systems result in impairments and inefficiencies such that the body does not perceive a postural threat or cannot respond quickly to it. Motor and nerve inefficiencies occur with aging due to reduced body water and inefficient neural transmission, whereas muscle wasting leads to reduced muscle strength, capacity, and reaction time. Gait, balance, and mobility in older adults are thus impaired, increasing the risk of falling. Foot issues such as bunions, calluses, and peripheral neuropathy reduce the sensory feedback through the feet, and foot pain impedes compensatory reactions. Poor vision due to cataracts enhances the risk of falling due to glare. Declining cognition (e.g., mild cognitive impairment) involves a reduced ability to identify, process, and react timely and correctly to a postural threat. Dehydration influences cognition by causing poor attention with resultant reduced visual input, and dehydration leads to inefficient neural and motor systems, all of which place one at greater risk for falling.

The environment, its objects, and time of day may heighten fall risk. Common environmental hazards include objects along pathways (e.g., throw rugs and pet dishes), stairs and steps, accessibility to objects that cannot be reached safely, and surface characteristics (e.g., uneven surface, slippery surface). Both dim lighting and glare reduce visibility, yielding an unsafe environment. Medications, as mentioned earlier, can facilitate falls. Darkness reduces visual feedback both early in the day and in the evening. As the day progresses, older adults may fatigue, lessening their ability to recover from a perturbation.

The environmental features of society and policy also play a role in an older adult's ability to perform and participate in community activity safely. For example, closure of public water fountains during a pandemic can lead to dehydration, orthostatic hypotension, and falling during a person's postural changes when in the community. Public bathroom closures may result in urinary urgency with rushed mobility leading to a fall upon arrival at home. The enforcement of the American with Disabilities Act regarding visual impairment may include sidewalk intersections with tactile paving (raised bumps), creating an uneven surface that requires lots of energy and postural balance to traverse, thereby impeding safe mobility and increasing fall risk.

Common activities that precede a fall include walking, vigorous activities, and climbing. For institutionalized older adults, activities that are more likely to end with a fall are walking during activities of daily living (ADLs) and transfers (Cameron et al, 2018). Activity location is another potential hazard, for example, institutionalized older adults tend to fall in bathrooms or their room (Cameron et al, 2018). Poor behavior choices may lead to increased risk for falling, such as dietary selection (including alcohol use), footwear choice (e.g., wearing high heels), and failing to exercise. In addition, a fear of falling increases fall risk when the person avoids physical activity, leading to deconditioning and weakness

from disuse, inability to adjust to postural challenges, smaller limits of stability (distance reached while maintaining one's balance), and less tolerance for perturbations. Fall risk factors incrementally increase depending on whether the person has experienced a fall (or not), fallen once, or is a recurrent faller (Porto et al, 2020). The chance of falling also heightens as the number of fall risk factors increase.

Outcomes of falling may include injuries, debility, occupational deprivation, and/or death. Injuries often involve bruises, contusions, lacerations, sprains, fractures, and traumatic brain injuries. Fallers may develop a fear of falling and self-limit participation in activities leading to occupational deprivation. In a retrospective study of 2,909 hospitalized patients admitted with a hip fracture, 32.7% died within 2 years of admission (Barceló et al, 2020). Death can occur soon after the fall due to a traumatic brain injury (e.g., cranial bleed) or a bit later from complications involving subsequent debility.

Assessment of Older Adult Falls

Postural balance evaluation is a multifactorial process best addressed by an interprofessional team and includes an annual postural balance screen, physical examination, vision examination, and physician (pharmacist) medication review (Eckstrom et al, 2021). The CDC's Stopping Elderly Accidents, Deaths and Injuries (STEADI) initiative is an interdisciplinary care plan with resources to prevent older adults from falling (Eckstrom et al, 2021). It is similar to world guidelines (Montero-Odasso et al, 2022) and based on recommendations from the American and British Geriatrics Societies. STEADI involves healthcare providers screening older adults for falls, assessing fall risk factors, and initiating interventions to prevent falling (Figure 7-2). The initiative includes information for both older adults and caregivers (e.g., care plan) along with guidance on fall monitoring and reporting (see Box 7-1 Resources). STEADI provides a brief screen of three key questions to ask older adult community clients annually:

- Have you fallen in the past year?
- Do you feel unsteady when standing or walking?
- Do you worry about falling? (Eckstrom et al, 2021)

One "yes" answer indicates the need for further assessment and a likely fall risk. STEADI's Stay Independent screen consists of 12 questions. A score of 4 or higher indicates a fall risk and need for further evaluation, and this screen reveals some client-specific fall risk factors (e.g., orthostatic hypotension, vision, medications) for possible attention (Eckstrom et al, 2021).

Occupational therapy has a role in older adult falls evaluation by conducting an occupational profile, history, and fall screen. Addressing the multifactorial nature of falls, the occupational therapist might gather the following:

- Full medication list
- Information on the corresponding circumstances of the fall

RESOURCE
Algorithm
for Fall Risk Screening, Assessment, and Intervention

As a healthcare provider, you are already aware that falls are a serious threat to the health and well-being of your older patients.

More than one out of four people 65 and older fall each year, and over 3 million are treated in emergency departments annually for fall injuries.

The CDC's STEADI initiative offers a coordinated approach to implementing the American and British Geriatrics Societies' clinical practice guideline for fall prevention. STEADI consists of three core elements: **Screen**, **Assess**, and **Intervene** to reduce fall risk.

The **STEADI Algorithm for Fall Risk Screening, Assessment, and Intervention** outlines how to implement these three elements.

Additional tools and resources include:

- Information about falls
- Case studies
- Conversation starters
- Screening tools
- Standardized gait and balance assessment tests (with instructional videos)
- Educational materials for providers, patients, and caregivers
- Online continuing education
- Information on medications linked to falls
- Clinical decision support for electronic health record systems

You play an important role in caring for older adults, and you can help reduce these devastating injuries.

CDC's STEADI tools and resources can help you screen, assess, and intervene to reduce your patient's fall risk. For more information, visit www.cdc.gov/steadi.

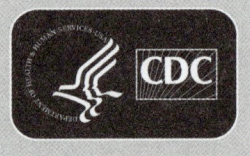

Centers for Disease Control and Prevention
National Center for Injury Prevention and Control

2019

STEADI — Stopping Elderly Accidents, Deaths & Injuries

FIGURE 7-2 The STEADI algorithm chart is a decision chart that depicts an algorithm for screening and evaluating falls risk in older adults and identifies subsequent intervention strategies. *(From https://www.cdc.gov/steadi/pdf/Steadi-Coordinated-Care-Plan.pdf)*

STEADI Algorithm for Fall Risk Screening, Assessment, and Intervention among Community-Dwelling Adults 65 years and older

START HERE → **1 SCREEN** for fall risk yearly, or any time patient presents with an acute fall.

Available Fall Risk Screening Tools:
- **Stay Independent**: a 12-question tool [at risk if score ≥ 4]
  - **Important**: If score < 4, ask if patient fell in the past year (if YES → patient is at risk)
- **Three key questions** for patients [at risk if YES to any question]
  - Feels unsteady when standing or walking?
  - Worries about falling?
  - Has fallen in past year?
    » If YES ask, "How many times?" "Were you injured?"

SCREENED NOT AT RISK

PREVENT future risk by recommending effective prevention strategies.
- Educate patient on fall prevention
- Assess vitamin D intake
  - If deficient, recommend daily vitamin D supplement
- Refer to community exercise or fall prevention program
- Reassess yearly, or any time patient presents with an acute fall

SCREENED AT RISK

2 ASSESS patient's modifiable risk factors and fall history.

Common ways to assess fall risk factors are listed below:

Evaluate gait, strength, & balance
Common assessments:
- Timed Up & Go
- 30-Second Chair Stand
- 4-Stage Balance Test

Identify medications that increase fall risk (e.g., Beers Criteria)

Ask about potential home hazards (e.g., throw rugs, slippery tub floor)

Measure orthostatic blood pressure (Lying and standing positions)

Check visual acuity
Common assessment tool:
- Snellen eye test

Assess feet/footwear

Assess vitamin D intake

Identify comorbidities (e.g., depression, osteoporosis)

3 INTERVENE to reduce identified risk factors using effective strategies.

Reduce identified fall risk
- Discuss patient and provider health goals
- Develop an individualized patient care plan (see below)

Below are common interventions used to reduce fall risk:

Poor gait, strength, & balance observed
- Refer for physical therapy
- Refer to evidence-based exercise or fall prevention program (e.g., Tai Chi)

Medication(s) likely to increase fall risk
- Optimize medications by stopping, switching, or reducing dosage of medications that increase fall risk

Home hazards likely
- Refer to occupational therapist to evaluate home safety

Orthostatic hypotension observed
- Stop, switch, or reduce the dose of medications that increase fall risk
- Educate about importance of exercises (e.g., foot pumps)
- Establish appropriate blood pressure goal
- Encourage adequate hydration
- Consider compression stockings

Visual impairment observed
- Refer to ophthalmologist/optometrist
- Stop, switch, or reduce the dose of medication affecting vision (e.g., anticholinergics)
- Consider benefits of cataract surgery
- Provide education on depth perception and single vs. multifocal lenses

Feet/footwear issues identified
- Provide education on shoe fit, traction, insoles, and heel height
- Refer to podiatrist

Vitamin D deficiency observed or likely
- Recommend daily vitamin D supplement

Comorbidities documented
- Optimize treatment of conditions identified
- Be mindful of medications that increase fall risk

FOLLOW UP with patient in 30-90 days.
Discuss ways to improve patient receptiveness to the care plan and address barrier(s)

Centers for Disease Control and Prevention
National Center for Injury Prevention and Control

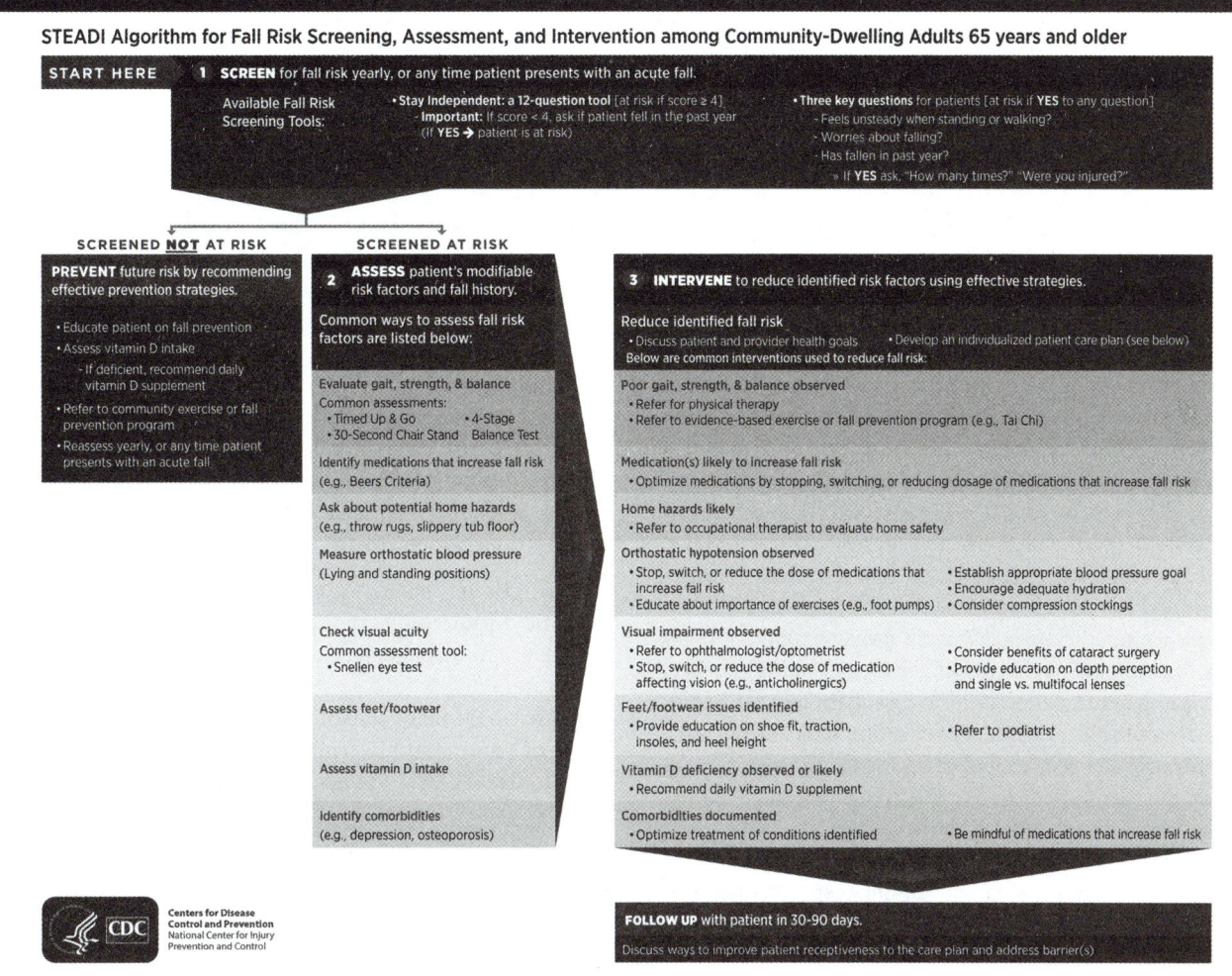

FIGURE 7-2—cont'd

- Current physical activity and functional mobility (e.g., basic and instrumental ADL performance)
- Psychological state, including reaction to falling
- Performance of underlying balance components (e.g., motor, sensory, and cognitive systems; postural alignment; **reactive control** [maintaining balance after a perturbation or a limits of stability challenge]; functional limits of stability; and static and dynamic balance)
- Interior and exterior evaluation of the home

In addition, assessment of other risk factors can be conducted by the team (physician, nurse, occupational therapist, or physical therapist) for feet and footwear, visual acuity, blood pressure during supine-sitting-standing, and vitamin D levels and intake. Based on this information, the therapist identifies a list of potential fall assessment tools that best match the client.

There are many fall assessment tools. Mancini and Horak (2010) conducted a systematic review regarding the psychometrics of balance assessment tools and identified a tool with good psychometrics that examines self-perception of balance, the Activities-specific Balance Confidence questionnaire. The clients rate themselves on their ability to perform everyday tasks (e.g., likelihood of falling). Marques-Vieira et al (2016) found that another self-rating tool, the Falls Efficacy Scale-International includes socially demanding tasks, uses language that is well understood by various cultures, measures fear of falling, and is psychometrically validated for international participants. Mancini and Horak (2010) also identified evidence-based tools aligned with performance testing: the Tinetti Balance and Gait Test, the Berg Balance Scale, Timed Up & Go (TUG), and the Functional Reach Test (FRT). The Multi-Directional Reach Test assesses limits of stability (distance reached while maintaining one's balance) during reaching—as does the FRT—but does so in four directions and not merely forward. Franc et al (2020) found validity in the Sock Test for Sitting Balance, an occupation-based tool for older adult community dwellers and hospitalized patients. The Elderly Mobility Scale assesses mobility and function for older adults (e.g., supine-sit-stand, walk, reach). Cut-off scores indicate independence level (ADLs) and living assistance needs, but scores are poorly predictive of single fallers (Shirley Ryan Abilitylab, 2019).

The STEADI initiative includes evidence-based tools, namely TUG, the 30-Second Chair Stand, and the 4-Stage Balance Test. For home hazards, the Home Falls and

Accidents Screening Tool (Home FAST), In-Home Occupational Performance Evaluation (I-HOPE), Safety Assessment of Function and the Environment for Rehabilitation-Health Outcome Measurement and Evaluation (SAFER-HOME) and the Westmead Home Safety Assessment are a few tools that involve client performance at the home (see Chapter 15). Both indoor and outdoor environments should be assessed (e.g., indoor: kitchen, bedroom, bathroom, main living area, floors, stairs and steps; outdoor: sidewalks, steps, patios and decks, gardens, mailbox), with consideration given to time of day and seasons of the year. Collaboration with physical therapy is vital to a comprehensive balance evaluation and intervention plan due to time constraints impeding each discipline. This may involve a coevaluation or shared assessment results. Physical therapists and occupational thearpists conduct multiple balance assessments with a variety of evidence-based tools (Sibley et al, 2011), and through systematic observational assessment during ADLs, IADLs, and occupation. Observing balance when the client is reaching high and low for clothing in a closet, opening a kitchen drawer, opening the refrigerator to procure food, carrying objects, walking on varied surfaces, and performing transfers with clothing management yields critical data about the older adult's dynamic balance, limits of stability, and possibly reactive control. The occupational therapist can provide a push (pull) on the client's body to test reactive control if the natural environment does not provide the opportunity.

For balance problems involving vestibular issues, there should be an assessment by an audiologist. Occupational therapy practitioners need further training beyond entry level to be skilled in assessment and intervention for vestibular issues. Some evidence-based vestibular balance assessments include the Dizziness Handicap Inventory, the Vestibular Disorders Activities of Daily Living Scale, and clinical testing for the vestibulo-ocular reflex (Gronski & Neville, 2017). The Clinical Test of Sensory Interaction on Balance is a low cost assessment of sensory input on postural control in which the therapist puts the client through a series of balance activities on challenging surfaces (Cohen et al, 1993; Shirley Ryan Abilitylab, 2023).

Implications for the Older Adult in Treatment: Falls

Montero-Odasso et al (2022) present an algorithm using their world guidelines, similar to STEADI, for prevention and management of falls. First, all older adults should be informed about preventing falls and given information on being physically active. Second, the authors recommend that fall risk needs to be graded or stratified with corresponding intervention strategies pertinent to a specific client. For example, people who have not fallen and have good balance and gait would benefit from low fall risk intervention including education about fall prevention and exercise for general health. Whereas for those who have fallen once or have impaired gait or balance, intermediate fall risk interventions would be beneficial involving the previous strategies plus targeted exercise or physical therapy referral to improve balance and muscle strength, as appropriate, and reduce fall risk. High fall risk intervention is needed if someone has had one of the following: a fall with an injury, two or more falls in the past year, frailty, loss of consciousness (syncope), or inability to get up off the floor. High-risk fall intervention should include offering a multifactorial risk assessment with codeveloped goals with the client and personally tailored interventions based on the risk assessment and on the client's beliefs, attitudes, priorities, and preferences.

Multifactorial interventions incorporate at least two components, are unique for each client, and are based upon the client's fall risk factors. Consistently effective components are exercise coupled with environmental modification. The world guidelines list effective component strategies based upon strong evidence, such as:

- Strength and balance exercise, medication review, orthostatic hypotension and cardiovascular disease management, and management of underlying disease (acute and chronic)
- Nutritional management, environmental hazard assessment and modification, and individual education (Montero-Odasso et al, 2022)

Interventions with weak evidence or considered expert recommendations include telehealth and technology (smart home system), managing vestibular issues, assistive device training, optimizing vision and hearing (e.g., refraction, avoidance of multifocal lens use outdoors, cataract surgery, hearing aid), vitamin D supplementation if levels are low, managing foot problems, appropriate footwear, continence management, and pain interventions (Montero-Odasso et al, 2022).

The guidelines highlight context as critical for determining appropriate falls intervention. All older adults in care homes and hospital settings are at high risk for falls. The world guidelines identify strong evidence that hospitalized patients benefit from tailored fall-prevention education and single or multicomponent strategies based on identified personal risk factors, behaviors, or situations. Cameron et al (2018) found low-quality evidence that multifactorial interventions reduce the rate of falls for hospitalized patients when the patient was in the rehabilitation or geriatric ward, but there was an uncertain effect on the risk of falling. Montero-Odasso et al (2022) identify strong evidence that in care home settings, multicomponent interventions, avoidance of physical restraints, optimizing nutrition, and exercise training are effective for falls management. Their guidelines address low- and middle-income countries, where consideration of context is particularly necessary for intervention and strongly supported by evidence in addition to the previously stated strategies. The guidelines address medical conditions. Strong evidence supports: (a) exercise training for persons with mild cognitive impairment or dementia, (b) personalized and graded exercise post hip fracture to improve mobility and balance, and (c) personalized exercise consisting of balance and resistance training. Balance and resistance training is recommended for persons with mild and mid-stage Parkinson disease (including mild or no cognitive impairment), as is supervised exercise focused on balance and strength for someone with complex-phase Parkinson disease.

Molitor et al (2022) conducted a systematic review of evidence for occupational therapy interventions. For the outcome of fall prevention and reduction:

- Low-strength evidence was found for interventions addressing a single risk factor or using customized programs focusing on multiple risk factors.
- Moderate-strength evidence indicated that falls were reduced for participants receiving a structured program (e.g., A Matter of Balance) in a community center setting that was non-customized but addressed multiple risk factors such as the environment and person.

Regarding community discharge and reintegration, there was low strength of evidence when intervention included education or physical activity with other strategies (Molitor et al, 2022).

The occupational therapy intervention process for falls intervention should be codeveloped with the client to address the present and future for enabling continued independence, staying safe at home, and being safe in the community. The plan involves the client's fall risk factors, environmental and activity modifications, fall risk and prevention education (e.g., influence of balance and muscle strength, medication effects and timing), strengthening and balance activities, and self-monitoring.

Environmental modifications for fall prevention include:

- Removing tripping hazards and clutter
- Adding grab bars both inside and outside the tub/shower and next to the toilet
- Placing railings on both sides of stairs
- Having nonslip mats in the tub/shower
- Providing adequate nonglare light (e.g., night light, light sensors, battery-operated lamp if no outlet)
- Having a contrasting stripe to delineate the edge of steps
- Using a bedside commode for nocturia to prevent falls (CDC, 2021d).

Activity modification may involve being seated for a task; using a step stool to reach objects rather than overstretching to reach; using a cart on wheels to carry objects; wearing low profile, well-fitting shoes that secure around the heel (no flip flops); and avoidance of bifocals for outdoor activities. Additional activity modifications require the older adult to be intentional during the activity, such as standing slowly and pausing before taking a step to enable blood pressure to stabilize and observing one's surroundings for obstacles and hazards when walking. For community safety, the client should identify navigation strategies including where they desire to go, how they currently get there, and future plans for when mobility may be compromised, as is covered in the MyMobility Plan (see Box 7-1 Resources). Espiritu (2013) found that a self-management approach (e.g., self-monitoring, problem-solving, strategy and goal generation, and finding and using resources) for medical conditions, life roles, and emotional control was key for fall prevention. An evidence-based 8-week balance program called A Matter of Balance: Managing Concerns About Falls focuses on reducing fear of falling and increasing activity participation for ambulatory community dwellers. Of note is that older adults tend to use fewer strategies than they used previously, so it is important for occupational therapists to help the client widen their current repertoire of successful aging strategies. AOTA provides resources for fall prevention and assessment within the Quality Toolkit (see Box 7-1 Resources).

CASE STUDY (CONTINUED)

Assessment and Intervention

Solveig was likely frail due to her weakness, fatigue, and unintentional weight loss. Given her confusion, the medical team reviewed her medications. Although her physician had appropriately prescribed her medications for high blood pressure, her medical team suspected that Solveig may not have been taking her medications at the correct frequency or safely in conjunction with her other medications. Solveig's occupational therapist had her practice reading the bottle labels, completing a daily schedule around meals, and filling her pillbox. The therapist cued Solveig to check that only one pill dropped into the pillbox compartment and to know the difference between pills that looked the same. Solveig realized that she had been taking two of the same pill instead of one each of two different pills daily. The occupational therapist relayed Solveig's self-assessment to the team.

Knowing Solveig had not been eating well, her occupational therapist inquired if Solveig had any pain with chewing or difficulty with her oral hygiene. Fortunately, Solveig did not have any trouble chewing or caring for her teeth. After being on IV antibiotics for a urinary tract infection, Solveig's confusion cleared. She had less burning with urination. The nurses continued to encourage her to drink liquids to flush the bacteria out of her urinary tract. In the last 15 years, Solveig began to have sudden and frequent urges to urinate. She typically made it to the toilet in time and would manage by not drinking as much when she went out. But with her blood pressure medications, she would get lightheaded if she did not drink water throughout the day.

Questions

1. How do the assessment results inform your interventions? What are Solveig's risks for performing daily activities? Use the assessment results for laboratory

values (e.g., urinalysis) and body readings (e.g., blood pressure, SpO_2, weight, height) to analyze Solveig's results and reveal her risks for performing daily activities to inform intervention.

2. What are two or three evidence-based, occupation-centered interventions that address the assessment results pertaining to at-risk daily activities? What assistive technologies or environmental modifications would you recommend?

3. What contextual elements from Solveig's occupational therapy profile influence your treatment planning?

Answers

1. All the results indicate a high risk of falling during activity participation. Laboratory values indicate she has a UTI, which may explain her confusion. Dehydration as noted by serum water osmolality is accompanied by reduced visual attention for tasks, orthostatic hypotension, and poor balance. Body readings indicate orthostatic hypotension, which impedes safe position changes (sit–stand) for bedroom and bathroom transfers due to fainting. Weight loss contributes to weakness, leading to falls during ambulation and transfers. Intervention needs to address these risks.

2. Please refer to the Implications section for each special concern for more information. Assessment results indicated high fall risk during ADLs and occupational participation due to reduced visual attention (related to dehydration), orthostatic hypotension, and poor balance (related to dehydration and poor medication management); confusion (related to UTI); and weakness (related to impaired oral health, malnutrition, and dehydration). Interventions may include having the client purposefully use vision to attend to the environment and its objects, creating a routine of drinking preferred beverages and scheduling regular toileting throughout the day, and training in medication management and oral health (using tools as needed).

3. Solveig has a number of contextual resources. Within her social context, Solveig has strong support from her adult children, two of whom live locally, and a church community. Her physical home environment includes a disability-accessible apartment and a community dining room. However, Solveig does live alone. Discharge planning will require ongoing assessment of her occupational performance, determination of whether her occupational performance fits her contextual environment, and indicated recommendations for additional support and assistance within her home while she recovers.

SUMMARY

The aging process presents special concerns for older adults that do not apply to other age groups. Due to impaired body structures and inefficient body functions with aging, an older adult's response to the challenges encountered in everyday life requires more effort and higher cognitive load to maintain function. In addition, the complex transactional network of body systems easily leads to a cascade of dysfunction starting with only one body structure or body function decline. When an environmental challenge or a person impairment occurs along with aging, the negative impact of these special concerns on occupational performance is amplified and likely will increase the risk for frailty and falling. Occupational therapists need to incorporate the influence of aging in the occupational therapy process with older adult clients.

Critical Thinking Questions

1. Discuss how each of the areas of concern discussed in the chapter can serve as a barrier and the supports that influence an older adult client's ability to resume their valued occupations.

2. How does aging affect interventions for an older adult with special concerns?

REFERENCES

Adila, F., & Walpola, R. L. (2021). Medicine self-administration errors in the older adult population: A systematic review. *Res Social Adm Pharm, 17*(11), 1877–1886. https://doi.org/10.1016/j.sapharm.2021.03.008

American Geriatrics Society Beers Criteria® Update Expert Panel (AGS). (2019). American Geriatrics Society updated Beers Criteria for potentially inappropriate medication use in older adults. *J Am Geriatr Soc, 67,* 674–694. https://doi.org/10.1111/jgs.15767

American Occupational Therapy Association (AOTA). (2017). Occupational therapy's role in medication management. *Am J Occup Ther, 71*(Suppl. 2), 7112410025. https://doi.org/10.5014/ajot.716S02

Atchison, K. A., & Dolan, T. A. (1990). Development of the Geriatric Oral Health Assessment Index. *J Dent Educ, 54*(11), 680–687. https://doi.org/10.1002/j.0022-0337.1990.54.11.tb02481.x

Avery, K., Donovan, J., Peters, T. J., Shaw, C., Gotoh, M., & Abrams, P. (2004). ICIQ: A brief and robust measure for evaluating the symptoms and impact of urinary incontinence. *Neurourol Urodyn, 23,* 322–330. https://doi.org/10.1002/nau.20041

Barceló, M., Torres, O. H., Mascaró, J., & Casademont, J. (2020). Hip fracture and mortality: Study of specific causes of death and risk factors. *Arch Osteoporos, 16*(15), 1–8. https://doi.org/10.1007/s11657-020-00873-7

Bongue, B., Buisson, A., Dupre, C., Beland, F., Gonthier, R., & Crawford-Achour, É. (2017). Predictive performance of four frailty screening tools in community-dwelling elderly. *BMC Geriatr, 17*(1), 1–9. https://doi/10.1186/s12877-017-0633-y

Bray, P., & Bonder, B. (2018). Considerations for medical care of older adults. In B. Bonder, & V. Dal Bello-Haas, (Eds.), *Functional performance in older adults* (4th ed., pp. 263–276). FA Davis. https://fadavispt.mhmedical.com/content.aspx?bookid=2302&sectionid=179707933

Cameron, I. D., Dyer, S. M., Panagoda, C. E., Murray, G. R., Hill, K. D., Cumming, R. G., & Kerse, N. (2018). Interventions for preventing falls in older people in care facilities and hospitals. *Cochrane Database Syst Rev.* https://doi.org/10.1002/14651858.cd005465.pub4

Carlson, M. C., Fried, L. P., Xue, Q. L., Tekwe, C., & Brandt, J. (2005). Validation of the Hopkins Medication Schedule to identify difficulties in taking medications. *J Gerontol A Biol Sci Med Sci, 60*(2), 217–223. https://doi.org/10.1093/gerona/60.2.217

Centers for Disease Control and Prevention (CDC). (2021a). *Disparities in oral health.* https://www.cdc.gov/oralhealth/oral_health_disparities/index.htm

Centers for Disease Control and Prevention (CDC). (2021b). *Oral health tips.* https://www.cdc.gov/oralhealth/basics/adult-oral-health/tips.html

Centers for Disease Control and Prevention (CDC). (2021c, April 30). *Nutrition: Micronutrients.* https://www.cdc.gov/nutrition/micronutrient-malnutrition/resources/index.html

Centers for Disease Control and Prevention (CDC). (2021d, August 6). *Older adult fall prevention: Facts about falls.* https://www.cdc.gov/falls/facts.html

Centers for Disease Control and Prevention (CDC). (2022, April 6). *Oral health conditions.* https://www.cdc.gov/oralhealth/conditions/index.html

Clegg, M. E., & Williams, E. A. (2018). Optimizing nutrition in older people. *Maturitas, 112,* 34–38. https://doi.org/10.1016/j.maturitas.2018.04.001

Cleveland Clinic. (2020, March 7). *Urinary tract infections.* https://my.clevelandclinic.org/health/diseases/9135-urinary-tract-infections

Cobey, C. (2022). *Incontinence impact questionnaire.* Shirley Ryan Abilitylab. https://www.sralab.org/rehabilitation-measures/incontinence-impact-questionnaire

Cohen, H., Blatchly, C. A., & Gombash, L. L. (1993). A study of the clinical test of sensory interaction and balance. *Physical Therapy, 73*(6), 346–354. https://doi.org/10.1093/ptj/73.6.346

Dal Bello-Haas, V. D., & MacIntyre, N. J. (2018). Neuromuscular and movement function: Falls. In B. Bonder & V. Dal Bello-Haas, (Eds.), *Functional performance in older adults* (4th ed., pp. 249–261). FA Davis. https://fadavispt.mhmedical.com/content.aspx?bookid=2302&sectionid=179707834

Dumoulin, C., Cacciari, L. P., & Hay-Smith, E. J. C. (2018). Pelvic floor muscle training versus no treatment, or inactive control treatments, for urinary incontinence in women. *Cochrane Database Syst Rev.* https://doi.org/10.1002/14651858.CD005654.pub4

Eckstrom, E., Parker, E. M., Shakya, I., & Lee, R. (2021). *A coordinated care plan to prevent older adult falls,* Edition 1.1. National Center for Injury Prevention and Control, Centers for Disease Control and Prevention. https://www.cdc.gov/steadi/pdf/Steadi-Coordinated-Care-Plan.pdf

Espiritu, E. W. (2013, September 9). Standing tall: A self-management approach to fall prevention intervention. *OT Practice,* 14–18. https://www.aota.org/-/media/Corporate/Files/Practice/Aging/Resources/Focus-On-Falls-Prevention-Home-Mod-Booklet.pdf

Fisher, S. R., Harmouche, I., & Kilic, G. S. (2022). Prevalence and predictors of increased fall risk among women presenting to an outpatient urogynecology and pelvic health center. *Female Pelvic Med Reconstr Surg, 28*(2), e7–e10. https://doi.org/10.1097/SPV.0000000000001118

Franc, I. A., Baxter, M. F., Mitchell, K., Neville, M., & Chang, P. F. (2020). Validity of the Sock Test for sitting balance: A functional sitting balance assessment. *OTJR (Thorofare NJ), 40*(3), 159–165.

Fried, L. P., Tangen, C. M., Walston, J., Newman, A. B., Hirsch, C., Gottdiener, J., Seeman, T., Tracy, R., Kop, W. J., Burke, G., McBurnie, M. A., & Cardiovascular Health Study Collaborative Research Group. (2001). Frailty in older adults: evidence for a phenotype. *The Journals of Gerontology. Series A, Biological Sciences and Medical Sciences, 56*(3), M146–M156. https://doi.org/10.1093/gerona/56.3.m146

Fritz, H., Seidarabi, S., Barbour, R., & Vonbehren, A. (2019). Occupational therapy intervention to improve outcomes among frail older adults: A scoping review. *Am J Occup Ther, 73*(3), 7303205130p1–7303205130p12. https://doi.org/10.5014/ajot.2019.030585

Gronski, M., & Neville, M. (2017). Vestibular impairment, vestibular rehabilitation, and occupational performance. *Am J Occup Ther, 71*(S2), 7112410055p1–7112410055p1. https://doi.org/10.5014/ajot.2017.716s09

Hooper, L., Abdelhamid, A., Ali, A., Bunn, D. K., Jennings, A., John, W. G., Kerry, S., Lindner, G., Pfortmueller, C. A., Sjöstrand, F., Walsh, N. P., Fairweather-Tait, S. J., Potter, J. F., Hunter, P. R., & Shepstone, L. (2015a). Diagnostic accuracy of calculated serum osmolarity to predict dehydration in older people: Adding value to pathology laboratory reports. *BMJ Open, 5*(10), e008846. https://doi.org/10.1136/bmjopen-2015-008846

Hooper, L., Abdelhamid, A., Attreed, N. J., Campbell, W. W., Channell, A. M., Chassagne, P., Culp, K. R., Fletcher, S. J, Fortes, M. B., Fuller, N., Gaspar, P. M., Gilbert, D. J., Heathcote, A. C., Kafri, M. W., Kajii, F., Lindner, G., Mack, G. W., Mentes, J. C., Merlani, P., ... Hunter, P. (2015b). Clinical symptoms, signs and tests for identification of impending and current water-loss dehydration in older people. *Cochrane Database Syst Rev.* https://doi.org/10.1002/14651858.CD009647.pub2

Iinuma, T., Arai, Y., Abe, Y., Takayama, M., Fukumoto, M., Fukui, Y., Iwase, T., Takebayashi, T., Hirose, N., Gionhaku, H., & Komiyama, K. (2015). Denture wearing during sleep doubles risk of pneumonia in the very elderly. *J Dent Res, 94*(3 Suppl), 28S–36S. https://doi.org/10.1177/0022034514552493

Institute of Medicine (IOM). (2010). *Providing healthy and safe foods as we age: Workshop summary.* National Academies Press. https://doi.org/10.17226/12967

Jafarinasabian, P., Inglis, J. E., Reilly, W., Kelly, O. J., & Ilich, J. Z. (2017). Aging human body: Changes in bone, muscle and body fat with consequent changes in nutrient intake. *J Endocrinol, 234*(1), R37–R51.

Jimoh, O. F., Brown, T. J., Bunn, D., & Hooper, L. (2019). Beverage intake and drinking patterns—clues to support older people living in long-term care to drink well: DRIE and FISE studies. *Nutrients, 11*(2): 447, 1–14. https://doi.org/10.3390/nu11020447

Kaiser, M. J., Bauer, J. M., Ramsch, C., Uter, W., Guigoz, Y., Cederholm, T., Thomas, D. R., Anthony, P., Charton, K. E., Maggio, M,. Tsai, A. C., Grathwohl, D., Vellas, B., & Sieber, C. C. (2009). Validation of the Mini Nutritional Assessment Short-Form (MNA®-SF): A practical tool for identification of nutritional status. *J Nutr Health Aging, 13*(9), 782–788.

Kannan, P., Hsu, W. H., Suen, W. T., Chan, L. M., Assor, A., & Ho, C. M. (2022). Yoga and Pilates compared to pelvic floor muscle training for urinary incontinence in elderly women: A randomised controlled pilot trial. *Complement Ther Clin Pract, 46*(2022), 101502. https://doi.org/10.1016/j.ctcp.2021.101502

Kwon, J. H., Fausone, M. K., Du, H., Robicsek, A., & Peterson, L. R. (2012). Impact of laboratory-reported urine culture colony counts on the diagnosis and treatment of urinary tract infection for hospitalized patients. *Am J Clin Pathol, 137*(5), 778–784. https://doi.org/10.1309/AJCP4KVGQZEG1YDM

Lacey, J., Corbett, J., Forni, L., Hooper, L., Hughes, F., Minto, G., Moss, C., Price, S., Whyte, G., Woodcock, T., Mythen, M., & Montgomery, H. (2019). A multidisciplinary consensus on dehydration: Definitions, diagnostic methods and clinical implications. *Ann Med, 51*(3–4), 232–251. https://doi.org/10.1080/07853890.2019.1628352

Lasak, A. M., Jean-Michel, M., Le, P. U., Durgam, R., & Harroche, J. (2018). The role of pelvic floor muscle training in training in the conservative and surgical management of female stress urinary incontinence: Does the strength of the pelvic floor matter? *PM&R Journal, 10*(2018), 1198–1210. https://doi.org/10.1016/j.pmrj.2018.03.023

Law, M., Cooper, B., Strong, S., Stewart, D., Rigby, P, & Letts, L. (1996). The Person-Environment-Occupation Model: A transactive approach to occupational performance. *Canadian J Occup Ther, 63,* 9–23. https://doi.org/10.1177/000841749606300103

Maleta, K. (2006). Undernutrition. *Malawi medical journal: The journal of medical association of Malawi, 18*(4), 189–205. https://www.ncbi.nlm.nih.gov/pmc/articles/PMC3345626/

Mancini, M., & Horak, F. B. (2010). The relevance of clinical balance assessment tools to differentiate balance deficits. *Eur J Phys Rehabil Med, 46*(2), 239.

Marques-Vieira, C. M. A., Sousa, L. M. M., Severino, S., Sousa, L., & Caldeira, S. (2016). Cross-cultural validation of the Falls Efficacy Scale

International in elderly: Systematic literature review. *J Clin Gerontol Geriatr, 7*(3), 72–76. https://doi.org/10.1016/j.jcgg.2015.12.002

Mayne, S., Bowden, A., Sundvall, P., & Gunnarson, R. (2019). The scientific evidence for a potential link between confusion and urinary tract infection in the elderly is still confusion-a systematic literature review. *BMC Geriatrics, 19*(32), 1–15. https://doi.org/10.1186/s12877-019-1049-7

Mayo Clinic. (2020, February 14). *Periodontitis.* https://www.mayoclinic.org/diseases-conditions/periodontitis/symptoms-causes/syc-20354473

Mayo Clinic. (2021a). *Urinary tract infection (UTI).* https://www.mayoclinic.org/diseases-conditions/urinary-tract-infection/symptoms-causes/syc-20353447

Mayo Clinic. (2021b, December 17). *Urinary incontinence.* https://www.mayoclinic.org/diseases-conditions/urinary-incontinence/symptoms-causes/syc-20352808

Meraz, R. (2019). Medication nonadherence or self-care? Understanding the medication decision-making process and experiences of older adults with heart failure. *J Cardiovasc Nurs, 35*(1), 26–34. https://doi.org/10.1097/JCN.0000000000000616

Molitor, W. L., Feldhacker, D. R., Lohman, H., Lampe, A. M., & Jensen, L. (2022). Occupational therapy and the IMPACT Act: Part 1. A systematic review of evidence for fall prevention and reduction, community discharge and reintegration, and readmission prevention interventions. *Am J Occup Ther, 76*(1). https://doi.org/10.5014/ajot.2022.049044

Molitor, W. L., & Nadeau, M. (2020). Occupational therapy for older women with urinary incontinence. *SIS Quarterly Practice Connections, 5*(3), 24–26. https://www.aota.org/publications/sis-quarterly/productive-aging-sis/pasis-8-20

Montero-Odasso, M., van der Velde, N., Martin, F. C., Petrovic, M., Tan, M. P., Ryg, J., Aguilar-Navarro, S., Alexander, N., Becker, C., Blain, H., Bourke, R., Cameron, I., Camicioli, R., Clemson, L., Close, J., Delbaere, K., Duan, L., Duque, G., Dyer, S., Freiberger, E., ... the Task Force on Global Guidelines for Falls in Older Adults. (2022). World guidelines for falls prevention and management for older adults: A global initiative. *Age Ageing, 51*(9), 1–36. https://doi.org/10.1093/ageing/afac205

Moon, S., Chung, H. S., Kim, Y. J., Kim, S. J., Kwon, O., Lee, Y. G., Yu, J. M., & Cho, S. T. (2021). The impact of urinary incontinence on falls: A systematic review and meta-analysis. *PLoS One, 16*(5): e0251711.https://doi.org/10.1371/journal.pone.0251711

Murphy, M. C., Somerville, E., Keglovits, M., Hu, Y. L., & Stark, S. (2017). In-home medication management performance evaluation (HOME-RX): A validity study. *Am J Occup Ther, 71,* 7104190020. https://doi.org/10.5014/ajot.2017.022756

National Institute of Dental and Craniofacial Research (NIDCR). (2018, July). *Oral cancer.* https://www.nidcr.nih.gov/health-info/oral-cancer

National Institutes of Health Office of Dietary Supplements (NIH). (2022, April 28). *Vitamin D fact sheet for health professionals.* https://ods.od.nih.gov/factsheets/VitaminD-HealthProfessional/

Op het Veld, L. P. M., van Rossum, E., Kempen, G. I. J. M. et al. (2015). Fried phenotype of frailty: Cross-sectional comparison of three frailty stages on various health domains. *BMC Geriatr* 15, 77. https://doi.org/10.1186/s12877-015-0078-0

Ouslander, J. G., Griffiths, P. C., McConnell, E., Riolo, L., Kutner, M., & Schnell, J. (2005). Functional incidental training: A randomized, controlled, crossover trial in Veterans Affairs nursing homes. *J Am Geriatr Soc, 53,* 1091–1100. https://doi.org/ 10.1111/j.1532-5415.2005.53359.x

Parker, M. L., Thornton-Evans, G., Wei, L., & Griffin, S. O. (2020). Prevalence of and changes in tooth loss among adults aged ≥50 years with selected chronic conditions–United States, 1999–2004 and 2011–2016. *MMWR Morb Mortal Wkly Rep, 69*(21), 641–646. https://doi.org/10.15585/MMWR.MM6921A1

Patel, U. J., Godecker, A. L., Giles, D. L., & Brown, H. W. (2022). Updated prevalence of urinary incontinence in women: 2015–2018 National Population-Based Survey data. *Female Pelvic Med Reconstr Surg, 28*(4), 181–187. https://doi.org/10.1097/SPV.0000000000001127

Porto, J. M., Iosimuta, N. C. R., Júnior, R. C. F., Braghin, R. D. M. B., Leitner, É., Freitas, L. G., & de Abreu, D. C. C. (2020). Risk factors for future falls among community-dwelling older adults without a fall in the previous year: A prospective one-year longitudinal study. *Arch Gerontol Geriatr, 91,* 104161. https://doi.org/10.1016/j.archger.2020.104161

Purba, J. (2021). Effectiveness of pelvic floor muscle training and yoga on the quality of life in perimenopausal women with urinary incontinence. *Nurse Media J Nurs, 11*(1), 85–93. https://doi.org/10.14710/nmjn.v11i1.32156

Rice, C. (2017). Occupational therapy's role in promoting hydration habits and routines of older adults. *SIS Quarterly Practice Connections, 2*(4), 19–21. https://www.aota.org/Publications-News/SISQuarterly/productive-aging-practiceconnections/GSIS-11-17.aspx

Rice, C. G. (2018). *Exploration of the hydration habits, morning balance, and morning blood pressure of institutionalized older adults* [Doctoral dissertation, Texas Woman's University]. Proquest Dissertations & Theses Global.

Rockwood, K., & Mitnitski, A. (2007). Frailty in relation to the accumulation of deficits. *J Gerontol A Biol Sci Med Sci.* 62:722–727. https://doi.org/10.1093/gerona/62.7.722

Rogowski, A., Krowicka-Wasyl, M., Chotkowska, E., Kluz, T., Wróbel, A., Berent, D., Mierzejewski, P., Sienkiewicz-Jarosz, H., Wichniak, A., Wojnar, M., Samochowiec, J., Kilis-Pstruskinska, K., & Bienkowski, P. (2021). Psychiatric history and overactive bladder symptom severity in ambulatory urogynecological patients. *J Clin Med. 10,* 3988.https://doi.org/10.3390/jcm10173988

Rolfson, D. B., Majumdar, S. R., Tsuyuki, R. T., Tahir, A., Rockwood, K. (2006). Validity and reliability of the Edmonton frail scale. *Age Ageing.* 35:526–29. https://doi.org/10.1093/ageing/afl041

Ruscin, J. M., & Linnebur, S. A. (2021a, July 21). *Aging and drugs.* Merck Manual. https://www.merckmanuals.com/home/older-people%E2%80%99s-health-issues/aging-and-drugs/aging-and-drugs

Ruscin, J. M., & Linnebur, S. A. (2021b, July 21). *Pharmacodynamics in older adults.* Merck Manual. https://www.merckmanuals.com/professional/geriatrics/drug-therapy-in-older-adults/pharmacodynamics-in-older-adults?query=pharmacodynamics

Ruscin, J. M., & Linnebur, S. A. (2022, September). *Pharmacokinetics in older adults.* Merck Manual. https://www.merckmanuals.com/professional/geriatrics/drug-therapy-in-older-adults/pharmacokinetics-in-older-adults

Salinas, T. J. (2017, November). *How do I clean dentures?* Mayo Clinic. https://www.mayoclinic.org/denture-care/expert-answers/faq-20058375#:~:text=Brush%20your%20dentures%20at%20least,food%2C%20plaque%20and%20other%20deposits

Sanchez, P., Everett, B., Salamonson, Y., Ajwani, S., Bhole, S., Bishop, J., Lintern, K., Nolan, S., Rajaratnam, R., Redfern, J., Sheehan, M., Skarligos, F., Spencer, L., Srinivas, R., & George, A. (2017). Oral health and cardiovascular care: Perceptions of people with cardiovascular disease. *PLoS One, 12*(7): e0181189. https://doi.org/10.1371/journal.pone.0181189

Saunders, J., Smith, T., & Stroud, M. (2011). Malnutrition and undernutrition. *Medicine, 39*(1), 45–50. https://dx.doi.org/10.7861%2Fclinmedicine.10-6-624

Schwartz, J. K., & Smith, R. O. (2017). The issue is—Integration of medication management into occupational therapy practice. *Am J Occup Ther, 71,* 7104360010. https://doi.org/10.5014/ajot.2017.015032

Shirley Ryan Abilitylab. (1 July, 2019). *Elderly mobility scale.* https://www.sralab.org/rehabilitation-measures/elderly-mobility-scale

Shirley Ryan Abilitylab. (2023). *Clinical test of sensory interaction on balance.* https://www.sralab.org/rehabilitation-measures/clinical-test-sensory-interaction-balance

Shumaker, S. A., Wyman, J. F., Uebersax, J. S., McClish, D. Fanti, J. A. (1994). Health-related quality of life measures for women with urinary incontinence: The incontinence impact questionnaire and the urogenital distress inventory. *Qual Life Res, 3*(5), 291–306. https://doi.org/10.1007/BF00451721

Sibley, K. M., Straus, S. E., Inness, E. L., Salbach, N. M., & Jaglal, S. B. (2011). Balance assessment practices and use of standardized balance

Sirls, L. T. (2008). Chapter 12–Measurement of urinary symptoms, health-related quality of life, and outcomes of treatment for urinary incontinence. In S. Raz, L. V. Rodriguez (Eds), *Female urology* (8th ed., pp. 147–157). W.B. Saunders. https://doi.org/10.1016/B978-1-4160-2339-5.50061-6

Smaje, A., Weston-Clark, M., Raj, R., Orlu, M., Davis, D., & Rawle, M. (2018). Factors associated with medication adherence in older patients: A systematic review. *Aging Med, 1*, 254–266. https://doi.org/10.1002/agm2.12045

Somerville, E., Massey, K., Keglovits, M., Vouri, S., Hu, Y.-L., Carr, D., & Stark, S. (2019). Scoring, clinical utility, and psychometric properties of the In-Home Medication Management Performance Evaluation (HOME–Rx). *Am J Occup Ther, 73*, 7302205060. https://doi.org/10.5014/ajot.2019.029793

Stanford University Health Care. (2021). *Urinary incontinence causes.* https://stanfordhealthcare.org/medical-conditions/primary-care/urinary-incontinence/causes.html

Tancock, K., & Roberts, J. (Editors). (2019). *Living well through activity in care homes: The tool kit.* College of Occupational Therapists. https://www.rcot.co.uk/about-occupational-therapy/living-well-care-homes-2019/balancing-risk-and-choice

Timsina, L. R., Willetts, J. L., Brennan, M. J., Marucci-Wellman, H., Lombardi, D. A., Courtney, T. K., & Verma, S. K. (2017). Circumstances of fall-related injuries by age and gender among community-dwelling adults in the United States. *PLoS One, 12*(5), e0176561. https://doi.org/10.1371/journal.pone.0176561

Travers, J., Romero-Ortuno, R., Bailey, J., & Cooney, M. T. (2019). Delaying and reversing frailty: A systematic review of primary care interventions. *Br J Gen Pract, 69*(678), e61–e69.

U.S. Department of Agriculture & U.S. Department of Health and Human Services (USDA & USHHS). (2020, December). *Dietary guidelines for Americans, 2020–2025.* 9th Edition. https://www.dietaryguidelines.gov/

Venkatesan, A. V. A., Ramalingam, S., Seenivasan, M. K., & Narasimhan, M. (2020, March 20). Evaluation of oral health status using the Geriatric Oral Health Assessment Index among the geriatric population in India: A pilot study. *Cureus, 12*(3): e7344. https://doi.org/10.7759/cureus.7344

Volkert, D., Beck, A. M., Cederholm, T., Cruz-Jentoft, A., Goisser, S., Hooper, L., Kiesswetter, E., Maggio, M., Raynaud-Simon, A., Sierver, C. C., Sobotka, L., van Asselt, D., Wirth, R., & Bischoff, S. C. (2018). ESPEN guideline on clinical nutrition and hydration in geriatrics. *Clin Nutr, 38*(1), 10–47. https://doi.org/10.1016/j.clnu.2018.05.024

World Health Organization. (2001). *International Classification of Functioning, Disability and Health (ICF).* World Health Organization. https://www.who.int/standards/classifications/international-classification-of-functioning-disability-and-health

World Health Organization. (2017). Evidence profile: Urinary incontinence. World Health Organization. https://www.who.int/ageing/health-systems/icope/evidence-centre/ICOPE-evidence-profile-urinary-incont.pdf

World Health Organization. (2021, June 9). *Malnutrition.* https://www.who.int/news-room/fact-sheets/detail/malnutrition

Wu, A., Alwawi, D., & Branson, B. (2016). Tooth-brushing ability after left stroke. *Am J Occup Ther, 70*(4)(Suppl. 1), 7011500041p1. https://doi.org/10.5014/ajot.2016.70S1-PO4055

Xu, F., Laguna, L., & Sarkar, N. (2018). A ging-related changes in quantity and quality of saliva: Where do we stand in our understanding? *J Texture Stud, 50*, 27–35. https://doi.org/10.111/itxs.12356

Yip, S. O., Dick, M. A., McPencow, A. M., Martin, D. K., Ciarleglio, M. M., & Erekson, E. A. (2013). The association between urinary and fecal incontinence and social isolation in older women. *Am J Obstet Gynecol, 208*(2), 146.e1–146.e1467. https://doi.org/10.1016/j.ajog.2012.11.010

Zartman, A. L., Hilsabeck, R. C., Guarnaccia, C. A., & Houtz, A. (2013). The Pillbox Test: An ecological measure of executive functioning and estimate of medication management abilities. *Arch Clin Neuropsychol, 28*(2013), 307–319. https://doi.org/10.1093/arclin/act014

CHAPTER 8

Metabolic Conditions

Suzanne Perea Burns, PhD, OTR/L ■ Emily Kringle, PhD, OTR/L ■
Jessica Salazar Sedillo, MSW, MOT, OTR

"My mother always used to say, 'The older you get, the better you get. Unless you're a banana.'"

—Betty White (1922-2021)

LEARNING OUTCOMES

By the end of this chapter, readers will be able to:

8-1. Summarize metabolic syndrome (MetS) and its relationship to cardiovascular disease (CVD), diabetes, cancer, and other chronic conditions.

8-2. Describe the relationship between MetS and aging with respect to CVD, diabetes, cancer, and other chronic conditions.

8-3. Compare different theories and practice frameworks that can be applied to addressing health and wellness interventions in older adults.

8-4. Discuss lifestyle factors and how they can be addressed through self-management treatments for older adults.

8-5. Select appropriate, evidence-based practice interventions to address lifestyle factors in older adults.

8-6. Analyze the role of occupational therapy working with interprofessional colleagues to address health and wellness goals in older adults.

Mini Case Study

Mr. Jenkins is a 68-year-old non-Hispanic white male. He has been overweight since childhood. He has smoked occasionally since his teens and is a social drinker. He separated from his wife 14 years ago and is estranged from his two adult children. He is in a positive relationship with a 70-year-old widower, Mike. Mr. Jenkins has severe arthritis in his knees, has uncontrolled hypertension, and is prediabetic. He drives a delivery truck part-time, which requires him to sit for prolonged periods of time and drive in dense urban traffic. He reports that he relaxes with a beer or two in front of the television when he gets home from work until he goes to bed. He also complains of sleep disturbances and has been diagnosed with sleep apnea. He reports that, due to his work conditions and sleeping issues, cooking meals for himself is a challenge and ordering takeout multiple times a week is more manageable.

Provocative Questions
1. What factors contribute to Mr. Jenkins's deconditioning and poor health?
2. Even without an exercise intervention, what benefit do you think addressing each unhealthy lifestyle behavior might have on his functional capacity?
3. How might you go about involving his partner into an exercise program for Mr. Jenkins?
4. How would you address his concern about cooking meals for himself?

Metabolic conditions are a growing burden worldwide. Although prevention and treatment approaches have demonstrated considerable progress, these conditions continue to be a major public health problem globally. Lifestyle-related factors such as smoking, dyslipidemia, hypertension, and obesity are major contributors to metabolic conditions, and interprofessional approaches are needed to lessen the risk of cardiometabolic diseases, including cardiovascular disease, diabetes, some cancers, and some gastrointestinal conditions. This chapter will address: (1) the metabolic system as it relates to typical age-related changes and atypical changes, (2) major health conditions influenced by MetS, (3) examples of theories and practice frameworks related to addressing metabolic conditions in older adults, (4) implications for treatment in older adults, and (5) an interprofessional approach to addressing metabolic conditions in this population.

Noncommunicable Diseases

Noncommunicable diseases (NCD) are a major public health problem and contribute to approximately 71% of deaths globally (World Health Organization [WHO], 2021a). Most NCD deaths are associated with **CVD,** followed by cancers, respiratory diseases, and diabetes, respectively. Although NCDs can influence health and disability outcomes across the life span, population aging is a major contributor to this problem. Rapid globalization of unhealthy lifestyles is another prime contributor to this global public health issue. For instance, lack of physical activity and unhealthy diets can lead to hypertension, increased blood glucose levels, elevated blood lipid levels, and obesity. Lifestyle-related effects to health are often referred to as metabolic risk factors (WHO, 2021a) and can contribute to morbidity and mortality. Table 8-1 provides the mortality rates for people of all ages in 2020.

MetS is defined by the co-existence of cardiometabolic risk factors, which increase the risk of CVD, type 2 diabetes mellitus, cancer, and other chronic health conditions. WHO defines this pathological condition as being characterized by abdominal obesity, insulin resistance, hypertension, and hyperlipidemia. With the global spread of the Western lifestyle, often characterized as (1) the consumption of high-calorie, low-fiber fast food and (2) decreased physical activity and greater sedentary behavior, NCDs related to MetS are becoming increasingly problematic. In fact, MetS contributes to conditions such as type 2 diabetes, coronary disease, and stroke (Saklayen, 2018). Additionally, MetS has been linked to mental health conditions such as major depressive disorder, anxiety disorders, and emotional distress related to chronic conditions (Hoffmann et al, 2021; Kuniss et al, 2021; Limon et al, 2020).

National survey data from a U.S. population collected between 2011 and 2016 suggest that approximately 35% of all adults and 48.6% of adults older than 60 years have MetS (Hirode & Wong, 2020). This is particularly concerning when addressing the needs of older adults because several health consequences are related to MetS. Refer to Table 8-2 for the relationship between health behaviors and health conditions described in this chapter.

Older adults are at risk for lifestyle-related health conditions that contribute to health outcomes, functional decline, and disability.

Advanced age leads to the exacerbation of systemic chronic inflammation, oxidative stress, DNA damage, decline of mitochondrial function, cellular senescence, and tissue dysfunction, all conditions which contribute to generate metabolic disorders (Longo et al, 2019 p. 1; Tchkonia & Kirkland, 2018).

When working with older adults, promoting positive health and wellness behaviors can support improved health and functional outcomes. In rehabilitation, primary,

TABLE 8-1 Leading Causes of Death in the United States, 2020

CAUSE OF DEATH	RANK	DEATHS
All causes		3,358,814
Heart disease	1	660,882
Cancer	2	598,932
COVID-19	3	345,323
Unintentional injuries	4	192,176
Stroke	5	159,050
Chronic lower respiratory diseases	6	151,637
Alzheimer's disease	7	133,382
Diabetes	8	101,106
Influenza and pneumonia	9	53,495
Kidney disease	10	52,260
Suicide	11	44,834

Source: National Center for Health Statistics. National Vital Statistics System: Mortality statistics. (https://www.cdc.gov/nchs/data_access/vitalstatsonline.htm#Mortality_Multiple). Data for 2020 are final.

TABLE 8-2 Lifestyle-Related Noncommunicable Diseases That Are Associated With Poor Health Practices, Including a Sedentary Lifestyle and Low Levels of Activity

RISK FACTOR	CVD	COPD	STROKE	TYPE 2 DM	CANCER	GASTROINTESTINAL DISORDERS
Smoking	X	X	X	X	X*	X
Physical inactivity	X		X	X	X	X
Obesity	X	X	X	X	X	X
Nutrition	X	X	X	X	X	X
High blood pressure	X		X	X		X
Dietary fat[†]/blood lipids	X		X	X	X	X
Elevated glucose levels	X		X	X	X	X
Alcohol[‡]	X		X	X	X	X

CVD, Cardiovascular disease; COPD, chronic obstructive pulmonary disease; DM, diabetes mellitus.
*An increased risk of all-cause cancer. Smoking is related not only to cancer of the nose, mouth, airways, and lungs, but also increases the risk of all-cause cancer.
†Partially saturated, saturated, and trans fats are the most injurious to health.
‡Alcohol can be protective in moderate quantities, particularly red wine. Adapted from Goldstein et al (2011); Siteman Cancer Center (n.d.).

secondary, and tertiary prevention interventions are used within interprofessional teams to address lifestyle-related health conditions. Self-management is one approach occupational therapists can use with clients when addressing lifestyle-related health conditions. Specifically, "self-management is the intrinsically controlled ability of an active, responsible, informed and autonomous individual to live with the medical, role and emotional consequences of his chronic condition(s) in partnership with his social network and the healthcare provider(s)" (Van de Velde et al, 2019, p. 10). Such interventions are discussed in greater detail later in the chapter.

Given the number of older adults with MetS, it is expected that occupational therapists working with this population will have the opportunity to address lifestyle and self-management across the continuum of care.

CASE STUDY

OT Profile

Mrs. Jaramillo is a 73-year-old Hispanic woman who works as a part-time cashier at the local dollar store. She is the primary caregiver for her husband, who was diagnosed with Parkinson disease 5 years ago. Mrs. Jaramillo values being able to care for her husband, despite her own chronic conditions. She has a 43-year-old daughter who comes over to help with caregiving once weekly, including dropping off groceries and attending various medical appointments. Unfortunately, Mrs. Jaramillo must use her paid time off (PTO) from her part-time job to attend the multiple medical appointments she and her husband have. Previously, Mrs. Jaramillo would play bridge with her church friends every week.

Medical History (Body Structures and Functions)

- Overweight (body mass index = 28.9 kg/m²)
- Hypertension (takes medication to manage her blood pressure)
- Prediabetes (hemoglobin A_{1c} = 6.3%)
- Osteoarthritis (affects her back and knees)
- Depression (Patient Health Questionnaire-9 score = 13, moderate depression)
- Intermittent claudication
- Nonsmoker

Problem Areas

- Pain and fatigue affect her community mobility and work tolerance.
- Time limitations interfere with her ability to manage activities of daily living and instrumental activities of daily living (meal preparation, leisure participation).
- Stress of pain, fatigue, time limitations, financial situation, current and future caregiving contribute to her depression.

Strengths

- Has family support (daughter)
- Views work as a positive social activity that she enjoys and brings in a little extra income
- Willingness to find and use resources, positive outlook that her family can "make" this work and improve her situation

Questions

1. As an occupational therapist, what performance areas and body functions/structures should be assessed?
2. How would the occupational therapist engage Mrs. Jaramillo in self-management activities?

Answers

1. Areas to assess include daily routines and specific problems (meal preparation, work, household maintenance, and financial management), endurance and activity tolerance, medication management for her and husband, home accessibility and fall risk, pain levels during daily activities and methods of pain management, current use of community resources. See section on Implications for Older Adults in Treatment. LO 8-5
2. Encourage Mrs. Jaramillo to discuss challenges and barriers to self-management, and create a plan of action together to address each barrier. SMART (specific, measurable, actionable/attainable, relevant, time bound) goal setting can also be used to promote better self-management and lead to achievable outcomes by creating short-term and long-term goals for managing her care needs and accessing resources. When incorporating self-management into occupational therapy interventions, the occupational therapist teaches the client problem-solving skills and increases Mrs. Jaramillo's participation and self-efficacy. See section on Theories and Frameworks for Practice. LO 8-4

Understanding the Metabolic System

CVD and Aging

Although cardiovascular disease CVD can affect people across the life span, it is the leading cause of death and disability for people age 65 years or older (Tsao et al, 2022). Aging is associated with a progressive decline in several physiological processes, which contributes to an increased risk of health complications. Specifically, aging has a substantial effect on the heart and arterial system, which contributes to an increase in CVD, including atherosclerosis (buildup of fats, cholesterol, and other substances in arterial walls), hypertension (high blood pressure), myocardial infarction (heart attack), and stroke. Aging tissues within the cardiovascular system can have pathological changes, such as **hypertrophy** (an adaptive response to pressure or volume stress that results in enlargement of an organ or tissue due to increased cell size) and alterations to left ventricular diastolic and systolic function (Chiao et al, 2016; North & Sinclair, 2012). When the vasculature ages, changes such as arterial thickening, arterial stiffness, and endothelium dysfunction can occur, which contribute to increased systolic blood pressure. This change to systolic blood pressure is a risk factor for the development of atherosclerosis, hypertension, stroke, and atrial fibrillation (Chiao et al, 2016; North & Sinclair, 2012). The heart also undergoes major changes with aging. Even slight changes in the heart can have major implications. In general, progressive degeneration of cardiac structures contributes to a loss of elasticity, fibrotic changes in the heart valves, and infiltration of amyloid (i.e., buildup of plaques of protein byproduct) in the heart muscle. Box 8-1 provides a depiction of the cardiovascular system in both a young and an aged person (North & Sinclair, 2012).

MetS risk factors such as abdominal obesity, impaired glucose tolerance, hypertension, hyperlipidemia, and hypertriglyceridemia are independent risk factors of CVD. Cumulatively, these risk factors can increase the rate and severity of CVD (Tune et al, 2017).

Obesity contributes to heart failure and coronary heart disease through body composition changes that affect hemodynamics, which can physically alter the heart's structure. For example, although the association is not entirely understood, increased visceral fat mass can contribute to low-grade systemic inflammation, and some inflammatory markers have been shown to induce cardiac dysfunction (Carbone et al, 2019). Adipose tissue, fatty tissue that is connective and composed of adipocytes (fat cells), can contribute to the buildup of atherosclerotic plaque and impair cardiac systolic and diastolic function. A Western diet has high saturated fat and sugar content, which also contribute to inflammation. Weight gain is associated with increased blood pressure, which can lead to arterial hypertension, a leading cause of heart failure (Carbone et al, 2019).

Smoking is another risk factor that can damage the cardiovascular system. It contributes to coronary artery disease, which is a leading cause of having a heart attack. Smoking can contribute to hypertension, limits one's ability to engage in physical activity, increases the likeliness of blood clots, and lowers high-density lipoprotein (HDL) cholesterol levels, all of which increase the risk for heart attacks and stroke. Smoking can also cause poor blood flow, leading to peripheral vascular disease, and can decrease the body's ability to heal from injuries and cuts (American Cancer Society, 2020).

CVD is closely linked with diabetes. Diabetes is associated with macrovascular (large arteries) and microvascular (small arteries and capillaries) disease. Chronic **hyperglycemia** (an excess of blood glucose in the bloodstream) and insulin resistance are related to vascular complications, such as the increased formation of advanced glycation end products (harmful products formed when proteins or lipids become glycated when exposed to sugar in the bloodstream), **oxidative stress** (an imbalance between free radicals and antioxidants in the body), and inflammation. Individuals with diabetes also have increased inflammatory markers, particularly C-reactive protein (CRP), which contributes to endothelial dysfunction and vascular health. Additionally, CRP may increase the uptake of low-density lipoprotein (LDL; Leon & Maddox, 2015). Poor glycemic control is associated with poor cardiovascular outcomes. However, evidence on very tight glycemic control guidelines and the effect on CVD is conflicting. A potential reason for this conflict is that the concurrent CVD risk factor profile in diabetics may overpower the benefit of the hyperglycemia treatment (Leon & Maddox, 2015). Individuals with diabetes frequently have

---

BOX 8-1 Examples of Age-Related Changes to the Cardiovascular System

- **Slower heart rate.** An age-related reduction in maximal heart rate is due to a decrease in the number of cells in the sinoatrial node. This can contribute to a reduction in the tolerance of cardiac exertion and slower aerobic performance.
- **Blood changes.** The blood exhibits some slight changes with aging because there is less fluid in the bloodstream and thus blood volume decreases. With increased stress, red blood cell production can slow, which creates a slower response to blood loss. White blood cells remain relatively unchanged with exception to neutrophil production. Neutrophils are related to immunity and decreased production can reduce the ability to resist infections.
- **Stiffening and thickening of heart valves, aorta, and capillaries.** The heart valves control and influence the direction of blood flow and the heart wall. Stiffening and thickening of the valves can decrease the tolerance for stress and exercise on the heart itself. Age-related increase in circumference can be observed in all four valves (aortic semilunar, semilunar, bicuspid, tricuspid) with greatest changes occurring in the aortic valve. Less flexibility in the aorta can contribute to a rise in blood pressure and an increase in how hard the heart is working. Capillary walls can undergo slight thickening, which can slow the rate of exchange for waste and nutrients.
- **Subcellular changes.** Mitochondria can have changes in size, shape, crystal pattern, and matrix density. These changes reduce functional surface area. The cytoplasm also undergoes changes, such as fatty infiltration or degeneration and accumulation of pigments of lipofuscin. Changes to subcellular compartments can result in decreased cellular activities, such as homeostasis and protein synthesis.

additional risk factors, including obesity, hypertension, and **dyslipidemia,** an imbalance between lipids in the bloodstream such as cholesterol, LDL cholesterol, triglycerides, and HDL cholesterol.

Hypertension is a remediable risk factor for CVD. However, only 28% of people with hypertension are controlling their blood pressure according to studies that used <140/90 mm Hg clinical targets (Patel et al, 2018; Mills et al, 2016). It is noteworthy that a systolic blood pressure of 120 to 139 mm Hg or diastolic blood pressure of 80 to 89 mm Hg was previously referred to as prehypertension. New guidelines have been set by the American Heart Association for healthy and unhealthy blood pressure ranges. The new ranges are

- Normal: Less than 120 mm Hg systolic and less than 80 mm Hg diastolic
- Elevated: 120 to 129 mm Hg systolic and less than 80 mm Hg diastolic
- High blood pressure (hypertension) stage 1: 130 to 139 mm Hg systolic or 80 to 89mm Hg diastolic
- High blood pressure (hypertension) stage 2: 140 mm Hg or higher systolic or 90 mm Hg or higher diastolic
- Hypertensive crisis: Greater than 180 mm Hg and/or greater than 120 mm Hg diastolic

Medication adherence is a major concern with hypertension control. For example, one study found that 25% of patients initiating antihypertensive therapy never fill their initial prescription (Berra et al, 2016; Lackland et al, 2018). Furthermore, only one in five patients is sufficiently adherent to drug therapy, limiting its benefits (e.g., stroke prevention) (Lackland et al, 2018). For many adults there is no identifiable cause of high blood pressure (essential hypertension), which develops gradually over time. Secondary hypertension tends to appear more suddenly and can be brought on by health conditions and medications, such as renal disease, adrenal gland tumors, thyroid problems, congenital birth defects, medications such as birth control, and decongestants. The use of illicit drugs, such as cocaine and methamphetamine, may also cause hypertension. Refer to Box 8-2 for a list of modifiable and nonmodifiable risk factors of hypertension.

Hypertension can cause damage to various organs dependent on healthy vasculature. Damage can occur to the (1) brain, which may include transient ischemic attack, stroke, dementia, and mild cognitive impairment; (2) kidneys, including scarring and renal failure; (3) eyes, including retinopathy, fluid buildup under the retina (choroidopathy), and optic neuropathy (nerve damage from blocked blood flow); (4) sexual dysfunction; and (5) hypertensive emergencies, which can result in blindness, pregnancy complications, aortic dissection, sudden loss of kidney function, and other major complications (Mayo Clinic, 2022).

Hypertension is a critical factor to consider when addressing stroke risk reduction. Multiple trials have demonstrated that the management of hypertension can reduce the risk of stroke. Recent guideline changes suggest a systolic blood

> **BOX 8-2** **Modifiable and Non-Modifiable Risk Factors for Hypertension (WHO-B, 2021)**
>
> - Modifiable risk factors:
>   - Unhealthful diets (excessive salt consumption, a diet high in saturated fat and trans fats, low intake of fruits and vegetables)
>   - Physical inactivity
>   - consumption of tobacco and alcohol
>   - Being overweight or obese
> - Nonmodifiable risk factors:
>   - Family history of hypertension,
>   - 65 years-of-age and older
>   - Coexisting diseases such as diabetes or kidney disease.
> - Hypertension places stress on the cardiovascular system including:
>   - Damaging cells in arterial lining contributing to less elasticity and narrowed arteries thus limiting blood flow
>   - Over time, blood moving through weak arteries can cause an aneurysm or bulge which can rupture
>   - Decreased blood flow through narrowed and damaged arteries to the heart can lead to angina, arrhythmias, or myocardial infarction
>   - Hypertension forces the heart to work harder to pump the blood causing the left ventricle to thicken enhancing risk of heart failure, myocardial infarction, and sudden cardiac death
>
> From *Hypertension*, by World Health Organization, August 25, 2021
> https://www.who.int/news-room/fact-sheets/detail/hypertension

pressure goal of less than 130/80 mm Hg for patients with hypertension who are at risk for CVD and stroke (Lackland et al, 2018). With the stricter guidelines in place, Lackland and colleagues (2018) recommend the following strategies:

> *...improvement of lifestyle modification using behavioral and motivational strategies, addressing drug nonadherence, employment of team-based care, greater utilization of health information technology, including electronic health records and patient registries, and forming new connections for patients to their healthcare teams by telehealth.* (Lackland et al, 2018, p. 777).

Ischemic stroke risk increases with age and in relation to MetS. Risk factors tend to cluster among older adults. Although modifiable risk factors can predict stroke across all age groups, older adults remain largely affected by stroke (Youssufuddin & Young, 2019). The presence of two or more chronic conditions, often referred to as comorbidity or multimorbidity, is prevalent in people with stroke. In fact, an estimated 89% of people with incident stroke older than 65 years have multimorbidity. Furthermore, comorbidities interact with risk factors and increase the risk of hospital readmission, functional recovery, and mortality (the number of deaths that result from an illness or condition), which is already heightened in older adults (Youssufuddin & Young, 2019). Refer to Box 8-3 for modifiable and controllable stroke risk factors.

CVD has also been associated with depression, panic disorder, specific phobias, posttraumatic stress disorder, and alcohol use disorders. Moreover, the greater number of mental health disorders a person experiences over a lifetime, the higher their risk for heart disease (Scott et al, 2013). According to the American Heart Association, depression should be recognized as a risk factor for coronary heart disease. CVD and depression have a bidirectional relationship. About 15% to 30% of people with CVD also have a co-occurring diagnosis of depression (Khawaja et al, 2009). Depression can affect a person's mood; disrupt their engagement in daily occupations, including medication management; and impact social relationships. Therefore, it is important to assess the effect of both CVD and mental health on a person's quality of life and engagement in daily occupations.

Cancer and Aging

Aging is a well-known risk factor for developing cancer. Biological changes that occur with aging influence the development of cancer in older adults. As the population continues to age, the proportion of older adults with cancer is increasing as well. Unfortunately, older adults also experience more side effects from anticancer treatments. Several specific factors associated with aging have been identified that may contribute to higher cancer incidence in older age (Berben et al, 2021). Refer to Box 8-4 on aging factors and the development of cancer.

Berben and colleagues (2021) acknowledge that biological age differs from chronological age and may be better reflected by frailty status (see Chapter 7 for further discussion of frailty). They further describe the relationship between aging, frailty, tumor development, and cancer

---

BOX 8-3 Modifiable or Controllable Stroke Risk Factors

Stroke risk is far from being well-controlled and remains a major public health problem. Modifiable risk factors or risk factors that can be controlled for stroke include:

- Hypertension
- Smoking
- Diabetes
- Diet (particularly those high in saturated fats, trans fat, cholesterol, sodium, and calorie, which lead to obesity)
- Physical inactivity
- Obesity
- High blood cholesterol
- Carotid artery disease
- Peripheral artery disease
- Atrial fibrillation
- Other heart diseases

BOX 8-4 Aging Factors and Cancer Development

- **Accumulation of oxidative stress and DNA damage.** Older adults have an accumulation of oxidative stress and DNA damage over time which is caused by exposure to metabolic insults like free radicals and environmental factors such as UV radiation and foods. These factors can lead to cellular-level changes and tumor development.
- **Senescent cell accumulation.** Senescent cells accumulate with aging and they secrete inflammatory mediators that may promote the growth of tumors.
- **Progressive decay of immune function.** As immune function declines in the aging process, so too does the effective immune response against developing tumors.

---

treatment decisions and how all of these inform clinical decision-making to support outcomes.

Most cancers directly or indirectly affect the cardiopulmonary and cardiovascular systems. The risk factors for cancer are well documented and include genetic and physiological factors, viral infections (e.g., hepatitis C), environmental and behavioral factors including inactivity, poor nutrition (high intake of fats and refined foods), poor air quality and smoking, psychological factors, and ingestion of and exposure to chemicals. Smoking has been implicated as a risk factor for many cancers, not only those involving the respiratory tract (American Cancer Society, 2020).

MetS has been associated with various cancer types and increases the risk of cancer development (Batelli et al, 2019). Though MetS does not cause cancer, a relationship with poorer cancer outcomes, including recurrence and mortality, has been identified (Micucci et al, 2016). MetS can increase risk for certain cancers and multiple risk factors, such as those present in MetS, may increase the risk of adverse outcomes compared with risk factors presenting individually. MetS and cancer both involve chronic inflammation and oxidative stress, which may promote abnormal growth of cells or tissues in the body (Batelli et al, 2019).

Obesity is a risk factor for cancer development and is associated with a poor prognosis for various tumor types. Systemic changes resulting from obesity include altered levels of insulin, insulin-like growth factor-1 (IGF-1), leptin, adiponectin, steroid hormones, and **cytokines** (proteins that stimulate or slow the immune system). These changes promote an environment that may facilitate tumor development and progression (Hopkins et al, 2016). Similarly, in people with diabetes, **hyperinsulinemia** (excess levels of insulin in the blood relative to glucose) increases the bioactivity of IGF-1 and may be a feasible explanation of carcinogenesis. Chronic inflammation may explain the increased risk of cancer in people with diabetes. Although diabetes treatment medications can modify cancer risk, managing diabetes can be a daunting challenge for individuals (Xu et al, 2014). Increased serum cholesterol levels are related to a higher risk of cancer development. Hypercholesterolemia and a high-fat/high-cholesterol diet have been shown to influence cancer development (Ding et al, 2019). People with MetS and cancer are at a higher risk of mortality than those without MetS. The majority of cancer survivors are older adults, and this population tends to be more susceptible to metabolic diseases in general.

Functional outcomes in older cancer survivors have been described in both clinical and population-based observational studies. Although it is unclear about the causal role of carcinogens and cancer treatments altering both physical and cognitive aging trajectories, biological rationale for accelerated aging trajectories in older adults is clear (Kobayashi et al, 2022). For instance, radiation and chemotherapies are known to induce cellular-level changes, which reflect the factors that influence the development of cancer in older adulthood, such as inflammation, cellular senescence (a process where cells age and stop dividing but do not die), DNA damage, and epigenetic (nongenetic influences on gene expression) alterations. Additionally, social factors may also perpetuate functional aging outcomes, such as psychosocial stress, financial stressors and costs, and disrupted social relationships (Kobayashi et al, 2022).

It has been reported that patients receiving cancer treatment can appear older and frailer. In fact, a growing body of literature describes the effects of cancer treatments on accelerated aging in people who have survived cancer.

Pulmonary Diseases and Aging

Age-associated changes occur in respiratory and pulmonary systems. Some of the changes include decreased volume of the thoracic cavity, reduced lung volume, and changes in the muscles that aid in respiration. Volume changes of the thoracic cavity are often due to narrowing of the intervertebral disk spaces which may cause kyphosis. The change in curvature of the spine can decrease the amount of space between the ribs leading to a smaller size of the chest cavity. Changes in musculature occur during the aging process and respiratory muscles decline, which can lead to difficulty or an inability to ventilate (Lowery et al, 2013; Schneider et al, 2021). Reduction in inspiratory and expiratory muscle strength occurs with age, and some evidence suggests that cellular level changes (i.e., reduction in mitochondrial adenosine triphosphate reserve) occur. Therefore, infections, including pneumonia, are more likely to lead to respiratory failure in older adults due to the physiological changes that occur with aging. Older adults may have more difficulty clearing mucus from the lungs due to reduction in cough strength and changes in the way that the body clears particles from airways (Lowery et al, 2013; Schneider et al, 2021). Advanced age also may contribute to immune dysfunction. Elevated inflammatory markers and heightened levels of cytokines without any infection targets may contribute to reduced elasticity and deterioration of lung parenchyma (Lowery et al, 2013; Schneider et al, 2021).

Chronic lower respiratory tract diseases such as asthma, emphysema, chronic bronchitis, and chronic obstructive pulmonary disease (COPD) can be particularly problematic in older adults. COPD is the third leading cause of death worldwide (WHO, 2021b), and 86% of deaths from COPD occur in people 65 years of age or older (American Lung Association, 2021). Cigarette smoking is the greatest risk factor for developing COPD. Long-term smokers have higher rates of all-cause morbidity and mortality (Centers for Disease Control and Prevention [CDC], 2020). Men who smoke are 17 times more likely to die of bronchitis and emphysema and are 23 times more likely to die of cancer of the trachea, lung, and bronchus. Women smokers are 12 times more likely to die of bronchitis and emphysema and the aforementioned cancers (CDC, 2020).

A link has been identified between MetS and lung diseases such as COPD and restrictive lung diseases (when the lungs cannot fill completely with air). First, elevated insulin levels during fetal development and lung maturation or even later in life can reduce lung function and increase bronchial hyperreactivity. It has also been identified that chronic elevation of insulin levels can reduce lung function in patients with diabetes (Baffi et al, 2016). Hyperlipidemia is associated with poor respiratory outcomes and triglyceride levels are associated with hyperresponsiveness of airways and wheezing which is initiated in adulthood. Obesity has a strong association with lung dysfunction (Baffi et al, 2016). For instance, people who are obese may have heightened levels of inflammatory markers and adipokines in visceral fat. Abdominal adiposity can lead to subepithelial fibrosis, smooth muscle hyperplasia of the airway, and bronchial hyperresponsiveness (Baffi et al, 2016).

Diabetes and Aging

Type 2 diabetes is a serious multisystem condition that has rapidly become pandemic in Western countries and some other countries where, previously, its incidence was minimal. Prevalence of diagnosed and undiagnosed diabetes mellitus in Americans over 65 years of age is estimated at 29.2% or 15.9 million (American Diabetes Association, 2019). With regards to aging, several factors may influence the risk of developing type 2 diabetes. First, aging has been associated with inflammatory markers. Body composition also changes with age which leads to an increase in fat mass, specifically visceral adiposity (abdominal fat), and a decrease in muscle mass. Furthermore, changes in insulin secretion and insulin sensitivity can lead to problems with glucose tolerance and potentially type 2 diabetes.

Formerly known as adult-onset diabetes, type 2 diabetes is increasingly diagnosed in children. Unfortunately, data shows that youth onset type 2 diabetes leads to early and severe effects and major public health implications (Today Study Group, 2021). This predisposes them to blindness, ischemic heart disease, stroke, renal disease, peripheral neuropathies, vascular insufficiency, and amputations. The primary consequences of type 2 diabetes include pathological changes to the macrovasculature and microvasculature and to nerve endings. Impaired glucose tolerance is a marker of vascular complications in the large and small blood vessels, independent of an individual's progression to diabetes. Early detection of glucose intolerance allows intensive dietary and exercise modifications, which may benefit from lifestyle interventions, to reduce the progression to diabetes (Ibrahim et al, 2018).

Individuals with type 2 diabetes are at an increased risk for CVD compared with individuals without diabetes, so lifestyle-based interventions may be particularly useful. Lifestyle has been established as a leading contributor to developing diabetes; hence, behavioral lifestyle practices need to be targeted foremost (Hivert et al, 2016). For example, cigarette smoking is an independent risk factor for type 2 diabetes (Kim et al, 2014) and is particularly dangerous for individuals with diabetes (Pan et al, 2015). Furthermore, physical activity has many beneficial effects on health for people with type 2 diabetes, including

- Improved insulin sensitivity
- Reduction in glycosylated hemoglobin A_{1c}
- Increased peak oxygen consumption
- Improved glycemic parameters
- Improved lipid profile
- Reduced blood pressure

These changes can support health outcomes in people with an existing diagnosis. For instance, progression of diabetic retinopathy can be reduced by as much as 40% when moderate physical activity is implemented 30 minutes per day, 5 days per week (Bryl et al, 2022). Weight reduction counters the effects of MetS and may counter the associated hypertension and dyslipidemia. Studies have shown that weight loss achieved by intensive health management programs, including diet and exercise, can lead to the remission of type 2 diabetes in as many as 80% of obese patients (Magkos et al, 2020).

In addition to its serious physical and functional consequences, people with type 2 diabetes have poor health-related quality of life, a high rate of depression (Zurita-Cruz et al, 2018), and diabetes-related emotional distress (Kuniss et al, 2021). Diabetes has been shown to increase emotional distress related to fear of serious complications related to a diabetes diagnosis and fear of elevated hemoglobin A_{1c} levels. Additionally, people with diabetes experience stress related to disruptions in daily routines due to diabetes self-management care. Another area of concern for people managing diabetes is social interference and dissatisfaction with support received from family and friends (Kuniss et al, 2021).

Gastrointestinal Disorders and Aging

It is well-accepted that aging affects virtually all functions of the gastrointestinal system, which includes gastric motility, enzyme and hormone secretion, digestion, and absorption of nutrients. When considering overall nutrition, it is important to first consider the oral cavity. In addition to poor fitting dentures, medication side effects, and other benign diseases, older adults may experience oral sensorial complaints such as dry mouth and taste disturbances that are explained by a decrease in the quality and quantity of salivary secretions (Dumic et al, 2019). Examples of esophageal conditions associated with aging include dysphagia (difficulty with swallowing), painful swallowing, and gastroesophageal reflux disease and its prolonged effects (e.g., Barrett's columnar-lined esophagus). The stomach can have decreased blood flow, decreased mucus (protective), altered gastric microbiota, and problems with repair mechanisms, all of which make older adults more susceptible to diseases like gastric ulcers, peptic ulcers, and *Helicobacter pylori* infections. Hormone secretion and absorption by the small intestine also changes with age, which can cause result in mesenteric ischemia, small intestinal overgrowth, and small bowel bleeding. The aging process can increase colon transit time, negatively affecting motility. Constipation, diverticular disease, irritable bowel syndrome, inflammatory bowel disease, and *Clostridioides difficile* colitis may be particularly problematic in this population (Dumic et al, 2019).

The gastrointestinal tract may contain as many as 1,000 bacterial species. The typical gut flora maintains an important role in digestion, fermentation, immunity, and the synthesis of vitamins and enzymes. Furthermore, the intestinal microbiota is associated with obesity and MetS (Parekh et al, 2015). MetS is associated with several gastrointestinal diseases and conditions such as cancer, inflammatory bowel disease, gastric and duodenal ulcers, and likely infections such as *H. pylori* (Metwaly et al, 2022; Parekh et al, 2015; Refaeli et al, 2018). Furthermore, the gastrointestinal tract can impact MetS.

In summary, older adults can experience both normal age-related decline and MetS leading to the development of metabolic conditions. Regardless of the cause, occupational therapy can contribute to transdisciplinary objectives of reducing morbidity and mortality associated with various conditions. Although occupational therapy most frequently receives referrals for individuals with these conditions in acute and postacute care settings, opportunities exist in prevention and primary care as well. Occupational therapists can address prevention and management for achieving improved health and well-being. This is often done through transdisciplinary approaches meaning that various disciplines may be working toward the same goal. Although occupational therapists often receive referrals to work with clients with diseases and conditions where secondary and tertiary prevention may be frequently addressed, opportunities for primary prevention and primary care also exist. Specific approaches are discussed later in this chapter.

Theories and Practice Frameworks

Occupational therapists are an important part of the interprofessional team to address clients with MetS and metabolic conditions. Since the primary focus for reducing metabolic risk factors includes lifestyle-related changes, it is important that occupational therapists utilize theories and models that specifically focus on behavioral changes to guide the therapeutic process when working with clients. There are several nonoccupation-based and occupation-based theories and models that occupational therapists can use with clients to incorporate behavior and lifestyle changes, promote healthy behavioral changes, and increase engagement in self-management of diseases. Nonoccupation-based theories and models that focus on behavior change include the Transtheoretical Model (TTM) and Health Belief Model (HBM). These models have been widely used in healthcare settings to promote healthy behavior change. Additionally, occupational therapists can use the Model of Human Occupation and Person-Environment-Occupation-Performance (PEOP) Model that focus on client factors, environmental factors, and engagement in occupation to assist clients with increasing healthy lifestyle behaviors.

Examples of Nonoccupation-Based Theories and Models

The Transtheoretical Model

The TTM of behavior change is a commonly used model that states that behavior change is a process and focuses intervention based on a person's readiness for change. The model includes five stages: precontemplation (client not currently thinking about or planning behavior change), contemplation (client deciding to make behavior change within next 6 months), preparation (client planning on making behavior change in immediate future), action (client actively engaging in behavior change within the last 6 months), and maintenance (client working toward relapse prevention). The model emphasizes that behavior change is not a linear process and happens over time, therefore a person may move forward and backward from stage to stage while engaging in behavior change (Prochaska & Velicer, 1997). Occupational therapists can use this model to identify the client's current stage and provide specific interventions to address the needs and barriers of the client at that current stage. Occupational therapists can also work with clients to provide interventions that support clients when they move back to a previous stage. For example, if the client is currently in the action stage but discontinues a newly established health behavior, they may have moved back into the preparation stage. Occupational therapists can provide education to the client that this is a normal part of the process in behavior change and can assist clients with moving back into the action stage through the use of therapeutic use of self and identifying barriers and challenges that led the client to discontinue the new health behavior.

Research has shown that the TTM increases positive health-related behavior changes in clients, including healthy eating, physical activity, and health-related management skills (Hashemzadeh et al, 2019; Jiménez-Zazo et al, 2020; Tseng et al, 2017). In addition, the TTM has been shown to improve medication adherence in clients with chronic conditions (Imeri et al, 2022).

Health Belief Model

The HBM can be used by occupational therapists to predict health behaviors with a focus on prevention among clients with MetS and chronic conditions. The HBM is an effective approach to providing comprehensive health education to clients. The HBM proposes that individuals will engage in lifestyle changes and healthy behaviors that decrease their risk of disease and illness if (1) they perceive themselves as susceptible to a certain disease or illness (perceived susceptibility) and (2) there is a potential for severe consequences due to the disease or illness (perceived severity). In addition, clients will be more likely to engage in specific health behaviors that will reduce the burden and consequences of the disease or illness if they believe that these health behaviors will provide benefits (perceived benefits) and believe any barriers to engaging in the specific health behavior are limited (perceived barriers; Rosenstock et al, 1988). The HBM also places emphasis on the self-efficacy of the client and cues to action that may influence the client's engagement in behavior change. Occupational therapists can utilize the HBM to provide specific interventions and education that addresses the client's perceptions of their chronic condition and how it affects them. If a client believes that the barriers to implementing a lifestyle change are greater than the benefits, they may not be motivated to change. However, occupational therapists can address these barriers and challenges the client is facing and provide them with education on how the lifestyle change can benefit the client and decrease the effect of the client's chronic condition.

The HBM has been effective to use with clients who have a diagnosis of a chronic condition. The HBM has been shown to increase client's engagement in self-care tasks to manage symptoms of their diabetes (Shabibi et al, 2017). Additionally, the HBM can be a tool that occupational therapists use to educate clients on the benefits of physical activity and address barriers to incorporating physical activity in the client's routine (Khodaveisi et al, 2021).

Examples of Occupation-Based Theories and Models

Model of Human Occupation

The Model of Human Occupation is an occupation-focused model that can be utilized with clients to increase participation in healthy lifestyle behaviors. This model comprises four components (volition, habituation, performance capacity, and environment) and explains that people's engagement in occupation is based on the dynamic interaction of each of the four components (Yamada et al, 2017).

Volition encompasses personal causation (a person's perception of their capacity and effectiveness), values (what a person finds meaningful), and interests (what a person finds enjoyable and interesting) (Yamada et al, 2017). Volition drives what occupations clients choose to do in their day-to-day life and plays a large part in what motivates clients to engage in certain occupations. Habituation is defined as "an internalized readiness to exhibit consistent patterns of behavior guided by our habits and roles and fitted to the characteristics of routine temporal, physical, and social environments" (Yamada et al, 2017, p. 17). For people to make sustaining health behavior changes, they must be able to incorporate these changes into their day-to-day routines. Performance capacity involves a person's physical and mental capacities to engage in occupations. These capacities include musculoskeletal, cardiopulmonary, neurological, and other body systems that impact function, as well as a person's mental and cognitive abilities. Through the evaluation process, occupational therapists can identify a client's barriers and strengths in relation to the components of their unique performance capacity and incorporate interventions to address these barriers. Environment is where occupations occur and can include both the physical environment and social environment in which a person completes their occupations. Both the physical and social environments, including access to healthy foods and resources, social support from family and friends, and safe and healthy places for people to exercise, can increase or decrease the ability for a person to successfully make health-related behavior changes.

Person-Environment-Occupation-Performance

The Person-Environment-Occupation-Performance (PEOP) Model is a systems model that centers the client within the context of their environment. PEOP considers three domains that impact engagement including client factors (a person's capacities and barriers), environment factors (physical, social, cultural, and political), and factors related to the occupation (activities, tasks, and roles) (Baum et al, 2015). In addition to these three domains, PEOP focuses on occupational performance which is "the doing of meaningful activities, tasks, and roles through complex interactions between the person and environment" (Baum et al, 2015, p. 50). Occupational performance supports participation and well-being for clients. Occupational therapists can use the PEOP Model with clients with MetS and other chronic conditions to evaluate how engagement in healthy occupations are impacted by the person factors, environment, and factors related to the occupation. For example, if a client has a goal of incorporating an exercise routine into their weekly routine, an occupational therapist can use the PEOP Model to guide the therapeutic process. The occupational therapist would evaluate the client's ability to complete this occupation based on the client factors (physical and cognitive abilities to safely engage in the physical activity). Additionally, the occupational therapist would assist the client with identifying strategies and barriers to incorporating exercise into their weekly routines and identify places in the client's home and community that they can exercise safely.

Implications for the Older Adult in Treatment

Nonpharmacological interventions that facilitate healthy lifestyle behaviors are an important component of treatment for older adults with MetS (Marcos-Delgado et al, 2021; van Namen et al, 2019). Healthy lifestyle behaviors include adherence to a nutritious diet, engagement in regular physical activity and reduced sedentary behavior, managing medication routines, maintaining healthy sleep routines, and participating in interventions to address emotional distress and mental health concerns. Normal aging processes can influence physiological, sensorimotor, social, and environmental components of each lifestyle behavior. Older adults seeking treatment to address cardiometabolic conditions may benefit from occupational therapy assessment and intervention to identify and address components of these behaviors.

Nutritious Diet

Adherence to healthy dietary patterns is important throughout the life span. "Dietary patterns" refers to the combination of specific types of foods, nutrients, and beverages that an individual consumes. Dietary patterns that are associated with reduced signs of MetS (e.g., lower blood pressure, total and LDL cholesterol, hemoglobin A_{1c}, insulin resistance, body weight), and reduced risk of CVD, stroke, and coronary heart disease include the Healthy U.S.-Style Dietary pattern (U.S. Department of Agriculture and U.S. Department of Health and Human Services, 2020), the Mediterranean-style dietary pattern (Davis et al, 2015; Godos et al, 2017; Papadaki et al, 2020), and the Dietary Approaches to Stop Hypertension (DASH) dietary pattern (Akhlaghi, 2020; Chiavaroli et al, 2019; Siervo et al, 2015). A brief description of each diet pattern is included in Box 8-5. A growing body of evidence suggests that plant-based diets may be associated with cancer prevention (DeClercq et al, 2022). As adults age, their need for the nutrients included in these dietary patterns remains the same. In fact, adhering to healthy dietary patterns has been associated with maintenance of physical performance, lower risk of developing sarcopenia, and high quality of life among older adults (Bloom et al, 2018; Govindaraju et al, 2018). However, physiological changes associated with aging affect metabolic rate, oxidative stress, and the presence of stomach acid, all of which affect how the body processes food, and suggests a need to reduce calorie intake (Tittikpina et al, 2019). Age-related changes in the body's ability to absorb nutrients, reduced calorie needs, and elevated dietary protein needs, place older adults at high risk for protein-energy malnutrition (Norman et al, 2021). Therefore, it is important that older adults select nutrient-dense foods that align with healthy dietary patterns. Although making specific nutrition recommendations is outside the scope of occupational therapy practice, occupational therapists play an important role in identifying

BOX 8-5 Dietary Patterns

Dietary Approaches to Stop Hypertension

- Eat vegetables, fruits, whole grains, fat-free or low-fat dairy, fish, poultry, beans, nuts, seeds, vegetable oils.
- Limit fatty meats, full-fat dairy, sugar-sweetened beverages, sweets, sodium (salt).
- More information available at www.nhlbi.nih.gov/education/dash-eating-plan

Mediterranean Diet

- High intake of olive oil, vegetables, fruits, breads and cereals, legumes, nuts, fish, and seafood
- Moderate intake of eggs, poultry, dairy, and red wine
- Limit intake of red meat and sweets.
- More information available at: Davis, C., Bryan, J., Hodgson, J., Murphy, K. (2015). Definition of the Mediterranean Diet: A literature review. *Nutrients*, 7: 9139–53. https://doi.org/10.3390/nu7115459

Healthy U.S.-Style Dietary Pattern

- Eat vegetables (includes dark-green vegetables, red and orange vegetables, beans, peans, lentils, starchy vegetables, other vegetables), fruits, grains (whole grains, refined grains should be fortified), dairy (fat-free low-fat dairy and fortified soy alternatives), and protein foods (lean or low-fat meats, poultry, eggs, seafood, unsalted nuts, seeds, soy products).
- Limit foods and beverages with added sugars, saturated fat, sodium, and alcohol beverages.
- More information available at: U.S. Department of Agriculture and U.S. Department of Health and Human Services. *Dietary Guidelines for Americans, 2020–2025*. 9th Edition. December 2020. Available at www.DietaryGuidelines.gov

---

and addressing personal, occupational, and environmental factors that affect older adults' habits and routines associated with obtaining, preparing, and eating healthful foods. For instance, occupational therapists may be particularly skilled at understanding how impairments and disabilities influence engagement in food-related activities such as self-feeding and meal preparation. They can evaluate for assistive technologies and kitchen technologies that may be supportive of the client. Furthermore, they can evaluate how the environment (i.e., physical, social, cultural) is supporting or hindering healthful eating.

Unfortunately, many older adults experience food insecurity which limits their ability to reliably access and consume a sufficient quantity of affordable and healthful foods (Juckett & Robinson, 2019). "Occupational therapy practitioners can identify how food insecurity and health status influence older adults' independence and engagement in meaningful food-related activities and occupations in later life" (Juckett & Robinson, 2019, p. 2). Some suggested assessment tools for understanding nutrition and food insecurity in occupational therapy include the following:

- **The Canadian Occupational Performance Measure (COPM; Law et al, 1990).** The COPM can be used to guide conversations around food-related occupations to identify potential problems (e.g., insecurity, malnutrition).
- **Occupational Performance Measure of Food Activities (OPMF; Schmelzer & Leto, 2018).** The OPMF gathers information from the client on importance, performance, and satisfaction with the following food-related activities: shopping, cooking, eating, dining out, and eating healthfully.
- **The Individual Food Resource Profile (IFRP; Schmelzer & Leto, 2018).** The IFRP can be used to identify problems and develop interventions around community food resources, food habits and routines, skill level for managing food resources, dietary patterns, dietary restrictions, and access to common kitchen items.

Sensorimotor, social, and environmental factors influence older adults' nutrition behaviors. These behaviors encompass selecting, preparing, and eating healthful foods. Some older adults experience decreased acuity of olfactory and gustatory sensory function, which can be attributed to genetics, past persistent environmental exposures (e.g., work-related dust or smoke exposure), or primary medical conditions (Boesveldt et al, 2018). Medications can also affect the perception of flavors, and the use of dentures may affect the experience of food textures, influencing older adults' food choices (Regan et al, 2021). Current evidence suggests that enhancing the aroma and visual display and varying the texture of foods, in addition to bolstering the flavor of food may improve the sensory experience of eating (Boesveldt et al, 2018). Motor impairments, pain, and fatigue can also affect nutrition as it relates to both eating and meal preparation (Bennett et al, 2019). For example, older adults with Parkinson disease, a neurodegenerative disorder impacting oral and fine motor control, report challenges during eating, including difficulty manipulating utensils to bring food to the mouth, difficulty chewing particular textures, and concerns about choking during swallowing (Forsberg et al, 2022). This influences the selection and preparation of vegetables, which are a main food group represented across all healthy dietary patterns (Forsberg et al, 2022). In addition to impacting food intake, motor function, fatigue, pain, and cognitive changes may make cooking more difficult or less enjoyable than earlier in life (Bennett et al, 2019; Whitelock & Ensaff, 2018). Eating is frequently a social experience. However, older adults who are at risk for social isolation or who live alone may be less likely to prepare nutritious meals. In fact, meal satisfaction among older adults was reported to be higher when eating with their family than alone (Lee & Mo, 2019). Older adults may also experience food insecurity, or unreliable access to the type or amount of food that they need. Food insecurity is affected by both economic status (for example, living on a fixed income), and availability of food within one's own community or neighborhood. Being food insecure is associated with having chronic health problems, which further exacerbate food insecurity. By 2030, it is expected that over 73 million older adults in the United States will be living in a food insecure household (U.S. Census Bureau Population Division, 2017). Community-based programs can help to overcome food insecurity and nutrition-related challenges in the social and physical environment. Some examples of these programs include home meal (e.g., Meals on Wheels™) or grocery delivery services, community-based senior centers that offer congregate meals served in a social environment or dining rooms that serve meals in independent living facilities, government assistance programs (e.g., Supplemental Nutrition Assistance Program in the United States), and evidence-based programs on healthy nutrition offered through local community organizations (e.g., Area Agency on Aging) or health systems (Pooler et al, 2019). *Mr. Jenkins' eating habits are likely suboptimal as he orders takeout multiple times a week. He does this because it is a challenge for him to prepare meals for himself.* Occupational therapists can work with interprofessional teams (e.g., dietitians, physicians, nurses, speech language pathologists) to address nutrition and healthful eating. Refer to Table 8-3 for examples of interventions that can be used by occupational therapists integrating a person-environment-occupation perspective (Juckett & Robinson, 2019)

Physical Activity and Sedentary Behavior

Maintaining a physically active lifestyle and minimizing sedentary behavior is consistently associated with reduced risk for MetS (Amirfaiz & Shahril, 2019; Myers et al, 2019).

Further, engaging in moderate to vigorous intensity physical activity reduces the risk for CVD (Lavie et al, 2019), certain types of cancer (Patel et al, 2019), and all-cause and cardiovascular mortality (Cunningham et al, 2020) and improves the management of diabetes (Colberg et al, 2016) in older adults. The WHO updated its physical activity recommendations for older adults in 2020 to reflect the most recent evidence, recommending that older adults (1) engage in a minimum of 75 to 150 minutes of vigorous-intensity or 150 to 300 minutes of moderate-intensity aerobic activity each week, (2) complete muscle-strengthening activities that involve all major muscle groups 2 or more days per week, and (3) minimize sedentary behavior (waking time spent sitting) (Tremblay et al, 2017; WHO, 2020). For older adults who do not currently meet these guidelines, engaging in any intensity of physical activity, including light intensity physical activity, is better than no physical activity (Bakker et al, 2018; Ekelund et al, 2019).

Physical activity engagement and sedentary behavior are affected by the cardiorespiratory, sensorimotor, and cognitive changes that are common among older adults. Age-related changes in cardiopulmonary and cardiovascular function that affect physical activity engagement are described in detail in Chapter 9. Sarcopenia is an age-related syndrome that affects the musculoskeletal system and is characterized by reduced muscle mass, muscle function, and physical performance, including physical activity engagement (Meier & Lee, 2020). Sarcopenia is part of a vicious cycle whereby physical inactivity and time spent sedentary can lead to worsening symptoms of sarcopenia, which is associated with less physical activity and more sedentary time (Sánchez-Sánchez et al, 2019). Given the relationship between sarcopenia and physical activity, it is unsurprising that sarcopenia is associated with the components of MetS (Du et al, 2018). In addition to sarcopenia, older adults are also at risk for frailty and comorbid conditions (e.g., neurodegenerative disorders,

---

TABLE 8-3 ■ Examples of Occupational Therapy Interventions Across Person, Environment, and Occupation

	OCCUPATION	PERSON	ENVIRONMENT
Focus	Focus on food-related activities and occupations	Focus on existing limitations and use remedial and compensatory approaches	Focus on physical, social, and cultural contexts
Examples	■ Meal preparation ■ Shopping ■ Transporting food (e.g., from transportation to kitchen) ■ Food safety ■ Fall risk during food-related activities ■ Self-feeding ■ Oral-motor and swallowing ■ Budgeting and financial management on a fixed income ■ Community mobility for locating and purchasing healthful foods	■ Assistive technology implementation and training ■ Kitchen technology implementation and training ■ Adaptive techniques for various impairments (e.g., one-handed techniques for hemiparesis, strategies for low-vision)	■ Environmental modifications for kitchen access and safety ■ Establish connections with community resources (e.g., home-delivered meals, food pantries, congregate dining options at places like senior centers or churches) ■ Consider how food preferences are shaped by culture and provide training on maintaining cultural food preferences while prioritizing nutritious eating

vestibular disorders, low vision, neuropathy, cognitive disorders including dementia) that can affect balance, fear of falling, and contribute to restricted engagement in the activities that comprise physical activity engagement (Denkinger et al, 2015; Hoang et al, 2017). Thus, these comorbid conditions elevate not only the risk for poor functional outcomes associated with the condition itself, but also of metabolic conditions associated with low physical activity levels.

Physical and social environments also play an important role in older adults' physical activity and sedentary behavior. When residing in private residences, the neighborhood environment may support or restrict engagement in active lifestyles. For example, parks or walking trails that are safe and well-suited to physical activity for older adults are associated with engagement in light intensity physical activity and walking activity in older adults (Van Cauwenberg et al, 2018). Access to recreational facilities that are designed with older adults' needs in mind and that includes physical fitness trainers who are knowledgeable about older adults' physical activity needs and abilities can also serve as a facilitator for maintaining physically active lifestyles while aging (Fragala et al, 2019; Van Cauwenberg et al, 2018). Further, social isolation can play an important role in maintaining physically active lifestyles. Recent evidence suggests that older adults who receive social support for physical activity from family or friends (Lindsay Smith et al, 2017) and those older adults who participate in group-based exercise programs with peers of a similar age (Beauchamp et al, 2018) are more physically active than those without social support. Older adults who reside in supportive living environments, such as assisted living facilities, group homes, and skilled nursing facilities, are at high risk of excessive sedentary behavior and extremely low levels of physical activity (Leung et al, 2021; Park et al, 2017). These facilities are frequently designed to prioritize safety and convenience over physical activity (Kotlarczyk et al, 2020). Modifying the physical environment in these spaces may provide opportunities to increase physical activity and contribute to enhanced cardiometabolic health.

Sleep

The National Sleep Foundation recommends that adults, including older adults, should strive to sleep for 7 to 8 hours per night (Hirshkowitz et al, 2015). Sleep duration, sleep quality, circadian rhythm disruption, and sleep disorders are associated with risk for MetS and health outcomes associated with MetS (Xie et al, 2021). Importantly, both too little (less than 6 hours) and too much (more than 9 hours) sleep are associated with incident MetS and individual components of MetS: visceral adipose tissue, insulin resistance, glycemic control, hypertension (Koren et al, 2016; Xie et al, 2021). Further, common sleep disorders such as obstructive sleep apnea and insomnia are associated with outcomes of MetS, including obesity and CVD (Koren et al, 2016; Y. Zhang et al, 2021). The Occupational Therapy Practice Framework specifies *sleep and rest* as an area of occupation within the scope of occupational therapy practice (American Occupational Therapy Association, 2020). Assessing and intervening to improve sleep among older adults is particularly important among older adults who are at elevated risk for MetS.

Age-related changes in sleep quality and circadian rhythm begin before the age of 60 years and persist through older adulthood (Miner & Kryger, 2020; Ohayon et al, 2004). Sleep quality is measured using sleep parameters, which are defined in Box 8-6. Age-related changes in these parameters include decreased sleep efficiency, total sleep time, proportion of time spent in slow wave sleep, and rapid eye movement sleep, and increased time awake after sleep onset, number of arousals from sleep, and sleep latency (Li et al, 2018; Ohayon et al, 2004). These changes in sleep quality are attributed to changes in neuroendocrine function and affect the secretion of sleep-related hormones (growth hormone, cortisol, prolactin, thyroid stimulating hormone, melatonin, and sex hormones) (Li et al, 2018). In addition to changes in sleep quality, Circadian disruption also occurs with aging and is associated with MetS (Koren et al, 2016). The term *circadian rhythm* is used to describe the physiological processes that are associated with the sleep-wake cycle. Age-related changes associated with circadian rhythm often result in feeling tired earlier in the evening and awakening earlier in the morning (Li et al, 2018). In addition to these normal age-related changes in sleep, older adults' sleep may also be impacted by comorbid chronic conditions that disrupt sleep (e.g., pain, depression, anxiety, digestive disease, cancer). Over 50% of older adults with one to three chronic conditions report sleep problems, including insomnia and daytime sleepiness (Miner & Kryger, 2020).

The social and physical environment can also affect older adults' sleep. Because older adults often retire from work, daily routines become much more flexible and provide opportunities for daytime napping. Evidence is mixed regarding whether daytime napping confers positive or negative effects on sleep quality, health-related quality of life, and MetS in older adults (Z. Zhang et al, 2020). Further, flexible daily routines offer opportunities for inconsistent bedtime and morning waking times. Older adults who serve

BOX 8-6 Sleep Parameters

- Total sleep time: The duration of time spent sleeping
- Sleep efficiency: The total number of hours spent sleeping divided by the number of hours spent in bed, multiplied by 100 to derive a percentage
- Wake after sleep onset: The duration of time spent awake after falling asleep for the night
- Arousals from sleep: The number of times awoken after falling asleep for the night
- Sleep latency: The length of time required to move from fully awake to fully asleep

as caregivers for their spouses or other family members may experience poor sleep quality related to stress or anxiety associated with providing care (McCurry et al, 2015). In addition, bereavement (the process of grieving loss) is commonly experienced among older adults who lose spouses, siblings, friends, and other loved ones. Bereavement increases the risk for sleep problems, particularly among those who may be experiencing a condition called complicated grief (Lancel et al, 2020). Finally, older adults who reside in institutional environments, such as an assisted-living facility, group home, or skilled nursing home, must establish a new sleep routine, such as adjusting to new noises and loss of control over routines which can affect sleep (Capezuti et al, 2018; Štefan et al, 2018). Occupational therapy can play a role in delivering nonpharmacological interventions, such as physical activity (Vanderlinden et al, 2020), cognitive-behavioral therapy for sleep (Mitchell et al, 2019), and multicomponent interventions, which aim to establish consistent sleep habits and routines by addressing behavioral and environmental factors (Leland et al, 2014). Multicomponent interventions in occupational therapy can be delivered in one-on-one or group settings and may include cognitive-behavioral therapy, sleep hygiene education, progressive relaxation, physical activity, social activities, goal setting, self-monitoring, and/or problem-solving (Smallfield & Molitor, 2018).

Mental Health

Several lifestyle behaviors already discussed in this chapter such as physical activity and sleep can have a positive impact on mental health. However, there are additional interventions that have been shown to improve mental health symptoms for people with MetS and chronic conditions. Mindfulness-based interventions, stress-reduction and relaxation techniques, cognitive-behavioral therapy, and problem-solving and goal setting activities have been demonstrated as effective intervention strategies for people experiencing co-occurring MetS/conditions and mental health diagnoses.

Mindfulness-based interventions and stress-reduction and relaxation techniques can positively impact individuals with chronic conditions. Mindfulness is a cognitive intervention that assists practitioners with moderating habitual responses to life situations. Additionally, practicing mindfulness can increase attention and focus, promote relaxation, and reduce the impact of stress. Mindfulness has been shown to improve symptoms of MetS for patients with CVD. Mindfulness contributed to a decrease in stress, increased regulation of emotions, self-awareness, and attention, and decreased rumination behaviors and judgment for events and issues (Shahbazi et al, 2021). Relaxation techniques such as deep breathing, biofeedback, progressive muscle relaxation techniques, yoga, and meditation can also be deployed with clients with chronic conditions. These techniques can be beneficial for managing stress, reducing blood pressure, and increasing client's engagement in self-management (Younge et al, 2015).

Cognitive behavioral therapy is another intervention approach that can be used to address mental health concerns for clients with MetS and chronic conditions. Cognitive restructuring is a technique where clients identify intrusive and negative thoughts and attempt to restructure. Cognitive restructuring can help decrease behaviors such as rumination and catastrophizing. Both rumination and catastrophizing can lead to increased stress and avoidance behaviors (Akyirem et al, 2022).

Interventions that promote problem-solving and goal setting can also decrease the negative impact of mental health diagnoses for people with diabetes and other chronic conditions. Problem-solving allows individuals to anticipate real-life situations or problems that may occur and create plans for solving them. Additionally, teaching problem-solving skills can increase a person's participation in self-management by allowing them to discuss challenges and barriers to self-management and create a plan of action to address each barrier. Goal setting can also be used with clients to promote better self-management. Occupational therapists can assist clients with creating short-term and long-term goals for managing their care needs and accessing resources. Both problem-solving and goal setting have been effective interventions for people with chronic conditions (Akyirem et al, 2022). Occupational therapists should consider mental health concerns for people with MetS and conditions. Occupational therapists are trained in working with clients to establish healthy habits and routines and should deploy interventions to address client's mental health concerns.

Energy-Balance Behaviors: Implications for the Older Adult

Nutrition, physical activity, sedentary behavior, and sleep are interwoven and interacting lifestyle behaviors that collectively contribute to energy balance and impact metabolic disorders (Al Khatib et al, 2017; Romieu et al, 2017). Interventions that aim to modify nutrition, physical activity, sedentary behavior, and sleep leverage behavior change strategies selected based on the theory underlying the intervention. For example, an intervention guided by the TTM may use a decisional balance scale to support or enhance the client's readiness to modify a particular routine (Hutchison et al, 2009; Prochaska et al, 2015). The Behaviour Change Wheel provides a framework for describing additional behavior change techniques (Michie et al, 2013). Examples of these techniques are provided in Promoting Best Practice 8-1. Further, the interconnected nature of these energy balance behaviors has led to the development of evidence-based lifestyle-based interventions that can be tailored to address the specific needs of older adult clients. The Chronic Disease Self-Management Program (CDSMP) (Lorig, 1993) is one example of an evidence-based program that may address multiple interconnected lifestyle behaviors. Based in social cognitive theory (Bandura, 2004), the CDSMP is a community-based program through which clients build knowledge, set goals, and engage in problem-solving to self-manage chronic conditions (Allegrante et al, 2019). Clients set goals related to self-identified problems, and these may include physical activity, nutrition, medication management, and sleep-related goals. The CDSMP is delivered in a group setting by trained facilitators and may be offered through community centers, healthcare centers, churches or religious organizations, or other community-based settings. The CDSMP is one program supported by the National Council on Aging as an evidence-based, packaged program that improves metabolic health among older adults. Additional programs may be identified through the National Council on Aging's evidence-based programs database (https://ncoa.org/evidence-based-programs). Similar to the CDSMP, these programs are often delivered through public health agencies (e.g., Area Agency on Aging) and community organizations (e.g., local senior centers, YMCA). Occupational therapists are well qualified to pursue training to facilitate these programs to support improved metabolic health among older adult clients.

PROMOTING BEST PRACTICE 8-1

Examples of behavior change techniques to change lifestyle behaviors based on Michie et al (2013) Behaviour Change Wheel:

- Goal setting: Establishing a mutually agreed upon goal defined by either the behavior to be achieved (e.g., walk for exercise three times per week), or the outcome to be achieved (e.g., lose 5 lb of body weight)
- Problem-solving: Identifying barriers to the desired behavior, brainstorming potential solutions, and selecting a solution to implement
- Action planning: Establishing a detailed plan for achieving a desired behavior
- Self-monitoring: Documenting or tracking a desired behavior (e.g., wearing an activity tracker and writing down daily step count) or outcomes (e.g., documenting weight daily)
- Social support: Provision of practical or emotional support to engage in the behavior by friends, relatives, colleagues, or staff to provide
- Demonstration of the behavior: Observing another person as they perform the desired behavior (sometimes called modeling)
- Reward: Delivering a reward based on preestablished criteria related to either the desired behavior or the outcome

Medication Management

If aggressive lifestyle-based interventions are not enough, individuals with metabolic conditions are often prescribed medications to control the effects and progression of their specific conditions or diseases. Occupational therapists are uniquely positioned to understand and address factors related to medication adherence because of their skilled task analysis. Taking medications is a daily occupation for many individuals with metabolic conditions. Medication management is addressed by several professions, with each discipline bringing forward their unique lens to solve problems with medication management. Professions addressing medication adherence goals include prescribers, nurses, pharmacists, occupational therapists, and therapy technicians and assistants (Schwartz & Smith, 2017). Each discipline has an essential role in medication management that can be inherently complex yet necessary to support health.

To manage one medication, the following actions are required:

- Meet with a physician to negotiate the prescription and gain an initial understanding of its purpose.
- Fill the prescription with a pharmacy.
- Interpret the information on how to safely take the medication as prescribed.
- Take the medication as prescribed.
- Refill the medication so no lapses occur before the prescription is refilled.

With aging, medication management can become one of the most complex instrumental activities of daily living. The complexity of this process is perpetuated by problems such as poor health literacy, misunderstanding the need for or nature of the medication, socioeconomic status and medication costs, health conditions or existing impairments that influence ability to manage medications (e.g., arthritis, living with the effects of stroke), fear of potential side effects, lack of symptoms, mistrust in pharmaceutical companies and the medical system, taking several different medications or medications with high dosing frequency, worry, and depression. Often, barriers to medication adherence are not identified and it is recommended that understanding and addressing these barriers can facilitate improved performance (Murphy et al, 2017).

Although various occupational therapy intervention protocols have been developed, we describe a three-step process by Schwartz and colleagues (2017) called the Integrative Medication Self-Management Intervention in Promoting Best Practice 8-2.

PROMOTING BEST PRACTICE 8-2

Integrative Medication Self-Management Intervention (IMedS)

1. The occupational therapist and client reflect on past experiences and performance of medication management. They do this by reviewing a 2-week medication diary and adherence questionnaire.
2. The occupational therapist collaborates with the client on setting a medication management goal. The client generates the goal that can be related to any element of medication management (e.g., refilling the prescription in a timely manner, taking a percentage of medications accurately).

3. The occupational therapist uses therapeutic use of self and motivational interviewing techniques to support the client in self generation of new medication management strategies.

In addition, the IMedS protocol prompts the occupational therapist to consider facilitating strategy development in six different areas: (1) modifying or altering the activity, (2) advocacy, (3) education, (4) assistive technology, (5) environmental modifications, and (6) timely refills.

Interprofessional Colleagues

Collaboration and Referrals

Many chronic conditions related to MetS are complex and can involve multiple body structures; therefore, a multi-modal and team-based approach to care is important for ensuring better client outcomes. The WHO defines interprofessional collaboration as "when multiple health workers from different professional backgrounds work together with patients, families, [caregivers], and communities to deliver the highest quality of care across settings" (2010, p. 7). Although occupational therapists have specific skills and competencies related to health management, routine, and habit formation, health assessment and health promotion interventions are shared competencies among other healthcare professionals. Healthcare professionals on an interprofessional team that addresses MetS and other chronic conditions include primary care physicians, specialty care physicians, nurses, occupational therapists, physical therapists, dietitians, social workers, and community health workers among other healthcare professionals.

Moreover, interprofessional teams utilize different team-based approaches to healthcare in clinical practice. Multidisciplinary care, interprofessional care, and transdisciplinary care are team-based approaches that are sometimes used interchangeably, however they each offer a distinct approach to patient care. A transdisciplinary approach to care is defined as "... the integration and transformation of fields of knowledge from multiple perspectives in order to define, address, and resolve complex real-world problems" (Transdisciplinary understanding and training on research-primary health care, n.d.). A transdisciplinary approach to care promotes an environment where professionals from multiple disciplines share knowledge, skills, and decision-making to promote efficient patient care and better patient outcomes (Rosenfield, 1992; Van Bewer, 2017).

Occupational therapists contribute to the interprofessional team by implementing nonpharmacological interventions with their clients. Additionally, occupational therapists help the interprofessional team "understand how the client's motor, process, and social skills converge with the client's habits, routines, roles, and rituals to affect health outcomes" (Johnson, 2017). Therefore, occupational therapists can shift the focus of care from a predominantly "illness" system to a "health" system. Due to this focus on health management and prevention, occupational therapists can contribute to better health outcomes in older individuals and people with chronic conditions.

CASE STUDY (CONTINUED)

Assessment and Intervention
Activity and Participation Limitations
- **Community mobility to get to work and run errands.** Mrs. Jaramillo walks to the bus stop and rides the bus. Because of pain in her legs and hips, she bought a single-point cane at the corner shop a couple of weeks ago to use when walking to the bus and sometimes forgets to take it with when she leaves her house.
- **Work as a cashier.** Mrs. Jaramillo fatigues during her long shifts and experiences pain when standing. She has irregular mealtimes based on when she can take her lunch break. She typically takes quick breaks for snacks that tend to be highly processed and do not include healthful foods like fruits and vegetables.
- **Caregiving.** Mrs. Jaramillo is a caregiver for her husband because his mobility has declined. He has difficulty with showering in the tub, which is situated in a small bathroom. The stress and time commitment between caregiving and work restrict Mrs. Jaramillo from playing bridge with her church friends.
- **Meal preparation.** Mrs. Jaramillo does not have time to cook healthy meals, so she typically prepares microwave meals or picks up fast food (high-sodium meals) to enjoy with her husband.

Environmental Factors
- Fast food locations are a short walk from Mrs. Jaramillo's home. The closest grocery store is two bus rides away, requiring a transfer.
- The Jaramillo's have lived in the same two-story house for the past 50 years. Although the home is well-cared for, there have been minimal updates for aging-in-place made (e.g., the tub-shower combination is in the upstairs bathrooms).
- The Jaramillo's live on a fixed income. They live paycheck to paycheck and experience substantial stress with unexpected expenses.
- The Jaramillo's keep to themselves. They do have an adult child who visits weekly.

Questions
1. How do the assessment results inform your interventions?
2. What are two or three evidence-based, occupation-centered exemplar interventions that address the case study client's priorities?
   a. What assistive technologies or environmental modifications would you recommend?

3. How can the occupational therapist work with the interprofessional team to improve outcomes?

Answers

1. The assessments reveal the daily routines and identify areas for intervention including modifying lifestyle, home assessment, and exploration of resources. See Section Implications for Older Adults in Treatment. LO 8-5.
2. Using the PEOP Model, the occupational therapist will consider the client's ability for changes and adaptation of behaviors, environmental factors including her home and community, and desired occupations, including caregiving, work, home maintenance, and playing bridge. See section on PEOP Model. LO 8-3. 8-5.

   A second intervention would incorporate the technique of Behaviour Change Wheel. The steps would include:

   a. Mrs. Jaramillo would begin by setting goals. Specific goals might include packing healthy snacks for break time at work and scheduling for daughter to stay with father so she can play bridge once weekly.
   b. Problem-solving how to accomplish these goals, including learning about healthy snacks, shopping for snacks and looking for sales, arranging a bridge game when their daughter can come over, or inviting friends to play at her house
   c. Making detailed plan to meet goals
   d. Monitoring goal achievement: what worked, what didn't?
   e. Seeking support by sharing with daughter and coworkers the goals of healthy eating and being with friends to play bridge
   f. Recognizing goal achievement and new goals

   See section Promoting Best Practice 8-1. LO 8-3, 8-5.
3. The occupational therapist will work with Mrs. Jaramillo's physician and nurse to assure client is taking meds as prescribed and communicate if there are any issues. The physical therapist can be consulted regarding balance, fall risk, endurance, and exercise, the dietitian can assist with healthy and budget friendly meal planning and snacks, and the social worker can assist with finding resources to assist Mrs. Jaramillo with financial needs and finding resources to help with home modifications for aging in place. See section on Collaboration and Referrals. LO 8-5, 8-6.

SUMMARY

In this chapter we highlighted the relationship between MetS and CVD, diabetes, cancer, pulmonary conditions, and gastrointestinal disorders in older adults. MetS is a global public health problem that is most prevalent in older adults. With the older adult population growth expected in coming years, an increased demand for rehabilitation services will undoubtedly have important implications for occupational therapy working with this population. Occupational therapists are important contributors to interprofessional teams addressing metabolic conditions in older adults. Integrating theory and having a foundational understanding about the relationship between MetS and aging can support the assessment and intervention development process in occupational therapists working with this population.

Critical Thinking Questions

1. You are a home health therapist working with an older woman, Juanita, who has a medical history of type 2 diabetes and CVD. You discover that she is not taking her medications as prescribed. How would you approach Juanita to learn why she is not taking her medications? What solution to this would you propose?
2. You are an occupational therapist working in a primary care. You have a new client referral for an older man, Steve, who had a stroke 6 months prior. He wants to reduce his risk of having another stroke and is ready to start making some lifestyle changes. How can you use the TTM to guide your intervention planning?

REFERENCES

Akhlaghi, M. (2020). Dietary Approaches to Stop Hypertension (DASH): Potential mechanisms of action against risk factors of the metabolic syndrome. *Nutrition Research Reviews, 33*(1), 1–18. doi: 10.1017/S0954422419000155

Akyirem, S., Forbes, A., Wad, J. L., & Due-Christensen, M. (2022). Psychosocial interventions for adults with newly diagnosed chronic disease: A systematic review. *Journal of Health Psychology, 27*(7), 1753–1782. http://doi.org/10.1177/1359105321995916

Al Khatib, H., Harding, S., Darzi, J., & Pot, G. (2017). The effects of partial sleep deprivation on energy balance: A systematic review and meta-analysis. *European Journal of Clinical Nutrition, 71*(5), 614–624. doi: 10.1038/ejcn.2016.201

Allegrante, J. P., Wells, M. T., & Peterson, J. C. (2019). Interventions to support behavioral self-management of chronic diseases. *Annual Review of Public Health, 40*, 127–146. 10.1146/annurev-publhealth-040218-044008

American Cancer Society. (2020, October 28). *Health risks of smoking tobacco*. https://www.cancer.org/healthy/stay-away-from-tobacco/health-risks-of-tobacco/health-risks-of-smoking-tobacco.html#:~:text=How%20smoking%20tobacco%20affects%20your,people%20in%20the%20United%20States

American Diabetes Association. (2019). *Statistics about diabetes*. Statistics. https://diabetes.org/about-us/statistics/about-diabetes#:~:text=Diagnosed%20and%20undiagnosed%3A%20Of%20the,seniors%20(diagnosed%20and%20undiagnosed)

American Lung Association. (2021). *Lung capacity and aging*. https://www.lung.org/lung-health-diseases/how-lungs-work/lung-capacity-and-aging

American Occupational Therapy Association. (2020). Occupational therapy practice framework: Domain and process - fourth edition. *American Journal of Occupational Therapy, 74*(7412410010), 1–87.

Amirfaiz, S., & Shahril, M. R. (2019). Objectively measured physical activity, sedentary behavior, and metabolic syndrome in adults: Systematic review of observational evidence. *Metabolic Syndrome and Related Disorders, 17*(1), 1–21. doi: 10.1089/met.2018.0032

Baffi, C. W., Wood, L., Winnica, D., Strollo Jr, P. J., Gladwin, M. T., Que, L. G., & Holguin, F. (2016). Metabolic syndrome and the lung. *Chest, 149*(6), 1525–1534. doi: 10.1016/j.chest.2015.12.034

Bakker, E. A., Sui, X., Brellenthin, A. G., & Lee, D.-c. (2018). Physical activity and fitness for the prevention of hypertension. *Current Opinion in Cardiology, 33*(4), 394–401. doi: 10.1097/HCO.0000000000000526

Bandura, A. (2004). Health promotion by social cognitive means. *Health Education & Behavior, 31*(2), 143–164. doi: 10.1177/1090198104263660

Battelli, M. G., Bortolotti, M., Polito, L., & Bolognesi, A. (2019). Metabolic syndrome and cancer risk: The role of xanthine oxidoreductase. *Redox Biology, 21*, 101070. doi: 10.1016/j.redox.2018.101070

Baum, C. M., Christiansen, C. H., & Bass, J. D. (2015). The person-environment-performance (PEOP) model. In C. H. Christiansen, C. M. Baum, & J. D. Bass (Eds.), *Occupational therapy: Performance, participation, and well-being, fourth edition.* (pp. 47–55). SLACK Incorporated.

Beauchamp, M. R., Ruissen, G. R., Dunlop, W. L., Estabrooks, P. A., Harden, S. M., Wolf, S. A., Liu, Y., Schmader, T., Puterman, E., Sheel, A. W., & Rhodes, R. E. (2018). Group-based physical activity for older adults (GOAL) randomized controlled trial: Exercise adherence outcomes. *Health Psychology, 37*(5), 451. doi: 10.1037/hea0000615

Bennett, R., Demmers, T. A., Plourde, H., Arrey, K., Armour, B., Ferland, G., & Kakinami, L. (2019). Identifying barriers of arthritis-related disability on food behaviors to guide nutrition interventions. *Journal of Nutrition Education and Behavior, 51*(9), 1058–1066. doi: 10.1016/j.jneb.2019.06.030

Berben, L., Floris, G., Wildiers, H., & Hatse, S. (2021). Cancer and aging: Two tightly interconnected biological processes. *Cancers, 13*(6), 1400. doi: 10.3390/cancers13061400

Berra, E., Azizi, M., Capron, A., Høieggen, A., Rabbia, F., Kjeldsen, S. E., Staessen, J. A., Wallemacq, P., & Persu, A. (2016). Evaluation of adherence should become an integral part of assessment of patients with apparently treatment-resistant hypertension. *Hypertension, 68*(2), 297–306.

Bloom, I., Shand, C., Cooper, C., Robinson, S., & Baird, J. (2018). Diet quality and sarcopenia in older adults: A systematic review. *Nutrients, 10*(3), 308. doi: 10.1161/HYPERTENSIONAHA.116.07464

Boesveldt, S., Bobowski, N., McCrickerd, K., Maître, I., Sulmont-Rossé, C., & Forde, C. G. (2018). The changing role of the senses in food choice and food intake across the lifespan. *Food Quality and Preference, 68*, 80–89. https://doi.org/10.1016/j.foodqual.2018.02.004

Bryl, A., Mrugacz, M., Falkowski, M., & Zorena, K. (2022). The effect of diet and lifestyle on the course of diabetic retinopathy—a review of the literature. *Nutrients, 14*(6), 1252. doi: 10.3390/nu14061252

Capezuti, E., Sagha Zadeh, R., Pain, K., Basara, A., Jiang, N. Z., & Krieger, A. C. (2018). A systematic review of non-pharmacological interventions to improve nighttime sleep among residents of long-term care settings. *BMC Geriatrics, 18*(1), 1–18. doi: 10.1186/s12877-018-0794-3

Carbone, S., Canada, J. M., Billingsley, H. E., Siddiqui, M. S., Elagizi, A., & Lavie, C. J. (2019). Obesity paradox in cardiovascular disease: Where do we stand? *Vascular Health and Risk Management, 15*, 89. doi: 10.2147/VHRM.S168946

Centers for Disease Control and Prevention. (2020, April 28). *Tobacco-related mortality. Smoking & Tobacco Use.* https://www.cdc.gov/tobacco/data_statistics/fact_sheets/health_effects/tobacco_related_mortality/index.htm

Chiao, Y. A., Lakatta, E., Ungvari, Z., Dai, D. F., & Rabinovitch, P. (2016). Cardiovascular disease and aging. *Advances in Geroscience,* 121–160. https://doi.org/10.1007/978-3-319-23246-1_5

Chiavaroli, L., Viguiliouk, E., Nishi, S. K., Blanco Mejia, S., Rahelić, D., Kahleová, H., Salas-Salvadó, J., Kendall, C. W., & Sievenpiper, J. L. (2019). DASH dietary pattern and cardiometabolic outcomes: An umbrella review of systematic reviews and meta-analyses. *Nutrients, 11*(2), 338. doi: 10.3390/nu11020338

Colberg, S. R., Sigal, R. J., Yardley, J. E., Riddell, M. C., Dunstan, D. W., Dempsey, P. C., Horton, E. S., Castorino, K., & Tate, D. F. (2016). Physical activity/exercise and diabetes: a position statement of the American Diabetes Association. *Diabetes Care, 39*(11), 2065–2079. https://doi.org/10.2337/dc16-1728

Cunningham, C., O'Sullivan, R., Caserotti, P., & Tully, M. A. (2020). Consequences of physical inactivity in older adults: A systematic review of reviews and meta-analyses. *Scandinavian Journal of Medicine & Science in Sports, 30*(5), 816–827. doi: 10.1111/sms.13616

Davis, C., Bryan, J., Hodgson, J., & Murphy, K. (2015). Definition of the Mediterranean diet: A literature review. *Nutrients, 7*(11), 9139–9153. doi: 10.3390/nu7115459

DeClercq, V., Nearing, J. T., & Sweeney, E. (2022). Plant-based diets and cancer risk: What is the evidence? *Current Nutrition Reports,* 1–16. doi: 10.1007/s13668-022-00409-0

Denkinger, M. D., Lukas, A., Nikolaus, T., & Hauer, K. (2015). Factors associated with fear of falling and associated activity restriction in community-dwelling older adults: A systematic review. *American Journal of Geriatric Psychiatry, 23*(1), 72–86. doi: 10.1016/j.jagp.2014.03.002

Ding, X., Zhang, W., Li, S., & Yang, H. (2019). The role of cholesterol metabolism in cancer. *American Journal of Cancer Research, 9*(2), 219.

Du, Y., Oh, C., & No, J. (2018). Associations between sarcopenia and metabolic risk factors: A systematic review and meta-analysis. *Journal of Obesity & Metabolic Syndrome, 27*(3), 175. doi: 10.7570/jomes.2018.27.3.175

Dumic, I., Nordin, T., Jecmenica, M., Stojkovic Lalosevic, M., Milosavljevic, T., & Milovanovic, T. (2019). Gastrointestinal tract disorders in older age. *Canadian Journal of Gastroenterology and Hepatology, 2019.* doi: 10.1155/2019/6757524

Ekelund, U., Tarp, J., Steene-Johannessen, J., Hansen, B. H., Jefferis, B., Fagerland, M. W., Whincup, P., Diaz, K. M., Hooker, S. P., Chernofsky, A., Larson, M. G., Spartano, N., Vasan, R. S., Dohrn, I. M., Hagströmer, M., Edwardson, C., Yates, T., Shiroma, E., Anderssen, S. A., & Lee, I. M. (2019). Dose-response associations between accelerometry measured physical activity and sedentary time and all cause mortality: Systematic review and harmonised meta-analysis. *BMJ, 366,* l4570. doi: https://doi.org/10.1136/bmj.l4570

Forsberg, S., Olsson, V., Bredie, W. L., & Wendin, K. (2022). Vegetables for older adults–general preferences and smart adaptations for those with motoric eating difficulties. *International Journal of Gastronomy and Food Science, 66,* 10.29219/fnr.v66.8269. https://doi.org/10.29219/fnr.v66.8269

Forsberg, S., Westergren, A., Wendin, K., Rothenberg, E., Bredie, W. L., & Nyberg, M. (2022). Perceptions and attitudes about eating with the fingers-an explorative study among older adults with motoric eating difficulties, relatives and professional caregivers. *Journal of Nutrition in Gerontology and Geriatrics,* 1–27. doi: 10.1080/21551197.2022.2025970

Fragala, M. S., Cadore, E. L., Dorgo, S., Izquierdo, M., Kraemer, W. J., Peterson, M. D., & Ryan, E. D. (2019). Resistance training for older adults: Position statement from the national strength and conditioning association. *Journal of Strength & Conditioning Research, 33*(8). doi: 10.1519/JSC.0000000000003230

Godos, J., Zappalà, G., Bernardini, S., Giambini, I., Bes-Rastrollo, M., & Martinez-Gonzalez, M. (2017). Adherence to the Mediterranean diet is inversely associated with metabolic syndrome occurrence: A meta-analysis of observational studies. *International Journal of Food Sciences and Nutrition, 68*(2), 138–148. doi: 10.1080/09637486.2016.1221900

Goldstein, L. B., Bushnell, C. D., Adams, R. J., Appel, L. J., Braun, L. T., Chaturvedi S., Creader, M. A., Culebras, A., Eckel, R. H., Hart, R. G., Hinchey, J. A., Howard, V. J., Jauch, E. C., Levine, S. R., Meschia J. F., Moore, W. S., Nixon J. V., & Pearson, T. A. (2011). Guidelines for the primary prevention of stroke: A guideline for healthcare professionals from the American Heart Association/American Stroke Association. *Stroke, 42,* 517–584. http://dx.doi.org/10.1161/STR.0b013e3181fcb238

Govindaraju, T., Sahle, B. W., McCaffrey, T. A., McNeil, J. J., & Owen, A. J. (2018). Dietary patterns and quality of life in older adults: A systematic review. *Nutrients, 10*(8), 971. doi: 10.3390/nu10080971

Hashemzadeh, M., Rahimi, A., Zare-Farashbandi, F., Alavi-Naeini, A. M., & Daei, A. (2019). Transtheoretical model of health behavioral change: A systematic review. *Iranian Journal of Nursing and Midwifery Research, 24*(2), 83–90. doi: 10.4103/ijnmr.IJNMR_94_17

Hirode, G., & Wong, R. J. (2020). Trends in the prevalence of metabolic syndrome in the United States, 2011–2016. *Journal of the American Medical Association, 323*(24):2526–2528. doi:10.1001/jama.2020.4501

Hirshkowitz, M., Whiton, K., Albert, S. M., Alessi, C., Bruni, O., DonCarlos, L., Hazen, N., Herman, J., Adams Hillard, P. J., Katz, E. S., Kheirandish-Gozal, L., Neubauer, D. N., O'Donnell, A. E., Ohayon, M., Peever, J., Rawding, R., Sachdeva, R. C., Setters, B., Vitiello, M. V., & Ware, J. C. (2015). National Sleep Foundation's updated sleep duration recommendations. *Sleep Health, 1*(4), 233–243. doi: 10.1016/j.sleh.2015.10.004

Hivert, M. F., Christophi, C. A., Franks, P. W., Jablonski, K. A., Ehrmann, D. A., Kahn, S. E., Horton, E. S., Pollin, T. I., Mather, K. J., Perreault, L., Barrett-Connor, E., Knowler, W. C., Florez, J. C., & Diabetes Prevention Program Research Group. (2016). Lifestyle and metformin ameliorate insulin sensitivity independently of the genetic burden of established insulin resistance variants in diabetes prevention program participants. *Diabetes, 65*(2), 520–526. doi.org/10.2337/db15-0950

Hoang, O. T. T., Jullamate, P., Piphatvanitcha, N., & Rosenberg, E. (2017). Factors related to fear of falling among community-dwelling older adults. *Journal of Clinical Nursing, 26*(1–2), 68–76. doi: 10.1111/jocn.13337

Hoffmann, M. S., Brunoni, A. R., Stringaris, A., Vianag, M. C., Andrade Lotufo, P., Martins Bensenor, I., & Abrahao Salum G. (2021). Common and specific aspects of anxiety and depression and the metabolic syndrome. *Journal of Psychiatric Research, 137*, 117–125. https://doi.org/10.1016/j.jpsychires.2021.02.052

Hopkins, B. D., Goncalves, M. D., & Cantley, L. C. (2016). Obesity and cancer mechanisms: Cancer metabolism. *Journal of Clinical Oncology, 34*(35), 4277. doi: 10.1200/JCO.2016.67.9712

Hutchison, A. J., Breckon, J. D., & Johnston, L. H. (2009). Physical activity behavior change interventions based on the transtheoretical model: A systematic review. *Health Education & Behavior, 36*(5), 829–845. doi: 10.1177/1090198108318491

Ibrahim, M., Tuomilehto, J., Aschner, P., Beseler, L., Cahn, A., Eckel, R. H., Fischl, A. H., Guthrie, G., Hill, J. O., Kumwenda, M., Leslie, R. D., Olson, D. E., Pozzilli, P., Weber, S. L., & Umpierrez, G. E. (2018). Global status of diabetes prevention and prospects for action: A consensus statement. *Diabetes/Metabolism Research and Reviews, 34*(6), e3021. doi: 10.1002/dmrr.3021

Imeri, H., Toth, J., Arnold, A., & Barnard, M. (2022). Use of the transtheoretical model in medication adherence: A systematic review. *Research in Social and Administrative Pharmacy, 18*, 2778–2785. https://doi.org/10.1016/j.sapharm.2021.07.008

Jiménez-Zazo, F., Romero-Blanco, C., Castro-Lemus, N., Dorado-Suarez, A., & Aznar, S. (2020). Transtheoretical model for physical activity in older adults: Systematic review. *International Journal of Environmental Research and Public Health, 17*, 9262. http://doi:10.3390/ijerph17249262

Johnson, C. E. (2017). Understanding interprofessional collaboration: An essential skill for all practitioners. *OT Practice, 22*(11), CE-1–CE 8.

Juckett, L. A., Robinson, M. L. (2019). The occupational therapy approach for addressing food insecurity among older adults with chronic disease. *Geriatrics, 4*(1), 1–10. https://doi.org/10.3390/geriatrics4010022

Khawaja, I. S., Westermeyer, J. J., Gajwani, P., & Feinstein, R. E. (2009). Depression and coronary artery disease: The association, mechanisms, and therapeutic implications. *Psychiatry, 6*(1), 38–51.

Khodaveisi, M., Azizpour, B., Jadidi, A., & Mohammadi, Y. (2021). Education based on the health belief model to improve the level of physical activity. *Physical Activity and Nutrition, 25*(4), 017–023. https://doi.org/10.20463/pan.2021.0022

Kim, S., Jee, S., Nam, J. M., Cho, W. H., Kim, J., & Park, E. (2014). Do early onset and pack-years of smoking increase risk of type II diabetes? *BMC Public Health, 14*, 178–188. doi:10.1186/1471-2458-14-178

Kobayashi, L. C., Westrick, A. C., Doshi, A., Ellis, K. R., Jones, C. R., LaPensee, E., Mondul, A. M., Mullins, M. A., & Wallner, L. P. (2022). New directions in cancer and aging: State of the science and recommendations to improve the quality of evidence on the intersection of aging with cancer control. *Cancer, 128*(9), 1730–1737. doi: 10.1002/cncr.34143

Koren, D., Dumin, M., & Gozal, D. (2016). Role of sleep quality in the metabolic syndrome. *Diabetes, Metabolic Syndrome and Obesity: Targets and Therapy, 9*, 281. doi: 10.2147/DMSO.S95120

Kotlarczyk, M. P., Hergenroeder, A. L., Gibbs, B. B., Cameron, F. D. A., Hamm, M. E., & Brach, J. S. (2020). Personal and environmental contributors to sedentary behavior of older adults in independent and assisted living facilities. *International Journal of Environmental Research and Public Health, 17*(17), 6415. doi: 10.3390/ijerph17176415

Kuniss, N., Kramer, G., Müller, U. A., Wolf, G., & Kloos, C. (2021). Diabetes related distress is high in inpatients with diabetes. *Diabetology & Metabolic Syndrome, 13*(40), 1–8. https://doi.org/10.1186/s13098-021-00659-y

Lackland, D. T., Carey, R. M., Conforto, A. B., Rosendorff, C., Whelton, P. K., & Gorelick, P. B. (2018). Implications of recent clinical trials and hypertension guidelines on stroke and future cerebrovascular research. *Stroke, 49*(3), 772–779. https://doi.org/10.1161/STROKEAHA.117.019379

Lancel, M., Stroebe, M., & Eisma, M. C. (2020). Sleep disturbances in bereavement: A systematic review. *Sleep Medicine Reviews, 53*, 101331. https://doi.org/10.1016/j.smrv.2020.101331

Law, M., Baptiste, S., McColl, M., Opzoomer, A., Polatajko, H., & Pollock, N. (1990). The Canadian occupational performance measure: An outcome measure for occupational therapy. *Canadian Journal of Occupational Therapy, 57*(2), 82–87.

Lavie, C. J., Ozemek, C., Carbone, S., Katzmarzyk, P. T., & Blair, S. N. (2019). Sedentary behavior, exercise, and cardiovascular health. *Circulation Research, 124*(5), 799–815.

Lee, K. H., & Mo, J. (2019). The factors influencing meal satisfaction in older adults: A systematic review and meta-analysis. *Asian Nursing Research, 13*(3), 169–176. doi: 10.1161/CIRCRESAHA.118.312669

Leland, N. E., Marcione, N., Niemiec, S. L. S., Kelkar, K., & Fogelberg, D. (2014). What is occupational therapy's role in addressing sleep problems among older adults? *OTJR: Occupation, Participation and Health, 34*(3), 141–149. doi: 10.3928/15394492-20140513-01

Leon, B. M., & Maddox, T. M. (2015). Diabetes and cardiovascular disease: Epidemiology, biological mechanisms, treatment recommendations and future research. *World Journal of Diabetes, 6*(13), 1246–1258. doi: 10.4239/wjd.v6.i13.1246

Leung, K.-C. W., Sum, K.-W. R., & Yang, Y.-J. (2021). Patterns of sedentary behavior among older adults in care facilities: A scoping review. *International Journal of Environmental Research and Public Health, 18*(5), 2710. doi: 10.3390/ijerph18052710

Li, J., Vitiello, M. V., & Gooneratne, N. S. (2018). Sleep in normal aging. *Sleep Medicine Clinics, 13*(1), 1–11. doi: 10.1016/j.jsmc.2017.09.001

Limon, V. M., Lee, M., Gonzalez, B., Choh, A. C., & Czerwinski, S. A. (2020). The impact of metabolic syndrome on mental health-related quality of life and depressive symptoms. *Quality of life Research, 29*, 2063–2072. http://doi.org/10.1007/s11136-020-02479-5

Lindsay Smith, G., Banting, L., Eime, R., O'Sullivan, G., & Van Uffelen, J. G. (2017). The association between social support and physical activity in older adults: A systematic review. *International Journal of Behavioral Nutrition and Physical Activity, 14*(1), 1–21. doi: 10.1186/s12966-017-0509-8

Longo, M., Bellastella, G., Maiorino, M. I., Meier, J. J., Esposito, K., & Giugliano, D. (2019). Diabetes and aging: from treatment goals to pharmacologic therapy. *Frontiers in Endocrinology, 10* (45/), 1–12. https://doi.org/10.3389/fendo.2019.00045

Lorig, K. (1993). Self-management of chronic illness: A model for the future. *Generations: Journal of the American Society on Aging, 17*(3), 11–14. https://www.jstor.org/stable/44877774

Lowery, E. M., Brubaker, A. L., Kuhlmann, E., & Kovacs, E. J. (2013). The aging lung. *Clinical Interventions in Aging, 8,* 1489–1496. https://doi.org/10.2147/CIA.S51152

Magkos, F., Hjorth, M. F., & Astrup, A. (2020). Diet and exercise in the prevention and treatment of type 2 diabetes mellitus. *Nature Reviews Endocrinology, 16*(10), 545–555. doi: 10.1038/s41574-020-0381-5

Marcos-Delgado, A., Hernández-Segura, N., Fernández-Villa, T., Molina, A. J., & Martín, V. (2021). The effect of lifestyle intervention on health-related quality of life in adults with metabolic syndrome: A meta-analysis. *International Journal of Environmental Research and Public Health, 18*(3), 887. doi: 10.3390/ijerph18030887

Mayo Clinic. (2022). *High blood pressure dangers: Hypertension's effects on your body.* https://www.mayoclinic.org/diseases-conditions/high-blood-pressure/in-depth/high-blood-pressure/art-20045868

McCurry, S. M., Song, Y., & Martin, J. L. (2015). Sleep in caregivers: What we know and what we need to learn. *Current Opinion in Psychiatry, 28*(6), 497–503. doi: 10.1097/YCO.0000000000000205

Meier, N. F., & Lee, D. C. (2020). Physical activity and sarcopenia in older adults. *Aging Clinical and Experimental Research, 32*(9), 1675–1687. doi: 10.1007/s40520-019-01371-8

Metwaly, A., Reitmeier, S., & Haller, D. (2022). Microbiome risk profiles as biomarkers for inflammatory and metabolic disorders. *Nature Reviews Gastroenterology & Hepatology,* 1–15. https://doi.org/10.3389/fmolb.2020.603740

Michie, S., Richardson, M., Johnston, M., Abraham, C., Francis, J., Hardeman, W., Eccles, M. P., Cane, J., & Wood, C. E. (2013). The behavior change technique taxonomy (v1) of 93 hierarchically clustered techniques: Building an international consensus for the reporting of behavior change interventions. *Annals of Behavioral Medicine, 46*(1), 81–95. doi: 10.1007/s12160-013-9486-6

Micucci, C., Valli, D., Matacchione, G., & Catalano, A. (2016). Current perspectives between metabolic syndrome and cancer. *Oncotarget, 7*(25), 38959. doi: 10.18632/oncotarget.8341

Mills, K. T., Bundy, J. D., Kelly, T. N., Reed, J. E., Kearney, P. M., Reynolds, K., Chen, J., & He, J. (2016). Global disparities of hypertension prevalence and control: A systematic analysis of population-based studies from 90 countries. *Circulation, 134*(6), 441–450. doi: 10.1161/CIRCULATIONAHA.115.018912

Miner, B., & Kryger, M. H. (2020). Sleep in the aging population. *Sleep Medicine Clinics, 15*(2), 311–318. doi: 10.1016/j.jsmc.2016.10.008

Mitchell, L. J., Bisdounis, L., Ballesio, A., Omlin, X., & Kyle, S. D. (2019). The impact of cognitive behavioural therapy for insomnia on objective sleep parameters: A meta-analysis and systematic review. *Sleep Medicine Reviews, 47,* 90–102. doi: 10.1016/j.smrv.2019.06.002

Murphy, M. C., Somerville, E., Keglovits, M., Hu, Y. L., & Stark, S. (2017). In-home medication management performance evaluation (HOME-RX): A validity study. *American Journal of Occupational Therapy, 71*(4), 7104190020p1–7104190020p7.

Myers, J., Kokkinos, P., & Nyelin, E. (2019). Physical activity, cardiorespiratory fitness, and the metabolic syndrome. *Nutrients, 11*(7), 1652. https://doi.org/10.5014/ajot.2017.022756

Norman, K., Haß, U., & Pirlich, M. (2021). Malnutrition in older adults—Recent advances and remaining challenges. *Nutrients, 13*(8), 2764. PMID: 34444924

North, B. J., & Sinclair, D. A. (2012). The intersection between aging and cardiovascular disease. *Circulation Research, 110*(8), 1097–1108. doi: 10.1161/CIRCRESAHA.111.246876

Ohayon, M. M., Carskadon, M. A., Guilleminault, C., & Vitiello, M. V. (2004). Meta-analysis of quantitative sleep parameters from childhood to old age in healthy individuals: Developing normative sleep values across the human lifespan. *Sleep, 27*(7), 1255–1273. doi: 10.1093/sleep/27.7.1255

Pan, A., Wang, Y., Talaei, M., & Hu, F. B. (2015). Relation of smoking with total mortality and cardiovascular events among patients with diabetes mellitus: A meta-analysis and systematic review. *Circulation, 132,* 1795–1804.

Papadaki, A., Nolen-Doerr, E., & Mantzoros, C. S. (2020). The effect of the Mediterranean diet on metabolic health: A systematic review and meta-analysis of controlled trials in adults. *Nutrients, 12*(11), 3342. doi: 10.1161/CIRCULATIONAHA.115.017926

Parekh, P. J., Balart, L. A., & Johnson, D. A. (2015). The influence of the gut microbiome on obesity, metabolic syndrome and gastrointestinal disease. *Clinical and Translational Gastroenterology, 6*(6), e91. doi: 10.1038/ctg.2015.16

Park, S., Thøgersen-Ntoumani, C., Ntoumanis, N., Stenling, A., Fenton, S. A., & Veldhuijzen van Zanten, J. J. (2017). Profiles of physical function, physical activity, and sedentary behavior and their associations with mental health in residents of assisted living facilities. *Applied Psychology: Health and Well-Being, 9*(1), 60–80. doi: 10.1111/aphw.12085

Patel, A. V., Friedenreich, C. M., Moore, S. C., Hayes, S. C., Silver, J. K., Campbell, K. L., Winters-Stone, K., Gerber, L. H., George, S. M., Fulton, J. E., Denlinger, C., Morris, G. S., Hue, T., Schmitz, K. H., & Matthews, C. E. (2019). American College of Sports Medicine roundtable report on physical activity, sedentary behavior, and cancer prevention and control. *Medicine and Science in Sports and Exercise, 51*(11), 2391. doi: 10.1249/MSS.0000000000002117

Patel, P., Ordunez, P., Connell, K., Lackland, D., DiPette, D., & Network, P. (2018). Standardized hypertension management to reduce cardiovascular disease morbidity and mortality worldwide. *Southern Medical Journal, 111*(3), 133. doi: 10.14423/SMJ.0000000000000776

Pooler, J. A., Hartline-Grafton, H., DeBor, M., Sudore, R. L., & Seligman, H. K. (2019). Food insecurity: A key social determinant of health for older adults. *Journal of the American Geriatrics Society, 67*(3), 421. doi: 10.1111/jgs.15736

Prochaska, J. O., Redding, C. A., & Evers, K. E. (2015). The transtheoretical model and stages of change. In K. Glanz, B. Rimer, & K. Viswanath (Eds.), *Health behavior: Theory, research, and practice* (5 ed., pp. 125–148). San Francisco: Jossey-Bass.

Prochaska, J. O., & Velicer, W. F. (1997). The transtheoretical model of health behavior change. *American Journal of Health Promotion, 12*(1), 38–48. doi: 10.4278/0890-1171-12.1.38

Refaeli, R., Chodick, G., Haj, S., Goren, S., Shalev, V., & Muhsen, K. (2018). Relationships of *H. pylori* infection and its related gastroduodenal morbidity with metabolic syndrome: A large cross-sectional study. *Scientific Reports, 8*(1), 1–7. https://doi.org/10.1038/s41598-018-22198-9

Regan, E., Feeney, E., Hutchings, S., O'Neill, G., & O'Riordan, E. (2021). Exploring how age, medication usage, and dentures effect the sensory perception and liking of oral nutritional supplements in older adults. *Food Quality and Preference, 92,* 104224. https://doi.org/10.1016/j.foodqual.2021.104224

Romieu, I., Dossus, L., Barquera, S., Blottière, H. M., Franks, P. W., Gunter, M., Hwalla, N., Hursting, S. D., Leitzmann, M., Margetts, B., Nishida, C., Potischman, N., Seidell, J., Stepien, M., Wang, Y., Westerterp, K., Winichagoon, P., Wiseman, M., Willett, W. C., & IARC Working Group on Energy Balance and Obesity. (2017). Energy balance and obesity: What are the main drivers? *Cancer Causes & Control, 28*(3), 247–258. doi: 10.1007/s10552-017-0869-z

Rosenfield, P. L. (1992). The potential of transdisciplinary research for sustaining and extending linkages between the health and social sciences. *Social Science & Medicine, 35*(11), 1343–1357. https://doi.org/10.1016/0277-9536(92)90038-r

Rosenstock, I. M., Strecher, V. J., & Becker, M. H. (1988). Social learning model and the Health Belief Model. *Health Education Quarterly, 15*(2), 175–183. doi: 10.1177/109019818801500203

Saklayen, M. G. (2018). The global epidemic of the metabolic syndrome. *Current Hypertension Reports, 20*(2), 1–8. doi: 10.1007/s11906-018-0812-z

Sánchez-Sánchez, J. L., Mañas, A., García-García, F. J., Ara, I., Carnicero, J. A., Walter, S., & Rodríguez-Mañas, L. (2019). Sedentary behaviour, physical activity, and sarcopenia among older adults in the TSHA: Isotemporal substitution model. *Journal of Cachexia, Sarcopenia and Muscle, 10*(1), 188–198. doi: 10.1002/jcsm.12369

Schmelzer, L., & Leto, T. (2018). Promoting health through engagement in occupations that maximize food resources. *The American Journal of Occupational Therapy, 72*(4), 1–9. https://doi.org/10.5014/ajot.2018.025866

Schneider, J. L., Rowe, J. H., Garcia-de-Alba, C., Kim, C. F., Sharpe, A. H., & Haigis, M. C. (2021). The aging lung: Physiology, disease, and immunity. *Cell, 184*(8), 1990-2019. https://doi.org/10.1016/j.cell.2021.03.005

Schwartz, J. K., & Smith, R. O. (2017). Integration of medication management into occupational therapy practice. *American Journal of Occupational Therapy, 71*(4), 7104360010p1-7104360010p7. doi: 10.5014/ajot.2017.015032

Schwartz, J. K., Grogan, K. A., Mutch, M. J., Nowicki, E. B., Seidel, E. A., Woelfel, S. A., & Smith, R. O. (2017). Intervention to improve medication management: Qualitative outcomes from a Phase I randomized controlled trial. *American Journal of Occupational Therapy, 71*(6), 7106240010p1-7106240010p10. https://doi.org/10.5014/ajot.2017.021691

Scott, K. M., de Jonge, P., Alonso, J., Viana, M. C., Liu, Z., O'Neill, S., Aguilar-Gaxiola, S., Bruffaerts, R., Caldas-de-Almeida, J. M., Stein, D. J., de Girolamo, G., Florescu, S. E., Hu, C., Taib, N. I., Lépine, P-J., Levinson, D., Matschinger, H., Medina-Mora, M. E., Piazza, M., Posada-Villa, J. A., Uda, H., Wojtyniak, B. J., Lim, C. C. W., & Kessler, R. C. (2013). Associations between DSM-IV mental disorders and subsequent heart disease onset: Beyond depression. *International Journal of Cardiology, 168*, 5293–5299. http://dx.doi.org/10.1016/j.ijcard.2013.08.012

Shabibi, P., Zavareh, M. S. A., Sayehmiri, K., Qorbani, M., Safari, O., Rastegarimehr, B., & Mansourian, M. (2017). Effect of educational intervention based on the Health Belief Model on promoting self-care behaviors of type-2 diabetes patients. *Electronic Physician, 9*(12), 5960–5968. http://doi.org/10.19082/5960

Shahbazi, K., Taghvaei, M. H., Solati, S. K., Khaledifar, A., & Shahnazari, M. (2021). Effectiveness of mindfulness-based stress reduction on hypertension among patients with metabolic syndrome. *Avicenna Journal of Neuro Psycho Physiology, 8*(4): 192–198. http://doi.org/10.32592/ajnpp.2021.8.4.104

Siervo, M., Lara, J., Chowdhury, S., Ashor, A., Oggioni, C., & Mathers, J. C. (2015). Effects of the dietary approach to stop hypertension (DASH) diet on cardiovascular risk factors: A systematic review and meta-analysis. *British Journal of Nutrition, 113*(1), 1–15. doi: 10.1017/S0007114514003341

Siteman Cancer Center, Barnes-Jewish Hospital, Washington University School of Medicine. (n.d.). *Your disease risk initiative.* http://www.yourdiseaserisk.wustl.edu/YDRDefault.aspx?ScreenControl=YDRGeneral&ScreenName=YDRAbout

Smallfield, S., & Molitor, W. L. (2018). Occupational therapy interventions addressing sleep for community-dwelling older adults: A systematic review. *The American Journal of Occupational Therapy, 72*(4), 1–8. https://doi.org/10.5014/ajot.2018.031211

Štefan, L., Vrgoč, G., Rupčić, T., Sporiš, G., & Sekulić, D. (2018). Sleep duration and sleep quality are associated with physical activity in elderly people living in nursing homes. *International Journal of Environmental Research and Public Health, 15*(11), 2512. doi: 10.3390/ijerph15112512

Tchkonia, T., & Kirkland, J. L. (2018). Aging, cell senescence, and chronic disease: Emerging therapeutic strategies. *Journal of the American Medical Association, 320*(13), 1319–1320. doi: 10.1001/jama.2018.12440

Tittikpina, N. K., Issa, A.-R., Yerima, M., Dermane, A., Dossim, S., Salou, M., Batobayena, B., Aboudoulatif, D., Yao, P., & Diop, Y. M. (2019). Aging and nutrition: Theories, consequences, and impact of nutrients. *Current Pharmacology Reports, 5*(4), 232–243. doi: 10.1007/s40495-019-00185-6

TODAY Study Group. (2021). Long-term complications in youth-onset type 2 diabetes. *New England Journal of Medicine, 385*(5), 416–426. doi: 10.1056/NEJMoa2100165

Transdisciplinary understanding and training on research-primary health care [TUTOR-PCH]. (n.d.). *Definitions.* https://www.uwo.ca/fammed/csfm/tutor-phc/aboutus/definitions.html

Tremblay, M. S., Aubert, S., Barnes, J. D., Saunders, T. J., Carson, V., Latimer-Cheung, A. E., Chastin, S. F. M., Altenburg, T. M., Chinapaw, M. J. M., & SBRN Terminology Consensus Project Participants. (2017). Sedentary behavior research network (SBRN)–terminology consensus project process and outcome. *International Journal of Behavioral Nutrition and Physical Activity, 14*(75). https://doi.org/10.1186/s12966-017-0525-8

Tsao, C. W., Aday, A. W., Almarzooq, Z. I., Alonso, A., Beaton, A. Z., Bittencourt, M. S., ..., & American Heart Association Council on Epidemiology and Prevention Statistics Committee and Stroke Statistics Subcommittee. (2022). Heart disease and stroke statistics—2022 update: A report from the American Heart Association. *Circulation, 145*(8), e153–e639. https://doi.org/10.1161/CIR.0000000000001052

Tseng, H. M., Liao, S., Wen, Y., & Chuang, Y. (2017). Stages of change concept of the transtheoretical model for healthy eating links health literacy and diabetes knowledge to glycemic control in people with type 2 diabetes. *Primary Care Diabetes, 11*(1), 29–36. http://dx.doi.org/10.1016/j.pcd.2016.08.005

Tune, J. D., Goodwill, A. G., Sassoon, D. J., & Mather, K. J. (2017). Cardiovascular consequences of metabolic syndrome. *Translational Research, 183*, 57–70. doi: 10.1016/j.trsl.2017.01.001

U.S. Census Bureau Population Division. (2017). Projected 5 year age groups and sex composition: Main projections series for the United States, 2017–2060: National population projections tables. Washington, DC. Retrieved on 4/25/2022. https://www.census.gov/data/tables/2017/demo/popproj/2017-summary-tables.html

U.S. Department of Agriculture and U.S. Department of Health and Human Services. (2020). Dietary guidelines for Americans, 2020–2025. 9th edition. www.DietaryGuidelines.gov

Van Bewer, V. (2017). Transdisciplinarity in health care: A concept analysis. *Nursing Forum, 52*(4), 339–347. https://doi.org/10.1111/nuf.12200

Van Cauwenberg, J., Nathan, A., Barnett, A., Barnett, D. W., & Cerin, E. (2018). Relationships between neighbourhood physical environmental attributes and older adults' leisure-time physical activity: A systematic review and meta-analysis. *Sports Medicine, 48*(7), 1635–1660. doi: 10.1007/s40279-018-0917-1

Van de Velde, D., De Zutter, F., Satink, T., Costa, U., Janquart, S., Senn, D., & De Vriendt, P. (2019). Delineating the concept of self-management in chronic conditions: A concept analysis. *BMJ Open, 9*(7), e027775. doi: 10.1136/bmjopen-2018-027775

van Namen, M., Prendergast, L., & Peiris, C. (2019). Supervised lifestyle intervention for people with metabolic syndrome improves outcomes and reduces individual risk factors of metabolic syndrome: A systematic review and meta-analysis. *Metabolism, 101*, 153988. doi: 10.1016/j.metabol.2019.153988

Vanderlinden, J., Boen, F., & Van Uffelen, J. (2020). Effects of physical activity programs on sleep outcomes in older adults: A systematic review. *International Journal of Behavioral Nutrition and Physical Activity, 17*(1), 1–15. doi: 10.1186/s12966-020-0913-3

Whitelock, E., & Ensaff, H. (2018). On your own: Older adults' food choice and dietary habits. *Nutrients, 10*(4), 413. doi: 10.3390/nu10040413

World Health Organization. (2010). *Framework for action on interprofessional education and collaborative practice.* http://www.who.int/hrh/resources/framework_action/en/

World Health Organization. (2020). *WHO Guidelines on Physical Activity and Sedentary Behavior.* https://www.who.int/publications/i/item/9789240015128

World Health Organization. (2021a). *Noncommunicable diseases.* https://www.who.int/news-room/fact-sheets/detail/noncommunicable-diseases

World Health Organization. (2021b, June 21). *Chronic obstructive pulmonary disease (COPD).* https://www.who.int/news-room/fact-sheets/detail/chronic-obstructive-pulmonary-disease-(copd)

World Health Organization. (2021). *Hypertension.* https://www.who.int/news-room/fact-sheets/detail/hypertension

Xie, J., Li, Y., Zhang, Y., Vgontzas, A. N., Basta, M., Chen, B., Xu, C., & Tang, X. (2021). Sleep duration and metabolic syndrome: An updated systematic review and meta-analysis. *Sleep Medicine Reviews, 59*, 101451. doi: 10.1016/j.smrv.2021.101451

Xu, C. X., Zhu, H. H., & Zhu, Y. M. (2014). Diabetes and cancer: Associations, mechanisms, and implications for medical practice. *World Journal of Diabetes, 5*(3), 372. doi: 10.4239/wjd.v5.i3.372

Yamada, T., Taylor, R. R., Kielhofner, G. (2017). The person-specific concepts of human occupation. In R. R. Tayler (Ed.), *Kielhofner's Model of Human Occupation, fifth edition.* (pp. 11–23). Wolters Kluwer.

Younge, J. O., Gotink, R. A., Baena, C. P., Roos-Hesselink, J. W., & Myriam Hunink, G. M. (2015). Mind–body practices for patients with cardiac disease: A systematic review and meta-analysis. *European Journal of Preventive Cardiology, 22*(11) 1385–1398. http://doi.org/10.1177/2047487314549927

Yousufuddin, M., & Young, N. (2019). Aging and ischemic stroke. *Aging, 11*(9), 2542–2544. doi: 10.18632/aging.101931

Zhang, Y., Jiang, X., Liu, J., Lang, Y., & Liu, Y. (2021). The association between insomnia and the risk of metabolic syndrome: A systematic review and meta-analysis. *Journal of Clinical Neuroscience, 89,* 430–436. doi: 10.1016/j.jocn.2021.05.039

Zhang, Z., Xiao, X., Ma, W., & Li, J. (2020). Napping in older adults: A review of current literature. *Current Sleep Medicine Reports, 6*(3), 129–135. doi: 10.1007/s40675-020-00183-x

Zurita-Cruz, J. N., Manuel-Apolinar, L., Arellano-Flores, M. L., Gutierrez-Gonzalez, A., Najera-Ahumada, A. G., & Cisneros-González, N. (2018). Health and quality of life outcomes impairment of quality of life in type 2 diabetes mellitus: A cross-sectional study. *Health and Quality of Life Outcomes,* 16(1), 1–7. doi: 10.1186/s12955-018-0906-y

CHAPTER 9

Cardiopulmonary and Cardiovascular Conditions

Samantha M. Barefoot, OTD, MOT, OTR/L, BCPR

"Be clear about your goal, but be flexible about the process of achieving it."

—Brian Tracy

LEARNING OUTCOMES

By the end of this chapter, readers will be able to:

9-1. Articulate age-related changes that are expected in cardiovascular and cardiopulmonary function and surgical versus nonsurgical interventions for cardiovascular and cardiopulmonary dysfunction.
9-2. Based on practice frameworks, prioritize the focus of assessment based on older adults with cardiovascular and cardiopulmonary dysfunction.
9-3. Design an intervention plan for the cardiovascular and cardiopulmonary population given associated theoretical and practice frameworks.
9-4. Connect the factors one should consider in prioritizing goals of an intervention plan with the cardiovascular and cardiopulmonary population.
9-5. Articulate a rationale for heart and pulmonary disease related to extrinsic factors, such as medical interventions and medications.
9-6. Distinguish the need for collaboration with interprofessional colleagues regarding the cardiovascular and cardiopulmonary population.
9-7. Evaluate the feasibility of providing education for the promotion of health and wellness in relation to disease management for the cardiovascular and cardiopulmonary population.
9-8. Differentiate the role of occupational therapy in providing evaluation and intervention to individuals within the cardiovascular and cardiopulmonary population.
9-9. Select appropriate intervention approaches to use when providing occupational therapy services for the cardiovascular and cardiopulmonary population.
9-10. Select proper intervention strategies and therapeutic outcomes for the cardiovascular and cardiopulmonary population when receiving occupational therapy services.

Mini Case Study

Jerilene Ruffin is a 73-year-old Hispanic woman who was diagnosed with chronic obstructive pulmonary disease (COPD) 1 year ago. She also has a previous medical history of diabetes, osteoporosis, and depression. She is a nonsmoker, but her husband smoked for 42 years. She currently is on 1 L of supplemental oxygen 24/7. She does not own adaptive equipment or durable medical equipment. She lives with and provides care for her husband, who has been on a disability pension for 12 years. They live in a one-story home with two steps to enter. Jerilene is able to complete her occupations independently, but she reports difficulty with initiating her morning routine. She states that she is able to complete necessary occupations with increased time and frequent rest breaks. She currently drives without difficulty. Jerilene works as a store attendant part-time 3 days a week. She reports that work has also become difficult for her, as she becomes quite fatigued when she stands for more than a few minutes.

Provocative Questions

1. In what ways are Jerilene's health and well-being compromised based on her current medical status?
2. With consideration of health and well-being, how will you identify and consider short- and long-term implications of her COPD diagnosis related to formulating an intervention plan?

Introduction

This chapter focuses on the cardiopulmonary and cardiovascular systems and the dysfunction that may occur within those systems. Occupational therapists assist older adults with cardiopulmonary and/or cardiovascular disease in maintaining and enhancing function that supports their ability to maintain independence while ultimately promoting their quality of life. The cardiopulmonary and cardiovascular systems are complex; it is vital to understand both the heart and lungs, as they are essential for maintaining homeostasis and health-related quality of life. The World Health Organization (WHO) recommends the use of the International Classification of Functioning, Disability, and Health (ICF) to comprehensively assess individuals living with specific health conditions, with considerations of their health experience related to the condition (WHO, 2022). Moreover, the WHO and ICF frame the importance of physical activity with respect to what an individual needs or wants to do, and their capacity for activity and participation.

Physical activity is key to offsetting age-related changes and maximizing function and health-related quality of life of older people. Physical activity reduces illness and disability, and its impact may mitigate side effects of medical treatment. Considering the needs of older adults, the exercise-based means of assessing cardiopulmonary and cardiovascular status are described across the spectrum of meeting minimal requirements for performing daily activities to having superior reserve capacity for increased physical capacity and functional independence. Irrespective of age, people have exercise conditioning potential that can be maximized, even in the presence of most chronic health conditions. Because exercise capacity is influenced by environment, ways in which an older person's environment might be modified to increase physical activity and reduce hazards—that is, by paying attention to contextual factors (environmental and personal in the ICF)—are outlined.

Theoretical Frameworks

On the basis of the WHO's definition of health, the ICF (WHO, 2022) has become a main framework and basis for assessment and defining goals and outcomes of intervention for occupational therapists. Each individual is viewed as a whole, such that their participation and quality of life are viewed distinctly and interdependently with the capacity to perform activities and the integrity of anatomic structure and physiological function. Specifically, the term activity includes activities of daily living (ADLs) and those activities associated with participation and engagement in living.

The ICF framework has particular relevance in health care today. First, this framework is consistent with a model of health versus illness care. Second, it is consistent with contemporary health-care priorities—namely, noncommunicable diseases that are lifestyle-related (e.g., ischemic heart disease, cancer, smoking-related conditions, hypertension and stroke, diabetes, and osteoporosis). The WHO has decreed that these conditions and their associated social and economic burdens are largely preventable (WHO, 2021; WHO, 2012). These conditions have achieved epidemic proportions. Furthermore, people are developing comorbidities earlier in their lives than in the past century because of unhealthy lifestyles. Because the biomedical model can maintain people's lives when threatened, people today experience long periods of morbidity—and particularly end-of-life morbidity—unless they pay attention to their lifestyle practices (specifically, nutrition, physical activity and exercise, smoking, sleep, and stress). Prolonged morbidity progressively limits a person's participation in or quality of life.

Cardiovascular Function and Age-Related Changes

The heart circulates blood to all the organs and the tissues of the body (Fig. 9-1). More specifically, the cardiovascular system is composed of the heart and vasculature. The left side of the heart is responsible for pumping blood that has been oxygenated in the lungs throughout the body to all the cells of the organ systems via the arterial vasculature. The venous vasculature is responsible for returning blood that has been partially deoxygenated and contains metabolic waste products, including carbon dioxide, to the right side of the heart when it is pumped through the lungs to be reoxygenated. Other metabolic waste products are cleared as the blood flows through the kidneys, gut, and liver. Clearance of such wastes and cellular debris is also facilitated by the lymphatic drainage system. Although loss of efficiency of the cardiovascular and lymphatic systems may occur with age, high levels of functioning of these systems can be maintained throughout the life cycle when lifestyles are optimized.

Electrical Behavior

Age-related fibrotic changes in the heart's specialized nerve conduction system may result in abnormal cardiac impulses. Electrocardiographic irregularities such as **premature ventricular contractions, atrial fibrillation,** and **heart blocks** are common in people over 65 years of age (Panizo et al, 2018; Fleg & Lakatta 2019; Perino et al, 2021). Medications can often help stabilize or regulate the heart's electrical activity; however, artificial pacemakers may be implanted when medications do not work.

Mechanical Behavior

The heart pumps less effectively with age due to changes in the mechanical properties of the cardiac muscle, which alter its length–tension and force–velocity relationships. Additionally, changes with age in both the integrity of the valves—the atrioventricular valves, the pulmonic valve, and the aortic valve—and variations in the aging cardiopulmonary and cardiovascular systemic circulations can result in less efficient pumping action of the heart (Strait & Lakatta, 2012). Histologically, the heart tissue becomes fattier, and both heart mass and volume increase. Amyloidosis, a histologic feature of aging observed in many organs including the heart and vasculature, is characterized by the progressive deposition of amyloid protein. This waxy protein infiltrates

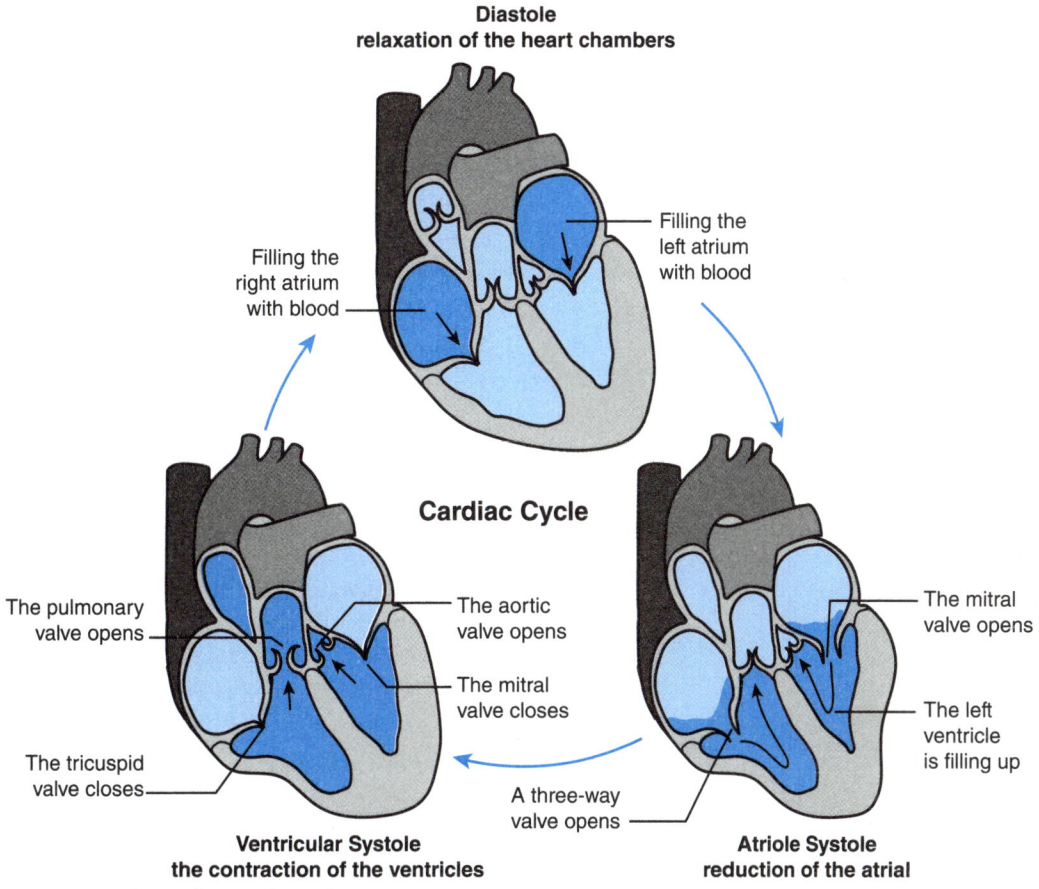

FIGURE 9-1 The cardiovascular cycle.

tissue, rendering it dysfunctional. In general, the walls of the heart become more compliant with age. The myocardial fibers no longer contract at optimal points on the length–tension or force–velocity curves, which reduces the efficiency of myocardial contraction and, in turn, the capacity for effective cardiac output.

Blood Vessels

Blood vessels require varying degrees of distensibility or compliance depending on their specific function. The forward motion of blood on the arterial side of the circulation is a function of the elastic recoil of the vessel walls and the progressive loss of pressure energy down the vascular tree. The decrease in elasticity of the arterial vessels with aging may result in chronic or residual increases in vessel diameter and vessel wall rigidity, which impair the function of the vessel. The reservoir function of the venous circulation is dependent on its being highly compliant to accommodate the greatest proportion of the blood volume at rest. Although the mechanical characteristics of venous smooth muscle have been less well studied compared with arterial smooth muscle, the efficiency of its contractile behavior can be expected to be reduced with aging. Furthermore, its electrical excitability and responsiveness to neurohumoral transmitters tend to be less rapid and less pronounced.

Blood

The ability of the vasculature to move blood through the vascular system and shift volumes of blood between vascular beds depending on need is diminished with aging; the rapidity with which these changes can be affected is correspondingly reduced. The ability to affect these vascular adjustments in response to gravity and exercise are tantamount to effective physical functioning.

Net Effects of Age-Related Cardiovascular Changes

The age-related anatomic and physiological changes of the heart and blood vessels result in reduced capacity for oxygen transport at rest and, in particular, in response to situations imposing an increase in oxygen demand of metabolically active tissue (particularly skeletal muscle) for oxygen (Table 9-1). Therefore, activities associated with a relatively low metabolic demand are perceived by older persons as physically demanding. Older adults may no longer be able to perform certain activities or may require rest periods to complete an activity. Many older people have electrical conduction abnormalities at rest and in the absence of clinical heart disease (Fleg & Lakatta, 2019), which have major implications for the mechanical behavior of the heart and

TABLE 9-1   Age-Related Changes in the Cardiovascular System and Its Function

MORPHOLOGICAL AND STRUCTURAL CHANGES	FUNCTIONAL SIGNIFICANCE
Heart - Fat constituents - Fibrous constituents - Mass and volume - Lipofuscin (byproduct of glycogen metabolism) - Amyloid content - Specialized nerve conduction tissue - Intrinsic and extrinsic innervation - Connective tissue and elastin - Calcification	- Excitability - Cardiac output - Venous return - Cardiac dysrhythmias
Blood Vessels - Loss of normal proportion of smooth muscle to connective tissue and elastin constituents - Rigidity of large arteries - Atheroma arterial circulation - Calcification - Dilation and tortuosity of veins	- Blood flow to oxygenate tissues - Blood flow and risk of clots in venous circulation - Cardiac output - Venous return

Note: Data from Strait & Lakatta (2012).

the regulation of cardiac output, particularly when stressed during activity and exercise.

Cardiopulmonary Function and Age-Related Changes

The pulmonary system maintains life by supplying oxygen to an individual's organs and tissues while removing carbon dioxide through the process of ventilation and respiration (Fig. 9-2). Aging has a direct effect on each component of the cardiopulmonary system, which includes the airways, lung **parenchyma** (connective and supportive tissue of an organ) and its interface with the circulation (the alveolar capillary membrane), chest wall, and respiratory muscles. Ventilation of the alveoli and oxygenation of venous blood depends on the anatomic and physiological integrity of these components (Koeppen & Stanton, 2018; West, 2012).

Airways

Aging is associated with a decrease in elastic tissue and an increase in fibrous tissue throughout the body's systems, including the cardiopulmonary system. Because the large airways are predominantly rigid connective tissue, few changes with aging are reported. Because the medium and small airways are composed of less connective tissue and more smooth muscle, a decrease in the elasticity of these structures occurs with aging, resulting in reduced structural integrity of the tissue and increased compliance (compliance = Δ volume/Δ pressure; increased compliance = increased stiffness).

Lung Parenchyma

The lung parenchyma is composed of spongy alveolar tissue that is designed to be ventilated and provide an interface with the pulmonary blood through the alveolar capillary membrane, which has a large surface area to promote the oxygenation of blood. Age-related increases in connective tissue and elastin disintegration reduce elastic recoil, the principal mechanism of normal expiration. The loss of normal recoil contributes to uneven distribution of ventilation, airway closure, air trapping, and impaired gas exchange. The

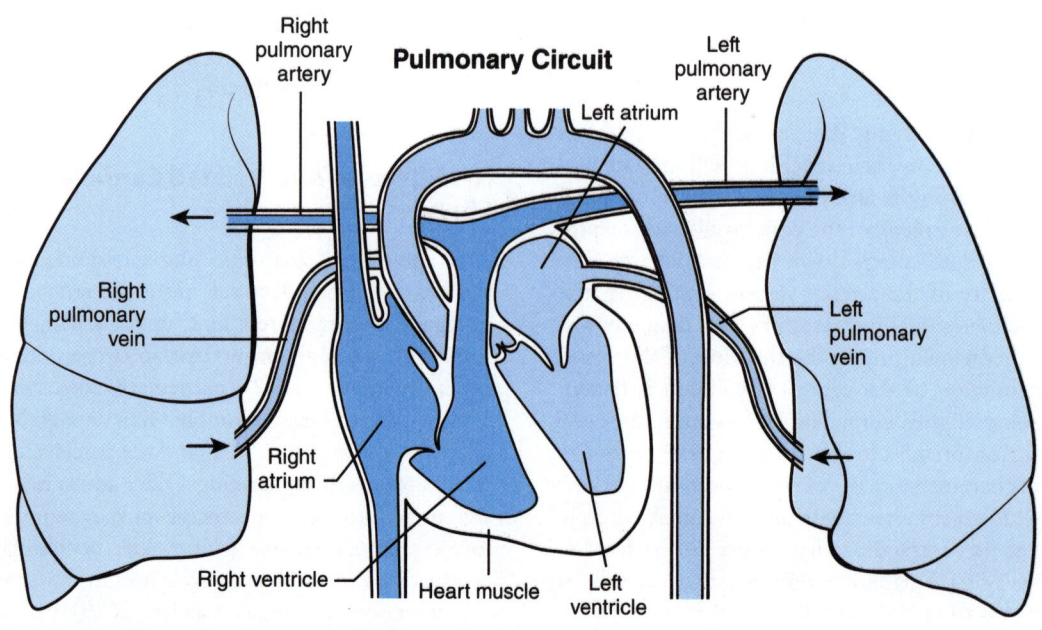

FIGURE 9-2 The cardiopulmonary cycle.

net result of these changes is a decrease in alveolar surface area, hence reduced efficient gas exchange.

Alveolar Capillary Membrane

The alveolar capillary membrane is uniquely designed to optimize the diffusion of gases between the alveolar air and the pulmonary circulation. The diffusing capacity, the ability of oxygen (O_2) to diffuse from the alveolar airspaces into the pulmonary capillary, progressively declines with age and has been attributed to reduced alveolar surface area, alveolar volume, and pulmonary capillary bed.

Chest Wall

The chest wall is composed of the structures separating the thorax from the head and neck, the diaphragm separating the thorax from the abdomen, the rib cage, the intercostal muscles, and the spinal column. With age, the joints of the thorax become more rigid, and cartilage becomes calcified; hence, the chest wall becomes less compliant. The chest wall becomes barrel shaped, the anteroposterior diameter increases, and the normal three-dimensional motion of the chest wall during the respiratory cycle is diminished.

Respiratory Muscles

The diaphragm, the principal muscle of respiration, becomes weaker with muscle atrophy. Loss of respiratory muscle mass parallels the age-related reduction in skeletal muscle mass in general. Loss of abdominal muscle strength reduces the force of coughing, which can contribute to impaired airway mucociliary clearance and aspiration.

Net Effect of Age-Related Cardiopulmonary Changes

These anatomic changes give rise to predictable physiological changes in pulmonary function after the cardiopulmonary system has matured (Table 9-2). Respiratory mechanics that largely reflect the resistance to airflow and the compliance of the chest wall and lung parenchyma are altered with aging. Specifically, both airflow resistance and lung compliance increase. With respect to cardiopulmonary function, forced expiratory volumes and flows and inspiratory and expiratory pressures are reduced. Functional residual capacity (the volume of air present in the lungs at the end of passive expiration) and **residual volume** (the amount of air remaining in the lungs after an individual fully exhales) are increased. These effects are further accentuated in recumbent positions. Arterial oxygen tension and saturation are also reduced linearly with age. Thus, progressively over the life cycle, the lung becomes a less efficient gas exchanger. Refer to Promoting Best Practice 9-1.

TABLE 9-2 Age-Related Changes in the Cardiopulmonary System and Its Function

MORPHOLOGICAL AND STRUCTURAL CHANGES	FUNCTIONAL SIGNIFICANCE
Thorax	
- Calcification of bronchial and costal cartilage - Stiffness of costovertebral joints - Anteroposterior diameter - Wasting of respiratory muscles	- Resistance to deformation of chest wall - Effective use of accessory respiratory muscles - Tidal volume - Exercise-induced hyperpnea - Maximal voluntary ventilation - Force of cough - Risk of aspiration or choking
Lung	
- Size of alveolar ducts - Supporting duct framework - Size of alveoli - Mucous glands - Alveolar compliance	- Surface area for gas exchange - Physiological dead space - Elastic recoil - Vital capacity - Inspiratory reserve volume - Expiratory reserve volume - Functional residual volume and residual volume - Ventilatory flow rates - Distribution of ventilation - Closure of dependent airways - Arterial desaturation - Resistance to airflow in small airways - Pulmonary capillary network - Distribution of perfusion - Impaired diffusion capacity - Fibrosis of pulmonary capillary intima - Ventilation to perfusion matching

Note: Data from Koeppen & Stanton (2018); West (2012).

PROMOTING BEST PRACTICE 9-1
Multiple Determinants of Health

In addition to addressing lifestyle factors, rehabilitation professionals need to appreciate the broader determinants of health, including social, political, economic, and environmental (Egger & Dixon, 2014).

Other intrinsic factors that affect cardiopulmonary and cardiovascular function include current and long-term lifestyle practices, such as level of physical activity, nutritional status, smoking history, and effectiveness of stress-management strategies. Regular exercise, in which the heart rate (HR) reflecting exercise intensity is within the training-sensitive HR zone, is essential for aerobic conditioning. Such conditioning ensures aerobic reserve capacity, which provides a cardiopulmonary protective effect if the person becomes ill or requires routine medical and surgical procedures. Also, years of active and passive smoking are well-known risk factors for chronic airflow limitation and cancer. Occupational environments over the long term can have significant long-term consequences (e.g., the occurrence of interstitial lung disease in workers exposed to toxic environmental agents and in farmers).

TABLE 9-3 ■ Subjective Scales of Exercise Responses

	PERCEIVED EXERTION	BREATHLESSNESS	DISCOMFORT/PAIN	FATIGUE
0	Nothing at all	Nothing at all	Nothing at all	Nothing at all
0.5	Very, very light	Very, very weak	Very, very light	Very, very weak
1	Very light	Very weak	Very light	Very weak
2	Light	Weak	Light	Weak
3	Moderate	Moderate	Moderate	Moderate
4	Somewhat strong	Somewhat strong	Somewhat strong	Somewhat strong
5	Hard	Strong	Hard	Strong
6				
7	Very strong	Very strong	Very heavy	Very strong
8				
9				
10	Very, very strong/maximal	Very, very strong/maximal	Very, very strong/maximal	Very, very strong/maximal

Note: Based on the Borg Rating of Perceived Exertion scale (Borg, 1982).

CASE STUDY

Occupational Therapy Profile

Uzoma Otieno is a 63-year-old African American male who has been living with congestive heart failure (CHF) for approximately 4 years. He has a previous medical history of hypertension, left ventricular hypertrophy, obesity, and diabetes mellitus. He currently lives with his wife in a one-story home with a ramped entrance. His wife is in good health and maintains the home to include the cooking, cleaning, laundry, etc. Uzoma's previous household role was to maintain the lawn and landscaping, but that has become increasingly difficult, and the maintenance of the outside of their home has been suffering. He does not own any adaptive equipment or durable medical equipment. He has difficulty performing functional mobility and everyday occupations; his wife assists him intermittently. He has difficulty with self-management and medication adherence to effectively manage his CHF.

He is currently on disability, and he was previously employed by the department of transportation. Uzoma was able to fulfill his work responsibilities until approximately 2 years ago, when the symptoms of his CHF made it too difficult to perform his work and he was placed on long-term disability. He has been referred to an outpatient cardiopulmonary rehabilitation center to improve his self-management skills and empower him to effectively manage his CHF. Uzoma is aware of his increasing activity limitations and has expressed his desire to improve his quality of life, as well as his independence, with meaningful occupations. He and his wife have also started the conversation of environmental modifications to their home to enable Uzoma's success within the home to maintain his independence as his disease progresses. You are the occupational therapist to assist Uzoma to promote health and wellness through community-based services.

Heart Disease

About 659,000 people die of heart disease every year, which is one in every four deaths (Centers for Disease Control and Prevention [CDC], 2021). This is of importance and significance, as many individuals do not recognize the presence of heart disease until they experience signs and symptoms of a major heart condition. Moreover, there are many risk factors associated with heart disease, some of which are controllable, whereas others are uncontrollable. Risk factors associated with disease include hypertension, diabetes, smoking, hyperlipidemia, physical inactivity, obesity, chronic alcohol use, improper diet, poverty, stress, and genetic disposition. With considerations of associated risk factors, prevalence of heart disease is growing rapidly and can range from a broad spectrum of diagnoses, including coronary artery disease, myocardial infarction (MI), arrythmias, and heart failure (Virani et al, 2021). These conditions will be discussed later in the chapter with implications for occupational therapy practice.

Major Cardiac Conditions

Coronary Artery Disease (CAD)

CAD, or ischemic heart disease, is the leading cause of death for individuals worldwide; it is also predicted to become the leading cause of global disability (ICF, 2017). CAD has associated physical and psychological symptoms, including angina (acute chest pain associated with inadequate oxygen to the heart), exercise intolerance, dyspnea (shortness of breath), depression, anxiety, irritability, and decreased quality of life. Treatment and decision-making related to ICF for individuals with CAD are focused on improving psychological symptoms and management of physical and physiological symptoms. CAD is commonly attributed to atherosclerosis, which is associated with thickening and/or hardening of the arteries. CAD is commonly diagnosed through a medical history, echocardiogram (a test that uses sound waves to assess how the heart is functioning and monitor how blood is pumping through the heart), cardiac catheterization, or angiogram. Interventions include coronary artery bypass graft (CABG) or coronary angioplasty.

Heart Failure (HF)/Congestive Heart Failure (CHF)

HF is a prevalent chronic disease in the United States, costing health-care systems an estimated $30.7 billion for associated healthcare services, medication to treat the disease, and lost work wages (CDC, 2020). According to the American Heart Association (AHA, 2017), HF occurs when there is either functional and/or structural impairment of ventricular filling or the reduction of ejection fracture. HF is diagnosed through ejection fraction, symptoms, and imaging, and it can be classified as shown in Box 9-1.

CHF commonly presents when there is dysfunction collectively with both sides of the heart. It is associated with an overall decrease of the heart's ability to effectively provide profusion to both sides and therefore causes congestion in the body's tissues. This type of HF is the most common form and is associated with clinical signs of edema in the extremities due to increased fluid pressure (AHA, 2017). Classifications and symptoms associated with heart failure are as follows (New York Heart Association, 2018; Bozkurt et al, 2021):

- At Risk for HF: Individuals who are at risk for HF but without current or prior symptoms/signs of HF and without structural or biomarkers that are indicative of heart disease
- Pre-HF: Individuals without current or prior symptoms/signs of HF but who have evidence of structural heart disease, abnormal cardiac function, or elevated peptide levels
- HF: Individuals with current or prior symptoms and/or signs of HF caused by structural and/or functional cardiac abnormality
- Advanced HF: Individuals with severe symptoms and/or signs of HF at rest, recurrent hospitalizations despite guideline-directed management and therapy, and requiring advanced therapies such as transplant, mechanical circulatory support, or palliative care

HF intervention and treatment is primarily focused on reducing the workload of the heart while increasing its efficiency. This is provided through nonsurgical intervention such as angiotensin-converting enzyme (ACE) inhibitors and diuretics; however, in extreme cases of HF, a heart transplant may be warranted.

Cardiomyopathy

Cardiomyopathy is an acquired or hereditary disease of the cardiac muscle that results in myocardium enlargement and dysfunction of the ventricle(s). Symptoms associated with cardiomyopathy are similar to those of HF and include dyspnea, lightheadedness, arrhythmia (abnormal cardiac rhythm), chest pain, dizziness, edema to the extremities, and fatigue. Depending on the extent of dysfunction, individuals with cardiomyopathy may be treated with nonsurgical intervention (e.g., ACE inhibitors, beta blockers, statins, or diuretics) or surgical intervention (e.g., cardiac catheterization, CABG, heart transplant, or implantable cardioverter-defibrillator).

Myocardial Infarction (MI)

MI is a type of acute coronary syndrome (ACS), a condition that results in a sudden reduction of blood flow or blockage to the heart. ACS is most often caused by plaque rupture or clot formation in the heart's arteries that ultimately leads to death of the cardiac tissue. Symptoms common to MI are severe left-sided chest pain (which can be described as crushing), arrhythmia, dyspnea, diaphoresis, and/or nausea. Some individuals will have no symptoms associated with MI. There are two types of MI: non-ST elevation MI (NSTEMI) and ST-elevation MI (STEMI). MI is typically diagnosed through medical history, completion of electrocardiogram (a test that assesses and evaluates the electrical system of the heart), and laboratory tests associated with cardiac enzymes. If cardiac enzymes are elevated, the MI is determined to have ST segment involvement and therefore is identified as STEMI. If diagnostics do not confirm ST elevation, the MI is diagnosed as NSTEMI. Treatment for MI is typically associated with intravenous medication such as vasodilation or thrombolytic drugs. Oxygen and aspirin may be administered as well. Prognosis is dependent on the extent of the damage to the cardiac tissue. Preventative measures include lifestyle modifications.

BOX 9-1 Classifications of Heart Failure

Right-sided HF is typically a result of left-sided HF. This is most commonly seen as increased fluid pressure and the retrograde flow of blood back into the lungs, damaging the right side of the heart.
   Left-sided HF can be either systolic HF or diastolic HF.

- Systolic HF: The left ventricle loses its ability to effectively contract and cannot push the blood with enough force out to the remainder of the body (AHA, 2017).
- Diastolic HF: The left ventricle loses its ability to relax normally, and it cannot fill with adequate blood supply during rest period (AHA, 2017).

Hypertension (HTN)

HTN is a result of chronically elevated blood pressure (BP) that causes the heart to work harder, as there is an increase in resistance within the vascular system. It is a common condition that is classified by a resting systolic BP of 140 mm Hg or higher and/or a diastolic BP of 90 mm Hg or higher (Frazier & Fuqua, 2021). This condition forces blood against the arterial walls at much too high of a level without associated symptoms. Many individuals with HTN are asymptomatic until the chronic dysfunction causes MI, CAD, or CHF. Treatment includes dietary modification, physical activity, stress management, management of risk factors, and medication (e.g., ACE inhibitor, diuretic, beta blocker, calcium channel blocker, and vasodilator).

Nonsurgical Intervention

Depending on the level of cardiovascular dysfunction, nonsurgical intervention may be appropriate to assist with management of the disease process. Common nonsurgical interventions listed within Box 9-2 are based on the cardiac conditions discussed previously.

Surgical Intervention

If nonsurgical intervention fails or if the cardiovascular condition worsens, cardiac surgery may be warranted as depicted in Box 9-3.

Functional Impairment Associated With Cardiovascular Conditions

Whether an individual has an acute or chronic cardiovascular condition, it can often limit function and participation

---

BOX 9-2 Cardiovascular Nonsurgical Interventions

- **Beta blockers** are known as blocking agents to reduce BP and block the effects of epinephrine. These medications cause the heart to beat more slowly and with less force while also widening veins and arteries to improve blood flow.
- **Statins** help lower cholesterol while also helping to stabilize the plaques on the walls of blood vessels to reduce the risk of blood clot formation.
- **ACE inhibitors** help relax the veins and arteries to lower BP and prevent production of the enzyme angiotensin, which narrows blood vessels.
- **Diuretics** promote increased production of urine to help rid the body of sodium and water. This subsequently decreases the amount of fluid flowing through the veins and arteries, which ultimately reduces BP.
- **Calcium-channel blockers** are known to lower BP and prevent calcium from entering the cells of the heart and arteries. Blocking the calcium channels allows blood vessels to relax and open.

BOX 9-3 Cardiovascular Surgical Interventions

- **Coronary artery bypass graft (CABG):** CABG is a surgical procedure that is performed to restore normal blood flow to an obstructed artery. A cardiothoracic surgeon will enter the heart via **sternotomy** to open the sternum and replace the occluded artery/arteries with arteries of vein grafts from a different part of the body. The preferred graft is an artery graft, as they last longer; however, grafts are typically taken from the legs, which are then vein grafts.
- **Valve replacements (aortic valve replacement or mitral valve replacement:** When the valves become damaged or diseased and do not work properly, they need to be repaired or replaced. These valves can be repaired or replaced via sternotomy or through minimally invasive techniques such as a thoracotomy or groin incision.
- **Left ventricular assist device (LVAD)** is a mechanical pump that takes the place in the left ventricular to take over the left-sided function of the heart. It is used for individuals who are at the end stage of HF and also can be used with an extremely sick person who is awaiting a heart transplant. LVADs can be used as a bridge to destination (individuals will have their LVAD for life), bridge to transplant, or bridge to recovery (an individual will wean off the pump after intervention to fix the acute damage to the heart, such as **cardiogenic shock,** a condition where the heart is unable to sufficiently pump blood based on the needs of the body). People who work with these individuals typically need special training before providing care.
- **Cardiac (heart) transplant** is a surgical procedure performed on individuals with an end-stage heart condition and is used when other medical and/or surgical interventions have failed. This operation entails the disease/failing heart to be removed and replaced with a healthier donor heart.
- **Pacemaker/defibrillator** is used to eradicate an arrythmia that is present in the heart. It can be single chamber (atrium or ventricle), dual chamber (lead in atrium and ventricle), or biventricular (leads in both left and right ventricle).
- **Intra-aortic balloon pump (IABP)** is a therapeutic device that helps the heart pump enough blood to the rest of the body. A catheter that is attached to a long balloon is inserted in the aorta, and the opposite end of the catheter is attached to a computer console to control and provide oxygenated blood to the arteries and vessels. Its use is common for unstable angina, MI, arrythmias, HF, and cardiogenic shock. The IABP gives the heart an opportunity to rest, with a goal of weaning off the pump to normal function.

---

in meaningful occupations. This is not specifically associated with nonsurgical or surgical intervention, as both can cause limitations to endurance, activity tolerance, independence with ADLs or instrumental activities of daily living (IADLs), work, leisure, etc. Moreover, when an individual undergoes open heart surgery, there are precautions associated with a sternotomy incision. These precautions last approximately 8 to 10 weeks and include (Cahalin et al, 2011):

- No lifting, pushing, or pulling anything that weighs more than 10 pounds
- Not bearing body weight on arms and no excessive twisting or turning
- Only raising the elbows above the head if it is done bilaterally; not raising unilateral arm above the head

Pulmonary Disease

Pulmonary disease is associated with decreased function of the lungs related to respiration and ventilation that can be associated with three concerns: airway dysfunction, disease of the lung tissue, and lung circulation disease. It is said that more than 35 million individuals have a diagnosis associated with a preventable lung disease. This is also the third leading cause of death, costing health systems more than $300 billion annually (American Lung Association, 2020). As with heart disease, there are many changeable and unchangeable predisposing factors associated with pulmonary disease, such as tobacco smoke, air pollutants, diet and nutrition, infection, physical inactivity, allergens, and occupational exposure (WHO, 2012).

Major Pulmonary Conditions

Chronic Obstructive Pulmonary Disease (COPD)

COPD is a major cause of disability, morbidity, and mortality worldwide that leads to dyspnea and limited capacity to participate in meaningful activities of daily life. COPD encompasses a number of obstructive diseases, such as chronic bronchitis, bronchiectasis, asthma, emphysema, cystic fibrosis, and pneumoconiosis. Other comorbidities are often associated with COPD, such as cardiovascular diseases, osteoporosis, limb muscle dysfunction, and psychological disorders. This consequently contributes not only to the limited capacity present with this disease but also to health-related quality of life. Dyspnea on exertion is the most common symptom associated with this disease, along with persistent cough, wheezing, and fatigue, which ultimately leads to ineffective exchange of respiratory gases (Bui et al, 2017; Frazier & Fuqua, 2021). Symptoms do not typically manifest with COPD until significant lung damage is already present. A diagnosis will likely be confirmed through a noninvasive pulmonary function test (PFT), chest x-ray, computed tomography (CT) scan, or arterial blood gas analysis, a test that measures the level of acidity or pH based on levels of oxygen and carbon dioxide in the blood from an artery. Management of COPD focuses on lifestyle changes and management of the symptoms associated with the disease. COPD is typically managed through nonsurgical intervention, which will be discussed later in this chapter. However, for acute exacerbations, immediate medical care is indicated and would be separate from primary management (Hancox et al, 2021).

Interstitial Lung Disease (ILD)

ILD is a group of disorders that cause progressive scarring (fibrosis) of the lung tissue and impede an individual's ability to breathe and provide sufficient oxygen to their bloodstream. ILD may be caused by long-term exposure to hazardous materials such as asbestos or coal dust, or it can be caused by an autoimmune disease, such as rheumatoid arthritis or scleroderma. Symptoms are associated with dyspnea, nonproductive cough, wheezing, and increased sputum production. **Sarcoidosis** and **pulmonary fibrosis** are common forms of ILD. Diagnostic testing typically involves a PFT and physical examination. Nonsurgical interventions such as supplemental oxygen or anti-inflammatory medications may be provided to manage the irreversible damage that is associated with ILD. In severe cases, surgical interventions such as lung transplantation may be required. Like many pulmonary conditions, ILD is chronic, and intervention is necessary to slow disease progression and preserve the quality of life.

Lung Cancer

Lung cancer is the most common cause of cancer-related deaths worldwide, accounting for almost 30% and affecting both men and women equally (Frazier & Fuqua, 2021). Common symptoms associated with lung cancer are cough (with or without sputum production), dyspnea, weight loss, and diffuse chest pain. The primary risk factor associated with lung cancer is cigarette smoking, which accounts for nearly 90% of cases. Other associated risk factors include exposure to secondhand smoke, radon, arsenic, air pollution, radiation therapy, and asbestos. Most individuals are symptomatic upon diagnosis which can be solidified through CT scan of the chest and tissue biopsy. Treatment is typically based on the type of lung cancer (small or nonsmall cell) and stage of the tumor itself. For nonsmall cell lung cancer (NSCLC), surgical resection (lobectomy or pneumonectomy) with or without radiation is common, whereas later stage NSCLC cannot be treated by surgical intervention alone and is typically combined with a modality such as chemotherapy, radiation, and/or palliative care for symptom management.

Acute Respiratory Distress Syndrome (ARDS)

ARDS is a type of acute lung injury categorized by severe pulmonary congestion, respiratory distress, hypoxemia, progressive hypercapnia, acidosis, septicemia, shock, or severe lung infection (**pneumonia**). Primary symptoms associated with this disease are classified as a medical emergency and include rales, rhonchi, wheezes, sudden and severe dyspnea, and shallow respirations. It is crucial that individuals with ARDS are admitted to the hospital to receive treatment, typically in the intensive care unit, to ensure constant monitoring and meticulous care. If ARDS is not addressed immediately through fluid management, supplemental oxygen, and medications such as vasodilators, further complications such as a **pneumothorax** (a collection of air or gas in the pleural cavity that results in a partially collapsed or collapsed lung) may present themselves. Depending on the swiftness of medical intervention and the severity of ARDS, recovery from this disease may be associated with residual physical and cognitive impairments requiring intervention related to quality of life and participation in meaningful activities.

Pulmonary Edema

Pulmonary edema is a common diagnosis, with more than 200,000 cases diagnosed per year. Pulmonary edema is usually caused by a cardiovascular dysfunction that ultimately leads to excess fluid in the lungs. Associated cardiovascular disease includes CAD, cardiomyopathy, heart valve dysfunction, HTN, and HF. Pulmonary edema may be noncardiogenic in nature as well as result from ARDS, **pulmonary embolism** (which occurs when a blood clot or other foreign material occludes an artery within pulmonary circulation), drug overdose, or aspiration (Lippincott, 2016). The fluid collects in the air sacs, making it difficult for individuals to breathe and can be mild to extreme. Other associated symptoms are cough, chest pain, and fatigue. Individuals with a diagnosis of pulmonary edema are typically provided supplemental oxygen and medications such as diuretics as treatment for this condition.

Nonsurgical Intervention

Similar to cardiovascular conditions, interventions related to cardiopulmonary conditions may be nonsurgical in nature. Common nonsurgical interventions are explained in Box 9-4.

Surgical Intervention

If nonsurgical interventions are deemed ineffective or if the cardiopulmonary condition worsens, surgical intervention may be necessary. Some of the common surgical interventions for this population are described in Box 9-5.

BOX 9-4 Cardiopulmonary Nonsurgical Interventions

Antibiotics are medicines that kill bacteria and are used to treat most cases of pneumonia. Antibiotics are not effective against viruses.

Bronchodilators are inhaled medicines that can help expand the airways (bronchi), which can reduce wheezing and shortness of breath in people with asthma or COPD.

Corticosteroids are inhaled or oral steroids that can reduce inflammation and improve symptoms in asthma or COPD. Steroids can also be used to treat less common lung conditions caused by inflammation.

Continuous positive airway pressure (CPAP)/bilevel positive airway pressure machines apply air pressure through a mask to keep the airways open. They are used at night to treat sleep apnea, but they are also helpful for some people with COPD. These devices offer a noninvasive form of therapy for patients suffering from sleep apnea.

Supplemental oxygen (O_2) therapy is a nonsurgical intervention that provides individuals with extra O_2 to promote normal organ function and is available through a prescription. Some individuals require supplemental O_2 for a brief period, whereas others use this treatment in a more permanent way. Supplemental O_2 is typically delivered through a nasal cannula or a face mask and can also attach to other medical equipment, such as a CPAP or ventilator.

Mechanical ventilation is a form of life support that takes over the work of the respiratory system for an individual who is having difficulty breathing on their own. This device delivers a high concentration of oxygen to the lungs, helps get rid of carbon dioxide, and decreases the amount of energy a person uses to breathe (American Thoracic Society, 2020). Oxygen from a ventilator is provided either through an endotracheal tube (through the nose or mouth) or as a tracheostomy (through the trachea/windpipe). This tube is then directly attached to the ventilator and controlled by a machine to provide the support an individual needs.

BOX 9-5 Cardiopulmonary Surgical Interventions

Lobectomy is the surgical removal of a lobe of the lung.

Wedge resection is the surgical removal of a small, wedge-shaped piece of lung tissue, usually a section that is diseased or damaged.

Pneumonectomy is a surgical procedure to remove one of an individual's lungs due to trauma or other conditions.

Pulmonary (lung) transplant is a surgical procedure in which one or both of the diseased or failing lungs is replaced by lungs from a healthy donor. This procedure is reserved for individuals who have attempted other nonsurgical and surgical interventions without success or improvement.

Thoracotomy is a surgery that enters the chest wall (thorax); it may be done to treat serious lung conditions or to obtain a lung biopsy.

Video-assisted thoracoscopic surgery (VATS) is a less-invasive chest wall surgery using an endoscope (flexible tube with a camera on its end). VATS may be used to treat or diagnose various lung conditions.

Thoracostomy is a surgical procedure in which an incision is made into the chest wall, usually followed by insertion of a tube between the pleurae and a system for draining fluid from that space.

Pleurocentesis is a procedure to place a needle into the chest cavity to drain fluid around the lung. A sample is usually examined to identify the cause.

Functional Impairment Associated With Cardiopulmonary Conditions

Individuals with cardiopulmonary conditions have associated dyspnea, chronic cough, and sputum production, as well as anxiety and depression that limit their participation in meaningful occupations. Persistent dyspnea and decreased ventilation also cause physiological dysfunction, which greatly affects an individual's ability to perform ADLs, IADLs, work, leisure, and eating. There is also functional impact on activity tolerance and endurance, along with a gradual increase in energy expenditure with chronic conditions. Refer to Promoting Best Practice 9-2.

PROMOTING BEST PRACTICE 9-2
"Health First" in Every Client Interaction

Occupational therapists are uniquely positioned to practice interprofessionally with respect to health behavior change competencies that need to be central in every health professional–client interaction (Leland et al, 2017; Dean & Lomi, 2022). With the context of health reform, it is important for occupational therapists to ensure individuals with chronic diseases are provided the skills and knowledge to promote health and well-being. Healthcare professionals are often siloed when interacting with clients who have a chronic disease, and therefore it can cause confusion and misinterpretation among the healthcare team and also lead to suboptimal care. Breaking down these silos has the potential to make changes to health behaviors while also improving the population's interactions with the interprofessional care team. When there are positive exchanges with healthcare professionals, individuals living with a chronic disease will have improved ratings of health professional–client interactions. This ultimately will decrease the burden on the healthcare systems and promote access for better self-management for the clients. Moreover, if the interprofessional team is consistent with their education and interactions, this can promote improved health and well-being for these individuals. Finally, occupational therapists can act as the liaison between the client and care team to ensure "health first" is at the forefront of the interprofessional teams' vocabulary when providing services to this population and can improve client interactions with healthcare professionals.

CASE STUDY (CONTINUED)
Assessment

Uzoma would benefit from endurance capacity assessments to address his cardiovascular dysfunction and his muscle endurance. Assessment results for the Modified Fatigue Impact Scale (MFIS) are as noted: Physical Subscale: 26, Cognitive Subscale: 0, Psychosocial Subscale: 5, and Total MFIS Score: 31. Assessment results for the Borg Rating of Perceived Exertion scale are 9 (very light) while resting and 17 (very hard) with functional activity such as yardwork and climbing stairs.

Questions
1. What assessments will you choose?
2. What more do you need to know that would be assessed by other members of the interdisciplinary team?
3. What assessments might others on the team complete?

Answers
1. ADL, IADL, and endurance assessments would be appropriate for this case (Box 9-6).
2. It would be beneficial to know the client's classification of heart failure (see section *Heart Failure [HF]/Congestive Heart Failure [CHF]*), medications the client is currently taking (see section *Heart Failure [HF]/Congestive Heart Failure [CHF]*), what type of HF (Box 9-1), and how the client's HF is being managed—nonsurgically (Box 9-2).
3. The interprofessional team would complete assessments within their scope of practice to develop a treatment plan addressing functional deficits considering the current diagnosis and medication intervention. Principal goals providing evaluation and intervention with this population focus on metabolic equivalent (MET) levels, effective breathing techniques, oxygen management, client education, ADL/IADL retraining, energy conservation/work simplification (ECWS), community and social support, and psychosocial factors (see section *Collaboration and Referrals* and *Promoting Best Practice 9-2*).

Practice Frameworks

To best serve clients with cardiovascular and/or cardiopulmonary conditions, occupational therapists must understand how to effectively and efficiently provide evaluation, assessment, and intervention to these individuals. Much revolves around maintaining and/or increasing function related to theories and practice frameworks. The WHO supports a framework that provides support to normative function and quality assurance principles with consideration of effective evaluation, assessment, and intervention (WHO, 2018). Occupational therapists rely on the Occupational Therapy Practice Framework (OTPF) to provide holistic and client-centered care to maximize an individual's functional capacity through education, advocacy of psychosocial support, lifestyle recommendations, and improved activity tolerance for performance of meaningful occupations. These services are provided across the continuum of care and in conjunction with the interprofessional team, which will be discussed later in this chapter. Moreover, the occupational therapist's role will be discussed in more depth after the presentation of frameworks. Specific considerations for individuals diagnosed with cardiovascular and/or cardiopulmonary conditions will be addressed. Occupational therapists must place considerations on environmental factors and context. These considerations will either enable or restrict a client's participation in meaningful occupations, which ultimately will become a barrier or support when providing occupational therapy services.

The occupational therapist's evaluation process should glean information from the occupational profile and the analysis of occupational performance to inform the intervention plan, as noted within the OTPF. The occupational therapist considers individual clients' medical and social history and also consults with the interprofessional team to ensure the patient's success. As part of the multidisciplinary team, occupational therapists are responsible for promoting quality of life and health in older adults with cardiovascular and/or cardiopulmonary conditions based on functioning, disability, environmental factors, and personal factors as presented in the ICF Framework (Shiota et al, 2021).

Common assessment and/or screening instruments for this population are presented in Box 9-6.

After performing the appropriate assessments, the occupational therapist develops an approach to intervention and an intervention plan. These approaches are primarily determined based on the level of care each individual requires, along with the occupation and activity demands associated with the interventions being provided. Box 9-7 further delineates approaches to intervention based on setting.

Implications for the Older Adult in Treatment

Occupational therapy has a unique role with cardiovascular and cardiopulmonary rehabilitation that has direct implications for the older adult. Occupational therapists have the ability to address multiple areas of intervention across the continuum of care. These include those noted previously in the chapter. Occupational therapy practitioners are well suited to provide interventions related to education strategies regarding occupation, health, and well-being. Moreover, occupational therapy practitioners can enable individuals with cardiovascular and/or cardiopulmonary dysfunction and their caregivers to acquire habits and behaviors to promote positive disease management (American Occupational Therapy Association [AOTA], 2020). Consequently, quality disease management can decrease healthcare costs and indirectly improve quality of life through increased participation in meaningful occupations both the client and their caregivers (Norberg et al, 2017; Schutt & Thompson, 2020; O'Toole et al, 2021).

As will be discussed, exercise increases the metabolic demand for oxygen and substrates. With aging, the oxygen transport system is less capable of responding to exercise stress as a consequence of the diminished efficiency of the various steps in the oxygen transport pathway, including oxidative metabolism at the cellular level as related to cardiovascular and cardiopulmonary disease (Vigorito & Giallauria, 2014; Sas et al, 2018). Despite the reported age-related

---

BOX 9-6 Common Screenings and Assessments

- ADLs
  - The Functional Independence Measure is a system to measure dysfunction and determines the level of assistance needed for an individual to perform ADL tasks that range from dependent to independent and are scored accordingly.
  - The Barthel Index can be used with this population to gather information regarding the level of success an individual will have performing ADLs safely and independently.
- ADLs/IADLs
  - The Canadian Occupational Performance Measure provides an evidence-based, patient-centered tool to assess the level of satisfaction an individual has with their performance of ADLs and IADLs.
- Cognition
  - The Mini-Mental State Examination can be used to assess cognition in the presence of illness and/or injury to estimate cognitive impairment, which is a consideration with this population based on the pathophysiology of the disease processes.
- Stress Management
  - An interest checklist is an effective way to gather information about an individual's strengths and interest in engagement to ultimately assist with development of motivation to actively participate in the intervention plan.
  - Stress Management Questionnaire is a reliable tool for gathering information regarding an individual's stressors, which are a common concern for those with cardiovascular and/or cardiopulmonary dysfunction. Information gathered with this tool can be used to promote healthy coping strategies to minimize symptoms associated with stress.
- Endurance/Activity Tolerance
  - The Borg CR10 Scale, also known as the modified Borg Scale, allows an individual to rate their perceived exertion and breathlessness during functional tasks. It provides the therapist with information regarding heart and respiration rate along with muscular exertion (refer to Table 9-3).

> **BOX 9-7 Occupational Therapy Practice Framework: Approaches to Intervention**
>
> - Acute Care
>   - Within acute care, most individuals have either had an exacerbation of their cardiovascular and/or cardiopulmonary condition or an associated surgery. These individuals typically present with an overall decrease in strength, activity tolerance, and ADL performance. Therefore, it is valuable to provide a remediation or restoration approach to intervention with these individuals. This will be discussed later in this chapter, but it typically is associated with pursed-lip breathing, O_2 management, diaphragmatic breathing, education on MET levels, and ADL retraining.
> - Inpatient Rehabilitation/Skilled Nursing Facility Rehabilitation
>   - Individuals who require extensive rehabilitation after an acute care stay may be transferred to an inpatient or skilled nursing facility for continued progression toward functional independence with performance of occupations. Within these facilities, it is common for the remediation or restoration intervention approach to continue, but more emphasis is placed on modification through compensation and adaptation to ensure successful performance of functional activities after discharge. This includes inventions related to the continuation of pursed-lip breathing, O_2 management, and diaphragmatic breathing and progresses to interventions related to ADL/IADL retraining along with patient education related to self-management and lifestyle changes.
> - Outpatient/Community
>   - After discharge from inpatient rehabilitation services, the patient is provided care at an outpatient cardiopulmonary facility and/or within the community. This is an influential and unique aspect to occupational therapy intervention, as much advocacy happens for individuals within this setting. Approaches to intervention are related to prevention, maintenance, and health promotion. Individuals are encouraged to bring knowledge of previous interventions forward to ensure successful disease management and promotion of engagement in meaningful occupations. Interventions are specifically associated with patient education for self-management and empowerment, increased understanding of MET levels and integration of energy conservation and work simplification, community resources, psychosocial supports, and lifestyle changes to support the intervention approaches within this setting.

changes, the considerable reserve capacity of the cardiopulmonary and cardiovascular systems tends to offset the potential functional consequences. The degree of this compensation, however, is highly variable among individual older persons. Although this variability reflects genetic factors to a considerable extent, fitness and lifestyle factors also have a significant role. That cardiopulmonary and cardiovascular reserve capacity is maximized with exercise irrespective of age has been known for several decades. Furthermore, age is not a limiter for the capacity to exhibit an exercise response (Sattelmair et al, 2011; Rebelo-Marques et al, 2018).

Moreover, cardiac and pulmonary rehabilitation is a standard of care that aims to improve patient condition, modify risk factors, and prevent progression and exacerbation of the many conditions discussed earlier (Swiatkiewicz et al, 2021). Occupational therapists are among the many healthcare professionals who have an ability to contribute to this standard of care and promote health and wellness with these populations.

Metabolic Equivalent (MET) Levels

The metabolic demand of an activity can be defined by a unit called the **metabolic equivalent** (MET). One MET is equal to 3.5 mL O_2/kg of body weight per minute, the normal basal metabolic demand for oxygen (Jette et al, 1990; Zientara et al, 2021). By convention, the metabolic demands of various activities are expressed as multiples of the basal metabolic rate. A list of typical activities with their associated METs can be found in Tables 9-4 and 9-5. Although scarce, research conducted over the past decade has found

TABLE 9-4 ■ MET Levels for Common Occupations

ADLS/IADLS	MET LEVEL
Grooming/bathing—seated	1.0–2.5
Bathing—standing	2.0–4.0
Dressing	1.0–4.0
Cooking	1.0–2.5
House cleaning	2.6–4.0
Gardening	2.6–4.0
Making a bed	1.0–2.5
Grocery shopping	2.0–7.0

Note: Based on Barefoot & Hayden (2021); Jette et al, (1990).

TABLE 9-5 ■ MET Levels for Common Physical Activity

PHYSICAL ACTIVITY	MET LEVEL
Walking (leisurely)	1.0–2.5
Walking (moderate effort)	2.6–4.0
Climbing stairs	6.0–10.0 (carrying groceries)
Running (moderate effort)	8.8
Various sports (basketball, baseball, wrestling, swimming, etc.)	8.0–12.0 (dependent on task analysis and performance of task)

Note: Based on Barefoot & Hayden (2021); Jette et al (1990).

that metabolic costs of daily activities and walking are substantially different in older adults (Knaggs et al, 2011; Corbett et al, 2017; Gupta et al, 2021) and that having mobility impairments increases metabolic cost (Knaggs et al, 2011; Gupta et al, 2021). It is thought that poor efficiency of movement, exacerbated by coactivation of antagonistic muscle groups, is partially responsible for elevated costs (Latash, 2018; Aguillar-Farias et al, 2019; Gupta et al, 2021). These differences are important for rehabilitation professionals to consider when prescribing activities and exercise for healthy and mobility-impaired older adults.

It can be difficult to know the metabolic cost of some activities. For example, the metabolic costs of sexual activity and the capacity to work have been relatively neglected in the literature, particularly with respect to older people. The metabolic cost of sexual activity in young people depends on the body position and other factors and is relatively low. Sexual activity is equivalent to 3 to 5 METs (climbing two flights of stairs or walking briskly for a short duration). Considering an older person's capacity for physical activity (Levine et al, 2012) and the variations in hemodynamic status that occur during sexual activity, it can be well tolerated for many older people (Steinke, 2014). If aerobically conditioned, an older person can perform sexual activity such as intercourse without excessive HR, BP, and overall exertion responses (Aguilar-Farias et al, 2019; Oliva-Lozano et al, 2022). However, sexual activity may be less well tolerated in older adults with cardiovascular conditions leading to heart palpitations, shortness of breath, and fatigue and is recommended only after a comprehensive evaluation of physical condition is completed (Jelavic et al, 2018). To minimize the metabolic demand and exercise stress, sexual encounters can be timed with medications and with energy peaks during the day, and body positions can be modified. For example, upright positions may be better tolerated than recumbency.

Progressive changes in the cardiopulmonary and cardiovascular systems, in conjunction with changes in the capacity for oxygen and substrate utilization in the musculature, result in less efficient oxygen transport in the older adult. With activity and exercise, the increased metabolic demand for oxygen and substrate requires a commensurate increase in ventilation and cardiac output. Both maximal ventilation and cardiac output decline linearly with age, and maximal oxygen consumption is correspondingly reduced. The extraction of oxygen at the tissue level, however, which is measured by the arteriovenous oxygen difference, does not change significantly with age. The degree of endurance needed to perform ADLs varies depending on the task. Those ADLs that are primarily skill based, such as dressing, toileting, grooming, shaving, bathing, and feeding, are associated with low metabolic demand and generally require little endurance. However, ambulation, climbing stairs and hills, yard work, housework, shopping, gardening, sexual activity, volunteer work, gainful employment, managing transportation, and social activities outside the home, which are associated with higher metabolic demand, require greater endurance and tend to reflect the status of the cardiopulmonary and cardiovascular systems. Tables 9-4 and 9-5 give examples of common occupations and the average MET level associated with that occupation.

Pursed-Lip Breathing, Dyspnea Control Postures, Diaphragmatic Breathing, and Oxygen Management

Many older adults with cardiovascular and cardiopulmonary conditions have associated dyspnea, which can lead to extreme fatigue, cough, and compensatory hyperventilation and ultimately impede overall quality of life and function (Ciubean et al, 2021). When treating individuals with cardiovascular and cardiopulmonary conditions, the occupational therapist should consider pursed-lip and diaphragmatic breathing, dyspnea control posturing, and O_2 management. Although these considerations apply specifically to patients with cardiopulmonary conditions as far as education, those with cardiovascular conditions can also benefit from this treatment, depending on their needs. When these intervention techniques are coupled with patient education, ADL/IADL retraining, and energy conservation techniques, they can improve the overall impact of treatment for older adults within these populations. Pursed-lip breathing decreases the workload on the pulmonary system while preventing tightness in the airway by providing resistance during expiration (Ciubean et al, 2021). Pursed-lip breathing is associated with inhaling through the nose and exhaling through the mouth with lips pursed as if blowing through a whistle. The exhalation should take about twice as long as the inhalation to effectively perform this breathing technique.

Dyspnea-controlled postures when paired with diaphragmatic breathing assists with managing dyspnea-related anxiety and compensatory hyperventilation through using accessory muscles for breathing, which is not as effective as using the diaphragm. An individual should be positioned for comfort or in a dyspnea-controlled position so diaphragmatic breathing techniques can be performed. These positions include erect postural sitting and semi-Fowler position (seated at a 45-degree angle). Once the individual is positioned in a dyspnea-controlled posture, diaphragmatic breathing education can be performed. The occupational therapy practitioner provides external tactile input to the abdomen and instructs the individual to inhale and exhale using the abdomen while incorporating pursed-lip breathing. It is also helpful for the occupational therapy practitioner to provide this tactile input in conjunction with the individual's hands being placed on their abdomen and sternal manubrium. This hand-over-hand technique is effective to ensure tactile feedback, which is necessary to promote carryover in education provided when client performs this technique on their own. Finally, the occupational therapy practitioner should provide O_2 management training, which will assist with ADL/IADL participation. Educating an individual to monitor their oxygen saturation (SpO_2), while also managing their O_2 at the same time they are performing various tasks will prolong their independent participation in meaningful occupations.

Client Education

Individuals with cardiovascular and cardiopulmonary conditions are at major risk for morbidity and mortality globally. To mitigate this risk, occupational therapists must provide education related to self-management and empowerment including secondary and tertiary prevention (Alcorn & Broome, 2014; Kahjoogh et al, 2016). By providing occupational performance coaching, the occupational therapist can empower individuals with these conditions to manage their chronic disease. Moreover, when occupational therapists are providing services within primary care, they can decrease the burden of care and strain on the healthcare system while also addressing the psychosocial components associated with this population (refer to Promoting Best Practice 9-3).

Education related to self-management and positive lifestyle changes can include poor diet, lack of physical activity, adherence to medical treatment, self-monitoring of symptoms associated with the chronic condition, and smoking cessation. Once this direct education is provided, it is then crucial for the occupational therapist to indirectly promote empowerment related to self-motivation, health, education, self-efficacy, and social support to shape and facilitate change through occupational performance coaching.

With occupational performance coaching, individuals are encouraged to develop and maintain autonomy related to well-being and disease management (Loizeau et al, 2021). Empowerment allows for creating a supportive environment that includes shared decision-making among the individual, their family, and the interdisciplinary care team, making the individual a key stakeholder in their chronic disease management. Empowerment can be exhibited on an individual basis or even based on community and social support. Community and social support could be provided in a number of contexts related to adaptation to responses, enabling a positive environment, enabling desired autonomy, and providing adaptation as appropriate related to empowerment as noted. For example, an individual with a cardiovascular and/or cardiopulmonary condition would benefit from occupational therapy education related to their ability to live safely within their environments. This could be completed through a community home evaluation to ensure necessary home modifications are in place for the individual to positively interact with their environment. Moreover, having the necessary adaptations in place, individuals can successfully perform ADLs/IADLs, which improves their ability to have a positive environment. When individuals can successfully perform their ADLs/IADLs and positively interact with their environment, this enables autonomy for them and promotes empowerment. Furthermore, with considerations of community and social support, it will enhance an individual's ability to be an active participant with the care team in relation to current societal and health trends. If an individual has appropriate social supports in place, they demonstrate the ability to effectively engage with the health professionals in their care team, which can promote disease management (Loizeau et al, 2021). Self-management of health is critical for cardiopulmonary health. Many individuals lack the skills and knowledge for successful self-advocacy, such as their ability to articulate their needs related to self-care, disease management, and organization of care (Loizeau et al, 2021). Therefore, occupational therapists have a role to increase their clients' abilities regarding health literacy and self-advocacy within the scope of the disease process. Through occupational performance coaching and empowerment, individuals within this population can increase their knowledge and skills to manage their condition more effectively.

ADL/IADL Retraining

Occupational therapists focus on improving occupational performance to enhance an individual's health-related quality of life (HRQOL) specifically through ADL/IADL retraining with an emphasis on energy conservation. Occupational therapists promote independent performance of ADLs/IADLs for all individuals. Moreover, the emphasis of traditional cardiovascular and cardiopulmonary rehabilitation on exercise modalities does not always translate to successful performance of ADLs/IADLs and promote the individual's sense of well-being (Saketkoo et al, 2021; Mahoney et al, 2020). ADL/IADL retraining through simulation is an effective way to promote enhancement of occupational performance for individuals. Also providing appropriate modifications and adaptations will assist individuals to maintain independence with ADLs/IADLs for a longer period while promoting education related to pursed-lip breathing, energy conservation, posturing, pacing, etc. Not only is this retraining important, but it also must be relevant and meaningful to the individuals receiving occupational therapy services.

The occupational therapist should first complete an occupational profile to explore the efficacy of adding ADL/IADL simulation to traditional cardiovascular and cardiopulmonary rehabilitation approaches. This can also be assessed through the common assessment/screening tools that were presented earlier in the chapter. A more holistic approach toward providing interventions with these populations will increase HRQOL and similarly enhance the multidisciplinary approach to providing care for these populations. Tailoring treatment to the individual patient by focusing on tasks they find difficult to manage will translate to carryover when they are no longer receiving occupational therapy services, which also supports the concepts of empowerment previously noted.

Energy Conservation/Work Simplification (ECWS)

ECWS is important and can be addressed with ADL/IADL simulation for effective carryover in intervention. Energy conservation is referred to as activities to be completed in a way that decreases muscle fatigue, joint stress, and pain

(Stromsdorfer, 2023). Occupational therapy practitioners serving this population emphasize ECWS techniques to allow for prolonged independence with participation in meaningful occupations on a daily basis and with disease progression. Occupational therapists can educate patients to incorporate ECWS into daily routines, including performing ADLs and/or IADLs. When considering ECWS techniques, it is crucial to understand the basic tenets: limit the amount of work it takes to complete the task, plan ahead, organize, use appropriate equipment, use effective biomechanical methods, and rest as needed (Duke University, n.d.).

Under the umbrella of ECWS, it is also key to understand the concept of MET levels. MET levels are based on the intensity of work and the energy expended to complete that work, as noted earlier. Occupational therapists use that knowledge to educate individuals on how to incorporate ECWS techniques to promote independence in planning their daily routine based on the amount of energy a task takes (refer to Tables 9-1 and 9-2). Training on ECWS techniques related to ADL participation prevents hyperventilation and enhances the patient's ability to perform tasks in a decreased amount of time with lower oxygen uptake compared with individuals who do not receive this training (Wingardh et al, 2020).

Caregiver Education

The cost of caregiving for individuals with cardiovascular and/or cardiopulmonary disease is projected to increase to $128 billion in 2035 (Dunbar et al, 2018). This does not include medical costs and productivity losses associated with burden and caregiving. It is occupational therapy's role to educate family, friends, and/or caregivers about the importance of caregiver burden and the effects of burnout (Rouch et al, 2021). This education and training should be embedded in outcome measures to promote increased payment models. Moreover, formalized training specific to the cardiovascular and/or cardiopulmonary condition their loved one is experiencing would be beneficial for the caregiver to recognize signs of exacerbation and have an effective strategy for management of those exacerbations before needing further care or hospitalization (Dunbar et al, 2018). Not only is it important for caregivers to recognize the needs of the individuals they are caring for, but it is also essential for them to understand their individual needs as well.

Training caregivers to recognize signs and symptoms of burnout is a crucial part of occupational therapy intervention. These signs and symptoms include withdrawal from family and friends; frequently acquiring illness; loss of interest in activities they previously enjoyed; feelings of self-harm; feeling irritable, hopeless, and/or helpless; emotional and/or physical exhaustion; changes in appetite, weight, or both; substance use; and changes in sleep patterns. If a caregiver is unable to recognize and address burnout, their ability to provide care will be negatively affected or even unsustainable. In addition, their own health and well-being will be affected (Rouch et al, 2021). Moreover, there is a need in current healthcare trends to provide more support and training to caregivers for development of coping and resilience skills to decrease their burden of care and ultimately improve their quality of life. It is also crucial to develop their self-confidence to provide care to their loved one who is experiencing a chronic condition that will require lifelong care (Subih et al, 2020). With little to no training, it is difficult for caregivers to participate in discharge planning and disease management. Therefore, they are unable to effectively cope with or manage situations and/or stressors associated with the systematic care their loved one may need, including surgical and nonsurgical interventions related to these populations (Agren et al, 2015; Subih et al, 2020).

Promoting Best Practice 9-3
Psychosocial Component With Cardiovascular and Cardiopulmonary Populations

Psychosocial components associated with cardiovascular and cardiopulmonary conditions include fear, anxiety, depression, decreased life satisfaction, and decreased life engagement. Individuals with chronic health conditions experience an overall decreased sense of well-being as the conditions progress, which in turn negatively affects them psychosocially (Janseen et al, 2022). Moreover, there is specific correlation between psychosocial factors and an individual's ability to effectively demonstrate self-management, which is then associated with disease burden and low self-efficacy. Because of this, occupational therapy practitioners need to identify those individuals who are at risk for poor self-management and incorporate education related to improving self-management abilities and empowerment (Hardman et al, 2022). Chronic disease management emphasizes the importance of addressing the emotional and psychosocial needs of patients to encourage and empower them (Loizeau et al, 2021).

Monitoring the Patient's Response to Activity/Intervention

To prevent complications when providing services to these populations, the occupational therapist must monitor the patient's response to interventions. Assessing vital signs is a top priority to be completed before, during, and after activity and/or intervention. Listed here are common considerations for monitoring patients during cardiovascular and/or cardiopulmonary rehabilitation. Moreover, there are contraindications that need to be evaluated, and interventions should be discontinued if individuals are experiencing chest pain, excessive fatigue, nausea and/or vomiting, diaphoresis, respiratory rate, discomfort/pain, and orthostasis. The occupational therapist should document these considerations and assessment considerations to track progress:

- HR needs to be monitored to ensure it is not outside parameters that have been set by the physician for activity.
- BP needs to be monitored to ensure it is within a therapeutic range and also not outside the parameters set forth by the physician.

- Perceived exertion through intermittent administration of the Modified Borg scale is effective as an objective measure of shortness of breath or dyspnea that an individual exhibits during performance of tasks during intervention (see Table 9-3). This will help provide information regarding how their body is responding to activity in conjunction with HR and BP.
- Arterial (oxygen) saturation that is measured using pulse oximetry (SpO_2) is necessary to monitor in addition to the individual's perceived exertion. Appropriate SpO_2 for activity should be considered and within the parameters recommended by the physician, typically to be greater than 90% when completing tasks.
- MET levels are fundamental to provide as an educational component for the individual(s) who are receiving intervention. As previously mentioned, MET levels are based on intensity of work and the energy expended to complete that work. Moreover, MET levels are used as a way to describe functional capacity or exercise tolerance of individuals and therefore would be helpful to monitor when providing intervention. Providing interventions that vary in task and activity through a range of MET levels may be helpful in being most effective for these populations. This will also ensure occupational therapy is within the parameters of activity tolerance as prescribed by the physician.
- Maximum aerobic heart rate (MAHR) provides a formula for exercise intensity that is appropriate to monitor with these populations while taking into consideration HR parameters prescribed by the physician. MAHR is an additional way to gauge exercise intensity along with other monitoring strategies previously discussed.
- Medications are consequential to monitor when providing intervention for these populations. If a change in medication has happened, it may influence symptoms that individuals are experiencing during intervention while also exhibiting changes to HR, BP, exertion, etc.

Interprofessional Colleagues

Collaboration and Referrals

The cardiovascular and cardiopulmonary populations benefit from an interprofessional approach to intervention that may include physicians, nurses, occupational therapists, physical therapists, social workers, psychologists, and dietitians to provide quality care. Although occupational therapists have unique competencies, health assessment and health promotion interventions are core shared competencies with other professionals. Occupational therapists practice largely nonpharmacologically and thus are in a unique position to shift focus of care from a predominantly "illness" system to a "health" system. Through their professional organizations, occupational therapists can help make a difference in outcomes of cardiovascular and pulmonary disease in addition to other conditions in older individuals (refer to Promoting Best Practice 9-2).

It is imperative to not only understand occupational therapy's role regarding education for improving self-management of the disease process but also understand the importance of the interdisciplinary care team. Moreover, interprofessional collaboration (IPC) among healthcare professionals is an integral part of patient satisfaction and success (Maree et al, 2017). IPC has the potential to improve the quality of healthcare (Shah et al, 2018; Maree et al, 2017). Providing patient-centered education through IPC not only allows for collaboration among healthcare professionals, but it also shows efficacy in improving patient care (Reeves et al, 2017). Additionally, occupational therapists have a distinct role within IPC to address environmental and context factors, roles and performance patterns, decreased ADL function, lifestyle changes, psychosocial adjustments, and prioritizing meaningful occupations to provide holistic and patient-centered care.

CASE STUDY (CONTINUED)

Intervention

Uzoma would benefit from self-management, energy conservation and work simplification strategies, lifestyle modifications, medication regimen adherence, participation in ADLs and IADLs, and empowerment (patient monitoring, diet adherence, symptom recognition, and management). It would also be beneficial to provide caregiver education along with social and emotional support, as this assists individuals with CHF to sustain lifestyle changes in managing their disease.

Questions

1. How do the assessment results inform your interventions?
2. What are two or three evidence-based, occupation-centered exemplar interventions that address the case study client's priorities?
3. What assistive technologies or environmental modifications would you recommend?
4. What contextual elements from the case study's occupational therapy profile influence your treatment planning?

Answers

1. Assessment results can assist with creating appropriate intervention plans for this case. Common interventions for this population include METs, pursed-lip breathing, dyspnea control postures, diaphragmatic breathing and oxygen management, client education, ADL/IADL retraining, ECWS, caregiver education, and monitoring client's response to activity/intervention (see section *Implications for the Older Adult in Treatment*).

2. Exemplar interventions include MET levels, pursed-lip breathing, dyspnea control postures, diaphragmatic breathing, O₂ management, client education (self-management, empowerment, and lifestyle changes), ADL/IADL retraining, ECWS, and caregiver education. Have students locate evidence-based articles based on chosen occupation-centered intervention (see section *Implications for the Older Adult in Treatment*).
3. Assistive technologies or environmental modifications would be recommended based on response to common interventions, which include METs, pursed-lip breathing, dyspnea control postures, diaphragmatic breathing, oxygen management, client education, ADL/IADL retraining, ECWS, caregiver education monitoring client's response to activity/intervention (see section *Implications for the Older Adult in Treatment*).
4. Contextual elements would be related to client education (self-management, empowerment, and lifestyle changes) (see section *Implications for the Older Adult in Treatment*). Factors to consider include: the client does not own any adaptive equipment or durable medical equipment, the client is on long-term disability, the client and his wife are open to environmental modifications, and his wife is in good health. Context should be related to environmental and personal factors influencing engagement and participation in occupation. Environmental factors related to the natural environment, technology, support and relationships, attitudes, services, systems, and policies. Personal factors should be related to age, sexual orientation, gender identity, race and ethnicity, cultural identification and attitudes, social background and socioeconomic status, upbringing and life experiences, habits and behavioral patterns, education, profession and professional identity, lifestyle, and health conditions and fitness status (AOTA, 2020).

SUMMARY

Individuals with cardiovascular and/or cardiopulmonary dysfunction or disease can benefit from occupational therapy services to maintain and enhance function to support their ability to maintain independence and promote quality of life. Moreover, individuals with chronic health conditions, such as cardiovascular and/or cardiopulmonary disease, are in need of comprehensive care for better self-management to maximize living with those conditions. Principal goals providing evaluation and intervention with this population focus on MET levels, effective breathing techniques, oxygen management, client education, ADL/IADL retraining, ECWS, community and social support, and psychosocial factors while incorporating an interprofessional team. Due to the complex nature of these various diagnoses, occupational therapists must have a high level of expertise and knowledge in these given areas to provide an appropriate assessment when establishing an intervention plan for this unique population. Finally, having the ability to provide holistic and patient-centered care in accordance with practice and theoretical frameworks will promote best practice, while improving client outcomes for this population as well.

Critical Thinking Questions

1. What are appropriate intervention approaches when providing occupational therapy services for people with cardiovascular and/or cardiopulmonary conditions?
2. What kinds of intervention activities would be appropriate to provide to individuals with a cardiovascular and/or cardiopulmonary condition?
3. How might IPC serve the cardiovascular and/or cardiopulmonary patient populations?

REFERENCES

Agren, S., Stromberg, A., Jaarsma, T., & Luttik, M. A. (2015). Caregiving tasks and caregiver burden; effects of a psycho-educational intervention in patients of patients with post-operative heart failure. *Heart Lung, 44*, 270–275, https://doi.org/10.1016/j.hrtlng.2015.04.003

Aguillar-Farias, N., Brown, W. J., Skinner, T. L., & Peeters, G. M. (2019). Metabolic equivalent values of common daily activities in middle-age and older adults in free-living environments: A pilot study. *J Phys Act Health, 16*, 222–229. https://doi.org/10.1123/jpah.2016-0400

Alcorn, K., & Broome, K. (2014). Occupational performance coaching for chronic conditions: A review of literature. *N Z J Occup Ther, 61*(2), 49–56.

American Heart Association. (2017, May 31). Types of heart failure. https://www.heart.org/en/health-topics/heart-failure/what-is-heart-failure/types-of-heart-failure

American Lung Association. (2020, May 13). *Estimated prevalence and incidence of lung disease.* https://www.lung.org/research/trends-in-lung-disease/prevalence-incidence-lung-disease

American Occupational Therapy Association. (2020). Occupational therapy practice framework: Domain and process (4th ed.). *Am J Occup Ther, 74*(Suppl. 2), 7412410010. https://doi.org/10.5014/ajot.2020.74S2001

American Thoracic Society. (2020). *Mechanical ventilation.* https://www.thoracic.org/patients/patient-resources/resources/mechanical-ventilation.pdf

Barefoot, S., & Hayden, C. (2021). Heart to heart: Occupational therapy for individuals living with heart failure. *OT Practice*, 1–11. https://myaota.aota.org/shop_aota/product/CEA1021

Borg, G. (1982). Psychophysical basis of perceived exertion. *Med Sci Sports Exerc, 14*, 377–381. http://dx.doi.org/10.1249/00005768-198205000-00012

Bozkurt, B., Coats, A. J. S., Tsutsui, H., Abdelhamid, C. M., Adamopoulos, S., Albert, N., Anker, S. D., Atherton, J., Böhm, M., Butler, J., Drazner, M. H., Michael Felker, G., Filippatos, G., Fiuzat, M., Fonarow, G. C., Gomez-Mesa, J. E., Heidenreich, P., Imamura, T., Jankowska, E. A., Januzzi, J., ... Zieroth, S. (2021). Universal definition and classification of heart failure: A report of the Heart Failure Society of America, Heart Failure Association of the European Society of Cardiology, Japanese Heart Failure Society and Writing Committee of the Universal Definition of Heart Failure. *J Card Fail, 27*(4), 387–413.

Bui, K. L., Nyberg, A., Maltais, F. Z, & Saey, D. (2017). Functional tests in chronic obstructive pulmonary disease, part 1: Clinical relevance and links to the international classification of functioning, disability, and health. *Ann Am Thor Soc, 14*(5), 778–784.

Cahalin, L. P., LaPier, T. K., & Shaw, D. K. (2011). Sternal precautions: is it time for change? Precautions versus restrictions—a review of literature and recommendations for revision. *Cardiopulm Phys Ther J, 22*(1), 5–15. http://doi.org/PMC3056839

Centers for Disease Control and Prevention. (2020, September 8). *Heart failure.* https://www.cdc.gov/heartdisease/heart_failure.htm

Centers for Disease Control and Prevention, Division for Heart Disease and Stroke Prevention. (2021, September 27). *Heart Disease.* https://www.cdc.gov/heartdisease/about.htm

Ciubean, A. D., Ciortea, V. M., Ungur, R. A., Borda, I. M., Dogaru, B. G., Popa, T., & Irsay, L. (2021). Occupational therapy intervention in pulmonary rehabilitation—an update in the COVID-19 era. *Balneo and PRM Research Journal, 12*(4), 439–444. https://dx.doi.org/10.12680/balneo.2021.476

Corbett, D. B., Wanigatunga, A. A., Valiani, V., Handberg, E. M., Buford, T. W., Brumback, R., Casanova, R., Janelle, C. M., & Manini, T. M. (2017). Metabolic cost of daily activity in older adults (Chores XL) study: Design and methods. *Contemp Clin Trials Commun, 6,* 1–8. http://doi.org/10.1016/j.conctc.2017.02.003

Dean, E., & Lomi, C. (2022). A health and lifestyle framework: An evidence-informed basis for contemporary physical therapist clinical practice guidelines with special reference to individuals with heart failure. *Physiother Res Int.* http://doi.org/10.1002/pri1950

Dunbar, S. B., Khavjou, O. A., Bakas, T., Hunt, G., Kirch, R. A., Leib, A. R., Morrison, R. S., Poehler, D. C., Roger, V. L., Whitsel, L. P. (2018). Projected costs of informal caregiving for cardiovascular disease: 2015 to 2035. *Circulation, 137,* 558–577. https://doi.org/10.1161/CIR0000000000000570

Egger, G., & Dixon, J. (2014). Beyond obesity and lifestyle: A review of 21st century chronic disease determinants. *BioMed Res Int, 2014,* 731685.

Fleg, J. L., & Lakatta, E. G. (2019). Normal aging of the cardiovascular system. In W. S. Aronow & J. L. Fleg (Eds.), *Cardiovascular disease in the elderly* (6th ed.). New York: Informa Healthcare USA.

Frazier, M. S., & Fuqua, T. (2021). *Essentials of human diseases and conditions* (7th ed.). Elsevier.

Gupta, S. D., Bobbert, M., Faber, H., Kistemaker, D. (2021). Metabolic cost in health fit older adults and young adults during overground and treadmill walking. *Eur J Appl Physiol, 121*(10), 2787–2797. https://doi.org/10.1007/soo421-021-04740-2

Hancox, R. J., Jones, S., Baggott, D. Chen, D., Corna, N., Davies, C., Fingleton, J., Hardy, J., Hussain, S., Poot, B., Reid, J., Travers, J. Turner, J., & Young, R. (2021). New Zealand COPD guidelines: Quick reference guide. *N Z Med J, 134*(1530), 76–110

Hardman, R., Begg, S., Spelten, E. (2022). *Exploring the ability of self-report measures to identify risk of high treatment burden in chronic disease patients: A cross-sectional study, 22*(1). https://doi.org/10.1186/s12889-022-12579-1

International Classification of Functioning, Disability, and Health (ICF). (2017). *ICF core set for chronic ischaemic heart disease.* https://www.icf-research-branch.org/icf-core-sets-projects2/cardiovascular-and-respiratory-conditions/icf-core-set-for-chronic-ischaemic-heart-disease

Janseen, I., Powell, L. H., Everson-Rose, S. A., Hollenberg, S. M., El Khoudary, S. R., Matthews, K. A. (2022). Psychosocial well-being and progression of coronary artery calcification in midlife women. *J Am Heart Assoc, 11*(5), e023937. https://doaj.org/article/88be8f5f66344a01a6e5370a6ec5d7f6

Jelavic, M. M., Krstacic, G., Perencevic, A., Pintaric, H. (2018). Sexual activity in patients with cardiac diseases. *Acta Clinica Croatica, 57*(1), 141–148. https://doi.org/10.20471/acc.2018.57.01.18

Jette, M., Sidney, K., & Blumchen, G. (1990). Metabolic equivalents (METS) in exercise testing, exercise prescription, and evaluation of functional capacity. *Clin Cardiol, 13,* 555–565. https://doi.org/10.1002/clc.4960130809

Kahjoogh, M. A., Rassafiani, M., Dunn, W., Hosseini, S. A., & Akbarfahimi, N. (2016). Occupational performance coaching: A descriptive review of literature. *N Z J Occup Ther, 63*(2), 45–49.

Knaggs, J. D., Larkin, K. A., & Manini, T. M. (2011). Metabolic cost of daily activities and effect of mobility impairment in older adults. *J Am Geriatr Soc, 59,* 2118–2223. http://doi.org/10.1111/j.1532-5415.2011.03655.x

Koeppen, B. M., & Stanton, B. A. (2018). *Berne & Levy physiology* (7th ed.). Philadelphia: Elsevier.

Latash, M.L. (2018). Muscle coactivation: Definitions, mechanisms, and functions. *J Neurophysiol, 120*(1), 88–104. https://doi.org/10.1152/jn.00084.2018

Leland, N.E., Fogelberg, D.J., Halle, A.D., & Mroz, T.M. (2017). Occupational therapy and management of multiple chronic conditions in the context of health care reform. *Am J Occup Ther, 71*(1). https://doi.org/10.5014/ajot/2017.711001

Levine, G. N., Steinkez, E. E., Bakaeen, F. G., Bozkurt, B., Cheitlin, M. D., Conti, J. B., Foster, E., Jaarsma, T., Kloner, R. A., Lange, R. A., Lindau, S. T., Maron, B. J., Moser, D. K., Ohman, E. M., Seftel, A. D., & Stewart, W. J.; American Heart Association Council on Clinical Cardiology; Council on Cardiovascular Nursing; Council on Cardiovascular Surgery and Anesthesia; Council on Quality of Care and Outcomes Research. (2012). American Heart Association Council on Clinical Cardiology; Council on Cardiovascular Nursing; Council on Cardiovascular Surgery and Anesthesia; Council on Quality of Care and Outcomes Research. Sexual activity and cardiovascular disease: A scientific statement from the American Heart Association. *Circulation, 125,* 1058–1072. https://doi.org/10.1161/CIR.0b013e3182447787

Lippincott (2016). *Pathophysiology made incredibly visual!* (Vol. 3rd). Wolters Kluwer Health.

Loizeau, V., Morvillers, J. M., Bertrand, D. P., Kilpatrick, K., & Rothan-Tondeur, M. (2021). Defining an enabling environment for those with chronic disease: An integrative review. *BMC Nurs, 20*(252). https://doi.org/10.1186/s12912-021-00741-w

Mahoney, K., Pierce, J., Papo, S., Imran, H., Evans, S., & Wu, W. (2020). Efficacy of adding activity of daily living simulation training to traditional pulmonary rehabilitation on dyspnea and health-related-quality-of-life. *PLoS One, 15*(8). https://doi.org/10.1371/journal.pone.0237973

Maree, C., Bresser, P., Yazbek, M., Engelbrecht, L., Mostert, K., Viviers, C., & Kekana M. (2017). Designing interprofessional modules for undergraduate healthcare learners. *African Journal of Health Professions Education, 9*(4), 185–188. https://doi.org/10.7196/AJHPE.2017.v9i4.853

New York Heart Association. (2018). The stages of heart failure. *Specifications Manual for Joint Commission National Quality Measures.* https://manual.jointcommission.org/releases/TJC2018A/DataElem0439.html

Norberg, E., Lofgren, B., Boman, K., Wennberg, P. Brannstrom, M. (2017). A client-centred programme focusing on energy conservation for people with heart failure. *Scand J Occup Ther, 24*(6), 455–467. https://doi.org/10.1080/11038128.2016.1272631.

Oliva-Lozano, J. M., Alacid, F., Lopez-Minarro, P. A., & Muyor, J. M. (2022). What are the physical demands of sexual intercourse? A systematic review of the literature. *Arch Sex Behav, 51,* 1397–1417. https://doi.org/10.1007/s10508-02246-8

O'Toole, L., Connolly, D., Bolan, F., & Smith, S. M. (2021). Effect of the OPTIMAL programme on self-management of multimorbidity in primary care: A randomized controlled trial. *Br J Gen Pract, 71*(705). https://doi.org/10.3399/bjgp20X714185

Panizo, J. G., Barra, S., Mellor, G., Heck, P., & Agarwal, S. (2018). Premature ventricular complex-induced cardiomyopathy. *Arrhythm Electrophysiol Rev, 7*(2), 128–134. https://doi.org/10.15420/aer.2018.23.2

Perino, A. C., Gummidipundi, S. E., Lee, J., Hedlin, H., Garcia, A., Ferris, T., Balasubramanian, V., Gardner, R. M., Cheung, L., Hung, G., Granger, C. B., Kowey, P., Rumsfeld, J. S., Russo, A. M., True Hills, M., Talati, N., Nag, D., Tsay, D., Desai, S., Desai, M., ... Perez, M. V. (2021). Arrhythmias other than atrial fibrillation in those with an irregular pulse detected with a smartwatch: Findings from the apple heart study. *Circ Arrhythm Electrophysiol, 14*(10). https://doi.org/10.1161/CIRCEP.121.010063

Rebelo-Marques, A., Sousa Lages, A. D., Andrade, R., Riberio, C. F., Mota-Pinto, A., Carrilho, F., & Espregueira-Mendes, J. (2018). Aging hallmarks: The benefits of physical exercise. *Front Endocrinol, 9.* https://doi.org/10.3389/fendo.2018.00258

Reeves, S., Pelone, F., Harrison, R., Goldman, J., & Zwarenstein, M. (2017). Interprofessional collaboration to improve professional practice and healthcare outcomes. *Cochrane Database Syst Rev, 6.* https://doi.org/10.1002/14651858.CD000072.pub3

Rouch, S. A., Fields, B. E., Alibrahim, H. A., Rodakowski, J., & Leland, N. E. (2021). Evidence for the effectiveness of interventions for caregivers of people with chronic conditions: A systematic review. *Am J Occup Ther, 75*(4). https://doi.org/10.5014/ajot.2021.042838

Saketkoo, L. A., Russell, A. M., Jensen, K., Mandizha, J., Tavee, J., Newton, J., Rivera, F., Howie, M., Reese, R., Goodman, M., Hart, P., Strookappe, B., De Vries, J., Rosenbach, M., Scholand, M. B., Lammi, M. R., Elfferich, M., Lower, E., Baughman, R. P., Sweiss, N., Judson, M. A., & Drent, M. (2021). Health-related quality of life (HRQoL) in sarcoidosis: Diagnosis, management, and health outcomes. *Diagnostics (Basel), 11*(6), 1089. https://doi.org/10.3390/diagnostics11061089

Sas, K., Szabo, E., & Vecsei, L. (2018). Mitochondria, oxidative stress and the kynurenine system, with a focus of ageing and neuroprotection. *Molecules, 23*(1). http://doi.org/10.3390/molecules23010191

Sattelmair, J., Pertman, J., Ding, E. L., Kohl, H. W. 3rd, Haskell, W., & Lee, I. M. (2011). Dose response between physical activity and risk of coronary heart disease: A meta-analysis. *Circulation, 124,* 789–795. https://doi.org/10.1161/CIRCULATIONAHA.110.010710

Schutt, S., & Thompson, K. N. (2020). Effectiveness of self-management programs to reduce occupational deprivation in older adults. *Critically Appraised Topics, 9.* https://doi.org/commons.end.edu/cat-papers/9

Shah, B., Forsythe, L., & Murray, C. (2018). Effectiveness of interprofessional care teams on reducing hospital readmissions in patients with heart failure: A systematic review. *Medical-surgical Nursing, 27*(3), 177–185.

Shiota, S., Naka, M., Kitagawa, T., Hidaka, T., Mio, N., Kanai, K., Mochizuki, M., Kimura, H., & Kihara, Y. (2021). *Selection of comprehensive assessment categories based on the international classification of functioning, disability, and health for elderly patients with heart failure: A delphi survey among registered instructors of cardiac rehabilitation.* https://doi.org/10.1155/2021/6666203

Steinke, E. E. (2014). Integrative review: Sexual dysfunction common in people with coronary heart disease, but few cardiovascular changes actually occur during sexual activity. *Evidence Based Nursing, 18.* Retrieved from http://ebn.bmj.com/content/18/1/19. doi: 10.1136/eb-2014-101787

Strait, J. B., & Lakatta, E. G. (2012). Aging-associated cardiovascular changes and their relationship to heart failure. *Heart Fail Clin, 8,* 143–164. https://doi.org/10.1016/j.hfc.2011.08.011

Stromsdorfer, S. (2023). my OT SPOT: Educating your patients about energy conservation techniques. https://www.myotspot.com/energy-conservation-techniques/

Subih, M., AlBarmawi, M., Bashir, D. Y., Jacoub, S. M., Syyah, N. S. (2020). Correlation between quality of life of cardiac patients and caregiver burden. *PLoS One, 15*(8), https/doi.org/10.1371/journal.pone.0237099

Swiatkiewicz, L., DiSomma, S., DeFazio, L., Mazzilli, V., Taub, P. R. (2021). Effectiveness of intensive cardiac rehabilitation in high-risk patients with cardiovascular disease in real-world practice. *Nutrients, 13,* 3883, http://doi.org/10.3390/nu13113833

Vigorito, C., & Giallauria. F. (2014). Effects of exercise on cardiovascular performance in the elderly. *Front Physiol, 20,* 51. https://doi.org/10.3389/fphys.2014.00051

Virani, S. S., Alonso, A., Aparicio, H. J., Benjamin, E. J., Bittencourt, M. S., Callaway, C. W., Carson, A. P., Chamberlain, A. M., Cheng, S., Delling, F. N., Elkind, M. S., Evenson, K. R., Ferguson, J. F., Gupta, D. K., Khan, S. S., Kissela, B. M., Knutson, K. L., Lee, C. D., Lewis, T. T., Liu, J., ...Tsao, C. W. (2021). Heart disease and stroke statistics—2021 update. *Circulation* 143(8), 254–743. https://doi.org/10.1161/CIR.0000000000000950

West, J. B. (2012). *Respiratory physiology: The essentials* (7th ed.). Lippincott Williams & Wilkins.

Wingardh, A. S., Goransson, C., Larsson, S., Slinde, F., & Vanfleteren, L. E. (2020). Effectiveness of energy conservation techniques in patients with COPD. *Respiration,* 99, 409–416. https://doi.org/10.1159/000506816

World Health Organization. (2012). *Assessing national capacity for the prevention and control of NCDs: Report of the 2010 global survey.* http://www.who.int/chp/knowledge/national_prevention_ncds/en

World Health Organization. (2018). *Evaluating WHO's normative function.* https://cdn.who.int/media/docs/default-source/documents/evaluation/evalbrief-normativefunction-15jan18.pdf?sfvrsn=bf320621_2

World Health Organization. (2021, June 11). *Cardiovascular diseases (CVDs).* https://www.who.int/news-room/fact-sheets/detail/cardiovascular-diseases-(cvds)

World Health Organization. (2022). *International classification of functioning, disability, and health (ICF).* https://www.who.int/standards/classifications/international-classification-of-functioning-disability-and-health

Zientara, A., Schwegler, I., Dzemali, O., Brujen, H., Bernheim, A., Dick, F., Attigah, N. (2021). Evaluation of metabolic equivalents of task (METs) in the preoperative assessment in aortic repair. *BMC Surg, 21*(1). https://doi.org10.1186/s12893-021-01143-0

CHAPTER 10

Sensory Function and Health Conditions

Sarah E. Blaylock, PhD, OTR/L ■ Megan Bewernitz, PhD, OTR/L, ECHM

"There are children playing in the streets who could solve some of my top problems in physics, because they have modes of sensory perception that I lost long ago."

– J. Robert Oppenheimer

LEARNING OUTCOMES

By the end of this chapter, readers will be able to:

10-1. Apply knowledge of vision changes that occur in older adults with resultant physical and behavioral compensation.

10-2. Analyze how common age-related hearing changes affect function in the older adult.

10-3. Evaluate how chemosensory changes affect functional performance in the aging population.

10-4. Relate the common presentations of the somesthesis and integumentary systems of the older adult to functional performance and lifestyle issues.

10-5. Evaluate pain presentations in older adults and assess pain's impact on functional performance.

10-6. Create assessment and intervention strategies that serve to improve function for older adults with sensory impairment.

Mini Case Study

Shirley Rosen is 75 years old. She retired at age 62 from her position as a receptionist at an office within walking distance from her home. When her husband died 5 years ago, she returned to part-time work at her previous place of employment and shares a position with another woman who works part-time. Typically, Mrs. Rosen walks the two blocks to work when the weather permits; otherwise, she drives herself to work. Recently, she has begun requesting rides to work due to intermittent pain and numbness in her lower extremities making it difficult to walk long distances and drive. Mrs. Rosen's coworkers notice she frequently asks people to repeat themselves when on the telephone, and she is often squinting when looking at the computer. Sometimes Mrs. Rosen wears a wool jacket during the summer months, because she finds the office too cold with the air conditioning. Judy Johnson, a long-time friend, has noted that when they go out to lunch, Mrs. Rosen takes small bites of her food, does not eat all her meal, and seems to have lost pleasure in eating. Often, when Judy makes a comment to Mrs. Rosen, she will smile and nod her head, but this response does not match Judy's comment. Judy wonders if Mrs. Rosen is developing dementia.

Provocative Questions

1. How might a sensory impairment influence how others perceive an older adult's (such as Mrs. Rosen's) cognitive and psychological health?
2. How does the social and physical environment of an older adult (such as Mrs. Rosen) support or hinder function in the context of pain or sensory changes due to aging?
3. How might impaired sensory conditions affect dietary choices and, consequently, overall health?

Introduction

Our bodies receive sensory information about the physical world through generalized and specialized sensory receptors. These receptors begin functioning in utero in most cases and, beginning in early adulthood, start a slow and progressive decline (Cech & Martin, 2012). The "senses" (vision, hearing, touch, taste, smell), or systems of sensation, send information via a sensory modality in the peripheral nervous system to the central nervous system (CNS), where the information is comprehended. Perception, a higher sensory function and a middle ground between sensation and comprehension, enables the organism to receive and perceive that a stimulus has occurred, process the information, and attach meaning to it (Albright, 2015).

The parietotemporal and parietooccipital areas of the cerebral cortex, important sensory areas, are responsible for the integration, or association, of information regarding sensory modalities. Sensory information does not travel through a direct route of monosynaptic connections from receptor cells to the CNS. Rather, somatosensory input and sensory fiber tracts travel through several relay stations, or integrating centers, in the brainstem reticular system and the thalamus (Grow, 2018). Any neuronal degeneration in these integrative and relay structures reduces the quality of information received at the CNS level.

The information contained in this chapter should be viewed in the context of the many typical changes that take place in the aging nervous system, as sensory and sensory integrative changes reflect these systemic changes. Age-related changes in the sensory systems (summarized in Table 10-1) can have a major impact on the social, psychological, and physical functions of the older person. This chapter also explores how some health conditions of older adults affect the sensory systems and how these conditions affect functional performance. See Promoting Best Practice 10-1.

TABLE 10-1 ■ Summary of Effects of Age-Related Sensory Changes on Functional Activities

SENSORY SYSTEM	PRIMARY CHANGES RELATED TO AGING	FUNCTIONAL RESULTS
Vision	Loss of subcutaneous fat around the eye Decreased tissue elasticity and tone Decreased strength of the eye muscles Decreased corneal transparency Degeneration of sclera, pupil, and iris Increase in density and rigidity of lens Increased frequency of disease processes Slowing of CNS information processing	Decreased near vision Poor eye coordination Distortion of images Blurred vision Compromised night vision Loss of color sensitivity; especially green, blue, and violet shades Difficulty with recognition of moving objects, items with a complex figure, or items that appear in and out of light quickly
Hearing	Loss or damage to sensory hair cells of cochlea and the lower basal turn of the inner ear Nerve cell diminution of cochlear ganglia Degeneration in central auditory pathways Loss of neurotransmitters	Difficulty in hearing higher frequencies, tinnitus Diminished ability for pitch discrimination Reduced speech recognition and reception Loss of speech discrimination
Taste	Decrease in taste buds Varicose enlargement	Higher thresholds for identification of substances
Smell	Degeneration of sensory cells of nasal mucosa	Decline in suprathreshold sensitivity for odors
Superficial sensation	Slower nerve conduction velocities	Decreased response to tactile stimuli Alterations in perception of pain Adversely affected by thermal extremes

PROMOTING BEST PRACTICE 10-1

How Sensory Impairments Affect Perceptions of Discrimination Among Older Adults

Research examining the relationship of vision impairments, hearing impairments, and dual sensory impairments on everyday discrimination suggests that older adults with these impairments experience higher perception of discrimination during daily life than those with neither hearing loss nor vision loss (Shakarchi et al, 2020). Additionally, those with both sensory and visual impairments perceived more discrimination than those with either visual impairments or hearing impairments. These results highlight the need to address the psychosocial effects of sensory loss when treating older adults.

CASE STUDY

Presenting Situation

Mrs. Aleka Spiros is an 81-year-old woman who has been referred for occupational therapy evaluation at a skilled nursing facility.

Occupational Profile

While completing the occupational profile, the occupational therapist learns the following information. Before admission, Mrs. Spiros lived with her son and daughter-in-law. She recently experienced a fall that has worried the family, making them feel nervous about providing proper care. The family reports that Mrs. Spiros often appears to wince as if in pain when walking and changing positions (e.g., sit to stand). They were hoping she could receive rehabilitation and then return to their home, although they worry she might fall again or that they cannot meet her needs if her pain increases further. Mrs. Spiros is from Greece, has only been in the United States for 2 years since her husband died, and speaks very little English. She often relies on her family members to communicate, although her son and daughter-in-law have work schedules conflicting with the ability to translate as often as needed. During the initial interaction, Mrs. Spiros demonstrates poor endurance and discomfort with movement, and she needs assistance to walk and move from chair to bed. Mrs. Spiros and her family report she loves cooking, although she has not been participating much in cooking activities since her move from Greece. They report no concerns with cognition but that people often think she is confused due to her language barrier.

Medical History

The review of the client's medical record reveals she has lived with peripheral vascular disease (PVD) and congestive heart failure (CHF) for approximately 2 years. She was referred to the skilled nursing facility after a fall within her son's home while trying to ambulate to the bathroom. She landed on her right side, and although she reported pain the day of the fall, there was no evidence of fracture. Her oxygen saturation readings were low, so she was monitored within the hospital for 3 days until stabilized. There is no evidence of her having a primary care physician or any other recent medical care other than her care at the emergency department for the fall.

Evaluation

The therapist decides to observe Mrs. Spiros eating in the facility dining room, where she is placed in a section with the other residents who need assistance with feeding. The therapist locates Mrs. Spiros, who is seated in a semi-reclined position, at a table with a white tablecloth. Mrs. Spiros appears to squint at her food: mashed potatoes and chicken with canned pears, all served on a white china plate. When the certified nursing assistant tries to help Mrs. Spiros feed herself, Mrs. Spiros turns her head away, grabbing her napkin to cover her face. The nursing assistant, fearful that Mrs. Spiros will starve without eating, tells her, "You have to eat. Your son will ask me about how much you have eaten of your lunch, and I can't lie to him." Despite this, Mrs. Spiros still does not eat, and her plate is sent back to the kitchen basically untouched. Mrs. Spiros is now agitated and groaning, and she appears to try to reach down to rub her feet. The therapist decides to discuss the observation of Mrs. Spiros's feeding session with the charge nurse, who knows that Mrs. Spiros's refusal to eat has been an ongoing situation. The nurse mentions the option of discussing a feeding tube with the physician.

Questions

1. Based on the information presented, what assessments will you choose to learn more about Mrs. Spiros's function?
2. What more do you need to know that would be assessed by other team members? What assessments might others on the team complete?

Answers

1. Pain assessment during activities of daily living (ADLs). Vision assessments: She is squinting at food, and the table setting has low contrast. She may have difficulty distinguishing food from the plate and table. (See section *Age-Related Visual System Changes* and section assessments.) Review of Olfactory and Taste sensation (See section on *Implications for the Older Adult in Treatment*.) Cognitive assessment—See section on assessment.) Home (See section on assessment.) LO 10.1, 10.3
2. Fall risk and balance could be evaluated by physical therapy or occupational therapy, and safe swallowing and communication should be evaluated by speech therapy. (See section on *Interprofessional Communication*.) LO 10.6

Visual System

Because of various structural changes in the eye, older adults experience a decrease in visual ability as they age. Although the older adult may not be acutely aware of the changes because they occur gradually and people can often adapt to them, visual problems are of great significance for many older adults. The relationship between vision impairments, activity limitations, and participation restrictions—along with depression, psychological distress, and decreased quality of life—has been well documented (Barstow et al, 2015; Demmin & Silverstein, 2020).

Age-related changes can affect many functional components of the visual system. Changes often reduce overall visual acuity, or the ability to see the environment clearly, in middle-aged and older adults. Bifocals, progressive lenses, or reading glasses are often prescribed for **presbyopia,** an age-related refractive error leading to difficulty clearly focusing on objects up close. Furthermore, visual changes due to aging can affect contrast sensitivity (Owsley et al, 2018). In its simplest terms, contrast sensitivity refers to the ability of the visual system to distinguish between an object and its background. For example, imagine milk served in a white cup (low contrast) versus black coffee served in a white coffee cup (high contrast). Age-related changes can also lead to difficulty adjusting to moving from sudden changes in illumination, making it difficult to see when traveling from well-lit areas into darkened spaces (and vice versa). Researchers have linked poor visual acuity, contrast sensitivity, and poor dark adaptation to accidents, falls, fractures, and mortality (Crews et al, 2016).

Age-Related Visual System Changes

Age-related changes occur in the support structures of the eye and the visual pathway. See Figure 10-1 for an illustration of a healthy eye. Changes in the support structures include loss of subcutaneous fat and decreased tissue elasticity and tone, all of which may make the eyes appear sunken or result in redundancy of the skin of the eyelids and eyelid malpositions. Tear production may decrease, causing symptoms of foreign body sensation and burning and, for some, corneal ulceration (Brodie & Francis, 2017; Esenwah et al, 2014). With aging, the jelly-like vitreous body filling the eye's central cavity begins to liquify, often leading to the development of spots that appear in a person's vision called floaters (Brodie & Francis, 2017; Chader & Tayler, 2015).

Additional changes in the eye begin at the cornea, where light first enters. The cornea thickens, flattens, and becomes less smooth and more rigid after age 60, causing or increasing astigmatism, which is a defect caused by a deviation from the spherical curvature, resulting in distorted or blurred images as light rays are prevented from meeting at a common focus. A ring of opaqueness also forms in the cornea of some individuals and a deposit of pigment occurs in most corneas.

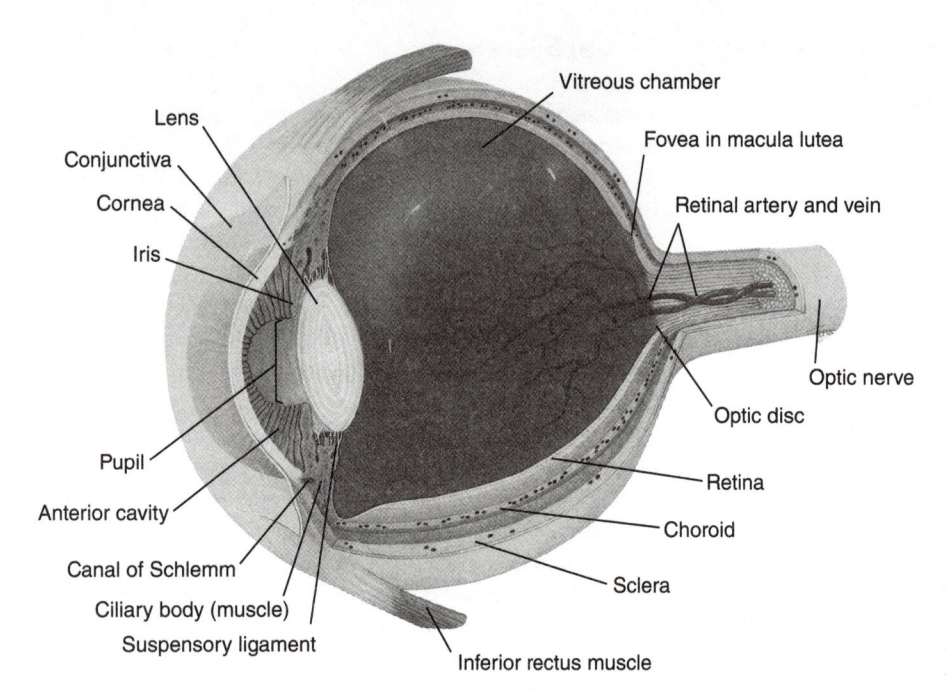

FIGURE 10-1 Internal anatomy of the eyeball. *(From Scanlon, V. C., & Sanders, T. [2007]. Essentials of anatomy and physiology: 5th. Ed. F.A. Davis Co., p. 205, with permission.)*

These changes result in a reduced corneal transparency limiting the amount of light reaching the retina and may reduce the visual field. In addition, decreased corneal sensitivity may cause older adults to be less aware of injury or infection within the eye (Brodie & Francis, 2017; Esenwah et al, 2014).

Other degenerative changes can occur in the sclera, pupil, and iris. The scleral tissue loses water and fatty deposits increase, causing a yellow cast and decreased opacity (Brodie & Francis, 2017; Esenwah et al, 2014). The pupil decreases in size and becomes more fixed (senile miosis) due to atrophy of the muscle controlling dilation. This restricts the amount of light falling on the retina. Senile miosis may affect depth perception, and objects may appear farther in the distance than they really are. The iris decreases in dilation ability because of several processes, including an increase of connective tissue, sclerosis of the blood supply, and muscle weakness. Because the maximum size of the pupil is decreased, the pupil cannot dilate to the same extent in response to reduced light, and less light gets to the retina. Thus, a gradual loss of visual acuity occurs, and older adults have more difficulty seeing clearly in low-light situations (Brodie & Francis, 2017; Esenwah et al, 2014).

The lens also changes with age, resulting in a decrease in the eye's ability to transmit and focus light. Cellular changes cause an increase in density and rigidity of the lens, which may compromise near and far vision. These changes in the lens may also contribute to filtering of the color spectrum, resulting in a loss of color sensitivity across the total spectrum but especially for green, blue, and violet shades (Brodie & Francis, 2017; Esenwah et al, 2014). As the lens ages, elasticity decreases, resulting in reduced ability of the lens to change shape (accommodate) in response to the distance of the object being viewed. Difficulty focusing on near objects, presbyopia, makes it difficult to read print and perform close-vision tasks. In addition, accommodation loss further reduces overall visual acuity. Bifocals, progressive lenses, or reading glasses are often prescribed for presbyopia (Kaldenberg & Smallfield, 2020).

The central area of the retina, the macula, has a concentration of cone cells (visual sensory receptors) allowing for color vision and fine-detail discrimination. Rod cells that are extremely sensitive to light are responsible for peripheral vision (the ability to perceive stimuli beyond the area of immediate focus) and night vision. However, rod density has been found to decrease by up to 30% with advancing age (Sugita et al, 2020). As the retina ages, it gradually loses neurons, and the retinal nerve fiber layer has been found to thin with increased age (Patel et al, 2014).

In addition to changes in the structures of the eye, older adults are often slower at processing visual stimuli and need to see stimuli longer before accurately identifying them. Some of these visual perception changes may occur because of degeneration along the optic pathway or in areas of the cortex responsible for processing visual information. Such changes result in slowed information processing and increased perceptual inflexibility that affects image recognition (Guest et al, 2015). This slowed processing translates into difficulty recognizing moving objects, items with a complex figure or ground, and items that appear in and out of light quickly. Personal care tasks and instrumental tasks such as driving, housekeeping, and meal preparation often depend on such recognition.

A variety of communication and environmental strategies and modifications can be implemented to assist the older adult in safe occupational function despite these age-related changes (Box 10-1).

> **BOX 10-1 Examples of Communication Strategies and Environmental Modifications for Older Persons With Low Vision**
>
> Use voice or touch to get attention.
> Face the older adult.
> Ensure adequate lighting in the room (note: high levels of illumination my result in glare).
> Direct the light source from behind the older adult or on the side of the better seeing eye for reading or writing to reduce glare.
> Remove clutter and limit the number of objects in the environment.
> Avoid visual clutter in the environment (e.g., decrease number of prints, posters, or pictures on the walls; use solid colors for background surfaces).
> Enlarge educational/reading materials.
> Provide written instructions on non-glossy paper; use high contrast print and paper and at least 18-point font (may need even greater font size for people with very poor visual acuity).
> Use a large black felt marker for written instructions.
> Enhance contrast (e.g.):
>   Add strips of contrasting tape to the edge of steps.
>   Mark light switches with contrasting fluorescent tape.

Major Conditions: Pathological Changes of the Visual System

According to the eleventh revision of the International Classification of Diseases (World Health Organization [WHO], 2019), there are four levels of visual impairment classified by acuity measurement: mild, moderate, severe, and blindness. The accuracy of vision is usually referred to as "Snellen acuity" after Dutch ophthalmologist Herman Snellen (1834 to 1908). Snellen created the chart now commonly used to measure visual acuity. In some countries (e.g., Canada, United States), 20/20 vision indicates "normal" vision. This refers to the ability to see an object clearly when the individual is 20 feet away from the object. In other countries, 6/6 may designate normal vision, where 6 refers to 6 meters versus 20 feet. Therefore, 6/6 vision is the same concept as 20/20 vision (Vimont, 2020).

Low Vision

Low vision (moderate or severe visual impairment) is generally defined as a loss of sight that is not correctable through medical intervention and interferes with the functioning of the individual. When ordinary eyeglasses, contact lenses, medication, or surgery cannot provide clear vision, a person is said to have low vision. Although reduced central or reading vision is common, low vision also includes decreases in peripheral, upper, or lower visual fields, the reduction or loss of color vision, or the eye's inability to properly adjust to light, contrast, or glare (National Eye Institute, 2022). Although visual impairment can affect individuals of any age, most are age 50 and older (WHO, 2021). In the United States, an estimated 4.2 million people have a permanent visual impairment (Centers for Disease Control and Prevention [CDC], 2020a). With the aging of the population, the total number of low vision cases is expected to double by about 2050 (Varma et al, 2016).

The term low vision implies that an individual has some vision remaining (National Eye Institute, 2022). In other words, a person with low vision has some usable vision, but the visual loss is significant enough to affect functional performance. In some countries, governments use a separate term, typically *legally blind*, to define a person whose degree of sight loss entitles them to special benefits. **Legal blindness** is defined as (1) visual acuity of 20/200 or less in the better eye after best possible standard correction *or* (2) a visual field of no greater than 20 degrees in the better eye (U.S. Social Security Administration, 2022). Visual acuity of 20/200 means that a person can see a letter at a distance of 20 feet that can be seen by a person with normal sight at a distance of 200 feet. It is important to note that legal blindness is not the same as total blindness (a complete loss of vision).

Cataracts

With advancing age, the lens of the eye may undergo protein degeneration and aggregation. This degeneration is referred to as lenticular opacity, a cataract, which reduces light transmission to the retina and causes the lens of the eye to appear cloudy and yellowish (Boyd, 2021; National Health Service, 2016). The most common cause of loss of useful vision worldwide is cataracts. According to the National Eye Institute (2019), roughly 24.4 million people currently have cataracts. It is projected that by 2050, the number will have doubled to 50 million. Individuals with cataracts experience the following: decreased acuity, hazy or blurred vision, altered color perception, increased sensitivity to glare, difficulty driving at night, difficulty seeing low-contrast objects, and image distortion (straight lines that appear wavy) (Boyd, 2021; National Health Service, 2016).

When the cataract interferes with vision to such an extent that functional activities are affected, cataract extraction and lens prosthesis implantation may be performed (Boyd, 2021). Although treatment for the removal of cataracts is widely available, access barriers, such as insurance coverage, treatment costs, patient choice, or lack of awareness, prevent many people from receiving the proper treatment (CDC, 2020a).

Age-Related Macular Degeneration

In 2020, approximately 196 million people were living with **age-related macular degeneration** (AMD), and this number is expected to increase to an estimated 288 million by 2040 (Saunier et al, 2018). AMD is characterized by retinal atrophy and scarring, along with hemorrhages in the macula, resulting in a gradual loss of the central field of vision. Risk factors associated with AMD include being a white female, smoking, having light iris color, living with hypertension, and having a family history of the disease (American Macular Degeneration Foundation, n.d.-a).

There are two types of AMD (American Macular Degeneration Society, n.d.-b):

1. Dry AMD (non-exudative): This type of AMD is characterized by yellow deposits of extracellular material (drusen) in the macula. Areas of retinal atrophy lead to vision loss over time. Dry AMD is the most common type of AMD.
2. Wet AMD (exudative): This type of AMD progresses more rapidly and is characterized by a proliferation of abnormal blood vessels that leak blood and fluid into the macula.

Wet AMD can sometimes be treated in the early stages of the disease with laser surgery (photocoagulation) to cauterize the new blood vessels and stop their development (CDC, 2020a; Brodie & Francis, 2017). Other treatments include medications injected directly into the eye and photodynamic therapy, which involves shining a special laser into the eye to activate a medication that has been administered intravenously. Though medical interventions can slow the progression of AMD, no known treatment prevents macular degeneration or can reverse the visual loss (Daniel et al, 2016).

Central vision loss can have very negative psychological and social effects. Because the macula is responsible for fine-detail vision, reading, needlework, writing, and recognizing faces become difficult. Problems with distance and depth cues and color and contrast perception are also evident. As a result, a reluctance to participate in social activities can appear, and limitations with ADLs, instrumental activities of daily living, work, and leisure are common (Gopinath et al, 2014; Warren et al, 2016).

Glaucoma

Glaucoma is a group of diseases characterized by progressive optic nerve damage secondary to increased pressure within the eye. Resultant vision loss progresses from the periphery toward the central field as it advances, and glaucoma can result in blindness. Glaucoma is the second leading cause of blindness worldwide, with a prevalence of approximately 3 million in the United States (CDC, 2020b). Within the black population, glaucoma presents at a younger age with higher intraocular pressures (IOPs), is more difficult to control, and is the main irreversible cause of blindness (Owsley et al, 2015). It is estimated that the number of people with glaucoma worldwide will increase to 111.8 million by 2040, disproportionately affecting people residing in Asia and Africa (Tham et al, 2014). There are several types of glaucoma. The two most common in older adults are as follows:

1. Primary open-angle glaucoma (POAG) has a slow and insidious onset. The major risk factor for developing POAG is raised IOP. The increased IOP may cause permanent loss of peripheral vision before the individual notes a change in vision, and blindness occurs if left untreated (Glaucoma Research Foundation, 2016).
2. Angle-closure glaucoma (ACG) is an acute condition resulting from a sudden blockage of aqueous fluid outflow and acute elevation of IOP. Gradual increase in lens size, with advancing age or because of cataracts, predisposes the eye to ACG. Symptoms include severe pain, blurry vision, and halos around lights. ACG is a medical emergency (Murray, 2018). Angle closure can appear suddenly and is painful. Visual loss can progress quickly, but the pain and discomfort usually lead patients to seek medical attention before permanent damage occurs (CDC, 2020b).

Glaucoma is treated medically or surgically, depending on the type and stage of the diagnosis. Regular eye examinations are essential, because early detection and treatment can prevent the visual loss that occurs if glaucoma is left untreated (Brodie & Francis, 2017; CDC, 2020b). Medical treatment consists of either focused topical medications, such as eye drops, or systemic medications that will lower the IOP. If pressure is not relieved enough or if medications are not effective or tolerated, surgery (e.g.., filtration surgery, laser trabeculectomy) is used to help remove the blockage and increase fluid drainage (Brodie & Francis, 2017; CDC, 2020b).

The effect of the loss of peripheral vision is great. The individual may not see objects in a path and bump into objects in the periphery, making functional and community mobility unsafe. Objects or people outside the person's peripheral field of view may suddenly appear, startling the individual. In addition, reading and writing may be problematic, because only a small portion of the page can be seen at once (Park et al, 2015).

Diabetic Retinopathy

Diabetic retinopathy (DR) is the leading cause of blindness among U.S. working-age adults ages 20 to 74 years. An estimated 4.1 million Americans are affected by retinopathy (CDC, 2020a). Although DR can affect individuals of all ages, damage to the blood vessels of the retina due to diabetes is a common cause of retina changes in the older adult.

DR is a complication of diabetes, and the incidence of this eye disease typically increases with the length of time a person has diabetes. The degree and rate of progression of the retinopathy strongly correlate with the level and duration of elevated blood sugars. Thus, good control of insulin levels is essential to prevent DR and delay its progression (CDC, 2020a). DR occurs in stages. In the initial stage (nonproliferative stage), microaneurysms form but are reabsorbed by the retina. With time, the retinal capillaries begin to leak fluid into the surrounding tissue, causing retinal edema and producing exudate, which leads to decreased visual acuity. In the later stage (proliferative stage), new blood vessels grow in the retina (neovascularization). These blood vessels easily rupture, bleeding into the eye. **Scotomas**, or blind spots, throughout the visual field often occur (Brodie & Francis, 2017; CDC, 2020a).

Symptoms of DR include fluctuating and blurred vision, decreased contrast sensitivity, problems with driving at night, difficulty with color discrimination, "spotty" visual field losses, and complete blindness. The degree of activity limitations and participation restrictions resulting from DR varies greatly and is dependent on time of diagnosis and severity of the disease. Medical management is dependent on the stage and may include laser surgery to treat the microaneurysms or vitrectomy, a procedure used to remove blood and scar tissue from the vitreous (Brodie & Francis, 2017; CDC, 2020a). The risks of DR are reduced through disease management that includes good control of insulin levels, blood pressure, and lipid abnormalities. Early diagnosis of DR and timely treatment reduce the risk of vision loss; however, as many as 50% of people with diabetes are not getting their eyes examined or are diagnosed too late for treatment to be effective (CDC, 2020a).

Parkinson and Alzheimer Diseases

Parkinson disease (PD) can also cause visual impairments. Visual complications in people with PD are not typically evident on routine eye examination, because the visual acuity score—the most commonly used measure of vision—remains unaffected in patients with PD if the impairment is well corrected with glasses. Contrast sensitivity measurement often shows specific changes, and older adults with PD often experience dry eyes due to diminished blink rate (Rimona et al, 2016). **Saccades**, continuous eye movements that occur in response to a sudden change of visual fixation, are also impaired by PD, leading to difficulty focusing on objects of interest within the environment (Rimona et al, 2016).

Alzheimer disease can lead to visuospatial deficits that appear primarily as difficulties with reading, problems in discriminating form and color, inability to perceive contrast, difficulties in visual–spatial orientation and motion detection, agnosia, and difficulty developing visual strategies, which may impair functional performance of everyday activities (Quental et al, 2013).

Treatment Implications for the Older Adult With Vision Changes

Evidence strongly supports the use of low vision interventions to address functional deficits among those with visual impairment. The American Occupational Therapy Association's (AOTA) Practice Guidelines for Older Adults With Low Vision outlines the evidence linking occupational therapy intervention services to improved functional independence (Kaldenberg & Smallfield, 2020). To meet the functional needs of older adults with visual impairment, it is important to understand common functional deficits to address these needs properly. Vision loss of any type can affect the life of an older adult—not only to the individuals but also their families, their communities, and the healthcare system.

Whether acute or gradual in onset and whether partial or full loss, any visual change can threaten the functional independence older adults strive to maintain. Older adults with visual impairment are approximately four times more likely to experience difficulty with daily function compared with those with normal vision (Warren, 2011).

Individuals with vision loss are a vulnerable subset of the population and often require greater assistance for safe occupational performance. Older adults with visual impairment often need three times more lighting than younger people to see clearly when performing daily activities (U.S. Department of Health and Human Services, 2017). Acuity problems can cause issues with reading, and practical day-to-day tasks such as housekeeping, shopping, and clothing selection can be quite frustrating. Color discrimination of critical items such as food and medication can be challenging. Common leisure activities such as card playing, sports requiring eye–hand coordination, television viewing, and needlepoint can become extremely difficult for the older adult with age-related visual changes. Glare and sudden illumination contrasts can compromise vision because of slower adaptation, and night vision may be poor, curtailing many activities, including driving (Barstow et al, 2015; Demmin & Silverstein, 2020; Park et al, 2015). In addition, older adults with visual impairment are often less safe during functional tasks due to being at a higher risk for falls than those with typical vision (Crews et al, 2016).

Although changes in vision affect functioning in daily activities, they can also affect the psychological health of the older adults. How an older adult adapts to vision changes varies and relates to personal factors such as personality characteristics and individual coping strategies, timing and degree of loss, and use of compensatory strategies. Older adults with vision loss may have to stop doing things they enjoy and may feel more isolated and vulnerable, often leading to depression (Renaud & Bédard, 2013). It is important to note that the sensitivity of others and environmental modifications can assist the older adult in facing visual changes. Adaptation to age-related visual changes is positively affected by support received from one's social network, coping strategies, and knowledge of and access to rehabilitation services (Barstow et al, 2015; Demmin & Silverstein, 2020).

Assessment

In treating older adults, it is important to screen and evaluate vision because of the strong influence it has on function. Assessment can focus on specific components of visual function (e.g., acuity [distance and reading], contrast sensitivity, and visual field). A Snellen chart is the most commonly used method of assessing distance acuity (Vimont, 2020). Many assessments exist to assess reading acuity, for example the MNREAD, with most consisting of a card with text that must be read at a close, specified distance from the client's face (Calabrèse et al, 2016).

The Mars Contrast Sensitivity Test is used to assess contrast sensitivity function by having the individual identify letters as contrast gradually decreases (Dougherty et al, 2005). Confrontation testing is a common way to assess a person's visual field, with a therapist presenting fingers and having the client identify the number of fingers in differing areas of the visual field (Johnson & Baloh, 1991). The Brain Injury Visual Assessment Battery for Adults is a collection of assessments for individuals—specifically those post brain injury—and includes multiple assessments including ones for acuity, contrast sensitivity, and visual field (Warren, n.d.). If a therapist has any concerns regarding an older adult's vision status, it is important that the client receives a referral to an optometrist or ophthalmologist for a thorough examination.

Visual disability questionnaires can also be used to examine the impact of visual impairment on overall function for older adults. Assessments with established psychometrics that can be used with older adults include the Revised Self-Report Assessment of Functional Visual Performance (Snow et al, 2018), the Visual Activities Questionnaire (Sloane et al, 1992), the Activities of Daily Vision Scale (Mangione et al, 1992), the Visual Function Index (VF-14) (Steinberg et al, 1994), the Visual Disability Assessment (Pesudovs & Coster, 1998), and the National Eye Institute Visual Functioning Questionnaire 25 (Mangione et al, 2001).

Environmental modification can increase functional independence for individuals with low vision. One study completed by Barstow et al (2011) highlighted the lack of comprehensive home assessments for individuals with visual impairment. The authors reported the need to address lighting, contrast, visual distractions, glare, and compensation strategies in addition to including components of existing environmental assessments. Perlmutter et al (2013) developed the Home Environment Lighting Assessment (HELA). For clients with low vision, the HELA provides a structured tool to describe the quantitative and qualitative aspects of home lighting environments. The assessment, which has high interrater reliability and moderate test–retest reliability, can be used to plan lighting interventions and has the potential to affect assessment and intervention practices of rehabilitation professionals in the area of low vision and improve near-task performance of people with low vision.

Occupational therapy practitioners should be aware that many cognitive assessments rely on intact vision for valid results. Therefore, it is important that therapists screen/assess visual function before the selection of cognitive tests. For example, the original Mini-Mental State Exam (MMSE; Folstein et al, 1975) would not be appropriate for cognitive testing because it requires intact vision. The MMSE and the Montreal Cognitive Assessment do have versions developed specifically for individuals with vision loss (Dawes et al, 2019; de Haan et al, 2020) found the Trail Making Test (Reitan, 1992)—a neuropsychological test of visual attention and attention or task switching that provides information about visual search speed, scanning, speed of processing, and mental flexibility—can be administered to those with vision acuity of up to 20/100 without visual impairment affecting performance.

Interventions

The AOTA low vision practice guidelines outline multiple articles regarding improving functional performance for those with low vision and discuss commonly used intervention strategies that are supported for clinical use based on study outcomes (Kaldenberg & Smallfield, 2020). The guidelines suggest a combination of evidence-based interventions, practice experience, and input of client and family often lead to the best functional outcomes for clients.

Evidence best supports the use of multicomponent interventions, or interventions composed of two or more strategies, to improve function for those with low vision (Kaldenberg & Smallfield, 2020). Visual impairment can have a complex effect on functional performance, leading to a common need of addressing many issues simultaneously through rehabilitation services. A review of available evidence led to the recommendation of using a combination of education regarding the relevant health conditions, teaching how to appropriately use low-vision devices (e.g., magnifiers), environmental modification, home practice to improve reading, and vision therapy services if available (Kaldenberg & Smallfield, 2020).

Environmental modification is a common and often beneficial intervention strategy to promote safer function. Improving lighting throughout the home, including introducing task lighting onto commonly used work surfaces while avoiding glare, often promotes occupational performance for those with vision loss. A therapist can increase contrast within the home, for example having dishware that is a different color of food and drink, ensuring light switches do not blend with wall color, and providing bright markers on the dials of appliances. Maintaining an organized home can improve an older adult's ability to locate items that are important for functional tasks and prevent falls by removing clutter. Having simple, plain colors versus intricate patterns on surfaces promotes ease of locating items. For navigating electronic devices, a therapist can use the accessibility features to improve screen contrast, increase font size, etc. (Kaldenberg & Smallfield, 2020; Warren & Barstow, 2011).

Low-vision rehabilitation is a growing specialty area for occupational therapists, and practitioners can become certified as low-vision specialists or undertake graduate-level training or a certificate program. Although multiple interventions are reported, the authors highlight the need for additional research to add to the body of evidence. See examples of occupational therapy interventions for older adults with visual impairment in Box 10-2. Table 10-2 lists some common optic devices for older adults with vision loss.

Auditory System

More than 5% of the world's population has a disabling hearing loss (WHO, 2015). The number of adults with hearing loss has doubled in recent years, in part because of the aging population. Hearing loss is the third most prevalent common condition in the United States: 25% of those ages 65 to 74 and 50% of those who are 75 and older have disabling hearing loss (National Institute on Deafness and Other Communication Disorders, 2016a). Vision and hearing—along with speech—contribute to human communication. Like the visual system, the auditory system likely undergoes many central and peripheral changes with age. This fact becomes critical when we consider the importance of hearing for speech and older adult functional living.

Age-Related Auditory System and Hearing Changes

Presbycusis, or age-related hearing loss, is a typical degradation of the hearing sensory system associated with age. Unique to the hearing system, the classification of "normal" (with aging) is often associated with some level of change. For younger people, normal hearing is measured by a standard decibel level (loudness) at selected frequencies (pitch) based on published normative data. Hearing loss of older adults is typically measured in an audiogram and recorded as the bilateral loss of high-frequency sounds. Contextually, the results of the audiogram measure the difficulty with hearing very high-pitched sounds, and if this loss extends to just slightly lower frequencies, the impact can be difficulty hearing normal speech. Changes in hearing are exacerbated by situational contexts such as loud and busy environments or poor positioning of speakers (Weinstein, 2017).

Audiologists, professionals who test hearing and treat hearing loss, usually divide hearing loss into conductive, sensorineural, and mixed loss. **Conductive hearing loss,** or blockage of acoustic energy that prevents the conduction of sound to the inner ear, may occur because of problems in the external or middle ear (Fig. 10-2). External ear infections or too much cerumen (wax) buildup in the external canal may cause blockage of sound. The middle ear may be filled with fluid from Eustachian tube dysfunction or upper respiratory disease, preventing the three bones of the middle ear from conducting sound efficiently past the eardrum. Diseases of the middle ear that affect bone movement, such as tumors, also can affect the mechanical transmission of energy (Weinstein, 2017). Interestingly, people with conductive hearing loss can hear better in noisy surroundings (Hanson & Gantz, 2018; Weinstein, 2017). Conductive-related problems can often be corrected by ear cleaning, medication, or surgery. Unfortunately, conduction loss is not the primary cause of hearing loss in the older population.

BOX 10-2 The Role of the Therapist When Working With Older Adults With Visual Impairment

- Educate the older adult, family members, and caregivers about low vision.
- Modify environments to support performance (e.g., increasing contrast, decreasing clutter, promoting organization).
- Teach the older adult how to use his or her prescribed optical and non-optical devices (common optic devices used for older adults with vision loss are listed in Table 10-2).
- Teach the older adult how to function more effectively within the context of the vision loss.
- Assist the older adult in developing appropriate adaptive techniques to expand their visual and physical capabilities.
- Educate the older adult about vision substitution techniques.
- Educate the older adult and the family about general compensation strategies and environmental modifications, such as management of lighting, contrast, and glare.
- Address any psychosocial issues.
- Refer the older adult to community resources.

Note: From Warren & Barstow (2011).

TABLE 10-2 ■ Common Optic Devices Used for Older Adults With Vision Loss

DEVICE	DESCRIPTION AND CONSIDERATIONS
Strong prescription reading glasses	Objects appear in focus only when held very close to the eyes.
Magnifiers	Amount of magnification is determined by one's visual acuity. Different magnification strengths used for different purposes. Enlarge objects held at a normal distance. Can be handheld (for spot reading), attached to a stand (for continuous reading), head-mounted, or attached to glasses (for hands-free work). Handheld devices require good hand control, and one hand is always in use.
Telescopes	Can be handheld or mounted onto a pair of glasses. Can be monocular or binocular. Used to view distant objects. Stronger telescopes allow only a small field of view—leads to the older adult getting "lost" trying to find the object of interest.
Electronic magnification	Can be achieved through closed-circuit television, video magnification, or computer software in which images are enlarged and contrast is enhanced. Provides very high magnification. Often expensive and not very portable.

Note: Magnification devices can cause nausea and dizziness. Postural support and ergonomics are important aspects to consider. Adapted from VisionAware, 2016; Kaldenberg & Smallfield, 2020.

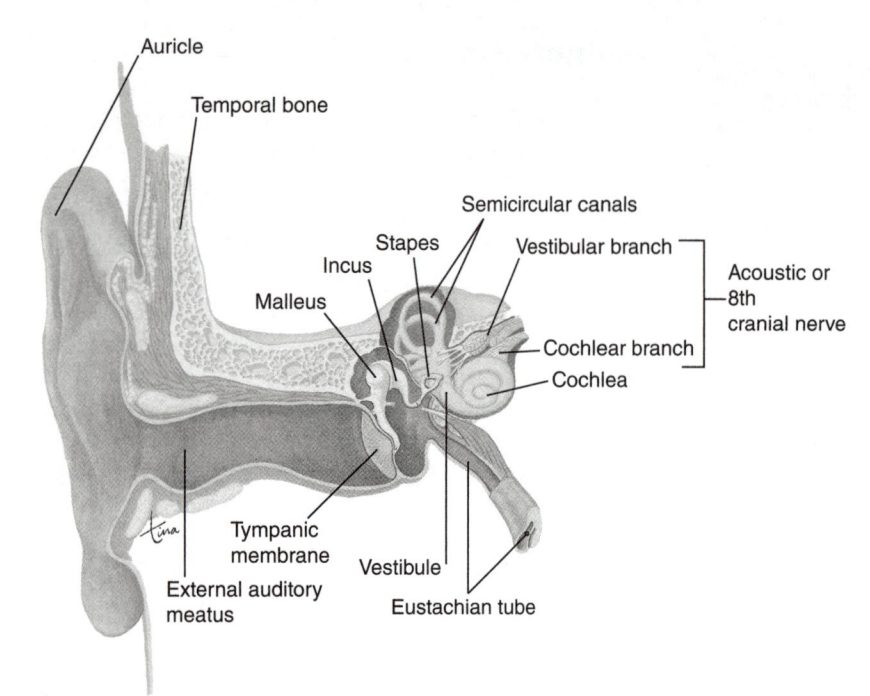

FIGURE 10-2 Outer, middle, and inner ear structures. *(From Scanlon, V. C., & Sanders, T. [2007]. Essentials of anatomy and physiology: 5th. Ed. F.A. Davis Co., p. 211, with permission.)*

Sensorineural hearing loss, the most common cause of hearing loss, results from loss or damage to the sensory hair cells of the cochlea, a pea-sized snail-shaped organ of the inner ear (Fig. 10-3), or to the nerve cells of the cochlear ganglion, brainstem tracts, or cortex or a combination of any of these. Presbycusis, medications, noise, acoustic neuroma, and Meniere disease can all cause sensorineural hearing loss (Weinstein, 2017). At the current time, sensorineural loss due to age-related changes is not correctable, but compensation with a hearing aid is possible.

The hair cells of the cochlea are slowly lost and may be associated with the progressive high-frequency hearing loss of old age (National Institute on Deafness and Other Communication Disorders, 2106a). Damage to the hair cells and degenerative changes in the organ of Corti, the band containing hair cells, can occur from exposure to a variety of drugs or noise. Although damage to the hair cells technically is not age related, as a person ages, increased opportunity for exposure to these noxious factors occurs. There are likely age-related factors that may alter the stiffness of the cochlear basilar membrane or changes in the fluid of the cochlea. These changes can be considered mechanical cochlear changes that affect older adult hearing (National Institute on Deafness and Other Communication Disorders, 2016a).

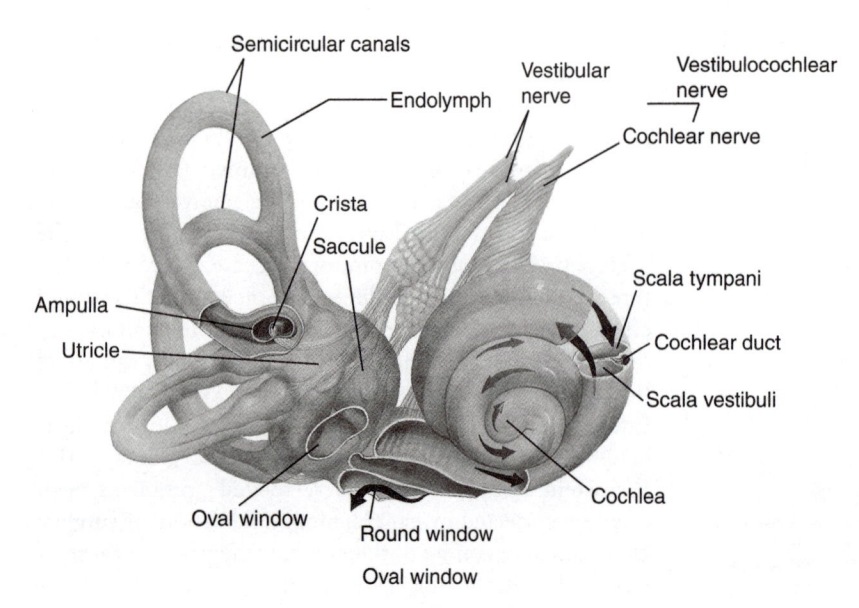

FIGURE 10-3 Inner ear structures. *(From Scanlon, V. C., & Sanders, T. [2007]. Essentials of anatomy and physiology: 5th. Ed. F.A. Davis Co., p. 212, with permission.)*

Major Conditions: Pathological Changes of the Auditory System

A common but often unrecognized cause of hearing loss in the older adult is central auditory processing disorder. The typical pathology is either in the central neuronal connections or auditory cortex; however, the peripheral mechanisms are intact. Hearing loss is often associated with accelerated cognitive decline, and the presence of dementia may lead to a perception of increased impairment when not managed correctly. Communication impairments, including hearing loss, can lead to social isolation, which has also been highly linked with the incidence of dementia (Goman & Lin, 2018; Bauer, 2018).

An ever-increasing common problem in older adults is tinnitus, or the perception of sound in the absence of an acoustic stimulus. Tinnitus is unilateral in about 50% of cases and is perceived as buzzing, whistling, or ringing in the ears. The prevalence of tinnitus is correlated with both age-related hearing loss and noise-induced hearing loss (Bhatt et al, 2016). Tinnitus is caused by several factors, including medications and metabolic and vascular diseases, and it is difficult to treat.

Auditory Implications for the Older Adult in Treatment

Whether the hearing loss older adults experience is only age-related (presbycusis) or from and in combination with other causes—such as noise exposure (sociocusis), ototoxic drugs, disease, or genetics—is difficult to determine. Regardless, the impact on function and occupation is typically significant. As noted previously, few older adults have conductive hearing loss primarily or at all. Instead, a majority have sensorineural hearing loss alone or in combination with conductive hearing loss (mixed loss). The sensorineural component affects both hearing sensitivity and speech understanding in complex ways. Hearing sensitivity appears to change with age. For example, as age increases, hearing loss increases.

The most dramatic difficulty for older adults is in hearing the higher frequencies, such as those greater than 400 Hz. In addition, there appear to be changes in pitch discrimination and auditory reaction time. The older adult's ability to detect small changes in pitch, a skill important for the understanding of both music and speech, may begin to diminish as early as the fourth decade. Beyond the mid-50s, the ability to detect small pitch changes decreases as a linear function of age and becomes more problematic in the higher frequencies (National Institute on Deafness and Other Communication Disorders, 2016a). Like pitch discrimination, auditory reaction time changes with age. Because older adults are more cautious in responding to auditory stimuli, changes in both pitch discrimination and auditory reaction time should be evaluated as part of broader changes in perception and cognition that may affect behavioral responses.

One of the most life-altering effects of hearing loss is on speech perception. This complex skill is related to several abilities: speech reception, speech discrimination, and speech understanding in stressful situations. A reduction or inability to understand speech is the most common reported symptom among older hearing-impaired individuals presenting to an audiology clinic. Speech reception and recognition are reduced with age, which typically correlates with decreased hearing sensitivity (Ruth, 2017). Gaeth (1948) first described this concept as phonemic regression—as a person ages, he or she has less ability to understand phonemes, which are units of sound that distinguish one word from another.

A closely related auditory skill is speech discrimination. A common characteristic of age-related hearing loss is the decreased ability to hear high-frequency sounds—in particular, *th* and *f*, resulting in poor speech recognition or discrimination (Ruth, 2017; Stender & Groth, 2014). This poor discrimination acuity can affect speech understanding of older adults and can restrict their speech intelligibility input to a narrower range. This leads to the common complaint described by Mascia (1994) as, "I can hear you, but I can't understand you." Speech may be difficult to understand or may not sound clear, and similar words may be confused—*pat* and *bat* or *dinner* and *thinner* (Ruth, 2017; Stender & Groth, 2014).

Social Consequences of Hearing Loss

When working with older adults, it is important to be able to recognize behaviors that may indicate a hearing loss and the functional consequences that may occur because of the loss. These behaviors include:

- Making repeated requests for a person to speak louder or to repeat what was said
- Not responding to verbal questions or conversation
- Giving non-pertinent or inappropriate responses to questions
- Directing questions to spouse, family, or caregiver
- Leaning forward, tilting head to one side
- Showing distress or irritation; becoming disoriented or confused during conversations
- Withdrawing in social situations

Understanding speech during stressful listening conditions is often troublesome for the typical older adult. Stressful listening conditions exist daily and everywhere, such as in the car, a room with background noise, or in a group-speaking situation. Although speech understanding in the older population is markedly decreased in the presence of these stressful listening conditions, it should be noted that variability exists among older adults. Each difficult listening condition does not result in the same degree of perceptual difficulty in every older person (Lee, 2015).

Untreated hearing loss can cause isolation, anxiety, depression, and paranoia and can have a significant negative impact on quality of life (Gopinath et al, 2014; National Council on Aging, 2013). The embarrassment caused by misunderstanding others may lead to social withdrawal, and poor hearing may lead the older adult to think others are mumbling. Family relationships may be strained, enjoyment of daily activities and occupations may be limited, social interactions may decrease, and the emotional and physical health of the spouse can be affected (Genther et al, 2013; National Council on Aging, 2013). In people with existing mental health or behavioral problems, such as depression or Alzheimer disease, a hearing loss may result in increased disability (Goman & Lin, 2018).

Investigators have noted that poor understanding of speech may appear to others as related to cognitive decline, when in fact it is more likely a consequence of hearing loss (Goman & Lin, 2018). Safety may also be a concern if the older adult cannot hear alarms or if someone is moving toward them; this may increase feelings of vulnerability. At a basic level, older adults may no longer have access to familiar sounds in the environment—for example, they may not hear birds chirping or footsteps approaching—which produces one more strain on a person already adjusting to changes. Several attitude or perception scales exist for use with older adults with hearing loss, and an audiologist typically administers these instruments.

Treating the hearing loss can result in significant clinical improvement in the older person's functioning—in particular, improved ability to attend to, understand, and respond to speech. A variety of adaptation techniques, accommodations, and devices are available that can make communication easier (Box 10-3).

Several kinds of hearing aids are available:

1. Behind-the-ear (BTE) fits behind the ear and has a small ear hook that extends over the top of the auricle into the ear canal. A new kind of BTE aid is an open-fit hearing aid, which is small and fits behind the ear completely, with only a narrow tube inserted into the ear canal, enabling the canal to remain open.
2. In-the-ear (ITE) fits completely inside the outer ear and is used for mild to severe hearing loss. Some ITE aids may have a telecoil, a small magnetic coil that allows sound to be received through the circuitry of the hearing aid rather than through its microphone, making it easier to hear conversations over the telephone.
3. In-the-canal (ITC) is nearly invisible because it is so small and is inserted into the canal. There are two types. The ITC aid is made to fit the size and shape of a person's ear canal. A completely in-canal aid is nearly hidden in the ear canal. Both types are used for mild to moderately severe hearing loss. Because they are small, ITC-type aids may be difficult for an older person to adjust and remove (National Institute on Deafness and Other Communication Disorders, 2016b).

Most hearing aids work best in a quiet environment because they amplify all sounds equally; thus communication with a hearing aid can be frustrating because background noise is picked up. Assistive listening devices (ALDs), which consist of headphones, earphones, or earbuds and a microphone, amplify the primary signal and not the competing noise (Fig. 10-4 A, B).

> **BOX 10-3** Examples of Communication Strategies and Environmental Modifications for Older Persons With Hearing Loss
>
> Communication
>   Face the older adult directly.
>   Get visual attention before speaking.
>   Speak clearly using a low-tone voice and moderate rate of speech.
>   Approach the older adult from the front to avoid startling.
>   Reduce glare and ensure adequate lighting to enhance visual and nonverbal cues.
>   Do not shout.
>   Rephrase if the message is not understood.
> Television, radio, music
>   Have the older adult use closed captioning, assisted listening devices, and remote controls to select programming.
>   Have the older adult avoid running the television or radio constantly.
> Background noise
>   Have the older adult use carpeting on floors, acoustical tiles on ceiling, drapes on windows, and upholstered furniture (rather than wood and metal furniture and banners from high ceilings) to absorb sound.
>   Have the older adult sit away from distracting background noises, windows, and plaster walls.
>   Have the older adult avoid crowded areas.
> Safety
>   Have the older adult use alerting devices (e.g., flashing lights or vibro-tactile devices) or lower-pitched rings for smoke detectors, doorbells, and telephones.
>   Have the older adult use volume controls for telephones.
> Other
>   Have the older adult use amplified doorbells, voice recognition, and telephone ringers.

Thus, ALDs are more advantageous when background noise exists (Cook & Polgar, 2015). Telephone amplification, personal communication devices, and room amplification systems with individual receivers are examples of technologies that may be of benefit for older adults with hearing loss.

Chemosensory System

Although taste and smell together make up the chemosensory system, they are quite different mechanisms anatomically. They are considered together because of their functional link to the flavor of food. Taste and smell change with age but are also very sensitive to environmental effects such as smoking.

Age-Related Taste and Olfactory Changes

Both smell and taste complaints are common in older persons. "Chemosensory impairments may be classified in

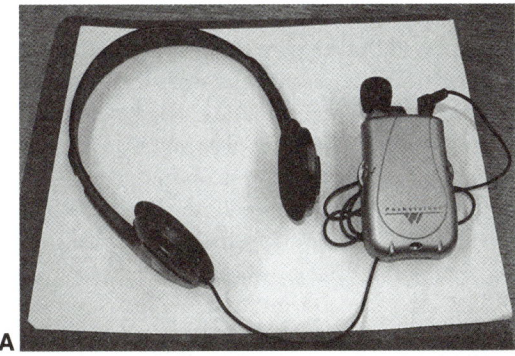

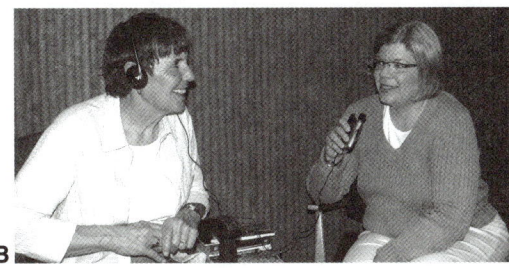

FIGURE 10-4 An assistive listening device, consisting of (A) a headphone and (B) a microphone, improves the ease of communication. *(Courtesy of the Rural and Remote Memory Clinic, Saskatoon, Saskatchewan, Canada.)*

several categories: **anosmia** (lack of smell), hyposmia (decrease in smell), dysosmia (distortion of smell), **ageusia** (absence of taste), hypogeusia (decreased sensitivity of taste) and dysgeusia (distortion of taste)" (Seiberling & Conley, 2004, p. 1209). Malaty & Malaty (2013) have since added two additional categories: phantosmia (smell hallucination) and phantogeusia (taste hallucination).

Taste changes relatively little with age compared with smell, which undergoes more significant change; thus, chemosensory complaints and associated disturbances of older adults are more likely due to olfactory changes rather than alterations in taste (Heft & Robinson, 2014). One explanation of the stronger decline in the olfaction (smell) than gustation (taste) is the rapid turnover of the taste receptors. In addition, several cranial nerves (VII, IX, and X) with robust innervation of taste receptors are responsible for detecting taste. In comparison, olfaction is mediated by one cranial nerve (cranial nerve I—olfactory nerve), and the receptors have a much slower turnover rate. Thus, disorders related to taste are much less common than other sensory disorders (Heft & Robinson, 2014). Interestingly, older men, on average, have larger and earlier age-related declines in odor perception than women (Sorokowski et al, 2019).

Various reasons have been reported for age-related decline in olfactory function, including higher detection thresholds (lowest intensity where a stimulus can be detected), a decline in suprathreshold (a stimulus above the specified threshold), sensitivity for odors, impaired ability to identify and discriminate odor, deficits in the ability to identify odors and taste on the basis of taste and smell, and distorted taste or smell (Attems et al, 2015; Sergi et al, 2017). Changes in the olfactory tract and bulb are similar to overall CNS changes, for example, generalized atrophy with a loss of neurons. Degeneration of the nasal mucosa sensory cells has been documented, such that by the ninth decade, the olfactory threshold increases by about 50%, contributing to poor smell recognition (Dharmarajan & Ugalino, 2000). Smell identification is impaired with increased age, even in generally healthy individuals. It appears that the ability to identify odors correctly increasingly deteriorates with age, especially in men (Malaty & Malaty, 2013; Pence et al, 2014).

For taste, common changes found in the mouth tissue of older adults include decline in thickness and dryness of the oral mucosa, decline and replacement of the acini (where secretions are produced) components of the salivary glands with fibrous adipose tissue, and decreased density of taste buds on the tongue (Imoscopi et al, 2012). The ability to detect, identify, and discriminate among sweet, sour, salty, bitter, and umami tastes also deteriorates as one ages (Sergi et al, 2017), with the biggest declines in the ability to taste salt followed by sour, umami, and bitter. The least decline is for sweetness (Sergi et al, 2017). These changes may result in poorer flavor discrimination and a decreased ability to identify foods in the mouth. However, because food flavor arises largely from olfactory stimulation, it is possible these changes are more likely related to age-related declines in smell.

Olfactory and Taste Implications for the Older Adult in Treatment

Taste and smell changes are functionally important for older adults. Because of taste and flavor changes, eating may be less pleasurable, leading to alterations in food choices, decreased appetite, and decreased food intake (Fluitman et al, 2021). Older adults who need specific dietary restrictions (e.g., reduced salt intake because of high blood pressure) may not adhere to those regimens. As a result, subsequent exacerbation of disease risk, weight loss, and nutritional and immune deficiencies can occur (Malaty & Malaty, 2013). In addition, older adults with chemosensory decrements may be at greater risk for food poisoning or overexposure to environmentally hazardous chemicals that might otherwise be detected by taste and smell (Pence et al, 2014). Olfaction plays a major role in safety. It provides early warning of dangers, such as fire, dangerous fumes, leaking gas, spoiled foods, and polluted environments. Thus, not only can smell dysfunction significantly diminish quality of life, but it can also be life-threatening (Pence et al, 2014).

For older individuals with chemosensory loss, several interventions can be implemented: (1) flavor amplification, which is adding concentrated essence of foods to meals; (2) providing various flavors, textures, and temperatures in one setting to improve intake; and (3) ensuring good oral care before meals. Additionally, counseling should be considered, as chemosensory disorders significantly affect an individual's overall well-being (Olofsson et al, 2021).

CASE STUDY (CONTINUED)

Assessment

After the observations, the occupational therapist plans the assessments for Mrs. Spiros to complete while family is present to translate. Pain appears to be affecting her function, so it is essential to determine the location and intensity of the pain. The Wong–Baker Faces Pain Rating Scale (Wong-Baker FACES Foundation, 2020) could be useful in determining the level of pain, coupled with range of motion (ROM) assessment of joint motion to locate the source. General assessment of sensation and edema of the extremities will assist in determining the effects that PVD and CHF have on the client's function. The Functional Reach Test (Duncan et al, 1990) can assess current fall risk, which is important due to Mrs. Spiros's history of falling. She demonstrates difficulty seeing her environment, so a functional low vision assessment is essential. After the evaluation of pain, ROM, and functional reach, the therapist decides to have Mrs. Spiros complete grooming tasks with included elements of visual assessment (e.g., visual identification of items in her environment, location of low-contrast items) and functional mobility. The therapist includes a pulse oximeter to monitor oxygen saturation throughout all assessments and monitors blood pressure before and after the activity. Because family will be present, it is also a good time to ask additional questions regarding vision, pain, and food preferences.

Assessment Results

Mrs. Spiros presents with full active ROM of her extremities. With most ROM of bilateral ankles and toes (especially when weight bearing), she grimaced and provided a pain score of 6/10. During the Functional Reach Test, Mrs. Spiros was able to reach 7 inches, indicating that she is a moderate fall risk (Duncan et al, 1990). Her legs and ankles present with edema, and she has difficulty feeling light touch through her feet. While performing the grooming activity, the therapist notices that the client appears to have difficulty seeing fine details both near and far during the task, indicating a possible acuity deficit, and she loses her brown comb on the dark color table, indicating decreased contrast sensitivity. Her family reports that Mrs. Spiros typically wears glasses and that she has not visited an optometrist in years. The practitioner recommends the family bring her glasses for her to wear and discuss making an appointment to have an optometrist check her visual status. Mrs. Spiros required mod assist to sit/stand for the grooming activity, but she was able to stand with standby assist twice for approximately 2 minutes each time to complete the functional reach and grooming tasks. Her oxygen saturation fluctuated around 85% when standing, though the percentage returned to above 90% once she was instructed to perform pursed-lip breathing. Her blood pressure remained stable—137/83 before and 139/84 after activity. The family reported the measure as typical.

Through further discussions with the client and her family, the therapist learns that Mrs. Spiros does have difficulty seeing the food on her plate and that she is nervous to eat without knowing what is on her plate. The family also reports a significant overall decline in hunger over the past month. The family further reports that she enjoys eating traditional Greek dishes, fresh fruit, and vegetables. Mrs. Spiros confirms that her pain is becoming significant in her lower extremities, especially with movement or when she sits for long durations. A main concern of Mrs. Spiros and her family is her decreased endurance and that she "tires so quickly."

Interprofessional Communication

The occupational therapist communicates concerns regarding Mrs. Spiros's pain level, lower extremity edema and decreased sensation, fall risk, and oxygen saturation during the interprofessional team meeting. The occupational therapist also reports the need for a referral for a comprehensive vision assessment. Barriers to successful communication due to the language barrier are also discussed. The therapist collaborates with physical therapy to organize a treatment plan to decrease fall risk and with speech therapy regarding safe eating and effective communication. In addition, a list of foods and snacks that Mrs. Spiros enjoys is shared with the kitchen staff in the hopes of improving intake.

Questions

1. What contextual elements from the case study's occupational therapy profile influence your treatment planning?
2. How do the assessment results inform your interventions?

Answers

1. The language barrier needs to be minimized to build a therapeutic relationship. Meals should be client-centered, including individual food preferences. Meals should be served in a pleasing environment. Treatment should include a simulated home environment so the client can learn adaptations and modifications to prevent falls and promote safety. Family education will be critical to build confidence if the client is to discharge back to her home. See section on Occupation-based interventions. LO 10.6
2. The assessment helps to identify strengths and weaknesses that can be used in treatment planning. Knowing the client's vision, cognition, taste, fall risk, and level of communication can inform client-centered treatments. See section Interventions and Case Study Interventions. LO 10.3, 10.5, 10.6

Somesthesis and Integumentary System

Somesthesis includes the sensations that arise from light and deep touch of the skin and the viscera, vibration, pain, and temperature, as well as kinesthesis, the sensation and awareness of active or passive movement. Similar to other sensory modalities, age-related somesthesis changes occur, but environmental effects cannot be ruled out. For example, neuropathies and structural changes in the skin (e.g., thinning) make age-related changes difficult to detect in the purest sense (Kazanci et al, 2017; Tobin, 2017).

The skin consists of three layers: the epidermis (outermost layer), the dermis (middle layer), and hypodermis or subcutaneous (innermost layer). The major functions of skin include immunity, temperature regulation, nutrient storage, sensory reception, communication, and excretion (Kazanci et al, 2017; Tobin, 2017). The epidermis, the thinnest layer, gives the skin its waterproofing barrier properties and protects against ultraviolet light. Within the epidermal layer are melanocytes, which provide skin color, and Langerhans cells, which play an immune-surveillance role. The dermis layer forms the bulk of the skin and is responsible for perception of environment, thermoregulation via sweat glands, immunological defense via mast and macrophage cells, and water storage. This layer also contains the proteins collagen and elastin, which provide structural stability and resilience. The innermost layer, the hypodermis, stores lipids to provide thermal insulation and a protective cushion against trauma. Finally, dispersed throughout the skin are the cutaneous appendages, which include eccrine glands (sweat), apocrine glands (scent), sebaceous glands (oil), and hair follicles (Thomas & Burkemper, 2013; Voegeli, 2012).

Age-Related Somesthesis and Integumentary System Changes

As adults age, atrophic changes occur at each of the three layers of the skin, which affects the sensations of touch and pressure, pain, and temperature, among other functions of the skin. The epidermis becomes thinner, drier, and stiffer. The overall thickness of the dermis also decreases, and along with degeneration of Pacinian and Meissner corpuscles, impairs the sensation of light touch and pressure. Further, the reduction of the number and size of sweat glands impedes proper thermoregulation. The decreased production of collagen and elastin and weak and decreased blood vessels make the skin frail and prone to bruises, damage, and wrinkles. Finally, the hypodermis layer stores less subcutaneous fat, reducing cushioning and impairing thermoregulation, both of which increase the risk of skin breakdown and hypothermia (Balmain et al, 2018; Cowdell & Radley, 2012; Voegeli, 2012).

Aging causes a decrease in collagen, a connective tissue making up a large part of the dermis that prevents tearing of the skin when it is stretched. Neurosensory perception of superficial pain is diminished both in intensity and speed of perception (increasing the risk of thermal injury); deep tissue pain, however, may be enhanced. A decline in lipid content as the skin ages inhibits the permeability of nonlipophilic compounds, reducing the efficacy of some topical medications. Allergic and irritant reactions are blunted, as is the inflammatory response, compromising the ability of the aged skin to affect wound repair. These functional impairments (although a predictable consequence of intrinsic structural changes) have the potential to cause significant morbidity in older adults and may also be greatly exacerbated by extrinsic factors like photodamage (Kazanci et al, 2017; Tobin, 2017).

Skin changes may lead to a heightened risk of medical problems such as dermatitis (skin irritation) and pruritus (excessive itching), **xerosis** (dry skin), pressure sores, and skin infections and infestations (Kazanci et al, 2017; Tobin, 2017). These skin disorders are often compounded by comorbidities, for example, diabetes, PVD, incontinence, polypharmacy, and other consequences of the aging process, such as reduced mobility and dexterity, general frailty, and cognitive decline (Kazanci et al, 2017; Tobin, 2017). Poor healing of chronic wounds, largely seen in the older population, is more often related to comorbid conditions rather than age alone (Thomas & Burkemper, 2013).

Touch and Pressure

Pacinian and Meissner corpuscles, the skin receptors responsible for the perception of pressure and light touch, undergo structural changes and decline in number and density (García-Piqueras et al, 2019). In addition, the sensory fibers innervating the peripheral receptors undergo changes and decline, and the speed, quantity, or quality of information processing may be affected (Bernard & Lacour, 2017; García-Piqueras et al, 2019). Decreased response to tactile stimuli, higher touch threshold (e.g., firmer stimulation of the skin is required before the stimulus is detected), and decreased ability to detect touch and pressure have been reported in some older adults (McIntyre et al, 2021). Poorer hand sensibility has been found to be associated with problems grasping or handling, independent of grip strength. Similarly, decreased foot sensation was related to balance problems, independent of tandem stand performance (Bernard & Lacour, 2017; García-Piqueras et al, 2019). It is important to note that the degree of change is highly variable amongst individuals.

Temperature

There are three mechanisms through which the skin assists in thermoregulation: blood vessel constriction or dilation, producing sweat from eccrine glands, and contraction of the erector pili muscles that surround the hair follicles (Kazanci et al, 2017; Tobin, 2017). Thermoreceptors, which are sensitive to external and internal changes in the surrounding environment, help to regulate and maintain a constant body temperature. Cold and heat receptors are found in the skin, spinal cord, and hypothalamus, and the skin receptors provide the hypothalamus with important information about the need to generate, converse, or dissipate heat (McLaferty, 2010). Part of the inability to cope with environmental temperature extremes is related to the decrease in perception of the thermal environment due to changes in the skin with aging, including reduction in the number of thermoreceptors and their function (McLaferty, 2010).

Aging causes a decline in the number of sweat glands and also decreases the functional efficiency of the remaining sweat glands. Therefore, less sweat is produced, leading to impaired ability to dissipate heat. Older women, who sweat less, are less likely to lose heat by sweating compared with older men. To sweat adequately, optimal hydration is required, and older adults may have suboptimal hydration levels due to decreased ability to concentrate urine, reduced thirst sensation, and limiting fluid intake as a way to manage urine incontinence (Balmain et al, 2018). Furthermore, older adults are not able to increase cutaneous blood flow as effectively as younger adults to lose heat through radiation (Balmain et al, 2018). In response to cold environments, older adults have a reduced ability to generate heat. The shivering response and the cutaneous vasoconstrictor response are less effective. The decreased amount of subcutaneous fat stored in the hypodermis reduces the body's insulation against heat loss. Finally, the hair on the body becomes thin, reducing the ability of the erect hair caused by the erector pili muscles around the hair follicles to trap air to support heat retention (Kazanci et al, 2017; Tobin, 2017). Research on thermal extremes of hot and cold indicates that older adults have increased thresholds in the hand and foot compared with younger adults (Riley et al, 2014). Interestingly, central body regions lost sensitivity more slowly compared with the extremities, which showed the greatest and earliest change with age.

Somesthesis and Integumentary Implications for the Older Adult in Treatment

Healthcare providers and caregivers must take precautions when transferring, bathing, and dressing older clients due to the possibility of skin tearing. In addition, skin tears in the older population may be slow to heal and therefore cause infection. It is necessary to assess clients' skin integrity and be aware of the chronic conditions that may compromise skin healing. Interaction with a client in a healthcare setting may provide an opportunity for a comprehensive assessment, which includes general skin health and inspection of the condition of the skin.

Touch provides important information about one's environment and is an important prerequisite for adequate performance of manual tasks (Kazanci et al, 2017; Tobin, 2017). Older adults who experience loss or a decrease in tactile acuity or sensitivity will have difficulty localizing and identifying stimuli. Response time may be decreased, as the speed and intensity in which the stimuli are perceived are reduced. An older person must take special care to avoid injury from prolonged pressure on the skin. Changes in tactile sensitivity result in increased reliance on other sensory systems for information, a problem for older adults with vision loss.

Age-related changes may make it more difficult for the older adult to detect a difference between cool and cold or warm and hot, and decreased temperature sensitivity increases the risk of injuries, such as burns, frostbite, and hypothermia. The physiological deficits could be compensated for by conscious behavioral responses, including wearing appropriate clothing layers, moving to a cooler or warmer environment as needed, and decreasing or increasing activity level as needed. However, due to perception deficits, implementation of preventative measures may not be seen as necessary (Balmain et al, 2018). Because older adults are more adversely affected by extremes of hot or cold, many social service agencies have special programs for the elderly population during the very hot or cold times of the year.

Several tools exist to assess the skin. For example, the Braden Scale for Predicting Pressure Sore Risk (Bergstrom et al, 1987) assesses risk for developing pressure sores and comprises six indicators: sensory perception, moisture, activity, mobility, nutrition, and friction or shear. The total score can range from 6 to 23, with a lower score indicating a higher risk. Older adults with a Braden Scale score below 18 (or any low subscale score) require intervention, and the care team should be consulted. The level of risk dictates the intervention strategies that should be used.

Pain

Pain is an unpleasant sensory and emotional experience associated with actual or potential tissue damage (International Association for the Study of Pain, 2017). Unrelieved pain has significant functional, cognitive, emotional, and societal consequences (Lagueux et al, 2018). For example, pain from fall-related injuries may result in decreased functional performance, which in turn may lead to deconditioning, fear of falling, and balance and mobility disturbances. Pain can lead to sleep deprivation, which may decrease pain thresholds, limit daytime energy, increase the incidence and severity of depression and mood disturbances, and decrease overall sense of well-being in older adults.

Aging and Pain

The nociceptive pathways of older adults undergo numerous and widespread changes in morphology, electrophysiology, neurochemistry, and function with aging. Although some studies of experimental pain support the view that pain thresholds to short-duration noxious stimuli are increased in older adults (e.g., the older adult can tolerate a more extreme stimulus without perceiving it to be painful), research has yielded inconsistent findings. Explanations for these contradictory findings could be related to research methodology, the tools used to assess pain, or the hypothesis that human endogenous pain-regulatory systems may be degenerating for some older adults as they age. Older adults with functioning endogenous pain-regulatory systems may be able to produce a greater analgesic response similar to younger adults, whereas older adults with a degenerating system may exhibit higher pain ratings and reduced habituation on repeated stimuli (Bruckenthal, 2017; Kemp et al, 2014).

Sensory fibers A-delta and C are also responsible for pain detection. The A-delta fibers are myelinated and sense short, localized, sharp pain sensation, and the C fibers are unmyelinated and sense dull and burning pain that outlasts the stimulus. The demyelination and reduced density of the A-delta fibers suggests that some older individuals rely on the C fiber input to respond to noxious stimulation (Bruckenthal, 2017). Riley et al (2014) concluded that such sensory changes in the skin of older adults increase the pain threshold and decrease tolerance, which reduces the "purposeful reserve between the onset of pain and the beginning of injury" (p. 279).

Although pain perception, particularly deep pain perception, may decrease in older adulthood (Bruckenthal, 2017; Kemp et al, 2014), pain in older adults is often underrecognized—with healthcare professionals often viewing pain as an inherent part of aging—and underreported, which in turn leads to undertreatment (Lehti et al, 2021). Chronic pain in later life can have a profound impact on an older adult's quality of life, social, physical, and occupational function, and independence and emotional well-being (Lagueux et al, 2018). Health professionals cannot ignore the nonphysiological aspects of pain and need to consider the psychological, sociological, cultural, and contextual factors that may all play a role in pain perception and pain expression in older adults. A summary of the structural and biochemical changes affecting pain perception in older adults is provided in Box 10-4.

Pain Implications for the Older Adult in Treatment

The experience of pain is important for occupational therapists to consider, because it may affect an older person's engagement in functional performance. All healthcare providers must be educated that pain in the absence of disease is not a normal part of aging, yet pain may be experienced daily by a majority of older adults. Older adults are at high risk for undertreatment of pain due to a variety of barriers, including lack of adequate education of healthcare professionals, cost concerns, and other obstacles related to the healthcare system, along with individual factors, such as reluctance to report pain or take analgesics (Bruckenthal, 2017; Reid et al, 2015).

Older adults' attitudes, such as stoicism, beliefs (e.g., "pain is a necessary part of aging") and external barriers generated by health professionals are determinants of whether an older adult decides to seek help for pain. Personality and perceived importance

---

BOX 10-4 Structural and Biochemical Changes Affecting Pain Perception in Older Adults

Decreased density of unmyelinated fibers by age 60
  Selective loss of unmyelinated fibers (1.2–1.6 mm in diameter)
Decreased density of myelinated fibers
  Decrease in large-diameter and finely myelinated afferent fibers (0.1–5.0 mm)
Peripheral nerves
  Decreased nerve conduction velocity
Wallerian degeneration
Marked reduction in substance P in aged human skin and in the thoracic and lumbar dorsal root ganglion cells
Dorsal horn sensory neurons
  Decrease in number and size of sensory neurons in dorsal root ganglia
  Marked loss of myelin
  Signs of damage including axonal involvement especially in the medial lemniscal pathways
  Altered spinal neurochemistry specifically age-related loss of serotonergic and noradrenergic neurons in the dorsal horn
Cortex, midbrain, brainstem
  Decreased numbers of opiates and decreased efficacy of opiate mediated antinociception
  Neuronal death, loss of dendritic arborization, neurofibrillary abnormalities
  Decreased synthesis, axonal transport, uptake, and receptor binding of neurotransmitters

Note: From McMahon et al (2013).

---

of independence were also found to influence help-seeking behaviors (Gammons & Caswell, 2014). Lower rates of pain treatment have been found for the oldest-old and for those with cognitive and communicative disorders. Identifying pain in the cognitively impaired older adult depends heavily on knowing the individual and paying attention to changes in behavior (Lazaridou et al, 2018). Poorly treated pain not only negatively affects the older adult directly, but it also has significant consequences for healthcare professionals and institutions. In the United States, national standards and guidelines for pain management that apply to all healthcare settings, including long-term care, have been published, and failure to adequately comply with the standards in the assessment and treatment of pain can lead to loss of accreditation for the institution. Important roles for occupational therapists include adequately assessing for pain, providing appropriate interventions, and referring older adults to pain specialists as needed.

Pain Assessment

A thorough pain assessment is critical to guiding the therapeutic process. Pain management among older adults is complicated by multiple, concomitant causes and locations of pain (Booker & Herr, 2016; Bruckenthal, 2017), making it difficult to distinguish acute pain caused by a new health condition from that of an old condition. Knowing the older adult's baseline level of functioning and taking a focused history assists in making this differentiation. Communication skills are critical to effective pain assessment, which in turn is dependent on the healthcare provider's ability to recognize sensory and cognitive impairments. Decreased hearing and vision may limit verbal communication and use of written pain assessment tools. Some older adults require extra time to consider the posed question and formulate an appropriate answer, so it is important to be patient. In turn, the healthcare provider may need to adapt the method of communication, for example, by speaking more slowly or ensuring a quiet setting (Booker & Herr, 2016).

Without any known biological markers or diagnostic tests to detect pain, self-report remains the most reliable indicator of the existence of pain and its intensity. Family members or caregivers may provide information about the older adult's baseline cognitive and physical functioning and validate history when cognition or communication are barriers (Booker & Herr, 2016). Individuals who cannot provide a self-report of pain should be directly observed for pain behaviors, and a proxy should be used where appropriate. Pain behavior includes agitation, confusion, social withdrawal, or apathy; facial expressions (grimacing, frowning); vocalization (shouting, moaning); body movements (pacing, rocking); changes in interpersonal interactions (eating alone, easily annoyed); changes in activity (no longer exercising, protecting a body part); and mental status changes (increased confusion, new agitation). Pain rating scales, such as the Wong-Baker Faces Pain Rating Scale (2020), can be used for older adults with mild to moderate cognitive impairment. The Royal College of Physicians, British Geriatrics Society, and British Pain Society provide a complete description of standardized pain assessments with copies for clinicians to use (Schofield, 2018).

Pain Interventions

Occupational therapists need to be aware of the medications that have been prescribed to treat pain, as many cause side effects and can affect safe functional performance. The goals of pharmacological therapy in the older adult include relief of pain, prevention and early management of adverse effects of analgesics, and enhanced quality of life. Useful pharmacological therapies for older adults include nonopioids (e.g, acetaminophen and nonsteroidal anti-inflammatory drugs), opioids, and adjunct drugs. Ablative procedures, such as nerve blocks and other invasive techniques, may be indicated in select cases (Ali et al, 2018).

Nonpharmacological treatments (NPTs) include various physical and emotional therapies for both acute and persistent pain, such as physical movement, heat, cold, massage, acupuncture or acupressure, and transcutaneous electrical nerve stimulation. NPTs are most effective when paired with analgesic medications and function as adjuvant pain treatment.

Selection of the appropriate NPT depends on the individual and the family, the type of pain being experienced, and preexisting medical problems. Research on the use of NPTs in older adults has been sparse, and results are inconclusive. Claims of dramatic pain relief from any NPT must be viewed with caution, and an important role for therapists includes educating seniors about the validity of such claims (Tang et al, 2019).

Physical movement such as sports, dance, or tai chi decreases pain from syndromes such as osteoarthritis, fibromyalgia, or PVD. Activity improves joint function and flexibility, increases muscle strength for improved alignment and reduced muscle spasms, and promotes collateral circulation, minimizing symptoms of claudication. Exercise improves well-being and preserves function and therefore is highly recommended in older adults who can participate safely (Tang et al, 2019).

The application of heat or cold may be beneficial as well (Chen et al, 2021). Care must be taken to avoid skin damage or burns in the susceptible older adult population. Cold is appropriate for acute injuries, especially during the first 48 hours post injury. Cold therapy is also appropriate to decrease bleeding or hematoma formation, edema, and chronic back pain. Heat works well for relief of muscle aches and abdominal cramping. Massage offers many therapeutic effects that reduce pain, including release of muscle tension, improved circulation, increased joint mobility, and decreased anxiety. A systematic review found acupuncture to be associated with significant reductions in pain intensity and improvement in functional mobility and quality of life (Manyanga et al, 2014). Therapy practitioners should be aware of the potential for these modalities to relieve pain and need to consider safety precautions in the use of heat and massage with older adults, whose skin is delicate.

Cognitive-based NPTs, such as guided imagery and relaxation, can be effective but require the ability to learn new skills and the motivation to practice these techniques (Knoerl et al, 2016). Once learned, guided imagery and active relaxation can be practiced individually or with the aid of a coach and are effective in reducing pain by relieving anxiety and reducing muscle tension (Chang et al, 2015). A systematic review by Ball et al (2017) revealed that mindfulness meditation improved psychological aspects of pain, including associated depression and quality of life. Cognitive behavior therapy–based pain self-management and exercise programs have been found to be more effective than exercises alone and usual care in older adults with chronic pain (Nicholas et al, 2013).

Interprofessional Practice

Addressing sensory changes associated with normal aging requires communication and collaboration among healthcare professionals. Loss of sensory abilities that are common among older adults require that occupational therapists collaborate with physicians, nurses, nutritionists, optometrists, nurse practitioners, speech and language therapists, physical therapists, and others. Collaboration with community service (e.g., Meals on Wheels) and government agencies at all levels and with private-sector organizations and charitable groups can assist with organizing needed environmental changes that enhance safety and function. Community and faith-based agencies bring more resources to clients, such as transportation (which can, for example, help older individuals participate in religious services).

CASE STUDY (CONTINUED)

Interventions

Based on the evaluation results and consultation with Mrs. Spiros and her family, the occupational therapist plans for the intervention sessions to address Mrs. Spiros's barriers to occupational performance, including pain, decreased endurance, edema, impaired sensation, and visual deficits.

Occupation-based interventions. Completing ADLs and cooking activities while simulating Mrs. Spiros's home environment will address many of the client's deficits within the context of occupation. While performing the occupations, the therapist plans to implement education and training in energy conservation, breathing techniques, and general safety (e.g., communication and environmental strategies and modifications) (see Box 10-1).

Environmental modification. The occupational therapist organizes a plan to increase function within the skilled nursing environment. Mrs. Spiros can have two sets of dishes (light/dark), and the kitchen staff can place the food on the plate with the most contrast. Providing a plain, darkly colored placemat to highlight the light silverware will also assist Mrs. Spiros in locating food items and utensils. The therapist also notes to make sure that there is adequate lighting within all skilled nursing rooms to promote function. Additionally, contrast should be increased within Mrs. Spiros's room for items of importance (e.g., placing high contrast markers on the call button, television controls, telephone buttons).

Pain management. The therapist decides to incorporate joint protection and task modification to reduce the pain experienced with movement. Education regarding the importance of functional mobility in managing PVD and CHF side effects may assist in addressing pain. The therapist will also ensure Mrs. Spiros and family are aware of positioning to decrease pain (e.g., not crossing the legs and elevating the feet below heart level with presenting edema).

Caregiver education. All staff interacting with Mrs. Spiros need to understand her language barrier and that she may not understand or respond to communication. The therapist organizes a list of translation services that can be used to strengthen communication when family is not present. An in-service regarding tips for improving function with patients who have low vision will assist not only Mrs. Spiros but all clients with visual impairment within the facility.

Question

1. What are two or three additional evidence-based, occupation-centered exemplar interventions that address the client's priorities?

Answer

1. Cooking activities to use her interest in cooking and can help build endurance. Pain management while performing ADLs, including teaching modifications and use of adaptive equipment, energy conservation, and breathing techniques. See section Interventions and Case Study Interventions. See also Chapters 15 and 20. LO 10-6

SUMMARY

The impact of sensory abilities on an older adult's functional performance must be emphasized in all rehabilitation and clinical settings. All senses are important sources of information about one's environment and play an important role in function, particularly in the social and cognitive domains. Sensory deprivation may lead to confusion, disorientation, social isolation, and the appearance of dementia. If not addressed, an older adult may become frail and this, potentially, will limit quality and span of life. All healthcare professionals must use their observation skills and assessments at their disposal to determine whether clients require special referrals to, for example, audiologists, eye care professionals, nutritionists, physical therapists, occupational therapists, pain specialists, and neurologists.

Critical Thinking Questions

1. How might changes in sensory systems affect the older adult's behavior? Are any changes generally more devastating than others? Why or why not?

2. How might an older adult change their daily activities because of sensory changes?

3. What dangers might an older adult face because of changes in taste, smell, or superficial sensations?

REFERENCES

Albright, T. D. (2015). Perceiving. *Daedalus, 144*(1), 22–41. https://doi.org/10.1162/DAED_a_00315

Ali, A., Arif, A. W., Bhan, C., Kumar, D., Malik, M. B., Sayyed, Z., Akhtar, K. H., & Ahmad, M. Q. (2018). Managing chronic pain in the elderly: An overview of the recent therapeutic advancements. *Cureus, 10*(9), e3293. https://doi.org/10.7759/cureus.3293

American Macular Degeneration Foundation. (n.d.-a). Risk factors for macular degeneration. Retrieved from https://www.macular.org/risk-factors

American Macular Degeneration Foundation. (n.d.-b). Dry versus wet age-related macular degeneration. Retrieved from https://www.macular.org/dry-vs-wet-macular-degeneration

Attems, J., Walker, L., Jellinger, K. A. (2015). Olfaction and aging: A mini-review. *Gerontology, 61*(6), 485–490. doi: 10.1159/000381619

Ball, E. F., Nur Shafina Muhammad Sharizan, E., Franklin, G., & Rogozinska, E. (2017). Does mindfulness meditation improve chronic pain? A systematic review. *Curr Opin Obstet Gynecol, 29*(6), 359–366. https://doi.org/10.1097/GCO.0000000000000417

Balmain, B. N., Sabapathy, S., Louis, M., & Morris, N. R. (2018). Aging and thermoregulatory control: The clinical implications of exercising under heat stress in older individuals. *BioMed Res Int, 2018*, 8306154. https://doi.org/10.1155/2018/8306154

Barstow, B. A., Bennett, D. K., & Vogtle, L. K. (2011). Perspectives on home safety: Do home safety assessments address the concerns of clients with vision loss? *Am J Occup Ther, 65*(6), 635–642. https://doi.org/10.5014/ajot.2011.001909

Barstow, B. A., Warren, M., Thaker, S., Hallmna, A., & Batts, P. (2015). Client and therapist perspectives on the influence of low vision and chronic conditions on performance and occupational therapy intervention. *Am J Occup Ther, 69*(3), 6903270010. doi: 10.5014/ajot.2015.014605

Bauer C. A. (2018). Tinnitus. *N Engl J Med, 378*(13), 1224–1231. https://doi.org/10.1056/NEJMcp1506631

Bergstrom, N., Braden, B. J., Laguzza, A., & Holman, V. (1987). The Braden Scale for predicting pressure sore risk. *Nurs Res, 36*, 205–210. http://dx.doi.org/10.1097/00006199-198707000-00002

Bernard, D. L., & Lacour, M. (2017). The fall in older adults: Physical and cognitive problems. *Curr Aging Sci, 10*(3), 185–200. https://doi.org/10.2174/1874609809666160630124552

Bhatt, J. M., Lin, H. W., & Bhattacharyya, N. (2016). Prevalence, severity, exposures, and treatment patterns of tinnitus in the United States. *JAMA Otolaryngol Head Neck Surg, 142*(10), 959–965. https://doi.org/10.1001/jamaoto.2016.1700

Booker, S. Q., & Herr, K. A. (2016). Assessment and measurement of pain in adults in later life. *Clin Geriatr Med, 32*(4), 677–692. https://doi.org/10.1016/j.cger.2016.06.012

Boyd, K. (2021). What are cataracts? *American Academy of Ophthalmology.* https://www.aao.org/eye-health/diseases/what-are-cataracts

Brodie, S. E., & J. H. Francis. (2017). Aging and disorders of the eye. In R. C. Tallis, H. M. Fillit, & J. Young (Eds.), *Brocklehurst's textbook of geriatric medicine and gerontology* (8th ed., pp. 799–810). Philadelphia: Elsevier, Inc.

Bruckenthal, P. (2017). Pain in the older adult. In R. C. Tallis, H. M. Fillit, & J. Young (Eds.), *Brocklehurst's textbook of geriatric medicine and gerontology* (8th ed., pp. 799–810). Philadelphia: Elsevier, Inc.

Calabrèse, A., Owsley, C., McGwin, G. & Legge, G. E. (2016). Development of a reading accessibility index using the MNREAD acuity chart. *JAMA Ophthalmol, 134*(4), 398–405.

Cech, D. J., & Martin, S. (2012). *Functional movement development across the lifespan* (3rd ed.). Philadelphia: W.B. Saunders.

Centers for Disease Control and Prevention. (2020a). *Common eye disorders.* Retrieved from https://www.cdc.gov/visionhealth/basics/ced/index.html

Centers for Disease Control and Prevention. (2020b). *Vision health initiative: don't let glaucoma steal your site!* Retrieved from https://www.cdc.gov/visionhealth/resources/features/glaucoma-awareness.html#:~:text=About%203%20million%20Americans%20have,know%20they%20have%20the%20disease

Chader, G. J., & Tayler, A. (2015). Preface: The aging eye: Normal changes, age-related diseases, and sight-saving approaches. *Invest Ophthalmol Vis Sci, 54*, ORSF1–ORSF4. https://doi.org/10.1167/iovs.13-12993

Chang, K. L., Fillingim, R., Hurley, R. W., & Schmidt, S. (2015). Chronic pain management: Nonpharmacological therapies for chronic pain. *FP Essent, 432*, 21–26. https://europepmc.org/article/med/25970869

Chen, W. S., Thiru, M. A., Yang, W., Wang, T. G., Kwon, D. R., & Chou, L. W. (2021). Physical agent modalities. *Braddom's physical medicine and rehabilitation,* (6th edition). Elsevier, Inc. https://doi.org/10.1016/B978-0-323-62539-5.00017-5

Cook, I. M., Polgar, J. M. (2015). Sensory aids for persons with auditory impairment. In A.M. Cook, J. M. Polgar (Eds.). *Assistive technologies* (352–374). https://doi.org/10.1016/B978-0-323-09631-7.00014-4

Cowdell, F., & Radley, K. (2012). Maintaining skin health in older people. *Nursing Times, 108*(49), 16–20. Retrieved from http://libaccess.mcmaster.ca.libaccess.lib.mcmaster.ca/login?url=http://search.proquest.com.libaccess.lib.mcmaster.ca/docview/1242448807?accountid=12347

Crews, J. E., Chou, C., Stevens, J. A., & Saaddine, J. B. (2016). Falls among persons aged ≥65 years with and without severe vision impairment—United States, 2014. *Morbid Mortal Wkly Rep, 65*, 433–437. doi: http://dx.doi.org/10.15585/mmwr.mm6517a2

Daniel, E., Shaffer, J., Ying, G., Grunwald, J. E., Martin, D. F., Jaffe, G. J., & Maguire, M. G. (2016). Outcomes in eyes with retinal angiomatous proliferation in the Comparison of Age Related Macular Degeneration Treatments Trials (CATT). *Ophthalmol, 123*, 609–616. doi.org/10.1016/j.ophtha.2015.10.034

Dawes, P., Pye, A., Reeves., W. K., Sheikh, S., Thodi, C., Charalambous, A. P., Gallant, K., Nasreddine, Z., & Leroi, I. (2019). Protocol for the development of versions of the Montreal Cognitive Assessment (MoCA) for people with hearing or vision impairment. *Br Med J, 9*, e026246. doi: 10.1136/bmjopen-2018-026246

de Haan, G.A., Tucha, O., & Heutink, J. (2020). Effects of low visual acuity on neuropsychological test scores: A simulation study. *Clin Neuropsychol, 34*(1), 140–157. doi: 10.1080/13854046.2019.1596315

Demmin, D.F., & Silverstein, S.M. (2020). Visual impairment and mental health: Unmet needs and treatment options. *Clin Opthalmol, 2020*(14), 4229–4251. 10.2147/OPTH.S258783

Dharmarajan, T. S., & Ugalino, J. T. (2000). The aging process. In D. Dreger & B. Krumm (Eds.), *Hospital physician geriatric medicine board review manual* (Vol. 1, Part 1, pp. 1–12). Wayne, PA: Turner White Communications. doi: 10.1186/s12939-015-02138

Dougherty, B.E., Flom, R.E., & Bullimore, M.A. (2005). An evaluation of the Mars Letter Contrast Sensitivity Test. *Optometr Vis Sci. 82*(11), 970–975. doi: 10.1097/01.opx.0000187844.27025.ea

Duncan, P.W., Weiner, D.K., Chandler, J., & Studenski, S. (1990). Functional reach: A new clinical measure of balance. *J Gerontol, 45*(6), 192–197. doi: 10.1093/geronj/45.6.m192. PMID: 2229941.

Esenwah, E. C., Azuamah, Y. C., Okorie, M. E., & Ikoro, N. C. (2014). The aging eye and vision: A review. *Int J Health Sci Res, 4*, 218–224.

Fluitman, K. S., Hesp, A. C., Kaihatu, R. F., Nieuwdorp, M., Keijser, B. J. F., IJzerman, R. J., & Visser, M. (2021). Poor taste and smell are associated with poor appetite, macronutrient intake, and dietary quality but not with undernutrition in older adults. *J Nutr, 151*(3), 605–614. https://doi.org/10.1093/jn/nxaa400

Folstein, M. F., Folstein, S. E., & McHugh, P. R. (1975). "Mini-mental state": A practical method for grading the cognitive state of patients for the clinician. *J Psych Res, 12*, 189–198.

Gaeth, J. (1948). *A study of phonemic regression in relation to hearing loss.* Unpublished doctoral dissertation, Northwestern University, Evanston, IL.

Gammons, V., & Caswell, G. (2014). Older people and barriers to self-reporting of chronic pain. *British Journal of Nursing, 23*, 274–278. http://dx.doi.org/10.12968/bjon.2014.23.5.274

García-Piqueras, J., García-Mesa, Y., Cárcaba, L., Feito, J., Torres-Parejo, I., Martín-Biedma, B., Cobo, J., García-Suárez, O., & Vega, J. A. (2019). Ageing of the somatosensory system at the periphery: Age-related changes in cutaneous mechanoreceptors. *J Anat, 234*(6), 839–852. https://doi.org/10.1111/joa.12983

Genther, D.J., Frick, K.D., Chen, D., Betz, J., & Lin, F. R. (2013). Association of hearing loss with hospitalization and burden of disease in older adults. *J Am Med Assoc, 309*, 2322–2324.

Glaucoma Research Foundation. (2016). *High eye pressure and glaucoma.* Retrieved from www.glaucoma.org/gleams/high-eye-pressure-and-glaucoma.php

Goman, A., & Lin, F. (2018). Hearing loss in older adults—from epidemiological insights to national initiatives. *Hear Res, 369*, 29–32. https://doi.org/10.1016/j.heares.2018.03.031

Gopinath, B., Liew, G., Burlutsky, G., & Mitchell, P. (2014). Age-related macular degeneration and 5-year incidence of impaired activities of daily living. *Maturitas, 77*(3), 263–266. https://doi.org/10.1016/j.maturitas.2013.12.001

Grow, W. A. (2018). The cerebral cortex. In Duane E. Haines & Gregory A. Mihailoff (Eds.), *Fundamental neuroscience for basic and clinical applications* (pp. 468–479). Philadelphia: Elsevier, Inc.

Guest, D., Howard, C. J., Brown, L. A., & Gleeson, H. (2015). Aging and the rate of visual information processing. *J Vis, 15*, 1–25. doi: 10.1167/15.14.10

Hanson, M., & Gantz, B. (2018). Types of hearing impairment. University of Iowa Hospitals and Clinics: University of Iowa Healthcare. https://uihc.org/health-topics/types-hearing-impairment

Heft, M. W., & Robinson, M. E. (2014). Age differences in suprathreshold sensory function. *Age, 36*, 1–8. doi: 10.1007/s11357-013-9536-9

Imoscopi, A., Inelmen, E. M., Sergi, G., Miotto, F., & Manzato, E. (2012). Taste loss in the elderly: Epidemiology, causes and consequences. *Aging Clin Exp Res, 24*, 570–579. doi: 10.3275/8520

International Association for the Study of Pain. (2017). *Taxonomy*. Retrieved from https://www.iasp-pain.org/Taxonomy

Johnson, L. N., & Baloh, F. G. (1991). The accuracy of confrontation visual field test in comparison with automated perimetry. *J Nat Med Assoc, 83*(10), 895–898. https://www.ncbi.nlm.nih.gov/pmc/articles/PMC2571584/

Kaldenberg, J., & Smallfield, S. (2020). Practice guidelines—Occupational therapy practice guidelines for older adults with low vision. *Am J Occup Ther, 74*, 7402397010. https://doi.org/10.5014/ajot.2020.742003

Kazanci, A., Kurus, M., & Atasever, A. (2017). Analyses of changes on skin by aging. *Skin Res Technol, 23*(1), 48–60. https://doi.org/10.1111/srt.12300

Kemp, J., Despres, O., Pebayle, T., & Dufour, A. (2014). Differences in age-related effects on myelinated and unmyelinated peripheral fibres: A sensitivity and evoked potentials study. *Eur J Pain, 18*(4). doi: 10.1002/j.1532-2149.2013.00388.x

Knoerl, R., Lavoie Smith, E. M., & Weisberg, J. (2016). Chronic pain and cognitive behavioral therapy: An integrative review. *West J Nurs Res, 38*(5), 596–628. doi: 10.1177/0193945915615869

Lagueux, É., Dépelteau, A., & Masse, J. (2018). Occupational therapy's unique contribution to chronic pain management: A scoping review. *Pain Res Manag, 5378451*. https://doi.org/10.1155/2018/5378451

Lazaridou, A., Elbaridi, N., Edwards, R. R., & Berde, C. B. (2018). Pain assessment. In T. Honorio, Benzon, T., N. R. Srinivasa, S. S. Liu, S. M. Fishman, & S. P. Cohen (Eds.), *Essent Pain Med* (39–46). https://doi.org/10.1016/B978-0-323-40196-8.00005-X

Lee, J. Y. (2015). Aging and speech understanding. *J Audiol Otol, 19*(1), 7–13. https://doi.org/10.7874/jao.2015.19.1.7

Lehti, T. E., Rinkinen, M. O., Aalto, U., Roitto, H. M., Knuutila, M., Öhman, H., Kautiainen, H., Karppinen, H., Tilvis, R., Strandberg, T., & Pitkälä, K. H. (2021). Prevalence of musculoskeletal pain and analgesic treatment among community-dwelling older adults: Changes from 1999–2019. *Drugs Aging, 38*(10), 931–937. https://pubmed.ncbi.nlm.nih.gov/34386937/

Malaty, J., & Malaty, I. A. C. (2013). Smell and taste disorders in primary care. *Am Fam Phys, 88*, 852–859. Retrieved from http://europepmc.org/abstract/med/24364550

Mangione, C. M., Lee, P. P., Gutierrez, P. R., Spritzer, K., Berry, S., & Hays, R. D. (2001). Development of the 25-item National Eye Institute Visual Function Questionnaire. *Arch Opthalmol, 119*, 1050–1058.

Mangione, C. M., Phillips, R. S., Sedon, J. M., Lawrence, M. G., Cook, E. F., Dailey, R., & Goldman, L. (1992). Development of the "Activities of Daily Vision Scale." A measure of visual functional status. *Med Care, 30*, 1111–1126.

Manyanga, T., Froese, M., Zarychanski, R., Abou-Setta, A., Friesen, C., Tennenhouse, M., & Shay, B. L. (2014). Pain management with acupuncture in osteoarthritis: A systematic review and meta-analysis. *BMC Complement Altern Med, 14*, 312–316. doi: 10.1186/1472-6882-14-312.

Mascia, J. (1994). Understanding age-related hearing loss among older adults. In S. E. Boone, D. Watson, & M. Bagley (Eds.). *The challenge to independence: Vision and hearing loss among older adults* (pp. 93–98). Little Rock: University of Arkansas Rehabilitation Research and Training Center for Persons Who Are Deaf or Hard of Hearing.

McIntyre, S., Nagi, S. S., McGlone, F., & Olausson, H. (2021). The effects of ageing on tactile function in humans. *Neuroscience*, (464), 53–58. https://doi.org/10.1016/j.neuroscience.2021.02.015

McLafferty, E. (2010). Prevention and management of hyperthermia during a heatwave. *Nursing Older People, 22*, 23–27. http://dx.doi.org/10.7748/nop2010.09.22.7.23.c7946

McMahon, S., Koltzenburg, M., Tracey, I., & Turk, D. C. (2013). *Wall & Melzack's textbook of pain*. Elsevier/Saunders.

Murray, D. (2018). Emergency management: Angle-closure glaucoma. *Commun Eye Health, 31*(103), 64. doi: https://www.ncbi.nlm.nih.gov/pmc/articles/PMC6253313/

National Council on Aging. (2013). *Hearing loss: It's a family affair*. Retrieved from http://www.ncoa.org/improve-health/community-education/hearing-loss-its-a-Family.html #sthash.0CVjAd7r.dpuf

National Eye Institute. (2019). *Cataracts*. Retrieved from https://nei.nih.gov/eyedata/cataract#5

National Eye Institute. (2022). *Low vision*. Retrieved from https://www.nei.nih.gov/learn-about-eye-health/eye-conditions-and-diseases/low-vision

National Health Service. (2016). *Age-related cataracts*. Retrieved from www.nhs.uk/conditions/cataracts-age-related/pages/introduction.aspx

National Institute on Deafness and Other Communication Disorders. (2016a). *Age-related hearing loss*. Retrieved from https://www.nidcd.nih.gov/health/age-related-hearing-loss

National Institute on Deafness and Other Communication Disorders. (2016b). *Hearing aids*. Retrieved from: https://www.nidcd.nih.gov/health/hearing-aids#hearingaid_04

Nicholas, M., Asghari, A., Blyth, F., Wood, B., Murray, R., McCabe, R., Brnabic, A., Beeston, L., Corbett, M., Sherrington, C., & Overton, S. (2013). Self-management intervention for chronic pain in older adults: A randomised controlled trial. *Pain, 154*, 824–835.

Olofsson, J. K., Ekström, I., Larsson, M., & Nordin, S. (2021). Olfaction and aging: A review of the current state of research and future directions. *i-Perception, 12*(3), 20416695211020331. https://doi.org/10.1177/20416695211020331

Owsley, C., Ghate, D., & Keday, S. (2018). Vision and aging. In M. Rizzo, S. Anderson, & B. Fritzsch (Eds.) *Aging mind brain*. https://doi.org/10.1002/9781118772034.ch15

Owsley, C., Rhodes, L. A., McGwin, G., Jr., Mennemeyer, S. T., Bregantini, M., Patel, N., Wiley, D. M., LaRussa, F., Box, D., Saaddine, J., Crews, J. E., & Girkin, C. A. (2015). Eye care quality and accessibility improvement in the community (EQUALITY) for adults at risk for glaucoma: Study rationale and design. *Int J Equity Health, 14*, 135–149.

Park, S., Kho, Y. L., Kim, H. J., Kim, J., & Lee, E. H. (2015). Impact of glaucoma on quality of life and activities of daily living. *H K J Occup Ther, 25*, 39–44. https://doi.org/10.1016/j.hkjot.2015.04.002

Patel, N. B., Lim, M., Gajjar, A., Evans, K. B., & Harwerth, R. S. (2014). Age-associated changes in the retinal nerve fiber layer and optic nerve head. *Invest Opthalmol Vis Sci, 55*, 5134–5143. https://doi.org/10.1167/iovs.14-14303

Pence, T., Reiter, E., DiNardo, L., & Costanzo, R. (2014). Risk factors for hazardous events in olfactory-impaired patients. *JAMA Otolaryngol Head Neck Surg 140*(10), 951–955. doi:10.1001/jamaoto.2014.1675

Perlmutter, M. S., Bhorade, A., Gordon, M., Hollingsworth, H., Engsberg, J. E., & Baum, M. C. (2013). Home lighting assessment for clients with low vision. *Am J Occup Ther, 67*, 674–682. http://dx.doi.org/10.5014/ajot.2013.006692

Pesudovs, K., & Coster, D. J. (1998). An instrument for assessment of subjective visual disability in cataract patients. *Br J Opthalmol, 82*, 617–624. professionals/whatisot/pa/facts/low-vision-fact-sheet.pdf

Quental, N. B. M., Brucki, S. M. D., & Bueno, O. F. A. (2013). Visuospatial function in early Alzheimer's disease—the use of the Visual Object and Space Perception (VOSP) Battery. *PLoS One, 8*, e68398. doi: 10.1371/journal.pone.0068398

Reid, M. C., Eccleston, C., & Pillemer, K. (2015). Management of chronic pain in older adults. *BMJ (Clinical research ed.), 350*, h532. https://doi.org/10.1136/bmj.h532

Reitan, R. (1992). *Trail making test: Manual for administration and scoring*. Tucson, AZ: Reitan Neuropsychological Laboratory.

Renaud, J., & Bédard, E. (2013). Depression in the elderly with visual impairment and its association with quality of life. *Clin Interv Aging, 8*, 931–943. http://doi.org/10.2147/CIA.S27717

Riley, J. L., Cruz-Almeida, Y., Glover, T. L., King, C. D., Goodin, B. R., Sibille, K. T., Bartley, E. J., Herbert, M. S., Sotolongo, A., Fessler, B. J., Redden, D. T., Staud, R., Bradley, L. A., & Fillingim, R. B. (2014). Age and race effects on pain sensitivity and modulation among middle-aged and older adults. *J Pain, 15*, 272–282. http://dx.doi.org/10.1016/j.jpain.2013.10.015

Rimona S. W., Schrag, A. E., Warren, J. D., Crutch, S. J., Lees, A. J., & Morris, H. R. (2016). Visual dysfunction in Parkinson's disease, *Brain, 139*(11), 2827–2843. https://doi.org/10.1093/brain/aww175

Ruth, M. A. (2017). The prevalence and impact of vision and hearing loss in the elderly. *N C Med J, 78*(2), 118–120. https://www.ncmedicaljournal.com/content/ncm/78/2/118.full.pdf

Saunier, V., Merle, B., Delyfer, M. N., Cougnard-Grégoire, A., Rougier, M. B., Amouyel, P., Lambert, J. C., Dartigues, J. F., Korobelnik, J. F., & Delcourt, C. (2018). Incidence of and risk factors associated with age-related macular degeneration: Four-year follow-up from the ALIENOR Study. *JAMA Ophthalmol, 136*(5), 473–481. https://doi.org/10.1001/jamaophthalmol.2018.0504

Schofield, P. (2018). The assessment of pain in older people: UK national guidelines. *Age Ageing, 47*(suppl_1), i1–i22. https://doi.org/10.1093/ageing/afx192

Seiberling, K. A., & Conley, D. B. (2004). Aging and olfactory and taste function. *Otolaryngol Clin N Am, 37*, 1209–1228. http://dx.doi.org/10.1016/j.otc.2004.06.006

Sergi, G., Bano, G., Pizzato, S., Veronese, N., & Manzato, E. (2017). Taste loss in the elderly: Possible implications for dietary habits. *Crit Rev Food Sci Nutr, 57*(17), 3684–3689. https://www.tandfonline.com/doi/abs/10.1080/10408398.2016.1160208

Shakarchi, A. F., Assi, L., Ehrlich, J. R., Deal, J. A., Reed, N. S., & Swenor, B. K. (2020). Dual sensory impairment and perceived everyday discrimination in the United States. *JAMA Ophthalmol, 138*(12). 1227–1233. doi:10.1001/jamaophthalmol.2020.3982

Sloane, M. E., Ball, K., Owsley, C., Bruni, S. R., & Roenkar, D. L., (1992). The visual activities questionnaire: Developing an instrument for assessing problems in everyday visual tasks. In *Everyday visual tasks. Technical digest of the noninvasive assessment of the visual system* (Vol. 1, pp. 26–29). Washington, DC: Optical Society of America.

Snow, M., Warren, M., & Yuen, H. K. (2018). Revised Self-Report Assessment of Functional Visual Performance (R-SRAFVP)-Part II: Construct validation. *Am J Occup Ther, 72*(5). doi: 10.5014/ajot.2018.030205

Sorokowski, P., Karwowski, M., Misiak, M., Marczak, M. K., Dziekan, M., Hummel, T., & Sorokowska, A. (2019). Sex differences in human olfaction: A meta-analysis. *Front Psych, 10*, 242. https://doi.org/10.3389/fpsyg.2019.00242

Steinberg, E. P., Teilsch, J. M., Schein, O. D., Javitt, J. C., Sharkey, P., Cassard, S. D. (1994). The VF-14: An index of functional impairment in patients with cataract. *Arch Opthalmol, 112*, 630–638.

Stender, T., & Groth, J. (2014). Evidence-based and practical considerations when fitting sound shaper for individual patients. *Hearing Rev*. Retrieved from https://hearingreview.com/inside-hearing/research/evidence-based-practical-considerations-fitting-sound-shaper-individual-patients

Sugita, Y., Yamamoto, H., Maeda, Y., & Furukawa, T. (2020). Influence of aging on the retina and visual motion processing for optokinetic responses in mice. *Front Neurosci, 14*(586013). doi: 10.3389/fnins.2020.586013

Tang, S. K., Tse, M. M. Y., Leung, S. F., & Fotis, T. (2019). The effectiveness, suitability, and sustainability of non-pharmacological methods of managing pain in community-dwelling older adults: A systematic review. *BMC Public Health, 19*. https://doi.org/10.1186/s12889-019-7831-9

Tham, Y. C., Li, X., Wong, T. Y., Quigley, H. A., Aung, T., & Cheng, C. Y. (2014). Global prevalence of glaucoma and projections of glaucoma burden through 2040. *Ophthalmol, 121*, 2081–2090.

Thomas, D. R., & Burkemper, N. M. (2013). Aging skin and wound healing. *Clin Geriatr Med, 29*. Xi–xx. doi: http://dx.doi.org/10.1016/j.cger.2013.02.001

Tobin, D. J. (2017). Introduction to skin aging. *J Tissue Viability, 26*(1), 37–46. https://www.sciencedirect.com/science/article/abs/pii/S0965206X16000280

U.S. Department of Health and Human Services, National Institutes of Health. (2017). NIH news in health, your aging eyes. Retrieved from https://newsinhealth.nih.gov/sites/nihNIH/files/Special-Issues/Seniors.pdf

U.S. Social Security Administration. (2022). If you're blind or have low vision-How we can help. Retrieved from https://www.ssa.gov/pubs/EN-05-10052.pdf

Varma, R., Vajaranant, T., Burkemper, B., Wu, S., Torres, M., Hsu, C., Choudhury, F., & McKean-Cowdin, R. (2016). Visual impairment and blindness in adults in the United States: Demographic and geographic variations from 2015 to 2050. *JAMA Ophthalmol, 134*(7), 802–809. doi:10.1001/jamaophthalmol.2016.1284

Vimont, C. (2020). All about the eye chart. *American Academy of Ophthalmology*. Retrieved from https://www.aao.org/eye-health/tips-prevention/eye-chart-facts-history

VisionAware. (2016). *What are low vision optical devices?* Retrieved from www.visionaware.org/info/everyday-living/helpful-products/overview-of-low-vision-devices/low-vision-optical-devices/1245

Voegeli, D. (2012). Understanding the main principles of skin care in older adults. *Nursing Standard, 27*, 59–68. http://dx.doi.org/10.7748/ns2012.11.27.11.59.c9414

Warren, M. (2011). *Occupational therapy's role with persons with visual impairment*. American Occupational Therapy Association. https://www.aota.org/-/media/corporate/files/aboutot/

Warren, M. (n.d.). THE biVABA (Brain Injury Visual Assessment Battery for Adults). https://www.visabilities.com/bivaba.html

Warren, M., & Barstow, E. A. (Eds.). (2011). *Occupational therapy interventions for adults with low vision*. AOTA Press.

Warren, M., DeCarlo, D. K, & Dreer, L. E. (2016). Health literacy in older adults with and without low vision. *Am J Occup Ther, 70*(3), 1–7. doi: 10.5014/ajot.2016.017400

Weinstein, B. (2017). Disorders of hearing. In R. C. Tallis, H. M. Fillit, & J. Young (Eds.), *Brocklehurst's textbook of geriatric medicine and gerontology* (8th ed., pp. 811–818). Philadelphia: Elsevier, Inc.

Wong-Baker FACES Foundation. (2020). Wong-Baker FACES® Pain Rating Scale. Retrieved with permission from http://www.WongBakerFACES.org. Originally published in *Whaley & Wong's Nursing Care of Infants and Children*.

World Health Organization. (2015, February 27). 1.1 billion people at risk of hearing loss. Retrieved from http://www.who.int/mediacentre/news/releases/2015/ear-care/en/

World Health Organization. (2019). *ICD-11: International classification of diseases* (11th revision). Retrieved from https://icd.who.int/

World Health Organization. (2021). *Blindness and vision impairment*. Retrieved from https://www.who.int/news-room/fact-sheets/detail/blindness-and-visual-impairment

CHAPTER 11

Musculoskeletal Function and Health Conditions

An T. Nguyen, OTD, OTR/L ■ Marianne Capps, OTD, OTR/L ■ Madison Tate, OTD, OTR/L

> *"Aging is not lost youth but a new stage of opportunity and strength."*
> —Betty Friedan (1921-2006), American writer and activist

LEARNING OUTCOMES

By the end of this chapter, readers will be able to:

11-1. Differentiate between typical and atypical age-related changes in the musculoskeletal system.
11-2. Describe the signs, symptoms, and risk factors of age-related musculoskeletal health conditions that commonly affect older adults.
11-3. Discuss the relationship between age-related musculoskeletal changes and their impact on occupational performance in older adults.
11-4. Explain occupational therapy assessment considerations for the older adult and the procedures for assessing musculoskeletal system factors, including joint ROM and muscle strength.
11-5. Select and justify use of specific assessments for the musculoskeletal system.
11-6. Identify occupational therapy interventions to address the impact of age-related musculoskeletal changes on occupational performance in older adults.

Mini Case Study

Ms. Ford is a 72-year-old African American woman who lives with her dog, a golden retriever named Sammy. Ms. Ford and Sammy live in a two-story townhouse home. There are four steps that lead into the house with a railing on one side of the steps. There are 15 steps (no railing) from the main floor to the second floor, where Ms. Ford's bedroom and bathroom are located. Ms. Ford's medical history includes osteoarthritis (OA), hypertension, diabetes mellitus (DM), hyperlipidemia, and asthma. Her medications include amlodipine 5 mg daily, metformin 500 mg twice daily, glyburide 10 mg daily, simvastatin 10 mg daily, albuterol 2 puffs as needed, and acetaminophen 325 mg daily for the past 3 months for pain.

Ms. Ford was diagnosed with OA 10 years ago. She has severe pain in her hands that causes problems during dressing, primarily with the fine motor coordination needed for buttons and zippers. In addition, food preparation is difficult (e.g., cutting food and opening containers). Ms. Ford has identified pain in her right hip that has progressively worsened to the point where she has difficulty negotiating stairs and can no longer take long walks with Sammy. Prior to her diagnosis of OA, Ms. Ford was a very active woman. She volunteered at a local animal shelter twice weekly; however, she is now only able to volunteer once every other week due to hip pain. Ms. Ford loves to garden but, because of the pain in her hip and hands, she minimizes the work by maintaining only the flower boxes in the front of her house.

Provocative Questions
1. What are some changes in the musculoskeletal system that may be affecting Ms. Ford's occupational performance?
2. How have Ms. Ford's meaningful occupations been affected by age-related changes and health conditions affecting the musculoskeletal system?
3. On the basis of the information provided about Ms. Ford, what should be the main areas of focus for occupational therapy intervention? What additional information or assessments might be useful to inform the occupational therapist's clinical judgment?

Various tissues comprise the musculoskeletal system, including muscle, tendon, ligament, bone, and cartilage. The musculoskeletal system is directly affected by age-related body structure and function changes, such as changes in strength, balance, and range of motion (ROM), thereby increasing the risk of occupational performance impairments in older adults. Older adults may experience a gradual decline in physical abilities and have difficulty performing daily occupations as they age. As with other body systems, the aging process in the musculoskeletal system varies greatly from one person to another. However, for some individuals, age-related changes may contribute to the development of several chronic conditions that are more commonly seen in older adults. In addition, changes secondary to disuse, other system pathologies, and personal factors (e.g., lifestyle, nutrition) may contribute to or magnify the effects of aging on the musculoskeletal system. This chapter will:

- Describe typical and atypical age-related changes in the musculoskeletal system that may lead to occupational performance impairments and affect occupational participation in the older adult.
- Discuss the effects of aging on muscle strength and power, joint flexibility, posture, and the resultant effects on the older adult's occupational performance and participation.
- Explain considerations for assessing musculoskeletal system function, including joint ROM and muscle strength for the older adult.
- Identify occupational therapy interventions that may be used to address the impact of age-related musculoskeletal changes on occupational performance and participation in older adults.

Typical Age-Related Changes in the Musculoskeletal System

Typical age-related tissue changes have been conceptualized as an accumulation of microinsults resulting in damage to or changes in body tissues, eventually leading to the diminution of physiological systems (Frontera, 2017; Jin, 2010). These tissue and system changes affect older adults' function, mobility, and ability to interact with the environment. Some of the most salient age-related changes in the musculoskeletal system include the following:

- Decreased muscle strength and power
- Marked loss of skeletal muscle mass
- Lower muscle quality with increases in fat and connective tissue
- Decreased number of functional motor units
- Decreased percentage of type II (fast twitch) fibers
- Changes in postural alignment
- Bone and cartilage changes
- Changes in balance and gait
- Decreased maximal speed of movement and initiation of responses
- Impaired muscle excitation-contraction coupling
- Decreased proprioception

Many alterations in the musculoskeletal system occur with the passage of time. However, aging is a personal and unique experience, not only because older adults differ from one another with respect to their personal and environmental factors but also because their physiological systems age at different rates. The rate of physiological change and resultant impact on function is highly individualized, and individual differences among older adults become strikingly more apparent with increasing age.

Musculoskeletal system functioning among older adults exists along a continuum (International Council on Active Aging, n.d.; Spiduso et al, 2005) (Fig. 11-1). At the highest level of the physical-performance hierarchy, *physically elite* older adults train on a daily basis, compete in sports competitions, or continue to work in a physically demanding occupation, such as firefighting or ski instruction. Although not many can continue working in these occupations into very old age, some do. Those who do represent older individuals with maximal musculoskeletal system functioning. *Physically fit* individuals may still participate in work activities and continue to exercise on a regular basis for their health and well-being. *Physically independent* older adults are those individuals whose musculoskeletal system functioning allows them to independently perform activities of daily living (ADLs) and instrumental activities of daily living (IADLs). Many continue to be active in hobbies, leisure, and social activities. Although these individuals may have one or more chronic conditions, but they are still able to function independently, they tend to engage in less physically demanding activities than those who are physically fit. *Physically frail* older adults can perform ADLs but may have a debilitating condition or disease that presents physical challenges on a daily basis. They can live independently with human or environmental assistance but may be unable to engage in certain IADLs due to physical limitations, such as yard work or heavy housekeeping tasks. *Physically dependent* older adults cannot perform some or all basic ADLs, such as bathing, toileting, or dressing, because of acute or chronic conditions that severely limit occupational performance skills and impair body functions, such as musculoskeletal impairments, cognitive impairments, or cardiopulmonary impairments. Lifestyle factors and behaviors may also contribute to physical dependence, such as physical inactivity, smoking-related impairments, or increased weight. Having more than one chronic condition, also known as multimorbidity, is a risk factor for physical dependence in ADLs (Bao et al, 2019). Physically dependent individuals require institutional care or full-time caregiver assistance (Bao et al, 2019). Considering the heterogeneity of aging and the continuum of musculoskeletal functioning among older adults, it is important to remember that although age-related changes do occur, deterioration in physical abilities and functioning is not inevitable for all older adults (Fig. 11-2). Occupational therapists and occupational therapy assistants must be aware of the variety of age-related changes that can significantly impact older adults' occupational performance, participation, and well-being.

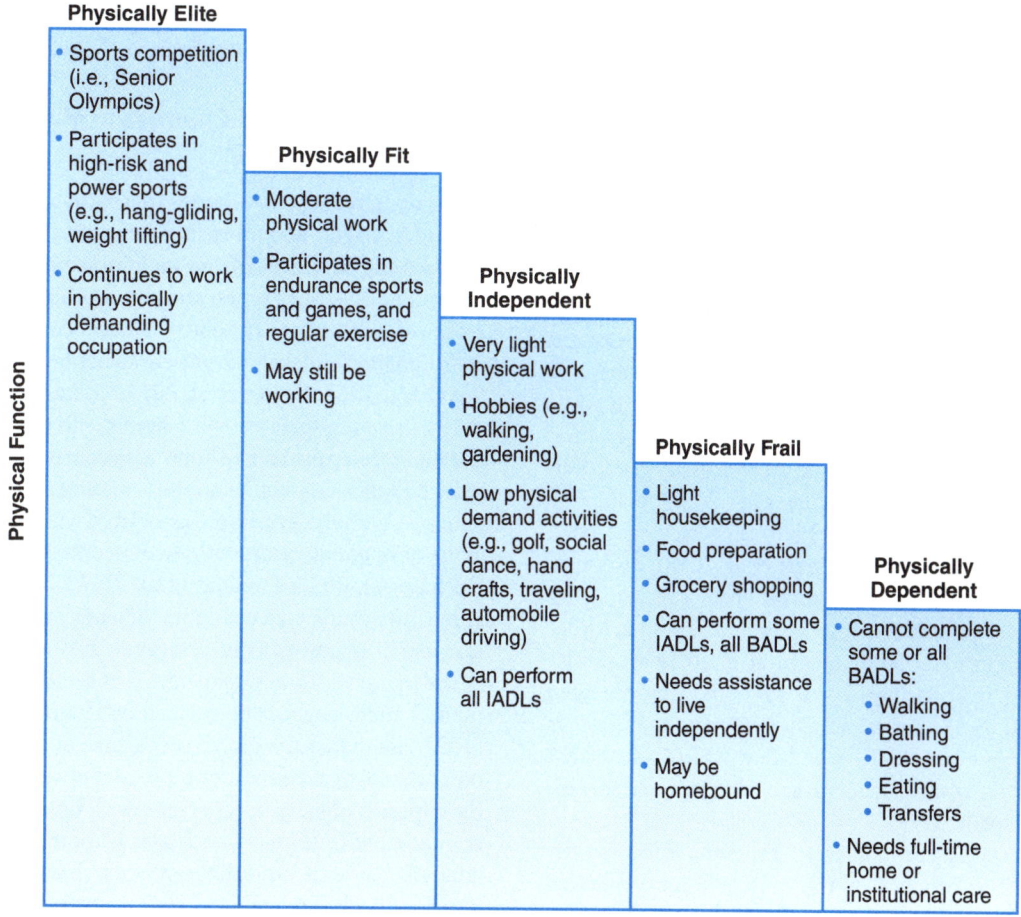

Physically Elite
- Sports competition (i.e., Senior Olympics)
- Participates in high-risk and power sports (e.g., hang-gliding, weight lifting)
- Continues to work in physically demanding occupation

Physically Fit
- Moderate physical work
- Participates in endurance sports and games, and regular exercise
- May still be working

Physically Independent
- Very light physical work
- Hobbies (e.g., walking, gardening)
- Low physical demand activities (e.g., golf, social dance, hand crafts, traveling, automobile driving)
- Can perform all IADLs

Physically Frail
- Light housekeeping
- Food preparation
- Grocery shopping
- Can perform some IADLs, all BADLs
- Needs assistance to live independently
- May be homebound

Physically Dependent
- Cannot complete some or all BADLs:
  - Walking
  - Bathing
  - Dressing
  - Eating
  - Transfers
- Needs full-time home or institutional care

BADLs = basic activities of daily living; IADLs = instrumental activities of daily living.

FIGURE 11-1 The continuum of physical function for older adults. *BADL,* Basic activities of daily living; *IADL,* instrumental activities of daily living. *(Adapted from Spirduso & MacRae, 2005, with permission.)*

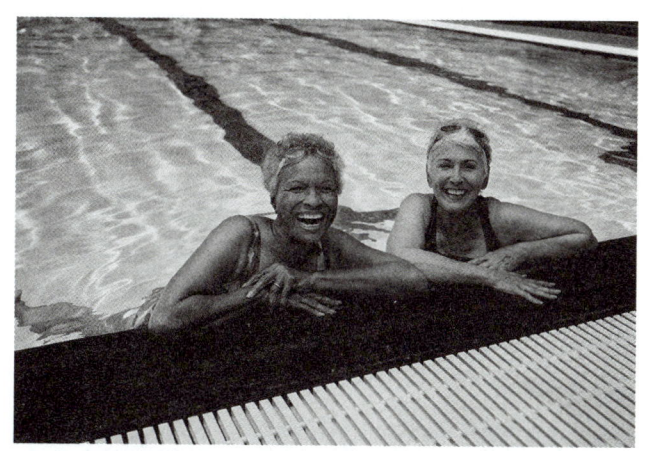

FIGURE 11-2 These older adults continue to be vigorous and active as they age. *(Jupiterimages/Stockbyte/Getty Images.)*

Typical Age-Related Changes in Muscle Strength and Power

Muscle size and function change dramatically across the life span, with rapid initial growth-related increases and aged-related declines later on. It is thought that maximal muscle strength, the amount of force produced in a single maximum contraction of a muscle or muscle group, is generally achieved in the second or third decade and then declines. For example, during tasks that require handgrip force, older adults produce a maximum handgrip force that is lower and is achieved at a slower rate compared with younger age groups (Correa et al, 2020). The effects of aging on muscle strength have been examined by investigating various factors, including type of strength loss (isometric, isotonic, or isokinetic), location of strength loss, and physical activity level and comorbidities of the individuals assessed.

Isometric strength, the maximum force that can be generated without changing the length of a muscle, has been found to change insignificantly until about the sixth decade, when it decreases approximately 1% to 1.5% yearly from age 50 to 70 years by about 3% each year hereafter (Vandervoort, 2002). Concentric strength, the maximum force that can be generated through shortening the length of a muscle, decreases in a pattern similar to isometric strength, with the most dramatic losses occurring after 70 years of age, with upper extremity muscles tending to demonstrate less decline than the lower-extremity muscles (Amaral et al, 2014). Eccentric strength is the maximum force that can be generated through increasing the length of a muscle as it contracts to resist an opposing force, such as when the biceps brachii elongates to lower a dumbbell weight in a biceps curl. Interestingly, eccentric strength declines are not as dramatic as concentric strength changes with age (Vandervoort, 2002) (Fig. 11-3).

Isokinetic strength is the maximum force, or torque, that can be generated through a specific joint ROM at a preestablished velocity of limb movement and is measured using an isokinetic dynamometer. Adults age 60 years or older been found to have 25% to 35% less isokinetic knee extension strength than do younger adults (younger than 60 years), with women experiencing greater losses compared with men (Charlier et al, 2015; Miller et al, 2021). Isokinetic handgrip strength decreases of 20% to 25% have also been reported after 60 years of age (Forrest et al, 2018). However, there is significant variability in the response to aging between different population subgroups. For example, Miller et al (2021) reported that handgrip strength was similar between young women (age 20 to 39 years), middle-aged women (age 40 to 59 years), and older women (age 60 years or older). Forrest et al (2018) found that whites and blacks had higher handgrip strength with age when compared with Asians and Hispanics.

Muscle power is the ability to generate force rapidly (calculated as the product of the muscle force generated multiplied by the velocity of movement) and thus is a combination of both force and speed. Generating peak power requires timing and coordination. Strength and power are separate but related muscle attributes. Measuring muscle power requires more sophisticated and expensive instrumentation and thus is evaluated less frequently in clinical settings. Age-related declines in muscle power are greater than declines in muscle strength, but age-related absolute power and relative power (scaled to body mass) decrease at similar rates: approximately 6% to 11% per decade and 6% to 8% per decade, respectively (Wiegmann et al, 2021).

Typical Age-Related Changes in Muscle Structure

Why do strength and power decrease with aging? Both muscle strength and muscle power are dependent on the number and diameter of the myofibrils within muscle cells, specific muscle fiber types, and the coordination of the neurological elements that control muscle contraction. A variety of changes in skeletal muscle structure occur with aging (Frontera, 2017; Power et al, 2013) (Box 11-1). The loss of muscle mass associated with aging, **sarcopenia,** is one of the main determinants of musculoskeletal impairments and reduced function in older adults (Fielding et al, 2011). Sarcopenia is a complex syndrome associated with muscle mass loss alone or in conjunction with increased fat mass (Petermann-Rocha et al, 2022; Fielding et al, 2011). The prevalence of clinically significant sarcopenia increases with age. Although sarcopenia is prevalent in both men and women, some evidence suggests that sarcopenia is more prevalent in older men. A meta-analysis performed by Petermann-Rocha et al (2022) estimated the global prevalence of sarcopenia among older adults over the age of 60 to be between 10% and 27%. **Sarcopenic obesity** is characterized by low muscle mass combined with high fat mass and is more common in older adults because of typical age-related changes in body composition. Both sarcopenia and sarcopenic obesity are significantly associated with higher levels of functional impairment and lower quality of life (Tyrovolas et al, 2015).

Sarcopenia should not be confused with muscle atrophy, which results from a lack of physical activity, also known as **disuse atrophy.** Sarcopenia is present in healthy, independent older adults and occurs even in elite athletes who maintain very high levels of physical activity, suggesting that typical age-related changes to muscle tissue are the primary cause of muscle mass loss associated with sarcopenia (Cruz-Jentoft, et al, 2014). With sarcopenia, the amount of the muscle mass that is able to contract decreases, resulting in a decrease in strength. This loss in muscle mass is clearly evident when comparing the cross-sectional muscle area between a young adult and an older adult (Fig. 11-4). High correlations between muscle mass and strength have been found in both longitudinal and cross-sectional studies (Wiegmann et al, 2021).

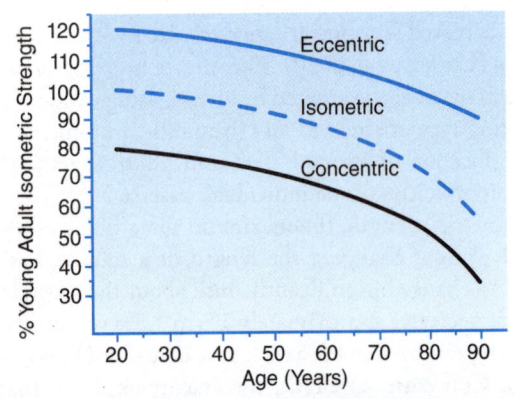

FIGURE 11-3 Effect of age on maximal strength throughout the human lifespan. The shape and height of the schematic curves depend on the type of strength being measured: isometric, concentric, or eccentric. *(From Vandervoort, A. A. [2002]. Aging of the human neuromuscular system. Muscle and Nerve, 25, 17–25, with permission.)*

> ### BOX 11-1 Typical Age-Related Changes in Muscle Morphology
>
> - Decline in the total number of muscle fibers
> - Atrophy of some fibers, hypertrophy of other fibers
> - Loss of muscle mass
> - Increased fatty and connective tissue
> - Myofibrillar degeneration
> - Denervation of muscle fibers

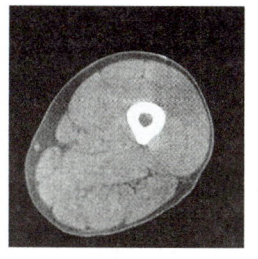

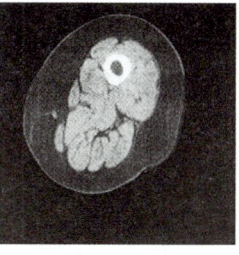

FIGURE 11-4 Magnetic resonance images through the midthigh of a healthy 25-year-old *(left)* and a healthy 75-year-old *(right)*, illustrating sarcopenia. The older adult's image shows smaller muscle mass *(light gray)*, more subcutaneous fat *(dark gray)*, and increased intramuscular fat (dark gray lines). *(From Roubenoff, R. [2003]. Sarcopenia: Effects on body composition and function. Journal of Gerontology: Series A. Biological Sciences and Medical Sciences, 58, 1012–1017, with permission.)*

Decreases in muscle mass are consistent with respect to timing and magnitude of strength loss, with aging and directly or indirectly affect weakness (Gheller et al, 2016). However, in older adults, the rate of muscle weakness exceeds the rate of muscle mass loss (Wiegmann et al, 2021). Although sarcopenia accounts for a large amount of strength loss in older adults, clearly it does not fully explain the strength loss picture. The underlying cause of decreased muscle strength and function is multifactorial, with the extent of contributions and interactions of diverse factors likely varying among individual older adults (Fig. 11-5).

Muscle fibers are characterized as slow- or fast-twitch fibers. Slow-twitch fibers (type I) contract very slowly, are fatigue resistant, and are recruited when muscle contractions must be maintained for long periods (e.g., maintaining an upright position). Fast-twitch fibers (type II) contract very rapidly and develop high tension that can only be sustained for short periods. Type IIb (fast glycolytic) fibers are recruited for activities that require rapid and powerful contractions, whereas type IIa fibers (fast oxidative-glycolytic) contract at an intermediate speed. Studies of age-related changes to the microstructure of muscle, including fiber size, number, and arrangement, have found that there is an overall loss of muscle fibers, types I and II, and a significant decrease in the average size and proportion of type II fibers with age (Frontera, 2017; Power et al, 2013). Age-related muscle weakness may also be attributable to a decrease in muscle force, specifically the amount of force each muscle fiber can produce.

Increases in fat and connective tissue have also been found in aging muscle, resulting in decreased muscle quality (Tieland et al, 2018; Wiegmann et al, 2021). The accumulation of fat within and around muscle tissue is associated with muscle weakness, mobility limitations, and an increased risk of hip fractures, suggesting that these age-related changes in muscle composition contribute to slowness and incoordination of muscle contractions (Tieland et al, 2018). This replacement of muscle tissue with fat tissue is important because it may disrupt the normal orientation of the myofilaments. Loss of muscle tissue in combination with a decline in skeletal muscle fiber numbers reduces the tension a contracting muscle can generate.

Muscle fibers are innervated by motor neurons, and all of the muscle fibers innervated by one motor neuron comprise the motor unit. Approximately 1% of the total number of motor neurons is lost each year beginning in the third decade of life, with this rate increasing after 60 years of age (Power et al, 2013). While age-related loss of motor neurons preferentially affects type II motor units, age-related decreases in motor axon conduction velocity also occur (Power et al, 2013; Tieland et al, 2018). These changes result in a decreased ability to generate muscle force in general and to generate force rapidly.

Skeletal muscle function relies on protein metabolism. Decreased rates of myofibrillar protein synthesis and increased protein turnover associated with aging may be responsible for increased muscle fatigability and decreased type II fibers, respectively (Tan et al, 2020). Diets low in protein have been shown to lead to decreased muscle mass and function in older individuals (Tan et al, 2020). Although decreased nutrition may be more prevalent in older adults in hospitals or institutions, community-dwelling older adults may also have inadequate intakes of protein and energy requirements for a variety of reasons, including age-related changes in the digestive and sensory systems, depression, social isolation, and functional losses secondary to acute and chronic health problems (Corish & Bardon, 2019).

Another factor that may influence age-related changes in muscle strength is the decreased number of capillaries per muscle fiber. The greater the number of capillaries per muscle fiber or the greater the number of capillaries that surround a muscle fiber, the better the oxygen exchange capacity. These decreases may also contribute to age-related changes in muscle structure and strength (Power et al, 2013). Different muscles in an older adult change to different degrees, with respect to reduction in the numbers of fibers. Despite these typical age-related changes, several studies have found that older individuals who have high levels of physical activity

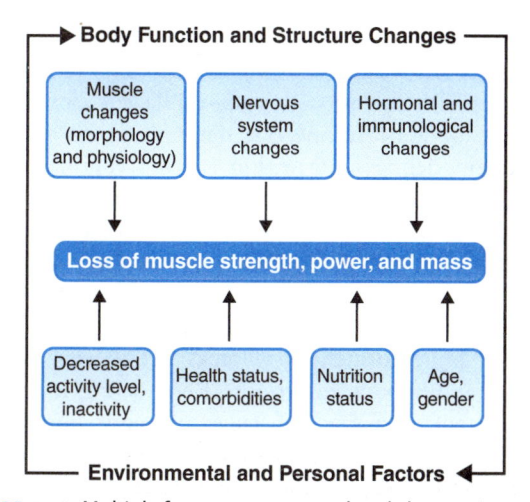

FIGURE 11-5 Multiple factors cause age-related changes in muscle strength and power.

tend to preserve their muscle structure and performance and experience only moderate losses in muscle strength and physical function (Ciolac, 2013).

Typical Age-Related Muscle Changes and Occupational Performance

Muscle strength is one of the main determinants of functional mobility when performing ADLs. An estimated 13% of men age 65 to 74 years and 40% age 85 years or older are unable to perform at least one of the following activities: lift a 10-pound weight, stoop or kneel down, reach overhead, write or grasp small objects, or walk two to three blocks. Among women, 19% of those age 65 to 74 years and 53% of those age 85 years or older are unable to perform at least one of these activities (Federal Interagency Forum on Aging-Related Statistics, 2016). Skeletal muscle weakness can lead to impaired mobility and occupational performance, decreased walking speed, loss of independence, poor balance, increased risk of falls, hospitalization, and mortality (Federal Interagency Forum on Aging-Related Statistics, 2016; Tieland et al, 2018). Typical age-related decreases in lean body mass and a concomitant increase in fat mass combined with displacement of the body, such as during walking, will place a greater metabolic load on muscle fibers, causing an increase in the energy cost of walking (Malatesta et al, 2003). Hence, sarcopenia not only leads to decreased muscle strength but is also associated with increased metabolic cost of movement.

Muscle power may be even more influential than muscle strength on an older adult's mobility, physical function, and functional performance (Gerstner et al, 2017). This is extremely relevant because functional mobility and most ADLs require the generation of power in addition to strength. Lower-extremity muscle power has been shown to be correlated with balance problems and falls in older adults (Winger et al, 2022).

The pooled results of 45 studies in a meta-analysis showed there are important reasons to maintain or increase muscle strength and power in older adults because there is a link between strength impairments and the development of activity limitations and restrictions in occupational participation (Wang et al, 2020). For example, impaired balance is a predictor of disability, with the risk increasing when combined with muscle weakness. Slow gait speed, decreased lower-extremity muscle strength, lower handgrip strength, and lower muscle mass are predictors of ADL and IADL performance limitations (Wang et al, 2020).

Typical Age-Related Changes in the Skeletal System

Next, we describe the ways in which the skeletal system forms and then changes in later life. The skeletal system functions to:

- Provide a stable framework (mechanical support) that enables muscle contractions to generate force and movement (e.g., act as a lever system for muscle action)
- Protect soft tissues and vital organs
- Serve as a reservoir for calcium homeostasis and a site for red blood cell production
- Trap toxic minerals

Late-life changes affect the extent to which the skeletal system functions effectively. Peak bone mass (PBM) is achieved during young adulthood; after the third decade, bone mass decreases (Watts et al, 2021). Initially, the rate of bone loss is slow and similar for men and premenopausal women. It is important to note that the balance between bone formation and bone resorption differs not only in different bones (e.g., weight-bearing versus non–weight-bearing bones) but also in different types of bone tissue (e.g., cortical tissue versus trabecular tissue). Trabecular bone tissue is the inner spongy bone tissue found in joints and vertebrae, whereas cortical bone tissue is the dense bone tissue found in the long bones of the arms and legs that covers the trabecular bone tissue of joints and vertebrae. From midlife onward, trabecular bone tissue is lost at a steady rate, while the rate of cortical bone tissue loss increases (Chen et al, 2013). Between the ages of 60 and 90 years, total trabecular bone volume decreases by an estimated 25% in the spinal vertebrae, femoral neck, and distal radius, with cortical bone thickness decreasing 3% to 5% per decade (Chen et al, 2013). During menopause, women experience rapid bone loss, at a rate of 2.5% to 3.0% of total bone volume each year, as well as greater losses in cortical bone thickness than men over a lifetime (Chen et al, 2013; Goltzman, 2019). After about 10 years, the rate of loss slows to match that of men. For both men and women, PBM is tightly controlled by genetics, and bone loss due to temporary perturbations, such as prolonged bedrest, may be prevented or quickly recovered after successful rehabilitation (Goltzman, 2019; Kramer et al, 2017). For older adults, the consequence of the age-related bone loss depends on PBM, the extent and rate of bone turnover, and the quality of the bone tissue.

Adult bone undergoes continuous repair, accrual, and release of mineral stores and adaptive shaping (or reshaping) of the skeleton. Bone remodeling is the primary process through which the adult skeleton repairs and adapts and is the process responsible for bone shape. The rate of bone turnover is determined by the number of remodeling units within a given volume of bone at a given time. The major types of bone cells activated in a coordinated fashion within each remodeling unit are osteocytes, cells embedded in mineralized bone that direct remodeling when mechanical stressors in the environment are detected. Osteoblasts are cells responsible for bone formation, whereas osteoclasts are cells responsible for bone resorption. Remodeling is initiated on the bone surface. Trabecular (spongy) bone tissue, found in the spine, flat bones, and ends of long bones, has greater surface area than the less porous cortical bone tissue surrounding the trabecular bone and marrow. Because of this, more remodeling units are active in the trabecular bone tissue, which explains the greater loss of trabecular bone by midlife. Bone remodeling becomes less active and more unbalanced during the second half of life, with increased bone resorption and decreased bone formation resulting in a net loss of bone (Sfeir et al, 2022). Nevertheless, with aging, isolated osteoblast activity on the outer surface of long bone cortical compartments results in bone mineral spatial distribution such that the mechanical strength is preserved to some extent as bone is lost.

Bone health is affected by nonmodifiable factors such as age, sex, race, ethnicity, and genetics (e.g., cellular regulation, family history of disease) and by modifiable factors such as nutrition (e.g., calcium and Vitamin D intake), physical activity, body weight, smoking, alcohol consumption, socioeconomic status, and hormones (Wilson-Barnes et al, 2022; Zhu & Zheng, 2021). After achieving PBM, strategies for increasing bone mass have limited success (Zhu & Zheng, 2021). However, the rate at which bone is lost may be attenuated by targeting modifiable factors (Wilson-Barnes et al, 2022). Bone mineral was redistributed in the region that is weakest for resisting bending; therefore, the small change in mineral placement associated with hormone replacement therapy and high-impact progressive resistance exercise may have significant effects on the strength of the aging skeleton. Bone, muscle, and fat are derived from the same mesenchymal stem cells (MSCs), and the development of MSCs depends to some extent on environmental conditions. Studies have shown that bouts of low-intensity vibration stimulate bone and muscle formation, increase muscle force activity, and promote MSC differentiation into osteoblasts rather than fat cells (Sen et al, 2011).

Typical Age-Related Changes in Cartilage, Joints, and Tendons

Age-related changes in cartilage, tendons, and joints are associated with alterations in collagen and elastin extensibility and decreases in various proteins found in cartilage (Table 11-1). Connective tissue is found nearly everywhere in the body, and all types of connective tissue have similar features. Collagen is the basic protein component in fibrous connective tissue found in bone, tendon, ligaments, and cartilage. Collagen fibers are arranged in crisscrossing bundles that are chemically linked *(cross-linkage)* to form structure in the body and are strong and flexible in the younger years. As a person ages, there is increased cross-linkage of fibers, resulting in more dense matrices. As these matrices become denser, the collagen structures become stiffer, and the cellular movement of nutrients and waste materials becomes impaired (Burr, 2019). Elastin molecules also have a specific arrangement *(a lattice-type network)* that allows connective tissue to return to its original shape after being stretched. With aging, the amount of elastin also decreases, further affecting the elasticity of connective tissues. Many of the cellular changes seen with aging are also seen in cases of inactivity or when the effects of weight-bearing are limited, such as bedrest. Thus, lack of physical activity can accentuate the normal effects of aging on connective tissue (Mavropalias et al, 2022).

TABLE 11-1 ■ Normal Age-Related Changes That Affect Bone, Cartilage, Tendons, and Joints

	DESCRIPTION, STRUCTURE, AND FUNCTION	CHANGES WITH AGING	FUNCTIONAL IMPLICATIONS
Collagen	The main protein of connective tissue and main component of cartilage, ligaments, tendons, and bone Arranged in crisscross pattern to provide structure and tensile strength to connective tissue	Increased cross-linkage of fibers Increased shortening and distortion of collagen fibers that become more dense and stiff	Increased stiffness of tissues Decreased mobility of tissues Decreased hydration Decreased tensile strength
Elastin	A connective tissue protein Lattice-type network arrangement allows elastin to return to its original shape after being stretched	Progressive decrease in amount of elastin	Decreased elasticity of tissues Decreased ease of movement of tissues
Hyaluronic acid	Secreted by connective tissue ribosomes, especially those in cartilage Helps regulate viscosity of tissue Decreases amount of friction	Decrease in hyaluronic acid secretion Decrease in hyaluronic acid molecule size	Decreased tensile strength Tissue degradation
Glycoproteins	Small molecules of soluble protein Produces osmotic force in extracellular matrix, which helps maintain fluid content of tissues	Decreased production and release of glycoproteins	Decreased hydration of tissues
Proteoglycans	Made up of a core protein to which chains of glycosaminoglycans are attached Resist complete compression of cartilage during joint motion	Aggrecan (large proteoglycan found in articular cartilage) molecules become smaller and structurally altered.	Decreased hydration of tissues

Synovial joints are typically found at the end of long bones of the upper and lower extremities. The ends of the bones in synovial joints are covered with hyaline cartilage, which acts as a shock absorber and, along with synovial fluid, greatly decreases the amount of friction during synovial joint movement. Cartilage is a unique connective tissue that is avascular. Rather, blood flow in adjacent bones and synovial fluid provides the nutrients to chondroblasts in cartilage. Chondroblasts secrete glycoproteins and hyaluronic acid that lubricate the joint. The joint capsule that surrounds the synovial joint is composed of a thick layer of dense connective tissue, and a synovial membrane lines most of the joint cavity. The membrane produces synovial fluid that fills the joint cavity and provides lubrication, nourishes the articular cartilage, and acts as a shock absorber when the joint is compressed. With aging, the cartilage that normally covers the joints thins and deteriorates, especially in the weight-bearing joints. Decreases in water content of the cartilage, decreased hydration of the joint, decreased elasticity of the joint capsule, and increased fibrous growth contribute to increased joint stiffness (Li et al, 2013). In addition to the muscle structure and characteristic changes described previously in this chapter, muscle tissue becomes less flexible and more rigid secondary to a decrease in elastin and an increase in collagen cross-linkages. Tendons and ligaments also become less resilient to length changes (Marcucci & Reggiani, 2020).

Joint ROM and flexibility depend on the condition of the soft tissues of the joints, tendons, ligaments, and muscles and are specific to each joint of the body. Maximum ROM gradually decreases with age. Older adults tend to be less flexible than their younger counterparts, though women are typically being more flexible than men (Milanović et al, 2013). However, the effect of age on ROM is nonuniform, affecting specific joints and specific movements differently. Descriptive data on age-related differences in flexibility in a large cross-sectional sample of male and female community-dwelling older adults age 55 to 86 years suggest a decrease in flexibility of the shoulder and hip joints by approximately 6° per decade (Stathokostas et al, 2013). Inadequate ROM and inflexibility in older adults can affect occupational performance (e.g., ADLs such as dressing), IADL performance (e.g., reaching into the cupboard to put away groceries), and motor skills (e.g., walking, bending, stair climbing). Loss of flexibility and ROM have important implications for older adults because these impairments can contribute to an increased risk of falls, such as when an older individual is unable to quickly react to recover from a loss of balance (Marcucci & Reggiani, 2020).

CASE STUDY

Presenting Situation

Mr. Martinez is a 78-year-old man who is 2 days postsurgical open reduction/internal fixation for a right proximal femur fracture. Mr. Martinez states that he was getting in and out of his bathtub after taking a shower when his right leg gave way. He felt immediate, intense pain. Mr. Martinez dragged himself to the living room and called the emergency medical system using his cell phone. Physician orders in the hospital for Mr. Martinez included "occupational therapy for discharge home" and "ambulation weight-bearing as tolerated."

Occupational Profile

Mr. Martinez lives with his wife, whom he met and were married in Mexico City, Mexico. They emigrated to the United States in their early 30s to seek new job prospects. They have two sons, both of whom live nearby with their families in a rural county. Mr. Martinez retired from cattle farming at age 70, when he decided he would "take life easy and let my son do all the hard work."

Medical History

Mr. Martinez has a history of hypertension, coronary artery disease, obesity, OA in both hips, obstructive sleep apnea, depression, and cataracts. He has difficulty with driving at night and is planning to have cataract surgery in the near future. His medications include two antihypertensives, an antilipemic, and an antidepressant.

Questions

1. What assessments will the occupational therapist perform?
2. What further information is needed that will be assessed by other team members?

Answers

1. In acute care, the clinician's primary role is to prepare the client for safe discharge. Occupational therapy assessments focus on obtaining an occupational profile to assess the patient's physical home environment, caregiver support, prior level of function, and current level of function. This will help inform the care team to plan the safest location for discharge. Useful assessments of the musculoskeletal system include screening for ROM, grip strength, and gross motor strength using manual muscle tests. The Borg Rating of Perceived Exertion (RPE) scale may be useful to assess the client's activity tolerance. Other functional tests may include the Activity Measure for Post Acute Care, Functional Independence Measure, or Modified Barthel Index LO 11-4, LO 11-5.
2. It may be useful to know the client's scores on balance assessments, such as the Berg Balance Scale, and ability to ascend steps and stairs as assessed by a physical therapist. It will also be useful to know the client's vital signs throughout the stay, including blood pressure, heart rate, and oxygen saturation, which are regularly assessed by nurses and nursing

assistants. It will also be important to examine the client's recent laboratory values (e.g., hemoglobin and hematocrit levels) for contraindications to participation in therapeutic activity after surgery (See Management of Musculoskeletal Impairments; LO 11-4, 11-5).

Atypical Age-Related Changes in the Musculoskeletal System

Next, we focus on some of the common health conditions that affect the musculoskeletal system in older adults. The two most prevalent musculoskeletal health conditions in older adults, OA and osteoporosis, are described. Because limb amputation may occur in older adults, often due to DM and vascular disease–related complications, limb amputation in the context of the age-related changes is described.

Musculoskeletal health conditions that cause loss of mobility and physical independence can be particularly devastating for older adults, both physically and psychologically. The importance of physical activity in managing ailments associated with aging is largely recognized in healthcare, but difficult for older adults to obtain when they are managing a painful musculoskeletal condition. There is a strong correlation between painful musculoskeletal conditions and a reduced capacity to participate in physical activity, which results in frailty, a general functional decline, and reduced independence (Briggs et al, 2016).

Osteoarthritis

OA is characterized by the degradation and loss of articular cartilage and active bone remodeling. With OA, the cartilage becomes thinner, tears, and disrupts the joint capsule. As the cartilage wears, eburnation (erosion of cartilaginous tissue), spur formation (osteophytes), synovitis, and thickening of the capsule occur, all resulting in decreased joint integrity. Individuals with OA commonly report joint pain, stiffness, swelling, decreased ROM, and crepitus (grating, grinding, cracking sensation) with movement. Pain is usually relieved by rest; paradoxically, most individuals with OA report a period of morning stiffness.

OA is the most common form of joint disease, globally affecting over 500 million people. It is one of the leading causes of disability in older adults, with women at greater risk. Rates of OA have increased 114% between 1990 and 2019 (Hunter et al, 2020). Hip and knee OA ranked as the 11th highest contributor to global disability and the 38th highest in disability-adjusted life years of 291 conditions investigated (Cross et al, 2014). Clearly, with the aging of the world's population and the increasing incidence of obesity globally, occupational therapy practitioners must be prepared for a large increase in the health service demands for older adults with OA.

Risk Factors, Signs, and Symptoms of Osteoarthritis

According to Johnson & Hunter (2014), OA is believed to be the result of a combination of mechanical, cellular, and biochemical factors interacting to cause OA in any given individual. Risk factors for OA include nonmodifiable factors such as increased age, genetics, and sex, with females being more susceptible to OA than men. As individuals age, joint tissues lose their ability to adapt to biomechanical stress and insults, and tissue integrity is compromised by cellular senescence and age-related sarcopenia (Johnson & Hunter, 2014). Although racial minorities account for only 3 million of the total 30 million OA cases in the United States, African Americans with OA tend to have the most severe forms of joint pain, functional and activity limitations, and decreases in mobility (Vina et al, 2018). African Americans with lower socioeconomic status have demonstrated even more severe pain compared with African Americans of middle and high economic status or white individuals, suggesting these disparities may be partly due to socioeconomic factors. African Americans also experience higher levels of stress related to their OA, which may affect their ability to effectively manage their pain (Booker et al, 2020).

Modifiable risk factors for OA include obesity, high physical workload occupations, and participation in high-impact sports, such as heavy weightlifting or long-distance running. Individuals have a higher risk of developing OA in their hands if they frequently engage in tasks that require repetitive fine motor movements. A dose-response relationship has been observed between body mass index (BMI) and OA, with a 35% increased risk of OA in the knees for every 5-unit increase in BMI (Johnson & Hunter, 2014). OA can occur in any joint, but most often affects the hips, knees, and joints of the hands.

Management of OA

Interventions to manage OA are typically directed at multiple levels. One of the most important aspects of management is the reduction or modification of risk factors, especially obesity. Exercise has also been found to improve symptoms and restore function, including gentle exercises such as tai chi and patient-directed activity programs (Buelt & Narducci, 2021). Although patient education on joint protection is a key element to an OA management plan, it has been found that patient education is often lacking in OA management by medical professionals, possibly due to discrepancies between the views of OA management among different professions (Ackerman et al, 2021).

Occupational therapy practitioners are well equipped to educate older adults on joint protection strategies and adaptive equipment that facilitate older adults' participation in meaningful occupations. OA in the joints of the hand can make completing daily tasks challenging and painful. Assistive devices with built-up handles or large grips can make holding onto small objects easier, such as writing utensils and kitchen tools. For example, kitchen tools that are ergonomically designed to reduce the force and endurance required can be recommended to complete cooking tasks. For individuals with OA in the joints of the hands, a certified hand therapist, who could be either an occupational or physical therapist, can provide pain relief modalities, ROM exercises, and individualized joint protection strategies. Strength training and physical fitness exercises are strongly recommended to improve function and decrease pain and disability in all affected joints but are often underutilized by individuals with OA (Ackerman et al, 2021).

It has also been found that cognitive behavioral therapy and balance training can improve OA symptoms in some patients and that acupuncture and thermal modalities result in slight improvements in symptoms and function (Buelt & Narducci, 2021). Pharmacological management consists of analgesics, nonsteroidal anti-inflammatory medications, topical agents, and glucosamine, which manage symptoms well in the short term (Buelt & Narducci, 2021). Of note, opioids are routinely prescribed for individuals with OA, despite this treatment not being listed in the guidelines from the American College of Rheumatology and Arthritis Foundation. In the United States between 2007 and 2014, opioids were prescribed for 13% of patients with hip OA and 16% with knee OA (Ackerman et al, 2021). Intraarticular injection of corticosteroids and arthroscopic surgery to remove loose cartilage or large osteophytes is often beneficial for patients with advanced OA. As a last resort, joint replacement is performed for patients with intractable pain or severely compromised function who have not responded well to conservative treatments.

Total joint replacements are highly effective in restoring function and quality of life for individuals with end-stage OA, with a success rate of 90% (Hafkamp et al, 2020). However, only 28% of patients report satisfaction with the results of their surgery, likely due to patients having high expectations for an immediate improvement in symptoms and function shortly after surgery. It is also possible that patients misremember themselves having a higher level of function before the surgery than they actually had. Conversely, high expectations of a total joint replacement can actually encourage positive results, as patients are motivated to reach their expectations after surgery (Hafkamp et al, 2020). Thus, management of expectations is an important component of therapeutic interventions after total joint replacement surgery.

After a total joint replacement surgery, occupational therapy practitioners can help older patients reach their highest level of function during their recovery while maintaining joint precautions. For example, occupational therapy practitioners can instruct patients on moving their affected joint safely while completing ADLs, such as dressing and bathing, and using adaptive equipment as needed. Occupational therapy practitioners can further facilitate patients' recovery through functional mobility training during daily tasks and IADLs. For example, occupational therapy practitioners can instruct patients on safe mobility and transfer techniques using a walker or other ambulation device while completing more complex tasks, such as cooking or laundry.

Activity pacing as well as land- and water-based therapeutic exercise programs are beneficial for people with OA. Education about activity pacing has been found to reduce joint stiffness, fatigue, and pain in people with hip and knee OA; individualized interventions were also found to be effective (Buelt & Narducci, 2021). Therapeutic exercise programs consisting of traditional muscle strengthening, functional training, and aerobic fitness exercise have been found to reduce pain and improve physical function among people with symptomatic hip OA and in people with knee OA (Fransen et al, 2014, 2015). Aquatic exercise decreases pain and disability and improves quality of life in people with knee and hip OA (Bartels et al, 2016). Aquatic exercises can be particularly beneficial for those with OA because movement in water applies less strain on the joints. There is some evidence suggesting that tai chi can increase lower-extremity strength and improve overall balance, thus lowering patients' risk of falls, though results are highly dependent on session duration, frequency, and intensity (Yang & Liu, 2021).

Because there are discrepancies between the views of OA management among different professions, there is the potential for interprofessional collaboration to improve patient outcomes (Ackerman et al, 2021). For example, because of their convenient locations in pharmacies throughout communities, pharmacists are in an ideal position to contribute to patients' management of their OA symptoms (McLachlan et al, 2021). Pharmacists are trained to counsel patients on medications to manage OA. Additionally, they are well positioned to bridge the gap that is often present between what a patient is told by their healthcare providers and what they understand about the management of their OA symptoms, allowing the patient to significantly improve self-management of OA symptoms (McLachlan et al, 2021). Occupational therapy practitioners can collaborate with pharmacists and advise patients to talk with a pharmacist regarding questions about managing their medications and symptoms of OA, such as pain. See Promoting Best Practice Box 11-1.

PROMOTING BEST PRACTICE 11-1
Occupational Therapy Intervention After Joint Replacement

After total joint replacement surgery, best practice in occupational therapy includes:

- Education on modified mobility during performance of ADLs
- Education on adaptive equipment to complete ADLs and practice with equipment
- Functional performance of IADLs, including cooking, laundry, housekeeping, and car transfers
- Instruction and practice with the use of mobility devices during functional activities including how to carry items while using a walker or cane
- Education and practice of activity pacing during the performance of daily activities
- Therapeutic exercises such as aquatic therapy, aerobics, and tai chi

- Encouragement of patients to self-manage their OA, including educating them on the pathology and encouraging discussions with doctors and pharmacists regarding disease management
- The performance of a falls assessment to address specific fall risks

Osteoporosis, Falls, and Fractures

Falls are the leading cause of fatal and nonfatal injuries among adults age 65 years or older (Bergen et al, 2016). A fall can be defined as an event which results in a person resting unintentionally on a lower level (World Health Organization, 2021). According to the Centers for Disease Control and Prevention, approximately 27,000 older adults in 2014 died in fall-related incidents, with 2.8 million people being treated in emergency departments for injuries from falls (Bergen et al, 2016). In 2014 alone, 28.7% of older adults reported falling within 1 year, with an estimated 29 million falls. Although falls are incredibly common within the older adult population, it is estimated that only half of older adults who fall discuss it with their healthcare provider (Bergen et al, 2016). Fall risk and fall prevention can be difficult to discuss with individuals who fear stigmatization surrounding the topic. Many older adults fear being labeled a "faller" by healthcare providers and family members. These fears often coincide with ageist assumptions, that older adults are feeble, unsafe, and cannot be trusted alone. Others may fear that falling is a sign of aging and therefore a threat to their identity, while others wish to not be perceived as cognitively impaired (Hoffman et al, 2018). Because of this, it is important that healthcare providers recognize the stigma associated with falling and reframe questions to normalize the experience of falls. One way to normalize the discussion of falls is to reframe questions from "Have you fallen?" to "Have you experienced a fall, even if the cause was accidental?" It is also important that healthcare providers and surveyors clearly define a fall to include incidences such as "tripping" and "stumbling", which many individuals do not include in the category of falls (Hoffman et al, 2018). These strategies can help healthcare providers obtain a clearer understanding of fall risk and implement appropriate fall prevention interventions.

Key risk factors for falls include abnormal gait, balance, and muscle strength. Other risk factors include reduced ability to stand on one leg, decreased walking speed, diminished grip strength, and difficulty transferring from sitting to standing. Cognition is also a key contributor to falls. Older adults with a moderate to severe cognitive impairment are more likely to fall and are at greater risk of serious injury than individuals without cognitive impairment. Factors such as slower processing speed and impaired executive function skills can increase fall risk, but the use of high-risk medications and other substances (e.g., alcohol) can interact with baseline cognitive impairments, further increasing fall risk.

A 2016 population-based study found that participants experiencing injury from a fall were "more likely to be older, women, have fewer years of formal schooling, have chronic diseases, use fall-increasing drugs, be less physically active, have lower body mass index, and have experienced a previous injurious fall" (Welmer et al, 2017). Finally, environmental hazards are an important risk factor for falls. Environmental hazards in an older adult's home may include clutter, unclear floors or pathways, low lighting, lack of handrails for stairs, and uneven flooring. The interaction between environmental hazards and an older adult's physical abilities and cognition can further increase the risk of falls (Montero-Odasso & Speechley, 2018).

Older individuals with lower-extremity OA are more likely to experience a fall than their peers without OA. It is estimated that 30% of community-dwelling older adults will sustain a fall each year, whereas 45% of older adults with lower-extremity OA will sustain a fall (Hunter et al, 2020). In persons with OA of the lower extremities, fall risk factors include pain, lower-limb weakness, slower reactions to disruptions of balance, and impaired functional ability (e.g., ability to rise from a chair). Additionally, the risk of falls and fractures is elevated in older adults prescribed narcotics to control OA pain, such as low-level opioids like tramadol (Musich et al, 2021). An individual's risk of falling has been shown to be positively correlated with the number of arthritic joints they have: people with OA in one joint have a 53% greater risk of falling, people with two arthritic joints have a 74% greater risk, and those with three or four joints with OA have an 85% great risk of falling (Doré et al, 2015). Arnold & Gyurcsik (2012) developed a conceptual integrated framework for fall-risk screening and assessment of people with OA based on the American Geriatrics Society's and British Geriatrics Society's 2011 clinical practice guideline for prevention of falls in older persons (Panel on Prevention of Falls in Older Persons, 2011). These adapted clinical practice guidelines for persons with OA underscore the importance of including fall prevention interventions in the care of older adults with musculoskeletal health conditions.

Falls can create a multitude of injuries for older adults, including fracture, soft tissue injuries, bruises, lacerations, dislocations, functional decline, decreased activity level, functional dependence, depression, and death (Terroso et al, 2012). Fractures in older adults are often attributed to a combination of falls and osteoporosis (Morrison et al, 2012). Osteoporosis, which manifests as a fragility fracture, is a growing public health problem throughout the world, in part because of the increasing number of people living beyond age 65 years. **Osteoporosis** is defined as a skeletal disorder characterized by compromised bone strength, predisposing a person to an increased risk of fracture (NIH Consensus Development Panel on Osteoporosis Prevention, 2001). Low bone mass and microarchitectural deterioration in bone tissue lead to bone fragility and a resultant increased risk of fractures among older adults with osteoporosis

(NIH Consensus Development Panel on Osteoporosis Prevention, 2001). Even a minor fall can result in a lifestyle-altering fracture. The most common skeletal sites for osteoporotic fractures are the vertebral body and proximal femur (Warriner et al, 2011).

Management of Osteoporosis

For older adults with osteoporotic vertebral fracture, consultation with an occupational therapist is recommended to ensure safe and appropriate performance of ADLs and activities (Giangregorio et al, 2015). It is also recommended that individuals with osteoporosis engage in a multicomponent exercise program that includes resistance training in combination with balance training (Giangregorio et al, 2015). Furthermore, it is recommended that individuals with osteoporosis not engage in aerobic training to the exclusion of resistance or balance training. For older adults with osteoporosis, physical activity can address some of the factors that contribute to risk of spinal injury, such as body weight and posture, spine curvatures, muscle forces, and neuromuscular control. However, not all risk factors (e.g., vertebral height and disc degeneration) can be addressed through exercise. Exercise prescription can also address impairments to improve body mechanics during daily activities. It is unsafe for people with or at risk for osteoporotic fracture to (1) repeatedly flex the spine forward without using a hip-knee-ankle strategy, (2) rotate the upper spine with respect to the pelvis (or vice versa) past midline, (3) hold loads unevenly or away from the midline of the body, and (4) perform activities or movements in a way that puts the body off balance (MacIntyre et al., 2014; Recknor et al, 2013). The main goals of therapeutic exercise for individuals with osteoporosis include fall prevention, safe movement, reduced rate of bone loss, and pain control as required.

Common across all these goals is the aim of maintaining or increasing muscle strength, power, and endurance and preventing future fragility fractures. A tailored multimodal treatment program, which includes patient and caregiver education, ADL/IADL retraining, functional mobility training, and appropriate referrals to other healthcare professionals may be beneficial to restore and maintain function and occupational performance.

Physical activity guidelines for older adults—such as those issued by the Canadian Society for Exercise Physiology, Centers for Disease Control and Prevention, and American College of Sports Medicines—recommend 150 minutes of moderate to vigorous intensity aerobic physical activity per week for general health benefits (Chodzko-Zajko et al, 2009). Meta-analysis determined that at least 2 hours per week of exercise that includes challenging balance exercises was most effective for fall prevention (Sherrington et al, 2011). If time is limited, resistance and balance training should take priority over aerobic exercise. See Box 11-2 for guideline recommendations for people with osteoporosis and no fragility fracture (Giangregorio et al, 2015).

> **BOX 11-2** Too-Fit-to-Fracture Initiative Exercise Recommendations for People With Osteoporosis and No Fragility Fracture
>
> - Weight-bearing aerobic activity preferable
> - Progressive resistance training designed to increase muscle strength
> - 8–12 repetitions
> - Intensity rating of 5 to 8 on a 0 to 10 scale for perceived exertion
> - Balance training strongly recommended
> - 2 hours per week or 20 minutes per day
> - Daily exercise to increase muscular endurance in spinal extensors

For people with osteoporosis and one or more vertebral fractures, with or without pain, and hyperkyphosis, consensus was that the guidelines in Box 11-2 are not appropriate (Giangregorio et al, 2015). The following is recommended instead:

- At least 150 minutes per week of moderate-intensity aerobic activity in bouts of 10 minutes or more
- Vigorous aerobic activity may not be appropriate
- Progressive resistance training designed to increase muscle strength, with emphasis on form and alignment instead of intensity
- Balance training strongly recommended—2 hours per week or 20 minutes per day
- Daily exercises to increase muscular endurance of spinal extensors, in positions in which the spine is least loaded, when possible (supine < standing < seated)
- Education by physical or occupational therapists about appropriate positioning and alignment, body mechanics, transitions, use of assistive aids, and pain control

It is recognized that when applying this information in the rehabilitation setting, occupational therapy practitioners should consider important factors such as the prevalence of osteoporosis within each clinic, therapeutic goals, and client-specific factors, such as history of and time since fracture, comorbid conditions that affect bone biology, medication use (e.g., length of time on bone-sparing medication), physical performance, and the client's motivation and goals for participating in a rehabilitation program.

Occupational therapy interventions for fall-related fractures will follow the physician's plan of care for managing the fracture. There are numerous treatment options that physicians may adopt including conservative treatment, internal or external fixation procedures, and partial or complete joint replacements (Baertle et al, 2020). Rehabilitation protocols may also be influenced by postsurgical protocols for exercise and weight-bearing, which vary depending on the surgeon and individual client's needs.

For upper-extremity fractures, exercises may include shoulder pendulum exercises and active-assisted ROM exercises, following physician protocols. Occupational therapy practitioners can provide education to the client regarding the importance of adhering to these protocols to reduce further injury, decrease pain and stiffness, and improve mobility in the affected limb. When choosing occupation-based interventions after a fracture, it is important to obtain an occupational profile to assess which areas of occupation need to be modified to allow for safe participation. Examples include training on strategies to perform transfers to a bedside commode with one nonweightbearing lower extremity, strategies to don and doff a shirt with an affected upper extremity, and strengthening of the unaffected extremities to improve safety with functional mobility. A recommendation for durable medical equipment may also be necessary to improve the client's ability to perform ADLs and IADLs safely and independently at home and in the community (Wong et al, 2018).

Amputation in Older Adults

Determining an accurate estimation of the incidence and prevalence of limb amputation worldwide is challenging due to conflicting published data. An estimated 57.7 million people were living with limb amputation due to traumatic causes worldwide in 2017 (McDonald et al, 2020). However, traumatic causes of amputations, such as falls and other mechanical forces, account for the minority of lower-extremity amputations. Up to 75% of all lower-extremity amputations are performed due to complications with diabetic foot disease, and it is estimated that over 50% of all limb amputations can be attributed to complications related to peripheral artery disease (PAD). This is because DM is known to both increase the incidence of PAD as well as accelerate the progression of PAD. The incidence of DM and circulatory diseases increase with age, and globally, the prevalence of DM rose to 8.8%, or 415 million people, in 2015 (Narres et al, 2017). The incidence of comorbidities such as DM, PAD, kidney disease, and other associated diseases, accompanied by poorer preoperative functional status, put older adults at an increased risk of morbidity and mortality related to limb amputation (Pandit et al, 2020). In the United States, the number of patients undergoing lower-extremity amputation is growing, and the amputation rates in those over age 65 years is expected to continue to rise with the aging U.S. population (Narres et al, 2017).

Racial and ethnic disparities are associated with amputation, with African Americans and Hispanic Americans having a higher prevalence of DM, PAD, and other comorbidities than nonHispanic whites. Amputation risk secondary to associated comorbidities is two to three times higher in Hispanics than non-Hispanic whites. African Americans also have a higher incidence of comorbidities, risk of amputation, and postamputation mortality (Pandit et al, 2020).

Amputation and Occupational Performance

Amputation can have significant effects on the occupational performance and well-being of older adults. Lower-extremity amputation in older adults with DM puts clients at risk for reduced quality of life, increased medical costs, and mortality (Narres et al, 2017). Depending on the location of the amputation, an amputation can affect functional mobility, self-care, fine motor tasks, and tasks that require bilateral upper or lower-extremity gross motor coordination. For older adults experiencing muscle weakness, cognitive changes, and other medical comorbidities, amputation can impact their recovery and may result in decreased independence. For example, amputation may negatively affect functional status, living situations, work status, and family and caregiver dynamics, putting additional strain on clients and their families. It is common for older adults to have negative emotions and thoughts after an amputation. Changes in habits and loss of independence can create feelings of burden and inadequacy. Denial, depression, anxiety, and suicidal thoughts may be present. In addition to coping with the loss of a limb and resultant loss of function, clients may also have to cope with negative perceptions of body image. Changes in other people's behavior toward a person after an amputation can greatly affect an individual's self-image, resulting in embarrassment and fear of being pitied (Şimsek et al, 2020). Loss of a body part can lead to grief and bereavement, similar to what may be experienced after the loss of a loved one (Sagar et al, 2016). For many, amputation is a long-term and traumatic experience that affects an individuals' roles, habits, routines, and sense of self.

Management of Limb Amputation in Older Adults

It is critical that postamputation management begin immediately after surgery once the patient is medically stable to participate. Successful rehabilitation for older adults after amputation is multifaceted because of age-related changes and the multimorbidity that accompanies aging. Thus, a variety of health professionals, with medical, surgical, nursing, rehabilitation, prosthetic, nutrition, psychological and vocational expertise, and a team approach are essential (Giangarra & Manske, 2017). Positive effects on functional outcome have been found when appropriate medical, surgical, and rehabilitative care are provided (Giangarra & Manske, 2017). It is particularly important to comprehensively evaluate rehabilitation potential of the older adult preoperatively to estimate functional prognosis and establish realistic rehabilitation goals (Schoppen et al, 2003).

Depending on rehabilitation potential, goals may vary from patient to patient, including the comfort of returning to independence in daily living, physical, vocational, and recreational and leisure activities. Cognitive impairment may influence not only the ability to regain functioning but may also interfere with residual and remaining limb care (e.g., checking for signs of ulceration or infection). Thus, those with cognitive impairments are at higher risk of future amputation (Fleury et al, 2013). Chronic health conditions, including congestive heart failure, coronary artery disease, diabetes, hypertension, osteoarthritis, peripheral vascular disease, and stroke, can reduce the potential for prosthetic wear and use, resulting in compounded adjustment problems. Although rehabilitation outcomes can be poorer in adults age 80 years or older, comorbidities, general health status, and level of amputation are more closely associated with outcomes than age (Fleury et al, 2013).

Interventions

Occupational therapy interventions for the older adult postamputation will include a variety of intervention strategies that require an interdisciplinary approach for implementation. Occupational therapy practitioners should obtain an occupational profile to establish realistic goals and to inform intervention planning for increasing safety and independence in performing meaningful occupations. Interventions include pain and contracture management, pre- and postprosthetic management, strengthening and ROM activities, and compensatory strategies for adapting occupations and daily routines.

Preprosthetic and postsurgical management after an amputation is multifaceted, with a focus on managing the surgical recovery of the residual limb as well as preparing it for a prosthetic. Edema is a common symptom after surgical intervention, and swelling of the residual limb can reoccur well after immediate postsurgical care. Common interventions to relieve swelling include positioning, cold therapy, taping, and limb elevation. Additionally, elastic shrinkers are often used to manage edema and shape the limb. Limb shaping is especially important in the early stages of recovery to prevent deformities from occurring during the healing process and to prepare the limb for prosthetic fitting. In addition to these interventions, occupational therapy practitioners can educate the client and caregivers on scar management and massage as well as strategies to promote and manage healthy skin integrity to prevent pressure injury. If the amputation is a result of vascular disease, wound healing can be severely compromised by the underlying disease or because of skin closure under tension.

Management of acute pain symptoms after surgery begins immediately with education to the client on positioning techniques to reduce pain. This is especially important for below-knee and below-elbow amputations, where education on positioning the joint in an extended position is necessary to prevent flexion contractures. Desensitization via weightbearing, rubbing, or massage may also be warranted for clients experiencing sensitivity at the incision site. After an amputation, chronic forms of pain and altered sensation can persist years after surgery and can be debilitating for clients. Phantom limb sensation, which is sensation in the amputated limb as if it were still intact, can cause discomfort and confusion. Phantom limb pain is pain in the amputated limb, which is typically described as a cramping or squeezing sensation or a shooting or burning pain. Phantom limb pain can cause debilitating pain and discomfort, negatively affecting the client's ability to participate in daily tasks (Giangarra & Manske, 2017). The cause of phantom limb pain is unclear, but mirror therapy is effective for reducing pain intensity in patients with phantom limb pain in the short term (Xie et al, 2022). A mirror is placed at groin or chest level (dependent on amputation level). The residual limb is placed behind the mirror, so that the view of this limb is obstructed. The intact limb is placed in front of the mirror, such that the client can see the reflection. The client is asked to position the intact limb in the position of the residual limb. This progresses to the client moving the residual limb to "mirror" the intact limb. This process can provide a short-term analgesic effect that can last hours.

Strengthening postamputation will take different forms, depending on the client's individual presentation and needs. Exercise in various forms can benefit the client in various ways by improving oxygen consumption, functional performance through strengthening, and circulation, which can in turn improve surgical wound healing. Strengthening exercises can include the residual limb, unaffected extremities, and core to improve functional mobility, balance, and postural control. Weightbearing with a prosthesis can strengthen surrounding muscles, resulting in increased prosthesis control. Functional mobility training can improve activity tolerance for daily tasks. ROM exercises may also be necessary for the residual limb and other joints to prevent flexion contractures (Ulger et al, 2018).

Adjusting to an amputation and prosthetic involves taking time and may require further training. In addition to training on care, maintenance, and use of a prosthetic, occupational therapy practitioners are uniquely qualified to educate and instruct on adaptive strategies for managing daily activities and routines. In addition to providing adaptive strategies for self-care skills with or without a prosthetic, occupational therapy practitioners provide education regarding positioning for activities, transfer training, bed mobility, wheelchair mobility, and home management skills. Compensatory strategies may include energy conservation, work simplification, environmental modifications, durable medical equipment, and education regarding the use of assistive devices and technologies. Occupational therapy practitioners should prioritize safety at all times because older adults with amputations are particularly vulnerable to falls (Ülger et al, 2010).

As part of an interprofessional team, discharge planning and care planning are important parts of the postamputation rehabilitation process. Interventions may include caregiver training, referral to community resources, vocational training, and community mobility training. Occupational therapy practitioners can collaborate with other professionals, including but not limited to social workers and neuropsychologists, to address the emotional and psychosocial symptoms that may accompany an amputation.

Prevention of Amputation

Prevention of amputation is a primary public health goal globally, particularly through DM prevention, management, and care. The majority of lower-limb amputations are preceded by a foot ulcer, and persons with DM have an estimated 30 times greater lifetime risk of having an amputation than do people without DM (Moxey et al, 2011). Comprehensive, multidisciplinary team-based programs that address DM self-management (e.g., blood sugar control), wound management, vascular disease, and infection have been shown to be effective in reducing amputation rates among patients with diabetic foot ulcers (Musuuza et al, 2020).

Implications for Occupational Therapy Practice With Older Adults: Assessment of the Musculoskeletal System

A comprehensive assessment provides the occupational therapy practitioner with the necessary information to design appropriate intervention and management programs. However, because the older adult may present with typical age-related changes in addition to changes related to chronic illnesses or comorbidities, assessment may be more challenging, and differentiating between changes due to typical aging and atypical changes due to pathology may not be straightforward.

ROM and Flexibility Assessment

Measurement of joint ROM is commonly assessed using a universal standard goniometer or through observation of functional movement, noting deficits in function based on joint range. Comparisons are also made with the uninvolved limb or with age and sex norms expected for each joint. Comparison to standard norms is not appropriate unless the norms include older groups, as studies have found differences in ROM in older subjects compared with younger subjects and differences among older adults by age groups (Milanović et al, 2013). These differences should be kept in mind when developing goals. While ROM may be functional for most everyday tasks, the practitioner should consider tasks and activities requiring movements that might be limited in the older adult. Some movements include reaching overhead, reaching behind the back and head to tuck in shirt, don a bra, or brush hair (interanal and external rotation). Further, ROM limitations can impact a person's participation in meaningful activities such as gardening, car repair, home repairs, and shopping thus affecting the individual's quality of life. Flexibility is a measure of the extent to which joint ROM is limited by the extensibility of joint soft tissues as well as tendons and muscles. Lower- and upper-extremity flexibility can be measured by the "sit-and-reach test" (Nieman, 2003) and the "back-scratch test" (Rikli & Jones, 2001), respectively. These tests should be administered only after measuring and confirming normal individual joint ROM (e.g., hip flexion allowing the knee to simultaneously flex, and elbow flexion with the arm at rest by the side). With the *sit-and-reach test*, the individual completes a warm-up activity such as walking or cycling and then sits facing a flexibility box with shoes off, knees fully extended, and feet flat against the box. The individual is instructed to reach directly forward as far as possible along a measuring scale four times, and the distance point reached on the fourth trial is measured (Nieman, 2003). Rikli & Jones's (2001) "chair sit-and-reach test" is a modification of the sit-and-reach test, which allows the older adult to remain seated in a chair for testing. The individual is instructed to reach toward their toes keeping the knee extended, and the distance the person can reach beyond the toes is recorded. Limitation of reach indicates shortness in hamstring muscle group inhibiting full hip flexion and decreased flexibility in the posterior ligaments and muscles of the vertebral column. The *back-scratch test* is administered by instructing the individual to reach one hand over the shoulder and one up the middle of the back, and the distance between the extended middle fingers is recorded (Rikli & Jones, 2001). Limitation noted in this test points to shortened triceps in the upper extremity reaching over the shoulder or (and) shortness in the external rotators, posterior joint capsule, and scapular retractors of the extremity reaching up the back.

Muscle Strength and Power Assessment

Assessing strength is an important element in the overall assessment of the older adult, and baseline measurements are necessary before the initiation of an intervention program to determine who would most benefit from an intervention and to quantify the outcome of the intervention. Muscle strength can be assessed in clinical settings using various methods including manual techniques, instrumentation, and functional activities. It is important to note that with some older adults, it may be necessary to modify the methods that are commonly used when performing these procedures because of pain, joint deformities, or limitations in endurance and flexibility. The more sophisticated and expensive dynamometers that measure isokinetic torques also have their place in testing muscle force in older adults. One of the greatest advantages of isokinetic testing is that it can be used to determine movement capability at different speeds and thus may be better able to quantify age-related changes than manual muscle testing. Assessing dynamic strength is important in older adults because common ADLs and functional mobility activities (e.g., walking, rising from a chair) require speed and the generation of power in addition to strength. Other methods that have been developed to assess lower-extremity muscle power in older individuals include vertical jump on a force platform, unloaded leg extensor power evaluation, and evaluating muscle power output using lower-extremity pneumatic resistance training equipment (Callahan et al, 2007). Therapists should be aware that isokinetic testing velocities are still significantly lower than many everyday movements (Kisner & Colby, 2012). Caution should be used, especially when testing older adults with osteoporosis or when testing the upper extremities of older, frail individuals because testing the isokinetic strength of these muscles may cause an exaggerated blood pressure response (Boreskie et al, 2020). The use of large isokinetic dynamometers is limited because they are not transportable, compared with portable hand-held dynamometers.

As an alternative to more standardized tests for muscle weakness, an older adult's performance of a functional activity can be used to assess strength, for example, as an individual rises from a chair, climbs stairs, or walks. A functional test might indicate that the individual is able to ascend six steps without assistance but needs minimal assistance to complete a total of 12 steps. The *sit-to-stand test* is a measurement of the time taken to complete several chair stands and examines lower-extremity strength (Csuka & McCarty, 1985; Macrae et al, 1992). Multiple variations of the sit-to-stand test exist, including measurement of the number of times taken to complete 10 chair stands (or five chair stands), or the number of chair stands completed in 30 seconds (or 10 seconds). For older adults, this kind of assessment may be the most relevant because it measures function rather than absolute strength. It is not unusual for an older adult to be more functional than might be expected based on manual muscle testing or dynamometer testing because motivation and other factors work in combination with muscle strength to produce movement. These functional concerns are of greatest importance in working with older adults as they manage their daily lives.

Management of Musculoskeletal Impairments in Older Adults

Positive aging equates to sustaining a high quality of life, supported through the maintenance of functional independence. Participation in physical activities may help control chronic conditions and decrease the impact of age-related changes. Physical activity can attenuate age-related physiological changes, in addition to improving strength and function. Numerous benefits of participation in regular physical activity have been identified for older adults in recent decades. The extent to which changes related to aging, such as decreased muscle mass and strength, can be ameliorated with interventions, including specific physical activity and exercise programs, has been the focus of numerous research studies.

Examination of positive aging reveals the degree to which factors extrinsic to aging and disease process (nutrition, lifestyle and daily routine, degree of social support, amount of exercise, and sense of autonomy and control) play a strong, positive role in enabling older individuals to maintain their health and independence. Research has shown that remaining active and productive is a critical component of healthy aging (Cherry et al, 2013; Lin et al, 2016;

Nilsson et al, 2015). Occupational therapy practitioners can play key roles in promoting healthy lifestyles in older adults (Box 11-3).

Health and quality of life can be promoted through specific exercise programs, chronic disease self-management plans, and occupation-based interventions that include meaningful choices of activities and productive activities (Fig. 11-6). A variety of factors have been found to influence adherence to exercise programs in older adults. Some of these increase adherence (motivators), whereas others decrease adherence (barriers). One of the strongest motivators affecting exercise adherence in older adults is self-efficacy, a person's belief that they are capable of controlling their own behavior (Resnick, 2001; Resnick & Spellbring, 2000). Outcome expectation, the belief that specific consequences will result from specific personal actions, is another strong motivator of exercise adherence (Resnick, 2001; Resnick & Spellbring, 2000). Barriers to exercise adherence for older adults include fear of falling or injury; lack of time, social support, a physical space to exercise, or transportation to the exercise site; and insufficient resources either to buy exercise equipment or to join an exercise facility (Spiteri et al, 2019). In addition, stress, depression, increased age, decreased health status, and lack of enjoyment while exercising are associated with poor exercise adherence (Spiteri et al, 2019).

Older adults may have specific needs or goals when seeking to work with an occupational therapy practitioner or when beginning an exercise program, and these client-specific needs must be considered when developing an intervention plan. For

---

BOX 11-3 Lifestyle-Based Occupational Therapy Intervention Promotes Well-Being in Older Adults

A randomized controlled trial investigated the effectiveness of a lifestyle-based occupational therapy intervention in promoting well-being among older people living in the community. The Well Elderly 2 study recruited ethnically diverse (37% white, 32% African American, 20% Hispanic or Latino, 4% Asian, and 6% "other") adults aged 60 to 95 years and randomly assigned them to a lifestyle-based occupational therapy intervention or no intervention. The intervention comprised 6 months of small group (6–8 people) and individual sessions led by a trained occupational therapist and included identification and implementation of feasible and sustainable activity-relevant changes, developing plans to overcome obstacles to participating in activities (e.g., pain or lack of transport), and participation in selected activities, and rehearsal and repetition of changes to everyday routine. Older adults in the intervention group had significantly greater improvements than those in the control group in several quality of life domains: bodily pain, vitality, social function, mental health, as well as improvement in life satisfaction and decreased depression. The intervention was also deemed cost-effective (Clark et al, 2012).

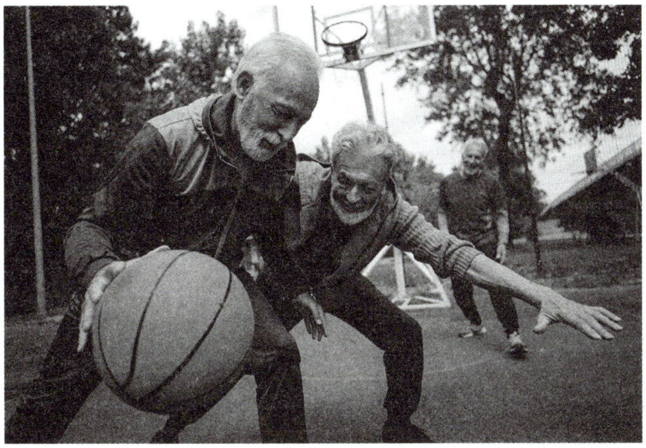

FIGURE 11-6 Regardless of physical abilities or function, exercising and remaining physically active are key to successful aging, especially when activities are personally meaningful and enjoyable. *(Nastasic/E+/Getty Images.)*

- Institute short and graded exercise sessions, but apply the overload principle.
- Use a variety of muscle contractions: isometric, isokinetic, concentric, and eccentric.
- Establish an exercise program with a focus on multiple components (low-impact aerobics, muscular strength, power, endurance, flexibility, and balance).
- Monitor skin for signs of heat stress.
- Monitor blood pressure, respirations, and pulse rate in response to exercise.
- Exercise at an RPE of 12 to 14 ("somewhat hard") or use the *talk test:* the older adult should be able to engage in a conversation during the exercise.
- Exercises should be performed through pain-free ROM only.
- Movements should be controlled.
- Older adults may gain less absolute strength, gain strength slowly, fatigue more easily, and have increased susceptibility to injuries due to exercise.

example, some clients may want to address musculoskeletal changes that interfere with their ability to participate in desired activities, while others may want to prevent further decline. Some may seek to participate in an exercise program to improve overall fitness or for general health benefits. Others may be drawn to opportunities for social interactions offered by group exercise programs. Because of the variability in personal preferences, lifestyle, fitness levels, and potential or actual comorbidities, it is important that physical activity and exercise programs are tailored and appropriate for the older individual. Areas of focus for occupational therapy intervention should be based on the older adult's needs and interests to be meaningful and to promote adherence.

Because typical age-related changes in the musculoskeletal system can cause physical impairments, older adults are at risk for functional decline and may have difficulty performing their daily occupations. Occupational therapy intervention programs should be comprehensive and consider including exercises to increase or maintain strength, flexibility, postural stability, and endurance needed for participation in occupations. Activities should also be included that are tailored to the functional needs of the client. Any exercise or activity program should be designed to emphasize safety in addition to addressing the older adult's occupational performance goals. Individual- and age-related differences in response to physical activity and exercise need to be taken into consideration, and modifications may be required when developing an occupational therapy intervention program. Exercise prescription and training guidelines for older adults have been published (e.g., American College of Sports Medicine, 2009; World Health Organization, 2010). Physical activity and exercise considerations for the older adult include:

- Use simple directions and gestures.
- Ensure adequate warm-up and cool-down.
- Take into consideration current and potential musculoskeletal problems, chronic conditions, and functional limitations.

Strength and Resistance Exercises

Although there is no evidence to date suggesting that strength training halts the age-related loss of muscle fibers, it has been well documented that systematic strength training programs can improve skeletal muscle strength in the older adult population, including the young-old, the very-old, those who are frail (de Labra et al, 2015), and those who have sustained an injury, such as post hip fracture (Mangione et al, 2010) or injurious fall (Sherrington et al, 2011). Changes in the muscles of older adults following strengthening programs are similar to the gains observed in younger subjects who participate in exercise. In addition, various training methods, including endurance-training programs, have been used with varying degrees of success to accomplish an increase in strength in older persons (de Labra et al, 2015; Liu & Latham, 2009). See Box 11-4 for information about dosing in strength training.

Isometric, isotonic, and isokinetic muscle strengthening programs, simple active exercises using body weight as resistance, and walking and aerobic exercise programs have been found to be successful at increasing upper extremity and lower-extremity strength in older adults. Early strengthening studies focused on low-intensity programs. However, in the past decades the benefits of moderate- to heavy-resistance programs have been demonstrated, with remarkable gains. Strength gains achieved in the healthy, older adult are maintained for at least short periods after the formal exercise program is discontinued, and some studies have documented structural changes of the muscles, specifically increases in cross-sectional type IIb fiber areas, after the use of formal exercise programs by older individuals. In addition, there is evidence that frail older adults in long-term care or nursing home settings can tolerate heavy-resistance programs and can make similar gains as healthy, community-dwelling older adults. Improvements extend beyond impairments, with significant functional benefits reported (de Labra et al, 2015; Liu & Latham, 2009).

BOX 11-4 Importance of Dose in Strength Training Programs for Older Adults

Research across the globe on the effects of strengthening exercises for older adults has been summarized in systematic reviews of progressive resistance strength training (Papa et al, 2017; Liu & Latham 2009). Progressive resistance training was found to improve functional mobility, gait speed, static and dynamic balance, and muscle strength (Papa et al, 2017). Aerobic capacity also improved, and fall risk was reduced (Papa et al, 2017; Liu & Latham, 2009). In general, older adults were able to safely engage in a strength-training exercise program with supervision. Adverse events were not typically reported, but when they were, joint and muscle pain were the most common adverse events. Older adults who participate in strength-training research studies are typically carefully screened for risk factors and exercise contraindications, but some studies did not monitor and report adverse events, making it difficult to assess the risk of injury (Liu & Latham, 2009). Before the initiation of any vigorous exercise program, the older adult, especially if known cardiovascular risk factors are present, should undergo a medical evaluation and appropriate stress testing (American College of Sports Medicine, 2009). Strength training programs for older adults should match the frequency, intensity, and duration of exercise to the individual's abilities and goals (White et al, 2015).

It is worthwhile to remember that some older adults may not be particularly interested in traditional exercise programs. Identifying more functionally based activities, such as yoga, tai chi, cycling, or ballroom dancing, that the individual may find more enjoyable can promote greater health benefits because of the increased probability of actual participation. Determining what might appeal to the individual is an important area of collaboration between occupational therapy practitioners and interprofessional colleagues, including physical therapists and recreational therapists.

Flexibility (Stretching) Exercises

Flexibility exercises increase the length and elasticity of periarticular tissues and muscle, increase joint mobility, prevent soft tissue contractures, decrease risk of injury, and are important to overall joint ROM (Kisner & Colby, 2012). The following are types of flexibility exercises:

- Static—a position is assumed, held for a period of time, and then relaxed
- Ballistic—repetitive bouncing motions where the muscle is rapidly stretched and immediately relaxed
- Proprioceptive neuromuscular facilitation—alternating isometric muscle contraction (hold-relax), alternating isotonic muscle contraction (contract-relax) or passive stretching through a series of movements
- Dynamic—the joint is moved through full ROM repetitively, such as with dancing or Tai Chi

Studies have found that older adults who participate in a program of regular exercise or general exercise interventions can increase ROM of various joints (Stathokostas et al, 2012). Engaging in activities such as tai chi and dancing has also been found to improve flexibility, balance, and muscle strength (Manson et al, 2013; Sooktho et al, 2022). See Box 11-5 for interventions specific to improving flexibility of older adults.

CASE STUDY (CONTINUED)

Assessment and Intervention

Mr. and Mrs. Martinez live in a two-story home. There are five steps with no railings to enter the house, and their bedroom and bathroom are on the second level. Before admission, Mr. Martinez states he was independent with mobility and all ADLs except bathtub transfers, with which he needed minimal assistance from his wife. Mr. Martinez had difficulty getting up from low height soft surfaces and used arm pushups to facilitate rising from the chair with extra effort. He enjoyed helping his wife with the gardening in the summer but found it difficult to find things to do "to keep busy" in the winter. He has quit his recreational baseball team because he does not feel like he can keep up with his friends and is embarrassed that he might fall. His current hobbies include playing bridge once weekly.

Questions

1. How do the assessment results inform your interventions?
2. a. What are two or three evidence-based, occupation-centered exemplar interventions that address the case study client's priorities?
   b. What assistive technologies or environmental modifications would you recommend?

BOX 11-5 Flexibility-Specific Interventions Increase ROM in Older Adults

A systematic review suggests flexibility-specific interventions may have effects on ROM-related outcomes. However, the authors report that there is conflicting information regarding the relationship between flexibility interventions and functional outcomes or daily functioning. Because of the wide range of intervention protocols, body parts studied, and functional measurements, conclusive recommendations regarding flexibility training for older adults or the validity of flexibility training interventions as supplements to other forms of exercise, or as significant positive influences on functional ability, require further investigation (Stathokostas et al, 2012).

3. What contextual elements from the case study's occupational therapy profile influence your treatment planning?

Answers

1. ROM and manual muscle testing will inform the client's overall strength and physical capacity to participate in daily activities. The RPE scale can inform the clinician of the client's activity tolerance for performing daily activities. Occupational performance assessments, such as the Functional Independence Measure and Modified Barthel, are important for assessing how much assistance the client will need upon discharge (See Management of Musculoskeletal Impairments; LO 11-4, 11-5, 11-6).

2. **a.** Interventions for Mr. Martinez may include performing daily occupations such as practicing bed mobility, transferring out of bed, using adaptive equipment to perform lower body dressing, and standing at the sink to perform his grooming routine. Improving strength and standing tolerance will be important after this procedure, so standing activities (e.g., standing to perform card games) and other valued leisure activities can benefit the client in preparation for discharge (approximate location of answer: pages 23-28; learning outcomes: 11-6).

   b. Mr. Martinez may benefit from training in the use of adaptive equipment to facilitate safety and independence during self-care activities at home. For example, he may benefit from instruction on how to use long-handled adaptive equipment, including a reacher, sock aid, dressing stick, and long-handled sponge, to facilitate lower-body dressing. If he is discharged home and is unable to ascend the stairs to his bedroom and bathroom on the second floor, he may require a bedside commode and a hospital bed on his first floor. If he demonstrates decreased dynamic standing balance after surgery, he may benefit from using a tub transfer bench or shower chair while bathing (approximate location of answer: pages 23-28; 11-6).

3. Mr. Martinez's occupational profile indicates that recently he has had a decline in participation and function, which may have contributed to his recent fall. It will be useful to address this decline to prevent future falls and improve his level of function. Contextual knowledge that the fall occurred in the bathroom provides insight into the potential need for adaptive equipment to facilitate safety during bathing, such as a shower chair, bathtub transfer bench, grab bars in the shower area, and handheld showerhead. Knowledge of Mr. Martinez's home setup, including that his bedroom and bathroom are on the second floor, inform the potential need for daily activities to be modified if the client is not yet able to safely ascend stairs. Mr. Martinez also has good social support from his wife and two sons who live nearby, which can inform the need for caregiver education and training to assist Mr. Martinez to safely perform ADLs and IADLs at home (See Management of OA; LO 11-6).

SUMMARY

Changes that occur in the musculoskeletal systems with aging can have negative consequences on occupational performance and participation. There is no clear distinction between "normal" aging and what constitutes "disease" or "dysfunction." Most older adults manage their daily tasks quite well until some specific event, such as a fall or an acute illness, changes their physical status or an accumulation of small decrements or chronic disease impairments reach a breakpoint at which a particular activity or occupation becomes impossible to perform without assistance from another person. Although changes in the musculoskeletal system may be a major barrier to occupational performance and participation, factors other than musculoskeletal integrity may be equally or more important to address as part of a comprehensive intervention plan, such as the consequences of impaired vision, changes in cognition, or cardiorespiratory symptoms. This chapter discussed the typical age-related changes in the musculoskeletal systems and the resulting impact on functional performance. It is important to recognize that these generalizations about change reflect an average and that individual variability is great. Physically active older adults tend to have less disability than frail older adults who are homebound or get out only infrequently.

Although not all-inclusive, a variety of assessments and intervention strategies were presented in this chapter. An exercise program consisting of strength, flexibility, balance, and endurance training can improve functioning of the musculoskeletal system. The training response is dependent on a multitude of factors and requires a thorough understanding of all the subsystems involved. Several factors should be evaluated before establishing an appropriate program. If the goal of care is to return or to maintain the older adult at their highest level of functioning, it is paramount for occupational therapy practitioners to view each aging person as having unique life experiences, goals, and preferences that influence adherence to physical activity and exercise programs that can help to promote occupational performance and participation.

Many health conditions affect the musculoskeletal system and movement function as people age. It is important for occupational therapy practitioners to understand the pathology, risk factors, and signs and symptoms of these health conditions to effectively function in environments along the continuum of care for older adults within healthcare systems. OA and osteoporosis are common in older adulthood and can lead to significant impairments in occupational performance and participation. With the increasing incidence of chronic diseases, such as DM and vascular conditions, resultant complications can lead to limb amputation in older adults.

Ultimately, management of older adults with health conditions affecting the musculoskeletal system requires an interprofessional team approach to effectively address barriers to occupational performance, participation, and well-being.

Critical Thinking Questions

1. Your neighbor, Mrs. Elena Sampson, is a 73-year-old woman without chronic illness. How would you expect Mrs. Sampson's musculoskeletal system to differ from that of a 35-year-old individual? Be sure to include changes in both body structures and functions.

2. What are the implications of musculoskeletal system changes for occupational performance in older adults like Mrs. Sampson?

3. What should occupational therapy practitioners consider when prescribing and monitoring exercise programs for older adults compared with younger age groups?

REFERENCES

Ackerman, I., Barton, C., Brusco, N., Jennings, S., Kemp, J., Sherwood, J., Trivett, A., Wallis, J., & Young, K. (2021). Exploring views of orthopaedic surgeons, rheumatologists and general practitioners about osteoarthritis management. *Musculoskeletal Care, 19*, 524–532. https://doi.org/10.1002/msc.1549

Amaral, J. F., Alvim, F. C., Castro, E. A., Doimo, L. A., Silva, M. V., & Novo Júnior, J. M. (2014). Influence of aging on isometric muscle strength, fat-free mass and electromyographic signal power of the upper and lower limbs in women. *Brazilian Journal of Physical Therapy, 18*, 183–190. doi.org/10.1590/S1413-35552012005000145

American College of Sports Medicine. (2009). *Special communication: Position stand. Exercise and physical activity for older adults.* http://journals.lww.com/acsm-msse/Fulltext/2009/07000/Exercise_and_Physical_Activity_for_Older_Adults.20.aspx

Arnold, C. M., & Gyurcsik, N. C. (2012). Risk factors for falls in older adults with lower extremity arthritis: A conceptual framework of current knowledge and future directions. *Physiotherapy Canada, 64*, 302–314. http://doi.org/10.3138/ptc.2011-12BH

Baertl, S., Alt, V., & Rupp, M. (2020). Surgical enhancement of fracture healing—operative vs nonoperative treatment. *International Journal of the Care of the Injured, 52*(2), S12-S17.

Bao, J., Chua, K. C., Prina, M., & Prince, M. (2019). Multimorbidity and care dependence in older adults: A longitudinal analysis of findings from the 10/66 study. *BMC Public Health, 19*(1), 585. https://doi.org/10.1186/s12889-019-6961-4

Bartels, E. M., Juhl, C. B., Christensen, R., Hagen, K. B., Danneskiold-Samsøe, B., Dagfinrud, H., & Lund H. (2016). Aquatic exercise for the treatment of knee and hip osteoarthritis. *Cochrane Database of Systematic Reviews, 3*, CD005523. http://doi.org/10.1002/14651858.CD005523.pub3

Bergen, G., Stevens, M. R., & Burns, E. R. (2016). Falls and fall injuries among adults aged ≥65 years—United States, 2014. *Morbidity and Mortality Weekly Report, 65*(37), 993–998.

Booker, S., Tripp-Reimer, T., & Herr, K. (2020). "Bearing the pain": The experience of aging African Americans with osteoarthritis pain. *Global Qualitative Nursing Research, 7*. http://doi.org/10.1177/2333393620925793

Boreskie, K. F., Rose, A. V., Hay, J. L., Kehler, D. S., Costa, E. C., Moffatt, T. L., Arora, R. C., & Duhamel, T. A. (2020). Frailty status and cardiovascular disease risk profile in middle-aged and older females. *Experimental Gerontology, 140*, 111061. https://doi.org/10.1016/j.exger.2020.111061

Briggs, A., Cross, M., Hoy, D., Sanchez-Riera, L., Blyth, F., Woolf, A., & March, L. (2016). Musculoskeletal health conditions represent a global threat to healthy aging: A report for the 2015 World Health Organization World Report on Ageing and Health. *The Gerontologist, 56*(suppl 2), S243-S255. http://doi.org/10.1093/geront/gnw002

Buelt, A., & Narducci, D. M. (2021). Osteoarthritis management: Updated guidelines from the American College of Rheumatology and Arthritis Foundation. *American Family Physician, 103*(2), 120–121.

Burr D. B. (2019). Changes in bone matrix properties with aging. *Bone, 120*, 85–93. https://doi.org/10.1016/j.bone.2018.10.010

Busija, L., Bridgett, L., Williams, S. R., Osborne, R. H., Buchbinder, R., March, L., & Fransen, M. (2010). Osteoarthritis. *Best Practice & Research Clinical Rheumatology, 24*, 757–768.

Callahan, D., Carabello, R., Phillips, E., Frontera, W. R., & Fielding, R. A. (2007). Assessment of lower extremity muscle power in functionally-limited elders. *Aging Clinical and Experimental Research, 19*, 194–199.

Charlier, R., Mertens, E., Lefevre, J., & Thomis, M. (2015). Muscle mass and muscle function over the adult life span: A cross-sectional study in Flemish adults. *Archives of Gerontology and Geriatrics, 61*(2), 161–167. https://doi.org/10.1016/j.archger.2015.06.009

Chen, H., Zhou, X., Fujita, H., Onozuka, M., & Kubo, K. Y. (2013). Age-related changes in trabecular and cortical bone microstructure. *International Journal of Endocrinology, 2013*, 213234. https://doi.org/10.1155/2013/213234

Cherry, K. E., Marks, L. D., Benedetto, T., Sullivan, M. C., & Barker, A. (2013). Perceptions of longevity and successful aging in very old adults. *Journal of Religion, Spirituality & Aging, 25*(4), 288–310. https://doi.org/10.1080/15528030.2013.765368

Cherry, K. E., Walker, E. J., Brown, J. S., Volaufova, J., LaMotte, L. R., Welsh, D. A., Su, L. J., Jazwinski, S. M., Ellis, R., Wood, R. H., & Frisard, M. I. (2013). Social engagement and health in younger, older, and oldest-old adults in the Louisiana Healthy Aging Study (LHAS). *Journal of Applied Gerontology, 32*, 51–75. https://doi.org/10.1177/0733464811409034

Chodzko-Zajko, W., Schwingel, A., & Park, C. (2009). Physical activity and exercise for older adults. In J. M. Rippe (Ed.) *Encyclopedia of Lifestyle Medicine & Health* (pp. 901–902). Sage. https://doi.org/10.4135/9781412994149.n278

Ciolac, E. (2013). Exercise training as a preventive tool for age-related disorders: A brief review. *Clinics, 68*, 710–717. https://doi.org/10.6061/clinics/2013(05)20

Clark, F., Jackson, J., Carlson, M., Chou, C. P., Cherry, B. J., Jordan-Marsh, M., Knight, B. G., Mandel, D., Blanchard, J., Granger, D. A., Wilcox, R. R., Lai, M. Y., White, B., Hay, J., Lam, C., Marterella, A., & Azen, S. P. (2012). Effectiveness of a lifestyle intervention in promoting the well-being of independently living older people: Results of the Well Elderly 2 Randomised Controlled Trial. *Journal of Epidemiology and Community Health, 66*, 782–790. https://doi.org/10.1136/jech.2009.099754

Corish, C. A., & Bardon, L. A. (2019). Malnutrition in older adults: Screening and determinants. *The Proceedings of the Nutrition Society, 78*(3), 372–379. https://doi.org/10.1017/S0029665118002628

Corrêa, T., Donato, S., Lima, K., Pereira, R. V., Uygur, M., & de Freitas, P. B. (2020). Age- and sex-related differences in the maximum muscle performance and rate of force development scaling factor of precision grip muscles. *Motor Control, 24*(2), 274–290. https://doi.org/10.1123/mc.2019-0021

Costa, A. G., Wyman, A., Siris, E. S., Watts, N. B., Silverman, S., Saag, K. G., Roux, C., Rossini, M., Pfeilschifter, J., Nieves, J. W., Netelenbos, J. C., March, L., LaCroix, A. Z., Hooven, F. H., Greenspan, S. L., Gehlbach, S. H., Díez-Pérez, A., Cooper, C., Compston, J. E., Chapurlat, R. D., ... Adami, S. (2013). When, where and how osteoporosis-associated fractures occur: An analysis from the global longitudinal study of osteoporosis in women (GLOW). *PLoS ONE, 8*(12), e83306. https://doi.org/10.1371/journal.pone.0083306

Cross, M., Smith, E., Hoy, D., Nolte, S., Ackerman, I., Fransen, M., Bridgett, L., Williams, S., Guillemin, F., Hill, C. L., Laslett, L. L., Jones, G., Cicuttini, F., Osborne, R., Vos, T., Buchbinder, R., Woolf, A., & March, L. (2014). The global burden of hip and knee osteoarthritis: Estimates from the Global Burden of Disease 2010 Study. *Annals of the Rheumatic Diseases, 73*, 1323–1330. https://doi.org/ 10.1136/annrheumdis-2013-204763

Cruz-Jentoft, A. J., Landi, F., Schneider, S. M., Zúñiga, C., Arai, H., Boirie, Y., Chen, L. K., Fielding, R. A., Martin, F. C., Michel, J. P., Sieber, C., Stout, J. R., Studenski, S. A., Vellas, B., Woo, J., Zamboni, M., & Cederholm, T. (2014). Prevalence of and interventions for sarcopenia in ageing adults: A systematic review. Report of the International Sarcopenia Initiative (EWGSOP and IWGS). *Age and Ageing, 43*, 748–759. https://doi.org/10.1093/ageing/afu115

Csuka, M., & McCarty, D. J. (1985). Simple method for measurement of lower extremity muscle strength. *American Journal of Medicine, 78*, 77–81. http://dx.doi.org/10.1016/0002-9343(85)90465-6

de Labra, C., Guimaraes-Pinheiro, C., Maseda, A., Lorenzo, T., & Millán-Calenti, J. C. (2015). Effects of physical exercise interventions in frail older adults: A systematic review of randomized controlled trials. *BMC Geriatr BMC Geriatrics, 15*(1). https://doi.org/10.1186/s12877-015-0155-4

Doré, L., Golightly, Y., Mercer, V., Shi, X., Renner, J., & Nelson, A. (2015). Lower limb osteoarthritis and the risk of falls in a community-based longitudinal study of adults with and without osteoarthritis. *Arthritis Care Res, 67*(5), 633–639. https://doi.org/10.1002/acr.22499

Federal Interagency Forum on Aging-Related Statistics. (2016). *Older Americans 2016: Key indicators of well-being.* https://agingstats.gov/docs/LatestReport/Older-Americans-2016-Key-Indicators-of-WellBeing.pdf

Fielding, R. A., Vellas, B., Evans, W. J., Bhasin, S., Morley, J. E., Newman, A. B., Abellan van Kan, G., Andrieu, S., Bauer, J., Breuille, D., Cederholm, T., Chandler, J., De Meynard, C., Donini, L., Harris, T., Kannt, A., Keime Guibert, F., Onder, G., Papanicolaou, D., Rolland, Y., … Zamboni, M. (2011). Sarcopenia: An undiagnosed condition in older adults. Current consensus definition: Prevalence, etiology, and consequences. International Working Group on Sarcopenia. *Journal of the American Medical Directors Association, 12*, 249–256. https://doi.org/10.1016/j.jamda.2011.01.003

Fleury, A. M., Salih, S. A., & Peel, N. M. (2013). Rehabilitation of the older vascular amputee: A review of the literature. *Geriatrics & Grontology International, 13*, 264–273. https://doi.org/10.1111/ggi.12016

Forrest, K., Williams, A. M., Leeds, M. J., Robare, J. F., & Bechard, T. J. (2018). Patterns and correlates of grip strength in older Americans. *Current Aging Science, 11*(1), 63–70. https://doi.org/10.2174/1874609810666171116164000

Fransen, M., McConnell, S., Harmer, A. R., Van der Esch. M., Simic, M., & Bennell, K. L. (2015). Exercise for osteoarthritis of the knee. *Cochrane Database of Systematic Reviews Issue 1*, CD004376. https://doi.org/10.1002/14651858.CD004376.pub3

Fransen, M., McConnell, S., Hernandez-Molina, G., & Reichenbach, S. (2014). Exercise for osteoarthritis of the hip. *Cochrane Database of Systematic Reviews, Issue 4*, CD007912. https://doi.org/10.1002/14651858.CD007912.pub2

Frontera, W. R. (2017). Physiologic changes of the musculoskeletal system with aging: A brief review. *Physical Medicine and Rehabilitation Clinics of North America, 28*(4), 705–711. https://doi.org/10.1016/j.pmr.2017.06.004

Gerstner, G. R., Giuliani, H. K., Mota, J. A., & Ryan, E. D. (2017). Age-related reductions in muscle quality influence the relative differences in strength and power. *Experimental Gerontology, 99*, 27–34. https://doi.org/10.1016/j.exger.2017.09.009

Gheller, B. J., Riddle, E. S., Lem, M. R., & Thalacker-Mercer, A. E. (2016). Understanding age-related changes in skeletal muscle metabolism: Differences between females and males. *Annual Review of Nutrition, 36*, 129–156.

Giangarra, C. E., & Manske, R. C. (2017). *Clinical orthopaedic rehabilitation: A team approach.* Elsevier Health Sciences.

Giangregorio, L. M., McGill, S., Wark, J. D., Laprade, J., Heinonen, A., Ashe, M. C., MacIntyre, N. J., Cheung, A. M., Shipp, K., Keller, H., Jain, R., & Papaioannou, A. (2015). Too fit to fracture: Outcomes of a delphi consensus process on physical activity and exercise recommendations for adults with osteoporosis with or without vertebral fractures. *Osteoporosis International, 26*(3), 891–910. https://doi.org/10.1007/s00198-014-2881-4

Goltzman, D. (2019). The aging skeleton. *Advances in Experimental Medicine and Biology, 1164*, 153–160. https://doi.org/10.1007/978-3-030-22254-3_12

Hafkamp, F., Gosen, T., & Oudsten, B. (2020). Do dissatisfied patients have unrealistic expectations? A systematic review and best-evidence synthesis in knee and hip arthroplasty patients. *Efort Open Review, 5*(4), 226–240. https://doi.org/10.1302/2058-5241.5.190015

Hoffman, G., Ha, J., Alexander, N., Langa, K., Tinetti, M., & Min, L. (2018). Underreporting of fall injuries by older adults: Implications for wellness visit fall risk screening. *Journal of American Geriatric Society, 66*(6): 1196–1200.

Hunter, S., Bobos, P., Somerville, L., Howard, J., Vasarhelyi, E., & Lanting, B. (2020). Prevalence and risk factors of falls in adults 1 year after total hip arthroplasty for osteoarthritis. *American Journal of Physical Medicine and Rehabilitation, 99*(9), 853–857.

International Council on Active Aging. (n.d.). Continuum of physical function. https://www.icaa.cc/activeagingandwellness/functionallevels.htm

Jin, K. (2010). Modern biological theories of aging. *Aging and Disability, 1*, 72–74.

Johnson, V., Hunter, D. (2014). The epidemiology of osteoarthritis. *Best Practice and Research Clinical Rheumatology, 28*, 5–15.

Kisner, C., & Colby, L. A. (2012). *Therapeutic exercise: Foundations and techniques.* F.A. Davis.

Kramer, A., Gollhofer, A., Armbrecht, G., Felsenberg, D., & Gruber, M. (2017). How to prevent the detrimental effects of two months of bed-rest on muscle, bone and cardiovascular system: An RCT. *Scientific Reports, 7*(1), 13177. https://doi.org/10.1038/s41598-017-13659-8

Li, Y., Wei, X., Zhou, J., & Wei, L. (2013). The age-related changes in cartilage and osteoarthritis. *BioMed Research International, 2013*, 916530. https://doi.org/10.1155/2013/916530

Lin, P., Hsieh, C., Cheng, H., Tseng, T., & Su, S. (2016). Association between physical fitness and successful aging in Taiwanese older adults. *PLoS ONE, 11*(3). https://doi.org/10.1371/journal.pone.0150389

Liu, C. J., & Latham, N. K. (2009). Progressive resistance strength training for improving physical function in older adults. *Cochrane Database System Review, 3*, CD002759. https://doi.org/10.1002/14651858.CD002759.pub2

MacIntyre, N. J., Recknor, C. P., Grant, S. L., & Recknor, J. C. (2014). Scores on the safe functional motion test predict incident vertebral compression fracture. *Osteoporosis International, 25*, 543–550. https://doi.org/10.1007/s00198-013-2449-8

Macrae, P. G., Lacourse, M., & Moldavon, R. (1992). Physical performance measures that predict faller status in community-dwelling older adults. *Journal of Orthopaedic and Sports Physical Therapy, 16*, 123–128.

Malatesta, D., Simar, D., Dauvilliers, Y., Candau, R., Borrani, F., Pre'faut, C., & Caillaud, C. (2003). Energy cost of walking and gait instability in healthy 65- and 80-yr-olds. *Journal of Applied Physiology, 95*, 2248–2256. https://doi.org/10.1152/japplphysiol.01106.2002

Mangione, K. K., Craik, R. L., Palombaro, K. M., Tomlinson, S. S., & Hofmann, M. T. (2010). Home-based leg-strengthening exercise improves function 1 year after hip fracture: A randomized controlled study. *Journal of the American Geriatrics Society, 58*, 1911–1917. https://doi.org/10.1111/j.1532-5415.2010.03076.x

Manson, J., Rotondi, M., Jamnik, V., Ardern, C., & Tamim, H. (2013). Effect of tai chi on musculoskeletal health-related fitness and self-reported physical health changes in low income, multiple ethnicity mid to older adults. *BMC Geriatr BMC Geriatrics, 13*, 114. https://bmcgeriatr.biomedcentral.com/articles/10.1186/1471-2318-13-114

Marcucci, L., & Reggiani, C. (2020). Increase of resting muscle stiffness, a less considered component of age-related skeletal muscle impairment. *European Journal of Translational Myology, 30*(2), 8982. https://doi.org/10.4081/ejtm.2019.8982

Mavropalias, G., Boppart, M., Usher, K. M., Grounds, M. D., Nosaka, K., & Blazevich, A. J. (2022). Exercise builds the scaffold of life: Muscle extracellular matrix biomarker responses to physical activity, inactivity, and aging. *Biological Reviews of the Cambridge Philosophical Society,* 10.1111/brv.12916. Advance online publication. https://doi.org/10.1111/brv.12916

McDonald, C. L., Westcott-McCoy, S., Weaver, M. R., Haagsma, J., & Kartin, D. (2020). Global prevalence of traumatic non-fatal limb amputation. *Prosthetics & Orthotics International, 45*(2), 105–114. https://doi.org/10.1177/0309364620972258

McLachlan, A., Carrol, P., Hunter, D., Wakefield, T., & Stosic, R. (2021). Osteoarthritis management: Does the pharmacist play a role in bridging the gap between what patients actually know and what they ought to know? Insights from a national online survey. *Health Expectations,* 1–11. https://doi.org/10.1111/hex.13429

Milanović, Z., Pantelić, S., Trajković, N., Sporić, G., Kostić, R., & James, N. (2013). Age-related decrease in physical activity and functional fitness among elderly men and women. *CIA Clinical Interventions in Aging, 2013,* 549–556. https://doi.org/10.2147/cia.s44112

Miller, R. M., Freitas, E., Heishman, A. D., Peak, K. M., Buchanan, S. R., Kellawan, J. M., Pereira, H. M., Bemben, D. A., & Bemben, M. G. (2021). Muscle performance changes with age in active women. *International Journal of Environmental Research and Public Health, 18*(9), 4477. https://doi.org/10.3390/ijerph18094477

Montero-Odasso, M., & Speechley, M. (2018). Falls in cognitively impaired older adults: Implications for risk assessment and prevention. *Journal of the American Geriatrics Society, 66*(2), 367–375. https://doi.org/10.1111/jgs.15219

Moxey, P. W., Gogalniceanu, P., Hinchliffe, R. J., Loftus, I. M., Jones, K. J., Thompson, M. M., & Holt, P. J. (2011). Lower extremity amputations-A review of global variability in incidence. *Diabetic Medicine, 28*(10), 1144–1153. https://doi.org/10.1111/j.1464-5491.2011.03279.x

Musich, S., Wang, S., Schaeffer, j., Slindee, L., Kraemer, S., & Yeh, C. (2021). Safety events associated with tramadol use among older adults with osteoarthritis. *Population Health Management, 24*(1), 122–132. https://doi.org/10.1089/pop.2019.0220

Musuuza, J., Sutherland, B. L., Kurter, S., Balasubramanian, P., Bartels, C. M., & Brennan, M. B. (2020). A systematic review of multidisciplinary teams to reduce major amputations for patients with diabetic foot ulcers. *Journal of Vascular Surgery, 71*(4), 1433–1446.e3. https://doi.org/10.1016/j.jvs.2019.08.244

Narres, M., Kvitkina, T., Claessen, H., Droste, S., Schuster, B., Morbach, S., Rümenapf, G., Van Acker, K., & Icks, A. (2017). Incidence of lower extremity amputations in the diabetic compared with the nondiabetic population: A systematic review. *Plos One, 12*(8). https://doi.org/10.1371/journal.pone.0182081

Nieman, D. C. 2003. *Exercise testing and prescription: A health-related approach* (5th ed.). Boston: McGraw-Hill.

NIH Consensus Development Panel on Osteoporosis Prevention, Diagnosis, and Therapy. (2001). Osteoporosis prevention, diagnosis, and therapy. *Journal of the American Medical Association, 285,* 785–795. https://doi.org/10.1001/jama.285.6.785

Nilsson, I., Nyqvist, F., Gustafson, Y., & Nygård, M. (2015). Leisure engagement: Medical conditions, mobility difficulties, and activity limitations—a later life perspective. *Journal of Aging Research, 2015,* 1–8. https://doi.org/10.1155/2015/610154

Pandit, V., Nelson, P., Kempe, K., Gage, K., Zeeshan, M., Kim, H., Khan, M., Trinidad, B., Zhou, W., & Tan, T. W. (2020). Racial and ethnic disparities in lower extremity amputation: Assessing the role of frailty in older adults. *Surgery, 168*(3), 1075–1078. https://doi.org/10.1016/j.surg.2020.07.015

Panel on Prevention of Falls in Older Persons, American Geriatrics Society and British Geriatrics Society Panel on Prevention of Falls in Older Persons. (2011). Summary of the updated American Geriatrics Society/British Geriatrics Society clinical practice guideline for prevention of falls in older persons. *Journal of the American Geriatrics Society, 59,* 148–157.

Papa, E. V., Dong, X., & Hassan, M. (2017). Resistance training for activity limitations in older adults with skeletal muscle function deficits: A systematic review. *Clinical Interventions in Aging, 12,* 955–961. https://doi.org/10.2147/CIA.S104674

Petermann-Rocha, F., Balntzi, V., Gray, S. R., Lara, J., Ho, F. K., Pell, J. P., & Celis-Morales, C. (2022). Global prevalence of sarcopenia and severe sarcopenia: A systematic review and meta-analysis. *Journal of Cachexia, Sarcopenia and Muscle, 13*(1), 86–99. https://doi.org/10.1002/jcsm.12783

Power, G. A., Dalton, B. H., & Rice, C. L. (2013). Human neuromuscular structure and function in old age: A brief review. *Journal of Sport and Health Science, 2,* 215–226. https://doi.org/10.1016/j.jshs.2013.07.001

Recknor, C. P., Grant, S. L., Recknor, J. C., & MacIntyre, N. J. (2013). Scores on the safe functional motion test are associated with prevalent fractures and fall history. *Physiotherapy Canada, 65,* 75–81. https://doi.org/10.3138/ptc.2011-25BH

Resnick, B. (2001). Testing a model of exercise behavior in older adults. *Research in Nursing Health, 24,* 83–92. https://doi.org/10.1002/nur.1011

Resnick, B., & Spellbring, A. M. (2000). Understanding what motivates older adults to exercise. *Journal of Gerontological Nursing, 26,* 34–42. https://doi.org/10.3928/0098-9134-20000301-08

Rikli, R. E., & Jones, C. J. (2001). *Senior fitness test manual.* Human Kinetics.

Sagar, R., Sahu, A., Sarkar, S., & Sagar, S. (2016). Psychological effects of amputation: A review of studies from India. *Industrial Psychiatry Journal, 25*(1), 4. https://doi.org/10.4103/0972-6748.196041

Schoppen, T., Boonstra, A., Groothoff, J. W., de Vries, J., Göeken, L. N., & Eisma, W. H. (2003). Physical, mental, and social predictors of functional outcome in unilateral lower-limb amputees. *Archives of Physical Medicine & Rehabilitation, 84,* 803–811.

Sen, B., Xie, Z., Case, N., Styner, M., Rubin, C. T., & Rubin, J. (2011). Mechanical signal influence on mesenchymal stem cell fate is enhanced by incorporation of refractory periods into the loading regimen. *Journal of Biomechanics, 44,* 593–599. https://doi.org/10.1016/j.jbiomech.2010.11.022

Sfeir, J. G., Drake, M. T., Khosla, S., & Farr, J. N. (2022). Skeletal aging. *Mayo Clinic Proceedings, 97*(6), 1194–1208. https://doi.org/10.1016/j.mayocp.2022.03.011

Sherrington, C., Tiedemann, A., Fairhall, N., Close, J. C., & Lord, S. R. (2011). Exercise to prevent falls in older adults: An updated meta-analysis and best practice recommendations. *New South Wales Public Health Bulletin, 22,* 78–83.

Şimsek, N., Öztürk, G. K., & Nahya, Z. N. (2020). The mental health of individuals with post-traumatic lower limb amputation: A qualitative study. *Journal of Patient Experience, 7*(6), 1665–1670. https://doi.org/10.1177/2374373520932451

Sooktho, S., Songserm, N., Woradet, S., & Suksatan, W. (2022). A meta-analysis of the effects of dance programs on physical performance: Appropriate health promotion for healthy older adults. *Annals of Geriatric Medicine and Research, 26*(3), 196–207. https://doi.org/10.4235/agmr.22.0066

Spirduso, W. W., Francis, K., & MacRae, P. (2005). *Physical dimensions of aging.* Human Kinetics.

Spiteri, K., Broom, D., Bekhet, A. H., de Caro, J. X., Laventure, B., & Grafton, K. (2019). Barriers and motivators of physical activity participation in middle-aged and older-adults—A systematic review. *Journal of Aging and Physical Activity, 27*(4), 929–944. https://doi.org/10.1123/japa.2018-0343

Stathokostas, L., Little, R. M. D., Vandervoort, A. A., & Paterson, D. H. (2012). Flexibility training and functional ability in older adults: A systematic review. *Journal of Aging Research,* Article 306818. https://doi.org/10.1155/2012/306818

Stathokostas, L., McDonald, M. W., Little, R. M. D., Vandervoort, A. A., & Paterson, D. H. (2013). Flexibility of older adults aged 55–86 years and the influence of physical activity. *Journal of Aging Research,* Article 743843. http://dx.doi.org/10.1155/2013/743843

Tan, K. T., Ang, S. J., & Tsai, S. Y. (2020). Sarcopenia: Tilting the balance of protein homeostasis. *Proteomics, 20*(5–6), e1800411. https://doi.org/10.1002/pmic.201800411

Terroso, M., Rosa, N., Marques, A., & Simoes, R. (2013). Physical consequences of falls in the elderly: A literature review from 1995 to 2010. *European Review of Aging and Physical Activity. 11,* 51–59.

Tieland, M., Trouwborst, I., & Clark, B. C. (2018). Skeletal muscle performance and ageing. *Journal of Cachexia, Sarcopenia and Muscle, 9*(1), 3–19. https://doi.org/10.1002/jcsm.12238

Tyrovolas, S., Koyanagi, A., Olaya, B., Ayuso-Mateos, J. L., Miret, M., Chatterji, S., Tobiasz-Adamczyk, B., Koskinen, S., Leonardi, M., & Haro, J. M. (2015). The role of muscle mass and body fat on disability among older adults: A cross-national analysis. *Experimental Gerontology, 69,* 27–35. https://doi.org/10.1016/j.exger.2015.06.002

Ulger, O., Sahan, T., & Celik, S. (2018). A systematic literature review of physiotherapy and rehabilitation approaches to lower-limb amputation. *Physiotherapy Theory and Practice, 34* (11), 821–824.

Ülger, Ö., Topuz, S., Bayramlar, K., Erbahçeci, F., & Sener, G. (2010). Risk factors, frequency, and causes of falling in geriatric persons who has had a limb removed by amputation. *Topics in Geriatric Rehabilitation, 26,* 156–163. https://doi.org/10.1097/tgr.0b013e3181e85533

Vandervoort, A. A. (2002). Aging of the human neuromuscular system. *Muscle and Nerve, 25,* 17–25. https://doi.org/10.1002/mus.1215

Vina, E.R., Ran, D., Ashbeck, E.L., & Kwoh, C.K. (2018). Natural history of pain and disability among African Americans and whites with or at risk for knee osteoarthritis: A longitudinal study. *Osteoarthritis and Cartilage,* 28, 471–479.

Wang, D., Yao, J., Zirek, Y., Reijnierse, E. M., & Maier, A. B. (2020). Muscle mass, strength, and physical performance predicting activities of daily living: A meta-analysis. *Journal of Cachexia, Sarcopenia and Muscle, 11*(1), 3–25. https://doi.org/10.1002/jcsm.12502

Warriner, M., Patkar, N., Curtis, J., Delzell, E., Gary, L., Kilgore, M., & Saag, K. (2011). Which fractures are most attributable to osteoporosis? *Journal of Clinical Epidemiology, 64*(1): 46–53.

Watts, N. B., Binkley, N., Owens, C. D., Al-Hendy, A., Puscheck, E. E., Shebley, M., Schlaff, W. D., & Simon, J. A. (2021). Bone mineral density changes associated with pregnancy, lactation, and medical treatments in premenopausal women and effects later in life. *Journal of Women's Health, 30*(10), 1416–1430. https://doi.org/10.1089/jwh.2020.8989

Welmer, A., Rizzuto, D., Laukka, E., Johnell, K., & Fratiglioni, L. (2017). Cognitive and physical function in relation to the risk of injurious falls in older adults: A population-based study. *The Journals of Gerontology: Series A, 72*(5), 669–675.

White, N. T., Delitto, A., Manal, T., & Miller, S. (2015). The American Physical Therapy Association's top five Choosing Wisely recommendations. *Physical Therapy, 95,* 9–24. https://doi.org/10.2522/ptj.20140287

Wiegmann, S., Felsenberg, D., Armbrecht, G., & Dietzel, R. (2021). Longitudinal changes in muscle power compared to muscle strength and mass. *Journal of Musculoskeletal & Neuronal Interactions, 21*(1), 13–25.

Wilson-Barnes, S. L., Lanham-New, S. A., & Lambert, H. (2022). Modifiable risk factors for bone health & fragility fractures. *Best Practice & Research Clinical rheumatology, 36*(3), 101758. https://doi.org/10.1016/j.berh.2022.101758

Winger, M. E., Caserotti, P., Cauley, J. A., Boudreau, R. M., Piva, S. R., Cawthon, P. M., Orwoll, E. S., Ensrud, K. E., Kado, D. M., Strotmeyer, E. S., & Osteoporotic Fractures in Men (MrOS) Research Group. (2022). Lower leg power and grip strength are associated with increased fall injury risk in older men: The Osteoporotic Fractures in Men (MrOS) Study. *The Journals of Gerontology: Series A,* Advance online publication. https://doi.org/10.1093/gerona/glac122

Wong, C., Fagan, B., & Leland, N. (2018). Occupational therapy practitioners' perspectives on occupation-based interventions for clients with hip fracture. *The American Journal of Occupational Therapy, 72*(4), 7204205050p1-7204205050p7. https://doi.org/ 10.5014/ajot.2018.026492

World Health Organization. (2010). *Global recommendations on physical activity for health.* http://apps.who.int/iris/bitstream/10665/44399/1/9789241599979_eng.pdf

World Health Organization. (2021). *Falls.* https://www.who.int/news-room/fact-sheets/detail/falls

Xie, H. M., Zhang, K. X., Wang, S., Wang, N., Wang, N., Li, X., & Huang, L. P. (2022). Effectiveness of mirror therapy for phantom limb pain: A systematic review and meta-analysis. *Archives of Physical Medicine and Rehabilitation, 103*(5), 988–997. https://doi.org/10.1016/j.apmr.2021.07.810

Yang, F., & Liu, W. (2021). Individual analysis of dynamic stability for twenty-four tai chi forms among persons with knee osteoarthritis: A pilot study. *Gait & Posture,* 86, 22–26.

Zhu, X., & Zheng, H. (2021). Factors influencing peak bone mass gain. *Frontiers of Medicine, 15*(1), 53–69. https://doi.org/10.1007/s11684-020-0748-y

CHAPTER 12

Neuromuscular and Neuromotor Conditions

Cara L. Brown, PhD, OTReg(MB) ■ Vanina Dal Bello-Haas, PhD, Med, BSc(PT)

"Most old(er) people are young people in old bodies."

—Bernard Isaacs

LEARNING OUTCOMES

By the end of this chapter, readers will be able to:

12-1. Identify typical age-related neuromotor changes you may see in an older adult while they are conducting activities of daily living (ADLs).

12-2. Justify three precautions to be taken when working with a client with different neuromotor conditions in relation to physical motor performance.

12-3. Critique the use of traditional motor control theories in relation to modern task-oriented motor learning theories.

12-4. Develop an evidence-based assessment plan for physical performance of an older adult with a neuromotor condition that considers the stage of the health condition.

12-5. Develop an evidence-based intervention plan for task performance for an older adult with a neuromotor condition that considers the stage of the health condition.

12-6. Design a plan for referrals to your interprofessional team members for an older adult with a neuromotor condition including a rationale for each referral.

Mini Case Study

Mrs. Boupha Voeum is a 92-year-old widow who lives with her adult son (age 67) and his wife (age 73) and her 30-year-old grandson. All the bedrooms and the bathroom are on the second floor of the home. Mrs. Voeum is originally from Cambodia, and her favorite occupation is volunteering at her local church and immigrant community center. Mrs. Voeum has osteoporosis, macular degeneration, and diabetes. Until very recently, Mrs. Voeum either walked or took the bus to the locations where she volunteers. However, Mrs. Voeum has not attended her volunteering as regularly, as she has noticed that she is becoming increasingly unsteady on her feet and is afraid of falling if the bus driver does not wait for her to sit down. When walking, she is rarely able to make it through the crosswalk without the crossing sign changing from "Walk" to "Don't Walk." Mrs. Voeum has been using a cane that she bought at the local pharmacy in her right hand to feel steadier when she walks outside the home.

Mrs. Voeum is also getting discouraged with cooking—something she enjoys doing for the whole family. Her hands feel weak. She is struggling to do things like open jars and grasp a knife firmly when cutting large hard objects (like a squash), and she has almost dropped pots filled with water or food when carrying them between the stove, counter, sink, and table. She also notices that her coordination is not as good when she is doing things like chopping vegetables; it seems like it takes much longer than it used to.

Provocative Questions

1. What typical age-related changes are illustrated in this case study about Mrs. Voeum?
2. What adaptations could be made to support Mrs. Voeum with maintaining her volunteering and meal-preparation activities?

This chapter discusses the neuromotor system and functions, including typical aging processes and neuromotor conditions prevalent in older adults. Neuromotor function refers to the muscular and nervous system working together in concert to produce movement. All motor movement, even the simplest, is complex in terms of the neural communication between the central and peripheral motor and sensory systems to make that movement happen. A movement first starts as an idea in the motor planning areas of the brain. The message travels from the motor planning area to the motor cortex, where upper motor neurons are activated, and then descends to or through the brainstem and spinal cord to synapse with cell body of lower motor neuron. The axon of the lower motor neuron leaves the spinal cord, exits the vertebral column as a cranial or peripheral nerve, and travels to the neuromotor junction to activate the muscle fibers. There are different types of descending tracts—some that control automatic skeletal muscle activity (for example, to maintain balance) and others that control voluntary movement. The basal ganglia and the cerebellum provide refinement and control of the movements by adjusting activity in the descending tracts in response to feedback from the sensory system to control the amount and timing of muscle contraction. Be sure to consult a neuroanatomy/physiology textbook if you require a more fulsome review of the workings of the neuromotor system before reading this chapter.

This chapter reviews:

- Age-related changes in the neuromotor system that affect motor function
- Common health conditions that typically affect neuromotor function—traumatic brain injury, stroke, and Parkinson's disease
- Conceptual frameworks for approaching the assessment and intervention of neuromotor conditions
- Assessment and intervention considerations for physical function for older adults with neuromotor conditions
- Considerations for promoting participation in older adults with neuromotor conditions
- Interprofessional practice for working with older adults with neuromotor conditions

Although typical and pathological changes in the neuromotor system can have an impact on other areas of body functions, including mental and sensory functions, this chapter will focus specifically on changes in the neuromotor system.

Typical Age-Related Changes in the Neuromotor System and Related Functions

The natural aging process affects all the components of the neuromotor pathway and the systems that support movement (sensory systems) and has an impact on movement in older adulthood (Hou et al, 2019; Rozand et al, 2020). Research is ongoing to understand the underlying cellular changes related to aging that result in these neuromotor system changes. Cellular changes include oxidative DNA damage, telomere shortening, epigenetic modifications, interrupted balance between protein synthesis and degradation causing protein buildup, suboptimal mitochondrial functioning, and chronic inflammation (Hou et al, 2019). At the level of the motor unit (a motor neuron and the muscle fibers it innervates) (American Psychological Association [APA], 2022), aging results in fewer motor units innervating the muscle fibers. Having a single motor unit innervate a larger number of muscle fibers results in less capacity for sustained motor unit firing. The functional implication is a decrease in executing smooth, accurate, controlled movements.

Changes at the level of the muscle include a reduction of fast twitch fibers (type II fibers) and consequential decrease in muscle mass. Because these fibers help us with heavier loads for shorter durations (Merriam-Webster, n.d.), the reduction in fast twitch fibers affects the older adult's ability to perform activities such as climbing stairs or lifting heavy grocery bags as well as they did when they were younger.

Functional imaging studies provide evidence that the brain is used differently to conduct motor activities in older people than it is in young people. This is thought to be because older adults are using compensatory mechanisms to continue to support motor performance despite age-related brain changes like cerebral atrophy, reduced blood flow, and decreased effectiveness of neurotransmitter systems. These changes affect both physical and sensory systems along with important feedback loops between these systems that allow for smooth coordinated movement through adjustments to improve movement execution (Parthasharathy et al, 2022). Generally, functional imaging studies suggest that older adults use more widespread brain networks for accomplishment of motor tasks. An example is that older adults use greater activation of the visual cortex during motor tasks, suggesting that they require more visual feedback during motor tasks or that they use visual imagery to support their performance (Zapparoli et al, 2022). A summary of the neurological changes thought to be due to typical aging is too extensive to discuss in detail here, although some of these changes are summarized in Box 12-1.

Despite evidence of changes in the neuromotor system of older adults, these changes are not directly correlated with changes in motor function. In fact, the functional integrity of the nervous system in most healthy older adults is maintained despite these reported structural, biochemical, and metabolic changes. It is important to remember that each

---

BOX 12-1 Age-Related Changes of the Nervous System

- Cerebral atrophy
- Increased cerebrospinal fluid space
- Specific neuronal loss
- Reduced dendritic branching
- Cellular protein and lipid accumulation in nerve and muscle cells (e.g., lipofuscin)
- Increased plaques and neurofibrillary tangles in selective brain regions
- Decreased effectiveness of neurotransmitter systems; selectively reduced activities in dopaminergic, cholinergic, and noradrenergic systems
- Reduced cerebral blood flow
- Diminished glucose utilization
- Alterations in electroencephalogram
- Loss of motor nerve fibers
- Decreased number and size of motor units
- Slowing of nerve conduction velocities
- Biochemical and morphological changes in the neurons and receptors
- Defects in neuronal transport mechanisms
- Decreases in myelin, reducing the conduction velocity of nerves

Source: Hou et al, 2019; Moreno-Garcia et al, 2018; Rozand et al, 2020.

older individual responds to changes in the neuromotor system in a unique manner and that multiple factors contribute to motor function changes. For example, practice of a skill allows for prevention of age-related decline in that skill (Gölz et al, 2018) (Fig. 12-1). It is difficult to tease out all the potential biological, behavioral, nutritional, socioeconomic, and personal factors affecting motor function in older adults (Tieland et al, 2018). Thus, it is best to assume that the neurological changes of aging have a minimal impact—if at all—on neuromotor function during rehabilitation. It is likely that many if not most of the motor function problems in older adults are related to pathology rather than a manifestation of a generalized aging process.

However, this needs to be balanced with the knowledge that the brain is very susceptible to age-related changes, with neurodegenerative diseases like Parkinson's disease being very similar to typical aging processes in the brain (Hou et al, 2019). Although compensatory mechanisms can be effective at maintaining performance for some time, they do not tend to be effective in the long term, and thus measurable changes in motor performance do occur over time as compensatory strategies become less effective (Zapparoli et al, 2022).

Proprioception

Proprioception is the awareness of body segments in relationship to each other and in relationship to the environment (orientation) (APA, 2022). Proprioception plays an important role in providing information that is needed for the planning of precise and coordinated movements, in maintaining balance and controlling body posture, and stability and orientation of the body (Ferlinc et al, 2019). As described in Chapter 10, all sensory modalities decrease in acuity with age, and proprioception is no exception. Research has cited changes in joint position sense in the lower and upper extremities including the elbow, wrist, fingers, knee in older adults (Ferlinc et al, 2019). In addition, older adults may have impaired integration of the proprioceptive input that is necessary for the information to be used effectively (Henry & Baudry, 2019). Decreased awareness of the body or limbs in space, combined with other sensory losses or cognitive changes such as those described in Chapter 10 and 13, may affect safety during daily activities, transfers, and ambulation. Evidence suggests regular physical activity attenuates age-related decreases in proprioception (Henry & Baudry, 2019).

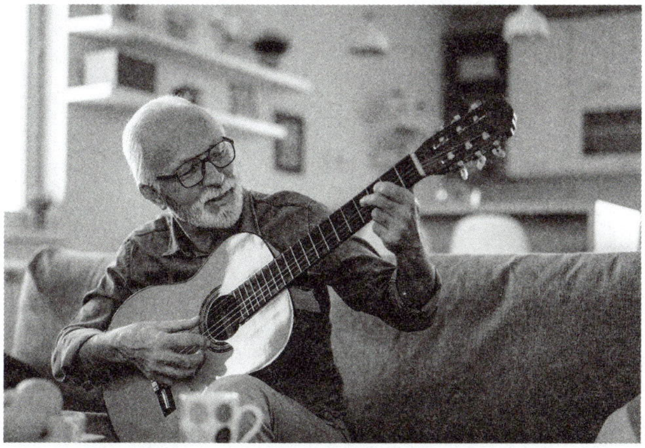

Balance

Balance is also known as postural control, which is the act of maintaining, achieving, or restoring a state of balance during any posture or activity. Postural control involves many different components, including maintaining alignment of the head and trunk in relation to gravity and maintaining postural stability during voluntary movements and in reaction to external perturbations. This building block to movement occurs through the complex interaction of many systems, including the somatosensory (sensory information from the muscles, joints, and tendons), vestibular, and visual systems, which provide input to subcortical and cortical brain regions (Osoba et al, 2019). To maintain balance, the center of mass must stay within the changing base of support. The brain monitors deviations from the desired stable posture and initiates messaging to the musculoskeletal system to make corrections (Stokkermans et al, 2022). The cerebellum is critical for coordinating limb and trunk movements and balancing opposing muscle forces when completing tasks. Box 12-2 provides an overview of the systems involved. Thus, although multiple systems are involved in postural control, the neurological system plays a primary role in postural control.

Age-related changes are seen in balance as early as in the fourth decade of life and include decreased postural stability and a higher sway velocity (sway in the trunk in quiet standing). Older adults compensate for the decreased postural stability and increased sway with proximal adjustments (such as at the hip) rather than with distal movements (such as foot adjustment, as is seen in younger people) (Osoba et al, 2019). For a comprehensive discussion about postural control from development to aging, see Shumway-Cook and Woollacott (2017).

Because balance and coordination rely on inputs from sensory systems, there are numerous age-related sensory changes occurring that influence balance performance. For example, the visual and vestibular systems work together to maintain body position at rest and in motion and to maintain a steady visual focus on objects when body position changes. Therefore, the numerous age-related changes in the visual and vestibular systems can negatively affect balance both in terms of detecting the sensory information and in processing it effectively (Chen et al, 2021a).

The extrapyramidal system, which refers to the basal ganglia and its connections (Lee & Muzio, 2021) also affects balance because of age-related changes. These changes result in a slowing of skilled movement **(bradykinesia)** (APA,

FIGURE 12-1 This older adult has maintained their ability to perform complex neuromotor movements, likely due to frequent and intense practice. *(PixelsEffect/E +/Getty Images.)*

> **BOX 12-2** Postural Control for Stability and Orientation Requires a Complex Interaction of Many Components and Systems
>
> - Joint range of motion, spinal flexibility, muscle properties, biomechanical relationships among linked body segments
> - Sensory information from muscles, joints, and tendons
> - Vestibular input from the inner ear
> - Visual input from the retina
> - Continuous integration of the proprioceptive, vestibular, visual, and mechanoreceptive information
> - Neuromuscular **synergies** (muscle activation of a set of muscles contributing to a particular movement)
> - Organization, coordination, and sequential activation of muscles and muscle groups
> - Adaptive mechanisms: Ability to integrate feedback rapidly to adapt to changes in the environment (e.g., an unstable surface)
> - Anticipatory mechanisms: Preparatory movements that position the body to be ready for movement
> - Higher-level neural processes to integrate information and react
> - Sensory and motor system modifications in response to changing task and environmental demands
> - Sensory and motor system pre-tuning based on previous experience and learning
> - Cognitive influences essential for mapping sensation to action and for adaptive and anticipatory mechanisms; internal representations
>
> Citation: Hsaio et al, 2020.

2022), alterations in gross movements, and tics or tremors that ultimately lead to impaired **postural stability** (inability to keep oneself from falling) (Appeadu & Gupta, 2020) in the older adult (Seidler et al, 2010).

Slowing of simple reaction time (SRT) is considered one of the most measurable and recognizable behavioral changes occurring with aging, and this adversely affects balance (Marusic et al, 2022). SRT is the total time that elapses between the presentation of a stimulus and the occurrence of a response in a task that requires a participant to perform an elementary behavior (e.g., pressing a key) whenever a stimulus (such as a light or tone) is presented (APA, 2022). Studies of choice reaction time suggest that as the task difficulty increases, the reaction times of older adults are significantly slower than the reaction times of those who are younger (Marusic et al, 2022). Slowed central processing is likely the primary factor leading to increased reaction time instead of other factors like slowed nerve conduction or muscle contraction. However, there is evidence that reaction time can potentially be preserved with the maintenance of activity (Marusic et al, 2022). See Box 12-3.

Coordination

Coordination depends on an intact neuromusculoskeletal system; inputs from visual, somatosensory, and vestibular systems; and sensorimotor processing. The ability to perform coordinated movement requires the integration of multiple muscle groups (muscle synergies) (APA, 2022) and involves afferent and efferent pathways (APA, 2022). Functional activities that require either gross- or fine-motor responses or a combination of these (e.g., getting

> **BOX 12-3** Considering the Effects of Cognitive Demand on Balance
>
> Balance requires attentional resources, and the cognitive demand of a task can affect a person's ability to maintain balance during the task. Older adults may need to stop or slow their movements to respond to a question or carry on a conversation. This cognitive demand for attention can put older adults at a greater fall risk. Simply observing an individual walk down a straight hallway (e.g., a clinic hallway or inpatient ward) does not adequately represent the balance demands of responding to natural environmental demands like walking down a sidewalk with small changes in incline and obstacles such as people and bicycles, processing crosswalk information, and maintaining the cognitive task of planning the route and maintaining orientation.
>
> There are many studies examining the impact of attention on balance (see Boisgontier et al, 2013, for a review). The dual-task Timed Up and Go (TUGDT) was developed to examine whether adding a secondary task to the Timed Up and Go (TUG) would increase the specificity and sensitivity of the TUG as a fall risk measure (Brauer et al, 2001). The TUGDT cognitive asks the older adult to complete the TUG while counting backward by threes, and the TUGDT manual asks the older adult to complete the TUG while carrying a cup of water. Although the TUG alone was found to be a sensitive and specific indicator of fall risk, the time to complete the TUGDT was significantly longer. This finding indicates that adding a secondary task may provide insight into how an older adult can maintain balance under multitasking conditions (Shumway-Cook et al, 2000).
>
> In observation of ADLs, the therapist should consider the cognitive demand of the task to fully understand the balance capacity of the older adult. For example, if the assessment is a part of a kitchen assessment, the older adult's balance may be affected by the cognitive planning occurring.

out of bed, buttoning and zipping clothing) are dependent on coordinated movements. Coordinated movements involve multiple joints and muscles that need to be activated at the appropriate time and with the appropriate force so the movement is accurate, smooth, and efficient (Shumway-Cook & Woollacott, 2017). The commands for muscle movement involve several different neurological structures, including the cerebellum. The cerebellum uses sensory feedback to determine needed changes to make movements smooth and includes providing information for adjustments to postural muscles, eye muscle movement, and gross- and fine-motor movements. The basal ganglia also play a key role in coordination; their primary role is to regulate muscle contraction, muscle force, and multijoint movements and the sequencing of movements. The basal ganglia predict movement and support that movement by inhibiting nondesired movement. For this reason, the basal ganglia and motor planning areas of the brain are closely connected. Changes in the ability to execute smooth, accurate, and controlled motor responses occur with normal aging for many of the reasons already discussed in this chapter (Zapparoli et al, 2022).

Upper Extremity Movement

Upper extremity neuromotor function is essential for performance of everyday tasks and is an important predictor of disability and mortality (Woytowicz et al, 2016). Completing upper extremity tasks requires many of the performance functions already discussed to work together efficiently. For example, to fold laundry, the individual needs to have intact postural control to stay upright during the task and to have intact coordination to be able to move the limbs smoothly. Fine-motor control, including precision grasp and manipulation, is essential for everyday activities like grooming (e.g., taking toothpaste lid off, applying toothpaste) and meal preparation (e.g., chopping, pouring). The descending neural pathway most responsible for fine-motor coordination is the lateral corticospinal tract. This tract allows for fractionation of movement—that is, the ability to activate individual muscles.

Upper extremity task performance generally declines with age, starting as early as the fourth decade. For example, tool use is slower, less complex, and less accurate overall. Several factors can contribute to changes, including proprioception and sensory loss, cortical thinning, central and peripheral demyelination, and slower reaction times and processing speeds (Hooyman et al, 2021). Upper and lower extremity movement can also be affected by visual processing resulting in slowed movement (Marusic et al, 2022).

An increase in tremors affects upper and lower extremity functioning for all older adults because of age-related changes (Khosa et al, 2019). This results in less accuracy in reaching for a target, such as when reaching into a cupboard for a dish or reaching for a light switch. Bilateral integration (using both sides of the body at the same time) and coordination (separating movements of the right and left hand to complete a task) also become less efficient with age, affecting bilateral tasks like typing, washing dishes, and drumming.

Age-related changes have been found to affect maximal muscle force (Rozand et al, 2020). A decrease in force production results in less steadiness in force production, difficulty regulating the force needed for tasks, using more force than needed, and a decline in overall muscle force capacity. Pethick and colleagues (2021) suggest that changes in force production can affect ADLs, particularly activities that are done against gravity and involve multijoint movements (Pethick et al, 2021). In addition, it has been found that force affects fine-motor skills because of a decreased ability to modulate fingertip force (Gölz et al, 2018). Further, decreased sensorimotor motor integration is linked to increases in falls and upper extremity injury of the shoulder (Overbeek et al, 2021).

Overall, older adults will perform bilateral tasks less accurately, require more time to do them, and do them with more movement variability than do younger people (Krehbiel et al, 2017). These changes may be due to changes in central nervous system processing (e.g., speed of processing, sensorimotor processing) or changes in the neuromusculoskeletal system (Zapparoli et al, 2022). However, it is important to note that continuous and deliberate practice can dampen this progressive decline in fine-motor performance (Gölz et al, 2018). An example is Charlie Watts, who was the drummer for the Rolling Stones until his death at age 80.

CASE STUDY

Mr. George is a 78-year-old man who lives with his wife in a two-story home with a basement utility room. Ten years ago, he noticed a slight tremor in his right hand and that it sometimes felt harder than normal to start walking, but he didn't really think much of it. Five years ago, the tremor got worse, to the point that he was having difficulty completing his favorite paper-and-pencil word puzzles and kept missing the correct buttons when trying to open an app or make a phone call on his smart phone. His wife noticed that his personality seemed different, because he didn't smile and laugh as much as he used to. She kept telling him to stand up straighter because he was hunched over when he walked, and he started having trouble keeping up with her when walking in the mall. They realized something was not right, and he was diagnosed with Parkinson's disease that year.

Last year, he had several falls at home, one of which resulted in a fractured wrist in his nondominant hand. Because Mr. George's wife was having trouble caring for him, their family physician enrolled them in home care to receive help with Mr. George's morning routine of bathing, getting dressed, and grooming.

Presenting Situation

Although Mr. George's wrist is healed, he continues to struggle to return to independence with his previous activities. The home care coordinator writes a referral to occupational therapy with the following information.

Mr. George has a very forward-stooped posture and seems to be unable to stand straight, making it difficult for him to see where he is going. Home care staff sometimes have to help him out of bed first thing in the morning or out of his chair, as he seems stiff and gets "stuck." He is furniture-walking in the home, with precarious balance. He is having trouble returning to his previous two-handed leisure activities like reading the paper and wood carving (his wife is afraid he is going to cut himself with this activity), seemingly because of a tremor. He has frequent spills (e.g., knocking over cup) at mealtimes.

Medical History

At the time of Mr. George's diagnosis of Parkinson's disease, he took one medication for high blood pressure. He also had some lingering back pain from working as a laborer in his career, but he was able to tolerate it or use various strategies he had learned over the years to manage it, like taking ibuprofen, using cold compresses, and distracting himself with his favorite mariachi music.

Problem Areas

1. Mr. George is having difficulty mobilizing in the home independently, potentially due to rigidity and muscular weakness as a result of his wrist fracture.
2. Mr. George is having trouble drinking from a glass without spilling due to intention tremor and potentially due to wrist weakness.
3. Mr. George is hesitant to re-engage in bowling because he worries that his poor balance will result in him falling while mobilizing in the community.
4. Mrs. George is not able to engage in her meaningful occupations outside the home because Mr. George requires her support for many ADLs.

Strengths

Mr. George has maintained strength despite his other physical limitations.
Mr. George has intact problem-solving abilities and learning capacity.
Mr. and Mrs. George have insurance that covers home care services for several hours/day as long as need is indicated.
Mr. and Mrs. George have social supports in their friends and one child who lives nearby.
Mr. George indicates motivation to engage in rehabilitation with a primary goal of being able to be home alone safely so his wife can go out and to return to bowling with his buddies.

Question

1. With the diagnosis of Parkinson's disease, what are two types of interventions the occupational therapy practitioner should consider when planning treatment?

Answer

1. Interventions should include environmental modifications and adaptation, activity adaptation, and physical exercise/activity to slow progression. (See sections on Theories and Practice Frameworks. LO 12-5)

Neuromotor Health Conditions Common in Older Adults

Many neuromotor conditions are known to affect older adults—too many to discuss here in detail. In this section, we discuss two acquired conditions that are common in older adults: stroke and head injury and the progressive condition Parkinson's disease. See Table 12-1 for a listing of neuromotor conditions that are common in older adults.

Stroke

Stroke is a broad term to include all brain or spinal cord injury with vascular origin (Sacco et al, 2013). Stroke is classified according to the underlying pathophysiology of the vascular injury. Refer to Chapter 9 for more information on heart health and stroke prevention. Depending on where the stroke occurred in the brain, persons will present with different sequelae. A stroke can affect cognitive and motor functions (see Chapter 13 for cognitive function). This chapter will focus on the impact of stroke on movement. See Figure 12-2 for motor areas of the brain that can be affected by stroke and Table 12-2 for an overview of anticipated impairment according to the vascular area compromised. Considering the anatomical region(s) of the brain affected by the stroke can be helpful to anticipate potential occupational issues that may be experienced by the person. For example, a right-middle cerebral artery stroke can result in the combination of left homonymous hemianopsia, left hemiplegia, left neglect, and impulsivity, putting the older adult at a very high risk of falls. This chapter will focus primarily on neuromotor rehabilitation specifically.

The most common neuromotor and neuromotor impairments after a stroke include:

- *Postural instability* is a tendency to fall or the inability to keep oneself from falling; imbalance (Apeadu & Gupta, 2020).
- *Apraxia* is the loss of the ability to execute or carry out skilled movements and gestures, despite having the desire and the physical ability to perform them (National Institute of Neurological Disorders and Stroke [NINDS], n.d.).
- *Impaired limb contralateral to the stroke* may present as limb weakness (hemiparesis) or paralysis (hemiplegia) contralateral to stroke (APA, 2022).

- *Ataxia* is an inability to perform coordinated voluntary movements that can be noted in upper limb movement or gait (APA, 2022).
- *Dysarthria* is a motor speech disorder characterized by difficulty speaking coherently (APA, 2022).
- *Change in muscle tone*
  - *Hypotonia* is decreased muscle tone, including flaccid paralysis, which is a complete loss of muscle tone (APA, 2022).
- *Hypertonia* is increased muscle tone, including spasticity, which occurs when muscles resist passive range of motion (APA, 2022), or hyperreflexivity, an exaggerated response of the deep-tendon reflexes (NINDS, n.d.).
- *Shoulder subluxation* is partial dislocation of the shoulder joint (Vitoonpong & Ke-Vin, 2022) and/or pain as a consequence of muscle tone and strength changes.

TABLE 12-1 Neuromotor Conditions Seen in Older Adults

CONDITION	BRIEF DESCRIPTION	ONSET AND COURSE
Amyotrophic Lateral Sclerosis (ALS)	ALS affects the neurons in the brain and spinal cord that control voluntary muscle movement. Most cases of ALS happen with no known cause, although a small percentage of cases are inherited.	ALS is a rapidly progressive, fatal disease. Motor neuron death results in loss of voluntary muscle movements, including those for swallowing and respiratory function. The typical course is 3 to 5 years but can be 10 years or more in some cases.
Motor Neuron Diseases (MND)	MND are a group of progressive neurological disorders that destroy motor neurons, the cells that control skeletal muscle activity such as walking, breathing, speaking, and swallowing. Many of these disorders have a typical onset in adulthood including ALS, progressive bulbar palsy, primary lateral sclerosis, progressive muscular atrophy, and postpolio syndrome.	These conditions are commonly acquired in middle age. The exact life expectancy and pattern of muscular weakness depends on the type of MND, with some affecting limbs more and some affecting swallowing more.
Myasthenia Gravis	Myasthenia gravis is a chronic autoimmune, neuromotor disease that causes weakness in the skeletal muscles that worsens after periods of activity and improves after periods of rest.	The onset of the disorder may be sudden, and symptoms often are not immediately recognized as myasthenia gravis. Onset is younger in females (20–30 years old) than males (50 years old). The degree of muscle weakness involved in myasthenia gravis varies greatly among individuals, and periods of remission are possible.
Multiple Sclerosis (MS)	MS is an unpredictable disease of the central nervous system that can range from relatively benign to highly disabling. It is commonly believed that MS is an autoimmune disease, although the pathophysiology is not fully understood. Any neurons in the central nervous system may be affected, and thus symptoms can include physical, cognitive, behavioral, autonomic and/or sensory symptoms. Physical symptoms range from weakness in extremities and difficulty with coordination and balance to paralysis in one or more of the extremities.	Most people experience their first symptoms of MS between the ages of 20 and 40 with the relapsing–remitting subtype, although the primary progressive subtype is typically diagnosed after age 40. The relapsing–remitting subtype waxes and wanes, whereas the primary progressive subtype results in steady progression of the disease. Life span is near normal.
Stroke	A stroke occurs when the blood supply to part of the brain is suddenly interrupted or when a blood vessel in the brain bursts, spilling blood into the spaces surrounding brain cells. Brain cells die when they no longer receive oxygen and nutrients from the blood or there is sudden bleeding into or around the brain. Therefore, symptoms can be physical, cognitive, behavioral, autonomic, and/or sensory.	Stroke is sudden in onset. Symptoms may or may not resolve, resulting in chronic stroke. Improvement in symptoms is possible for months after the stroke, especially with rehabilitation. Although stroke can affect anyone of any age, the average onset is at around 70 years of age.
Cerebral Palsy (CP)	CP is a group of neurological disorders that appear in infancy or early childhood and permanently affect body movement, muscle coordination, and balance. CP affects the part of the brain that controls muscle movements and may also be associated with other cognitive or behavioral symptoms.	The disorder isn't progressive, meaning that the brain damage typically doesn't get worse over time. For many people, the disorder does not affect life expectancy, and people with CP can live into old age.

Continued

TABLE 12-1 ■ Neuromotor Conditions Seen in Older Adults—cont'd

CONDITION	BRIEF DESCRIPTION	ONSET AND COURSE
Spinal Cord Injury (SCI)	SCI is damage to the spinal cord. Because the spinal cord contains both upper and lower motor neurons, some of the intervention techniques outlined in this chapter are relevant for upper motor nerve involvement.	SCI can occur at any age from traumatic or nontraumatic causes. In older adults, a common cause of SCI is a fall. This damage can result in temporary or permanent changes in sensation, movement, strength, and body functions below the site of injury. Some injuries that cause little or no cell death may allow for an almost complete recovery, whereas those that occur higher on the spinal cord can cause paralysis in most of the body.
Guillain-Barré Syndrome (GBS)	GBS is a rare neurological disorder in which the body's immune system attacks part of the peripheral nervous system. Initial symptoms include unexplained sensations such as tingling or pain in the feet or hands, followed by weakness on both sides of the body. The exact cause of GBS is unknown. It can occur a few days or weeks after the person has had symptoms of a respiratory or gastrointestinal viral infection.	GBS has a sudden and rapid onset, and 70% of people with GBS eventually experience full recovery. The weakness can increase in intensity over a period of hours to days to weeks until the muscles cannot be used at all and the person is almost totally paralyzed. If breathing muscles are affected, the person is often put on a ventilator. Most individuals, however, have good recovery from even the most severe cases of GBS, although some continue to have some degree of weakness.
Polymyositis	Polymyositis refers to a group of muscle diseases known as the inflammatory myopathies, which are characterized by chronic muscle inflammation accompanied by muscle weakness. Polymyositis affects skeletal muscles (those involved with making movement) on both sides of the body.	Polymyositis is rarely seen in persons under age 18; most cases are in adults between the ages of 31 and 60. Progressive muscle weakness starts in the proximal muscles (muscles closest to the trunk of the body) which eventually leads to difficulties climbing stairs, rising from a seated position, lifting objects, or reaching overhead. Most people respond fairly well to therapy, but some have a more severe disease that does not respond adequately to therapies and are left with significant disability.

Reference: National Institute of Neurological Disorders and Stroke, n.d.

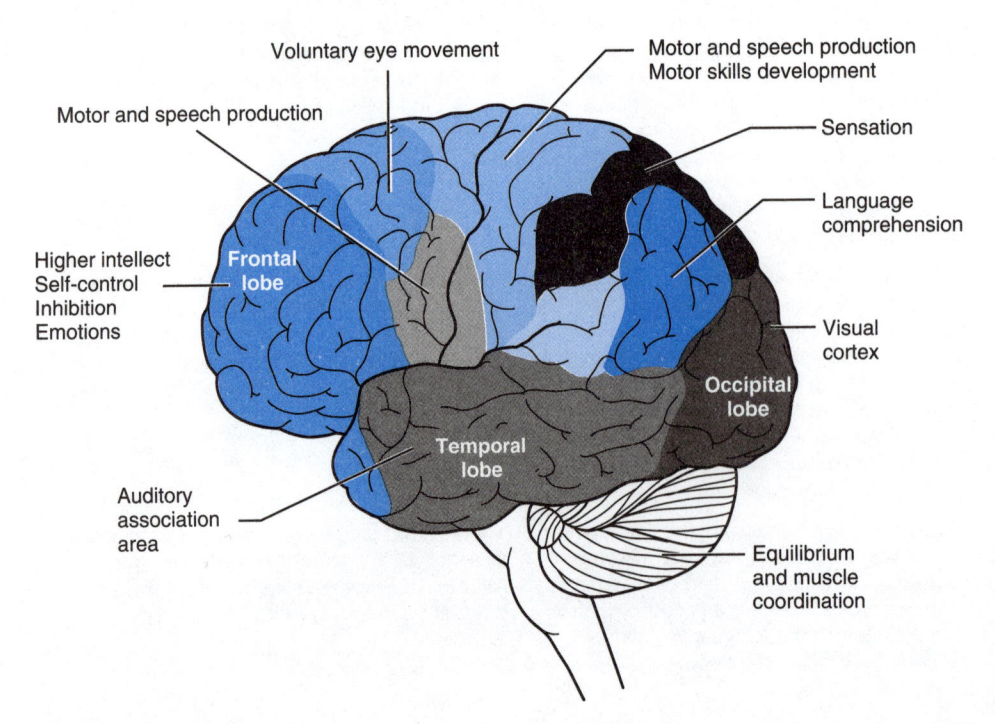

FIGURE 12-2 Motor areas of the brain that may be affected by stroke.

TABLE 12-2 ■ Stroke Signs and Symptoms by Vascular Territory/Distribution

Anterior Cerebral Artery

Less common type of stroke	Contralateral weakness, affecting the distal lower extremity more than upper extremity and face
	Apraxia

Middle Cerebral Artery (MCA)

Most common type of stroke	Contralateral hemiparesis/hemiplegia, affecting the lower part of the face, upper extremity and hand, largely sparing the lower extremity
Individual's laterality (e.g., dominance – right-handed vs. left-handed) and the division of the MCA affected determines signs and symptoms	
Superior division	Broca's aphasia (typically when left hemisphere affected)—motor/expressive aphasia, problem with output, e.g., speech is nonfluent, but comprehension is good
Inferior division	Less likely motor involvement

Posterior Cerebral Artery

Laterality (e.g., dominance) determines signs and symptoms	Involuntary movements
PCA stroke can affect the inferolateral and medial temporal lobe; lateral and medial occipital lobe, upper brainstem (e.g., midbrain, visual cortex, cerebral peduncles, thalamus, and splenium of the corpus callosum).	Hemiataxia, ataxia
	Intention tremor
	Ipsilateral oculomotor palsy
	Contralateral hemiparesis

Posterior Inferior Cerebellar Artery

Can affect the inferior cerebellum and lateral medulla	
Lateral medullary syndrome (Wallenberg Syndrome)	Ipsilateral limbs ataxia
	Nystagmus—rotatory or horizontal gaze
Ipsilateral medulla	Ataxia
Contralateral medulla	Dysphagia, dysarthria, hoarseness, vocal cord paralysis
Cerebellum	Ataxia
	Dyssynergia—impaired coordination
	Dysmetria—impaired measure, extent, and speed of intended movement
	Intention tremor
	Dysdiadochokinesis—difficulty with alternating movements
	Nystagmus
	Dysarthria

Vertebral Basilar Artery

Can affect the cerebellum, brainstem, or both	
Signs and symptoms dependent on what part of the medulla, midbrain pons is affected or if cerebellum is affected	
Cranial nerves	Facial muscle weakness

Small arteries penetrating the medial and basal portions of the brain and brainstem (lacunar syndromes)

Posterior limb of internal capsule/lower pons	Contralateral weakness of face, arm, and leg

Management of Neuromotor Manifestations of Stroke and Associated Complications

Stroke is an acute injury, and timely medical care is important after a stroke. Occupational and physical therapists are important members of the acute care team for promoting early mobility and movement, which will help prevent common complications such as deep vein thrombosis, pressure sores, and orthopedic contractures. Shoulder subluxation is very common post-stroke and affects up to two-thirds of individuals with paresis post-stroke (Fig. 12-3). Those with shoulder subluxation frequently experience shoulder pain, and the malpositioned joint results in a poor biomechanical position for optimal distal hand movements. Although there is no evidence on the best treatment for shoulder subluxation, its treatment needs to be carefully considered by the rehabilitation team to ensure the prevention of further pain and disability. (See Arya et al, 2018 for a systematic review of shoulder subluxation interventions.)

After the acute phase, the reduction of disability becomes the focus of management. The time for the initiation of

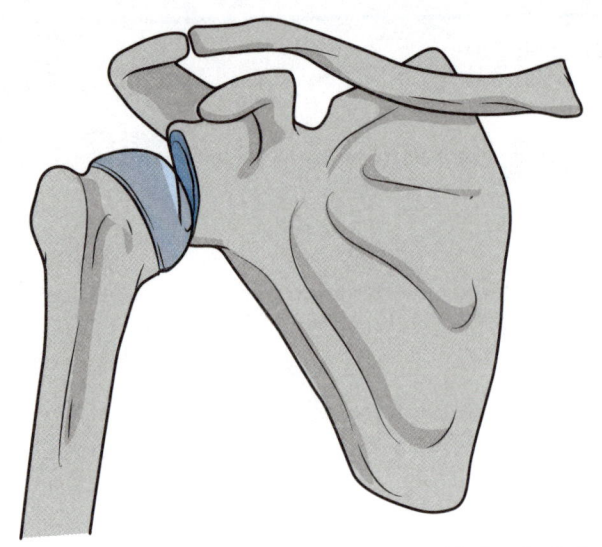

FIGURE 12-3 Shoulder subluxation is common with chronic stroke.

therapy is important. Earlier rehabilitation results in more positive outcomes, and evidence indicates that initiating intense rehabilitation 7 days postinjury can be well tolerated. Initiation of therapy in the acute care setting is associated with a higher rate of return to the community from inpatient rehabilitation, indicating the importance of early rehabilitation (Ikramuddin et al, 2022). However, caution needs to be exercised when initiating intense early rehabilitation within that period, as a large clinical trial found that initiating intensive mobilization within 24 hours of injury resulted in poorer outcomes (Langhorne et al, 2017). The therapist, therefore, should initiate early physical intervention but hold off on very early mobilization (within 24 hours) and intense therapy such as constraint-induced movement therapy (CIMT) until after the first 7 days post-stroke (Ikramuddin et al, 2022; Langhorne et al, 2017). In the postacute phase, disability is used as an outcome measure to determine progress. The Modified Barthel Index is a disability scale that could be used by an interprofessional team and has been validated for stroke with a mean age of 61 years (Yang et al, 2022).

Because many older adults survive the initial stroke, long-term impairments, activity limitations, and decreased participation greatly affect not only the person living with stroke but also the family. The best evidence for motor recovery suggests a task-based approach, with a high level of repetition and intensity to drive neuroplastic change and improve function (Chen et al, 2022). Recently published guidelines provide evidence-based recommendations for promoting motor recovery and participation following stroke (Teasell et al, 2020). Considering the world context regarding COVID-19, new guidelines on virtual rehabilitation of stroke can also support best practice by clinicians (Salbach et al, 2022).

Traumatic Brain Injury

Traumatic brain injuries (TBIs) are an alteration in brain function caused by an external mechanical force. Older adults have been reported to have higher rates of TBI than other age groups. TBI is a leading cause of morbidity and mortality in older adults. Older adults accounted for 38.4% of TBI-related deaths and 43.9% of all TBI-related hospitalizations in the United States in 2017 (Waltzman et al, 2022). The main causes of brain injury for older adults is falling from standing height or less (with peak incidence for those over 85 years of age) and motor vehicle collisions (Waltzman et al, 2022).

Management of Neuromotor Manifestations of Traumatic Brain Injury and Associated Complications

Physical manifestations like muscle weakness and poor balance can persist after brain injury but are less common than cognitive and behavioral manifestations (Oberholzer & Müri, 2019). Severe brain injury can result in paralysis or paresis and/or alterations in muscle tone, including spasticity. During the period of impaired consciousness that typically occurs in the first days after the brain injury, the therapist will need to monitor for complications that result from reduced mobilization, like contractures and pressure injuries. As with stroke, research indicates that early and ongoing rehabilitation promotes more positive outcomes (Oberholzer & Müri, 2019). Brain injury signs and symptoms will be related to the area of the brain affected. For older adults who have had a fall, the impact may be on the whole brain, due to the brain shaking inside the skull and interrupting axonal transmission throughout the entire cerebrum.

Parkinson's Disease

Parkinson's disease, a slowly progressive movement disorder, is one of the most common age-related neurodegenerative disorders, second in prevalence only to Alzheimer disease. Parkinson's disease is characterized by voluntary and involuntary movement dysfunction. A very common motor feature is **rigidity,** exhibited as difficulty initiating motion due to stiffness of the muscles. Other common motor symptoms are bradykinesia and **resting tremor**—trembling of limbs or trunk at rest (APA, 2022). See Figure 12-4 for a more thorough list of common motor symptoms in Parkinson's disease. Signs and symptoms associated with Parkinson's disease gradually progress over time; however, the rate of progression varies greatly among individuals. Common motor manifestations of Parkinson's disease are found in Table 12-3.

Management of Parkinson's Disease

Currently there is no known cure for Parkinson's disease. Instead, a combination of pharmacological interventions and rehabilitation is essential in the management of the disease (Kalia et al, 2015). Pharmacological interventions aim to increase the level of dopamine reaching the brain and to stimulate the parts of the brain where dopamine works. Levodopa is one of the main medications used to treat Parkinson's disease signs and symptoms and remains

Parkinson's Disease Symptoms

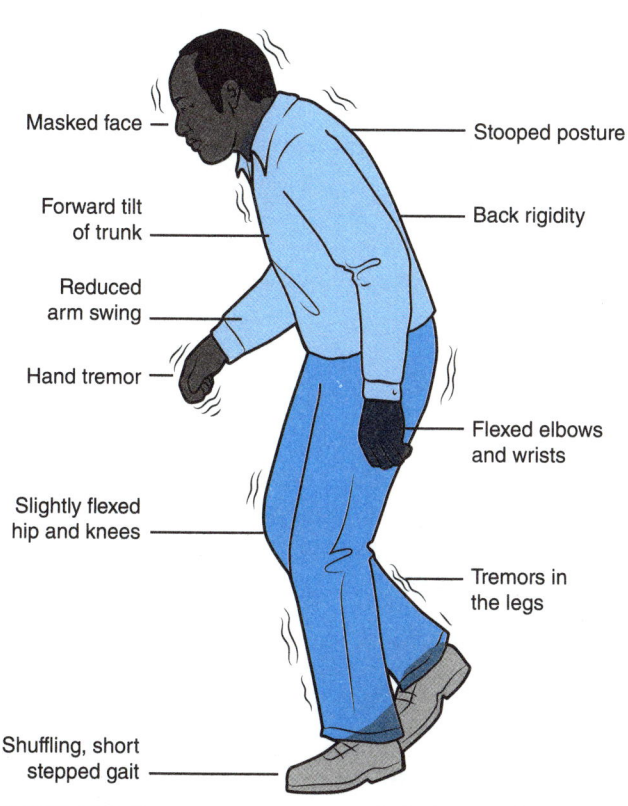

Figure labels: Masked face; Forward tilt of trunk; Reduced arm swing; Hand tremor; Slightly flexed hip and knees; Shuffling, short stepped gait; Stooped posture; Back rigidity; Flexed elbows and wrists; Tremors in the legs

FIGURE 12-4 Common motor symptoms in Parkinson's disease.

the most effective medication for the management of motor symptoms. A side effect of levodopa, particularly long-term use, is motor complications, such as dyskinesias, which are involuntary, jerky movements affecting the trunk, limbs or head, and motor fluctuations (APA, 2022).

Theories and Practice Frameworks

Motor control and motor learning frames of reference guide rehabilitation practice for addressing neuromotor and neuromotor conditions such as head injury, stroke, and Parkinson's disease (Cole & Tufano, 2020). Motor learning is the process of acquiring and perfecting motor skills and movements (APA, 2022). Traditional motor control frames—like Bobath's (1990) neurodevelopmental treatment (NDT) and Knott and Voss's (1956) proprioceptive neuromotor facilitation (PNF)—have been questioned more recently because of a lack of a robust body of research evidence to confirm their efficacy and because they are based on an old understanding of motor control as being hierarchical (Cole & Tufano, 2020; Díaz-Arribas et al, 2020). Newer theories of motor learning have evolved based on an understanding of the neurological system as a complex network that includes both bottom-up and top-down control. Although there continues to be some evidence generated that the older frameworks of motor control can have some positive impact, newer frameworks

TABLE 12-3 Common Motor Symptoms, Impairments, and Activity Limitations in People With Parkinson's Disease

SYMPTOM	CHARACTERISTICS, DESCRIPTION OF IMPAIRMENT
Rigidity	Characteristic feature of Parkinson's disease Increased resistance to passive movement • **Cogwheel rigidity,** jerky, fluctuating resistance to passive movement • **Lead pipe rigidity,** sustained resistance to passive movement Typically asymmetrical in the early stages Typically affects proximal muscles first
Bradykinesia	Characteristic feature of Parkinson's disease Slowness of movement Results from insufficient recruitment of muscle force during initiation of movement Decreased facial expressions **Micrographia,** writing becomes smaller and smaller **Hypokinesia,** slowed and reduced movement **Akinesia,** decreased spontaneous movement
Tremor	Characteristic feature of Parkinson disease Rhythmical, involuntary movement that affects a part of the body when at rest **Pill-rolling tremor,** a low-frequency, resting tremor • On observation, it appears the individual is trying to roll a pill between thumb and index finger **Action tremor,** a tremor that continues with movement Postural tremor, seen in antigravity muscles
Postural Instability	Rare in the early stage Abnormal and inflexible postural responses to destabilizing events Increased difficulty with dynamic destabilizing events Difficulty with regulating feedforward, anticipatory adjustments of postural muscles during voluntary movements Increased falls

Continued

TABLE 12-3 Common Motor Symptoms, Impairments, and Activity Limitations in People With Parkinson's Disease—cont'd

Gait Problems	More common in the later stages Decreased arm swing with asymmetry common **Festinating gait,** a progressive increase in speed with stride shortening • Can be anteropulsive, forward-festinating gait or retropulsive, backward-festinating gait
Fatigue	Difficulty sustaining activity Increased lethargy and weakness as the day progresses
Muscle Performance	Decreased strength • May be dopamine related, e.g., people on dopamine replacement medication demonstrate increased strength Antigravity muscle weakness leads to flexed, stooped posture (kyphosis)
Motor Function	Difficulty with motor planning Paucity of movement Decreased movement accuracy Difficulty with dual tasks Difficulty with motor skill learning
Dysphagia	Related to rigidity Often an early symptom Difficulty in all four phases of swallowing • Can lead to choking, aspiration pneumonia, nutritional deficiencies Decreased spontaneous swallowing • May lead to excessive drooling
Speech Impairments	Hypokinetic dysarthria • Characterized by decreased volume, monotonic or monopitch speech, imprecise/distorted articulation, uncontrolled speech rate Late disease stage may have loss of speech

Scherbaum et al, 2020.

of motor learning are more efficacious (Nowa et al, 2020). The most robust evidence available on neurological rehabilitation indicates that therapy should be based on the concepts of neuroplasticity and that attention to specificity, amount, intensity, and saliency of task practice is most effective for return to motor function (Chen et al, 2022; Scheets et al, 2021).

Motor Control Frame of Neurodevelopmental Theory

This traditional theory of motor control (NDT, PNF) is based on the belief that reflexes drive motor movement as a response to sensory input. Its use is not supported by evidence (Scheets et al, 2021), but we present it here because it is the theory to which newer theories are most related. It is important to understand that some components of motor control theory underly and include preparatory movement for occupation-based skilled voluntary movement (Cole & Tufano, 2020). In NDT, therapy focuses on building foundational skills such as postural stability and balance, which are then used as a foundation for voluntary skilled movements. These preparatory activities include facilitating symmetrical posture, ensuring good joint alignment for movement, facilitating typical movement patterns in the affected limbs, and promoting weight shifting to the affected limbs. Over time, the founders of the theory noted that the development of foundational skills did not necessarily transfer into daily living activities on their own, and so the founders started evolving the theory to include ADLs (Cole & Tufano, 2020). Examples include encouraging the use of the affected upper extremity to push up from an armchair while practicing sit to stand or encouraging use of the affected hand to grasp a knife to chop vegetables.

Occupational therapists who incorporate NDT in their practice may use it when there is little capacity for motor movement initially, limiting therapy options for task-oriented movement. NDT then provides a framework for promoting motor movement using sensory input. Occupational therapists tend to combine NDT with other frames of reference, acknowledging its limitations. Occupational therapists interested in learning about including NDT elements in their practice to promote regaining of motor skills after neurological injury should engage in advanced training and educate themselves on the extensive limitations of this approach before choosing it over contemporary motor learning task-oriented approaches.

Motor Learning Frames: Contemporary Task-Oriented Approaches

Contemporary task-oriented approaches to motor relearning are based on scientific knowledge of how motor learning occurs in the nervous system. The term *motor learning* applies to both the initial learning of and the reacquisition process of a motor skill that was lost (Cole & Tufano, 2020). For example, after a stroke, this may involve relearning how to use an affected upper extremity to complete functional bilateral tasks such as opening containers to complete grooming activities or zipping up a jacket. Motor learning is not the same as motor performance; motor performance involves the acquisition of a skill but not necessarily the retention of the skill. For motor learning to have occurred, the skill has been retained such that the learner can perform the skill later and under different conditions (e.g., in different environments), demonstrating transference of skill. Acquisition or refinement of motor skills involves both motor and cognitive processes. Although the initial learning of a new skill may involve the episodic memory system to some degree (e.g., the older adult can tell you that you taught them a specific stretching exercise) (APA, 2022), motor learning is nondeclarative and involves the procedural memory circuits, which are distributed and linked with the neural circuits underlying motor planning (premotor cortex), sensorimotor systems (primary somatosensory cortex and motor cortex), and coordination (cerebellum). In other words, procedural memory is performance-based (Janacsek & Nemeth, 2022).

Motor learning is complex; it cannot happen in isolation and involves the cognitive and sensory systems (Cole & Tufano, 2020). For example, walking requires attention to the environment to watch for obstacles, plan the route, and ignore distracting information (Chen et al, 2021b). All motor learning approaches acknowledge the importance of motor practice based on the individual's specific needs and goals (Scheets et al, 2021). Thus, the practice should be done in a variety of conditions to mimic the variability in everyday life.

Motor Learning and Motivation

Motor learning and relearning is very dependent on client motivation. "Research has demonstrated that meaningful tasks of the client's own choosing provide the greatest motivation for repeated efforts to recover and refine skilled voluntary movements in clients with acquired motor impairments" (Cole & Tufano, 2020, p. 309). The acquisition or reacquisition of a skill is highly influenced by the match between the person, the task demand, and the environment. Change consists of learning motor strategies by trial and error at first and later by practice and refinement of skilled movements. The occupational therapist needs to be highly skilled in task-demands analysis and in centering the treatment plan around the individual's interests and motivators for the just-right fit between person, environment, and occupation (Cole & Tufano, 2020).

Table 12-4 provides principles for motivational motor learning intervention. The therapist needs to work with the client to identify meaningful social and occupational roles to provide context for the skill development the individual is working toward. Motivation is enhanced by the client's selection of tasks that are at a just-right challenge and that are a priority for the client (Cole & Tufano, 2020). For example, for a client with dominant upper extremity weakness with a

TABLE 12-4 ■ Factors That Promote Skill Acquisition

CLIENT FACTORS	THERAPIST FACTORS
Match between task demands, environmental demands, and the client's abilities	Able to analyze the task, environment, person fit for a just-right challenge
Client understands what is to be achieved	Communicates clearly the expected motor performance and outcome
Able to problem-solve to find their optimal movement strategies	Encourages client problem-solving rather than being prescriptive about how the skill should be performed
In the later stages of learning, the client has the ability to self-evaluate their performance by focusing on feedback from their body and environment.	In the early stages of learning, provides summarized feedback on movement outcome (not detailed feedback on the motor movement itself).
Practices skills in daily routines	Encourages practice of whole, rather than parts of a task
Practice is done in daily routines and in varied natural settings and contexts.	

Cole & Tufano, 2020.

goal of folding the laundry, the intervention may start with folding smaller items with simple shapes resting on a tabletop and then progress by stages toward items that are heavier, with more complex shapes, and toward holding the items in space rather than having them rest on the table.

Fitts & Posner's Motor Learning Model (1967)

This three-stage model of motor learning provides a sequential framework for occupational therapists to adopt as they consider, plan, and organize learning strategies for older adults.

- *Cognitive* is the beginning learning process phase, in which the learner is working to develop an understanding of the skill. The learner must focus and pay attention; thus this stage involves many cognitive components, including executive functions, working and episodic memory, and intellectual abilities.
- *Associative* is the phase in which the skill improves with practice. Cognitive involvement decreases during this phase. This phase is characterized by more consistent performance, fewer errors, and slower gains.
- *Autonomous* is the stage in which processes become automatic, performance speed and efficiency improve, and cognitive functions involved in the cognitive phase are not required. As daily performance tasks are often "overlearned," they become automatic, and thus procedural memory is often maintained with aging.

Strategies to enhance learning in each of the three stages of skill/motor learning and motor learning variables are summarized in Table 12-5.

TABLE 12-5 Strategies to Enhance Learning in Each Stage of Fitts and Posner's Stages of Motor Learning

PHASE OF MOTOR LEARNING	STRATEGIES
Cognitive Stage	• Minimize distractions. • Emphasize purpose of the skill using meaningful and relevant contexts. • Use clear and concise instructions. • Break down complex skills into parts, if appropriate. • Make connections to other/previously learned skill(s). • Demonstrate ideal skill performance. • Use guidance and feedback.
Associative Stage	• Focus on fine-tuning the skill. • Increase the complexity of the skill. • Increase the level of environmental distractions. • Emphasize problem-solving. • Decrease feedback and guidance.
Autonomous Stage	• Focus on speed and efficiency. • Set up progressive and more challenging skills. • Practice the skill in a variety of environments and in more challenging environments.

Older adults have decreased rates of skill learning, and even when provided with protracted rehearsal and practice, they may not achieve the performance levels of young adults. However, evidence suggests that older adults *can* learn new motor skills despite age-related decrements in sensorimotor function and adaptation by using compensatory strategies such as environmental cues. Older adults may learn with more proficiency with implicit learning approaches, as explicit learning declines with aging (Poirier et al, 2021). Implicit learning is experiential and done without conscious processing. Learning to ride a bike is an example of implicit learning, as is repetitive practice of a motor movement by attempting to do it and acting on internal and external feedback, rather than following specific instructions in how to do the movement (Woytowicz et al, 2016). This is one reason that specific functional practice is an effective rehabilitation strategy for older adults.

Some older adults may never reach the autonomous stage. In a rehabilitation context, skill learning may include improvement of performance, adapting the activity, and/or retrieving a solution from a set of previously learned options. Although the older adult may not be able to perform the practice at the level of intensity or duration as a younger adult due to comorbidities or age-related strength limitations, therapy must be offered frequently to promote motor learning.

Specific Motor Learning Intervention Strategies

A specific intervention strategy commonly applied in motor relearning theory after a stroke or head injury is weight-bearing on the affected extremity. Weight-bearing within a task-oriented framework requires the weight-bearing to be completed within the context of a functional activity rather than it being the activity. Borrowing from its NDT roots, weight-bearing and weight-shifting are believed to help normalize tone and are helpful building blocks for motor skills that allow for ADLs like standing and putting away dishes, gait, and chair and bed mobility.

Another specific motor learning intervention used for hemiparesis of an upper extremity is CIMT. Although authors of a randomized controlled trial with older adults living with stroke did not find strong evidence to support using CIMT, it is seen as a promising approach, particularly after brain injury (Cole and Tufano, 2020). The intention of this approach is to force the use of the nonaffected limb, thus promoting neuroplastic changes resulting in neuroplastic changes in the brain. CIMT should be used early after the neurological injury, and therapists need to understand protocols (Cole and Tufano, 2020). Research indicates that 20% to 25% of people benefit from this approach after brain injury (Cole & Tufano, 2020).

Restoration Versus Adaptation

There is a continuum between restorative approaches (like motor learning to restore motor function) and rehabilitative/adaptive approaches (Cole & Tufano, 2020). In adaptive approaches, the focus is more firmly on the adaptation of the environment and the task rather than the improvement of motor performance. Examples of modification of the task include modifying the tools to do the task (e.g., built-up eating utensil handles for people with weak grip strength), changing the method of accomplishing the task (e.g., ordering groceries instead of going to the store), and modifying the positioning for the task (e.g., sitting instead of standing for a task).

Integrating Frameworks

Most typically, an occupational therapist will integrate multiple frameworks. For example, for someone who has had a stroke, therapy may begin with motor performance restoration using a task-oriented approach. Once there is a plateau in motor performance, the therapist and client may work together to develop adaptive approaches to tasks that are still challenging that the client wants to be able to perform to compensate for the lack of full return of motor function.

Occupational Therapy Assessment and Intervention With the Older Adult With a Neuromotor Condition

Although research has found links between older age and poorer outcomes for various neurological health conditions, the research is not definitive. It is important for the occupational therapist to understand the factors that may negatively affect the interventions provided and the overall care of the older adult, which in turn may influence outcomes. There is strong evidence that occupational therapy and other rehabilitation (such as physical therapy) improve outcomes. Although Parkinson's disease and many other neurological diseases are progressive and degenerative in nature, occupational and physical therapists have much to offer the older adult to maximize function and promote quality of life.

Assessment and intervention for neuromuscular and neuromotor conditions can be framed using the Person-Environment-Occupation Model. Through assessment, the therapist can determine whether outcomes would best be achieved with person-oriented interventions (like remediation of physical capacity) or with environmental adaptations or if the occupation itself should be adapted or changed. Whether to address the personal or environmental factors can depend on many things. One is the capacity of the individual for physical remediation. For example, in the early stages of Parkinson's disease, remediation may be effective in slowing the physical progression of the condition, whereas in late stages, environmental adaptation to support function may be indicated (e.g., a power wheelchair). Often the therapist is addressing both the person and the environment. For example, the therapist may be supporting a client after a stroke with regaining lost physical function while also providing adaptive aids to maximize independence and dignity with self-care activities. This section starts with person-oriented assessment and intervention strategies for body functions and then goes on to an overview of evidence-based strategies promoting participation and occupation that include a combination of Person-Environment-Occupation–based approaches.

In considering assessment and intervention strategies, the occupational therapist needs to apply knowledge of the specific health condition and its course. For example, although stroke and brain injury start with an acute injury followed by the potential for improvement, Parkinson's disease is an insidious and progressive condition. The therapist needs to adapt goal-setting strategies between condition types and according to the stage of the condition. Goals for a person with Parkinson's disease will be more focused on maintenance and prevention, whereas goals for a person in the initial stages post-stroke will focus on remediation.

Assessment of Body Structures and Functions for Neuromotor Conditions

There are a number of reliable and valid assessments for evaluating neuromotor conditions classified at the body function/structure, activity, and participation levels (van der Veen et al, 2022) that can be used to supplement nonstandardized assessment. Box 12-4 contains resources that can help therapists find and review standardized outcome measures. In using standardized assessment, the occupational therapist needs to be cognizant of the Eurocentric bias of standardized assessments, which can make them potentially

> **BOX 12-4** Web Sources for Finding and Reviewing Outcome Measures for Neurological Assessment
>
> Outcome measures for neurological assessment are constantly being developed, updated, and studied for their reliability and validity. Fortunately, there are web resources that summarize the outcome measures available to rehabilitation professionals in the assessment of performance components and participation for people with neurological disorders.
>
> Here are two high-quality websites that can support you in selecting outcomes measures that will be relevant to your population along with assessment and intervention goals.
>
> Stroke Engine provides the most current information about intervention and assessment tools specific to neurorehabilitation: https://strokengine.ca/en/
>
> Shirley Ryan AbilityLab Rehabilitation Measures Database is a resource for measuring benchmarks and outcomes in physical medicine and rehabilitation: https://www.sralab.org/rehabilitation-measures

irrelevant or inappropriate for Indigenous and other populations in North America (White & Beagan, 2020). Standardized assessments with an evidence base for neuromotor conditions can be found in Table 12-6.

Muscle Tone, Range of Motion, and Strength

Alterations in muscle tone—either high or low—are very common with neurological conditions and very important to assess, because tone alterations can impede functional movement and quickly result in contracture. Related to muscle tone is assessing muscle strength and range of motion, which should always be done with a neurological condition and is described further in Chapter 11. Tone can be assessed formally using the Modified Ashworth Scale (Figueiredo & Zeltzer, 2011) and the effect of tone on ADLs using the Arm Activity Measure (Ashford & Alexandrescu, 2016).

Balance Assessment

The ability to maintain balance is crucial for the successful performance of most ADLs. Impairment of balance is common in neurological conditions because of the neurological system's integral role in taking in multiple types of sensory information, interpreting it within the central nervous system, and then sending messaging for the head, trunk, and limb adjustments to maintain postural control and balance.

For neurological conditions, assessment needs to include all the components of a balance assessment, as would be done for musculoskeletal conditions, and it also needs to consider additional impairments that may be affecting balance that are more specific to the neurological system. For example,

TABLE 12-6 ■ Assessment of Body Structures and Body Functions: Neuromuscular and Neuromotor Conditions

This table lists assessments that have been found to be reliable and valid for neuromuscular and neuromotor conditions. It also provides information on type of assessment for each assessment (patient-oriented, performance) and the health conditions for which it is valid and reliable.

	ASSESSMENTS	TYPE	CONDITION
Body Structure or Function			
Range of Motion	Passive range of motion	O	All
	Active assisted range of motion		
	Active range of motion		
Tone	Modified Ashworth Scale	O	TBI; CP; SCI; stroke
	Arm Activity Measure	PO	
Strength	Manual muscle testing	PM	All
	Grip strength		
	Pinch strength		
Balance	FMA	O	Stroke
	CMSA		
	Berg Balance Scale (Berg et al, 1989)	O	Stroke
	Functional reach test and multidirectional reach test	PM	All
	TUG	PM	PD; SCI; stroke
	TUGDT	O	TBI; PD; SCI; stroke
	Activities-specific Balance Confidence Scale (Powell & Meyers, 1995)	O	PD
		PO	PD; stroke; TBI
Shoulder Pain	Chedoke-McMaster Stroke Assessment – Shoulder pain	O	Stroke
	Visual Analogue Scale	PO	All
Gait	Functional gait assessment	O	All
	Freezing of gait questionnaire	PO	PD
Coordination	Box and Block Test	O	All
	Nine-Hole Peg Test		
	Finger-nose test		
	Rapid alternating movement test		
Upper Extremity Function	FMA	O	Stroke
	CMSA	O	Stroke
Activities and Participation			
Kettle Test		PM	Stroke
Performance Assessment of Self-Care Skills		PM	All
Chedoke Arm and Hand Activity Inventory		PM	Stroke; movement disorders
COPM		PO	All
Rivermead Motor Assessment		PM	TBI; stroke
Physical Performance Test		O	All
Assessment of Motor and Process Skills		PM	All
Disabilities of the Arm, Shoulder and Hand Questionnaire		PO	MS
Stroke Impact Scale		PO	Stroke
Sickness Impact Profile		PO	All

All, Appropriate for most neuromotor conditions as validated on several neuromotor conditions as well as nonneuromotor conditions (e.g., heart failure; mental illness), but the therapist should confirm appropriateness of each assessment for the individual; *CP*, cerebral palsy; *MS*, multiple sclerosis; *O*, observed; *PD*, Parkinson's disease; *PM*, performance measure; *PO*, patient-oriented; *SCI*, spinal cord injury; *stroke*, stroke recovery; *TBI*, traumatic brain injury.

impairments specific to neurological injury in relation to balance include:

- Orienting one's trunk in space in static sitting and standing
- Difficulty processing and using the sensory information at the level of the central nervous system
- Inability to plan and send messages for initiation of motor adjustments
- Impaired or absent anticipatory or reactive responses

Chapter 11 describes typical balance impairment and assessments that can be done in relation to musculoskeletal conditions. Several balance measures have been validated for neurological conditions. For example, the Mini-Balance Evaluation Systems Test has been validated for people with multiple sclerosis (Cameron et al, 2014). Other assessments have been developed specifically for neurological conditions. The Fugl-Meyer Assessment of Sensorimotor Recovery After Stroke (FMA) (Fugl-Meyer & Jaasko, 1980) is an example of a stroke-specific measure that includes balance as one component of the assessment. When a balance assessment is being conducted, the older adult will be asked to perform various tasks that will cause instability and thus safety is essential—the therapist should closely guard and protect the person to prevent a fall. Occupational therapists can also assess balance more informally by observing the older adult engaging in ADLs. Evidence is emerging that indicates that ADLs can be an effective substitute for standardized assessments for balance (Box 12-5). For example, Rice and colleagues (2022) found that putting on a shirt requires the same amount of **postural sway** as the Multi-Directional Reach Test (Newton, 2001). In rehabilitation settings with a multidisciplinary team, formal balance assessment is often the role of the physical therapist, with the occupational therapist assessing the implications of balance instability during daily activities.

Coordination

A common challenge with coordination after traumatic neurological insult such as brain injury or stroke includes ataxia and hemiparesis or paralysis that interfere with coordination of unilateral and bilateral arm movements. In Parkinson's disease, the most common coordination challenges are **intention tremor** (trembling of body part near end of action) (APA, 2022), rigidity, bradykinesia, and dyskinesia. Gait assessments that have already been discussed can be used with careful observation for assessing ataxia in gait.

BOX 12-5 Assessing Balance in Context

Functional assessment of balance is essential, as evidence suggests that balance performance is task specific (Kiss et al, 2018) and very dependent on cognitive demands (Boisgontier et al, 2013). For example, a systematic review and meta-analysis suggest that a single fall risk assessment tool, such as the TUG, should not be used to identify community-dwelling older adults at increased risk of falls. Clinicians who assess older adults for risk of falling should ideally do so in a comprehensive manner rather than relying on a single test of mobility, and the multifactorial nature of falls should be taken into account (Barry et al, 2014). This affirms the importance of observational functional assessment in addition to standardized balance assessment. Noncontextual balance tests can be helpful to determine the safety of embarking on a more challenging assessment in a functional setting where there is less control over the environment or to find a "just right" challenge for intervention. But these tests cannot be used to predict the person's ability to manage functional activities in context. Contextual assessment allows for understanding of how all the components of balance (e.g., postural stability, cognition) are working together in concert. For example, having the older adult walk down a busy hallway allows the therapist to see if the older adult can process and react to environmental information.

Very easily administered coordination tests are the finger-nose test and rapid alternating movement test (Alouche et al, 2021). Standardized, valid, and reliable assessments of arm-hand function and motor coordination in older adults with neuromotor conditions are numerous and include the Nine-Hole Peg Test (Kellor et al, 1971) and the Box and Block Test (Desrosiers et al, 1994).

Upper Limb Function Assessment

Similar to gait, upper limb function requires the integration of many sensory, physical, and cognitive functions to work together. Following stroke, the FMA (Fugl-Meyer & Jaasko, 1980) can assist with determining the factors contributing to impairment in function, as it includes assessment of motor functioning (in the upper and lower extremities), sensory functioning, balance, joint range of motion, and joint pain.

Also, for stroke, the Chedoke-McMaster Stroke Assessment (CMSA) (Miller et al, 2008) arm and hand sections can be used to help categorize the affected upper extremity into low, intermediate, or high levels. For example, if the client is in the low level, intervention would focus on mastering stabilization tasks and moving toward level 2, which is manipulation tasks. High-level tasks include manipulation along with a focus on speed, accuracy, and quality of movement.

Interventions for Neuromotor Conditions

In this section, we cover interventions for neuromotor conditions with a focus on intervention practices in relation to older adults with musculoskeletal conditions. There is less high-level evidence on interventions with older adults. For example, although there is an increasing prevalence of older adults with TBI, there are few studies specific to older adult rehabilitation (Waltzman et al, 2022). However, there is no reason that these interventions cannot be implemented with older adults. Therefore, Table 12-7 provides an overview of interventions with strong evidence for addressing neuromotor conditions in adults—not just older adults—according to systematic reviews. As with all interventions, assessment needs to be done to identify issues that may impede safety during the intervention, and common issues in older adults, such as sensory and balance loss, should be assessed.

Muscle Tone, Range of Motion, Strength, and Associated Complications

Prevention of postural and limb deformities is a key occupational therapy role in working with people with neuromotor conditions, as they are common complications for people with altered muscle tone, weakness, and reduced range of motion. Limb contractures can quickly result when there is immobility of the limbs or a change in tone as a result of a neuromotor condition. Care should be taken to regularly assess and adapt the intervention plan for maintaining an improving range of motion in older adults—as one would with younger

TABLE 12-7 ■ Evidence-Based Interventions for Neuromotor Conditions

INTERVENTION	POPULATION(S)	POSITIVE OUTCOMES
Cooling (Kaltsatou & Flouris, 2019)	MS	Body functions (gait, grip strength, etc.)
Visual feedback intervention (Kearney et al, 2019)	PD	Balance/gait
Strength training (Cordner et al, 2021; Paolucci et al, 2020; Radder et al, 2020)	PD; stroke; MS; traumatic brain injury	Strength, mobility, gait
Bilateral functional task training (Chen et al, 2022)	Stroke	Coordination, active range of motion
Task-oriented intervention (Doucet et al, 2021)	PD	ADLs
Handwriting intervention (Foster et al, 2021)	PD	Handwriting
Individualized home-based task-specific training (Foster et al, 2021)	PD	Participation in daily tasks
Education and self-management (Rafferty et al, 2021)	Early-phase PD	Unspecified
Modification of activities and environment and use of adaptations to improve occupational performance (Rafferty et al, 2021)	Middle- and late-phase PD	Unspecified
Tai chi, Pilates, yoga, martial arts, social physical activity (e.g., dance) (Foster et al, 2021; Walter et al, 2022; Caron et al, 2021; Mazzarin et al, 2017; Radder et al, 2020)	Stroke, PD, MS	Functional balance, standing, static and dynamic balance, reaction time, maximum excursion, functional reach, dynamic gait, walking speed, improved aerobic endurance, fewer falls, instrumental ADLs
Neuromotor electrical stimulation in combination with other treatments (Hong et al, 2018)	Stroke	Lower limb motor function; gait speed, balance, spasticity, and range of motion
Multimodal exercise (including functional movement and tasks) and targeted exercise to body parts (e.g., hand) (Doucet et al, 2021)	PD	Unspecified
Mental imagery with conventional therapy (Park, 2022; Stockley et al, 2021)	Stroke	Upper limb activities performance on Fugl-Meyer Assessment
Virtual reality for gait training (De Keersmaecker et al, 2019)	Stroke	Functional gait, balance
Self-rehabilitation (Evarard et al, 2021)	Stroke	Motor function (grip strength, Fugl-Myer)

ADLs, Activities of daily living; *MS*, multiple sclerosis; *PD*, Parkinson's disease.

adults—using passive and active range of motion, occupations that challenge range of motion, and splinting as required.

For older adults with a condition affecting one side of the body, positioning recommendations need to account for positioning on the affected and unaffected side and need to consider common complications like shoulder pain. Figure 12-5 provides illustrations of positioning following stroke that supports the affected limbs to prevent complications. For older adults requiring a wheelchair for mobility, it is essential for the occupational therapist to complete a full seating assessment, including mat assessment, to provide recommendations for seating and positioning products and a wheelchair that will promote independent mobility as much as possible for the older adult. This can help prevent further postural issues, allow for optimal participation in daily living activities, and prevent complications such as pressure ulcers and respiratory issues.

Balance Intervention

Whenever possible, therapeutic intervention for balance in the older adult should be specific to the cause or causes of the problem and the impact on function. For example, after a stroke, an individual with poor postural stability and slowed reactionary reflexes would benefit from positioning feedback by using a mirror for visual feedback on trunk position and having their balance safely challenged by the therapist through activity to improve central processing. Even if there is no obvious alteration in gait from the neuromotor condition, comprehensive assessment and intervention should be done because of the high risk of falls for many older adults—even in absence of a health condition—and the myriad factors that can influence balance and fall risk in older adults.

For most older adults with neurological conditions, the root of the balance issue is multifactorial, and the older adult is often at high risk of falls. In most cases, a complex intervention is most appropriate, where the task and physical context are taken into account (Comber et al, 2021). Interventions may include altering footwear, lighting, or other environmental influences; applying a properly fitting orthosis; or using an assistive device.

An example of an evidence-based complex intervention is one that was developed by Comber and colleagues (2021)

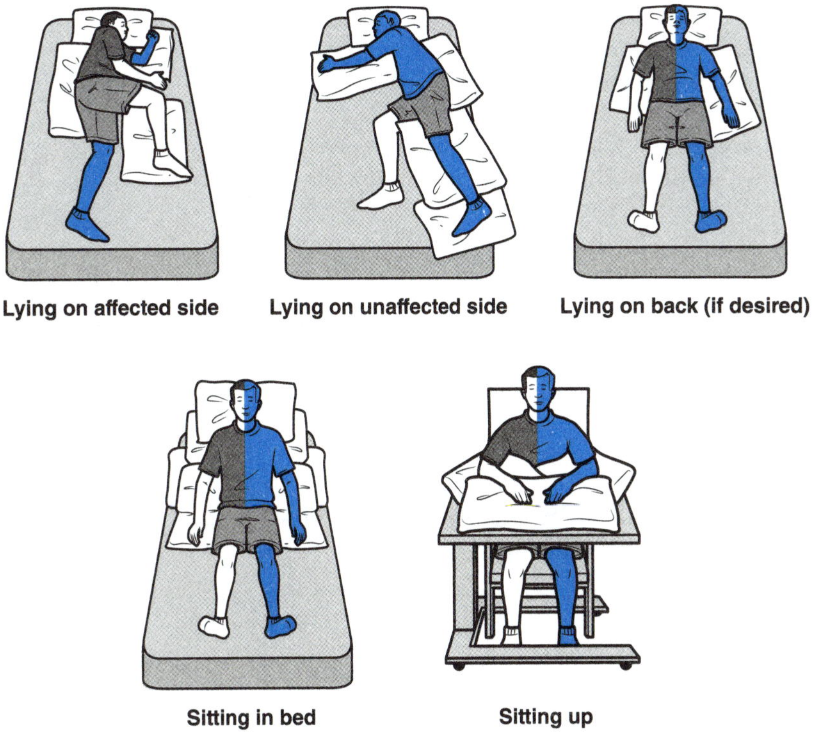

FIGURE 12-5 Positioning for stroke.

for people living with multiple sclerosis. Multiple sclerosis is progressive by nature, with balance issues requiring a remediation approach to progressive loss of balance skill from neurological impairment like slowed central processing and altered tone. The progressive nature also requires a focus on intervention for equipment (e.g., a walking aid) and environmental modification (e.g., ramp versus stairs) to reduce the risk of falls. The program developed by Comber and colleagues includes fall prevention education (environmental aspects, psychosocial and behavioral risk factors) and exercise. The exercises target the systems that contribute to balance, like the vestibular, visual, and proprioceptive systems, and challenge dual-task performance.

Balance intervention, just like all forms of motor relearning, should be task based and motivating for the individual. The therapist needs to carefully choose activities that sufficiently challenge the older adult's individual abilities to ensure improvement. If the individual needs to work on static balance (maintaining postural control with a static base of support), the therapist can work with the client to find a game or activity that can be done while standing that will challenge them through weight shifts and arm movement. Once the individual is ready for more dynamic movement, tasks can increase in difficulty gradually. For example, they could start with a kitchen task or craft at a counter, progress to doing things that require moving between two surfaces, and then progress to tasks with external support available, such as folding laundry while standing. Decreasing the size of the base of support, incorporating upper extremity and head movements during balance activities, altering sensory demands, changing directions suddenly, and changing speed during a balance activity are methods of challenging the individual's balance.

Coordination and Upper Extremity Intervention

Because requirements for accuracy create increasing demands for coordination, selecting functional tasks with increasing accuracy demands may also train coordination (Shumway-Cook & Woollacott, 2017). As with balance, the therapist is looking for a just-right fit between the individual and the task to ensure that the task will be interesting and motivating. For example, for an individual interested in cars, the task could progress from tasks requiring less accuracy—like working with large nuts and bolts—to tasks requiring more accuracy—like making model cars.

For traumatic neurological impairment (e.g., stroke, brain injury) in which restoration of function of the upper extremity can be promoted through neuroplasticity, it is important to focus on preventing learned nonuse of the affected limb in the first 3 months after injury. Because walking requires both limbs, use of both lower extremities is encouraged early in rehabilitation, and there tends to be better outcomes achieved for gait. A similar approach needs to be taken with the upper limbs to improve upper extremity outcomes. This will require more deliberate intervention, however, because many activities can be accomplished one handed, and therefore older adults may start to use compensatory strategies. The therapist needs to consider the pros and cons of teaching compensatory strategies, as they can encourage nonuse of the affected limb and reduce the potential for neuroplastic changes that will encourage restoration of function of the affected limb.

For individuals with neurological fatigue or limited cardiorespiratory reserve, addition of task-oriental mental practice has been found to improve upper limb coordination more than task training alone (Park, 2022). For progressive neurological conditions, such as middle to late Parkinson's disease, environmental modifications may be the most helpful approach, as there is less opportunity for neurological recovery. The therapist also should thoroughly understand the underlying health condition to be able to use condition-specific interventions. Example of these include cooling for multiple sclerosis (Campbell et al, 2019), interventions for essential and intention tremor in Parkinson's disease, and specialized dynamic orthotic intervention and robotics for stroke.

Assessing and Promoting Task Performance, Occupational Participation

Although the evidence for occupational therapy in high-quality studies such as randomized controlled trials is still limited, what is available confirms that occupational therapy is an effective nonpharmacological intervention for older adults with neuromuscular or neuromotor conditions (Stewart et al, 2018; Tofani et al, 2020). Most of the available research focuses on stroke and suggests that occupational therapy is one of the best nonpharmacological interventions post-stroke for improvement in ADLs, including basic, instrumental, and leisure activities. Evidence that is also building for Parkinson's disease suggests that occupational therapy that focuses on meaningful activities can improve self-perceived performance and that upper limb therapy improves function, at least in the short term (Welsby et al, 2019). Because occupational therapy is often a multicomponent intervention, the research does not indicate which occupational therapy approaches are best, aside from the literature on motor learning in relation to older adults (Walter et al, 2019) and literature on the effectiveness of environmental interventions for related outcomes, such as falls (Pighills et al, 2019). The occupational therapist also needs to consider the social, psychological, and environmental factors influencing recovery as described in Box 12-6.

Because motor learning is most effective when there is motivation for the achievement of the goals, a client-centered (Rodríguez-Bailón et al, 2022) goal-setting approach should be used. Goal attainment scaling has been found to be valid with older adults (Gordon & Rockwood, 1999), and the Canadian Occupational Performance Measure has been found to be sensitive to changes in geriatric rehabilitation settings (de Waal et al, 2022).

Maintenance of function is best when therapy is home based, suggesting that therapy should be context specific for the most long-term benefit, just as task-oriented theories suggest (Stewart et al, 2018). Additionally, it should be noted that satisfaction with performance is most related to the quality of life rather than the actual performance. Thus, an occupational therapy approach can be particularly helpful for working with clients to understand their goals and work toward those goals by considering different options, like modifying the environment or the task (Hultqvist et al, 2020). Occupational therapists can employ the many different intervention options and tools that they use for other types of health conditions with people with neuromotor conditions, such as:

- Recommendations for home modifications
- Prescription, education, and training for adaptive devices for daily living activities (e.g., handwriting, feeding, kitchen tasks)
- Community mobility and driving assessment
- Intimacy and sex positioning education
- Prescription, education and training for mobility devices (e.g., walking aids, wheelchairs)

Psychosocial and emotional intervention that can support well-being includes cognitive-behavioral therapy with education, goal-setting, performance skill training, practice, and feedback related to incorporating habits into daily life (Foster et al, 2021).

Bringing together the evidence on occupation-based approaches, task-specific frameworks, and aging research, it is evident that task-specific approaches are important for older adults. Older adults have been found to perform better in rehabilitation that is more task oriented for upper extremity movements like reaching, postural tasks, and gait (Walter et al, 2019). For occupational therapists, it is important to stay current with best practices for task-based upper extremity task rehabilitation because this is an area of special expertise for the profession (see Promoting Best Practice 12-1). Therefore, learning the older adult's goals and addressing these goals directly is the best evidence-based approach. For example, if the older adult is interested in regaining kitchen skills post-stroke, then regardless of the physical impairment, the rehabilitation should consist of practicing those specific kitchen skills. These may include chopping, washing, and stirring, with the therapist promoting movement and adapting the environment to promote successful task achievement, such as is pictured in Figure 12-6. The closer the intervention to the

---

BOX 12-6 Social, Psychological, and Environmental Factors

Therapists need to consider evidence specific to older adults that points to the importance of social, psychological, and environmental factors in recovery. Recent research supports the importance of recommendations for environmental support for older adults with a brain injury to facilitate a successful discharge to home. These include a safe home layout, meal and homemaking support, and a stimulating and creative social environment (Lafiatoglou et al, 2021). It also includes humanizing care in terms of including the older adult in decision-making and goal-setting, providing emotional support, and including families in the care (Lafiatoglou et al, 2021).

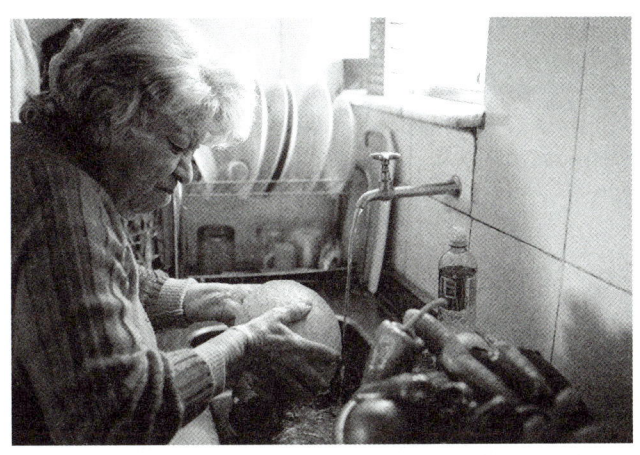

FIGURE 12-6 Complex motor activity intervention. This is a complex motor activity in which the individual needs to maintain postural control and balance while coordinating work of the bilateral upper extremities. This task-specific activity could be made simpler (sitting on stool) or more complex (locating the bowl of vegetables further from her body), depending on the therapeutic goals. *(Giselleflissak/E +/Getty Images.)*

task being performed, the better the functional improvement for ADLs (Doucet et al, 2021). For the health condition of stroke, evidence suggests that participation can improve for at least 12 months postinjury (Engel-Yeger et al, 2018).

PROMOTING BEST PRACTICE 12-1
Upper Extremity Task Training for Older Adults With Chronic Stroke

With our increased understanding of neuroplasticity, there have been many new innovative interventions developed for post-stroke rehabilitation. Some of these are showing very promising results in research trials. For example, in CIMT, the nonaffected limb is restrained to encourage motor movement in the affected limb. This reduces the opportunity for the nonaffected limb to compensate for the affected limb and theoretically can increase the opportunity for neuroplastic changes to favor returned use of the affected limb rather than rewiring to favor the unaffected limb. Another promising emerging practice for promoting rewiring is mirror therapy, wherein the nonaffected limb is hidden and the individual looks at the reflection of their nonaffected limb moving in a mirror, giving the brain the illusion that the affected limb is moving. Robotics is an emerging field where exoskeletons can promote movement in the affected limb.

Chen and colleagues (2022) conducted a review to better understand best practices for bilateral upper extremity restoration. They found bilateral functional training with adequate dosing demonstrated positive improvements in patient with stroke. Bilateral training recruits more areas of the cortex than unilateral training alone, so unilateral training will not necessarily transfer to bilateral activities. Taken together with the knowledge that older adults benefit from task-specific rehabilitation, it is clear that the best practice at this point in time is to promote bilateral task engagement (Walter et al, 2019). We also know that having a variety of interventions is typically more effective than use of one alone. Therefore, the therapist can incorporate some of the emerging best practices, such as mirror therapy, so long as bilateral task training is a crucial component of the rehabilitation plan. Essentially, the evidence supports the use of the contemporary task-oriented framework as discussed in this chapter to approach rehabilitation of bilateral upper extremity function.

Interprofessional Colleagues

The provision of therapy with an interprofessional team is the best practice for neuromotor conditions. Interprofessional intervention treatment performs better than a single professional treatment for improving ADLs (Doucet et al, 2021). This is not a complete review of all the professionals who may be able to support the older adult with a neuromotor condition. It is important for each team member to have a strong understanding of the health conditions they are working with and the evidence on how their profession can contribute to the rehabilitation plan, and to communicate their role to the team for an integrated rehabilitation plan. See the example of specialized team member contributions in Promoting Best Practice 12-2.

PROMOTING BEST PRACTICE 12-2
Team Member Contributions in Parkinson's Disease Intervention

Individualized interventions focused on health and wellness self-management and cognitive-behavioral strategies focused on lifestyle modifications and personal control positively affect quality of life in individuals with Parkinson's disease (Foster et al., 2021). This intervention is best delivered in a team. Physical therapists can support exercise and physical activity interventions that can improve impairments, such as muscle strength, motor performance and skills, mobility, balance, gait, and aerobic fitness. Speech language pathologists (SLPs) also play an important rehabilitation role with individuals with PD through interventions that address improvement of vocal loudness and pitch range; speech therapy programs, such as Lee Silverman Voice Treatment (www.lsvtglobal.com) to optimize speech intelligibility; and interventions that improve the safety and efficiency of swallowing to minimize the risk of aspiration. SLP practitioners also work to ensure an effective means of communication is maintained throughout the disease course, which may include prescribing assistive technologies. In people with PD, the intensity and complexity of physical activities and exercise were found to be critical for improvement in motor function, cognition, and quality of life and for decreased worsening of motor function in people with new-onset of the disease (Ferrazzoli et al., 2018; Scherbaum et al., 2020).

Physical Therapy Collaboration

Close collaboration with the physical therapist is very important in neuromotor rehabilitation. There are components of physical assessment for which the physical therapist has more expertise and can provide important information that can support intervention planning. For example, for postural control and balance, the physical therapist's expertise in assessing different components of balance—like the ability to prepare for movement and react to an outside force—can clarify the client's ability to maintain balance in uncontrolled settings, which is very important for making recommendations for supports at home. Gait is another area where physical therapy expertise can contribute greatly to assessment and intervention planning for the older adult.

Collaboration with physical therapy is highly important for promoting participation in exercise and physical activity, as it has numerous physiological and functional benefits for older adults with and without neuromuscular or neuromotor conditions (Luan et al, 2019). Engaging in physical activity and incorporating a comprehensive and safe exercise program tailored to the functional needs of older adults may be beneficial in preventing and managing the posture, coordination, balance, and gait problems associated with aging and neuromotor conditions. Working with a physical therapist can ensure the client receives individualized advice on appropriate and safe exercise prescription and progression that considers the primary diagnosis, associated limitations, and comorbidities such as diabetes.

Speech–Language Therapy Collaboration

Speech–language pathologists are essential professionals in the care of older adults with neuromotor conditions to ensure safety with eating, ensure adequate nutrition, and address speech and language impairments to maximize communication abilities. Aspiration pneumonia, where food or liquid is breathed into the airways or lungs, is a potential risk in all neuromotor conditions affecting the muscles of the face and throat that aid in a safe swallow. The speech–language pathologist will conduct a swallowing assessment to ensure that food is not being aspirated into the lungs and then make recommendations for safe swallowing, such as a recommendation for the safest food texture. The occupational therapist needs to be aware of the swallowing recommendations and precautions before embarking on a feeding or kitchen assessment.

The speech–language pathologist can also conduct assessments of language to determine whether the issue is related to cognitive or physical impairment, such as expressive and receptive aphasia (impairment in understanding or generating speech) (National Library of Medicine, 2022) or dysphagia (an impaired ability to swallow) (APA, 2022). The speech-language pathologist then can help with intervention of language through physical or cognitive exercises or the prescription and teaching of the use of assistive technology. In the area of assistive technology in particular, the occupational therapist and speech–language pathologist will work closely together to determine the positioning of the assistive device, particularly if the older adult is using a wheelchair for mobility.

Vision and Hearing Experts

Assessment and recommendations from vision and hearing experts such as audiologists, optometrists, and neuro-ophthalmologists are important for older adults with a neuromotor condition. This is because there are typical age-related changes to hearing and vision that need to be optimized through assistive technology like hearing aids and glasses to provide the older adult with the best opportunity for success in learning new skills.

Medical Staff – Physicians and Nurses

The occupational therapist needs to work closely with medical staff, particularly in acute care settings, to thoroughly understand the medical intervention and how it may affect activity and positioning restrictions. Specialties may be particularly helpful for providing information or recommendations that relate to ADLs. For example, nurses with expertise in bowel, bladder, and sexual function with neuromotor conditions can provide recommendations for optimizing function or for devices that may be helpful, and the occupational therapist can then work with the client to incorporate these recommendations into their daily activities.

Social Worker Collaboration

Social workers can support older adults with neuromotor conditions by addressing issues related to family dynamics, finances, and emotional adjustment. The social worker has an important role in the care of older adults, because the size of social circles and number of supports often become smaller for people as they enter older age. For example, social workers play a major role in supporting families to make decisions about long-term care and then helping with planning and supporting adjustment to long-term care. Families may need emotional and practical support for progressive neurological conditions like Parkinson's disease or amyotrophic lateral sclerosis (ALS), where future planning needs to be done with the anticipation of physical decline.

> ### CASE STUDY (CONTINUED)
> *Assessment and Intervention*
> Mr. George is really missing visiting with his bowling buddies. Although bowling had been getting more difficult, he was still able to join them at their game and visit. He stopped going when he broke his wrist, and now he

and his wife are afraid that he will fall if walking outside or in the bowling alley where there are changes in levels (e.g., stairs). His wife told the home care coordinator in confidence that she is struggling with feelings of resentment with caregiving, because the reciprocity between Mr. George and her is becoming imbalanced.

When Mr. George broke his wrist, a commode was set up on the main floor temporarily, because he previously used bilateral railings to get to the second-floor bathroom safely and could not hang on to the railing with his left hand with a cast on. Now, Mr. George is anxious about trying the stairs with his weakened wrist and what feels like worse balance. Mrs. George would like to return to some of the activities she was doing outside of the home before he broke his wrist, like attending her book club and taking care of her grandchildren two half-days per week. She is feeling nervous, though, about leaving Mr. George home alone lest he fall.

Mr. and Mrs. George seem to have both lost their zest from the broken wrist and long recovery and are having trouble finding joy with each other, which is atypical for them. They have always been proud of the life they had together and the family they created, with three children and now seven grandchildren. They are starting to wonder if they need to move to a personal care home, where they "won't be a bother."

Questions

1. What assessments will inform the occupational therapy treatment? Why?
2. What assessments from other healthcare professionals can inform intervention planning?
3. What three occupational therapy interventions are indicated based on this case? Consider the person-environment-occupation fit in planning interventions.

Answers

1. Canadian Occupational Performance Measure (COPM) to determine client's interests and priorities, Berg Balance Scale to learn more about Mr. George's fall risk, test of coordination (e.g., Box and Block Test, finger-nose test, Performance Assessment of Self-care Skills [PASS]) to determine cognitive functioning. (See sections on Assessing and Promoting Task Performance, Occupational Participation and Assessment of Body Structures and Functions for Neuromotor Conditions and Table 12-6. LO 12-4.)
2. Gait, balance, speech, swallowing, vision, hearing, bowel, bladder, sexual function, emotional adjustment. (See section on Interprofessional colleagues. LO 12-6.)
3. Person: Introduce an exercise/activity such as tai chi with focus on moves related to building balance for bowling. Environment: Explore adaptive equipment for drinking, eating, and other daily activities affected by tremors and consider home modifications including grab bars in the bathroom and entrances, if needed. Occupation: Explore with client modifications for bowling, including starting with virtual reality and/or video games. (See Table 12-7 and Occupational Therapy Assessment and Intervention With the Older Adult With a Neuromotor Condition section. LO 12-5.)

SUMMARY

This chapter has discussed the typical and expected age-related changes in the neuromotor system and typical neuromotor conditions seen in older adults. It has provided theoretical frameworks to support the assessment and intervention of neuromotor conditions and presented assessment and intervention strategies, drawing on older adult-specific research where available. It is important to recognize that the generalizations about typical age-related changes reflect an "average" and that individual variability is the norm. The occupational therapist is encouraged to do more reading on the specific health condition of the older adult they are working with, as this chapter cannot cover every health condition in detail.

Critical Thinking Questions

1. Georgia is an avid bird-watcher. She is having more difficulty with this activity as she ages. Name three reasons typical aging of the neuromotor system might be making this activity more challenging. For each reason, identify one remedial and one adaptive intervention to address the issue.

2. Considering motor control and motor learning theories, which of these should the therapist use in most clinical situations? Name one situation where a motor control approach might be a building block toward the use of motor learning theory.

3. Name, and using an example, explain at least one important difference between the occupational therapy approach for traumatic injuries, such as stroke and TBI, versus progressive disease, such as Parkinson's disease.

REFERENCES

Alouche, S. R., Molad, R., Demers, M., & Levin, M. F. (2021). Development of a comprehensive outcome measure for motor coordination; step 1: Three-phase content validity process. *Neurorehabilitation and Neural Repair, 35*(2), 185–193. https://doi.org/10.1177/1545968320981955

American Psychological Association. (2022, July 23). *APA dictionary of psychology.* Retrieved November 7, 2022 from https://dictionary.apa.org

Appeadu, M., & Gupta, V. (2020). Postural instability. In *StatPearls.* Treasure Island (FL), 19 Aug 2020.

Arya, K. N., Pandian, S., & Puri, V. (2018). Rehabilitation methods for reducing shoulder subluxation in post-stroke hemiparesis: A systematic review. *Topics in Stroke Rehabilitation, 25*(1), 68–81. https://doi.org/10.1080/10749357.2017.1383712

Ashford, S. R. J., & Alexandrescu, R. (2016). Rasch measurement: The Arm Activity measure (ArmA) passive function sub-scale. *Disability and Rehabilitation, 38*(4), 384–390. https://doi.org/10.3109/09638288.2015.1041613

Barry, E., Galvin, R., Keogh, C., Horgan, F., & Fahey, T. (2014). Is the Timed Up and Go test a useful predictor of risk of falls in community dwelling older adults: A systematic review and meta-analysis. *BMC Geriatrics, 14,* 14. doi: 10.1186/1471-2318-14-14

Berg, K. O., Wood-Dauphinee, S. L., Williams, J. I., & Maki, B. (1989). Measuring balance in the elderly: Preliminary development of an instrument. *Physiotherapy Canada, 41,* 304–311. doi: 10.3138/ptc.41.6.304

Bobath, B. (1990). *Adult hemiplegia: Evaluation and treatment* (3rd ed.). Heinemann Medical.

Boisgontier, M. P., Beets, I. A., Duysens, J., Nieuwboer, A., Krampe, R. T., & Swinnen, S. P. (2013). Age-related differences in attentional cost associated with postural dual tasks: Increased recruitment of generic cognitive resources in older adults. *Neuroscience & Biobehavioral Reviews, 37,* 1824–1837. doi:10.1016/j.neubiorev.2013.07.014

Brauer, S. G., Woollacott, M., & Shumway-Cook, A. (2001). The interacting effects of cognitive demand and recovery of postural stability in balance-impaired elderly persons. *The Journals of Gerontology: Series A. Biological Sciences and Medical Sciences, 56,* M478-M496. doi:10.1093/gerona/56.8.m489

Cameron, M., Mazumder, R., Murchison, C., & King, L. (2014). Mini Balance Evaluation Systems Test in people with multiple sclerosis: Reflects imbalance but may not predict falls. *Gait and Posture, 39*(1), 669. https://doi.org/10.1016/j.gaitpost.2013.08.009

Campbell, A., Killen, B., Cialone, S., Scruggs, M., & Lauderdale, M. (2019). Cryotherapy and self-reported fatigue in individuals with multiple sclerosis: A systematic review. *Physical Therapy Reviews, 24*(5), 259–267, doi: 10.1080/10833196.2019.1674546

Caron, L., Coquart, J., & Gilliaux, M. (2021). Effect of yoga on health-related quality of life in central nervous system disorders: A systematic review. *Clinical Rehabilitation, 35*(11), 1530–1543. https://doi.org/10.1177/02692155211018429

Chen, B., Liu, P., Xiao, F., Liu, Z., & Wang, Y. (2021a). Review of the upright balance assessment based on the force plate. *International Journal of Environmental Research and Public Health, 18*(5), 2696. https://doi.org/10.3390/ijerph18052696

Chen, H., Chen, H, Fu, S., Wang, C., & Hsieh, Y. (2021b). Attentional demands of cane-free walking and cane walking in subacute stroke patients who have just learned to walk without a cane. *International Journal of Rehabilitation Research, 44*(4), 377–381. https://doi.org/10.1097/MRR.0000000000000488

Chen, S., Qiu, Y., Bassile, C. C., Lee, A., Chen, R., & Xu, D. (2022). Effectiveness and success factors of bilateral arm training after stroke: A systematic review and meta-analysis. *Frontiers in Aging Neuroscience, 14,* 875794. https://doi.org/10.3389/fnagi.2022.875794

Cole, M., & Tufano, R. (2020). *Applied theories in occupational therapy: A practical approach* (2nd ed.). SLACK Incorporated.

Comber, L., Peterson, E., O'Malley, N., Galvin, R., Finlayson, M., & Coote, S. (2021). Development of the better balance program for people with multiple sclerosis: A complex fall-prevention intervention. *International Journal of MS Care, 23*(3), 119–127. DOI: 10.7224/1537-2073.2019-105

Cordner, T., Egerton, T., Schubert, K., Wijesinghe, T., & Williams, G. (2021). Ballistic resistance training: Feasibility, safety, and effectiveness for improving mobility in adults with neurologic conditions: A systematic review. *Archives of Physical Medicine and Rehabilitation, 102*(4), 735–751. https://doi.org/10.1016/j.apmr.2020.06.023

De Keersmaecker, E., Lefeber, N., Geys, M., Jespers, E., Kerckhofs, E., & Swinnen, E. (2019). Virtual reality during gait training: Does it improve gait function in persons with central nervous system movement disorders? A systematic review and meta-analysis. *NeuroRehabilitation, 44*(1), 43–66. doi: 10.3233/NRE-182551

de Waal, M. W., Haaksma, M. L., Doornebosch, A. J., Meijs, R., & Achterberg, W. P. (2022). Systematic review of measurement properties of the Canadian Occupational Performance Measure in geriatric rehabilitation. *European Geriatric Medicine, 13*(6), 1281–1298. https://doi.org/10.1007/s41999-022-00692-8

Desrosiers, J., Bravo, G., Hébert, R., Dutil, E., & Mercier, L. V. (1994). Validation of the Box and Block Test as a measure of dexterity of elderly people: Reliability, validity, and norms studies. *Archive of Physical Medical Rehabilitation, 75*(7):751–755. https://doi.org/10.1016/0003-9993(94)90130-9

Díaz-Arribas, M. J., Martín-Casas, P., Cano-de-la-Cuerda, R., & Plaza-Manzano, G. (2020). Effectiveness of the Bobath concept in the treatment of stroke: A systematic review. *Disability and Rehabilitation, 42*(12), 1636–1649. https://doi.org/10.1080/09638288.2019.1590865

Doucet, B. M., Franc, I., & Hunter, E. G. (2021). Interventions within the scope of occupational therapy to improve activities of daily living, rest, and sleep in people with Parkinson's disease: A systematic review. *American Journal of Occupational Therapy, 75*(3). doi: 10.5014/ajot.2021.048314

Engel-Yeger, B., Tse, T., Josman, N., Baum, C., & Carey, L. M. (2018). Scoping review: The trajectory of recovery of participation outcomes following stroke. *Behavioural Neurology, 2018,* 5472018. doi: 10.1155/2018/5472018

Everard, G., Luc, A., Doumas, I., Ajana, K., Stoquart, G., Edwards, M. G., & Lejeune, T. (2021). Self-rehabilitation for post-stroke motor function and activity-a systematic review and meta-analysis. *Neurorehabilitation and Neural Repair, 35*(12), 1043–1058. https://doi.org/10.1177/15459683211048773

Ferlinc, A., Fabiani, E., Velnar, T., & Gradisnik, L. (2019). The importance and role of proprioception in the elderly: A short review. *Materia Socio-medica, 31*(3), 219. doi: 10.5455/msm.2019.31.219–221

Figueiredo, S., & Zeltzer, L. (2011). Modified Ashworth Scale. In (Eds. Nicol Korner-Bitensky, & Elissa Sitcoff) *StrokeEngine.* https://strokengine.ca/en/assessments/modified-ashworth-scale/

Fitts, P. M., & Posner, M. I. (1967). *Human performance.* Brooks/Cole.

Foster, E. R., Carson, L. G., Archer, J., & Hunter, E. G. (2021). Occupational therapy interventions for instrumental activities of daily living for adults with Parkinson's disease: A systematic review. *The American Journal of Occupational Therapy, 75*(3), 7503190030p1–7503190030p24.

Fugl-Meyer, A. R., & Jaasko, L. (1980). Post-stroke hemiplegia and ADL-performance. *Scandinavian Journal of Rehabilitation Medicine, S7,* 140–152.

Gölz, C., Voelcker-Rehage, C., Mora, K., Reuter, E. M., Godde, B., Dellnitz, M., ... Vieluf, S. (2018). Improved neural control of movements manifests in expertise-related differences in force output and brain network dynamics. *Frontiers in Physiology, 9,* 1540. https://doi.org/10.3389/fphys.2018.01540

Gordon, P. C., & Rockwood, K. (1999). Goal attainment scaling as a measure of clinically important change in nursing-home patients. *Age and Ageing, 28*(3), 275–281. https://doi.org/10.1093/ageing/28.3.275

Henry, M., & Baudry, S. (2019). Age-related changes in leg proprioception: Implications for postural control. *Journal of Neurophysiology, 122*(2), 525–538. https://doi.org/10.1152/jn.00067.2019

Hooyman, A., Wang, P., & Schaefer, S. Y. (2021). Age-related differences in functional tool-use are due to changes in movement quality and not simply motor slowing. *Experimental Brain Research, 239*(5), 1617–1626. doi:10.1007/s00221-021-06084-x.

Hong, Z., Sui, M., Zhuang, Z., Liu, H., Zheng, X., Cai, C., & Jin, D. (2018). Effectiveness of neuromotor electrical stimulation on lower limbs of patients with hemiplegia after chronic stroke: A systematic review.

Archives of Physical Medicine and Rehabilitation, 99(5), 1011–1022.e1. https://doi.org/10.1016/j.apmr.2017.12.019

Hou, Y., Dan, X., Babbar, M., Wei, Y., Hasselbalch, S. G., Croteau, D. L., & Bohr, V. A. (2019). Ageing as a risk factor for neurodegenerative disease. *Nature Reviews Neurology, 15*(10), 565–581. https://doi.org/10.1038/s41582-019-0244-7

Hultqvist, J., Sahlström, T., Timpka, J., Henriksen, T., Nyholm, D., Odin, P., & Eklund, M. (2020). Everyday occupations and other factors in relation to mental well-being among persons with advanced Parkinson's disease. *Occupational Therapy in Health Care, 34*(1), 1–18. https://doi.org/10.1080/07380577.2019.1692269

Ikramuddin, F. S., Guarino, A. J., Siedel, E., Vonderhor, K., Larson, E., Battaglino, R., & Morse, L. (2022). Physical medicine and rehabilitation consultation for stroke patients in acute care setting may be associated with an increased rate of discharge to the community from the inpatient rehabilitation facility. *American Journal of Physical Medicine & Rehabilitation, 101* (5), 429–432. doi: 10.1097/PHM.0000000000001842

Janacsek, K., & Nemeth, D. (Eds). (2022). Procedural memory. The cognitive unconscious: The first half century. New York: NY. Oxford University Press. ISBN-10: 0197501575.

Kalia, L. V., Kalia, S. K., & Lang, A. E. (2015). Disease-modifying strategies for Parkinson's disease. *Movement Disorders, 30*(11), 1442–1450. https://doi.org/10.1002/mds.26354

Kaltsatou, A., & Flouris, A. D. (2019). Impact of pre-cooling therapy on the physical performance and functional capacity of multiple sclerosis patients: A systematic review. *Multiple Sclerosis and Related Disorders, 27,* 419–423. https://doi.org/10.1016/j.msard.2018.11.013

Kearney, E., Shellikeri, S., Martino, R., & Yunusova, Y. (2019). Augmented visual feedback-aided interventions for motor rehabilitation in Parkinson's disease: A systematic review. *Disability and Rehabilitation, 41*(9), 995–1011. doi:10.1080/09638288.2017.1419292

Kellor, M., Frost, J., Silberberg, N., Iversen, I., & Cummings R. (1971). Hand strength and dexterity. *American Journal of Occupational Therapy, 25,* 77–83.

Khosa, S., Trikamji, B., Khosa, G. S., Khanli, H. M., & Mishra, S. K. (2019). An overview of neuromotor junction aging findings in human and animal studies. *Current Aging Science, 12,* 28–34. doi: 10.2174/1874609812666190603165746

Kiss, R., Schedler, S., & Muehlbauer, T. (2018). Associations between types of balance performance in healthy individuals across the lifespan: A systematic review and meta-analysis. *Frontiers in Physiology, 9,* 1366. https://doi.org/10.3389/fphys.2018.01366

Knott, M., & Voss, D. E. (1956). *Proprioceptive neuromotor facilitation: Patterns and techniques.* Hoeber Medical Division, Harper & Row.

Krehbiel, L. M., Kang, N., & Cauraugh, J. H. (2017). Age-related differences in bimanual movements: A systematic review and meta-analysis. *Experimental Gerontology, 98,* 199–206. https://doi.org/10.1016/j.exger.2017.09.001

Lafiatoglou, P., Ellis-Hill, C., Gouva, M., Ploumis, A., & Mantzoukas, S. (2021). A systematic review of the qualitative literature on older individuals' experiences of care and well-being during physical rehabilitation for acquired brain injury. *Journal of Advanced Nursing, 78*(2), 377–394. https://doi.org/10.1111/jan.15016

Langhorne. P., Wu, O., Rodgers, H., Ashburn, A., & Bernhardt, J. (2017). A very early rehabilitation trial after stroke (AVERT): A phase III, multicentre, randomised controlled trial. *Health Technology Assessment, 21*(54), 1–120. https://doi.org/10.3310/hta21540

Lee, J., & Muzio, M. R. (2021). Neuroanatomy, extrapyramidal system. In *StatPearls.* Treasure Island (FL): StatPearls Publishing.

Luan, X., Tian, X., Zhang, H., Huang, R., Li, N., Chen, P., & Wang, R. (2019). Exercise as a prescription for patients with various diseases. *Journal of Sport and Health Science, 8*(5), 422–441. doi.org/10.1016/j.jshs.2019.04.002

Marusic, U., Peskar, M., De Pauw, K., Omejc, N., Drevensek, G., Rojc, B., ... Kavcic, V. (2022). Neural bases of age-related sensorimotor slowing in the upper and lower limbs. *Frontiers in Aging Neuroscience, 14,* 819576. https://doi.org/10.3389/fnagi.2022.819576

Mazzarin, C. M., Valderramas, S. R., de Paula Ferreira, M., Tiepolo, E., Guérios, L., Parisotto, D., & Israel, V. L. (2017). Effects of dance and of Tai Chi on functional mobility, balance, and agility in Parkinson disease: A systematic review and meta-analysis. *Topics in Geriatric Rehabilitation, 33*(4), 262–272. https://doi.org/10.1097/TGR.0000000000000163

Merriam-Webster. (n.d.). Fast-twitch. Retrieved November 7, 2022 from https://www.merriam-webster.com/dictionary/fast-twitch#:~:text=Definition%20of%20fast%2Dtwitch,requiring%20strength%20%E2%80%94%20compare%20slow%2Dtwitch

Miller, P., Huijbregts, M., Gowland, C., Barreca, S., Torresin, W., Moreland, J., ... Barclay-Goddard, R. (2008). *Chedoke-Mcmaster stroke assessment.* Hamilton, ON: Chedoke-McMaster Hospitals and McMaster University. https://www.sralab.org/sites/default/files/2017-07/CMSA%20Manual%20and%20Score%20Form.pdf

Moreno-García, A., Kun, A., Calero, O., Medina, M., & Calero, M. (2018). An overview of the role of lipofuscin in age-related neurodegeneration. *Frontiers in Neuroscience, 12,* 464. https://doi.org/10.3389/fnins.2018.00464

National Institute of Neurological Disorders and Stroke [NINDS]. (n.d.). Health information. National Institutes of Health. Bethesda: MD. Accessed on August 5, 2022 from https://www.ninds.nih.gov/health-information

National Library of Medicine. (2022, July 23). *Health topics.* Retrieved from National Library of Medicine: https://medlineplus.gov/healthtopics.html

Newton, R. A. (2001). Validity of the multi-directional reach test: A practical measure for limits of stability in older adults. *Journal of Gerontology: Medical Sciences, 56A,* M248-M252. doi: 10.1093/erona/56.4.M248.

Nowa, J., Franzsen, D., & Thupae, D. (2020). Comparison of motor relearning occupation-based and neurodevelopmental treatment approaches in treating patients with traumatic brain injury. *South African Journal of Occupational Therapy, 50*(3), 40–51. https://dx.doi.org/10.17159/2310-3833/2020/vol50no3a5

Oberholzer, M., & Müri, R. M. (2019). Neurorehabilitation of traumatic brain injury (TBI): A clinical review. *Medical Sciences, 7*(3), 47. https://doi.org/10.3390/medsci7030047

Osoba, M. Y., Rao, A. K., Agrawal, S. K., & Lalwani, A. K. (2019). Balance and gait in the elderly: A contemporary review. *Laryngoscope Investigative Otolaryngology, 4*(1), 143–153. https://doi.org/10.1002/lio2.252

Overbeek, C. L., Geurkink, T. H., Groot, F. A., Klop, I., Nagels, J., Nelissen, R. G. H. H., & Groot, J. H. (2021). Shoulder movement complexity in the aging shoulder: A cross-sectional analysis and reliability assessment. *Journal of Orthopaedic Research, 39*(10), 2217–2225. https://doi.org/10.1002/jor.24932

Paolucci, T., Sbardella, S., La Russa, C., Agostini, F., Mangone, M., Tramontana, L., ... Saggini, R. (2020). Evidence of rehabilitative impact of progressive resistance training (PRT) programs in Parkinson Disease: An umbrella review. *Parkinson's Disease, 2020,* 9748091. https://doi.org/10.1155/2020/9748091

Park, J. (2022). The effects of task-oriented mental practice on upper limb function and coordination in chronic stroke patients—Randomized controlled trial design. *British Journal of Occupational Therapy, 85*(3), 164–171. https://doi.org/10.1177/03080226211057838

Parthasharathy, M., Mantini, D., & Orban de Xivry, J. J. (2022). Increased upper-limb sensory attenuation with age. *Journal of Neurophysiology, 127*(2), 474–492. https://doi.org/10.1152/jn.00558.2020

Pethick, J., Winter, S. L., & Burnley, M. (2021). Physiological complexity: Influence of ageing, disease and neuromotor fatigue on muscle force and torque fluctuations. *Experimental Physiology, 106*(10), 2046–2059. https://doi.org/10.1113/EP089711

Pighills, A., Drummond, A., Crossland, S., & Torgerson, D. J. (2019). What type of environmental assessment and modification prevents falls in community dwelling older people? *BMJ, 364,* l880. https://doi.org/10.1136/bmj.l880

Poirier, G., Ohayon, A., Juranville, A., Mourey, F., & Gaveau, J. (2021). Deterioration, compensation and motor control processes in healthy aging, mild cognitive impairment and Alzheimer's disease. *Geriatrics, 6*(1), 33. doi.org/10.3390/geriatrics6010033

Powell, L. E., & Myers, A. M. (1995). The Activities-specific Balance Confidence (ABC) scale. *Journal of Gerontology: Series A. Biological Sciences and Medical Sciences, 50,* M28-M34. doi: 10.1093/erona/50A.1.M28

Radder, D. L. M., Silva de Lima, A., Domingos, J. M., Keus, S. H., Nimwegen, M. L., van Bloem, B., & de Vries, N. M. (2020). Physiotherapy in Parkinson's disease: A meta-analysis of present treatment modalities. *Neurorehabilitation and Neural Repair, 34*(10), 871–880. https://doi.org/10.1177/1545968320952799

Rafferty, M. R., Nettnin, E., Goldman, J. G., & MacDonald, J. (2021). Frameworks for Parkinson's disease rehabilitation addressing when, what, and how. *Current Neurology and Neuroscience Reports, 21*(3), 12. https://doi.org/10.1007/s11910-021-01096-0

Rice, C. G., Michaels, K., Patel, U., & Stahl, C. (2022). Balance relationships between the multidirectional reach test and upper body dressing. *The American Journal of Occupational Therapy, 76*(Supplement_1), 7610500015p1. doi: 10.5014/ajot.2022.76S1-PO15

Rodríguez-Bailón, M., López-González, L., & Merchán-Baeza, J. A. (2022). Client-centred practice in occupational therapy after stroke: A systematic review. *Scandinavian Journal of Occupational Therapy, 29*(2), 89–103. https://doi-org.uml.idm.oclc.org/10.1080/11038128.2020.1856181

Rozand, V., Sundberg, C. W., Hunter, S. K., & Smith, A. E. (2020). Age-related deficits in voluntary activation: A systematic review and meta-analysis. *Medicine and Science in Sports and Exercise, 52*(3), 549–560. https://doi.org/10.1249/MSS.0000000000002179

Sacco, R. L., Kasner, S. E., Broderick, J. P., Caplan, L. R., Connors, J. J., Culebras, A., ... Vinters, H. V. (2013). An updated definition of stroke for the 21st century: A statement for healthcare professionals from the American Heart Association/American Stroke Association. *Stroke, 44*(7), 2064–2089. doi.org/10.1161/STR.0b013e318296aeca

Salbach, N. M., Mountain, A., Lindsay, M. P., Blacquiere, D., McGuff, R., Foley, N., ... Yao, J. (2022). Canadian stroke best practice recommendations: Virtual stroke rehabilitation consensus statement 2022. *American Journal of Physical Medicine & Rehabilitation, 101*(11), 1076–1082. https://doi.org/10.1097/PHM.0000000000002062

Scheets, P. L., Hornby, T. G., Perry, S. B., Sparto, P., Riley, N., Romney, W., ... Nordahl, T. (2021). Moving forward. *Journal of Neurologic Physical Therapy, 45*(1), 46–49. https://doi.org/10.1097/NPT.0000000000000337

Scherbaum, R., Hartelt, E., Kinkel, M., Gold, R., Muhlack, S., & Tönges, L. (2020). Parkinson's disease multimodal complex treatment improves motor symptoms, depression and quality of life. *Journal of Neurology, 267*(4), 954–965. doi: 10.1007/s00415-019-09657-7.

Seidler, R. D., Bernard, J. A., Burutolu, T. B., Fling, B. W., Gordon, M. T., Gwin, J. T., ... Lipps, D. B. (2010). Motor control and aging: Links to age-related brain structural, functional, and biochemical effects. *Neuroscience & Biobehavioral Reviews, 34,* 721–733. doi:10.1016/j.neubiorev.2009.10.005

Shumway-Cook, A., Brauer, S., & Woollacott, M. (2000). Predicting the probability for falls in the community-dwelling older adults using the Timed Up & Go Test. *Physical Therapy, 80,* 896–903. Retrieved from: http://ptjournal.apta.org/content/80/9/896

Shumway-Cook, A., & Woollacott, M. H. (Eds.). (2017). *Motor control: Translating research into clinical practice* (5th ed.). Philadelphia: Lippincott, Williams & Wilkins.

Stewart, C., Subbarayan, S., Paton, P., Gemmell, E., Abraha, I., Myint, P. K., ... Soiza, R. L. (2018). Non-pharmacological interventions for the improvement of post-stroke activities of daily living and disability amongst older stroke survivors: A systematic review. *PloS One, 13*(10), e0204774–e0204774. https://doi.org/10.1371/journal.pone.0204774

Stockley, R. C., Jarvis, K., Boland, P., & Clegg, A. J. (2021). Systematic review and meta-analysis of the effectiveness of mental practice for the upper limb after stroke: Imagined or real benefit? *Archives of Physical Medicine & Rehabilitation, 102*(5), 1011–1027. https://doi-org.uml.idm.oclc.org/10.1016/j.apmr.2020.09.391

Stokkermans, M., Solis-Escalante, T., Cohen, M. X., & Weerdesteyn, V. (2022). Midfrontal theta dynamics index the monitoring of postural stability. *Cerebral Cortex, 33*(7), 3454–3466. https://doi-org.uml.idm.oclc.org/10.1093/cercor/bhac283

Teasell, R., Salbach, N. M., Foley, N., Mountain, A., Cameron, J. I., de Jong, A., ... Lindsay, M. P. (2020). Canadian stroke best practice recommendations: Rehabilitation, recovery, and community participation following stroke. Part one: Rehabilitation and recovery following stroke; 6th ed. update 2019. *International Journal of Stroke, 15*(7), 763–788. https://doi.org/10.1177/1747493019897843

Tieland, M., Trouwborst, I., & Clark, B. C. (2018). Skeletal muscle performance and ageing. *Journal of Cachexia, Sarcopenia and Muscle, 9*(1), 3–19. https://doi.org/10.1002/jcsm.12238

Tofani, M., Ranieri, A., Fabbrini, G., Berardi, A., Pelosin, E., Valente, D., ... Galeoto, G. (2020). Efficacy of occupational therapy interventions on quality of life in patients with Parkinson's disease: A systematic review and meta-analysis. *Movement Disorders Clinical Practice, 7*(8), 891–901. https://doi.org/10.1002/mdc3.13089

van der Veen, S., Evans, N., Huisman, M., Welch Saleeby, P., & Widdershoven, G. (2022). Toward a paradigm shift in healthcare: Using the International Classification of Functioning, Disability and Health (ICF) and the capability approach (CA) jointly in theory and practice. *Disability and Rehabilitation, 45*(14), 2382–2389.

Vitoonpong, T., & Ke-Vin Chang, K. (2022). Shoulder subluxation. In *StatPearls.* Treasure Island (FL), Aug 2022.

Walter, A. A., Van Puymbroeck, M., Bosch, P., & Schmid, A. A. (2022). Complementary and integrative health interventions in post-stroke rehabilitation: A systematic PRISMA review. *Disability and Rehabilitation, 44*(11), 2223–2232. doi.org/10.1080/09638288.2020.1830440

Walter, C. S., Hengge, C. R., Lindauer, B. E., & Schaefer, S. Y. (2019). Declines in motor transfer following upper extremity task-specific training in older adults. *Experimental Gerontology, 116,* 14–19. https://doi.org/10.1016/j.exger.2018.12.012

Waltzman, D., Haarbauer-Krupa, J., & Womack, L. S. (2022). Traumatic brain injury in older adults—A public health perspective. *JAMA Neurology, 79*(5), 437–438. https://doi.org/10.1001/jamaneurol.2022.0114

Welsby, E., Berrigan, S., & Laver, K. (2019). Effectiveness of occupational therapy intervention for people with Parkinson's disease: Systematic review. *Australian Occupational Therapy Journal, 66*(6), 731–738. https://doi.org/10.1111/1440-1630.12615

White, T., & Beagan, B. L. (2020). Occupational therapy roles in an Indigenous context: An integrative review. *Canadian Journal of Occupational Therapy, 87*(3), 200–210. https://doi.org/10.1177/0008417420924933

Woytowicz, E., Whitall, J., & Westlake, K. P. (2016). Age-related changes in bilateral upper extremity coordination. *Current Geriatrics Reports, 5*(3), 191–199. https://doi.org/10.1007/s13670-016-0184-7

Yang, C. M., Wang, Y. C., Lee, C. H., Chen, M. H., & Hsieh, C. L. (2022). A comparison of test-retest reliability and random measurement error of the Barthel Index and modified Barthel Index in patients with chronic stroke. *Disability and Rehabilitation, 44*(10), 2099–2103. https://doi.org/10.1080/09638288.2020.1814429

Zapparoli, L., Mariano, M., & Paulesu, E. (2022). How the motor system copes with aging: A quantitative meta-analysis of the effect of aging on motor function control. *Communications Biology, 5*(1), 79. https://doi.org/10.1038/s42003-022-03027-2

CHAPTER 13

Neurobehavioral Function and Health Conditions

Marsha Neville, PhD, OT

> *"Don't try to be young. Just open your mind. Stay interested in stuff. There are so many things I won't live long enough to find out about, but I'm still curious about them."*
>
> —Betty White

LEARNING OUTCOMES

By the end of this chapter, readers will be able to:

13-1. Evaluate the factors of normal cognitive aging that impact a person's occupational participation.
13-2. Choose and justify best practices for facilitation of cognitive function in normal aging including lifestyle, activity, and stimulation.
13-3. Design and support cognitive interventions using knowledge of theories of cognitive aging.
13-4. Compare and contrast assessments of cognitive functioning including assessments at level of body function and performance-based assessments.
13-5. Identify assessments and design interventions for an older adult with cognitive changes after a stroke.
13-6. Identify assessments and design interventions for older adults with dementia.
13-7. Identify assessments and design interventions for older adults with depression, anxiety disorders, schizophrenia, bipolar disorder, and substance use disorder.
13-8. Compare and contrast cognitive functioning in normal cognitive aging and cognitive functioning in persons with dementia.
13-9. Using knowledge of foundations of cognitive health, create treatment environments and programs for optimizing cognitive health for healthy older adults and those with neuropathologies.
13-10. Compare the different roles of interprofessional health team members working with older adults and considerations for a referral.

Mini Case Study

Henry Webster is a 70-year-old white male who lives alone after the recent death of his wife of 40 years. Henry has lived in the same home for 45 years in a large metropolitan city in the Midwest region of the United States. It is a single-story home with a basement. Before her death, Henry's mother lived with him and his wife. She had cancer and Alzheimer disease. Henry has three children: two sons and a daughter. One son and daughter live in the same city as Henry. They work full-time and have children age 4 to 16 years old. Both of these adult children visit their father regularly but are busy working and involved with their children. Henry retired 1 year ago from his career as a plant manager of a large production company. He and his wife enjoyed playing golf and taking trips to visit family and friends. Before the sudden death of his wife 8 months ago, they were planning on selling their home and living in an RV for 2 years before settling on where to live. Since his wife's death, he has joined a men's golf league but is not playing regularly. He has lost interest in swimming and does not enjoy walking in the park, only walking around his neighborhood. He is reconsidering selling his home and has not traveled to see family or friends in the past 8 months. Henry's children are concerned about Henry's occupational performance. He is missing appointments and is having difficulty following conversations. Other issues include poor housekeeping, including dirty floors. Henry's general health is good, taking medication only for high blood pressure, which is controlled. He has hearing loss but refuses hearing aids. He does have bifocals that he wears when driving. Henry's children have noticed changes in his personality, including grumpiness, decreased energy level, and weight loss. Some of Henry's family and friends think these changes are a passing phase due to the recent loss of his wife, while others think these may be early symptoms of something more serious.

Provocative Questions
1. What environmental factors could be contributing to the changes in Henry's occupational performance?
2. What are some personal factors that can facilitate or inhibit Henry's healthy aging?

3. What assessments and interventions might provide insights into the underlying factors Henry is experiencing?
4. What are some cultural factors that are affecting or could affect Henry's occupational performance and roles?

Cognitive processes include attention, memory, problem-solving, and decision-making. Changes in cognitive functioning begin as early as the fourth decade of life. Cognitive aging occurs over time and varies among individuals. Changes in cognitive functioning are not specifically caused by aging; factors such as general health, education, lifestyle, genetics, socioeconomics, and socialization can cause changes in individuals. These factors and the variability of cognitive changes must be considered when interacting with older adults. Cognition holds such primacy in society that people fear and are aware of any changes in cognitive functioning. The stereotype that older adults have fewer cognitive skills can lead to assumptions in relationships that could be less than ideal. This chapter will review typical changes in cognitive function during aging and neuropathologies, including stroke, dementias, and mental illnesses.

A Perspective on Cognition and Aging

A healthy brain, when stimulated, continues to learn and adapt. This is critical for sustaining cognitive functioning in older adults. While older adults may experience cognitive changes, the amount of change and impact on lifestyle is as variable in older adults as it is in other individuals. Studies of cognitive functioning comparing older and younger adults typically use language that disproportionately reflects negative aspects of the aging process, such as "deficits," "losses," "decrements," and "impairments." It is important to note these findings are based on laboratory experiments reflecting differences in reaction time (in the range of milliseconds) or decreases in accuracy (by one to two stimuli) between younger and older adults. These results and the language used to describe findings can be misleading when considering functioning in real-world versus clinical settings. It is therefore important to consider the implications of using potentially negative language that may have unintended consequences for older and younger adults, laypersons, clinicians and professionals, and policymakers. To illustrate, Marquet & colleagues (2019) studied 151 adults age 60 to 80 years and found that perceptions of discrimination and negative aging stereotypes were internalized among study participants, leading to lower self-esteem and negative perceptions of one's abilities. Older adults exposed to negative stereotypes showed changes in brain activity related to perceptions of self and error prevention. Those exposed to negative stereotypes had slower response times and more false alarms on episodic memory tasks (Nakamura et al, 2022). For these reasons, this chapter uses terms such as cognitive "changes" or "differences" and, when appropriate for describing the nature of these differences, "gains," "declines," and "stability" rather than negatively charged language.

Cognitive Processes and Implications for Older Adults

Changes and stability of cognitive functioning in older adults cannot be reduced to a single cognitive process. Cognitive processes are attention, memory, and executive functions, including problem-solving, reasoning, judgment, language, and speed of processing. Further cognitive functioning involves complex processes dependent on attention, memory, and executive functions. Intelligence, wisdom, and implicit and explicit processing influence cognitive functioning. This section will describe and provide evidence on how cognitive functioning changes and remains stable with aging. See Table 13-1 for a summary of cognitive processing.

Attention

Attention is the ability to focus on stimuli for the purpose of processing information. Attention requires effort and the ability to filter relevant and irrelevant stimuli. The ability to successfully make decisions, problem-solve, or think through an issue requires attentional resources. Attention is often described from the most basic to more complex:

- *Sustained (or focused) attention* is the ability to direct attentional resources to a single task or activity. An example is concentrating on reading a book.
- *Selective attention* is the ability to direct attentional resources to a task or activity while simultaneously directing attentional resources to ignore distracting information. An example is listening to a story someone is telling while others are talking around you.
- *Alternating attention* is the ability to direct or switch attentional resources between two or more tasks or activities. It is conceptually distinct from divided attention because tasks are performed one at a time with attentional resources switching back and forth between tasks. An example is when cooking, a person attends to stirring one item and then letting it cook, while they work on chopping and prepping another item. The person then shifts back and forth depending on the instructions.
- *Divided attention* is the ability to allocate attentional resources to two or more tasks or activities at the same time. An example, reading an e-mail while following a phone conversation. It is well documented that encoding of information into memory is degraded with the introduction of a secondary task and the more complex the task the greater the reduction (Greene et al, 2020).

Implications of Attention on Treatment of Older Adults

The ability to selectively attend and inhibit irrelevant information is foundational to cognitive functioning. In a study by Greene et al (2020), divided attention affected the encoding of both specific details and the gist of the event,

TABLE 13-1 Cognitive Processing and Older Adults

CHANGES IN OLDER ADULTS	STABLE IN OLDER ADULTS	CLINICAL CONSIDERATIONS
Selective attention - Divided attention	- Vigilance - Concentration	- Minimize distractors in environment. - Reduce clutter in home. - Ensure person has time to process information.
- Recognition - Recall of information events without cues	- Retains familiarity with events Example: - Person looks familiar - Recalls the gist of the conversations Example: - The doctor said I needed a follow-up appointment (not sure why). - Performing familiar procedures, including simple activities (e.g., dressing) to complex activities (e.g., sewing, car mechanics)	- Encourage strategies for ensuring storage of information in memory – ask person to repeat information. - Encourage use of lists, calendars, timers. - Ensure continued participation in meaningful activities.
- Learning and sequencing novel motor tasks - Example: How to get in and out of bathtub using equipment and hip precautions	- Performing familiar procedures including simple activities – dressing to complex activities – sewing, car mechanics	
- Complex planning for future (prospective memory). Example: Packing for a vacation; planning timing for preparing a meal	- Carrying out daily routines and habits Schedules that are well-rehearsed	- Recognize effort needed to modify routines. - Assist person in breaking down the task into smaller segments.
- Word-finding and tip-of-tongue experiences	- Knowledge of facts, rules, and language	- Allow time for person to generate language.

suggesting that decreased attention may affect recall of specific information. Clinicians must consider the client's ability to attend during treatment and implement strategies to enhance attention. Attention is foundational to higher-order cognitive processing such as problem-solving and decision-making. See Promoting Best Practice 13-1.

PROMOTING BEST PRACTICE 13-1
Optimizing Attention

Clinic scenario: Teaching bathroom safety and bathtub transfer to a 75-year-old client after total hip replacement surgery. The client is experiencing typical changes in cognitive functioning and has minor hearing loss.

Factors affecting a person's attention include the amount of distraction, relevance of the task, motivation, and fatigue. If the client has never had problems entering and exiting the bathtub, they may not appreciate why you are telling them to do it differently. A clinician must take responsibility for ensuring the client is motivated. This is particularly important for allied health professionals (e.g., occupational therapists, speech-language pathologists, physical therapists) who are developing goals and implementing treatment with clients. To increase engagement and treatment participation, it is critical to include the client in developing realistic and meaningful goals that are important to them.

1. Minimize all distractions. Remove unneeded equipment, ensure privacy.
2. Consider speed of processing. Slow the instruction if client needs more time to process.
3. Know the client's sensory processing abilities and ensure the client is understanding and seeing what you are doing. Asking the client for feedback is one way of checking their understanding.
4. Explain to the client your goal for the session and ask what they would like to get from the session. This can build meaning and set expectations.
5. Actively engage the client in the treatment. This can emphasize the meaning and relevance to the client. Engage the client with probes to describe their bathroom, talk about bathroom routines, and ask the client about their concerns. Engage the client in problem-solving. For example, ask the client if they have rugs in the bathroom. You explain that rugs can be a fall risk. Rather than tell the client they need to remove the rugs, you ask them to problem-solve how they might avoid tripping or catching their foot.
6. Use a "teach-back" method of instruction, asking the client to explain what was said and ask their opinion.
7. For learning transfers, repetition is needed. Engage in problem-solving for the client's learning.
8. Once the transfer is performed safely, you may introduce distractions to challenge the client and simulate a real-world environment, such as a busy home.
9. Review the session, address questions and concerns, and ask the client if the session met their expectations and what more is needed.
10. Handouts can be helpful to enhance learning. Some examples include pictures of equipment discussed, a bulleted list of common bathroom safety rules, and information on types and placement of grab bars.

Memory

Memory is a generic term used to describe types of memory including sensory memory, short-term memory, working memory, and several long-term memory systems, including declarative and procedural long-term memory.

- *Sensory memory* is the processing of information through the vestibular, visual, auditory, and tactile systems.
- *Short-term memory* can take on two forms. The first form, new information, is stored based on sensory inputs; the second form is memories that have been stored and retrieved through cueing such as smelling an odor and recalling a feeling or conversation (Baddeley, 2020).
- *Working memory* demands attention and requires the intentional use of strategies to manipulate, store, and maintain information. Working memory serves a vital role in facilitating higher-order cognitive processes such as language production and comprehension (Kemper & Mitzner, 2001), decision-making, problem-solving, and learning (Tulving & Craik, 2000). For more information see working memory in the section on Cognitive Theories of Aging.
- *Procedural or nondeclarative memory* is a nonverbal-based memory system that stores information for motor-based skills and behaviors (e.g., muscle memory), habits, emotional associations, priming, and classical conditioning. Retrieval of nondeclarative memories can occur with little effort or even conscious awareness. Examples of procedural memory include how to play a musical instrument, ride a bike, or perform a habitual task, such as brushing your teeth.
- *Prospective memory* enables individuals to remember future-oriented or scheduled tasks without the use of external memory aids (e.g., written note or list). Examples of prospective memory include remembering to take medications twice daily, wearing a brace to bed, stopping at the grocery store, or buying a birthday card for a friend.
- *Semantic memory* is the knowledge of language including words, phrases, definitions, and grammar. Understanding language and memory for facts is considered crystallized intelligence and remains relatively stable with aging. However, age-related differences can be found in the production of speech (Zhang et al, 2019).

Implications of Memory on Treatment of Older Adults

Directed attention and processing of sensory information are foundational to processing, storing, and retrieving memories. A person who has problems seeing or hearing may appear to have deficits in cognition. Thus, older adults may appear to have memory deficits when the primary problem is due to sensory deficits.

Procedural memory has minimal to no age-related declines (Ward, 2022). Age-related differences are more likely to be found when the complexity of the motor task increases. A clear trend from these findings is the role of task complexity and the subsequent need to use additional cognitive resources. An example of a complex task would be learning how to perform a bathtub transfer as illustrated in Promoting Best Practice 13-1.

Evidence suggests that older adults do have changes in prospective memory, but it is dependent on the complexity. However, these differences tend to be evident in laboratory studies, and the difference is less significant in naturalistic environments (Haas et al, 2022).

Executive Functioning

Executive functioning refers to higher-order cognitive processes such as reasoning, decision-making, problem-solving, judgment, abstract thought, cognitive flexibility, initiation, and inhibition (Burgess et al, 2000). Executive function underlies a person's ability to engage in everyday activities. A clinician must assess a client's executive function to determine effective treatment approaches. See the section on Functional Cognition for a list of assessments.

Implication of Executive Functions on Treatment of Older Adults

Older adults experience changes in executive functioning. Age-related longitudinal declines were found for four types of executive functioning-related processes (e.g., inhibition, manipulation, semantic and phonological retrieval, and task switching), whereas five executive functioning–related processes (e.g., abstraction, capacity, chunking, discrimination, and short-term memory) were maintained or showed improvements with age (Goh et al, 2012).

Intellectual Abilities

Conceptually, intelligence comprises two types of abilities: fluid intelligence and crystallized intelligence. **Fluid intelligence** is the ability to use abstract reasoning, flexibly shift one's mental set, and initiate and complete purposeful action. It includes the creative and flexible thinking required in novel situations and can be directly affected by physiological structure changes (Horn & Cattell, 1967). Speed of processing, memory recall, reasoning, and problem-solving use fluid intelligence (Sánchez-Izquierdo & Fernández-Ballesteros, 2021).

Crystallized intelligence is the accumulation of knowledge, experience, and acculturation that is highly representative of individual differences (Horn & Cattell, 1967). Knowledge of facts, rules, and verbal skills rely on crystallized intelligence (Sánchez-Izquierdo & Fernández-Ballesteros, 2021).

Implications of Intelligence on the Treatment of Older Adults

There is a decline in fluid intelligence and specifically speed of processing, working memory, long-term memory, and reasoning as people age. (For an illustration of the data, see Park & Bischof, 2022.) Crystallized intelligence, on the other hand, increases throughout the life span and is maintained in old age. In treatment, a clinician should recognize that the client has the knowledge to draw upon for new learning. However, adaptations and strategies need to be introduced to compensate for slower processing, working memory, and long-term memory (see Table 13-1).

Wisdom

Definitions of **wisdom** typically reflect knowledge gained through life experience, the ability to understand what others may not, and good sense or judgment (Merriam-Webster, http://www.merriam-webster.com/dictionary/wisdom). Wisdom develops from a person reflecting on challenging life experiences (Glück & Westrate, 2019). Jeste & Lee (2019) defined wisdom as a complex human trait that includes social decision-making, emotional regulation, prosocial behaviors, self-reflection, acceptance of uncertainty, decisiveness, and spirituality.

Implications of Wisdom on the Treatment of Older Adults

Wisdom is linked to well-being, physical and mental health, happiness, life satisfaction, and resilience (Ardelt & Jeste, 2018; Jeste & Lee, 2019). It is believed that wisdom increases with age. Older adults have been found to rely on wisdom for decision-making, while younger adults tend to use fluid intelligence when making decisions. It is suggested that older adults rely on life experience for reasoning and decision-making (Glück & Westrate, 2022).

Implicit and Explicit Processing

Implicit and explicit processing are two types of cognitive processes used to learn (or transfer) information from short-term to long-term memory and to retrieve information from long-term to short-term memory. **Implicit processing** is unintentional, occurs without awareness, and is effortless, requiring minimal cognitive resources. **Explicit processing** is intentional, occurs with awareness, and is effortful, requiring moderate to substantial cognitive resources. To illustrate both processes, imagine learning the lyrics to a song. You could learn the words to a song implicitly by listening to a song on the radio multiple times, or you could use explicit processing by deliberately practicing the song lyrics every night for 30 minutes.

Implications of Processing on the Treatment of Older Adults

Older adults experience changes in explicit processing and little to no changes in tasks and activities that require implicit processing (Yamamoto et al, 2022). Older adults may benefit from strategies to enhance explicit processing including increasing awareness of the need for effort and practice. Use of visual feedback is one strategy found to enhance processing in older adults (Yamamoto et al, 2022). In clinical practice, it is essential for the clinician to monitor the client's level of understanding when performing an activity, as a client may require more time and practice to learn a novice activity. For example, a client with a hand injury might better exercise their hand doing familiar activities rather than doing exercises. Some activities for the hand injury could include playing their guitar, buttoning buttons, opening jars, and working with tools.

Functional Cognition

Functional cognition is described as the cognitive ability to perform basic activities of daily living (BADLs) and instrumental activities of daily living (IADLs) incorporating the cognitive processes previously discussed in this chapter (Wesson et al, 2016; Giles et al, 2020). Because functional cognition is intrinsically linked to BADLs and IADLs, functional cognition should be assessed in the natural, real-world context in which the task is performed rather than a laboratory setting using standardized measures (e.g., tests of memory, attention, verbal fluency). For example, the differences found between younger and older adults on a variety of laboratory-based tasks are operationalized and quantified in milliseconds, measuring the speed of processing. Additionally, tasks used in cognitive aging research are designed to overload and tax participants' cognitive resources, resulting in decreased accuracy and increased reaction time. Further, the assessment can lack meaning and saliency, affecting a participant's interest in the test. Although theoretically informative and interesting, these results do not provide information regarding how older adults use cognitive resources daily.

A number of approaches are used to assess functional cognition, including self-report, informant reports, and performance-based assessments. Self-report measures have poor psychometrics (Wesson et al, 2016). Performance-based assessments simulate real-world environments. Performance-based executive function assessments specific to occupational therapy include the following:

- Assessment of Motor and Performance Skills (AMPS; Fisher, 1995)
- Cognitive Performance Test (CPT; Burns et al, 1994)
- Complex Task Performance Assessment (CTPA; Wolf et al, 2008)
- Multiple Errand Test (MET; Shallice & Burgess, 1991)
- Performance Direct Assessment of Functional Status (modified) (PDAFS; Rankin & Keefover, 1998)
- Executive Function Performance Test (EFPT; Baum, 2011)
- The Kitchen Task Assessment (KTA; Baum & Edwards, 1993)
- Large Allen's Cognitive Level Screen-5 (LACLS-5; Allen et al, 2007)
- Menu Task (Edwards et al, 2019)
- Performance Assessment of Self-Care Skills (PASS; Holm & Rogers, 2008)
- Weekly Planning Calendar Activity (WPCA; Toglia, 2015)

Implications of Functional Cognition on the Treatment of Older Adults

Older adults compensate for age-related differences in memory and attention when completing decision-making tasks by relying on their knowledge and experience with decision-making (Li et al, 2013). Older adults' ability to successfully use everyday cognition can be illustrated with research findings pertaining to work performance. Generally, significant age-related differences in job performance have not been found between younger and older adults (Kooij et al, 2015). Older adults can effectively use their prior experience and knowledge and specific strategies such as teamwork. Additional strategies facilitating effective job performance include job sharing, effective workstation design, and training or retraining (Kanfer et al, 2017).

As with other domains of cognition, certain everyday tasks may be more difficult for older adults, especially as task complexity increases. For example, novel activities that heavily use executive functioning processes may be more challenging for older adults. A common example can be seen with driving. Although much of driving is automatic or implicit, other parts, such as merging onto a busy freeway or finding a restaurant in a new city at night, require considerable cognitive resources and faster reactions. Specifically, changes in older adults' executive functioning and speed of processing may come into play in these types of real-world situations. Additional examples of real-world situations that may be more challenging for older adults include maintaining a complicated medication regime or remembering complex instructions from one's physician.

CASE STUDY

Tom is a 73-year-old retired fireman. He retired 5 years ago when diagnosed with dementia with Lewy bodies. Tom and his wife have been married for 45 years. His wife, Mandie, is a nurse and retired 1 year ago to take care of Tom. They have two children who live out of state. Tom is an only child and has no other family. Mandie has four siblings and is only in contact with one sister.

Occupational Profile

Tom was independent in BADLS and IADLS up to 2 years ago when he began to require supervision for IADLs. Tom's IADLs included managing the finances, automobiles, home maintenance, and his health care. He was driving, playing golf, and volunteered with a local nonprofit in doing home repairs for older adults. About 2 years ago his wife noted he was having difficulty organizing his routines and organizing his activities. He failed to pay a few bills, missed appointments, and neglected to do tasks around the house. He showed gradual declines in memory but was able to effectively use lists and reminders from his wife. About 1 year ago, Tom became more dependent on his wife. Mandie had to retire from nursing due to the demands of caring for Tom. His wife became his caretaker and was unable to leave him without him getting extremely anxious. He was independent in self-care (bathing, dressing, hygiene, toileting, and eating).

Medical History (physical, psychological)

Tom has a history of high blood pressure that is treated with medication. Aside from dementia and Parkinson symptoms, he has no other medical issues. He is 6'1" and weighs 190 lb.

List Problem Areas

- Declining cognitive function – memory, attention, executive function, functional cognition
- Dependent in IADLs and BADLs
- Difficulty handling utensils and needs modified diet for swallowing
- Does not recognize family members or friends
- Agitated, disoriented, paranoid

List Strengths

- Physical health/physically active
- Supportive family including wife who is a nurse
- A supportive community of retired firefighters
- Educated
- Many interests
- Access to healthcare providers
- Socioeconomically advantaged

Questions

1. What is the classical picture of dementia with Lewy bodies? Which of Tom's symptoms and behaviors align with the classical picture?
2. What is the prognosis for dementia with Lewy bodies and how might that affect planning for continued care of Tom and Mandie's caregiving experience?

Answers

1. The classical picture includes progressive dementia with Parkinson-related motor involvement diagnosed as early as 50 years old. Persons present with a range of impaired cognition, including attention, executive functions, visual perceptual, neuropsychiatric (hallucinations), sleep disorders, and autonomic symptoms. Tom has many of the signs of dementia with Lewy bodies, including cognitive changes and parkinsonian tremors. His cognitive changes include declines in memory, attention, executive function, functional cognition. (See section on dementia with Lewy bodies for specifics. L.O. 3-8)
2. Dementia with Lewy bodies is a progressive disease with an expected life span of 5 to 7 years. Tom was diagnosed 5 years ago. Considerations for Mandie will include planning for continued care as Tom

continues to progress. Additional considerations include modifying the environment for Tom's safety and continued mobility and consulting with a medical care team to meet his nutritional needs. (See Occupational Therapy Intervention for Persons with Dementia; L.O. 13-6.)

Cognitive Theories of Aging

Several models and theories have emerged attempting to explain why and how certain cognitive processes change across the life span. This section will review the current theories and focus on how each contributes to understanding age-related cognitive changes.

Speed of Processing

The speed of processing theory (Salthouse, 1996) proposes that generalized slowed processing is responsible for age effects on cognition over the life span. This theory suggests that age-related differences between younger and older adults on cognitive tasks can be attributed to a generalized slowing or decreased speed at which individuals are able to process information. With aging, cognitive resources and cognitive energy are diminished. It is theorized that the slowing in processing speed affects performance across a wide range of cognitive processes, including information processing, problem-solving, decision-making, attention, and working memory.

Sensory Deficit Theory

The sensory deficit hypothesis proposes that cognitive changes in older adults is due to changes in sensory processing, primarily visual and auditory information (Stine-Morrow et al, 2006). These declines in sensory functioning result in degraded (or poorer quality) information and are proposed to explain why older adults perform differently from younger adults on cognitive tasks.

Declines in hearing and vision have been linked to a decline in cognitive functioning. When comparing participants with and without hearing loss, the persons with hearing loss had a greater cognitive decline and the decline was related to the severity of the hearing loss (Lin et al, 2013). Declines in auditory and visual processing can also impact social participation, leading to loneliness and depression (Mick et al, 2018). Thus, if visual or auditory information is processed through a less-optimal system, subsequent cognitive processing of information may result in errors or slowed processing time. See Chapter 10 for more detail on sensory changes with aging.

Memory Deficit and Dual-Process

In this section, theories related to memory deficits will be explored. The review will include working memory, declarative memory, procedural memory, and dual process theory.

Working Memory

Working memory requires effortful attention and processing for the purpose of storing, maintaining, and actively manipulating incoming information. Working memory serves a vital role in facilitating higher-order cognitive processes, such as language production and comprehension (Kemper & Mitzner, 2001), decision-making, problem-solving, and learning (Tulving & Craik, 2000).

Older adults may have deficits in working memory due to slowed processing, changes in sensory processing, and decreased inhibition. Older adults may be more affected by interruptions during a task and have more difficulty than younger adults in resuming the task (Rösner et al, 2022). However, older adults with stimulating lifestyles are shown to have fewer white matter lesions (linked to decline in working memory) and perform better than expected on working memory assessment (Ducharme-Laliberté et al, 2022).

Dual-Process Theory

The dual-process theory proposes that recall of an event can take two different forms: recollection or familiarity (Yonelinas, 2002). Recollection of an event requires effort to recreate the "what", "where", and "when" of an event. Familiarity may occur without effort, triggered by an unexpected event (e.g., a song triggering a memory of a vacation). Older adults are more likely to have cognitive changes in recollection and no changes in familiarity (Koen & Yonelinas, 2016).

Structural Changes in Aging

Advances in magnetic resonance imaging (MRI) neuroimaging the past few decades have enabled scientists to examine living brains. Before these advances, scientists were only able to study the brain after death. Imaging has contributed to a greater understanding of structural changes occurring with aging, including grey matter volume and functional and structural connectivity. Brain weight and volume changes beginning in the third to fourth decade of life. While the initial change is slower, after the age of 70, brain volume decreases by 0.3% to 0.5% annually (Esiri, 2007). Changes in brain volume include both white and grey matter. MRIs reveal the greatest changes are in the frontal and temporal cortex, putamen, thalamus, and nucleus accumbens (Pomponio et al, 2020). Marner et al (2003) found that white matter increased into the sixth decade and then began to decline. By age 80 it declined by 40% compared with the brain volume of 20-year-olds. This is not to say that cognitive behavior declined at the same rate. Cognitive abilities are related to brain volume and structural connectivity, but cognitive abilities cannot be predicted only by measures of brain volume and connectivity.

Summary of Typical Cognitive Functioning in Older Adults

Older adults experience cognitive changes. Cognitive health is less a factor of chronological age than lifestyle, education, socioeconomic status, and access to health care. An older adult with greater cognitive reserve than age-matched adults will have a higher level of functioning. Older adults will have word-finding problems, slips of tongue, and at times conversations, appointments, and trouble remembering where the car was parked. Older adults may need more time to process verbal and written information, and new learning can require slowed, intentional instruction and simplification of the task. Despite these changes, older adults retain intelligence and wisdom that is used for problem-solving and reasoning. The brains of older adults are neuroplastic and benefit from a lifestyle, activities, and environment that promote the development of cognitive reserve. Older adults will benefit from vigorous exercise and activity, cognitive stimulation, and social participation. Most importantly, the exercise, activity, cognitive stimulation, and social participation must have meaning to the client. Mental health, medical, and rehabilitation professionals can greatly benefit from understanding normal changes in cognition and factors known to benefit cognitive health. In the clinical setting, clinicians can use this knowledge to provide treatment that facilitates cognitive health or adapt the environment and treatment to meet the client's needs (see Promoting Best Practice 13-2).

PROMOTING BEST PRACTICE 13-2
Optimizing Cognitive Capacity

From a clinical perspective, clinicians must consider the client's cognitive capacity and tailor treatment to ensure the best outcomes. Often clinical treatments involve verbal communication with the client. As the amount and complexity of information increases, it may be difficult for the client to maintain, organize, and process the relevant information. To minimize this difficulty,

- Break up instructions and check in with the client on the instructions to ensure client understanding.
- Provide information in handouts developed for the appropriate level of literacy. Review the handout with the client.
- Teach strategies such as keeping a calendar, making lists, posting instructions.
- Minimize distractions.
- Minimize multitasking (doing two or more tasks concurrently that require complex attention).
- Use teach-back methods to ensure the client understands the information.

Neuropathologies and Impact on Cognitive Functioning in Older Adults

Cognitive aging ranges from the normal changes as discussed above to debilitating, progressive neuropathologies. Neuropathologies include delirium, mild cognitive deficits and dementias, cerebrovascular accident (CVA) (e.g., stroke), and traumatic brain injury (TBI), and mental disorders. This section will review neuropathology's related to aging and the impact on occupational performance.

Delirium

Delirium is a syndrome with an acute onset of changes in attention, awareness, and cognition functioning. A person with delirium can present with psychotic thoughts and behaviors. Onset is as rapid as 1 or 2 hours and can last for days to months. Delirium is caused by a medical condition not related to a preexisting neurocognitive disorder. Causative factors include frailty, infections (e.g., urinary tract infections), prolonged illness, low sodium, medication reactions, alcohol, and surgery with anesthesia. Delirium often presents during daytime and worsens at night. Being in an unfamiliar environment can also exacerbate delirium (Wilson et al, 2020). The incidence of delirium in older adults in the hospital is as high as 30% for those having surgery and 40% to 60% for older adults in intensive care. Two thirds of older adults with delirium have underlying dementia (Anand & MacLullich, 2021). Assessments used to diagnose delirium in the hospital include the Rapid Clinical Test for Delirium Detection (Wilson et al, 2020), the Intensive Care Delirium Screening Checklist (ICDSC), and the Confusion Assessment Method for the Intensive Care Unit (CAM-ICU, Rains & Chee, 2017). Treatment of delirium consists of discovering the cause and intervening. Multi-intervention approaches including occupational and physical therapy have been effective in reducing the number of days with delirium. The D.E.L.I.R.I.U.M. mnemonic encompasses the key elements of current best practice in managing delirium (Rains & Chee, 2017).

- **D**rugs – remove any delirogenic medications including narcotics.
- **E**nvironment – reduce noise and excess stimulation, particularly during sleep times.
- **L**ight – use natural light that is appropriate for day and night. Limit lights during sleep time.
- **I**nitiate cognitive tasks – engage client in meaningful cognitively stimulating tasks.
- **R**outine – use clocks, schedules, and routines; include times for rest and sleep; and use a 24-hour approach.
- **I**ntegrate an interprofessional team approach, including occupational therapy, physical therapy, speech-language pathology, pharmacology, and psychotherapy.
- **U**nder hydration/nutrition – ensure food and fluid intake is sufficient and integrate in the client's routine.
- **M**obility – incorporate movement, including exercise and activity, in the client's daily routine.

Interprofessional Approach in Treatment of Delirium

Evidence suggests that an interprofessional approach in the treatment of delirium is critical. Collaboration between healthcare professionals is essential (Lee et al, 2022). As a member of the interprofessional team, occupational therapists play a critical role in the treatment of delirium and in creating an environment to reduce episodes of delirium (Cuevas-Lara et al, 2019). Essential to reducing episodes of delirium is strict adherence to schedules and routines (Rains & Chee, 2017). The health care team must work together to develop a client-centered treatment program addressing the client's specific habits and routines. As much as possible the client should engage in usual daily activities including ADLs, exercise, and activities. In addition, if the client has regular routines, such as reading a paper, watching a television show, or listening to certain music, these should be built into the schedule. When possible, the occupational therapist obtains an occupational profile from the client or family to establish the patients' typical routines and habits.

Treatment interventions incorporated into the daily schedule include cognitive stimulation, mobilization, assessment and augmentation of hearing and visual impairments, sleep hygiene practices, and assurance of adequate fluid and dietary intake. Below are suggestions for specific treatment interventions.

- Cognitive stimulation – Ensuring the client has access to a clock, schedule, and familiar items such as photos contributes to the client's orientation. Depending on the client's interests, this might include watching a news program and discussing the content, doing a crossword puzzle, discussing cooking recipes, discussing family rituals, talking about a person's hobby, making a photo album of family pictures and creating narratives, or an oral history.
- Mobility – Early mobilization facilitates joint mobility, strength, balance, motor control, and cognitive alertness. Early mobilization can include sitting at the edge of the bed to perform grooming, eating, and cognitive activities. When able, the client should have a schedule for when they will be out of bed and the duration of time. This schedule will progress as the client recovers.
- Vision and hearing augmentation – Vision and hearing should be assessed by team members, and the client should have the needed adaptations. If the client wore hearing aids and/or glasses, therapists must ensure the client has access to these devices. Make sure glasses are clean and there is a system in place for caring for hearing aids. Adaptations can include audio books, magnification, closed captions on the television, the use of tablets for communication, and augmented communication devices.
- Sleep enhancement – It is essential that the client have a sleep schedule that includes rest periods. For rest periods lights should be dimmed and minimal noise and disruptions. For extended sleep at night, the client should have a regular schedule and a routine to prepare for sleep. The nighttime routine may incorporate the client's typical routine, and lighting, temperature, noise, and disturbances must be considered. The client might benefit from learning relaxation techniques, listening to meditations, use of essential oils, and use of white or pink noise.
- Eating and fluid intake – Dietitians determine the client's nutritional needs. The healthcare team, including occupational therapy, can incorporate fluid and food intake in the context of treatments. Encouraging the client to drink liquids throughout treatment and incorporating snack breaks can facilitate meeting the client's nutritional needs. Ensuring that the client's specific food and beverage preferences are available can facilitate goal attainment.

Mild Cognitive Impairment

Mild cognitive impairment (MCI) affects 10% to 15% of adults over the age of 65. MCI is a transitional stage between healthy aging and dementia. The prevalence of MCI in older adults increases with age, lower level of education, and sex (higher in men) (Anderson, 2019). Diagnosis of MCI includes client history and cognitive testing, including the Montreal Cognitive Assessment (MoCA; Nasreddine et al, 2005). The progression of MCI is defined by the presence of amnesia and the number of areas affected by the amnesia, including attention, language, visuospatial, and executive functioning. MCI may lead to dementia. Current medications are shown to only slow progression (Jongsiriyanyong & Limpawattana, 2018).

Persons with MCI benefit from inclusion in exercise, client-centered activities, cognitive stimulation, and socialization. Client and family education is also critical in understanding the client and their behaviors. The occupational therapist can work with the client and caregivers to develop memory strategies including timers, calendars, and written or verbal cues. An example of a treatment intervention would be working with the client and caregivers on medication management. The therapist with the client and caregiver can problem-solve and devise a method for the client to adhere to daily medications.

Dementia

Dementia is a syndrome of cognitive impairment affecting cognitive processes and significantly affects a person's ability to independently perform BADLs and IADLs and participate in meaningful and fulfilling activities. Risk factors for dementia include the following:

- Less education
- Hypertension
- Hearing impairment
- Smoking
- Obesity
- Depression
- Physical inactivity
- Diabetes
- Excessive alcohol consumption
- TBI
- Air pollution
- Low social contact

Modifying risk factors may prevent or delay onset of dementia by up to 40% (Livingston et al, 2020). Dementia is the second largest cause of disability for individuals age 70 years or older, and the seventh leading cause of death (World Health Organization [WHO], n.d.). It is estimated that there are currently over 55 million people worldwide living with dementia. The number of people affected is set to rise to 139 million by 2050, with the greatest increases in low- and middle-income countries (Alzheimer's Disease International [ADI], n.d.-a).

Dementia can be classified as either reversible or irreversible. Reversible dementias are caused by health issues having a temporary and reversible effect on cognitive processes. Conditions include endocrine disorders, urinary tract infection, electrolyte imbalance, brain tumors, chronic bacterial meningitis, neurosyphilis, chronic infections (e.g., tuberculous meningitis, tuberculoma, herpes encephalitis, AIDS), drug use, depression, and normal-pressure hydrocephalus (Chari et al, 2015). Proper assessment and treatment of these conditions typically lead to the reversal of the cognitive symptoms, allowing individuals to regain their former level of cognitive functioning.

The next section will focus on irreversible dementia resulting in a progressive loss of functioning. Four types of dementia are Alzheimer disease, frontotemporal, Lewy body, and vascular.

Alzheimer Disease

Alzheimer disease is the most common type of dementia, accounting for approximately 60% to 70% of cases (WHO, n.d.). It is characterized by abnormal deposits of proteins forming amyloid plaques and tau tangles throughout the brain. Most cases are found in people in their 60s or older, though it can be diagnosed in younger adults. Death usually occurs within 8 to 10 years of diagnosis. Alzheimer disease symptoms are classified as mild, moderate, or severe. In the mild stages of the illness, individuals can continue their daily activities with minimal assistance. For example, individuals can complete self-care activities (e.g., bathing, dressing, toileting, grooming, and transferring); socialize and engage with friends and family; and continue to complete day-to-day activities that are familiar and well-practiced, such as driving a familiar route, playing a game of skill or a musical instrument, or participating in physical activity. As the illness progresses, individuals experiencing severe symptoms may require complete assistance for completing personal care activities and may no longer be able to effectively communicate or actively engage in certain activities because they are bed ridden (WHO, n.d.). Diagnosing Alzheimer disease is a process of excluding other conditions because there is not a specific test used for diagnosis or a specific biomarker that indicates the presence of Alzheimer disease (e.g., blood work, cerebrospinal fluid, results from functional MRI, or positron emission tomography [PET] scans). Subsequently, confirmation of Alzheimer disease as the official diagnosis is only available upon death via autopsy (Livingston et al, 2020).

Vascular Dementia

Vascular dementia is the second most commonly diagnosed form of dementia and is caused by an overall inefficient supply of oxygenated blood to the brain that may be caused by small transient ischemic attacks (e.g., small, unnoticeable strokes), major strokes, or untreated high blood pressure. Vascular dementia accounts for more than 15% to 20% of all dementias. Most interesting is vascular dementia has had a decline of about 20% per decade in the 20th century. This decline is attributed to advances in the treatment of vascular diseases (Wolters & Ikram, 2019). A primary risk factor for vascular dementia is a history of having one or more major strokes. Additional risk factors include hypertension, diabetes, and a history of smoking, all of which either directly or indirectly affect the body's ability to efficiently pump oxygenated blood to the brain (O'Brien & Thomas, 2015). Compared with individuals with Alzheimer disease, individuals with vascular dementia may not experience progressive cognitive changes across time but instead will typically experience daily fluctuations in their cognitive abilities, with symptoms becoming worse over the course of the day. Symptoms of vascular dementia can be similar to those of Alzheimer disease or may be more localized. For example, an individual with vascular dementia may have specific focal impairments in short-term memory and attentional processing but may retain executive functioning abilities, such as decision-making, reasoning, problem-solving, and judgment. Vascular dementia is typically diagnosed in people older than 65 years, and life expectancy is about 5 years after onset of initial symptoms.

Dementia With Lewy Bodies

Dementia with Lewy bodies is a progressive dementia and represents two related diagnoses: dementia with Lewy bodies and Parkinson disease dementia. Up to 80% of people with Parkinson disease will have dementia with Lewy bodies. Persons with Parkinson disease often experience motor involvement about 1 year before the onset of dementia (Taylor et al, 2020). Up to 85% of people with dementia with Lewy bodies experience motor difficulties. Dementia with Lewy bodies is diagnosed as early as 50 years old, and life expectancy is 5 to 7 years after onset of symptoms. Persons present with a range of cognitive changes including attention, executive functions, visual perceptual symptoms, neuropsychiatric symptoms (hallucinations), sleep disorders, and autonomic symptoms (syncope, dizziness) (Taylor et al, 2020). Diagnosing dementia with Lewy bodies includes a physical examination as well as brain imaging (e.g., computed tomography or PET scans); however, as in Alzheimer disease, conclusive diagnosis can only be made after death (Taylor et al, 2020).

Frontotemporal Dementia

Frontotemporal dementia is a hereditary neurodegenerative disorder with 30% of cases having a strong family history. Characteristics of frontotemporal dementia include changes in behavior (personality), language (progressive aphasia), and motor function (amyotrophic lateral sclerosis or Parkinson disease) (Greaves & Rohrer, 2019). Frontotemporal dementia is characterized by abnormal amounts or forms of tau and TDP-43 proteins accumulating inside neurons in the frontal and temporal lobes.

Factors Impacting Functioning for Persons Living With Dementia

A person with dementia, even mild dementia, requires assistance to perform daily activities. This section will address specific changes in cognition, communication, activities of daily living, and behavioral and psychological symptoms. See Table 13-2 for specific signs of dementia.

Cognition

Primary cognitive symptoms of dementia include difficulties with short-term memory; attention; orientation to time, place, and person; visuospatial processing; language production and comprehension; and executive functioning. Individuals with dementia also experience difficulties performing day-to-day activities, such as handling finances, grocery shopping, participating in leisure activities and hobbies, and performing self-care tasks.

Communication

Individuals with dementia often experience difficulties producing language (e.g., thinking of a specific word) or understanding what is being said to them (e.g., following a conversation or directions). With early dementia, the person often has difficulty naming a person or object. They often will replace one word with another (saying "fork" but meaning "spoon") (Klimova & Kuca, 2016). It is common for individuals with dementia to feel frustrated and confused when others do not understand them or they do not understand others. Other common communication issues include repeatedly asking the same question and retelling the same story or information within a short amount of time. It is suggested that these behaviors are due to changes in memory and poor recall (Klimova & Kuca, 2016).

Activities of Daily Living

Persons with mild dementia can complete BADLs without difficulty. Difficulty performing IADLs, which demand higher levels of cognitive processing, is seen early in the diagnosis of dementia. dePaula et al (2015) found relationships between such activities as medication management, shopping, laundry, telephone use, and meal preparation with declines in episodic memory and executive functioning.

Behavioral and Psychological Symptoms

Individuals with dementia may experience changes in their emotions and usual behaviors. Most people with even mild dementia will experience some changes in behavior. Severe changes or problematic behavioral changes lead to earlier institutionalization (Martin & Velayudhan, 2020). Behaviors such as aggression, paranoia, and wandering can make it unsafe for the person to stay at home. The range of emotions and behaviors includes delusions and hallucinations, feelings of frustration, anger, agitation, apathy, sleep–wake cycle disruptions, and appetite changes. These changes can occur during any stage of the illness. It is estimated that 90% of all individuals with dementia will experience behavioral and psychological symptoms (Martin & Velayudhan, 2020). See Table 13-2.

Individuals with dementia are at risk for experiencing symptoms of depression and anxiety, along with other negative outcomes such as strained family relationships, loss of self-identity, and feelings of isolation and embarrassment (Eddy et al, 2020).

Because there is no known cure for many dementias like Alzheimer disease and dementia with Lewy bodies, and current drug therapies do not dramatically improve symptoms or stop the progression of the illness, there is a growing emphasis on the development, implementation, and evaluation of nonpharmacological intervention programs that address the care needs of both the individual and his or her family members. The Alzheimer's Association is one of the leading social service agencies dedicated to providing individuals and their families with a wide range of educational and supportive service programs. Examples of resources and programs include a multitude of educational information and programs, the 24/7 Helpline, the Safe Return program, support groups for individuals and families, and online resources and message boards (ADI, n.d.-b).

Occupational Therapy Interventions for Persons With Dementia

Occupational therapy assessment and interventions must focus on promoting quality of life and participation for the client with dementia and the caregiver. With no cure for dementia and the progression of pathology, occupational therapy focuses on environmental and personal factors affecting the client and caregiver. Interventions are aimed at minimizing behavioral symptoms and enhancing functional status, cognition, and mood. Exercise, sensory-based treatments, cognitive stimulation, reminiscence therapy, validation therapy (accepting the person's reality), and simulated presence (videotape played of loved one) are interventions found to influence behaviors (Bessey & Walaszek, 2019). In a systematic review of nonpharmacological interventions for people with dementia, several interventions were investigated and had positive outcomes. Interventions addressed person factors (e.g., exercise, cognitive stimulation, music therapy) and environmental factors (e.g., socialization, mealtime routines). Based on the review, the strongest evidence for neuropsychiatric symptoms (aggression, outburst) was sensory stimulation, music, simulated presence, and validation therapy. Evidence supporting the promotion of physical and cognitive functioning included cognitive stimulation, reminiscence therapy, exercise, light therapy, and transcutaneous electrical stimulation. Evidence supporting interventions for

TABLE 13-2 ■ Signs of Alzheimer Dementia Compared With Typical Age-Related Changes

SIGNS OF ALZHEIMER DEMENTIA	TYPICAL AGE-RELATED CHANGES
Memory loss that disrupts daily life: one of the most common signs of Alzheimer dementia, especially in the early stage, is forgetting recently learned information. Others include asking the same questions over and over, and increasingly needing to rely on memory aids (for example, reminder notes or electronic devices) or family members for things that used to be handled on one's own.	Sometimes forgetting names or appointments, but remembering them later
Challenges in planning or solving problems: some people experience changes in their ability to develop and follow a plan or work with numbers. They may have trouble following a familiar recipe or keeping track of monthly bills. They may have difficulty concentrating and take much longer to do things than they did before.	Making occasional errors when managing finances or household bills
Difficulty completing familiar tasks: people with Alzheimer dementia often find it hard to complete daily tasks. Sometimes, people have trouble driving to a familiar location, organizing a grocery list, or remembering the rules of a favorite game.	Occasionally needing help to use microwave settings or record a television show
Confusion with time or place: people living with Alzheimer dementia can lose track of dates, seasons, and the passage of time. They may have trouble understanding something if it is not happening immediately. Sometimes they forget where they are or how they got there.	Getting confused about the day of the week but figuring it out later
Trouble understanding visual images and spatial relationships: for some people, having vision problems is a sign of Alzheimer dementia. They may also have problems judging distance and determining color and contrast, causing issues with driving.	Vision changes related to cataracts
New problems with words in speaking or writing: people living with Alzheimer dementia may have trouble following or joining a conversation. They may stop in the middle of a conversation and have no idea how to continue or they may repeat themselves. They may struggle with vocabulary, have trouble naming a familiar object, or use the wrong name (e.g., calling a watch a "hand clock").	Sometimes having trouble finding the right word
Misplacing things and losing the ability to retrace steps: people living with Alzheimer dementia may put things in unusual places. They may lose things and be unable to go back over their steps to find them. They may accuse others of stealing, especially as the disease progresses.	Misplacing things from time to time and retracing steps to find them
Decreased or poor judgment: individuals may experience changes in judgment or decision-making. For example, they may use poor judgment when dealing with money or pay less attention to grooming or keeping themselves clean.	Making a bad decision or mistake once in a while, such as neglecting to schedule an oil change for a car
Withdrawal from work or social activities: people living with Alzheimer dementia may experience changes in the ability to hold or follow a conversation. As a result, they may withdraw from hobbies, social activities, or other engagements. They may have trouble keeping up with a favorite sports team or activity.	Sometimes feeling uninterested in family and social obligations
Changes in mood, personality and behavior: the mood and personalities of people living with Alzheimer dementia can change. They can become confused, suspicious, depressed, fearful, or anxious. They may be easily upset at home, at work, with friends, or when out of their comfort zones.	Developing very specific ways of doing things and becoming irritable when a routine is disrupted

Adapted with permission from Alzheimer's Association: https://www.alz.org/media/Documents/alzheimers-facts-and-figures.pdf

emotional disorders included exercise, music therapy, psychological treatments, reminiscence, and validation therapy (Meyer & O'Keefe, 2020).

Interventions must also consider the needs of the caregivers. Caregiving duties can create a high level of burden affecting the caregiver's physical and mental health (Bessey & Walaszek, 2019). According to the WHO (2022), caregivers spent an average of 5 hours daily caregiving, and much of the caregiving is without pay. Caregivers have an increased risk of depression. In one study, 69.8% of the caregivers were depressed, and their depression was correlated with the severity of the client's dementia. While caregiving has some negative aspects, caregivers can also experience positive feelings about caregiving (Brodaty & Donkin, 2022). People act as caregivers for several reasons, including love, spiritual fulfilment, a sense of duty, guilt, social pressures, and finances. Interventions with caregivers focus on building knowledge and skills to enhance psychological and physical capacities and well-being (Gitlin et al, 2021) Studies suggest that skill-building education, mindfulness practices, and cognitive behavioral therapy (CBT) decreased depression, anxiety, and stress in caregivers (Cheng et al, 2020; Kishita et al, 2018). Two programs that have been extensively tested align with the WHO's press for dementia care involving the client and carers and promoting a reablement model. The Tailored Activity Program (TAP) is a program designed to reduce neuropsychiatric symptoms and functional dependence and enhance caregiver well-being. TAP matches a client's abilities and interests with activities tailored specifically for the client. Caregivers are provided education about dementia and the disease progression along with stress reduction techniques. In a randomized control trial, TAP did not have a clinically significant impact on neuropsychiatric symptoms but, functional dependence significantly decreased and caregiver well-being and confidence increased (Gitlin et al, 2021). The Care of People with Dementia in their Environments (COPE) model focuses on reducing environmental stressors to decrease sensory, physical, and cognitive demands and align the environment with the individual's capabilities. The goal is to enable the individual to reengage in functional activities and reduce the caregiver burden (Gitlin et al, 2010). COPE has been found to reduce functional dependence and increase activity participation. After completion of the program, individuals with dementia were significantly more engaged in functional activities, and carers had a significantly higher sense of well-being (Clemson et al, 2021).

Regardless of the type of dementia, it is important that individuals and their families receive the appropriate educational information and supportive resources for managing and coping with the symptoms of dementia. Family caregivers, home health nurses, doctors, and therapists (occupational, physical, and speech) are critical in providing care and support for a person to remain in their home. Providing care for a loved one with dementia typically rests on the shoulders of one individual, usually the spouse or the daughter/daughter-in-law (Livingston et al, 2020). It is imperative that the person living with dementia and their caregiver(s)/family are equipped to effectively manage and cope with the demands. It is the responsibility of the physician, nurse, therapists, and counselors to ensure that the person living with dementia and their caregivers receive evidence-based interventions to meet individual needs. For example, the individual may benefit from occupational therapy and counseling, whereas the family may benefit from receiving additional educational information about future care planning, information pertaining to adult day care services, and respite care.

Stroke

Stroke, CVA, has a rapid onset caused by either blocked vessels or bleeding in the brain. The effect of the stroke on functioning depends on the area of the brain where the stroke occurred. The chronicity of the stroke is dependent on the severity. The person may experience changes in cognitive functioning, hemiparesis or hemiplegia, emotional lability, and communication skills. This section will focus on cognitive changes occurring with a stroke.

It is well known that a stroke can affect cognitive functioning. Approximately 38.0% to 53.4% of persons with a stroke will have cognitive deficits in one or more areas including attention, language, executive function, visuospatial cognition, episodic, working memory, affect, and behavior (Sexton et al, 2019). In addition to affecting specific cognitive processes, a stroke affects functional cognition (Lau et al, 2022). Cognitive deficits, more so than physical deficits, have been linked to reduced quality of life (Stolwyk et al, 2021). Up to one third of persons with a severe stroke will have the onset of dementia within 1 year, with a stroke in the dominant hemisphere being more likely to result in dementia (Filipska et al, 2020).

Cognitive changes after a stroke impact the individual's recovery. Cognitive deficits after stroke affect independence in BADLs, IADLs, ability to perform meaningful activities, and participation. As discussed earlier in this chapter, participation, self-efficacy, and activity are critical for cognitive health. The cognitive deficits from a stroke create barriers to function. Because stroke affects not only cognition but motor skills, individuals must relearn and learn adaptive skills including walking, performing daily tasks with one hand and possibly the nondominant arm, operating a wheelchair, methods of transferring, etc. Stroke guidelines require all clients to undergo cognitive screening. Note: some screening assessments require credentialing. Screenings include:

- Patient Health Questionnaire (PHQ; Kroenke et al, 2003)
- Beck Depression Inventory (BDI; Beck et al, 1961)
- Montreal Cognitive Assessment (MoCA; Nasreddine et al, 2005)
- Mini-Mental State Examination (MMSE; Folstein et al, 1975)
- Saint Louis University Mental Status Examination (SLUMS; Morley & Tumosa, 2002)
- Short Blessed Test (SBT; Ball et al, 1999)

Occupational Therapy Assessment and Practice With Older Adults With Stroke

Occupational therapists provide treatment across all treatment environments (acute care, rehabilitation, outpatient, home health, and long-term care). Occupational therapists must screen for cognitive functioning and further assess cognitive processes depending on the outcomes of screenings and objective observation of the client during treatments. A recent systematic review reported the MMSE and MoCA as the most reported screening tool. The MoCA has been found to be more sensitive to mild cognitive deficits compared with the MMSE (Siqueira, et al, 2019). In addition to cognitive screening, persons with stroke experience vision changes affecting performance on cognitive tests and daily activities. See Chapter 10 for a detailed description of visual testing. Comprehensive assessments of cognition can be divided into those focusing on cognitive impairment and those focusing on performance and participation (functional cognition). For a list of performance and participation-based assessments, see the section in this chapter on Functional Cognition. Below is a list of commonly used impairment-based assessments.

- Motor Free Visual Perceptual Test (MVPT; Colarusso & Hammill, 1972)
- Behavioral Inattention Test (BIT; Wilson et al, 1987)
- Block Design Test (BDT; Wechsler, 1981)
- Letter Cancellation Test (Diller & Gordon, 1981)
- Digit Symbol Modalities Test (Smith, 1973)

- Trail Making Test (Reitan & Wolfson, 1985)
- Rey-Osterrieth Complex Figure Test (Barker-Collo et al, 2012)
- Clock Drawing Test (CDT; Friedman, 1991)
- Beck Depression Inventory (BDI; Beck et al, 1961)

Occupational therapy interventions will depend on the outcomes of skilled observations and assessments. The Multicontext Treatment Approach (MTA, Toglia, 1991) and the Cognitive Orientation to Daily Occupational Performance (CO-OP, Skidmore et al, 2015) provide guidelines for interventions for persons with stroke with cognitive deficits. The MTA provides guidelines for use of strategies in performing daily activities. A key component of MTA is promoting self-monitoring and increasing metacognition. Interventions use techniques such as guided anticipation, "stop and check," self-assessment, specific goal rating, and journaling. Metacognitive strategy interventions are evidence based and linked to increased executive functioning, self-awareness, and functional performance (Cicerone et al, 2019). MTA has been found to increase self-awareness, strategy use, and functional performance in persons with stroke (Nagelkop et al, 2021).

The CO-OP also focuses on improving performance using cognitive strategies. However, CO-OP focuses on skill acquisition. Cognitive Orientation is focused on orienting to problem-solving. Daily Occupational Performance is focused on performance of a skill, not the components. Foundations of CO-OP have evolved from motor learning theory, learning theory, and cognitive theories. CO-OP uses an approach that promotes self-direction and self-monitoring to identify problems when performing occupations. The process uses a "GOAL-PLAN-DO-CHECK" strategy, where the client sets the goal and then plans, does, and reflects on their performance. CO-OP has been found to be effective in the treatment of upper extremities after stroke and improved function in daily activities (Song et al., 2019). The COPM is widely used as an outcome measure with CO-OP.

Interprofessional Practice With Older Adults With Stroke

According to the Guidelines for Adult Stroke Rehabilitation and Recovery, stroke rehabilitation requires a highly sophisticated and coordinated effort by healthcare professionals (Winstein et al, 2016). Occupational therapists play a critical role on the team, and interventions are intricately woven with other disciplines on the team. Depending on their needs, stroke survivors typically require a combination of rehabilitation services that can include physical therapy, occupational therapy, speech-language pathology, and social work or counseling. When addressing cognitive deficits after stroke, occupational therapists can work with physical therapists, speech-language pathologists, and social workers for use of cognitive strategies for learning skills in each of the disciplines. A knowledge translation study showed that when CO-OP was introduced across disciplines at five rehabilitation hospitals, it resulted in increased rehabilitation for mild and moderate strokes (Linkewich et al, 2022). Clients benefit from integrated interventions for recovery of motor and cognitive deficits. Reinforcing use of cognitive strategies across all treatments has been shown effective in client outcomes. For example, the client may be having difficulty in physical therapy learning a specific transfer. The occupational therapist and speech-language pathologist can reinforce the treatment by doing the transfers as prescribed by the physical therapist. The occupational therapist can work with the physical therapist on problem-solving learning strategies such as breaking the transfer up into small parts (standing and turning, then reaching for chair arm and sitting). Cognitive strategies such as having the client teach back the skills can also be used. In occupational therapy, teach strategies, optimize the environment for learning, and focus on participation in occupations and activities.

Mental Health Conditions

Mental illness is a chronic condition affecting a person's cognitive functioning, mood, and behaviors. Mental illness impacts a person's ability to function and perform everyday activities and impacts relationships. Fifty percent of all mental illnesses are diagnosed by the age of 14 and 75% by the age of 24 (National Alliance on Mental Illness [NAMI], n.d.). One out of five persons older than age 65 has some form of mental illness (Bodner et al, 2018). In a study of 2,592 elderly adults across Europe, the MentDis_ICF65+ found that 47% of adults age 65 to 84 years were diagnosed with a mental disorder at some point in life. The rate of substance misuse was 18.2%, and the rate of affective disorders was 14.3% (Andres et al, 2022). Other mental disorders include severe conditions like major depressive disorder, bipolar disorder, or schizophrenia. As discussed earlier in this chapter, determinants of healthy cognitive aging include socialization, physical health, and cognitive stimulation. Older adults with mental illness are often isolated and have limited financial and human resources affecting opportunities for participation in healthy aging activities. Aging with mental illness can intensify challenges in maintaining health, performing daily activities, and managing social interactions (Jimenez et al, 2017).

Older adults with mental illness were found to have less physical activity, unhealthy diets, more use of medications, sleep disorders, and agitation (Houben et al, 2019). Mental illness can affect a person's ability to build relationships, marry, or have children. Individuals with mental illness often rely on close relatives and friends to assist with everyday activities and to provide socialization. With aging, the death of these supports is a source of great stress and trauma for persons with mental illness (O'Hare et al, 2017). This loss of support often results in the initialization of a person, leading to further problems with isolation. Aging persons with mental illness are more likely to experience insufficient and inappropriate support due to a lack of trained professionals and target programs addressing the complexity of aging and mental illness (Morgan et al, 2016). The following section will present specific mental conditions, general forms of medical interventions, and a review of specific occupational therapy and interprofessional interventions for this population.

Depression

Depression is one of the most common illnesses in older adults. Factors contributing to depression in older adults include chronic illness, loss of socialization, hearing loss, stressful life events, female sex, low resilience, decreased mobility, loss of loved ones, and limited income (Pilania et al, 2019). Depression is linked to decreased functioning and decreased life satisfaction in older adults. About 2% of adults older than 55 years have major depression, and 10% to 15% have clinical depression. The rate of major depression increases with age and for older adults who are in nursing homes or hospitalized (Kok & Reynolds, 2017). Depression occurs along a continuum, varying from mild symptoms to more severe conditions, such as major depressive disorder. Depression is thought to be caused by a combination of factors, including trauma, genetics, life stressors, changes in the pituitary gland and hypothalamus, substance abuse, and other medical conditions (e.g., chronic pain, sleep disorders, anxiety) (Kok & Reynolds, 2017).

Symptoms of depression range from loss of interest and pleasure in activities, change in appetite, sleep disturbances, feeling agitated, fatigue, low self-worth, difficulty concentrating, suicidal thoughts, hopelessness, sadness, and loss of energy (Kok & Reynolds, 2017). Depression also can affect an individual's cognitive abilities, resulting in memory loss, difficulties in concentration and attentional processes, problems with learning, and problems with executive functioning (Kok & Reynolds, 2017).

Treatment of depression in older adults includes pharmacological and behavioral components. Antidepressants are beneficial in treating depression. However, older adults often have comorbidities, such as heart disease, demanding attention to drug interactions. Some antidepressants (tricyclic antidepressants and selective serotonin reuptake inhibitors) are associated with an increased risk of falls and osteoporosis (Kok & Reynolds, 2017). In addition, monitoring changes in cognition, hypotension, or other issues (e.g., electrolyte imbalance) can assist clinicians. Because older adults metabolize or excrete many medications slower than younger individuals and because these medications can cause cognitive changes, careful monitoring is essential.

Anxiety Disorders

Generalized anxiety disorders are the most prevalent mental illness among older adults. In a large European study of adults 65 to 84 years old, the prevalence of generalized anxiety disorders was 17% (Canuto et al, 2018). However, 58.4% of adults in long-term care facilities were found to have generalized anxiety disorders (Atchison et al, 2022). Studies of anxiety and depression have found relationships between life stressors, loneliness, and health to exacerbate mental illness. Adults age 50 to 59 years were found to have high rates of anxiety, possibly due to life transitions and retirement (Curran et al, 2020). Anxiety triggers for older adults may include worries about their health, disability, and dependence, whereas anxiety triggers for younger adults center around work, finances, and family. Diagnosis and detection of generalized anxiety disorders in later life can be complicated by chronic medical conditions, cognition decline, life changes, and medication side effects.

Symptoms of anxiety can be manifested cognitively, emotionally, and/or physically. Examples of such manifestations include ruminating, excessive worry and fear, difficulty concentrating or focusing, restlessness, irritability, fatigue, body aches/pains, insomnia, and increased cardiovascular and respiratory responses (i.e., pounding heart, irregular breathing) (NAMI, n.d.). Risk factors related to developing an anxiety disorder in older adults include the loss of a spouse or loved one, physical illness, social isolation, low quality of life, and no religious affiliation (Andreas et al, 2022).

Evidence-based treatments for anxiety disorders include psychotherapy including CBT, medications, and complementary health approaches for stress reduction and relaxation. Benzodiazepines and anxiolytics can have negative effects on older adults and may not be recommended. Antidepressants are also used to treat anxiety disorders but, as discussed above, may not be tolerated by older adults (Atchison et al, 2022). Psychosocial interventions, including relaxation training, CBT, cognitive restructuring, and supportive therapy, appear helpful in reducing anxiety in older adults. However, the effects appear to be less than those found in younger adults (Curran et al, 2020). It will be important for researchers and therapists to develop more-effective anxiety interventions for older individuals.

Schizophrenia

Schizophrenia is considered a severe mental illness, affecting about 1 in 300 people worldwide (WHO, 2022). It is characterized by disturbances in thought processes, hallucinations, delusions, cognitive impairments, and deficits in daily functioning. Schizophrenia is typically diagnosed in young adults and is a chronic condition with premature mortality and characterized by severe dysfunction (Olfson et al, 2015). Older adults with schizophrenia often have comorbidities and dementia (Stroup et al, 2021). The severe dysfunction related to schizophrenia often leads to institutionalization, social isolation, and stress on family and friends. About 15% of older adults with schizophrenia are living in long-term care facilities. A systematic review found that 46.51% of the homeless population had some diagnosis of psychosis, highlighting the extensive public health needs of this population (Ayano et al, 2019).

Bipolar Disorder

Bipolar disorder is a serious mood disorder characterized by alternating elevated periods of mania (bipolar I mood disorder) and depression (bipolar II mood disorder). However, some individuals experience a mixed state in which manic, hypomanic, and depression are present concurrently. Eyler et al (2022) found that 70% of older adults with bipolar disorder had mixed manic and depressive symptoms. Older adults with bipolar disorder with severe mixed symptoms presented with disorders in language and thought, with irritability during the manic state, and with concentration problems, sadness, and anxiety during the depressive state. While the prevalence of bipolar disorder decreases with age, about 25% of persons with bipolar disorder are older than 60 years (Sajatovic et al, 2015).

Bipolar disorder has been found to be a predictor of Alzheimer disease. Neuroimaging in older adults with bipolar disorder has revealed similar structural changes as those individuals with neurodegenerative conditions. These structural changes are attributed to neuroprogression. Neuroprogression is caused by the biological changes linked to the frequency of changing mood states. With each episode of mania, depression, or hypomania, the brain is exposed to damaging biological changes, resulting in a decline in functioning. Older adults with bipolar disorder, especially mixed symptoms and frequent episodes, are likely to be more dependent in daily activities and cognitive functioning (Eyler et al, 2022). Cognitive problems are extensive in this population compared with age-matched healthy controls. Older adults with bipolar disorder presented with difficulty with attention, inhibition, immediate memory, working memory (storing and retrieving), processing speed, cognitive flexibility, verbal fluency, psychomotor function, executive functions, and recognition (Montejo et al, 2022).

Substance Use Disorders

Substance use disorders (SUDs) refer to the misuse of substances that result in physical and/or psychological addiction; these substances include alcohol, prescription drugs, nonprescription medications, and illicit drugs. Although older adults do have SUDs, relatively little is known about prevalence, etiology, or treatment. Between 2008 and 2018, older adults' rate of seeking first-time treatment for SUDs was proportionally higher than that of younger adults. The primary substances misused at admission by older adults were illicit drugs including opioids, heroin, and methamphetamine. There were fewer admissions for alcohol use compared with those for illicit drug use (Weber et al, 2022). This population is defined by the baby boomer generation, which had early exposure to a drug and alcohol culture. Risk factors contributing to SUD include chronic pain, poor overall health, polypharmacy, social isolation, history of abuse, loss of loved ones, no religious affiliation, single or divorced, and avoidant coping strategies (Jaqua et al, 2022).

SUD is a modifiable risk factor for dementia, with illicit drug and alcohol use associated with higher rates of dementia. Alcohol is neurotoxic, leading to brain damage. Heavy alcohol use is also linked to a thiamine deficiency causing Wernicke-Korsakoff syndrome (WKS). WKS is a neurological disorder with symptoms of mental confusion, vision problems, hypothermia, low blood pressure, and ataxia. WKS is linked to poor nutrition, found in adults with heavy alcohol use, eating disorders, and persons with cancer (Schwarzinger et al, 2018). Older adults who reported long-term recreational use of cannabis were found to have slowed processing speeds and impaired executive functioning compared with nonusers and short-term users (Stypulkowski & Thayer, 2022).

Treatment of SUD in older adults must consider the physiological changes associated with aging. Older adults are at risk of decline in renal and liver functions caused by SUD. Treatment programs such as detoxification must consider underlying medical conditions (Jaqua et al, 2022). Nonpharmacological treatments for SUD include psychotherapy, including CBT, self-help groups (e.g., Alcoholics Anonymous, Narcotics Anonymous), motivational interviewing, and group therapy (Jaqua et al, 2022).

Optimizing Cognitive Functioning in Older Adults

Cognitive functioning in older adults is affected by several factors. While many of these factors cannot be modified, others can be influenced by lifestyle. Genetics, socioeconomics, access to health care, and low education level have been linked to declines in cognitive function with aging. Education consistently predicts crystallized intelligence and memory (Roldán-Tapia et al, 2017). Factors such as participation in cognitively stimulating activities, physical activity and exercise, and socialization have been linked to facilitating enhanced cognitive reserve. **Cognitive reserve** is the amount of cognitive resources available after an individual engages in a task. Many physiological functions, including those involving the cardiovascular system and the brain, have a residual or reserve capacity. Cardiovascular reserve is the difference between one's maximum heart rate and current heart rate. The purpose of aerobic exercise is to increase cardiovascular endurance to perform at greater intensity and for longer periods. To increase cognitive reserve, a person must engage in brain exercises. Refer to Table 13-3 for information on Enhancing Cognitive Reserve.

Cognitive and Mental Stimulation

Through regular interactions during the rehabilitation process, therapists can integrate cognitively stimulating activities into the plan of care as well as educate the client on continuing these aspects of cognitive enrichment after formal rehabilitation. Participating in mentally stimulating and

TABLE 13-3 ■ Enhancing Cognitive Reserve

INTERVENTION	IMPACT ON AGING	BEST PRACTICE
Cognitive/mental stimulation	■ Continued cognitive functioning ■ Reduced risk of developing dementia	Stimulation should be: ■ Relevant ■ Meaningful ■ Challenging ■ Novel
Physical activity/exercise	■ Enhanced cognitive performance in executive function, controlled processing, speed of processing, visuospatial processing) ■ Enhanced balance (reducing falls)	Strength training Aerobic exercise Low impact exercise Effortful exercise Dance Sports
Socialization	■ Decrease in depression ■ Overall sense of well-being ■ Enhanced cognitive functioning	Ensure person has means to interact with family and friends (transportation, accessible telephone (considering hearing impaired). Social clubs – books, hobbies Contact with family

novel activities can include increasing the difficulty of cognitive tasks during therapy and educating patients to challenge themselves at home with new and unfamiliar tasks, such as learning a new language or activity. To be considered mentally stimulating, tasks should be novel and mentally challenging, as new learning facilitates neural growth, development, and plasticity (Chapman et al, 2015).

Physical Activity and Exercise

The aging brain is capable of neuroplastic changes. Regular physical exercise has been linked to changes in brain volume (Maass et al, 2015) due to the production of a protein called brain-derived neurotrophic factor. Brain-derived neurotrophic factor is linked to advancing neuroplasticity and is released in the blood during exercise. Regular vigorous exercise is linked to cognitive health and longevity (Gebel et al, 2015). Dance as a form of exercise has been linked to higher releases of brain-derived neurotrophic factor compared with that found with other types of exercise (Rehfeld et al, 2018).

Socialization

Socialization is paramount for healthy cognitive aging. Besser and colleagues (2017) found that socioeconomic status and distance to travel to community resources were linked to cognitive function. Specific neighborhood entities promoting socialization were found to include senior centers, eateries, and coffee shops. Participants valued engaging with others in the neighborhood, identifying opportunities for laughter, fun, and gossip (Finlay et al, 2021). More-diverse social networks have been linked to greater cognitive functioning (Ali et al, 2018).

Occupational Therapy Interventions for Mental Health

One theme has played out repeatedly in this chapter, whether talking of healthy cognitive aging, neuropathological conditions, or mental illness, cognitive functions are impacted by both modifiable and nonmodifiable risk factors. Genetics, early childhood stressors, education, socioeconomics, access to health care, nutrition, and environment affect healthy cognitive aging. While some of these risk factors can be argued to be modifiable, it will take a systems approach to provide services across groups of individuals. Modifiable risk factors include participation in cognitively stimulating activities, socialization, and physical exercise. The role of occupational therapists working with this population is to ensure an environment allowing for participation and facilitating participation using meaningful activities and occupations (AJOT, 2017). At the systems level, occupational therapy can advocate for the clients to have access to health care, healthy nutrition, and a healthy environment that is safe and promotes participation. Occupational therapists must reflect on prejudices, ageism, and discrimination and ensure each client is respected and specific attention is paid to promoting self-confidence and self-efficacy.

Treatment interventions must address the specific needs of the client. Treatment must be client centered, engaging the client in meaningful and valued occupations (Lai et al, 2020). Several challenges to productive aging have been identified, including health problems, side effects of medication, lack of purpose and boredom, and the loss of family and friends. A systematic review of occupational therapy interventions in mental illness identified five types of interventions: occupation-based interventions, psychoeducation, skills training, cognition-based interventions, and technology-supported interventions (D'Amico et al, 2018). Occupation-based, individualized, client-centered interventions focused on specific client goals yielded better outcomes in social participation and performance compared with individuals without individualized interventions. Occupation-based programs implemented by occupational therapists had better outcomes than treatment-as-usual groups (D'Amico et al, 2018).

Occupation-based interventions include individualized treatment plans within the client's environment. Interventions include life skills training, empowerment, BADL and IADL training, and affording opportunities for community participation. One evidenced-based manualized program is The Life Adaptations Skills Training (LAST). LAST manualized treatment was tested with adults with depression. The treatment uses strategies and skills to enhance occupational participation. Concepts and skills included in the program were living a balanced and satisfying life, appraising emotional expression, managing symptoms/illnesses, developing interpersonal relationships, and managing stress. Both groups had enhanced quality of life. The intervention group, however, had significantly reduced anxiety and depression compared with the control group (Chen et al, 2015). Several evidence-based manualized programs have been developed using psychoeducation to address BADL and IADL skills. Manualized treatments included adherence therapy (Chien et al, 2016) and the Illness Management and Recovery program (Salyers et al, 2014).

Participation in cognitively stimulating activities is linked to healthy cognitive aging. Cognitive stimulation is likened to physical exercise building endurance; cognitive exercise builds cognitive reserve. Ávila et al (2018) studied occupational therapy interventions with community-dwelling individuals with a diagnosis of Alzheimer disease. Client-centered, goal-specific occupational therapy was performed in the client's home. Interventions included orientation to space and time, participant-directed activities/tasks, specific BADL training, relaxation/breathing, and caregiver counseling. Participants had significant improvements in place and time orientation and attention and concentration. Given that Alzheimer disease is a progressive illness, this evidence supports continued therapy to maintain and enhance cognitive skills. Participants also had significant increases in performance of self-care activities (Ávila et al, 2018).

Social participation is associated with increased self-confidence, enhanced quality of life, and overall perceived health. A group of adults with MCI were found to benefit from volunteering in the community. Participants had a higher rated perceived health and greater sense of self-purpose (Lee et al, 2022).

Summary of Cognitive Functioning in Persons with Neuropathologies

Persons with neuropathologies become dependent on others due to a loss of executive functioning and can benefit from the adaptation of the environment, including reducing clutter, using signs to identify each room in the house, placing lists on a mirror for hygiene tasks, and using technology for reminders. In addition, programs teaching strategies and increasing self-awareness are effective in compensating for some cognitive changes. Despite the progression of some pathologies, persons with neuropathologies benefit from cognitive health practices including exercise and activity, social participation, and cognitive stimulation. The demand of caring for a person with neuropathologies can be stressful and disruptive to persons responsible for caregiving. Clinicians must ensure that the client receives the best care and that the caregiver's needs and goals are addressed in the care plan. As the condition progresses, persons with neuropathologies will often require institutionalization. Individuals will benefit from programs that provide activity and exercise, cognitive stimulation, and opportunities for socialization. While there are no cures for cognitive changes due to neuropathologies, clinicians can provide interventions and create environments that reduce negative effects such as feelings of frustration, agitation, isolation, confusion, and paranoia.

Interprofessional Practice

Clinicians working with older adults must consider normal cognitive changes such as speed of processing and changes in vision and hearing that can influence participation in treatment. Occupational therapists, physical therapists, speech-language pathologists, nursing, and social workers have a unique opportunity to facilitate optimal cognitive functioning in older adults. In a monograph discussing the cognitive enrichment of older adults, Hertzog et al (2021) outlined a set of principles for interventions to enhance older adults' memory. It is suggested that teaching metacognitive strategies can compensate for age-related changes and promote goal attainment in daily activities. Interventions and environments promoting exercise, socialization, and cognitive stimulation are shown to promote healthy cognitive functioning and reverse some cognitive decline (Rivera-Torres et al, 2019). In addition, rehabilitation professionals must be sensitive to attitudes and beliefs about aging, because one's perception about aging can influence the trajectory of the aging process. For example, if an older adult believes aging is predominantly a negative process, this can affect their performance on cognitive tasks. It is important that therapists discuss aging within a life span developmental framework, highlighting the gains, losses, and stability.

An example of professionals working together can be seen in the use of the CO-OP. The team can work together learning the best strategies for the individual client and then reinforcing the use of the strategies across activities. Nursing can use strategies in reinforcing medication management, hygiene, and toileting. Physical therapy can use the strategy in working with the client on motor skills and performing exercises, occupational therapy can use the strategy for performing a meaningful activity such as baking, and speech-language pathology can use the strategy when working with the client on processing a conversation. The team, working together, can create an environment where the client can experience success to promote self-confidence and ensure consistency of interactions to alleviate confusion.

> ### CASE STUDY (CONTINUED)
>
> *Assessment and Intervention*
>
> Mandie enrolled Tom in LSVT Big classes, and Tom participated for a few months. The disease led to him being paranoid during classes; his wife had to be in sight, and he was often disruptive. Mandie tried a day-care program for a few days a week to give her respite. After 2 weeks, Tom refused to go to day care, and the day care felt he was not adjusting. Tom continued to decline and now needs assistance with basic self-care, eating, and walking. Mandie is struggling with Tom's behavior around toileting, with accidents and some smearing. Tom requires a modified diet for swallowing and drools frequently. Tom no longer recognizes his adult children and sometimes does not recognize Mandie. He has night terrors and sometimes gets out of bed. Mandie realizes she is no longer able to care for Tom. She has mixed feelings about moving her husband to a long-term facility but feels she must do so for his safety and her health.
>
> ### Questions
>
> 1. What are two or three evidence-based, occupation-centered exemplar interventions that address Tom's priorities?
> 2. What are two evidence-based interventions for his wife?
>
> ### Answers
>
> 1. Sensory stimulation such as music therapy to reduce agitation, reminiscence therapy, and exercise. Implementing a COPE program. (See section on Occupational Therapy Interventions for Persons with Dementia. LO 13-3, 13-6.)
> 2. Education to build knowledge and skills for coping, implementing a TAP program for the caregiver. (LO 13-3, 13-6)

SUMMARY

Older adults and their families coping with neurocognitive and behavioral changes and mental health issues face unique challenges in providing care for and managing cognitive, functional, and behavioral symptoms. Older adults and older adults with mental illness face many barriers to participation. Ageism has a negative impact on health, well-being, and quality of life. Further, ageism among healthcare workers can result in inaccurate assumptions about cognitive and physical functioning (e.g., "An 87-year-old should not live alone"), withholding of some treatments, and discounting some behaviors as simply part of aging (e.g., depression, memory problems) (Burnes et al, 2019). An individual's self-esteem and self-efficacy are linked to perceived quality of life. Ageism and discrimination can contribute to poor self-esteem and self-efficacy.

In conclusion, older adults experience cognitive changes. Chronological age is less a predictor of cognitive functioning than are factors such as genetics, education, access to healthcare, early-life trauma, and socioeconomic status. There are several factors that facilitate cognitive functioning, such as access to healthcare and nutrition, an enriched environment with cognitively stimulating activities and exercise, and opportunities for socialization and participation. Creating a culture free of ageism and opportunities to enhance cognitive reserve are critical for promoting healthy cognitive aging.

Critical Thinking Questions

1. Identify barriers and facilitators for healthy cognitive aging (modifiable and nonmodifiable). Formulate some interventions that facilitate healthy cognitive functioning, addressing environments, occupations, and the person.

2. Older adults with and without neurodegenerative conditions have been found to have cognitive changes. Identify common cognitive changes in older adults. Propose what other conditions of aging may affect cognitive functioning. When interacting with older adults and when teaching an individual a new skill, what techniques should be used to adapt for cognitive changes and other factors affecting functioning?

3. Persons with dementia and other neurodegenerative conditions continue to decline with progressive loss of independence and an added burden of care. What should be included in the treatment of these individuals to ensure the highest level of functioning? What activities would be therapeutic for this population?

REFERENCES

Ali, T., Nilsson, C. J., Weuve, J., Rajan, K. B., & De Leon, C. F. M. (2018). Effects of social network diversity on mortality, cognition and physical function in the elderly: A longitudinal analysis of the Chicago Health and Aging Project (CHAP). *Journal of Epidemiology & Community Health, 72*(11), 990–996. https://doi.org/10.1136/jech-2017-210236

Allen, C. K., Austin, S. L., David, S. K., Earhart, C. A., McCraith, D. B., & Riska-Williams, L. (2007). *Allen Cognitive Level Screen–5 (ACLS–5) and Large Allen Cognitive Level Screen–5 (LACLS–5)*. ACLS and LACLS Committee.

Alzheimer's Disease International. (n.d.-a). *Alzheimer's disease facts and figures*. Retrieved September 2, 2022, from https://www.alz.org/media/Documents/alzheimers-facts-and-figures.pdf

Alzheimer's Disease International. (n.d.-b). *Dementia statistics*. Retrieved September 2, 2022, from https://www.alzint.org/about/dementia-facts-figures/dementia-statistics

American Journal of Occupational Therapy (AJOT). (2017). Mental health promotion, prevention, and intervention in occupational therapy practice. (2017). *American Journal of Occupational Therapy*, 71(Suppl. 2), 7112410035p1–7112410035p19. https://doi.org/10.5014/ajot.2017.716S03

Anand, A., & MacLullich, A. M. (2021). Delirium in older adults. *Medicine*, 49(1), 26–31. https://doi.org/10.1016/j.mpmed.2020.10.002

Anderson, N. (2019). State of the science on mild cognitive impairment (MCI). *CNS Spectrums*, 24(1), 78–87. https://doi.org/10.1017/S1092852918001347

Andreas, S., Schulz, H., Volkert, J., Lüdemann, J., Dehoust, M., Sehner, S., Suling, A., Wegscheider, K., Ausín, B., Canuto, A., Crawford, M. J., Da Ronch, C., Grassi, L., Hershkovitz, Y., Muñoz, M., Quirk, A., Rotenstein, O., Belén Santos-Olmo, A., Shalev, A., ... Härter, M. (2022). Incidence and risk factors of mental disorders in the elderly: The European MentDis_ICF65+ study. *Australian and New Zealand Journal of Psychiatry*, 56(5), 551–559. https://doi.org/10.1177%2F00048674211025711

Ardelt, M., & Jeste, D. V. (2018). Wisdom and hard times: The ameliorating effect of wisdom on the negative association between adverse life events and well-being. *The Journals of Gerontology: Series B*, 73(8), 1374–1383. https://doi.org/10.1093/geronb/gbw137

Atchison, K., Watt, J. A., Ewert, D., Toohey, A. M., Ismail, Z., & Goodarzi, Z. (2022). Non-pharmacologic and pharmacologic treatments for anxiety in long-term care: A systematic review and meta-analysis. *Age and Ageing*, 51(9), afac195. https://doi.org/10.1093/ageing/afac195

Ávila, A., De, R. I., Torres, G., Vizcaíno, M., Peralbo, M., & Durán, M. (2018). Promoting functional independence in people with Alzheimer's disease: Outcomes of a home-based occupational therapy intervention in Spain. *Health & Social Care in the Community*, 26(5), 734–743. https://doi.org/10.1111/hsc.12594

Ayano, G., Tesfaw, G., & Shumet, S. (2019). The prevalence of schizophrenia and other psychotic disorders among homeless people: A systematic review and meta-analysis. *BMC Psychiatry*, 19, Article 370. https://doi.org/10.1186/s12888-019-2361-7

Baddeley, A. (2020). Short-term memory. In *Memory* (pp. 41–69). Routledge.

Ball, L. J., Bisher, G. B., & Birge, S. J. (1999). A simple test of central processing speed: An extension of the Short Blessed Test. *Journal of the American Geriatrics Society*, 47(11), 1359–1363. https://doi.org/10.1111/j.1532-5415.1999.tb07440.x

Barker-Collo, S., Starkey, N., Lawes, C. M., Feigin, V., Senior, H., & Parag, V. (2012). Neuropsychological profiles of 5-year ischemic stroke survivors by Oxfordshire stroke classification and hemisphere of lesion. *Stroke*, 43(1), 50–55. https://doi.org/10.1161/STROKEAHA.111.627182

Baum, C. M. (2011). *Executive function performance test: Training manual*. Washington University. https://www.ot.wustl.edu/about/resources/executive-function-performance-test-efpt-308

Baum, C., & Edwards, D. F. (1993). Cognitive performance in senile dementia of the Alzheimer's type: The kitchen task assessment. *The American Journal of Occupational Therapy*, 47(5), 431–436. https://doi.org/10.5014/ajot.47.5.431

Beck, A. T., Ward, C. H., Mendelson, M., Mock, J., & Erbaugh, J. (1961). An inventory for measuring depression. *Archives of General Psychiatry*, 4(6), 561–571. https://doi.org/10.1001/archpsyc.1961.01710120031004

Besser, L. M., McDonald, N. C., Song, Y., Kukull, W. A., & Rodriguez, D. A. (2017). Neighborhood environment and cognition in older adults: A systematic review. *American Journal of Preventive Medicine*, 53(2), 241–251. https://doi.org/10.1016/j.amepre.2017.02.013

Bessey, L. J., & Walaszek, A. (2019). Management of behavioral and psychological symptoms of dementia. *Current Psychiatry Reports*, 21(8), Article 66. https://doi.org/10.1007/s11920-019-1049-5

Bodner, E., Palgi, Y., & Wyman, M. F. (2018). Ageism in mental health assessment and treatment of older adults. In L. Ayalon, & C. Tesch-Römer (Eds.), *Contemporary perspectives on ageism. International Perspectives on Aging*, vol 19. Springer, Cham. https://doi.org/10.1007/978-3-319-73820-8_15

Brodaty, H., & Donkin, M. (2022). Family caregivers of people with dementia. *Dialogues in Clinical Neuroscience*, 11(2), 217–228. https://doi.org/10.31887/DCNS.2009.11.2/hbrodaty

Burgess, P. W., Veitch, E., de Lacy Costello, A., & Shallice, T. (2000). The cognitive and neuroanatomical correlates of multitasking. *Neuropsychologia*, 38(6), 848–863. https://doi.org/10.1016/S0028-3932(99)00134-7

Burnes, D., Sheppard, C., Henderson Jr, C. R., Wassel, M., Cope, R., Barber, C., & Pillemer, K. (2019). Interventions to reduce ageism against older adults: A systematic review and meta-analysis. *American Journal of Public Health*, 109(8), e1–e9. https://doi.org/10.2105/AJPH.2019.305123

Burns, T., Mortimer, J. A., & Merchak, P. (1994). Cognitive performance test: A new approach to functional assessment in Alzheimer's disease. *Journal of Geriatric Psychiatry and Neurology*, 7(1), 46–54. https://doi.org/10.1177/089198879400700109

Canuto, A., Weber, K., Baertschi, M., Andreas, S., Volkert, J., Dehoust, M. C., Sehner, S., Suling, A., Wegscheider, K., Ausín, B., Crawford, M. J., Da Ronch, C., Grassi, L., Hershkovitz, Y., Muñoz, M., Quirk, A., Rotenstein, O., Santos-Olmo, A. B., Shalev, A., ... Härter, M. (2018). Anxiety disorders in old age: Psychiatric comorbidities, quality of life, and prevalence according to age, gender, and country. *The American Journal of Geriatric Psychiatry*, 26(2), 174–185. https://doi.org/10.1016/j.jagp.2017.08.015

Chapman, S. B., Aslan, S., Spence, J. S., Hart, J. J., Jr, Bartz, E. K., Didehbani, N., Keebler, M. W., Gardner, C. M., Strain, J. F., DeFina, L. F., & Lu, H. (2015). Neural mechanisms of brain plasticity with complex cognitive training in healthy seniors. *Cerebral Cortex*, 25(2), 396–405.

Chari, D., Ali, R., & Gupta, R. (2015). Reversible dementia in elderly: Really uncommon? *Journal of Geriatric Mental Health*, 2(1), 30–37. doi: 10.4103/2348-9995.161378

Chen, Y. L., Pan, A. W., Hsiung, P. C., Chung, L., Lai, J. S., Gau, S. S. F., & Chen, T. J. (2015). Life adaptation skills training (LAST) for persons with depression: A randomized controlled study. *Journal of Affective Disorders*, 185, 108–114. https://doi.org/10.1016/j.jad.2015.06.022

Cheng, S. T., Li, K. K., Losada, A., Zhang, F., Au, A., Thompson, L. W., & Gallagher-Thompson, D. (2020). The effectiveness of nonpharmacological interventions for informal dementia caregivers: An updated systematic review and meta-analysis. *Psychology and Aging*, 35(1), 55–77. https://doi.org/10.1037/pag0000401

Chien, W. T., Mui, J., Gray, R., & Cheung, E. (2016). Adherence therapy versus routine psychiatric care for people with schizophrenia spectrum disorders: A randomised controlled trial. *BMC Psychiatry*, 16, Article 42. https://doi.org/10.1186/s12888-016-0744-6

Cicerone, K. D., Goldin, Y., Ganci, K., Rosenbaum, A., Wethe, J. V., Langenbahn, D. M., Malec, J. F., Bergquist, T. F., Kingsley, K., Nagele, D., Trexler, L., Fraas, M., Bogdanova, Y., & Harley, J. P. (2019). Evidence-based cognitive rehabilitation: Systematic review of the literature from 2009 through 2014. *Archives of Physical Medicine and Rehabilitation*, 100(8), 1515–1533. https://doi.org/10.1016/j.apmr.2019.02.011

Clemson, L., Laver, K., Rahja, M., Culph, J., Scanlan, J. N., Day, S., Comans, T., Jeon, Y. H., Low, L. F., Crotty, M., Kurrle, S., Cations, M., Piersol, C. V., & Gitlin, L. N. (2021). Implementing a reablement intervention, "Care of People Dementia in their Environments (COPE)": A hybrid implementation-effectiveness study. *The Gerontologist*, 61(6), 965–976. https://doi.org/10.1093/geront/gnaa105

Colarusso, R. P., & Hammill, D. D. (1972). *Motor-free visual perception test*. Academic Therapy Publications.

Cuevas-Lara, C., Izquierdo, M., Gutiérrez-Valencia, M., Marín-Epelde, I., Zambom-Ferraresi, F., Contreras-Escámez, B., & Martínez-Velilla, N. (2019). Effectiveness of occupational therapy interventions in acute geriatric wards: A systematic review. *Maturitas*, 127, 43–50. https://doi.org/10.1016/j.maturitas.2019.06.005

Cullum, C. M., Saine, K., Chan, L. D., Martin-Cook, K., Gray, K. F., & Weiner, M. F. (2001). Performance-based instrument to assess functional capacity in dementia: The Texas functional living scale. *Neuropsychiatry, Neuropsychology, and Behavioral Neurology, 14*(2), 103–108.

Curran, E., Rosato, M., Ferry, F., & Leavey, G. (2020). Prevalence and factors associated with anxiety and depression in older adults: Gender differences in psychosocial indicators. *Journal of Affective Disorders, 267,* 114–122. https://doi.org/10.1016/j.jad.2020.02.018

D'Amico, M. L., Jaffe, L. E., & Gardner, J. A. (2018). Evidence for interventions to improve and maintain occupational performance and participation for people with serious mental illness: A systematic review. *The American Journal of Occupational Therapy, 72*(5), 7205190020p1–7205190020p11. https://doi.org/10.5014/ajot.2018.033332

de Paula, J. J., Diniz, B. S., Bicalho, M. A., Albuquerque, M. R., Nicolato, R., de Moraes, E. N., Romano-Silva, M. A., & Malloy-Diniz, L. F. (2015). Specific cognitive functions and depressive symptoms as predictors of activities of daily living in older adults with heterogeneous cognitive backgrounds. *Frontiers in Aging Neuroscience, 7,* Article 139. https://doi.org/10.3389/fnagi.2015.00139

Diller, L., & Gordon, W. A. (1981). Interventions for cognitive deficits in brain-injured adults. *Journal of Consulting and Clinical Psychology, 49*(6), 822–834. https://doi.org/10.1037//0022-006x.49.6.822

Ducharme-Laliberté, G., Mellah, S., & Belleville, S. (2022). Having a stimulating lifestyle is associated with maintenance of white matter integrity with age. *Brain Imaging and Behavior, 16*(3), 1392–1399. https://doi.org/10.1007/s11682-021-00620-7

Eddy, E., Heron, P., McMillan, D., Dawson, S., Ekers, D., Hickin, N., Littlewood, E., Shafran, R., Meader, N., & Gilbody, S. (2020). Cognitive or behavioural interventions (or both) to prevent or mitigate loneliness in adolescents, adults, and older adults. *Cochrane Database of Systematic Reviews.* 11, CD013791. https://doi.org/10.1002/14651858.CD013791

Edwards, D. F., Wolf, T. J., Marks, T., Alter, S., Larkin, V., Padesky, B. L., Spiers, M., Al-Heizan, M. O., & Giles, G. M. (2019). Reliability and validity of a functional cognition screening tool to identify the need for occupational therapy. *American Journal of Occupational Therapy, 73*(2), 7302205050p1–7302205050p10. https://doi.org/10.5014/ajot.2019.028753

Esiri, M. M. (2007). Ageing and the brain. *The Journal of Pathology, 211*(2), 181–187. https://doi.org/10.1002/path.2089

Eyler, L. T., Briggs, F. B. S., Dols, A., Rej, S., Almeida, O. P., Beunders, A. J. M., Blumberg, H. P., Forester, B. P., Patrick, R. E., Forlenza, O. V., Gildengers, A., Jimenez, E., Vieta, E., Mulsant, B. H., Schouws, S., Paans, N. P. G., Strejilevich, S., Sutherland, A., Tsai, S., & Sajatovic, M. (2022). Symptom severity mixity in older-age bipolar disorder: Analyses from the global aging and geriatric experiments in bipolar disorder database (GAGE-BD). *The American Journal of Geriatric Psychiatry, 30*(10), 1096–1107. https://doi.org/10.1016/j.jagp.2022.03.007

Filipska, K., Wiśniewski, A., Biercewicz, M., & Ślusarz, R. (2020). Are depression and dementia a common problem for stroke older adults? A review of chosen epidemiological studies. *Psychiatric Quarterly, 91*(3), 807–817. https://doi.org/10.1007/s11126-020-09734-5

Finlay, J., Esposito, M., Li, M., Kobayashi, L. C., Khan, A. M., Gomez-Lopez, I., Melendez, R., Colabianchi, N., Judd, S., & Clarke, P. J. (2021). Can neighborhood social infrastructure modify cognitive function? A mixed-methods study of urban-dwelling aging Americans. *Journal of Aging and Health, 33*(9), 772–785. https://doi.org/10.1177/08982643211008

Fisher, A. (1995). *The assessment of motor and process skills (AMPS).* Three Star Press.

Folstein, M. F., Folstein, S. E., & McHugh, P. R. (1975). "Mini-mental state": A practical method for grading the cognitive state of patients for the clinician. *Journal of Psychiatric Research, 12*(3), 189–198. https://doi.org/10.1016/0022-3956(75)90026-6

Friedman, P. J. (1991). Clock drawing in acute stroke. *Age and Ageing, 20*(2), 140–145. https://doi.org/10.1093/ageing/20.2.140

Gebel, K., Ding, D., Chey, T., Stamatakis, E., Brown, W. J., & Bauman, A. E. (2015). Effect of moderate to vigorous physical activity on all-cause mortality in middle-aged and older Australians. *JAMA Internal Medicine, 175*(6), 970–977. https://doi.org/10.1001/jamainternmed.2015.0541

Giles, G. M., Edwards, D. F., Baum, C., Furniss, J., Skidmore, E., Wolf, T., & Leland, N. E. (2020). Making functional cognition a professional priority. *The American Journal of Occupational Therapy, 74*(1), 7401090010p1–7401090010p6. https://doi.org/10.5014/ajot.2020.741002

Giles, G. M., Radomski, M. V., & Wolf, T. J. (2019). Cognition, cognitive rehabilitation, and occupational performance. *American Journal of Occupational Therapy, 73*(Suppl. 2), 7312410010p1–7312410010p25. https://doi.org/10.5014/ajot.2019.73S201

Gitlin, L. N., Marx, K., Piersol, C. V., Hodgson, N. A., Huang, J., Roth, D. L., & Lyketsos, C. (2021). Effects of the tailored activity program (TAP) on dementia-related symptoms, health events and caregiver wellbeing: A randomized controlled trial. *BMC Geriatrics, 21*(1), Article 581. https://doi.org/10.1186/s12877-021-02511-4

Gitlin, L. N., Winter, L., Dennis, M. P., Hodgson, N., & Hauck, W. W. (2010). A biobehavioral home-based intervention and the wellbeing of patients with dementia and their caregivers: The COPE randomized trial. *JAMA, 304*(9), 983–991. https://doi.org/10.1001/jama.2010.1253

Glück, J., Bluck, S., & Weststrate, N. M. (2019). More on the MORE life experience model: What we have learned (so far). *The Journal of Value Inquiry, 53*(3), 349–370. https://doi.org/10.1007/s10790-018-9661-x

Glück, J., & Weststrate, N. M. (2022). The wisdom researchers and the elephant: An integrative model of wise behavior. *Personality and Social Psychology Review, 26*(4), 342–374. https://doi.org/10.1177/10888683221094650

Goh, J. O., Yang, A., & Resnick, S. M. (2012). Differential trajectories of age-related changes in components of executive and memory processes. *Psychology and Aging, 27*(3), 707–719. https://doi.org/10.1037/a0026715

Greaves, C. V., & Rohrer, J. D. (2019). An update on genetic frontotemporal dementia. *Journal of Neurology, 266*(8), 2075–2086. https://doi.org/10.1007/s00415-019-09363-4

Greene, N. R., & Naveh-Benjamin, M. (2020). A specificity principle of memory: Evidence from aging and associative memory. *Psychological Science, 31*(3), 316–331. https://doi.org/10.1177/0956797620901760

Haas, M., Mehl, M. R., Ballhausen, N., Zuber, S., Kliegel, M., & Hering, A. (2022). The sounds of memory: Extending the age-prospective memory paradox to everyday behavior and conversations. *The Journals of Gerontology. Series B, Psychological Sciences and Social Sciences, 77*(4), 695–703. https://doi.org/10.1093/geronb/gbac012

Hertzog, C., Pearman, A., Lustig, E., & Hughes, M. (2021). Fostering self-management of everyday memory in older adults: A new intervention approach. *Frontiers in Psychology, 11,* 560056. https://doi.org/10.3389/fpsyg.2020.560056

Holm, M. B., & Rogers, J. C. (2008). Performance assessment of self-care skills (PASS). In B. J. Hemphill-Pearson (Ed.), *Assessments in Occupational Therapy Mental Health* (2nd ed., pp. 101–110). Slack Incorporated.

Horn, J. L., & Cattell, R. B. (1967). Age differences in fluid and crystallized intelligence. *Acta Psychologica, 26,* 107–129. https://doi.org/10.1016/0001-6918(67)90011-X

Houben, N., Janssen, E. P. C. J., Hendriks, M. R. C., van der Kellen, D., van Alphen, B. P. J., & van Meijel, B. (2019). Physical health status of older adults with severe mental illness: The PHiSMI-E cohort study. *International Journal of Mental Health Nursing, 28*(2), 457–467. https://doi.org/10.1111/inm.12547

Jaqua, E. E., Nguyen, V., Scherlie, N., Dreschler, J., & Labib, W. (2022). Substance use disorder in older adults: Mini review. *Addiction & Health, 14*(1), 62–67. doi: 10.22122/ahj.v14i1.1311

Jeste, D. V., & Lee, E. E. (2019). Emerging empirical science of wisdom: Definition, measurement, neurobiology, longevity, and interventions. *Harvard Review of Psychiatry, 27*(3), 127–140. https://doi.org/10.1097/HRP.0000000000000205

Jimenez, D. E., Schmidt, A. C., Kim, G., & Cook, B. L. (2017). Impact of comorbid mental health needs on racial/ethnic disparities in general medical care utilization among older adults. *International Journal of Geriatric Psychiatry*, *32*(8), 909–921. https://doi.org/10.1002/gps.4546

Jongsiriyanyong, S., & Limpawattana, P. (2018). Mild cognitive impairment in clinical practice: A review article. *American Journal of Alzheimer's Disease & Other Dementias*, *33*(8), 500–507. https://doi.org/10.1177/1533317518791401

Kanfer, R., Frese, M., & Johnson, R. E. (2017). Motivation related to work: A century of progress. *Journal of Applied Psychology*, *102*(3), 338–355. https://doi.org/10.1037/apl0000133

Kemper, S., & Mitzner, T. L. (2001). Language production and comprehension. In J. E. Birren & K. W. Schaie (Eds.), *Handbook of the psychology of aging* (5th ed., pp. 378–398). Academic Press.

Kishita, N., Hammond, L., Dietrich, C. M., & Mioshi, E. (2018). Which interventions work for dementia family carers? An updated systematic review of randomized controlled trials of carer interventions. *International Psychogeriatrics*, *30*(11), 1679–1696. https://doi.org/10.1017/S1041610218000947

Klimova, B., & Kuca, K. (2016). Speech and language impairments in dementia. *Journal of Applied Biomedicine*, *14*(2), 97–103. https://doi.org/10.1016/j.jab.2016.02.002

Koen, J. D., & Yonelinas, A. P. (2016). Recollection, not familiarity, decreases in healthy ageing: Converging evidence from four estimation methods. *Memory*, *24*(1), 75–88. https://doi.org/10.1080/09658211.2014.985590

Kok, R. M., & Reynolds, C. F (2017). Management of depression in older adults: A review. *JAMA*, *317*(20), 2114–2122. http://doi.org/10.1001/jama.2017.5706

Kooij, D. T. A. M., Tims, M., & Kanfer, R. (2015). Successful aging at work: The role of job crafting. In P. M. Bal, D. T. A. M. Kooij, & D. M. Rousseau (Eds.), *Aging workers and the employee-employer relationship* (pp. 145–161). Springer International Publishing. https://doi.org/10.1007/978-3-319-08007-9_9

Kroenke, K., Spitzer, R. L., & Williams, J. B. (2003). The Patient Health Questionnaire-2: Validity of a two-item depression screener. *Medical Care*, *41*(11),1284–1292. https://doi.org/10.1097/01.MLR.0000093487.78664.3C

Lai, D. W. L., Chan, K. C., Xie, X. J., & Daoust, G. D. (2020). The experience of growing old in chronic mental health patients. *Aging & Mental Health*, *24*(9), 1514–1522. https://doi.org/10.1080/13607863.2019.1609903

Lau, S. C., Connor, L. T., Heinemann, A. W., & Baum, C. M. (2022). Cognition and daily life activities in stroke: A network analysis. *OTJR: Occupation, Participation and Health*, *42*(4), 260–268. https://doi.org/10.1177/15394492221111730

Law, M., Baptiste, S., Carswell, A., McColl, M., Polatajko, H., & Pollock, N. (2014). *Canadian Occupational Performance Measure* (5th ed.). Ottawa: CAOT Publications.

Lee, H.-L., Hwang, E. J., Wu, S.-L., & Hsu, W.-C. (2022). Appraising psychiatric care from a different angle: Occupational therapy activities and cardiorespiratory fitness for inpatients with chronic mental illness. *American Journal of Occupational Therapy*, *76*(4), 7604205090. https://doi.org/10.5014/ajot.2022.049126

Li, Y., Baldassi, M., Johnson, E. J., & Weber, E. U. (2013). Complementary cognitive capabilities, economic decision making, and aging. *Psychology and Aging*, *28*(3), 595–613. https://doi.org/10.1037/a0034172

Lin, F. R., Yaffe, K., Xia, J., Xue, Q. L., Harris, T. B., Purchase-Helzner, E., Satterfield, S., Ayonayon, H. N., Ferrucci, L., Simonsick, E. M., & Health ABC Study Group. (2013). Hearing loss and cognitive decline in older adults. *JAMA Internal Medicine*, *173*(4), 293–299. https://doi.org/10.1001/jamainternmed.2013.1868

Linkewich, E., Rios, J., Allen, K. A., Avery, L., Dawson, D. R., Donald, M., Egan, M., Hunt, A., Jutzi, K., & McEwen, S. (2022). The impact of an integrated, interprofessional knowledge translation intervention on access to inpatient rehabilitation for persons with cognitive impairment. *PloS one*, *17*(9), e0266651. https://doi.org/10.1371/journal.pone.0266651

Livingston, G., Huntley, J., Sommerlad, A., Ames, D., Ballard, C., Banerjee, S., Brayne, C., Burns, A., Cohen-Mansfield, J., Cooper, C., Costafreda, S. G., Dias, A., Fox, N., Gitlin, L. N., Howard, R., Kales, H. C., Kivimäki, M., Larson, E. B., Ogunniyi, A., Orgeta, V., … Mukadam, N. (2020). Dementia prevention, intervention, and care: 2020 report of the Lancet Commission. *The Lancet*, *396*(10248), 413–446. https://doi.org/10.1016/S0140-6736(20)30367-6

Maass, A., Düzel, S., Goerke, M., Becke, A., Sobieray, U., Neumann, K., Lövden, M., Lindenberger, U., Bäckman, L., Braun-Dullaeus, R., Ahrens, D., Heinze, H. J., Müller, N. G., & Düzel, E. (2015). Vascular hippocampal plasticity after aerobic exercise in older adults. *Molecular Psychiatry*, *20*(5), 585–593. https://doi.org/10.1038/mp.2014.114

Marner, L., Nyengaard, J. R., Tang, Y., & Pakkenberg, B. (2003). Marked loss of myelinated nerve fibers in the human brain with age. *Journal of Comparative Neurology*, *462*(2), 144–152. https://doi.org/10.1002/cne.10714

Marquet, M., Chasteen, A. L., Plaks, J. E., & Balasubramaniam, L. (2019). Understanding the mechanisms underlying the effects of negative age stereotypes and perceived age discrimination on older adults' well-being. *Aging & Mental Health*, *23*(12), 1666–1673. https://doi.org/10.1080/13607863.2018.1514487

Martin, E., & Velayudhan, L. (2020). Neuropsychiatric symptoms in mild cognitive impairment: a literature review. *Dementia and Geriatric Cognitive Disorders*, *49*(2), 146–155. https://doi.org/10.1159/000507078

Meyer, C., & O'Keefe, F. (2020). Non-pharmacological interventions for people with dementia: A review of reviews. *Dementia*, *19*(6), 1927–1954. https://doi.org/10.1177/1471301218813234

Mick, P., Parfyonov, M., Wittich, W., Phillips, N., & Pichora-Fuller, M. K. (2018). Associations between sensory loss and social networks, participation, support, and loneliness: Analysis of the Canadian Longitudinal Study on Aging. *Canadian Family Physician*, *64*(1), e33–e41. https://www.ncbi.nlm.nih.gov/pmc/articles/PMC5962968/

Mitchell, M., & Miller, L. S. (2008). Executive functioning and observed versus self-reported measures of functional ability. *The Clinical Neuropsychologist*, *22*(3), 471–479. https://doi.org/10.1080/13854040701336436

Montejo, L., Torrent, C., Jiménez, E., Martínez-Arán, A., Blumberg, H. P., Burdick, K. E., Chen, P., Dols, A., Eyler, L. T., Forester, B. P., Gatchel, J. R., Gildengers, A., Kessing, L. V., Miskowiak, K. W., Olagunju, A. T., Patrick, R. E., Schouws, S., Radua, J., Bonnín, C. D. M., Vieta, E., … International Society for Bipolar Disorders (ISBD) Older Adults with Bipolar Disorder (OABD) Task Force. (2022). Cognition in older adults with bipolar disorder: An ISBD task force systematic review and meta-analysis based on a comprehensive neuropsychological assessment. *Bipolar Disorders*, *24*(2), 115–136. https://doi.org/10.1111/bdi.13175

Morgan, L. A., Perez, R., Frankowski, A. C., Nemec, M., & Bennett, C. R. (2016). Mental illness in assisted living: Challenges for quality of life and care. *Journal of Housing for the Elderly*, *30*(2), 185–198. https://doi.org/10.1080/02763893.2016.1162255

Morley, J. E., & Tumosa, N. (2002). Saint Louis University mental status examination (SLUMS). *Aging Successfully*, *12*(1), 4. https://doi.org/10.1037/t27282-000

Nagelkop, N. D., Rosselló, M., Aranguren, I., Lado, V., Ron, M., & Toglia, J. (2021). Using multicontext approach to improve instrumental activities of daily living performance after a stroke: A case report. *Occupational Therapy In Health Care*, *35*(3), 249–267. https://doi.org/10.1080/07380577.2021.1919954

Nakamura, J. S., Hong, J. H., Smith, J., Chopik, W. J., Chen, Y., VanderWeele, T. J., & Kim, E. S. (2022). Associations between satisfaction with aging and health and well-being outcomes among older US adults. *JAMA Network Open*, *5*(2), e2147797. https://doi.org/10.1001/jamanetworkopen.2021.47797

Nasreddine, Z. S., Phillips, N. A., Bédirian, V., Charbonneau, S., Whitehead, V., Collin, I., Cummings, J. L., & Chertkow, H. (2005). The Montreal Cognitive Assessment, MoCA: A brief screening tool for mild cognitive impairment. *Journal of the American Geriatrics Society*, *53*(4), 695–699. https://doi.org/10.1111/j.1532-5415.2005.53221.x

National Alliance on Mental Illness. (n.d.). *Mental health conditions*. Retrieved September 9, 2022, from https://www.nami.org/about-mental-illness/mental-health-conditions

O'Brien, J., & Thomas, A. (2015). Vascular dementia. *The Lancet*, *386*(10004), 1698–1706. https://doi.org/10.1016/S0140-6736(15)00463-8

O'Hare, C., Kenny, R. A., Aizenstein, H., Boudreau, R., Newman, A., Launer, L., Satterfield, S., Yaffe, K., Rosano, C., & Health ABC Study. (2017). Cognitive status, gray matter atrophy, and lower orthostatic blood pressure in older adults. *Journal of Alzheimer's Disease*, *57*(4), 1239–1250. https://doi.org/10.3233/JAD-161228

Olfson, M., Gerhard, T., Huang, C., Crystal, S., & Stroup, T. S. (2015). Premature mortality among adults with schizophrenia in the United States. *JAMA Psychiatry*, *72*(12), 1172–1181. https://doi.org/10.1001/jamapsychiatry.2015.1737

Park, D. C., & Bischof, G. N. (2022). The aging mind: Neuroplasticity in response to cognitive training. *Dialogues in Clinical Neuroscience*, *15*(1), 109–119. https://doi.org/10.31887/DCNS.2013.15.1/dpark

Pilania, M., Yadav, V., Bairwa, M., Behera, P., Gupta, S. D., Khurana, H., Mohan, V., Baniya, G., & Poongothai, S. (2019). Prevalence of depression among the elderly (60 years and above) population in India, 1997–2016: A systematic review and meta-analysis. *BMC Public Health*, *19*(1), Article 832. https://doi.org/10.1186/s12889-019-7136-z

Pomponio, R., Erus, G., Habes, M., Doshi, J., Srinivasan, D., Mamourian, E., Bashyam, V., Nasrallah, I. M., Satterthwaite, T. D., Fan, Y., Launer, L. J., Masters, C. L., Maruff, P., Zhuo, C., Völzke, H., Johnson, S. C., Fripp, J., Koutsouleris, N., Wolf, D. H., Gur, R., ... Davatzikos, C. (2020). Harmonization of large MRI datasets for the analysis of brain imaging patterns throughout the lifespan. *NeuroImage*, *208*, 116450. https://doi.org/10.1016/j.neuroimage.2019.116450

Rains, J., & Chee, N. (2017). The role of occupational and physiotherapy in multi-modal approach to tackling delirium in the intensive care. *Journal of the Intensive Care Society*, *18*(4), 318–322. https://doi.org/10.1177/1751143717720589

Rankin, E. D., & Keefover, R. W. (1998). Clinical cutoffs in screening functional performance for dementia. *Journal of Clinical Geropsychology*, *4*, 31–43.

Rehfeld, K., Lüders, A., Hökelmann, A., Lessmann, V., Kaufmann, J., Brigadski, T., Müller, P., & Müller, N. G. (2018). Dance training is superior to repetitive physical exercise in inducing brain plasticity in the elderly. *PLoS One*, *13*(7), e0196636. https://doi.org/10.1371/journal.pone.0196636

Reitan, R. M., & Wolfson, D. (1985). *The Halstead-Reitan neuropsychological test battery: Theory and clinical interpretation* (Vol. 4). Reitan Neuropsychology.

Rivera-Torres, S., Fahey, T. D., & Rivera, M. A. (2019). Adherence to exercise programs in older adults: Informative report. *Gerontology and Geriatric Medicine*, *5*, 2333721418823604. https://doi.org/10.1177/2333721418823604

Roldán-Tapia, M. D., Cánovas, R., León, I., & García-Garcia, J. (2017). Cognitive vulnerability in aging may be modulated by education and reserve in healthy people. *Frontiers in Aging Neuroscience*, *9*, 340. https://doi.org/10.3389/fnagi.2017.00340

Rösner, M., Zickerick, B., Sabo, M., & Schneider, D. (2022). Aging impairs primary task resumption and attentional control processes following interruptions. *Behavioural Brain Research*, *430*, 113932. https://doi.org/10.1016/j.bbr.2022.113932

Sajatovic, M., Strejilevich, S. A., Gildengers, A. G., Dols, A., Al Jurdi, R. K., Forester, B. P., Kessing, L. V., Beyer, J., Manes, F., Rej, S., Rosa, A. R., Schouws, S. N., Tsai, S. Y., Young, R. C., & Shulman, K. I. (2015). A report on older-age bipolar disorder from the International Society for Bipolar Disorders Task Force. *Bipolar Disorders*, *17*(7), 689–704. https://doi.org/10.1111/bdi.12331

Salthouse, T. A. (1996). The processing-speed theory of adult age differences in cognition. *Psychological Review*, *103*, 403–428. https://doi.org/10.1037/0033-295X.103.3.403

Salyers, M. P., McGuire, A. B., Kukla, M., Fukui, S., Lysaker, P. H., & Mueser, K. T. (2014). A randomized controlled trial of illness management and recovery with an active control group. *Psychiatric Services*, *65*(8), 1005–1011. https://doi.org/10.1176/appi.ps.201300354

Sánchez-Izquierdo, M., & Fernández-Ballesteros, R. (2021). Cognition in healthy aging. *International Journal of Environmental Research and Public Health*, *18*(3), 962. https://doi.org/10.3390/ijerph18030962

Schwarzinger, M., Pollock, B. G., Hasan, O. S. M., Dufouil, C., Rehm, J., & QalyDays Study Group. (2018). Contribution of alcohol use disorders to the burden of dementia in France 2008–13: A nationwide retrospective cohort study. *The Lancet Public Health*, *3*(3), e124–e132. https://doi.org/10.1016/S2468-2667(18)30022-7

Sexton, E., McLoughlin, A., Williams, D. J., Merriman, N. A., Donnelly, N., Rohde, D., Hickey, A., Wren, M. A., & Bennett, K. (2019). Systematic review and meta-analysis of the prevalence of cognitive impairment no dementia in the first year post-stroke. *European Stroke Journal*, *4*(2), 160–171. https://doi.org/10.1177/2396987318825484

Shallice, T. I. M., & Burgess, P. W. (1991). Deficits in strategy application following frontal lobe damage in man. *Brain*, *114*(2), 727–741. https://doi.org/10.1093/brain/114.2.727

Siqueira, G. S., Hagemann, P. D. M., Coelho, D. D. S., Santos, F. H. D., & Bertolucci, P. H. (2019). Can MoCA and MMSE be interchangeable cognitive screening tools? A systematic review. *The Gerontologist*, *59*(6), e743–e763. https://doi.org/10.1093/geront/gny126

Skidmore, E. R., Whyte, E. M., Butters, M. A., Terhorst, L., & Reynolds III, C. F. (2015). Strategy training during inpatient rehabilitation may prevent apathy symptoms after acute stroke. *PM&R*, *7*(6), 562–570. https://doi.org/10.1016/j.pmrj.2014.12.010

Smith, A. (1973). *Symbol digit modalities test* (p. 122). Western Psychological Services.

Song, C. S., Lee, O. N., & Woo, H. S. (2019). Cognitive strategy on upper extremity function for stroke: A randomized controlled trials. *Restorative Neurology and Neuroscience*, *37*(1), 61–70. https://doi.org/10.3233/RNN-180853

Stine-Morrow, E. A., Miller, L. M. S., & Hertzog, C. (2006). Aging and self-regulated language processing. *Psychological Bulletin*, *132*(4), 582–606. https://doi.org/10.1037/0033-2909.132.4.582

Stolwyk, R. J., Mihaljcic, T., Wong, D. K., Chapman, J. E., & Rogers, J. M. (2021). Poststroke cognitive impairment negatively impacts activity and participation outcomes: A systematic review and meta-analysis. *Stroke*, *52*(2), 748–760. https://doi.org/10.1161/STROKEAHA.120.032215

Stroup, T. S., Olfson, M., Huang, C., Wall, M. M., Goldberg, T., Devanand, D. P., & Gerhard, T. (2021). Age-specific prevalence and incidence of dementia diagnoses among older US adults with schizophrenia. *JAMA Psychiatry*, *78*(6), 632–641. https://doi.org/10.1001/jamapsychiatry.2021.0042

Stypulkowski, K., & Thayer, R. E. (2022). Long-term recreational cannabis use is associated with lower executive function and processing speed in a pilot sample of older adults. *Journal of Geriatric Psychiatry and Neurology*, *35*(5), 740–746. https://doi.org/10.1177/08919887211049130

Taylor, J. P., McKeith, I. G., Burn, D. J., Boeve, B. F., Weintraub, D., Bamford, C., Allan, L. M., Thomas, A. J., & O'Brien, J. T. (2020). New evidence on the management of Lewy body dementia. *The Lancet Neurology*, *19*(2), 157–169. https://doi.org/10.1016/S1474-4422(19)30153-X

Toglia, J. P. (1991). Generalization of treatment: A multicontext approach to cognitive perceptual impairment in adults with brain injury. *The American Journal of Occupational Therapy*, *45*(6), 505–516. https://doi.org/10.5014/ajot.45.6.505

Toglia, J. P. (2015). *Weekly calendar planning activity (WCPA): A performance test of executive function*. AOTA Press.

Tulving, E., & Craik, F. I. M. (2000). *The Oxford handbook of memory*. Oxford University Press.

Ward, E. V. (2022). Age and processing effects on perceptual and conceptual priming. *Quarterly Journal of Experimental Psychology*, *76*(1), 1–14. https://doi.org/10.1177/17470218221090128

Weber, A., Lynch, A., Miskle, B., Arndt, S., & Acion, L. (2022). Older adult substance use treatment first-time admissions between 2008 and 2018.

The American Journal of Geriatric Psychiatry, 30(10), 1055–1063. https://doi.org/10.1016/j.jagp.2022.03.003

Wechsler, D. (1981). The psychometric tradition: Developing the Wechsler Adult Intelligence Scale. *Contemporary Educational Psychology, 6*(2), 82–85. https://doi.org/10.1016/0361-476X(81)90035-7

Wesson, J., Clemson, L., Brodaty, H., & Reppermund, S. (2016). Estimating functional cognition in older adults using observational assessments of task performance in complex everyday activities: A systematic review and evaluation of measurement properties. *Neuroscience & Biobehavioral Reviews, 68*, 335–360. https://doi.org/10.1016/j.neubiorev.2016.05.024

Wilson, B., Cockburn, J., & Halligan, P. (1987). Development of a behavioral test of visuospatial neglect. *Archives of Physical Medicine and Rehabilitation, 68*(2), 98–102.

Wilson, J. E., Mart, M. F., Cunningham, C., Shehabi, Y., Girard, T. D., MacLullich, A. M. J., Slooter, A. J. C., & Ely, E. W. (2020). Delirium. *Nature Reviews Disease Primers, 6*(1), 1–26. https://doi.org/10.1038/s41572-020-00223-4

Winstein, C. J., Stein, J., Arena, R., Bates, B., Cherney, L. R., Cramer, S. C., Deruyter, F., Eng, J. J., Fisher, B., Harvey, R. L., Lang, C. E., MacKay-Lyons, M., Ottenbacher, K. J., Pugh, S., Reeves, M. J., Richards, L. G., Stiers, W., Zorowitz, R. D., & American Heart Association Stroke Council, Council on Cardiovascular and Stroke Nursing, Council on Clinical Cardiology, and Council on Quality of Care and Outcomes Research. (2016). Guidelines for adult stroke rehabilitation and recovery: A guideline for health care professionals from the American Heart Association/American Stroke Association. *Stroke, 47*(6), e98–e169. https://doi.org/10.1161/STR.0000000000000098

Wolf, T. J., Morrison, T., & Matheson, L. (2008). Initial development of a work-related assessment of dysexecutive syndrome: The Complex Task Performance Assessment. *Work, 31*(2), 221–228.

Wolters, F. J., & Ikram, M. A. (2019). Epidemiology of vascular dementia: Nosology in a time of epiomics. *Arteriosclerosis, Thrombosis, and Vascular Biology, 39*(8), 1542–1549. https://doi.org/10.1161/ATVBAHA.119.311908

World Health Organization (2022). Schizophrenia. https://www.who.int/news-room/fact-sheets/detail/schizophrenia

World Health Organization. (n.d.). *Dementia.* Retrieved September 2, 2022, from https://www.who.int/news-room/fact-sheets/detail/dementia

Yamamoto, R., Akizuki, K., Yamaguchi, K., Yabuki, J., & Kaneno, T. (2022). A study on how concurrent visual feedback affects motor learning of adjustability of grasping force in younger and older adults. *Scientific Reports, 12*, 10755. https://doi.org/10.1038/s41598-022-14975-4

Yonelinas, A. P. (2002). The nature of recollection and familiarity: A review of 30 years of research. *Journal of Memory and Language, 46*(3), 441–517. https://doi.org/10.1006/jmla.2002.2864

Zhang, H., Eppes, A., & Diaz, M. T. (2019). Task difficulty modulates age-related differences in the behavioral and neural bases of language production. *Neuropsychologia, 124*, 254–273. https://doi.org/10.1016/j.neuropsychologia.2018.11.017

PART III

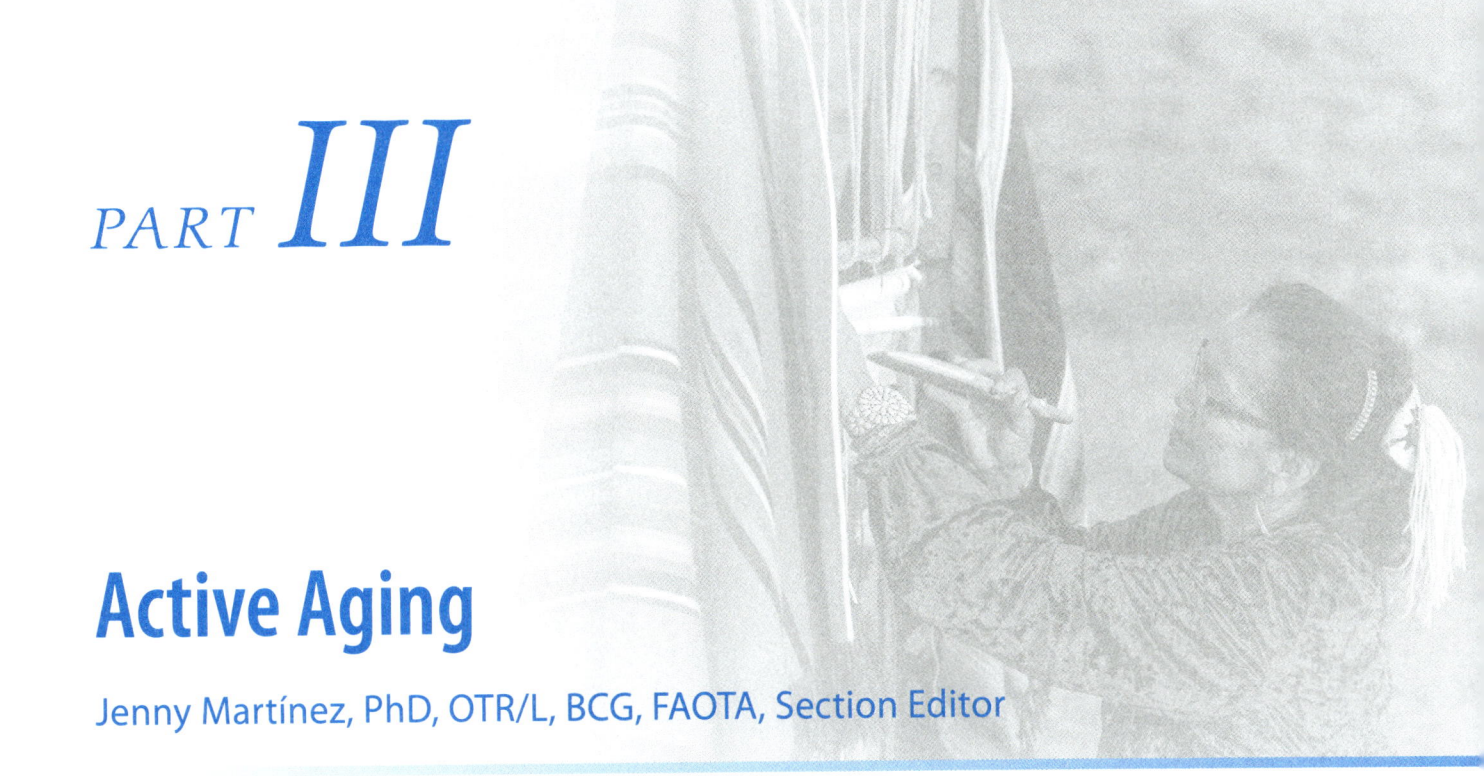

Active Aging

Jenny Martínez, PhD, OTR/L, BCG, FAOTA, Section Editor

By now it is clear that aging is a complex set of processes that occur within complex biological, environmental, and sociopolitical contexts. How older adults spend their time and what is meaningful to them occurs in equally dynamic systems and is individually determined. To this end, Part I introduced multiple contexts for aging. Part II followed with a discussion of body structures and body functions in aging.

As the number of older adults across the globe increases, healthy aging—the development and maintenance of functional abilities that enable well-being in older age—continues to be a priority (World Health Organization [WHO], 2020). Occupational therapy is uniquely positioned to promote healthy aging by facilitating occupational engagement and participation in those activities that individuals, families, and communities need and want to do. Through a lens that understands both the broader and individual experiences of aging, occupational therapists can partner with older adults and their caregivers to address occupational needs in client-centered and inclusive ways.

This part of the text explores important occupations in detail. The way occupations are enacted and interact for any one person is unique. Some individuals may prefer to receive help with self-care or homemaking occupations so that they have more energy for meaningful leisure or work occupations. Others may retain a fierce sense of independence about taking care of their basic needs. Of course, in addressing these preferences, consideration of context, personal priorities, and cultural meaning, among other factors is vital.

A new addition to the fifth edition of this book is the expansion of discussions about home management, health management, and sleep through inclusion of new chapters. Ensuring that caregivers and their needs are integrated into occupational therapy care is essential as well. Thus, the perspective of caregivers and how occupational therapy can support their needs is presented as a new chapter. Areas such as self-care, leisure, work, retirement, community mobility, and driving are also addressed in this part.

World Health Organization. (2020). *Healthy ageing and functional ability*. https://www.who.int/news-room/questions-and-answers/item/healthy-ageing-and-functional-ability

CHAPTER 14

Self-Care

Kristine Haertl, PhD, OTR/L, FAOTA, ACE

> *"The capacity to do something useful for yourself or others is key to personhood, whether it involves the ability to earn a living, cook a meal, put on shoes in the morning, or whatever other skill needs to be mastered at the moment."*
>
> —M. C. Bateson (1996, p. 11)

LEARNING OUTCOMES

By the end of this chapter, readers will be able to:

14-1. Examine self-care activities within the domains of everyday occupations.
14-2. Explain relevance of activities of daily living (ADLs) for health, wellness, and quality of life.
14-3. Examine impact of health conditions on self-care performance.
14-4. Describe the theories related to self-care performance and perceptions of competence and control.
14-5. Compare the roles of the occupational therapist with other healthcare professionals' role in self-care training.
14-6. Select common assessments of ADL used for older adults.
14-7. Apply evidence-based intervention strategies for enabling self-care performance.

Mini Case Study

Mr. Macarthur is a 75-year-old man recently diagnosed with Parkinson disease and mild cognitive impairment. He lives alone in his three-story home and until recently was able to manage with occasional help from friends. Over the past few months, Mr. Macarthur has developed tremors and difficulty with gross and fine motor movements, which affect his self-care activities. He is able to walk without using adaptive equipment but is slow and unsteady. Stairs have been difficult as have showering and dressing.

Mr. Macarthur is a retired high-school French teacher on a fixed income. His funds have recently diminished due to various medical costs and need for home adaptation. Historically, Mr. Macarthur was very active, loved to play tournament tennis, and traveled the world with his ex-wife and various friends. He has expressed frustration at his decreased motor abilities and increased forgetfulness. He has one son who lives in the same city but no other family nearby for support.

Mr. Macarthur's physician has recommended he consider moving to a home where he can more easily move about, but he fears leaving his community and friends he values.

Provocative Questions
1. How would an occupational therapist address Mr. Macarthur's health and personal well-being?
2. What are the current and potential future effects of Mr. Macarthur's diagnoses on his ability to complete self-care?
3. What assessments and interventions would address Mr. Macarthur's current needs?

A complete understanding of the functional performance of older adults includes recognizing the importance of daily activities and how they contribute to overall health and well-being. Self-care skills are affected by declining function, including sensory limitations, cognitive declines, reduced strength and agility, and restricted mobility. These often accompany chronic disease and are expected physiological changes that occur throughout the aging process. Emphasis is placed on preserving function and developing strategies to maximize quality of life throughout the performance of ADLs. This chapter considers self-care, a special category of the domain of everyday human activity that has important implications for the health and well-being of older adults.

The chapter begins with a definition of self-care and describes a framework for understanding how daily living tasks often present challenges to older adults as they attempt to fully engage in life and participate in society in order to achieve a sense of well-being. Within this framework, self-care may be viewed as a foundation to social participation. This discussion is followed by a brief review of common limitations to functional performance and how they can be assessed. The chapter concludes with a description of the possibilities for intervention, including requirements for assistance in performing self-care tasks.

Defining Self-Care

Self-care is daily activity composed of duties and chores ranging from basic or personal care (e.g., bathing, dressing, grooming) to personal business (e.g., using the telephone, managing medications, banking, or shopping for food). These tasks are fundamental to living in a social world; they enable basic survival and sustained health and create a sense of self-efficacy and greater life satisfaction. After conducting a comprehensive analysis of 139 definitions of self-care, Godfrey et al (2011) proposed the following definition: "Self-care involves a range of activities deliberately engaged throughout life to promote physical, mental, and emotional health, maintain life, and prevent disease. Self-care is performed by the individual on their own behalf, for their families and communities, and includes care by others" (p. 11). More recently, a comprehensive scoping review (Laposha & Smallfield, 2020) found that definitions of self-care in the occupational therapy literature are often ambiguous and though they include ADLs and independent ADLs, they do not always acknowledge all areas of well-being, including emotional, mental, and social health. For the purposes of this chapter, emphasis is placed on individual self-care activities that are sometimes referred to as **ADLs** or **instrumental activities of daily living** (IADLs) (American Occupational Therapy Association [AOTA], 2020). It should be noted, however, that self-care also includes additional occupations, such as health management, rest, and sleep (see Chapters 15 and 16), all of which affect an individual's well-being and overall level of functioning.

The *Practice Framework–OTPF 4th edition* (AOTA, 2020) classifies ADLs as actions "oriented toward taking care of one's own body and completed on a routine basis." They include bathing/showering, toileting and toileting hygiene, dressing, eating and swallowing, feeding, functional mobility, hygiene and grooming, and sexual activity. IADLs are those "activities to support life within the home and community" (AOTA, 2020). Health management and maintenance is separated out in this text but critical to personal self-care and maintaining health and wellness routines. Together basic or personal self-care activities (ADLs) and IADLs may be viewed as forming a foundation for survival and participation in the community.

Positive aging emphasizes the importance of personal choice and the capacity to participate in multiple domains, including that of personal care (Torregrosa-Ruiz et al, 2021). Not only is performing self-care ADLs a significant aspect of life satisfaction in older persons but continued participation in one's personal care routine is viewed as essential in maintaining physical and emotional health and well-being (Isik et al, 2020). These elements—the person, their transactions within the physical and social environment, and the successful performance of the specific tasks necessary to those interactions—are referred to repeatedly in the description of a general conceptual framework for self-care (e.g., Torregrosa-Ruiz et al, 2021).

CASE STUDY

Occupational Profile

Mr. Arkmadian is a 74-year-old man who was admitted to the acute care unit of the local hospital after his wife found him exhibiting slurred speech and significant weakness on the left side of his body. He stayed in the acute care unit for 9 days before being transferred to the inpatient rehabilitation unit for more intensive therapy to address his decreased ADL functioning. His medical history includes a right cerebrovascular accident (CVA) 7 years before this admission, hypertension, coronary artery disease, and mild dementia. Mr. Arkmadian presented to the inpatient rehabilitation unit with residual left limb weakness, left-sided paresis, incoordination, and slight left neglect. He stated that he was independent in ADLs before this hospitalization. Mr. Arkmadian lives with his wife and son in a one-story home with a ramped entry. He already had a raised toilet with arms, a handheld shower, and a wheelchair, as well as a tub bench and rolling walker that he does not use. Given his cognitive changes in recent years, his wife has slowly taken on the household IADLs, such as financial management and driving.

Identified Problem Areas Related to Self-Care

- Requires supervision with ADLs (needs help with lower-extremity dressing) and transfers
- Has decreased strength, balance, and endurance to perform basic ADLs
- Has decreased coordination (difficulty with snaps on a shirt)
- Needs verbal cues to use affected side and to modify actions when problems arise in task performance
- Some lack of awareness of safety, especially with relation to visual neglect

Identified Strengths

- Independent before hospitalization
- Home has some prior modifications
- Supportive spouse

Goals for Occupational Therapy

Mr. Arkmadian will

- Demonstrate safe stand pivot transfers for toilet, tub, wheelchair, and bed with supervision
- Perform feeding, grooming, dressing, and bathing with supervision and minimal cuing
- Demonstrate safe use of recommended assistive devices
- Assist with self-care activities

- Verbally communicate understanding of home exercise program
- Provide encouragement to attend to the affected side
- Encourage return to leisure interests and daily activity as able to do so safely

Questions

1. How does the family's understanding of the situation and the recovery process influence Mr. Arkmadian's potential for functional improvement?
2. What assessment tools could be used to assess this client's skills in self-care?

Answers

1. Mrs. Arkmadian has demonstrated being a supportive partner as she has already taken over some of the household responsibilities. She and their son will need to be educated about the impact of the stroke on Mr. Arkmadian's self-care activities, including training on different levels of assistance to promote his dignity and as much independence as possible. (LO14.2 Significance of self-care)
2. Assessment options include the Assessment of Motor and Process Skills (provided the therapist has the credential to use it) and the Barthel Index of Activities of Daily Living. A home safety assessment, such as those found in Chapter 15, is important to evaluate performance in the home context and physical environmental supports or barriers. (LO 14.6 Assessments for self-care)

Significance of Self-Care

Self-care is integral to individual function and public health (Narasimhan, 2019). Research has identified self-care activities as a contributing factor to healthy aging, subjective well-being and longevity (Gilbert et al, 2012; Ziedonis, 2019), and quality of life (Landa-Gonzalez & Molnar, 2012). Conversely, the inability or refusal to care for oneself is referred to as self-neglect and can negatively affect cognition, mood, and overall functioning (Rachey & Janssen, 2021). Personal neglect and lack of motivation for self-care may also be caused by mental health conditions such as depression (Deverajooh & Chinna, 2017). Decline in the ability to perform ADLs may lead to increased dependence on the healthcare system and increased need for in-home supports. Self-care factors including personal mobility, fall risk, malnutrition, and cognitive impairment have been shown to predict prolonged hospital stays in the older population (Lang et al, 2006). In addition, factors such as cognition, nutrition, fear of falling, poor mobility, depressive symptoms, and decreased strength have been associated with functional decline after hospitalization (Aarden et al, 2019), thus rehabilitation intervention involves special attention to ADLs. Consideration of individual capacity for self-care along with client and environmental factors are integral to the development of rehabilitation programs to address a client's self-care abilities (Imaginario et al, 2020).

The extent of an individual's ability to perform self-care tasks independently affects decisions about the need for personal care assistance or special environments, including the need for home health services, assistance from caregivers, or placement in long-term-care facilities. In Western countries, especially in the United States, approaches to caregiving often stress independence, whereas in other parts of the world, interdependence is more common, as cultures with kinship networks often have multiple generations living together and caring for one another.

For example, in the United States, a chronically ill individual is defined as having a condition lasting more than a year that may require medical attention, affect ADLs, or both (Centers for Disease Control and Prevention, 2021). As older adults experience a decline in function, increased assistance or a change in residence may be required to provide supports needed to manage daily self-care requirements. Yet in other countries and with other cultures, efforts may be made to maximize time spent at home and caring for kin. For instance, Asian cultures often emphasize caregiving and respect of elders (Chan, 2020), which may result in multiple generations living together; thus, consideration of caregiving in the context of self-care must take on a cultural lens. Promoting Best Practice 14-1 offers suggestions for caring for the caregiver.

PROMOTING BEST PRACTICE 14-1
Supporting Caregivers

Many older adults require assistance from a family caregiver during a period of illness or as self-care skills become more difficult later in life. Caregivers are often related to the individual and may need to balance the needs of their own family or manage their own health challenges as often occurs in spouses of older adults. Caregiving tasks often bring a blend of personal satisfaction in assisting the loved one, while at the same time, may add extra stress that affects the caregiver physically and emotionally. Kepic et al (2019) asserted the importance of providing services to help individuals through the caregiving process to help them (1) address their own grief, (2) maintain their own self-care, (3) find sources of support (e.g., support groups), and (4) advocate for resources.

Occupational therapists are well suited to provide services to caregivers in the abovementioned areas. In addition to general education on strategies for managing the caregiving tasks, tother areas can be addressed with caregivers, such as

- Time management
- Strategies to facilitate the caregiving occupation
- Sleep hygiene and relaxation
- Stress management

- Personal self-care, health and wellness
- Leisure exploration
- Life balance

Practical Importance of Self-Care: Health and Safety

Self-care activities are necessary for survival, safety, general health, and well-being. One of the primary health and survival requirements is adequate nutrition. Without nourishment, health declines rapidly. Good nutrition requires the ability to plan menus, prepare food, and eat independently (i.e., "self-feed"). In addition to having possible motor, sensory, and cognitive disabilities that limit meal preparation, some older adults have dental problems or lack the teeth to eat regular meals. Dental health not only influences adequate nutrition but is also an indicator of overall health status (Federal Interagency Forum on Aging Related Statistics, 2020).

Safety is another concern for older adults. According to the Centers for Disease Control and Prevention (2020), every second of the day a senior in the United States falls, with falls being the leading cause of fatal and nonfatal injuries in seniors. Care must be taken not only to maintain physical health and mobility but also to minimize environmental barriers that could contribute to falls or functional mobility deficits. See Chapter 7 for additional discussion on falls and fall prevention.

The inability to maintain a safe living environment may lead to injury. For instance, older adults must have the ability to prepare and cook healthy meals to maintain adequate nutrition. Research has demonstrated that lack of mobility in seniors and poor environmental setup often leads to safety hazards in the kitchen (Ibrahim & Davies, 2012). Care should be taken to minimize environmental hazards and teach compensatory and adaptation skills necessary for safe performance of ADLs and IADLs. Finally, the ability to perform self-care activities promotes better general health. Adequate personal hygiene and sanitation protect the individual from germs that spread disease. Laws protecting public health are based on the awareness that neglect of hygiene can contribute to poor health.

Self-care performance has practical importance because it enables people to maintain their personal health and the environments in which they live. It also has symbolic importance because it enables social relationships, fosters and reflects self-identity, and promotes psychological well-being.

Importance of Self-Care for Self-Identity and Socialization

Many cultures place value in meeting self-care needs and fitting in with society. Meeting social expectations requires role performance that extends to dress, appearance, speech, mannerisms, and other elements of symbolic communication in the culture. Functional capacity and personal self-care have been shown to relate to healthy self-esteem, life satisfaction (Li-Hsing et al, 2020), healthy aging (Gilbert et al, 2012), and psychological health (Isik et al, 2020). Self-care has also been shown to influence personal identity and perception of life situation (Sundsli et al, 2013). Maintaining function is necessary not only for performing daily living tasks but also for promoting an individual's self-esteem, social acceptance, and, ultimately, social well-being.

Unfortunately, during the COVID-19 pandemic, whether at home or in a long-term care facility, many seniors were isolated from loved ones. Such isolation affected physical, cognitive, and mental health (Amanzio et al, 2021) which had deleterious effects on seniors' personal identity and functional capacity. Studies show that the pandemic had a significant effect on personal health, increasing the risk of depression and anxiety and subsequently affecting self-care (Fiske et al, 2021). Continued focus on the effects of the pandemic on overall health and psychological well-being is important in order to develop effective strategies for the future.

Importance of Self-Care for Psychological Well-Being

Studies have shown that the inability to perform self-care tasks has a negative impact on psychological well-being (Luthfi et al, 2018). Drageset (2004) found that as competence in ADLs declined among older adults in nursing homes, their loneliness and social isolation tended to increase. Shea et al (2021) found that loneliness substantially increased during the pandemic and subsequently affected health and well-being. Difficulties with self-care affect self-efficacy and quality of life; thus, therapeutic approaches are aimed at facilitating a client's ability to perform daily self-care tasks (Orellano et al, 2012). In addition to individualized approaches, group interventions in care facilities have been shown to increase self-efficacy and psychological well-being (Toledano-Gonzalez et al, 2018). Such interventions may focus on self-care skills; coping and stress management skills; and sensorimotor, social, and cognitive skills. Additional rehabilitation approaches include preparing clients for a variety of housing options, including retirement communities, assisted-living facilities, and other alternative housing models to provide older adults with choice (Mayo et al, 2021). Physiological changes associated with the aging process often create conditions that decrease performance or enjoyment of daily activities. The following section addresses the effect of various impairments on daily functioning.

Prevalence and Type of Limitations of ADLs Among Older Adults

Data from the National Health Interview Survey (NHIS) in 2014 indicated that reliance on others for help increases with age and of those over age 75, 10.6% need assistance in ADLs and 18.8% need assistance in IADLs (Adams & Martinez, 2016). The 2018 National Health Interview

Survey found that 64% of older adults who lived at home with a care provider, but participated in adult day care services, needed assistance with three more ADLs (Lendon & Singh, 2021). Research from Japan and India (Chiu et al, 2022; Sharma et al, 2021) found that health condition comorbidities affect self-care performance and that older adults have more difficulty with IADLs than ADLs. The NHIS report and others found that older adults of low socioeconomic status are more likely to need assistance with ADLs and IADLs (Adams & Martinez, 2016; Liu & Wang, 2022; U. S. Department of Health and Human Services, 2012). Thus, in addition to individual and programmatic efforts to address self-care, occupational therapists are useful to inform public health and social efforts to promote health and well-being in older adults.

Impact of Health Conditions on Self-Care Performance

Rates of disability and associated functional limitations can increase with age and may be exacerbated by additional variables, including pain secondary to chronic conditions (Axon & Le, 2021; Song et al, 2020) and diseases, particularly the presence of multiple health conditions, often referred to as multimorbidity (Jindai et al, 2016). The following section covers specific conditions common in older adult populations and their effects on functioning. An awareness of the potential impact on self-care due to aging and disability is critical to the development of strategies for evaluation and intervention. For additional detail on these conditions, see individual chapters in Section 2—Aging: Body Structures/Body Functions.

Stroke

Cerebrovascular disease can result in weakness or paralysis of extremities on one side of the body, visual limitations, vestibular and sensory problems, and loss of the ability to communicate, all of which may have a devastating effect on an individual's ability to perform self-care tasks. Lee et al (2021) studied the individual and combined effects of cognition and stroke on ADLs and IADLs. The study found that stroke and cognitive deficits caused difficulties in both ADLs and IADLs; those with both CVA and cognitive deficits had more difficulty with higher level IADLs (e.g., use of phone, financial management) and those with both stroke and cognitive deficits had more difficulties in basic ADLs (e.g., dressing) than individuals with only cognitive deficits in absence of CVA.

Rehabilitation can help older adults gain functional performance in daily self-care tasks after stroke. Kristensen et al (2014) found that many individuals with mild stroke who had received inpatient rehabilitation regained independence in ADLs and IADLs; however, some required additional adaptations and special equipment, which suggests the importance of providing resources and strategies in functional recovery. Despite the improvements in ADLs and IADLs reported by the study participants, many participants reported increased fatigue, an area of importance for therapists to address in relation to self-care skills. Rehabilitation techniques to address stroke and improvement of self-care include not only remedial and adaptive strategies, but also prevention, education, and compensation. In addition, new advancements such as wearable technology have been found to help predict ADL function after stroke and may have potential future use in rehabilitation (Chen et al, 2021).

Cardiovascular Disease

Heart disease continues to be the leading cause of death globally (WHO, 2020) and has significant effects on daily self-care and overall function (Scott & Collings, 2012). Lack of energy, decreased fitness, lower limb swelling, and angina may all impair an individual's ability to perform daily self-care, especially in activities that require a significant amount of mobility or energy expenditure. Cardiovascular disease may also cause secondary cognitive decline, which further affects self-care and the performance of ADLs and IADLs (Norris, 2020). In a large community cohort study of persons with heart failure, Dunlay et al (2015) found that heart disease significantly affected ADL function, with individuals having a higher degree of difficulty with ADLs/self-care being at increased risk for hospitalization and death. Thus, addressing self-care skills is integral to cardiac rehabilitation.

Occupational therapists are part of an integral team designed to address functional limitations and improve ADL and IADL performance in cardiac rehabilitation (Hobbs, 2020). Therapists are not only integral to the evaluation of function during cardiac rehabilitation but use individualized and community-based approaches to improve self-care for those with heart disease (Riegel et al, 2017). Hobbs (2020) identified the importance of occupational therapists adjusting their evaluation and intervention approaches based on the phase of cardiac rehabilitation. Once a client is able to partake in consistent therapy, in addition to skill retraining, (e.g., basic dressing, hygiene, grooming), fatigue management and compensatory techniques are also used. Environmental adaptations are enacted in the home and community to help facilitate increased independence in performing ADLs and IADLs. Safety considerations, including oxygen management in the home environment and ability to maintain health precautions, are also considered when addressing self-care for those with heart conditions.

Neurocognitive Disorders and Cognitive Decline

Studies have indicated that cognition and memory play a critical role in the performance of everyday tasks, including ADLs and IADLs. A decline in cognitive functioning reduces the ability to perform ADLs and IADLs, with memory and executive functions shown to affect IADL performance and attention and executive functioning affecting ADLs (Wadley et al, 2021). The ability of individuals with dementia to complete ADLs and IADLs affects the levels of care needed and institutionalization (Eska et al, 2013). For instance, an older adult with a neurocognitive disorder who is unable to dress, bathe, and toilet may be more likely to need external supports and institutionalization than one who has retained these self-care activities. Often, ADLs such as dressing and grooming are retained longer than higher level IADLs (e.g., financial management) in early stages of neurocognitive impairment and decreases as the level of severity worsens (Mlinac & Feng, 2016). When this happens, external supports within the home may be needed, caregivers may take on extra responsibilities, or the individual may have to move to a supportive living and care residence. Amelia and Batchelor-Aselage (2014) developed the C3P (Change the Person, Change the People, Change the Place) model designed to work with caregivers and clients with dementia. This model, though originally designed for mealtimes, can be adapted to other self-care routines and emphasizes change and adaptation with the client, caregiver, and environment. Similar to other occupational therapy models, consideration of the impact of the interaction of the client, occupation (task), and environment are of key importance in working through cognitive change and functional decline.

Evaluation and intervention for those with neurocognitive disorders often includes an assessment of current functioning level, review of the living environment, and ability to follow through daily tasks with good safety and judgment. Consideration of resources available (e.g., caregivers in the home, environment) is crucial when making determinations related to cognitive dysfunction and prognosis for self-care. Therapeutic interventions and the approach of caregivers have been shown to influence ADL and IADL performance (Suzuki et al, 2019). A systematic review and meta-analysis (Bennett et al, 2019) demonstrated positive effects of occupational therapy interventions in ADLs and IADLs. The studies represented in the meta-analysis found that individuals with moderate levels of dementia who received 8 to 12 hours of occupational therapy in their home had significantly improved the ability to perform ADLs and IADLs and psychological performance. Additional discussion of intervention techniques can be found later in this chapter.

Joint Inflammation and Disease

Self-care activities are often affected in joint disease. Pain, limitations in mobility, and inflammation may all impact daily self-care. A 10-year follow-up within a National Retirement Study found that persons with arthritis were significantly more likely to have difficulties with functional mobility and ADLs than those without the condition (Covinsky et al, 2008). In addition, older adults with osteoporosis and osteoarthritis are significantly more likely to have difficulties with ADLs than those without the condition (Stamm et al, 2016). Clynes et al (2019) found that knee and hip osteoarthritis is associated with difficulties in mobility and ability to perform self-care. Their study also suggested that the locale of the joint disease may influence how ADLs and IADLs are affected, with hip osteoarthritis affecting mobility and self-care such as toileting and both hip and knee osteoarthritis impeding mobility in the kitchen and bathroom. Thus, occupational therapists must consider how the joint inflammation and disease affects not only the individual ADLs but also mobility within the environment.

Research also demonstrates that those with rheumatoid arthritis with higher levels of pain and disability have lower levels of agency (personal competency and follow through) with self-care (Ovayolu et al, 2012). Persons with rheumatoid arthritis who attend and follow through with a joint protection program may increase their long-term functional ability (Hammond & Freeman, 2004), and those in rehabilitation have been shown to improve ADL function (Ellegard et al, 2019) thus demonstrating the effectiveness of rehabilitation intervention for persons with joint disease.

Sensory Problems

Sensory impairment can present unique challenges for older adults and affect ADL performance. This section discusses sensory problems related to vision, hearing, touch, and taste and smell.

Vision

Vision impairment causes limitations in the ability to perform ADLs such as dressing, eating, (American Foundation for the Blind, 2020; Markowitz et al, 2008), and functional mobility (Cobb, 2013). Studies of elders indicate that visual impairment is correlated with the need for assistance in ADLs, resulting in higher levels of loneliness and poorer self-rated health (Peres et al, 2017). Studies demonstrate the effectiveness of rehabilitation and assistive devices to facilitate increased function in ADLs. AOTA has published practice guidelines for older adults with low vision (Kaldenberg & Smallfield, 2020) which provide important information of the evidence behind specific intervention techniques.

Hearing

The impact of hearing deficits on quality of life is well understood, but some evidence shows that hearing impairments can also influence performance of ADLs. One in three people over age 65 years have some hearing loss, with the severity often increasing with age (Stevens et al, 2019). Studies demonstrate that hearing loss correlates with higher levels of physical disability and difficulties with ADLs, IADLs, and leisure function (Yi et al, 2020). Dual sensory loss (vision and hearing) often has a greater impact on an individual's daily function compared with those in the general population of community-dwelling older adults (Davidson & Guthrie, 2017). In addition, the level of hearing loss affects the amount of difficulty with ADLs, as those with more severe hearing impairment have been shown to have significantly more difficulty with ADLs than those with moderate hearing loss (Yi et al, 2020). Because older adults may be unaware of or reluctant to report hearing loss, it is important for primary care providers and other health professions to advocate for assessment of hearing loss and educate clients on potential intervention options (Stevens et al, 2019). Occupational therapists are an integral part of an interprofessional team in addressing hearing loss. Environmental modifications may be made to improve acoustics, and a number of adaptive devices available for those with hearing loss. While compensatory strategies and Hearing Assistive Technologies (HAT) can help enhance an individual's independence in ADL and IADL (Chang, 2020), there is a need for increased education of occupational therapy students in this area (Chang, 2020; Wittig et al, 2017).

Touch

Diminished sense of touch may cause safety issues, such as lack of sensitivity to temperatures (e.g., in adjusting water temperature for the shower) and in fine motor tasks such as threading a needle. Neurological impairments and paresthesia may cause difficulty with fine motor skills, noticing temperature differences, or may cause safety concerns around stoves, sharp objects, or items needing temperature regulation. A thorough sensory evaluation with aging populations should include not only hearing and vision but discussion and evaluation of touch sensation as well (Ho et al, 2021). Sensory loss associated with conditions such as stroke requires strategies to facilitate coping and occupational adaptation (Williams & Murray, 2013). Techniques such as task modification, dressing aids, and sensory cues may facilitate increased self-care skills and improve tactile responsivity in older adults (Martinez, 2019).

Taste and Smell

The effect of declines in taste and smell on nutrition is readily apparent. If food is enjoyed less, appropriate intake may become problematic. Over 50% of persons 60 to 80 years old and over 75% of those older than 80 years have taste and smell deficits (Doty, 2018). Because of these sensory deficits, older adults may not take in adequate nutrition or may choose to put too many spices (e.g., salt) on their food (Saxon et al, 2010). Additionally, olfactory deficits can increase the risk of ingesting spoiled food, detecting toxic substances, or perceiving personal hygiene problems (Olofsson, 2021). Continued monitoring of nutrition intake is a critical part of the rehabilitation team's roles and responsibilities. In addition to working with the interdisciplinary team, the occupational therapist can educate the client on sensory sensitivities, identify through activity analysis areas that may be affected by olfactory and taste changes, and may work with the client and dietitian to develop habits and daily self-care routines, such as eating healthy meals, checking burners to ensure they are off, and keeping home fire/smoke alarms and carbon dioxide detectors in working order.

Theoretical Approaches

Many models in the social and behavioral sciences explain the factors that influence everyday actions. Most consider the individual person and environments in which a person transacts the business of living. Such "contextual or ecological" models are often described in terms of "person–environment fit." The implication is that people best meet the demands of living when their capabilities fit well with those demands (Deci & Ryan, 2011). Deci and Ryan's Self Determination Theory of Motivation proposes that individuals have innate tendencies to act in effective ways within everyday activity and that social context and psychological experiences affect behavior (Deci & Ryan, 2011). This theory emphasizes the innate properties of an activity or occupation that have intrinsic value and motivation.

Competence is defined as the ability to do something successfully or efficiently (Oxford University Press, 2021). Ecological or person–environment-fit models view competence as dependent both on the individual's capabilities and skills and on the nature of the task and the environment in which it is performed. The term *environment* includes not only physical aspects, such as natural terrain or the person-made, "built" environment (such as buildings, tools, and other objects), but also the less-apparent sociocultural environment that influences the attitudes and expectations of performance through policies, customs, or societal prejudices. In rehabilitation, emphasis is placed on considering person factors along with contextual aspects of the activity. Both physical context and social contextual factors (e.g., cultural, social, temporal) influence an individual's self-care performance. For instance, an older adult with increased weakness and spasticity after stroke will have varying ability to perform independent dressing skills based on person factors (e.g., motivation, area of stroke) along with contextual factors, such as the setup of the room, the type of clothing, and the adaptive equipment available.

Competence, Value, and Meaning in Self-Care

Competence involves physical, psychological, and social functioning, which are dependent on a host of underlying factors. In addition to the term *competence*, authors have suggested "capacity for ADL/IADL" as an important construct in measuring ability to perform self-care (e.g., Mlinac & Feng, 2016). Consideration of capacity may include both the person and environmental factors that affect daily self-care.

Personal value and meaning also affect occupational performance. In the context of self-care, someone who values personal appearance may take extra time and care dressing and grooming. The nature, type of dress, and context in which the grooming takes place is further affected by cultural norms and social expectations. The successful completion of dressing and grooming would therefore contribute to an individual's self-perception and personal satisfaction. It is important for occupational therapists to consider personal and sociocultural differences in addressing self-care. For instance, persons in the LGBTQIA+ community may prefer clothing choices that vary from gender stereotypes, and individuals from other cultures may have unique garments, such as hijabs, that require client-centered approaches when addressing self-care.

An individual's ability to perform daily activities competently is also affected by client factors, context, and task requirements. Personal competence is unique for each individual and is constantly changing. Although everyday competence may involve instrumental tasks that are viewed as mundane or as less meaningful than discretionary activities, these tasks are nonetheless foundations for participation in a social world and are important symbols of personal competence and efficacy.

Interprofessional Practice

Although occupational therapy practice heavily focuses on ADLs and IADLs, several professions are concerned with an individual's ability to perform daily self-care. Nurses may initially work with the client, especially in acute care, to ensure safe practices in transfer and daily care. Referrals will likely be made to occupational and physical therapy for additional rehabilitation. Occupational therapists generally conduct formal assessment in ADLs and IADLs and develop intervention plans guided toward successful rehabilitation and discharge (e.g., to the client's home). Physical therapists will often address strengthening and functional mobility required for self-care activities. For instance, after a client suffers a hip fracture, occupational therapy may address hip precautions and return to dressing, bathing, and other self-care, while physical therapy may emphasize strengthening and return to safe walking. Both may work on safe transfers and recommendations for the home environment.

Assessments for Self-Care

Self-care evaluations for older adults are performed for several reasons. Evaluation of self-care gives a better understanding of medical problems in older adults as a decline in function may be an early indicator of disease or illness. Self-care assessments also identify the level of impairment or disability. A brief discussion is provided here, with greater detail included in Chapter 21.

In addition to the occupational profile, the results of a self-care assessment as part of a comprehensive evaluation helps professionals identify the individual's current and potential level of functioning and develop effective interventions. Determining a person's ability to live independently and the supports (internal and external) needed to do so can be ascertained, in part, through an assessment of self-care skills. Gerontology literature has focused on prediction of ADL function to assist in determining the need for residential placement (Albert et al, 2014). There is somewhat less emphasis on measures that guide possible remediation or compensatory strategies, though remediation or compensation can help older adults avoid institutionalization. James & Pitonyak (2019) outlined a seven-step process for selection of assessments. Steps are as follows:

1. Identify the purpose of the evaluation.
2. Have clients identify personal needs, interests and perceived difficulties with ADLs and IADLs.
3. Explore the client's relevant ADLs and IADLs so they are operationally defined.
4. Estimate client factors that affect ADLs, IADLs, and the assessment process.
5. Identify contextual features that affect assessment.
6. Consider the features of assessment tools in selecting instruments.
7. Integrate information to select optimal activities of the tools before selection.

In addition to the process outlined above, because self-care activities are multifaceted, it is necessary to use assessment measures that are multidimensional in order to evaluate a number of self-care activities. For instance, the Kohlman Evaluation of Living Skills (Kohlman & Robnett, 2016) utilizes both self-report and observation. Thus, therapists often use multiple methods to gain a greater understanding of an individual's capabilities. A review of a person's history, interviews with the individual and the caregivers, and direct observation of task performance supply objective and subjective data and add detail about the individual's performance. When used with a variety of evaluation techniques, the sum of these methods leads to the clearest determination of where and why limitations in function occur.

In the event of functional challenges with a particular ADL, the complexity of everyday tasks necessitates that the evaluator pays careful attention to the factors underlying the individual's difficulty in performance. For example, an older adult involved in a cooking task may have difficulty following written directions because of visual impairment or with verbal directions due to hearing loss. The person may also have memory deficits that make it difficult to recall the correct sequence of steps to execute a task successfully. Persons with aphasia may have difficulty with reception or expression of language, causing poor comprehension or communication resulting in impaired daily function. For example, someone with receptive aphasia might be able to follow written, but not verbal, directions to fry an egg or vice versa. Determining the underlying cause of the functional deficit is necessary for successful intervention planning. See Chapter 21—Evaluation of Functional Performance With Older Adults.

Special Considerations in Evaluation of Self-Care

Many factors impact an older adult's ability to perform ADLs and the occupational therapy evaluation. The impact of sensory and sensorimotor deficits and cognitive impairment are discussed in the following section.

Sensory and Sensorimotor Deficits

The majority of self-care assessments require adequate vision. A test of ADLs for persons with visual impairment, the Melbourne Low Vision ADL Index, demonstrates satisfactory reliability and validity (Haymes et al, 2001). The test is not only a measure of ADL but is also useful for measuring the effect of disability on ADL performance (Haymes et al, 2001). In recent years, a Canadian-French version of the scale was developed and has been shown to have good reliability and validity (Duquette et al, 2020).

Hearing loss distorts any assessment process because of potential difficulty hearing the instructions and misinterpretation of the information. Various self-care instruments may be used to assess individuals with hearing impairment. In addition to tools designed by occupational therapy, research has demonstrated the validity of the WHO Disability Assessment Schedule 2.0 (WHODAS 2.0) (WHO, 2010) as an effective tool for assessing activity limitations, disability, and health. The 2010 WHO-DAS 2.0 manual is available from the WHO website.

Assessments for self-care skills often include tasks with motor components. These frequently require the manipulation of objects or the use of pen and paper, which may be difficult for older adults because of decreased flexibility, coordination, and other declines. The Assessment of Motor and Process Skills provides a highly standardized method for assessing observable motor and process skills during ADL and IADL performance (Fisher & Jones, 2014). This tool has utility in its comprehensive assessment of motor and process skills; however, the training and costs of administering this assessment limit its practicality in many settings. Another test, the A-One (Arnadottir, 1990) assesses neurobehavioral dysfunction within an ADL context and may be used to determine the extent a sensory motor dysfunction affects occupational performance. The associated A-One Neurobehavioral Scale helps therapists identify which neurobehavioral deficits affect ADL performance (Arnadottir et al, 2012) and thus may facilitate information for a comprehensive evaluation as well as intervention planning. The Quality of Life in Neurological Disorders (Neuro-QOL) is a set of standardized interdisciplinary quality of life tools that measure physical, mental, and social health factors that may impact self-care (National Institute of Neurological Disorders and Stroke, 2015). The Neuro-QOL addresses 11 domains including the ability to participate in social roles and activities, cognitive function, and positive affect and well-being, among others. There are translations in Spanish with efforts underway to validate the measure in a number of other languages.

Cognitive Impairment

In recent years, increased emphasis has been placed on functional cognition, the means by which individuals use their thought process in completing daily activities. Evaluation in this area uses functional tasks to assess a client's ability to safely complete self-care activities. AOTA (2021) asserts the importance of assessing functional cognition for intervention planning and to provide the necessary supports for clients both in the intervention and discharge environments. Addressing functional cognition may lower hospital readmission rates and improve client outcomes (Giles et al, 2020) and thus should be included in the occupational therapy process.

Measures such as the Executive Function Performance Test (Baum et al, 2003), the Kettle Test (Hartman-Maeir et al, 2009), the Performance Assessment of Self-Care Skills (Holm & Rogers, 2020), and the Cognitive Performance Test (CPT; Burns, 2018) may facilitate an understanding of the potential effects of cognitive decline and functional performance, yet therapists must be aware that mild cognitive impairment may be less likely to be detected in certain ADL measures. Therapists must understand the intent of the instrument and application to intervention planning. For instance, often practitioners mistake the CPT for an ADL test when the actual skills measure looks at information processing required for ADLs and IADLs. Burns and Haertl (2018) presented best practices for use of the CPT to include the use of the cognitive profiles that result from the scores in order to plan intervention. The emphasis is placed within the CPT on understanding the client's information processing, using the cognitive profile, and planning intervention based on the client's cognitive capacity along with additional physical and psychological considerations.

ADL Assessments

There are numerous tools available for assessing ADL performance in older adults. Two commonly used tools include the Katz Index of Daily Living and the Barthel Index. The Katz Index of Daily Living (Katz, 1983), assesses clients on six tasks of daily living: bathing, dressing, toileting, transferring, continence, and feeding. The Barthel Index measures 10 basic ADLs and facilitates therapists' decisions related to intervention and discharge planning; the scale has demonstrated reliability and validity (Collin et al, 1988). Another assessment, the Bristol Activities of Daily Living Scale (Bucks et al, 1996) was designed specifically for persons with dementia. The instrument consists of caregiver ratings for 20 ADLs. The scale's psychometric properties indicate satisfactory reliability, and it correlates well with the Mini Mental Status Examination. The Kohlman Evaluation of Living Skills 4th edition (Kohlman & Robnett, 2016) includes basic living skills and IADLs. This tool was revised and updated to include online forms and incorporate more of the therapist's clinical reasoning in the summary of results. In addition to other standardized tools, therapists often use informal observation to assess ADL performance; however, observations of a client at a hospital or transitional care unit may not reflect the client's ability to function in the home environment.

Assessing Environmental Factors

When assessing function in the older adult population, evaluators often overlook environmental factors—the physical environment (e.g., living space and the objects therein) and the social and cultural environments (e.g., group memberships and interactions) in which the individual performs life tasks. The level of assistance, support, and adaptations individuals require to perform self-care activities are also components of the environment. The availability of such support may enhance function, just as lack of support can hinder the individual's level of functioning. Assessing the environments in which specific tasks take place can be difficult because the environment is often a home, a workplace, or another location in the community.

Assessment of social environment concerns include the care receiver and the caregiver or care partner, which in this context can be defined as a knowledgeable person who is able to provide assistance to older adults and receive training in their care. It is important that the caregiver can manage caregiving needs and has a healthy attitude regarding functional independence, including supporting the older adult in participation and independence in self-care to the extent possible. Strategies for working effectively with informal caregivers are discussed in Chapter 20. Involvement of older adults in social activities may be compromised by a decline of independence, the inability to perform self-maintenance tasks, or poor mobility. Cultural factors, such as the individual's health, beliefs, values, roles, education, experiences, and family makeup, need to be taken into account to ensure that the assessment is relevant to the individual being assessed. It is also important to consider the reliability and validity of assessment tools available in working with persons of other cultures.

Several assessments are available to evaluate the effects of older adults' environments on their level of functioning and ability to maintain self-care. Because the environment is not an isolated component of everyday functioning, many assessments also address cognitive, self-care, and IADL performance. One such instrument is the Home and Community Environment Instrument (Keysor et al, 2005), which assesses home mobility, community mobility, mobility devices, communication devices, and attitudes. This assessment has shown promising psychometric properties for home evaluation. Additional examples of environmental assessments of the home can be found in Chapter 15.

Intervention for Self-Care Activities of Daily Living

As previously described, progression of normal aging, pathological conditions, and trauma can create impairments and limitations in function that interfere with the performance of self-care ADLs. In many cases, occupational therapy intervention techniques can address these difficulties. See Promoting Best Practice 14-2 for important questions to ask when setting self-care intervention goals.

PROMOTING BEST PRACTICE 14-2
Important Questions for Setting Self-Care Intervention Goals

- How important is the activity to the client and their well-being? Is it client-directed?
- Does the client feel the time and effort required for self-performance is worth the benefit?
- What assistive technologies are available to facilitate the task?
- Does the living environment support safe performance and quality of life?
- To what extent will the activity contribute to the individual's sense of identity and social participation?
- Have the perspectives of family members or caregivers been considered?
- What is the client–environment–task fit in developing the ADL and IADL goals?

For older adults, the limitations of function often are due to chronic and progressive disorders or injuries due to falls and accidents. Compensatory strategies may helpfully focus on adaptation of the environment, task, or the use of residual function. In changing the context of performance, the individual may be provided with assistive devices, or modifications may be made to the physical environment. If the current living situation does not promote optimal occupational performance, the individual may be able to move to a congregate home or an apartment complex designed for older adults or, in cases of significant functional deficits, to an assisted-living or skilled nursing facility.

Remediation strategies are directed at correcting the underlying pathology or physiological change. If this is accomplished successfully, performance of ADLs usually improves. This is an area in which involvement of the whole treatment team can help ascertain the potential prognosis and the most helpful course of action. For instance, if an individual has a cognitive impairment due to a stroke or head trauma resulting from a fall, the timing of the incident, the amount and type of damage, and physician prognosis for improvement have a bearing on intervention planning.

The following sections provide brief summaries of skill training, environmental changes, assistive technologies, and task modification approaches useful for enabling older adults to perform self-care tasks. The section is not meant to be exhaustive, but rather to summarize approaches that may be used in ADL interventions.

Skill Training

The use of skill training in older adult rehabilitation requires clinical discernment as to the client's functional capacity (e.g., cognition, physical status), goals, desired skills, prognosis, and projected living environment. For instance, an individual with a left CVA who has a good prognosis for recovery may go through fairly intensive physical and cognitive rehabilitation in hopes of returning to independent living in their home. However, skill training in high-level IADLs, such as financial management, would not likely be undertaken for someone with moderate to advanced stages of progressive neurocognitive conditions resulting in dementia. Thus, establish/restore approaches as outlined in the *Practice Framework* (AOTA, 2020) are usually used when prognosis for significant recovery is positive. Such approaches are generally used when it is expected that skills can transfer to the client's living environment (Latham, 2008). A study in New Zealand of restorative approaches in the home found improved functional performance and quality of life (Weir, 2018), but client factors and clinical reasoning must be incorporated when planning the intervention approach. Whereas a restorative approach is often used for those with a good prognosis, if the client's current and projected future skill level does not match the demands of the context (environment), modifications to the task or environment are often used to enhance functional performance.

Environmental Modifications

Environmental modifications may be individual or systems oriented. Such modifications range from adaptation of a home bathroom or entryway to curb cuts in sidewalks and major alterations in the design of rooms or dwellings for older adults. Environmental modifications for self-care activities related to mobility, food preparation and eating, toileting, and dressing can enhance ADL abilities. Environmental modifications may be particularly problematic in low-income areas or developing nations where other healthcare concerns take priority.

Mobility

Within the home, individuals with deficits affecting mobility often require ramps, widened doorways, or other accommodations for facilitating wheelchair access. In multistory homes, the conversion of downstairs rooms to bedrooms or bathrooms may be necessary. In general, safety can be enhanced by replacing rugs and carpets with tile, wood, or linoleum. Leg extenders can be added to low chairs or beds to improve the ease with which people can transfer to and from them. High legs on beds or chairs can be cut to lower the height; in recent years, motorized furniture is available to lift a person to standing if weak leg muscles make sit-to-stand movement difficult. For those in wheelchairs, simply removing interior doors may provide sufficient access. If privacy is not an issue, this approach avoids costlier modifications.

Bathroom and Dressing Areas

Bathroom modifications for safety and access include higher toilet seats and shallow sinks positioned in lowered counters (Fig. 14-1). Grab bars should be installed for showers and tubs, and insecure towel racks should be removed or replaced. Glass shower doors should be replaced with shower curtains. A tub chair (Fig. 14-2) and removable showerhead is often helpful for those with coordination and balance issues. All areas need adequate lighting and nonskid surfaces. For those with vision loss, increased contrast and experimenting with the wattage of lighting can facilitate function and help manage the glare an individual may experience in the environment (Willings, 2020). For those with physical limitations, cabinets may be lowered and cabinet doors removed to make them accessible. Adequate room must be ensured for transfers from wheelchair to bed. Electric beds that can be purchased or rented can improve accessibility to persons with physical limitations. Closets should have adequate reachable storage and access to clothing and other needed items. Control systems to operate lights, drapes, fans, televisions, stereos, and heat are available and can greatly reduce the physical demands of adjusting the environment.

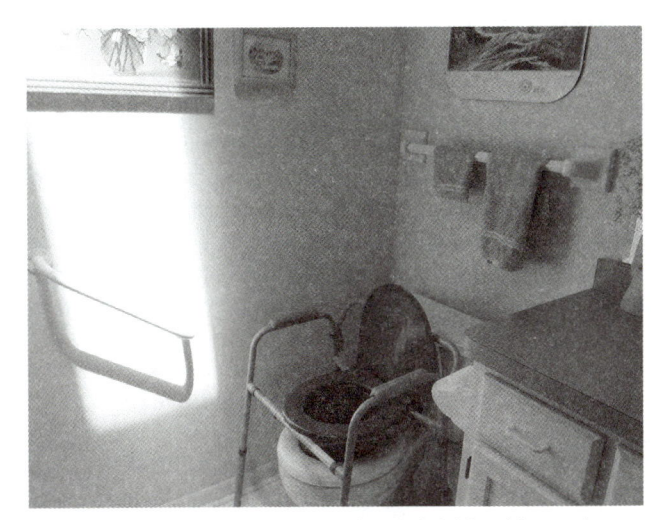

FIGURE 14-1 A raised toilet seat is often helpful for elders with mobility difficulties. *(Photo courtesy of Kristine Haertl.)*

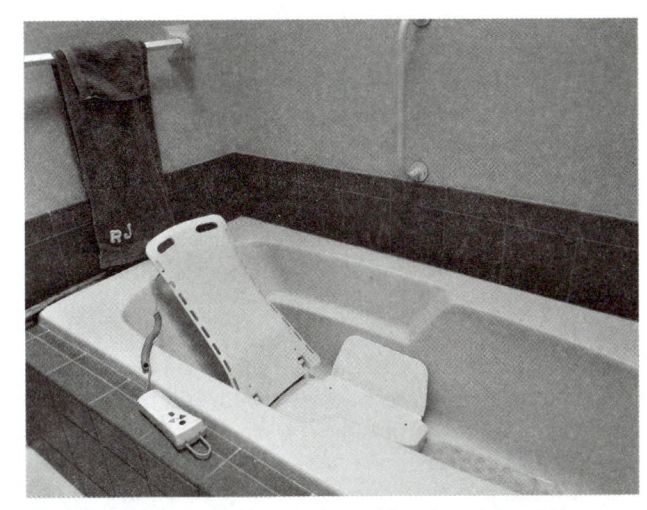

FIGURE 14-2 This reclining tub chair adds safety and mobility options for those who prefer taking baths instead of showers. *(Photo courtesy of Kristine Haertl.)*

Assistive Technology Devices for Self-Care

The use of assistive devices and smart home technology can help older adults overcome impairment, promote safety through the prevention of accidents, and enhance independence and quality of life. Such technology may be used not only to control environmental factors but may also monitor the status of the elder (e.g., falls) to detect health and safety concerns (Yu et al, 2019). Additional examples of assistive technologies that can support ADLs and minimize accidents include timers on stove burners, electronic sensors for turning on lights, and water temperature monitors. Research has demonstrated that although assistive technology can increase functional performance, older adults need support in learning how to work with assistive devices and getting accustomed to them (Skymne et al, 2012). Current advances have significantly broadened the scope, sophistication, and availability of assistive devices.

Task Modifications

Task modification (also known as compensation) strategies, a final category of intervention, may successfully address some self-care limitations in older adults with intact cognition and endurance who have caregiver support and the motivation to practice. Modification often refers to substituting one act for another or using a device or alternative technique to replace a lost ability. For example, adults who cannot reach or bend because of balance deficits or restricted range of motion may use a reacher to pick up objects on the floor. Use of the reacher, however, requires upper-extremity coordination, wrist and grip strength, and adequate cognitive skills.

Compensation or task modification strategies are often coupled with remediation strategies. In certain instances, remedial/restorative efforts take more time and effort than adaptation and thus care should be taken to consider the client's priorities and abilities when determining the approach. Teaching task modification requires adequate practice to facilitate automatic performance of ADLs (Flinn & Radomski, 2008). A simple alteration may include use of built-up utensils or an extended handle, whereas significant alterations may include learning to dress with one limb or perform a task with the nondominant hand. Significant alterations take more time and energy to master. The context must also be considered, as some modifications are easy to implement in the client's environment but may not be transferable to another setting (James & Pitonyak, 2019).

Task modifications are appropriate if the older adult desires or needs immediate success, if the therapist expects little or no improvement in the older adult's sensory or motor deficits, if the person prefers this method, or if the therapist identifies problems with safety. A simple example of self-task modification might be recommending that the older adult with limited standing tolerance sit down to perform activities typically performed while standing, such as washing dishes. Older adults with fatigue or limited endurance can perform more difficult self-care activities earlier in the day, thus avoiding exertion, stress, or cognitive errors when they have the least energy. Regardless of the intervention used, a client-centered focus is integral to the development of intervention goals and strategies for treatment.

CASE STUDY (CONTINUED)

Intervention Plan and Discharge Status

The intervention plan for Mr. Arkmadian's week and a half stay in the inpatient rehabilitation unit included an activity program implemented collaboratively by occupational and physical therapy. Occupational therapy focused on ADL training to address bilateral coordination and scanning of the left visual field. In addition, client and family education that emphasized safety awareness, guided supervision to Mr. Arkmadian during his daily activities, and recommended compensatory strategies and modifications that support Mr. Arkmadian's functional independence were provided. Physical therapy emphasized proper management of the left upper extremity for positioning, instruction and practice of safe transfers, and instruction and practice using mobility aids for ambulation.

Mr. Arkmadian was discharged to his home with his wife and son. Both his wife and son attended family education sessions before discharge to familiarize them with the home exercise program, provide information on the use of the recommended assistive devices, and make suggestions to assist with the supervision of self-care activities as well as modifications that may promote participation and independence in his desired leisure activities. Written and printed handouts that covered the material addressed in the family education sessions were provided.

Question

1. If Mr. Arkmadian indicated that he would not use the assistive devices that were recommended for him, what other strategies might assist him in his self-care?

Answer

1. Mr. Arkamadian has made some modifications to his home already, which may provide task supports. Alternative strategies could include modifying the task (e.g., he could sponge bathe until he is comfortable using a tub chair and handheld shower.) (LO 14.7; Interventions for self-care)

SUMMARY

The self-care activities of older adults discussed in this chapter are of vital importance to meaningful participation in the home environment and in the larger social world. The normal aging processes as well as various health conditions can cause sensory, motor, and cognitive losses that limit self-care performance, yet maintaining positive health and exercise can help delay the onset of difficulties with ADLs.

Assessment of an individual's performance in their environment can identify potential interventions to help older adults manage ADL performance. In addition to skill training, environmental modifications, assistive technologies, and modifications in task performance may reduce the need for institutionalization (and loss of control and self-identity) by preserving self-care functions. If, with this help, elders can successfully remain at home or can live productively in a community, these interventions may foster the self-esteem and sense of well-being that we all cherish as adults.

Critical Thinking Questions

1. Why is functional performance in ADLs important to health and wellness?
2. What assessment would you select if you were concerned about health factors influencing self-care performance?
3. How could environmental modifications increase or support performance of basic self-care for someone with mobility issues in the bathroom?

Acknowledgment

Special thanks to my friend and esteemed colleague, Charles Christiansen, EdD, OTR/L, FAOTA, who contributed significant portions of this chapter in the original editions and whom I had the pleasure of coauthoring with. I would also like to thank Catherine Sullivan, PhD, OTR/L, and Teresa Wickboldt, OTD, OTR/L, for their valuable input into the contents of the chapter.

REFERENCES

Aarden, J. J., van der Schaaf, M., van der Esch, M., Reichardt, L. A., van Seben, R., Bosch, J. A., Twisk, J. W., Buurman, B. M., Engelbert, R. H. (2019). Muscle strength is longitudinally associated with mobility among older adults after acute hospitalization: The hospital-ADL study. *PLoS ONE, 14*(7):e0219041. https://doi.org/10.1371/journal.pone.0219041

Adams, P. F., & Martinez, M. E. (2016). QuickStats: Percentage of adults with activity limitations by age group and type of limitation: National Health Interview Survey- 2014, United States. *CDC Weekly, 65*, 14.

Albert, S. M., Bear-Lehman, J., & Anderson, S. J. (2014). Declines in mobility and changes in performance in the instrumental activities of daily living among mildly disabled community-dwelling older adults. *Journals of Gerontology: Series A. Biological Sciences and Medical Sciences, 30*, 71–77. doi:10.1093/gerona/glu088

Amanzio, M., Canessa, C., Bartoli, M., Cipriani, G. E., Palermo, S., & Cappa, S. F. (2021). Lockdown effects on healthy cognitive aging during the Covid-19 pandemic: A longitudinal study. *Frontiers in Psychology, 12*, 685180. doi: 10.3389/fpsyg.2021.685180

Amelia, E. J., & Batchelor-Aselage, M. B. (2014). Facilitating ADLs by caregivers of persons with dementia: The CP3 model. *Occupational Therapy in Health Care, 28*, 51–61. doi: 10.3109/07380577.2013.867388

American Foundation for the Blind. (2020). *Key definitions of statistical terms.* https://www.afb.org/research-and-initiatives/statistics/key-definitions-statistical-terms

American Occupational Therapy Association. (2020). Occupational therapy practice framework: Domain and process (4th ed.). *American Journal of Occupational Therapy, 74*(Suppl. 2), 7412410010. https://doi.org/10.5014/ajot.2020.74S2001

American Occupational Therapy Association. (2021). *Role of occupational therapy in assessing functional cognition.* https://www.aota.org/Advocacy-Policy/Federal-Reg-Affairs/Medicare/Guidance/role-OT-assessing-functional-cognition.aspx

Arnadottir, G. (1990). *The brain and behavior. Assessing cortical dysfunction through activities of daily living.* Mosby.

Arnadottir, G., Lofgren., B., & Fisher, A. (2012). Neurobehavioral functions evaluated in naturalistic contexts: Rasch analysis of the A-ONE Neurobehavioral Impact Scale. *Scandinavian Journal of Occupational Therapy, 19*, 439–449. doi: 10.3109/11038128.2011.638674

Axon, D. R., & Le, D. (2021). Association of self-reported functional limitations among a national community based sample of older adults in the United States with pain: A cross sectional study. *Journal of Clinical Medicine, 10*(9). 1836. doi: 10.3390/jcm10091836

Bateson, M. C. (1996). Enfolded activity and the concept of occupation. In R. Zemke & F. Clark (Eds.), *Occupational science: The evolving discipline*, 5–12. F.A. Davis.

Baum, C. M., Edwards, D. F., Morrison, T. & Hahn, M. (2003). *Executive function performance test.* Washington University School of Medicine.

Bennett, S., Laver, K., Voigt-Radloff, S., Letts, L., Clemson, L., Graff, M., Wiseman, J., & Gitlin, L. (2019). Occupational therapy for people with dementia and their family carers provided at home: A systematic review and meta-analysis. *BMJ Open, 9*, e026308 doi: 10.1136/bmjopen-2018-026308

Bucks, R. S., Ashworth, D. L., Wilcock, G. K., & Siegfried, K. (1996). Assessment of activities of daily living in dementia: Development of the Bristol Activities of Daily Living Scale. *Age and Ageing, 25*, 113–120. doi:10.1093/ageing/25.2.113

Burns, T. (2018). *Cognitive performance test revised manual.* Maddock.

Burns, T., & Haertl, K. (2018). Cognitive performance test: Practical applications and evidenced based use. *SIS Practice Connections, 3*, 16–18. American Occupational Therapy Association.

Centers for Disease Control and Prevention. (2020). *Keep on your feet: Preventing older adult falls.* https://www.cdc.gov/injury/features/older-adult-falls/index.html

Centers for Disease Control and Prevention. (2021). *About chronic diseases.* https://www.cdc.gov/chronicdisease/about/index.htm

Chan, A. (2020). Asian countries do aged care differently: Here's what we can learn from them. https://theconversation.com/asian-countries-do-aged-care-differently-heres-what-we-can-learn-from-them-148089

Chang, K. M. W. (2020). *Hearing loss in older adults: Exploring occupational therapy's role.* Doctoral Project- St. Catherine University. https://sophia.stkate.edu/cgi/viewcontent.cgi?article=1021&context=otd_projects

Chen, P., Baune, N. A., Zwir, I., Wang, J., Swamidass, V., & Wong, A.W.K. (2021). Measuring activities of daily living in stroke patients with motion machine learning algorithms: A pilot study. *International Journal of Environmental Research and Public Health, 18*, 1634. https://doi.org/10.3390/ijerph18041634

Chiu, C-J., Li, M-L., & Chou, C-Y. (2022). Trends and biopsychosocial correlates of physical disabilities among older men and women in Taiwan: Examination based on ADL, IADL, mobility and frailty. *BMC Geriatrics, 22*, Article 148. https://doi.org/10.1186/s12877-022-02838-6

Clynes, M. A., Jameson, K. A., Edwards, M. H., Cooper, C., & Dennison, E. M. (2019). Impact of osteoarthritis on activities of daily living: Does joint site matter? *Aging Clinical and Experimental Research, 31*, 1049–1056. doi: 10.1007/s40520-019-01163-0

Cobb, S. M. (2013). Mobility restriction and comorbidity in vision-impaired individuals living in the community. *British Journal of Community Nursing, 18*, 608–613.

Collin, C., Wade, D., Davies, S., & Horne, V. (1988). The Barthel ADL Index: A reliability study. *International Disabilities Studies, 10,* 61–63.

Covinsky, K. E., Lindquist, K., Dunlop, D. D., Gill, T. M. & Yelin, E. (2008). Effect of arthritis in middle age on older age functioning. *Journal of the American Geriatrics Society, 56,* 23–28. doi:10.1111/j.1532-5415.2007.01511.x

Davidson, J. G., & Guthrie, D. M. (2017). Older adults with a combination of vision and hearing impairment experience higher rates of cognitive impairment, functional dependence, and worse outcomes across a set of quality indicators. *Journal of Aging and Health, 31,* 85–108. doi:10.1177/0898264317723407

Deci, E. L., & Ryan, R. M. (2011). Levels of analysis, regnant causes of behavior and well-being: The role of psychological needs. *Psychological Inquiry, 22,* 17–22. doi:10.1080/1047840X.2011.545978

Deverajooh, C., & Chinna, K. (2017). Depression, distress and self-efficacy: The impact on diabetes self-care practices. *PLoS ONE, 3,* :e0175096. https://doi.org/10.1371/journal.pone.0175096

Doty, R. L. (2018). Age related deficits in taste and smell. *Otolaryngetic Clinics of North America, 4,* 815–825. https://doi.org/10.1016/j.otc.2018.03.014

Drageset, J. (2004). The importance of activities of daily living and social contact for loneliness: A survey among residents in nursing homes. *Scandinavian Journal of Caring Sciences, 18,* 65–71. doi:10.1111/j.0283-9318.2003.00251.x

Dunlay, S. M., Manemann, S. M., Chamberlin, A. M., Cheville, A. L., Jiang, R., Weston, S. A., & Roger, V. L. (2015). Activities of daily living and outcomes in heart failure. *Circulation: Heart Failure, 8,* 261–267. doi: 10.1161/CIRCHEARTFAILURE.114.001542

Duquette, J., Loiselle, J., Frechette, D., Dery, L., Senecal, M.-J., Wittich, W., & Wanet-Defalque, M.-C. (2020). Reliability and validity of the Canadian-French ecological adaptation of the weighted version of the Melbourne Low Vision ADL Index. *Disability and Rehabilitation, 42,* 1021–1030. doi: 10.1080/09638288.2018.1516813

Ellegaard, K., von Bulow, C., Bartholdy, C., Hansen, I. S., Rifbjerg-Madsen, S., Henricksen, M., & Waehrens, E. E. (2019). Hand exercise for women with rheumatoid arthritis and decreased hand function: An exploratory randomized control trial. *Arthritis Research and Therapy, 21,* 158. https://doi.org/10.1186/s13075-019-1924-9

Eska, K., Graessel, E., Donath, C., Schwarzkoph, L., Lauterberg, J., & Holle, R. (2013). Predictors of institutionalization of dementia patients in mild and moderate stages: A 4-year prospective analysis. *Dementia and Geriatric Cognitive Disorders Extra, 3,* 426–445.

Federal Interagency Forum on Aging Related Statistics. (2020). *Older Americans: Key indicators of well-being.* https://agingstats.gov/docs/LatestReport/OA20_508_10142020.pdf

Fisher, A. G., & Jones, K. B. (2014). *Assessment of motor and process skills: User's manual (8th ed.).* Three Star Press.

Fiske, A., Schneider, A., McLennan, S., Kerapetyan, S., & Buyx, A. (2021). Impact of Covid-19 on patient health: A mixed method survey with German patients. *BMJ Open.* 11:e051167. doi:10.1136/bmjopen-2021-051167

Flinn, N. A., & Radomski, M. V. (2008). Learning. In M. V. Radomski & C. A. T. Latham (Eds.), *Occupational therapy for physical dysfunction,* 6, 382–401. Lippincott Williams & Wilkins.

Gilbert, C., Hagerty, D., & Taggert, H. M. (2012). Exploring factors related to healthy ageing. *Self-Care, Dependent Care Nursing, 19,* 20–25.

Giles, G. M., Edwards, D. F., Baum, C., Furniss, J., Skidmore, E., Wolf, T., & Leland, N. E. (2020). Health policy perspectives: Making functional cognition a professional priority. *American Journal of Occupational Therapy, 74.* https://doi.org/10.5014/ajot.2020.741002

Godfrey, C. M., Harrison, M. B., Lysaght, R., Lamb, M., Graham, I. D., & Oakley, P. (2011). Care of self—care by other—care of other: The meaning of self-care from research, practice, policy and industry perspectives. *International Journal of Evidenced-Based Healthcare, 9,* 3–24. doi:10.1111/j.1744-1609.2010.00196.x

Hammond, A., & Freeman, K. (2004). The long-term outcomes from a randomized controlled trial of an educational-behavioural joint protection programme for people with rheumatoid arthritis. *Clinical Rehabilitation, 28,* 520–528. doi:10.1191/0269215504cr766oa

Hartman-Maeir, A., Harel, H., & Katz, N. (2009). Kettle test: A brief measure of cognitive functional performance. Reliability and validity in stroke rehabilitation. *American Journal of Occupational Therapy, 63,* 592–599. https://doi.org/10.5014/ajot.63.5.592

Haymes, S. A., Johnston, A. W., & Heyes, A. D. (2001). A weighted version of the Melbourne low-vision ADL index: A measure of disability impact. *Optometry and Vision Science, 78,* 565–579.

Ho, I. C., Chenoweth, L., & Williams, A. (2021). Older people's experience of living with, responding to and managing sensory loss. *Healthcare, 9,* 329. https://doi.org/10.3390/healthcare9030329

Hobbs, M. (2020). *The role of occupational therapy in cardiac rehabilitation.* AOTA continuing education course. PDH Academy. Course OT-1709.

Holm, M. B., & Rogers, J. C. (2020). Performance assessment of self-care skills. In B. J. Hemphill-Pearson (Ed.), *Assessments in occupational therapy mental health: An integrative approach, 4,* 359–370. Slack.

Ibrahim, N. I., & Davies, S. (2012). Aging: Physical difficulties and safety in cooking tasks. *Work, 41,* 5152–5159. doi:10.3233/WOR-2012-0804-5152

Imaginario, C., Rocha, M., Machado, P., Antunes, C., & Martins, T. (2020). Functional capacity and self-care profiles of older people in senior care homes. *Scandinavian Journal of Caring Sciences, 34,* 69–77. doi: 10.1111/scs.12706

Isik, K., Cengiz, C., & Dogan, Z. (2020). The relationship between self-care agency in depression in older adults and influencing factors. *Journal of Psychosocial Nursing, 58,* 39–47. doi: 10.3928/02793695-20200817-02

James, A. B., & Pitonyak, J. S. (2019). Activities of daily living and instrumental activities of daily living. In B. Schell & G. Gillen (Eds.), *Willard and Spackman's Occupational Therapy, 13,* 714–752.

Jindai, K., Nielson, C. M., Vorderstrasse, B. A., & Quinones, A. R. (2016). *Multi-morbidity and functional limitations among adults 65 and older NHANES 2005–2012. Preventing Chronic Disease (CDC), 13.* https://www.cdc.gov/pcd/issues/2016/16_0174.htm

Kaldenberg, J., & Smallfield, S. (2020). Occupational therapy practice guidelines for older adults with low vision. *American Journal of Occupational Therapy, 74,* 1–23. doi: 10.5014/ajot.2020.742003

Katz, S. (1983). Assessing self-maintenance: Activities of daily living, mobility, and instrumental activities of daily living. *JAGS, 31,* 721–726.

Kepic, M., Randolph, A., & Hermann-Turner, K. M. (2019). Care for caregivers: Understanding the need for caregiver support. *Adultspan Journal,* https://doi.org/10.1002/adsp.12068

Keysor, J. J., Jette, A. M., & Haley, S. M. (2005). Development of the home and community environment (HACE) instrument. *Journal of Rehabilitation Medicine, 37,* 37–44.

Kohlman, L. K., & Robnett, R. H. (2016). Kohlman evaluation of living skills, 4th edition. American Occupational Therapy Association.

Kristensen, H., Post, A., Poulsen, T., Jones, D., & Minet, L. R. (2014). Subjective experiences of occupational performance of activities of daily living in patients with mild stroke. *International Journal of Therapy and Rehabilitation, 21,* 118–125.

Landa-Gonzalez, B., & Molnar, D. (2012). Occupational therapy intervention: Effects on self-care performance, satisfaction, self-esteem/self-efficacy and role functioning of older Hispanic females with arthritis. *Occupational Therapy in Health Care, 26,* 109–119. doi:10.3109/07380577.2011.644624

Lang, P. O., Heitz, D., Hédelin, G., Dramé, M., Jovenin, N., Ankri, J., Somme, D., Novella, J-L., Gauvain, J. B., Couturier, P., Voisin, T., De Wazière, B., Gonthier, R., Jeandel, C., Jolly, D., Saint-Jean, O., & Blanchard, F. (2006). Early markers of prolonged hospital stays in older people: A prospective multicenter study of 908 inpatients in French acute hospitals. *Journal of the American Geriatrics Society, 54,* 1031–1039.

Laposha, I., & Smallfield, S. (2020). Examining the occupational therapy definition of self-care: A scoping review. *Occupational Therapy in Health Care, 34,* 99–115. DOI: 10.1080/07380577.2019.1703238

Latham, C. A. T. (2008). Conceptual foundations for practice. In M. V. Radomski & C. A. T. Latham (Eds.), *Occupational therapy for physical dysfunction, 6,* 1–20. Lippincott Williams and Wilkins.

Lee, P., Yeh, T., Yen, H., Hsu, W., Chiu, V. J., & Lee, S. (2021). Impacts of stroke and cognitive impairment on activities of daily living in the Taiwan longitudinal study on aging. *Scientific Reports, 11,* Article 12199.

Lendon, J. P., & Singh, P. (2021). Adult day services center participant characteristics: United States, 2018. NCHS Data Brief, no 411. Hyattsville, MD: National Center for Health Statistics. https://dx.doi.org/10.15620/cdc:106697

Li-Hsing, L., Chia-Chan, K., & Ying, J. C. (2020). Functional capacity and life satisfaction in older adult residents living in long-term care facilities: The mediator of autonomy. *Journal of Nursing Research, 28,* pe102. doi: 10.1097/JNR.0000000000000362

Liu, H., & Wang, M. (2022). Socioeconomic status and ADL disability of older adults: Cumulative health effects, social outcomes, and impact mechanisms. *PLoS ONE.* https://doi.org/10.1371/journal.pone.0262808

Luthfi, M., Sukartini, T., & Efendi, F. (2018). The relationship of self-care with elderly well-being: A systematic review. *Proceedings of the 9th International Nursing Conference, 527–531.*

Markowitz, S. N., Kent, C. K., Schuchard, R. A., & Fletcher, D. C. (2008). Ability to read medication labels improved by participation in a low vision rehabilitation program. *Journal of Visual Impairment and Blindness, 102,* 774–777.

Martinez, L. (2019). *A professional's guide to sensory impairment. The OT practice experts in therapy.* https://www.theotpractice.co.uk/news/our-experts-blog/a-professional-s-guide-to-sensory-impairment

Mayo, C. D., Kenny, R., Scarapicchia, V., Ohlhauser, L., Syme, R., & Gawryluk, J. R. (2021). Aging in place: Challenges of older adults with self-reported cognitive decline. *Canadian Geriatrics Journal, 24,* 138–143. doi: 10.5770/cgj.24.456

Mlinac, M., E., & Feng, M. C. (2016). Assessment of activities of daily living, self-care and independence. *Archives of Clinical Neuropsychology, 31,* 506–516.

Narasimhan, M. (2019). It's time to recognize self-care as an integral component of health systems. *BMJ, 365,* 1403. doi: https://doi.org/10.1136/bmj.l1403

National Institute of Neurological Disorders and Stroke (NINDS). (2015). User manual for the Quality of Life in Neurological Disorders (Neuro-QoL) Measures, version 2.0. https://www.sralab.org/rehabilitation-measures/neuro-qol

Norris, J. (2020). Cognitive function in cardiac patients: Exploring the occupational therapy role in lifestyle management. *American Journal of Lifestyle Medicine, 14,* 61–70. doi: 10.1177/1559827618757189

Olofsson, J. K. (2021). Olfaction and aging: A review of the current state of the research and future directions. *Iperception, 12,* 20416695211020331. doi: 10.1177/20416695211020331

Orellano, E., Colon, W. I., & Arbesman, W. (2012). Effect of occupation and activity based interventions on instrumental activities of daily living performance among community dwelling older adults: A systematic review. *American Journal of Occupational Therapy, 66,* 292–300. doi: 10.5014/ajot.2012.003053

Ovayolu, O. U., Ovayolu, N., & Karadag, G. (2012). The relationship between self-care agency, disability levels and factors regarding these situations among patients with rheumatoid arthritis. *Journal of Clinical Nursing, 21,* 101–110. doi: 10.1111/j.1365-2702.2011.03710.x

Oxford University Press. (2021). Competence. *Oxford Lexico Dictionary Online.* https://www.lexico.com/en/definition/competence

Peres, K., Matharan, F., Daien, V., Nael, V., Edjolo, A., Bourdel-Marchasson, I., Ritchie, K., Tzourio, C., Delcourt, C., & Carriere, I. (2017). Visual loss and subsequent activity limitations in the elderly: The French three city cohort. *American Journal of Public Health, 107,* 564–569. doi: 10.2105/AJPH.2016.303631

Rachey, K., & Janssen, S. (2021). Self-neglect among older adults: The role of occupational therapy in interprofessional primary care teams. *OT Practice, September 2021, 15–17.*

Riegel, B., Moser, D. K., Buck, H. G., Dickson, V. V., Dunbar, S. B., Lee, C. S., Lennie, T. A., Lindenfeld, J., Mitchell, J. E., Treat-Jacobson, D. J., & Webber, D. E. (2017). Self-care for the prevention and management of cardiovascular disease and stroke. *Journal of the American Heart Association, 6,* e006997. https://doi.org/10.1161/JAHA.117.006997

Saxon, S. V., Etten, M. J., & Perkins, E. A. (2010). *Physical change and aging: A guide for the helping professions* (5th ed.). New York: Springer.

Scott, K. M., & Collings, S. C. (2012). Gender differences in the disability (functional limitations) associated with cardiovascular disease: A general population study. *Psychosomatics, 53,* 38–43. http://dx.doi.org/10.1016/j.psym.2011.05.005

Sharma, P., Priya, M., & Muhammad, T. (2021). Number of chronic conditions and associated functional limitations among older adults: Cross-sectional findings from the longitudinal aging study in India. *BMC Geriatrics, 21,* 664. https://doi.org/10.1186/s12877-021-02620-0

Shea, B. Q., Finlay, J. M., Kler, J., Joseph, C. A., & Kobayashi, L. C. (2021). Loneliness among U.S. adults aged >55: Findings from the Covid 19 coping study. *Public Health Reports, 136,* 754–764. doi: 10.1177/00333549211029965

Skymne, C., Dahlin-Ivanoff, S., Claesson, L., & Eklund, K. (2012). Getting used to assistive devices: Ambivalent experiences by frail elderly persons. *Scandinavian Journal of Occupational Therapy, 19,* 194–203. doi:10.3109/11038128.2011.569757

Song, Y., Anderson, R. A., Wu, B., Scales, K., McConnell, E., Leung, A. Y., & Corazzini, K. N. (2020). Resident challenges with pain and functional limitations in Chinese residential care facilities. *Gerontologist, 60,* 89–100. https://doi.org/10.1093/geront/gny154

Stamm, T. A., Pieber, K., Crevenna, R., & Dorner, T. E. (2016). Impairment in the activities of daily living in older adults with and without osteoporosis, osteoarthritis, and chronic back pain: A secondary analysis of population based health survey data. *BMC Musculoskeletal Disorders, 17,* 139. doi: 10.1186/s12891-016-0994-y

Stevens, M. N., Dubno, J. R., Wallhagen, M. I., & Tucci, D. L. (2019). Communication and healthcare: Self reports of people with hearing loss in primary care settings. *Clinical Gerontology, 42,* 485–494. doi: 10.1080/07317115.2018.1453908

Sundsli, K., Espnes, G. A., & Soderhamn, O. (2013). Being old and living alone in urban areas: The meaning of self-care and health on the perception of life situation and identity. *Psychology Research and Behavior Management, 6,* 21–27. http://dx.doi.org/10.2147/PRBM.S46329

Suzuki, Y., Nagasawa, A., Mochizuki, H., & Shimoda, N. (2019). Effects on activities of daily living independence in patients with Alzheimer's disease when the main nursing caregiver consciously provides only minimal nursing care. *Journal of Physical Therapy Science, 31,* 398–402. doi: 10.1589/jpts.31.398

Toledano-Gonzalez, A., Labajos-Monzaneras, T., & Romero-Ayuso, D. M. (2018). Occupational therapy, self-efficacy well-being in older adults living in residential care facilities: A randomized clinical trial. *Frontiers in Psychology, 9,* 1414. doi: 10.3389/fpsyg.2018.01414

Torregrosa-Ruiz, M., Gutierrez, M., Alberola, S., & Tomas, J. M. (2021). The successful aging model based on personal resources, self-care and life satisfaction. *Journal of Psychology: Interdisciplinary and Applied, 155,* 606–623. https://doi.org/10.1080/00223980.2021.1935676

U.S. Department of Health and Human Services. (2012). *Summary health statistics for the U.S. population National Health Interview Survey.* https://www.cdc.gov/nchs/data/series/sr_10/sr10_260.pdf

Wadley, V. G., Bull, T. P., Zhang, Y., Barba, C., Bryan, R. N., Crowe, M., Desiderio, L., Deutsch, G., Erus, G., Geldmacher, D. S., Go, G., Lassen-Greene, C. L., Mameva, O. A., Marson, D. C., McLauglin, M. Nasrallah, I. M., Owlsley, C., Passler, J., Perry, R. T., Pilonieta, G., Steward, K. A., & Kennedy, R. E. (2021). Cognitive processing speed is strongly related to driving skills, financial abilities, and other instrumental activities of daily living in persons with mild cognitive impairment and mild dementia. *Journals of Gerontology 76,* 1829–1838. https://doi.org/10.1093/gerona/glaa312

Weir, A. (2018). Effective restorative home support for older people living with dementia and their caregivers: A New Zealand case study. *InTechOpen Limited.* doi: 10.5772/intechopen.73165

Williams, S., & Murray, C. (2013). The lived experience of older adults' occupational adaptation following stroke. *Australian Occupational Therapy Journal, 60,* 39–47. doi:10.1111/1440-1630.12004

Willings, C. (2020). *Bathroom adaptations for individuals who are blind or visually impaired.* https://www.teachingvisuallyimpaired.com/bathroom-adaptations.html

Wittig, W., Jarry, J., & Barstow, E. (2017). Vision and hearing impairment and occupational therapy education: Needs and current practice. *British Journal of Occupational Therapy, 80,* 384–391. https://doi.org/10.1177/0308022616684853

World Health Organization. (2020). *Top 10 causes of death.* https://www.who.int/news-room/fact-sheets/detail/the-top-10-causes-of-death#:~:text=Leading%20causes%20of%20death%20globally&text=The%20world's%20biggest%20killer%20is,8.9%20million%20deaths%20in%202019

World Health Organization. (2010). *Measuring health and disability: Manual for the WHO Disability Assessment Schedule 2.0 (WHODAS 2.0).* https://www.who.int/publications/i/item/measuring-health-and-disability-manual-for-who-disability-assessment-schedule-(-whodas-2.0)

Yi, X., Zhu, D., Chen, S., & He, P. (2020). The association of hearing impairment and its severity with physical and mental health among Chinese middle aged and older adults. *Health and Quality of Life Outcomes, 18,* 155. https://doi.org/10.1186/s12955-020-01417-w

Yu, J., An, N., & Hassan, T. (2019). A pilot study on a smart home for elders based on continuous in-home unobtrusive monitoring technology. *Health Environments Research and Design Journal, 12,* 206–219. https://doi.org/10.1177/1937586719826059

Ziedonis, D. (2019). Looking for healthy aging pathways to subjective well-being: The road to personal empowerment and enhanced self-care. *International Psychogeriatrics, 31,* 451–453. doi: 10.1017/S1041610218002053

CHAPTER 15

Home Management

Elizabeth G. Hunter, PhD, MS, OTR/L
Hillary Richardson, MOT, OTR/L, DipACLM
Elizabeth K. Rhodus, PhD, MS, OTR/L
Carly Braun, MS, OTR/L

> *Instrumental activities of daily living (IADLs) are those activities that allow an individual to live independently in a community. Although not necessary for functional living, the ability to perform IADLs can significantly improve the quality of life.*
>
> —(Guo and Sapra, 2022, p. 1)

LEARNING OUTCOMES

By the end of this chapter, readers will be able to:

15-1. Describe types of home management activities and their relevance to health and quality-of-life outcomes for older adults.
15-2. Articulate the complexity of physical, environmental, and social factors involved in providing person-centered home management services for older adults.
15-3. Understand relevant theories and frameworks of reference relevant to home management in older adults.
15-4. Identify common assessments that can help occupational therapists assess performance related to home management for older adults.
15-5. Understand common occupational therapy intervention strategies for supporting home management performance in older adults.

Mini Case Study

Mrs. Wilson is 80 years old, lives alone in a large metropolitan area, and was recently widowed. She is a retired preschool teacher with two adult children, four grandchildren, and two pet cats. Mrs. Wilson is a breast cancer survivor who received surgery and chemotherapy and has been cancer free for 10 years. Her treatment did result in long-term peripheral neuropathy in both of her hands and feet. Mrs. Wilson has hypertension that is appropriately managed by medication; however, she reports the side effects of the medications cause occasional, minor dizziness. She also has arthritis that negatively influences her fine motor skills, mobility, and pain tolerance. Decreased mobility has led to reduced strength and fitness. Many aspects of her comorbidities have resulted in her diminished balance and high risk of falling. Two weeks ago, she had a fall in her home that resulted in a right distal ulnar fracture. After surgical treatment of the fracture, she was referred to occupational therapy due to an inability to independently complete home management tasks (e.g., driving, cooking, home cleaning, laundry).

Mrs. Wilson has lived in her apartment, the first floor of a row house, in a large city for all of her adult life. She has a daughter who lives one block away and has been a major support since the death of Mr. Wilson. However, her daughter is 60 years old and currently undergoing treatment for breast cancer, so she is not able to provide much support at this time. Mrs. Wilson's son lives out of town and can help financially but not physically. While Mrs. Wilson's goal is to age in place and remain in her home, there are factors involved that make this more difficult over time. The row house her apartment is in is old and has eight steps to reach the entry to the building. In addition, her neighborhood is not the safe neighborhood with a strong sense of community that it once was, and community support has disappeared due to her neighbors dying or moving away. Her children are worried for their mother's safety in the home.

Provocative Questions
1. What are the personal, environmental, and social factors affecting Mrs. Wilson's ability to engage in home management occupations and live independently?
2. What are the barriers and facilitators to Mrs. Wilson aging in her home? How might Mrs. Wilson's circumstances influence her home management performance?

This chapter includes information on key factors that can influence home management and related instrumental activities of daily living (IADLs). Guidelines are shared for understanding the complexity of providing services to older adults with the goal of improving or maintaining performance in home management tasks and helping to support their quality of life. This information is followed by a brief overview of common health conditions that might negatively influence home management performance among older adults, as well as common assessments and interventions to provide services. The chapter concludes with a clinical case study that illustrates the common processes a practitioner might take to address home management performance problems for older adults.

Defining Home Management

Home management, for the purposes of this chapter, is inclusive of home-based IADL occupations. For older adults, home management activities such as meal preparation, clothing care, safety and emergency maintenance, disaster preparedness, and care of others (including pets), are essential to maintaining roles, safety and independence. For example, being able to safely prepare meals and manage laundry needs are important activities to support living independently. The abilities to maintain the home in terms of upkeep and maintain a safe environment are other important factors that require support. Finally, many older adults perform caregiving roles, whether for a spouse, an adult child, or a pet. These relationships are important and need to be assessed to ensure an optimal fit for the person, activity, and environment. See Table 15-1: Home Management Activities for more information on home management activities for older adults.

CASE STUDY

Occupational Profile

Sybil is a 72-year-old woman who was referred to occupational therapy through an in-home outpatient program by her primary care physician after falling in her bathroom at home. Sybil's medical history is significant for high blood pressure and chronic obstructive pulmonary disease (COPD), major depressive disorder (MDD), and mild cognitive impairment (MCI). She lives with her 75-year-old wife in a single-story home in a rural area.

Sybil completes ADLs with independence to modified independence; her wife manages her medications and assists with IADLs and home management tasks. This is difficult for her wife due to her own diagnosis of arthritis. The interview revealed that Sybil has had difficulty sequencing steps for cooking and kitchen safety concerns due to her cognitive impairment, and she often feels fatigued during the day. They do not currently have an emergency plan in place, which is a concern because of the threat of severe weather in their area.

Identified Problem Areas Related to Home Management and IADLs: Assessment

After completing Sybil's occupational profile, the occupational therapist administered the Canadian Occupational Performance Measure (COPM), on which Sybil indicated high importance but low satisfaction with participation in laundry and meal preparation. The occupational therapist also administered the Allen's Cognitive Levels Screen (ACLS-5), a functional cognition screening tool (Allen et al, 2007). Sybil scored a 5.6, suggesting that having assistance to identify challenges or safety issues and plan for activities would likely be beneficial to supporting her participation in desired home management activities (Allen, 1991). The occupational therapist then concluded the evaluation by completing the Safety Assessment of Function and the Environment for Rehabilitation–Health Outcome Measurement and Evaluation (SAFER-HOME) and observed Sybil completing laundry and cold-meal preparation tasks.

The occupational therapist noted that Sybil's engagement in her desired home management activities was inhibited by MCI, impaired balance and fear of falling, fatigue and decreased activity tolerance due to COPD and MDD, and loss of participation in roles and habits due to MDD.

Identified Strengths

- Has social and caregiving support from her wife
- Receives assistance with medication use, IADLs, and home management from her wife
- Lives in a single-story home, which facilitates mobility and reduces need to climb stairs

Goals for Occupational Therapy

The occupational therapist collaborated with Sybil and her wife to identify goals. Sybil's goals included increasing her ability to complete laundry tasks, establishing and using an emergency plan, increasing the safety and frequency of meal preparation, and verbalizing satisfaction with her activity level and participation.

Impact of Health Conditions on Performance of Home Management Activities and Related IADLs

IADL performance is often one of the first areas of performance to begin to show changes due to a deterioration of skills (see Promoting Best Practice 15-1, Importance of Home Management and IADL Performance for Older Adults). This deterioration can be caused by a variety of factors, such as changes in cognition, vision, and fine motor

TABLE 15-1 ■ *Home Management Activities*

IADLs

TASK	DESCRIPTION	OLDER ADULTS
Care of Others	Providing care for others, arranging or supervising formal care (by paid caregivers) or informal care (by family or friends) for others	Many older adults have the responsibility of providing care to a partner. This is an important role that can be difficult.
Care of Pets and Animals	Providing care for pets and service animals, arranging or supervising care for pets and service animals	Having pets has been shown to be beneficial to people. This can be particularly true for older adults as they can alleviate depression and loneliness and may increase physical activity.
Financial Management	Using fiscal resources, including financial transaction methods (e.g., credit card, digital banking); planning and using finances with long-term and short-term goals	Older adults who live alone and are managing their own finances must have the ability and access resources (e.g., bank) to be successful at financial management. This task may be one that will need to be taken over by a support network member.
Home Establishment and Management	Obtaining and maintaining personal and household possessions and environments (e.g., home, yard, garden, houseplants, appliances, vehicles), including maintaining and repairing personal possessions (e.g., clothing, household items) and knowing how to seek help or whom to contact	Home management can entail many activities and some can be quite difficult. These tasks can be difficult for older adults and may be important for them to manage depending on the level of support they have.
Meal Preparation and Cleanup	Planning, preparing, and serving meals and cleaning up food and tools (e.g., utensils, pots, plates) after meals	Fully independent older adults need to be able to prepare nutritious meals safely and efficiently. Meal preparation and clean up may be tasks that can be fulfilled by social support networks.
Safety and Emergency Maintenance	Evaluating situations in advance for potential safety risks; recognizing sudden, unexpected hazardous situations and initiating emergency action; reducing potential threats to health and safety, including ensuring safety when entering and exiting the home, identifying emergency contact numbers, and replacing items such as batteries in smoke alarms and light bulbs	Living independently in the community requires that older adults have basic safety and a plan for managing unforeseen emergency situations. These may be related to keeping their homes safe or perhaps having a plan to having extra medications available if an emergency situation emerges.

(Adapted from AOTA, 2020, OTPF 4th edition.)

skills (Feger et al, 2020). Importantly, a decrease in the ability to manage the home and perform IADLs is common in the early decline of cognitive ability (Lahav & Katz, 2020). In this section, we will discuss factors that can influence home management performance and quality of life. There are many potential factors, but five are highlighted here: complexities of aging, age-related change, disease-related change, MCI, and safety issues.

PROMOTING BEST PRACTICE 15-1
Importance of Home Management and IADL Performance for Older Adults

Home management activities are complex tasks that are important for independent living. IADL performance can be an important sign of overall health and wellbeing in older adults. For example, it is common for older adults to exhibit difficulties with IADLs and home management as an early sign of physical and/or cognitive functional decline (Feger et al, 2020). Research has shown that those who report difficulty with IADLs and home management were more likely to be older and female and have lower overall health (Feger et al, 2020). IADL task categories, such as driving, handling finances, housework, managing healthcare and phone use, often reveal early functional changes related to age and illness (Tabira et al, 2020; Feger et al, 2020). Recognizing early difficulty in IADLs and home management may be one step toward minimizing future performance and safety problems.

Complexities of Aging: Physical, Environmental, and Social Factors

Aging is a complex dynamic that is closely related to a variety of factors, such as genetics, health behaviors, and social inequities (Colich et al, 2020; Martin, 2017; Rea et al, 2016). More specifically, older adults can be faced with physical, environmental, and social factors that influence their performance in home management tasks. Older adults have a high incidence of having multiple comorbidities, such as high blood pressure, diabetes, and arthritis (Fong, 2019; Wei et al, 2020). The interaction of multiple health problems is a burden on the individual, due to the complexity in treatment (Shippee et al, 2012). Additionally, many of the health problems faced by older adults are chronic and will most likely worsen over time. The potential burden, both physically and emotionally, from managing multiple chronic diseases can increase any problems that occur from an acute diagnosis being added to existing disease states. For example, side effects from medications needed for the chronic medical conditions, stress levels due to the burdens of self-management, potentially high fatigue levels, and possible caregiver burnout can make home management more difficult. The existence of chronic conditions can be complex to manage themselves, but they can exacerbate the situation when an acute injury or illness occurs.

In terms of environmental factors, the built environment is extremely important for older adults when it comes to safety and performance of home management tasks. There are both physical and emotional aspects to the built environment. **Aging in place** is an important goal for many people and describes one's ability to age in the environment or setting that they choose, most often at home in the community (Iecovich, 2014). While many older adults want to age in place, some do so because they cannot afford to move (AARP, 2021a). The American Association of Retired Persons (AARP) provides many useful materials for older adults, including an aging in place home checklist (AARP, 2021b). Having options to stay or move is dependent on the physical, financial, and social environments the older adults have, resulting in potential inequity in the ability to live in the best-fitting place of their choosing. Practitioners need to understand that a client's personal agency to choose where and with whom they live, as well as their personal and historical associations to their home, may be very important to them, even if the environment is not optimal.

Social influences on health and aging are found at multiple levels, from the societal to the individual (see Chapter 1 for more information on Social Determinants of Health). At the individual level, social support refers to the existence of a social network that can help people stay healthy, provide care, and/or cope with adverse events (Sherman et al, 2016; Dykstra, 2015; Thoits, 2011). **Social support** has been shown to be a powerful predictor of living a healthy and long life. There are four main types of social support: instrumental (tangible goods and services), informational (advice, information), emotional (love, caring), and appraisal (feedback to help self-evaluation) (Thoits, 2011). Assessing social support is important when working with older adults, and adequate social support can often alleviate many home management performance problems. Shopping, yard care, and bill paying are examples of tasks that may be supported by family members if needed. If there is limited social support, other options should be considered.

Common Physical Changes Influencing Home Management and IADL Performance

While aging is not synonymous with disease, biological changes do occur as one ages. These changes will influence how and if people can complete the tasks they need and want to do. Decreased muscle strength (sarcopenia), bone strength, and sensory changes that happen to everyone as they age can negatively influence home management and IADL performance. Refer to Chapters 7 through 13 for specific conditions and their impact on occupational performance.

Beyond normal age-related changes, the incidence of certain diseases or conditions increases with age (Centers for Disease Control and Prevention [CDC], n.d.). Important examples are arthritis, stroke, cardiovascular disease, glaucoma, cataracts, cancer, and mild to severe cognitive changes. These conditions significantly affect function. For example, arthritis may negatively influence a person's ability to make a bed, hold shopping bags, place items into or remove items from cabinets, walk the dog, and many others. Stroke may result in minor to severe changes in upper-extremity function, thereby decreasing the ability to manage one's home independently. Glaucoma or other vision-related problems can cause problems when writing checks or reading recipes. Vertigo can lead to diminished participation and falls. These age-related physical changes and many others present obstacles to the successful, safe, and satisfactory completion of many home management activities.

Cognitive changes are often first noticed in changes to functional ability related to home management. There are numerous types of cognitive changes, from mild to severe, that can happen as one ages. MCI, which may or may not be a sign of the onset of some type of dementia, is commonly connected to emerging problems with home management and safety performance. Executive processing skills required to complete home management tasks, such as planning, sequencing, and problem-solving, are particularly sensitive to prodromal and early stages of cognitive impairment. It does not always mean someone is developing dementia, and not all cognitive changes are permanent (Mayo Clinic, n.d.). Often a practitioner who is seeing a client for an acute problem such as a stroke will become aware of potential cognitive changes that need to be included in any treatment plan.

Theoretical Approaches

Theoretical approaches influence occupational therapy practice in home management. Environmental press theory, a theory that influenced occupational therapy theoretical approaches, is discussed first. The Person-Environment-Occupation-Performance model (PEOP) and task-oriented approach are also discussed.

Environmental Press Theory

Lawton's environmental press theory (Lawton, 1983) is a gerontological theoretical framework developed to understand how people and environments interact and adapt, coined *environmental press*. The model includes the person's competencies, the environmental variables, and the interaction between the two. The theory examines the interactions (press) between the variables and ultimately provides guidance as to where a practitioner can provide intervention. The optimal goal is a fit between the level of the person's competencies and the demand from their environment. If an older adult's competencies decline due to age and/or illness, their demand for environmental support will increase. The press can be too much, too little, or just right. If there is too much environmental press, the person has difficulty negotiating the current environment and their skills need to be improved, the task needs to be changed, or the environment modified. A lack of environmental press can result in poor outcomes as well as maladaptive behaviors, boredom, and occupational deprivation. The goal is to find the optimal level of press to support the personal competencies of each individual.

Person-Environment-Occupation-Performance (PEOP) Model

The PEOP model is a patient-centered model that reflects the complex interactions between the person's unique characteristics, the environment in which activities occur, and the tasks and roles that are meaningful to them (Baum et al, 2015). Examples of these components can be seen in Table 15-2: Aspects of the Person-Environment-Occupation-Performance (PEOP) Model.

The interaction among the three components can positively or negatively affect the performance outcome. This assessment helps guide practitioners to what parts of the components need to be modified or encouraged. This model requires a collaborative relationship between the client and practitioner. This system model is an important overarching model that can guide any occupational therapy practice.

Task-Oriented Approach

The task-oriented approach considers task performance in relation to a person's valued life roles. This approach includes both assessing important roles and activities, as well as using those activities to guide the intervention. The foundation of this approach is that occupational performance builds on the interaction of persons and their environments (Cohen & Coster, 2014). This systems-model, function-based approach suggests that motor learning and behavior emerge from the interaction of the person, the tasks and the environment (Mathiowetz et al, 2021). The task-oriented approach helps practitioners to clinically improve motor behavior. There is an underlying assumption that if the person is engaged in the process of setting goals for intervention based on their values and preferences, the person will engage more effectively in the intervention activities. Strong engagement and outcomes result when the following are considered:

1. Client's collaboration in setting goals
2. Client-centered functional and meaningful tasks
3. Intervention in the natural settings
4. Use of real objects versus rote exercises without objects (Mathiowetz et al, 2021)

TABLE 15-2 ■ *Aspects of the Person-Environment-Occupation-Performance (PEOP) Model*

MODEL COMPONENT	TYPES OF CHARACTERISTICS	IADL EXAMPLE
Person	Including physiological, psychological, motor, sensory/perceptual, cognitive, or spiritual	Participation in IADLs places physiological, sensory, and motor demands, including such things as activity tolerance for standing to cook a meal, strength and sensory input required to complete fine motor tasks such as opening prescription bottles, and maintaining balance when cleaning or doing laundry. Personal factors such as cognition, psychology, and spirituality also affect IADLs, in how a person processes and acts on information related to safety or household management, how they feel about their current roles and routines, and how they perceive themselves and their roles in the context of their faith or community.
Environment	Including cultural, social support, social determinants, and social capital, physical and natural environments, health education and public policy, assistive technology	Environment encompasses the context in which a person completes their IADLs. This can include the built environment such as the safety and accessibility of their home or structures they use in their communities, as well as social or cultural factors such as the overall safety of their community and the availability of resources for food or medical care.
Occupation	Characteristics of the activity, task, or role	Occupations may be performed individually or with others, and occur within the context of the person and the environment. For example, engaging in the IADL of shopping for groceries might differ depending on the community access to food sources, availability of transportation, and the individual's budget and food preferences.
Performance	The actual doing of the task	Occupations are performed in the context of the person, the environment, and the unique demands of the task. An occupation such as doing the dishes might be performed in different ways by different people, depending on their abilities and their environment. For example, for an individual experiencing difficulties with sequencing, the task might be completed in stages with a compensatory strategy such as prompting by a family member or by following steps in a list, whereas a person with COPD and limited activity tolerance might use a compensatory strategy of performing the activity while seated.

Assessments for Home Management and IADLs

Many assessments can be used to gather information about home management in older adults. Special considerations in assessment, the occupational profile and the Canadian Occupational Performance Measure (COPM), home management and IADL assessments, and home safety assessments are discussed below.

Special Considerations in Assessment

Assessment is important to understand the level of performance at the start of therapy as well as to follow therapy and assess levels of change in performance. The selection of assessments relevant to home management needs to include the reason for referral and the ability of the client to participate in the process. Optimally, the evaluation will occur in the natural environment of the client (e.g., home) for best task performance. A home-based evaluation can be in person or via telehealth and provides contextually accurate assessment results, including the opportunity to assess the environment in relationship to task performance (Carrington & Islam, 2022). This allows for recommendations for beneficial equipment, modifications, and adaptations.

Practitioners should use standardized, reliable, and valid assessments whenever possible. Assessment types include patient self-report, measurement tools, or observation. As home management is multifaceted, multidimensional assessment measures are needed. Performance-based assessment entails observing and measuring in some way the actual process of an individual taking part in home management activities. It is crucial that practitioners have a good understanding of their clients' experiences, beliefs, values, social context, and personal goals. Conducting an occupational profile interview (AOTA, 2020) is the first step in the occupational therapy evaluation process. Additionally, it is important to use person-centered assessments to start any clinical assessment. The information you gather in this initial step of the assessment process will drive the remainder of the assessments, goal setting and interventions. For more information about evaluation, see Chapter 21.

The Occupational Profile and the Canadian Occupational Performance Measure (COPM)

The evaluation process begins with the occupational profile, an interview to summarize the "client's occupational history and experiences, patterns of daily living, interests, values, needs, and relevant contexts" (AOTA, 2022). The COPM is an evidence-based, client-centered assessment tool that can be used in tandem with the interview process and can also measure outcomes in function and client satisfaction as the therapy plan of care progresses (Enemark et al, 2018; Law et al, 1990). Occupational therapists can use the COPM as a tool to assess and measure client goals in household management, personal care, functional mobility, community mobility, work, and leisure occupations. Use of the COPM enhances clinical decision making when working with older adults and increases client participation in goal setting (Capdevila, et al, 2020). The COPM provides the basis for setting intervention goals by capturing the client's self-perception of performance over time. It is used to set treatment goals, for reassessment, and at discharge from services to measure treatment outcomes. It allows the client to prioritize the areas they are most concerned with and assesses the level of satisfaction they currently have with their performance in these areas. Practitioners find this type of assessment useful to include during the evaluation of IADLs with older adults, in clinical practice settings such as home health, outpatient, inpatient rehabilitation or community-based practice.

Home Management and IADL Assessments

After completing the occupational profile interview and evaluating the goals of the client, practitioners should conduct some performance-based assessments of the client performing IADL tasks (e.g., meal planning, shopping, laundry, house cleaning, yard maintenance, use of communication technology). The observation of actual performance is important. There are a number of psychometrically sound assessments as described in Table 15-3: Assessments of Home Management and IADLs.

Home Safety Assessments

Overall safety is an important concern for older adults. An unsafe environment can lead to occupational disruption and injury. Vision changes may lead to a higher risk of falling and poorly organized environments can create safety hazards around the home (Ibrahim & Davies, 2012). Evaluating safety concerns in and around the home is important when providing services to older adults. Many resources exist to guide people related to safety issues and aging. Along with telerehabilitation, there is a growing practice and acceptance of virtual home safety assessment (Read et al, 2020). Table 15-4: Home Safety Assessments Identifies Common Assessments Of Home Safety.

Intervention for Home Management and IADLs

There are two important ways to approach interventions to address home management performance: establish/restore (remediation) and modify (adaptation/compensation) (AOTA, 2020). Establish/restore approaches are typically used when recovery is possible. However, as may be the case

TABLE 15-3 ■ Assessment of Home Management and IADLs

IADL ASSESSMENTS

Assessment Name	Brief Description
Lawton IADL Scale (Lawton & Brody, 1969)	Self-report assessment tool that is used to determine level of independence in IADLs
Texas Functional Living Scale (Cullum et al, 2001)	An ecologically valid, performance-based screening tool to assess IADLs and to identify the level of care an individual needs
Independent Living Scale (ILS) (Loeb, 1996)	Is used to gather information related to the individual's ability to achieve successful independent community living. There are five sub scales: memory orientation, managing money, managing home and transportation, health and safety, social adjustment.
Assessment of Motor and Process Skills (AMPS)	Standardized assessment tool to evaluate the quality of IADL performance, for activities that have been prioritized by the client. Special AMPS training is required to use this assessment.
Kohlman Evaluation of Living Skills (KELS) (Kohlman Thomas & Robnett, 2016)	An observation and interview-based assessment, testing 17 skills in the areas of self-care, safety, health, money management, community mobility, telephone, employment, and leisure participation
Executive Function Performance Test (Baum et al 2003)	Assessment for the execution of four basic tasks that are independent living: cooking, telephone use, medication management, and bill payment
Kitchen Picture Test (KPT) (Mansbach et al, 2014)	Assessment of practical judgment and basic cognitive problems through the use of pictures that the client describes, highlights safety problems and is tested on recall
Performance Assessment of Self-Care Skills (PASS) (Rogers et al, 2001)	A performance based criterion referenced, observation tool. PASS includes two IADL domains (physical and cognitive emphasis).

TABLE 15-4 ■ Home Safety Assessments

IADL ASSESSMENTS

Assessment Name	Brief Description
In Home Occupational Performance Evaluation (I-HOPE) (Stark et al 2010)	A performance-based measure that evaluates 44 activities in the home. Subscales include activity participation, client's rating of performance, client's satisfaction with performance, and severity of environmental barriers are sensitive to change in the environment.
Westmead Home Safety Assessment (WeHSA) (Clemson et al, 1999).	An assessment that systematically identifies fall hazards for clients at risk for falls. Checklist that identifies relevance of items to client and rates hazards.
SAFER-Home V3 (Chiu & Oliver, 2006)	Assesses client's ability to safely carry out functional activities in the home and evaluates effectiveness of modifications as an outcome measure. Using interview and observation of client participating in activity, assesses level of safety risk as scored on a 4-point scale
Cougar Home Safety Assessment (CHSA) (Fisher et al, 2019)	An assessment of the home through observation, testing and questioning client in the categories of fire and carbon monoxide hazards, emergency/medical, electrical/water temperature, flooring/hallways, kitchen, bathroom, closets/storage, parking areas, and entrances; marked as safe or unsafe with comments
Home Environment Assessment Protocol (HEAP) (Gitlin & Corcoran, 2005) (Struckmeyer et al, 2020) [HEAP-R]	An assessment specific to the home environment of caregivers and people who have dementia. Addresses safety hazards in eight areas of the house, rated through caregiver interview and direct observation of safety hazards and adaptations. Provides recommendations for home modification. A revised, shorter version, the HEAP-R is available.

with certain areas of home management performance for older adults, if the person's current functional ability level is not expected to improve but there is a goal of maintaining a functional level to participate, modify is the approach used. This entails potentially adapting the task, modifying the environment, or compensating with the use of assistive technology. Adaptation includes things like adapting the light on kitchen workstations to support safe productivity, or perhaps labeling drawers or cupboards in the kitchen as a memory device to support performance and decrease fatigue.

Modification includes changing the built environment, such as reorganizing the kitchen to improve the ergonomics or keeping a phone available at all times for safety. It can also include finding strategies or techniques that work around limitations. If a client has a diagnosis that will cause continued deterioration of function, modifying to improve home management performance might include managing fatigue and teaching energy conservation techniques, using a daily planner to compensate for a poor memory, or planning to grocery shop during less busy times. The following are common interventions that can address aspects of modifying or establishing/restoring tasks to support home management performance for older adults. Within all approaches, a person-centered approach is paramount (see Promoting Best Practice 15-2: Importance of Person-Centered Care for Older Adults).

PROMOTING BEST PRACTICE 15-2
Importance of Person-Centered Care for Older Adults

A basic tenet of occupational therapy is the provision of person-centered care. Person-centered care includes nine main components: empathy, respect, engagement, relationship, communication, shared decision-making, holistic focus, individualized focus, and coordinated care (Eklund et al, 2019). Practitioners integrate the importance of a client's personal goals, current habits/routines, beliefs, and values when designing a plan of care. Practitioners must clearly understand the specific context, needs, wants, supports, and barriers faced by older adults before providing services for occupational performance in the context of the home.

Task Adaptation

Analyzing and adapting tasks, including individual home management tasks, relies on an occupational therapist's skill to understand the full context of activities, including the cognitive, physical, environmental, personal, and interpersonal components, and the client's motivations for engaging in the activity. After understanding the full context of activities, it is then possible to observe a client performing tasks to identify any barriers to the client's desired participation.

When analyzing home management tasks, consider the following components and subcomponents:

- Environmental: Where does the activity occur and what types of structures are involved? How does the client navigate the environment?
- Cognitive: What are the demands of the activity related to sequencing, memory, problem-solving, judgment, and metacognition?
- Physical: What level of strength, coordination, and range-of-motion is required to complete the task? How does the client's mobility affect their ability to complete the task? What are the sensory demands of the task?
- Personal and interpersonal: How does this activity relate to the individual's conception of themselves? Is the activity an important factor in their roles in relation to other people?
- Motivations: Is this something the individual wants or needs to do? What is the underlying meaning of the activity to them, and how can that be used to support overcoming barriers to participation?

As discussed earlier in the chapter, home management may be some of the first types of occupations affected by cognitive or physical changes during the aging process. The ability to participate in home management is often closely tied to a client's roles and routines and may involve or affect partners, children, or other family members who have historically relied on the client to perform some of these tasks. However, keep in mind that the roles one held in the past may no longer be desired as future roles. Further, roles valuable to an older adult may not reflect societal expectations typically constructed around gender, age, relationship status, or any other aspect of one's identity. Thus, goal setting around home management activities should remain client-centered and collaborative.

For example, clients may value interdependence and collective collaboration with family or friends. In such cases, home management may be assisted or completed by others, including family members or care partners. This may be an acceptable solution and distribution of roles for all involved individuals instead of seeking one's independence. Analyzing the task within the multifactorial context of the client's life, environment, and experiences allows for collaboration on client-centered goals and intervention planning (Buckley & Poole, 2014).

Energy Conservation

Increased fatigue can be a normal part of aging. Older adults who have chronic illnesses or are recovering from a temporary condition may experience higher-than-normal levels of fatigue (De-Bernardi-Ojuel et al, 2021; Racine et al, 2019; Rijpkema et al, 2020). Chronic conditions may cause pain, which is another common cause of fatigue (AOTA, 2014). Increased fatigue levels often require temporary or permanent changes to daily routines. Occupational therapists are uniquely qualified to address energy conservation strategies, such as using adaptive equipment, modifying tasks, and making changes to the environment to accommodate increased fatigue (Vatwani & Margonis, 2019). Activities must be prioritized into categories of what the older adult *needs* to do versus what they *want* to do. Activities that need to get done need to be completed first. Rest breaks may need to be planned into an older adult's daily routine. Activities that require a large expenditure of energy (e.g., attending a family reunion, going to the doctor's office, pharmacy, or grocery store) may need to be scheduled on separate days to spread out the activity and allow time for rest in between.

Task-Specific Skill Training

Direct skill training provides the opportunity for the client to practice specific skills like planning for a grocery trip or organizing and paying bills. The direct practice ensures the person has the opportunity to improve performance and provides chances to experience success in their tasks thus building confidence. Providing skill training may require grading activities and helping the person improve and move forward until they are at their optimal performance level. An occupation can be both an intervention and an outcome. Repeated practicing of occupations is beneficial to improved outcomes (Wolf et al, 2015). When possible and appropriate, supporting the client in taking part in the actual activity of interest is an important component of task-specific skill training (see Promoting Best Practice 15-3: Task-Specific Skill Training).

PROMOTING BEST PRACTICE 15-3
Task-Specific Skill Training

Performance emerges from the interaction of the person, task, and environment; therefore, it is important to include all three factors to the best of a practitioner's ability and as realistically as possible to improve task performance (Kurahashi et al, 2011). Task-specific skill training uses everyday tasks as the therapeutic intervention for functional improvement (Dobkin & Carmichael, 2005). This entails goal-directed practice and repetition of a specific task, with feedback, as an intervention to improve the performance of that specific occupation (Teasell et al, 2008). The focus of this training is performance of a task versus something like increasing muscle strength (Hubbard & Parsons, 2009). It is optimal to provide interventions that are as similar to the actual activity in the actual environment in which it will occur. This is particularly true for older adults. Task-specific training interventions emerged from motor skill learning research (Schmidt & Lee, 2005; Hosp et al, 2013), which stemmed from animal models in the 1960s (Knapp et al, 1963) that then became the focus of psychological and motor research (Schmidt & Lee, 2005; Bosse et al, 2015). In the rehabilitation setting, interventions that are not meaningful and do not specifically connect with the performance of an occupation in which the client would like to improve performance should be avoided. For example, if an older adult is having difficulties preparing a meal, training by having them practice preparing a sandwich will be more beneficial than doing the motions needed without performing the task (e.g., fine motor exercises).

Assistive Technology

Technology is changing every day. It is important for occupational therapists to keep learning about new and existing assistive technology options that can help their older adult clients stay as safe and independent as possible. Some older adults who are not able to complete household tasks or stay safely by themselves any longer may be able to continue to function independently by adopting assistive technology into their daily routines.

Assistive technology can be used to address safety, cognition, and physical function and needs to be carefully selected to meet the needs of individual clients (Sriram et al, 2020). Assistive technology devices, such as smart speakers, can be used to make emergency calls through voice activation if an older adult has a fall in the home and cannot reach their phone. Smart watches can also be used to call for help in the case of an emergency. Not all clients may be able to afford such devices. States typically have assistive technology libraries that loan or lend assistive technology equipment to individuals with physical and cognitive disabilities. These programs can be connected to regional departments of developmental disabilities, universities, or other organizations. To find these programs, AACCESSIBLE has a database showing lending libraries within the United States (AACCESSIBLE, 2022).

Many forms of smart technology are now used regularly by individuals across the lifespan. Smart home technology such as automatic lighting, intercoms, video monitors, and voice activation may be useful to help older adults age well at home and allow for controlling their ambient home conditions (Wallock & Cerny, 2021). Intercoms, video monitors, and voice activation may be useful to help older adults age well at home. These can also be useful, when used with careful planning and ethical considerations related to privacy, to help caregivers monitor and support older adult loved ones (Brims & Oliver, 2019; Collins, 2018). It is important to keep up-to-date with the fast-paced changes in current technology options.

Home Environmental Modification

The home environment has a direct effect on mental and physical health and well-being (Park et al, 2021). The home environment is a very personal one, and any changes need to be agreed upon by the older adult. Although modifications can create better and safer home environments, many older adults do not have needed modifications or equipment installed (Meucci et al, 2016). The lack of modifications may be due to things such as the age of the home (e.g., cannot be retrofitted), cost of making changes, and lack of knowledge about types of adaptations. Any modifications need to align with the preferences and needs of the person.

There are many ways environmental modifications can enhance performance. For IADL performance, home adaptation can be important. Home adaptation can range from removing clutter to renovating a room. These changes are guided by the safety and performance needs of the client. Home adaptations often occur in the bathroom, kitchen, entry and exit from home, and stairways. Table 15-5 outlines common home management and IADL-oriented home adaptations.

Home safety can encompass the built environment to the social environment surrounding a person's home. It is important to assess the home situation to provide interventions that can support safety in the home. Occupational therapy practitioners often recommend home safety interventions to increase safety from the external surroundings (e.g., locks, lighting) and internal environment (e.g., trip hazards, access, lighting, handrails) and identify safety issues that may hinder a person exiting their home in a timely fashion (e.g., doors or windows that do not open, inaccessibility). Safe environments can become unsafe with function changes. A kitchen setup that has worked for decades may not be functional when new conditions, such as arthritis, a back injury, or balance issues, emerge. Moving often-used items to easy access spots or reducing the need to bend over to retrieve items may be necessary.

TABLE 15-5 ■ Common Home Management and IADL Type Home Adaptations

ADAPTATION	GOAL
De-Clutter Room	Facilitate access to rooms, cabinets, stairways, and to decrease fall risk.
Secure Carpets and Electrical Wiring	Decrease fall risk as people move around the environment.
Improve Lighting (general and task)	Adding task lighting in the kitchen can improve performance and increase safety in terms of preparing and cooking food. Lighting as a whole can decrease fall risk.
Provide Nonslip Mats, and/or Flooring	Could decrease risk of slipping and falling around the kitchen sink and dishwasher.
Provide Seating in Work Areas	If needed, this can improve performance and safety by reducing the physical demand and fatigue.
Adapt Counter Heights in Kitchen	For those who need to sit while working in the kitchen this will improve performance and safety.
Appliance Choice	Certain appliances are more easily accessible. Side by side refrigerator/freezers, raised front loading washers and dryers. Install a microwave oven to decrease or replace need for regular oven. These changes can improve performance and safety.
Lighting and Color Contrast in Kitchen, Office, etc.	Adapting can improve visibility without glare to improve performance, general safety, and decrease fall risk.
Pullout Drawers in Lower Cabinets	To reduce the need to bend down low and reach. Beneficial to protect the back and to increase efficiency and safety.
Changing Door and Cabinet Handles	Longer D shaped or lever shaped handles are easier to use and require less fine motor skills than small knobs.
Change Faucet in Kitchen	Lever or even hands-free type faucets reduce the need for strength and fine motor skills.

Disaster Preparedness

Being prepared in case of a disaster is crucial for independent, community-dwelling older adults. Unfortunately, research has shown that communities do not place a high priority on promoting disaster preparedness, and when preparedness activities did occur they were not tailored to older adults (Shih et al, 2018). Individuals may have to evacuate their home or shelter in place when there is a natural disaster. Depending on the disaster, there may not be a period of warning. Although a natural disaster is stressful and scary for everyone, for older adults there may be additional challenges (e.g., mobility problems, health conditions, lack of family support nearby). Additionally, sensory or cognitive changes may negatively affect an older adult in accessing, understanding, and responding to emergency instruction (CDC, n.d.). Resources are available to help older adults develop a disaster-preparedness plan. For example, the American Red Cross has many informational and useable products to help people understand what is needed (American Red Cross, n.d.). One resource is an Older Adult Disaster Preparation Booklet (American Red Cross, 2020). This booklet provides information related to becoming knowledgeable about emergency preparedness in an individual's community, assessing an individual's current supports and barriers, evaluating and developing a support network, creating a plan (including for pets), developing a communication/emergency contact list, gathering supplies, and preparing key documents. Occupational therapy practitioners are well-suited to help people prepare for emergencies and disaster (AOTA, 2017).

Care Partner Training

It is always important to understand and acknowledge that caregiving is an important role in the lives of many older adults (see Chapter 20). Care partners can be informal (family/friends) or formal (paid caregiver). When a client requires caregiver support, the occupational therapist must work with care partners as well, which can increase the complexity of service and requires strong communication skills as a practitioner. As IADL performance is typically addressed with older adults living in the community, care partners are often involved to some degree or another. The presence of a care partner can extend the length of time an older adult can continue participating in home management tasks. Occupational therapy practitioners can help facilitate skills such as communication, stress management, coping skills, problem-solving, skill training, healthy lifestyle management, support groups, and knowledge of available services (O'Sullivan, 2016). Occupational therapy practitioners must include the care partner as part of the team, give them the information and training they need, and help them manage daily details and promote self-care.

CASE STUDY (CONTINUED)

Intervention Plan

Sybil participated in 10 sessions of occupational therapy over 5 weeks. The occupational therapy intervention plan included development of personal goal and task lists, incorporation of her scrapbooking and journaling hobbies, energy conservation education, dual task training to improve balance and reduce fall risk, environmental and task compensations and adaptations to support meal preparation and laundry tasks, and task-specific training to use an emergency plan.

Discharge Status

Sybil met her goals within the initial 5-week intervention plan. She reported that she was less fearful of falling after improving her balance and incorporating the seated task adaptations to her home management activities, more satisfied with IADL performance, and experienced less fatigue after incorporating energy conservation techniques. Sybil and her wife reported satisfaction with the safety and emergency plans they currently have in place at home.

Questions

1. Why might the occupational therapist have used the chosen evaluation strategy and assessments?
2. Would other assessments have been appropriate to use with this client?
3. What other goals might be addressed with Sybil and why?
4. What factors should be considered when developing an intervention plan?
5. What assistive technology or environmental modifications could be recommended?
6. What factors support Sybil's performance of IADLs?

Answers

1. Evaluations and task observations in the client's natural environment provide an opportunity to evaluate tasks as well as how the environment supports or impairs function. The COPM was chosen because it allowed the occupational therapist to understand the IADLs and home management activities that were most important to the client and track progress toward her goals. The ACLS-5 was used to assist in understanding the type of cognitive support Sybil might need in developing an emergency plan and in structuring the task-specific training strategy as well as the compensatory and adaptive techniques used for home management. (See the section on Assessments for Home Management and IADLs and the case study section on assessment.)
2. Other assessments that might have been used with the client are the KELS and the Kitchen Picture Test. (See Table 15-4: Assessments for IADLs and Home Management.)
3. Beyond the IADLs and home management activities addressed in the case study, a full occupational therapy evaluation might reveal additional areas for intervention. Though the case study mentioned that she was independent in ADLs, one could imagine that Sybil might identify additional housekeeping tasks as specific goals or that her satisfaction with leisure and social participation might have been affected by MDD, MCI, or decreased activity tolerance. (See the case study section on the occupational profile.)
4. When developing an intervention plan, occupational therapists should consider the client's occupational profile and goals, historical information provided in the evaluation by the client and care partners, the analysis of assessment results, and environmental and social factors. Care should be given to design interventions that are personally meaningful to the client. (See the sections on Assessments and Interventions for Home Management and IADLs, and the case study sections on the occupational profile and assessments.)
5. Environmental modifications that could be beneficial to Sybil might include increasing the availability of seating throughout the home to compensate for decreased activity tolerance and adapting the laundry room by positioning machines to decrease the balance demands of the activity or adding a seat to conserve energy during the task. (See the Environmental modification section.)
6. Sybil has many supportive factors. She is motivated by her desire to return to her daily routines and home management tasks, she has self-awareness of safety concerns related to her cognition, and she has a supportive wife, both of whom have already collaborated on solutions to challenges such as transitioning the financial management duties and Sybil's fear of falling in the shower (see case study section on the occupational profile).

SUMMARY

Home management is important for older adults who wish to remain living in the community as independently as possible. Deficits in home management skills can be the first indicator of functional change. Helping older adults maintain or improve IADL performance can be strongly influenced by factors such as overall health, the burden of chronic condition management, level of social support, and supportiveness of the built and social environments in which they live. Social inequities throughout a lifespan may influence the trajectory of a person's aging and ultimately their ability to maintain function and independence.

Providing occupational therapy services requires a person-centered approach, including shared goal setting and prioritization as well as assessment of performance in an individual's own environment, if possible. Interventions can address remediation, adapting, modifying, and compensating the environment and home management tasks that the individual needs to perform. Helping older adults successfully live in the location of their choosing with the appropriate skills and supports in place can lead to better health outcomes and greater quality of life.

Critical Thinking Questions

1. In the mini case study, what aspects of Mrs. Wilson's current situation would be important for an occupational therapist to understand and consider when developing goals and a treatment plan?

2. Describe the process an occupational therapist would take when they start providing services to a community-dwelling older adult who is having problems performing home management tasks. What are key components of developing goals and a treatment plan? What decisions might be made in choosing the proper assessment(s) and intervention(s)?

REFERENCES

AACESSIBLE. (2022). *Lending libraries.* https://www.aaccessible.org/at-lending-libraries

Allen, C. K. (1991). Cognitive disability and reimbursement for rehabilitation and psychiatry. *Journal of Insurance Medicine, 23*(4), 245–247.

Allen, C. K., Austin, S. L., David, S. K., Earhart, C. A., McCraith, D. B, & Riska-Williams, L. (2007). *Manual for the Allen cognitive Level Screen-5 (ACLS-5) and Large Allen Cognitive Level Screen-5 (LACLS-5).* ACLS and LACLS Committee.

American Association of Retired Persons, & Davis, K. M. (2021a). *Despite pandemic, percentage of older adults who want to age in place stays steady.* https://www.aarp.org/home-family/your-home/info-2021/home-and-community-preferences-survey.html

American Association of Retired Persons, & Pajer, N. (2021b). *Your home checklist for aging in place.* https://www.aarp.org/home-family/your-home/info-2021/aging-in-place-checklist.html

American Occupational Therapy Association. (2022). *Domain and process: Evaluation and assessment.* https://www.aota.org/practice/domain-and-process/evaluation-and-assessment

American Occupational Therapy Association. (2020). Occupational therapy practice framework: Domain and process (4th ed.). *American Journal of Occupational Therapy, 74*(Suppl. 2), 7412410010. https://doi.org/10.5014/ajot.2020.74S2001

American Occupational Therapy Association. (2017). AOTA's societal statement on disaster response and risk reduction. *American Journal of Occupational Therapy, 71*(Suppl. 2), 7112410060p1–7112410060p3. https://doi.org/10.5014/ajot.2017.716S11

American Occupational Therapy Association. (2014). *Occupational therapy's role in pain rehabilitation fact sheet.* https://www.aota.org/~/media/Corporate/Files/AboutOT/Professionals/WhatIsOT/HW/Facts/Pain%20Rehabilitation%20fact%20sheet.pdf

American Red Cross. (n.d.). *How to prepare before a disaster occurs.* https://www.redcross.org/get-help/how-to-prepare-for-emergencies/older-adults.html

American Red Cross. (2020). *Disaster and emergency preparedness for older adults: A practical guide to help plan, respond, and recover.* https://www.redcross.org/content/dam/redcross/get-help/how-to-prepare/Older_Adults_Disaster_Prep_Booklet_07272020.pdf

Baum, C., Christiansen, C., & Bass, J. (2015). Person-environnement-occupations performance model. In C. Christiansen, C. Baum, J. Bass (Eds.), *Occupational therapy: Performance, participation, well-being.* (4th ed.). Slack.

Baum, C. M., Morrison, T., Hahn, M., & Edwards, D. F. (2003). *Test manual: Executive function performance test.* Washington University.

Bosse, H. M., Mohr, J., Buss, B., Krautter, M., Weyrich, P., Herzog, W., Junger, J., & Nikendei, C. (2015). The benefit of repetitive skills training and frequency of expert feedback in the early acquisition of procedural skills. *BMC Medical Education, 15,* 22. https://doi.org/10.1186/s12909-015-0286-5

Brims, L., & Oliver, K. (2019). Effectiveness of assistive technology in improving the safety of people with dementia: A systematic review and meta-analysis. *Aging & Mental Health, 23*(8), 942–951. https://doi.org/10.1080/13607863.2018.1455805

Buckley, K., & Poole, S. (2014). Occupation and activity analysis. In J. Hinojosa & M. Blount (Eds.), *The texture of life: Occupations and related activities* (pp. 55–104). American Occupational Therapy Association.

Capdevila, E., Rodríguez-Bailón, M., Kapanadze, M., & Portell, M. (2020). Clinical utility of the Canadian occupational performance measure in older adult rehabilitation and nursing homes: Perceptions among occupational therapists and physiotherapists in Spain. *Occupational Therapy International, 2020,* Article ID 3071405. https://doi.org/10.1155/2020/3071405

Carrington, M., & Islam, M. S. (2022). The use of telehealth to perform occupational therapy home assessments: An integrative literature review. *Occupational Therapy in Health Care, 31,* 1–16.

Centers for Disease Control and Prevention. (n.d.). *Promoting health for older adults.* https://www.cdc.gov/chronicdisease/resources/publications/factsheets/promoting-health-for-older-adults.htm#:~:text=Aging%20increases%20the%20risk%20of,death%2C%20and%20health%20care%20costs

Chiu, T., & Oliver, R. (2006). Factor analysis and construct validity of the SAFER-HOME. *OTJR: Occupation, Participation & Health, 26*(4), 132–142.

Clemson, L., Fitzgerald, M., & Heard, R. (1999). Content validity of an assessment tool to identify home fall hazards: The Westmead Home Safety Assessment. *British Journal of Occupational Therapy, 62*(4), 171–179.

Cohen, E. S., & Coster, W. J. (2014). Unpacking our theoretical reasoning. In B. A. Boyt Schell, G. Gillen, & M. E. Scaffa (Eds.), *Willard & Spackman's Occupational Therapy, 12th edition.* Wolters Kluwar/Lippincott Williams & Wilkins.

Colich, N. L., Rosen, M. L., Williams, E. S., & McLaughlin, K. A. (2020). Biological aging in childhood and adolescence following experiences of threat and deprivation: A systematic review and meta-analysis. *Psychological Bulletin, 146*(9), 721–764. http://doi.org/10.1037/bul0000270

Collins, M. E. (2018). Occupational therapists' experience with assistive technology in provision of service to clients with Alzheimer's disease and related dementias. *Physical & Occupational Therapy in Geriatrics, 36*(2–3), 179–188. https://doi.org/10.1080/02703181.2018.1458770

Cullum, C. M., Saine, K., Chan, L. D., Martin-Cook, K., Gray, K. F., & Weiner, M. F. (2001). The Texas functional living scale. *Neuropsychiatry Neuropsychology Behavioral Neurology, 14*(2), 103–108.

De-Bernardi-Ojuel, L., Torres-Collado, L., & García-de-la-Hera, M. (2021). Occupational therapy interventions in adults with multiple sclerosis or amyotrophic lateral sclerosis: A scoping review. *International Journal of Environmental Research and Public Health, 18*(4), 1432. https://doi.org/10.3390/ijerph18041432

Dobkin, B. H., Carmichael, T. S. (2005). Principals of recovery after stroke. In M. Barnes, B. H. Dobkin, & J. Bogouslavsky (Eds.), *Recovery after stroke* (pp. 47– 66). Cambridge University Press.

Dykstra, P. A. (2015). Aging and social support. https://www.academia.edu/77442223/Aging_and_Social_Support

Eklund, J. H., Holmstrom, I. K., Kumlin, T., Kaminsky, E., Skoglund, K., Hoglander, J., Sundler, A. J., Conden, E., & Meranius M. S. (2019). "Same same or different?" A review of reviews of person-centered and patient-centered care. *Patient Education and Counseling, 102*(1), 3–11. https://doi.org/10.1016/j.pec.2018.08.029

Enemark Larsen, A., Rasmussen, B., Christensen, J. R. (2018). Enhancing a client-centered practice with the Canadian occupational performance measure. *Occupational Therapy International, 2018,* Article ID 5956301. https://doi.org/10.1155/2018/5956301

Feger, O. M., Willis, S. L., Thomas, K. R., Marsiske, M., Rebok, G. W., Felix, C. & Gross, A. L. (2020). Incident instrumental activities of daily living difficulty in older adults: Which comes first? Findings from the Advanced Cognitive Training for Independent and Vital Elderly

Study. *Frontiers in Neurology, 11,* 550577. http://doi.org/10.3389/fneur.2020.550577

Fisher, G., Burgess, B., DiMassimo, H., Florenzo, C., Hymers, B., Kuchta, K., & Natale, O. (2019) *Cougar home safety assessment 5.0.* https://resources.finalsite.net/images/v1587754449/misericordia/ectokqd4oenv9yx8seau/chsa_50_April_11_2019.pdf

Fong, J. H. (2019). Disability incidence and functional decline among older adults with major chronic diseases. *BMC Geriatrics, 19,* 323–332. https://doi.org/10.1186/s12877-019-1348-z

Gitlin, L., & Corcoran, M. (2005). *Occupational therapy in dementia care.* American Occupational Therapy Association.

Guo, H. J. & Sapra, A. (2022). Instrumental activity of daily living. StatPearls. PMID: 31985920 Bookshelf ID: NBK553126

Hosp, J. A., Mann, S., Wegenast-Braun, B. M., Calhoun, M. E., Luft, A. R. (2013). Region and task-specific activation of Arc in primary motor cortex of rats following motor skill learning. *Neuroscience, 250*(10), 557–564. https://doi.org/10.1016/j.neuroscience.2013.06.060

Hubbard I., & Parsons, M. (2009). The conventional care of therapists as acute stroke specialists: A case study. *International Journal of Therapy and Rehabilitation, 14,* 357–362.

Ibrahim, N. I., & Davies, S. (2012). Aging: Physical difficulties and safety in cooking tasks. *Work, 41,* 5152–5159. https://doi.org/10.3233/WOR-2012-0804-5152

Iecovich, E. (2014). Aging in place: From theory to practice. *Anthropological Notebooks, 20*(1), 21–33.

Knapp, H., Taub, E., Berman, A. (1963). Movements in monkeys with deafferented forelimbs. *Experimental Neurology, 7,* 305–315.

Kohlman Thomas, L., & Robnett, R. (2016). *KELS Kohlman evaluation of living skills.* American Occupational Therapy Association.

Kurahashi, A. M., Harvey, A., MacRae, H., Moulton, C., Dubrowski, A. (2011). Technical skills training improves the ability to learn. *Surgery, 149* (1), 1–6. https://doi.org/10.1016/j.surg.2010.03.006

Lahav, O., & Katz, N. (2020). Independent older adult's IADL and executive function according to cognitive performance. *OTJR, Occupation, Participation and Health, 40*(3), 183–189. https://doi.org/10.1177/1539449220905813

Law, M., Baptiste, S., McColl, M., Opzoomer, A., Polatajko, H., Pollock, N. (1990). The Canadian occupational performance measure: An outcome measure for occupational therapy. *Canadian Journal of Occupational Therapy, 57*(2), 82–87. https://doi.org/10.1177/000841749005700207

Lawton, M. P. (1983). Environment and other determinants of well-being in older people. Robert W. Kleemeier Memorial Lecture. *Gerontologist, 23*(4), 349–357.

Lawton, M. P., & Brody, E. M. (1969). Assessment of older people: Self-maintaining and instrumental activities of daily living. *Gerontologist, 9*(3), 179–186.

Loeb, P. A. (1996). *The Independent Living Scales (ILS).* Pearson Assessment.

Mansbach, W. E., MacDougall, E. E., Clark, K. M., & Mace, R. A. (2014). Preliminary investigation of the Kitchen Picture Test (KPT): A new screening test of practical judgment for older adults. *Aging, Neuropsychology, and Cognition: A Journal on Normal and Dysfunctional Development, 21*(6), 674–692. https://doi.org/10.1080/13825585.2013.865698

Martin, G. M. (2017). The biology of aging: 1985–2010 and beyond. *FASEB Journal, 25*(11), 3756–3762. https://doi.org/10.1096/fj.11-1102.ufm

Mathiowetz, V., Nilsen, D., & Gillen, G. (2021) Task-oriented approach to stroke rehabilitation. In G. Gillen & D. M. Nilsen (Eds.), *Stroke rehabilitation: A function-based approach,* 5th edition. Elsevier.

Mayo Clinic. (n.d.). *Mild cognitive impairment.* https://www.mayoclinic.org/diseases-conditions/mild-cognitive-impairment/symptoms-causes/syc-20354578

Meucci, M., Gozalo, P., Dosa, D., & Allen, S. (2016). Variation in the presence of simple home modifications of older Americans: Findings from the National Health and Aging Trends Study. *Journal of the American Geriatric Society, 64*(10), 2081–2087. https://doi: 10.1111/jgs.14270

O'Sullivan, A. (2016). Community resources and living life to its fullest. In Vance, K. (Ed.), *Home health care: A guide for occupational therapy practice* (pp. 129–143). American Occupational Therapy Association.

Park, S., Kim, B., Amano, T., & Chen, Q. (2021). Home environment, living alone, and trajectories of cognitive function among older adults with functional limitations. *Environment and Behavior, 53*(3), 252–276. https://doi.org/10.1177/0013916519879772HOMETHERAPYSOLUTIONS, LLC

Racine, M., Jensen, M. P., Harth, M., Morley-Forster, P., & Nielson, W. R. (2019). Operant learning versus energy conservation activity pacing treatments in a sample of patients with fibromyalgia syndrome: A pilot randomized controlled trial. *Journal of Pain, 20*(4), 420–439. https://doi.org/10.1016/j.jpain.2018.09.013

Rea, I. M., Dellet, M., & Mills, K. I. (2016). Living long and ageing well: Is epigenomics the missing link between nature and nurture? *Biogerontology, 17,* 33–54. https://doi.org/ 10.1007/s10522-015-9589-5

Read, J., Jones, N., Fegan, C., Cudd, P., Simpson, E., Mazumdar, S., & Ciravegna, F. (2020). Remote home visit: Exploring the feasibility, acceptability and potential benefits of using digital technology to undertake occupational therapy home assessments. *British Journal of Occupational Therapy, 83*(10), 648–658. https://doi.org/10.1177/0308022620921111

Rijpkema, C., Duijts, S. F., & Stuiver, M. M. (2020). Reasons for and outcome of occupational therapy consultation and treatment in the context of multidisciplinary cancer rehabilitation; a historical cohort study. *Australian Occupational Therapy Journal, 67*(3), 260–268. https://doi.org/10.1111/1440-1630.12649

Rogers J. C., Holm M. B., Beach S., Schulz R., & Starz, T. W. (2001). Task independence, safety, and adequacy among nondisabled and osteoarthritis-disabled older women. *Arthritis & Rheumatology. 45*(5), 410–418. https://doi.org/ 10.1002/1529-0131(200110)45:5<410::aid-art359>3.0.co;2-y

Schmidt, R. A., & Lee, T. D. (2005). *Motor control and learning: A behavioural emphasis (4th edition).* Human Kinetics.

Sherman, S. M., Cheng, Y., Fingerman, K. L., & Schnyer, D. M. (2016). Social support, stress and the aging brain. *Social Cognitive and Affective Neuroscience, 11*(7), 1050–1058. https://doi.org/10.1093/scan/nsv071

Shih, R. A., Acosta, J. D., Chen, E. K., Carbone, E. G., Xenakis, L., Adamson, D. M., & Chandra, A. (2018). Improving disaster resilience among older adults: Insights from public health departments and aging in place efforts. *Rand Health Quarterly, 8*(1), 3.

Shippee, N. D., Shah, N. D., May, C. R., Mair, F. S., & Montori, V. M. (2012). Cumulative complexity: A functional, patient-centered model of patient complexity can improve research and practice. *Journal of Clinical Epidemiology, 65,* 1041–1051. https://doi.org/10.1016/j.jclinepi.2012.05.005

Sriram, V., Jenkinson, C., & Peters, M. (2020). Carers' experience of using assistive technology for dementia care at home: A qualitative study. *BMJ Open, 10*(3), e034460. http://dx.doi.org/10.1136/bmjopen-2019-034460

Stark, S. L., Somerville, E. K., & Morris, J. C. (2010). In home occupational performance evaluation (I-HOPe). *American Journal of Occupational Therapy, 64*(4), 580–589. https://doi.org/10.5014/ajot.2010.08065

Struckmeyer, L., Pickens, N., Brown, D., & Mitchell, K. (2020). Home Environmental Assessment Protocol-Revised (HEAP-R) initial psychometrics; a pilot study. *OTJR: Occupation, Participation, & Health, 40*(3), 175–182. doi: 10.1177/1539449220912186

Tabira, T., Hotta, M., Murata, M., Yoshiura, K., Han, G., Ishikawa, T., Koyama, A., Ogawa, N., Maruta, M., Ikeda, Y., Mori, T., Yoshida, T., Hashimoto, M., & Ikeda, M. (2020). Age-related changes in instrumental and basic activities of daily living impairment in older adults with very mild Alzheimer's disease. *Dementia and Geriatric Cognitive Disorders, 10,* 27–37. https://doi.org/10.1159/000506281

Teasell, R. W., Foley, N. C., Salter, K. L., & Jutai, J. W. (2008). A blueprint for transforming stroke rehabilitation care in Canada: The case for change. *Archives of Physical Medicine and Rehabilitation, 89,* 575–578. https://doi.org/10.1016/j.apmr.2007.08.164

Thoits, P. A. (2011). Mechanisms linking social ties and support to physical and mental health. *Journal of Health and Social Behavior, 52*(2), 145–161. https://doi.org/10.1177/0022146510395592

Vatwani, A., & Margonis, R. (2019). Energy conservation techniques to decrease fatigue. *Archives of Physical Medicine and Rehabilitation, 100*(6), 1193–1196. https://doi.org/10.1016/j.apmr.2019.01.005

Wallock, K. E. & Cerny, S. L. (2021). Benefits of smart home technology for individuals living with Amyotrophic Lateral Sclerosis. *Assistive Technology Outcomes and Benefits, 15*(1), 132–138.

Wei, M. Y., Levine, D. A., Zahodne, L. B., Kabeto, M. U., & Langa, K. M. (2020). Multimorbidity and cognitive decline over 14 years in older Americans. *Journals of Gerontology: Medical Sciences, 75*(6), 1206–1213. https://doi.org/10.1093/erona/glz147

Wolf, T. J., Chuh, A., Floyd, T., McInnis, K., & Williams, E. (2015). Effectiveness of occupation-based interventions to improve areas of occupation and social participation after stroke: An evidence-based review. *American Journal of Occupational Therapy, 69*(1), 6901180060p1–6901180060p11. https:// doi.org/10.5014/ajot.2015.012195

CHAPTER 16

Health Management and Sleep

Stacy Smallfield, DrOT, OTR/L, BCG, FAOTA
Katelyn Mwangi, OTD, MSOT, OTR/L ▪ Isabelle Laposha, OTD, OTR/L

"Health is, therefore, seen as a resource for everyday life, not the objective of living."

—Ottawa Charter for Health Promotion

LEARNING OUTCOMES

By the end of this chapter, readers will be able to:

16-1. Articulate the relationship between health management, sleep, and occupational therapy with older adults.
16-2. Relate age-related changes and common health conditions in older adulthood to health management and sleep.
16-3. Apply theoretical knowledge to health management and sleep in older adults.
16-4. Select common occupational therapy assessments to use when addressing health management and sleep for older adults.
16-5. Create occupational therapy interventions supported by evidence that promote health management and sleep for older adults.
16-6. Apply knowledge of health management and sleep to a case scenario.

Mini Case Study

Gladys is a 78-year-old Asian American female who uses she/her pronouns, with diagnoses of diabetes, hypertension, and diabetic retinopathy. Gladys sustained a cerebral vascular accident (CVA) 5 years ago, with residual left-sided weakness, decreased balance, and mild cognitive deficits. Since her CVA and progressive visual impairment, Gladys receives assistance with community mobility, mostly for doctors appointments and grocery shopping. Gladys also receives assistance for instrumental activities of daily living (IADLs), including cooking, cleaning, and check-ins on her medication management.

Before the pandemic, Gladys enjoyed spending time with family and friends, socializing at the senior center, and living a healthy lifestyle with her partner. Gladys lived with her partner of 30 years in a one-bedroom apartment until they recently passed away due to COVID-19.

With the pandemic and the passing of her partner, Gladys has experienced decreased mood with disruptions to her sleep and social participation. Gladys's partner drove her to medical appointments, but since her passing, Gladys has missed several follow-up visits and medication refills. She attempted to use telehealth but has found the use of technology frustrating. Gladys has also found exercising and healthy eating to be challenging. Gladys feels unsafe walking around her neighborhood due to her balance but also feels she does not have the space to exercise in her apartment. Her partner cooked most of their meals, because Gladys has a difficult time reading ingredient labels and recipes. Gladys is now eating one meal a day because of challenges with cooking and financial difficulty since the passing of her partner.

This chapter will provide you with the knowledge, assessment tools, and interventions to address Gladys' concerns with managing her health.

Provocative Questions
1. What factors of health management and sleep is Gladys demonstrating difficulty with during her daily routine?
2. What occupational therapy assessment and intervention strategies could address Gladys's management of her health conditions?

Health is a complex concept that consists of many factors, including physical, mental, social, and spiritual wellness. Presence of chronic conditions and poor health affect quality of life and occupational performance; therefore, effective health management routines are critical for older adults to achieve high levels of wellness (Barile et al, 2013). **Health management** includes managing medications and health appointments, engaging in physical activity, consuming adequate nutrition, and maintaining one's mental health. Effective engagement in these occupations, in addition to getting adequate sleep and rest, not only promotes health and wellness but also enables participation in other categories of occupations, including ADLs, leisure, and social participation. As individuals age and health complications become more prevalent, occupational therapy practitioners can play a role in promoting effective health management and sleep routines.

This chapter begins by conceptualizing health and health management, incorporating both a global perspective and specific definitions used in the occupational therapy profession. From these definitions, the text examines the connection between health conditions in older adulthood and managing health, including changes in vision, hearing, cognition, and mobility. Sleep and sleep patterns in older adulthood are defined, including the relationship between sleep and chronic health conditions and the impact of poor-quality sleep on occupational performance. In addition to person factors, this chapter discusses the impact of environmental factors on managing health and sleep, such as social support, social determinants of health, and environmental modifications. Using a theoretical foundation, readers will learn about assessments and interventions to address sleep and health management in clinical practice. The chapter concludes with a case study, in which readers are encouraged to apply their knowledge of sleep and health management.

Defining Health

Before describing health management occupations further, it is important to define the concept of health. The World Health Organization (WHO, 2006) defines health as "a state of complete physical, mental, and social well-being and not merely the absence of disease or infirmity" (p. 1). However, this definition has faced criticism due to its emphasis on complete well-being, which excludes older adults and individuals with chronic conditions (Card, 2017; Leonardi, 2018). By this definition, most older adults would be considered unhealthy. Experts have proposed new definitions related to health that prioritize the subjective experience and individual perception of one's own wellness. These experts base the concept of healthy living on an individual's resilience, including the ability to adapt, cope, self-manage, and maintain one's wellness in the face of challenging circumstances (Card, 2017; Huber et al, 2011; Leonardi, 2018). They describe health as a dynamic process that changes across one's lifetime (Leonardi, 2018).

This redefined understanding of health has important implications for older adults. As established in previous chapters, changes in the body caused by aging make individuals more vulnerable to some health conditions. Consequently, managing one's health becomes more challenging. In the face of decreased physical functioning, older adults must alter their health management routines to maintain their overall health and wellness; if they are able to do this effectively, older adults can still subjectively experience high levels of health. This idea is consistent with data from the 2018 National Health Interview Survey (Centers for Disease Control and Prevention [CDC]) in which 41.4% of adults age 75 and older rated their health as excellent or very good, 32.5% rated their health as good, and only 26% rated their health as fair or poor, despite the physical deconditioning and chronic conditions that accompany aging. Older adults report that they place less value on physical functioning. Instead, they report that health and aging well are more strongly influenced by mental well-being, life purpose and satisfaction, independence, social engagement, and remaining active (Halaweh et al, 2018; Spuling et al, 2015). When working with older adults in clinical practice, it is important to apply a holistic definition of health that not only addresses physical functioning but also addresses mental, social, and spiritual health, as this reflects the values reported by this population.

Health Management

In the Occupational Therapy Practice Framework, health management is defined as "activities related to developing, managing, and maintaining health and wellness routines, including self-management, with the goal of improving or maintaining health to support participation in other occupations" (American Occupational Therapy Association [AOTA], 2020a, p. 32). Health management includes seven different occupations:

- Social and emotional health promotion and maintenance
- Symptom and condition management
- Communication with the healthcare system
- Medication management
- Physical activity
- Nutrition management
- Personal care device management (AOTA, 2020a)

These occupations reflect a more holistic definition of health, including physical, social, and emotional components. Effective engagement in these health management occupations promotes overall health and wellness and supports occupational performance and participation. Refer to Table 16-1 for examples of health management occupations.

From a global perspective, the International Classification of Functioning, Disability and Health (ICF) does not define the concept of health management; instead, it describes the activity of "looking after one's health" (WHO, 2001, d570). This activity involves managing one's physical and mental health and includes "maintaining a balanced diet, and an appropriate level of physical activity, keeping warm or cool, avoiding harms to health, following safe sex practices... getting immunizations and regular physical examinations" (WHO, 2001, d570).

Looking after one's health is divided into three components. The first, ensuring one's physical comfort, includes regulating one's body position, lighting, moisture, and temperature. The second component involves managing one's nutrition and fitness, which aligns with *the Framework* (AOTA, 2020a). The final component, maintaining one's health, involves following medical advice and avoiding health risks, including injury, drug-taking, and sexually transmitted disease.

TABLE 16-1 ■ Examples of Health Management Occupations

HEALTH MANAGEMENT OCCUPATIONS	EXAMPLES
Social and emotional health promotion and maintenance	Regulating emotions, expressing one's needs; developing self-identity, engaging in social and leisure activities that support wellness
Symptom and condition management	Managing pain; managing chronic conditions; tracking fluctuations in symptoms; using coping strategies for illness, trauma history or societal stigma; using emotion-regulation strategies
Communication with the healthcare system	Expressing and obtaining oral, written, or digital communication with healthcare practitioners, organizations, and insurance providers; advocating for oneself to the healthcare system
Medication management	Filling/refilling prescriptions, adhering to medication routines, understanding medication instructions, understanding and managing medication side effects
Physical activity	Engaging in cardiovascular exercise, strength training, or balance training that promotes health
Nutrition management	Preparing meals that support one's health goals, following hydration and nutrition recommendations
Personal care device management	Obtaining and maintaining personal care devices such as hearing aids, glasses, orthotics, mobility devices, adaptive equipment, glucometers, personal alert systems, or dentures

Note: Table adapted from *the Framework* (AOTA, 2020a).

Social Determinants of Health

In 1986, WHO published the Ottawa Charter for Health Promotion, an international agreement that proposed new ideas related to health promotion. WHO described health as "a resource for everyday life, not the object of living" (p. 1). From this perspective, health is a means to living well, which highlights the impact of health management on successful performance and participation in other categories of occupation. In addition, WHO identified fundamental resources that must be present in order to improve one's health. These prerequisites for health are peace, shelter, education, food, income, a stable ecosystem, sustainable resources, social justice, and equity. Thus, it is important to remember that older adults must feel secure in these foundational needs before they can address or improve their health and well-being.

Since the Ottawa Charter for Health Promotion was published, WHO has also defined the concept of social determinants of health. WHO defines social determinants as "the conditions in which people are born, grow, work, live and age and their access to power, money and resources" (WHO, 2021, p. 1). These conditions affect a variety of health, wellness, and quality of life outcomes. Examples of social determinants of health include education access and quality, access to safe housing and transportation, job opportunities, influence of political and economic systems, pollution, social inclusion, food security, and access to quality healthcare services. Social determinants of health strongly influence health outcomes, including how individuals engage in health management occupations. For example, older adults may struggle to eat nutritious food if they do not live close to a grocery store, and they may not engage in physical activity if they feel unsafe where they live. Because social determinants of health are a barrier to occupational participation and performance, occupational therapy practitioners must address these barriers in the lives of the patients, communities, and populations they serve.

Accessing and Using Health Care Services

Older adults undergo a variety of physical and cognitive changes that have an impact on their ability to manage their health effectively. Because of these changes and the prevalence of chronic conditions, older adults spend more time accessing healthcare services than other age groups (CDC, 2009). Access to healthcare services is highly influenced by demographic characteristics, including socioeconomic status. Cost is a barrier to health management, as 23% of older adults in the United States reported that they skipped accessing healthcare services in the previous year due to high cost (Osborn et al, 2017). A scoping review by McGilton et al (2018) studied healthcare needs of older adults with multiple chronic conditions and their care partners. Healthcare barriers included lack of information such as explanations from healthcare practitioners regarding conditions, medication, and treatment. They reported struggling with poor coordination of care and services, including lack of specialists, long wait times, and poor communication among multiple providers (McGilton et al, 2018). These environmental barriers negatively affect the ability of older adults to effectively manage their health.

Healthcare providers report that patient education level and health literacy are also barriers to effective health management of older adults (McGilton et al, 2018). There are different types of health literacy, and each influences one's ability to communicate with the healthcare system. **Personal health literacy** is an individual's ability to obtain, interpret, and use information to make appropriate decisions regarding health. **Organizational health literacy** is the degree to which organizations enable individuals to obtain, interpret, and use information to make health-related decisions (U.S. Department of Health and Human Services, 2021). Thus, healthcare systems and providers, including occupational therapy practitioners, have the responsibility to use clear language and share information equitably to empower clients to make decisions that support their health and wellness.

Many healthcare systems now rely on electronic communication with patients. Experts have proposed the concept of eHealth literacy as distinct from other types of health literacy. **eHealth literacy** is defined as the ability to seek, appraise, and understand health information from electronic sources and apply this knowledge to solve problems related to one's health (Norman & Skinner, 2006). Monkman and colleagues (2017) found that there is not a relationship between health literacy and eHealth literacy; an older adult may have a high level of health literacy, but this skill may not translate to electronic sources. Nguyen & Roberts (2021) found older adults are at increased risk for decreased participation in health management using electronic technologies. Occupational therapy practitioners can educate older adults on the use of electronic sources to increase their independence with health management.

Impact of Health Conditions on Health Management

Many older adults live with chronic health conditions, which often affect their ability to manage their health. The National Council on Aging (2021b) reported that 80% of older adults have at least one chronic condition, and nearly 70% have two or more conditions. The following paragraphs explore how age-related sensory changes, cognitive decline, and mobility challenges influence older adults' ability to manage their health.

Impact of Sensory Changes on Health Management

Sensory changes can affect older adults' ability to manage health. The roles of vision and hearing in this process are described next.

Vision

Older adults with low vision are more likely to demonstrate occupational performance difficulties with ADLs, IADLs including driving, and social interaction (Brown et al, 2014). Additionally, older adults with low vision have increased difficulty managing their own health conditions, including difficulties with healthy meal preparation, appropriately managing their medications, and accessing healthcare services. Individuals living with low vision are more likely to be diagnosed with depression and anxiety (Kempen et al, 2012). Visual impairment among older adults is associated with an increase in chronic health conditions and higher incidence of stroke and heart disease (Crews et al, 2006). (See Chapter 10 for more information on sensory impairments.)

Hearing

For adults, age is the highest predictor for loss of auditory function; the prevalence of hearing loss is up to two-thirds of older adults over the age of 70 (Hoffman et al, 2017; Lin et al, 2011). More than 22 million older adults in the United States with hearing loss do not use hearing aids (Chien & Lin, 2012). Older adults living with hearing loss are less likely to engage in social participation, increasing the likelihood of isolation and possible emotional disturbances (National Council on Aging, 2021a). When looking at overall quality of life and health, 39% of older adults with hearing impairment felt they had excellent health, compared with 68% of age-matched peers without hearing impairment (Monzani et al, 2008). Hearing loss can affect an older adults' ability to communicate with the healthcare system, especially with interpersonal interactions that require hearing. This can be further complicated for adults living with dual sensory impairment that affects both the auditory and visual systems, occurring in up to 23% of adults over the age of 81 (Bergman & Rosenhall, 2001). (See Chapter 10 for more information on sensory impairments.)

Impact of Cognitive Changes on Health Management

The number of individuals worldwide living with dementia is around 50 million, with the frequency increasing as the population ages (Alzheimer's Disease International, 2018). Adults over the age of 65 with dementia on average live with four comorbidities, which is double that of age-matched peers without dementia (Poblador-Plou et al, 2014). In addition to dementia, around 30% of older adults develop age-related cognitive changes and 15% develop mild cognitive impairment, often affecting their executive functioning and higher-level cognitive abilities (Swanson & Carnahan, 2007). These cognitive changes can significantly impair the ability to care for one's health, including social and emotional health, communication with the healthcare system, medication and nutrition management, and physical activity.

Depression is commonly found in individuals with dementia and age-related cognitive changes and can significantly influence emotional well-being (Bennett & Thomas, 2014). Research has found a correlation between an increase in social isolation and worsening cognitive functioning in individuals with dementia (Shankar et al, 2013). This social isolation and depression in older adults with cognitive deficits could lead to difficulties in social engagement and participation, therefore affecting overall emotional health and well-being.

Older adults with cognitive impairments may experience difficulty with activities requiring higher level cognitive skills. Poor medication adherence has been found to correlate with cognitive dysfunction in up to 40% of older adults, specifically memory and executive functioning skills, making cognitive functioning the number one contributor to medication nonadherence (Suchy et al, 2020; Sumida et al, 2019). Executive functioning and working memory are two necessary components of cognitive functioning for proper medication management; both skills are significantly affected by dementia (Insel et al, 2006). Older adults with mild cognitive impairment have the same degree of confidence in their medication management skills compared with age-matched peers without cognitive deficits, indicating a decrease in awareness and insight related to performance skills (Sumida et al, 2019). In addition to dementia and mild cognitive impairment, several chronic health conditions prevalent in older adulthood—including heart disease, stroke, diabetes mellitus, arthritis, cancer, and kidney disease—can affect cognition. Cognitive impairment may limit the ability to effectively manage chronic health conditions with appropriate medications, exercise, and nutritional eating, further contributing to declines in health (CDC, 2020). (See Chapter 13 for more information on cognition and neurobehavioral conditions.)

Impact of Mobility on Health Management

Around one in four adults over the age of 65 sustains a fall each year (CDC, 2021). Older adults have an increased risk of falling due to age-related changes in the musculoskeletal system that affect strength and mobility of the lower extremities. In addition, older adults are more likely to be affected by visual conditions, vitamin deficiencies, and side effects of medications that cause dizziness or imbalance (CDC, 2021). Immonen et al (2020) found that older adults with chronic health conditions, including conditions such as diabetes mellitus, rheumatoid arthritis, Parkinson disease, and chronic obstructive pulmonary disease, are more likely to experience falls compared with those without chronic disease. Falling once increases the probability of sustaining another fall, potentially leading to serious medical complications, including fractures and traumatic brain injury (CDC, 2021). A fear of falling has been found to negatively affect performance of daily occupations, including self-care, community mobility, and IADLs (Liu et al, 2021). This fear can lead to social isolation, influencing an older adult's emotional and social well-being. Additionally, many older adults who have experienced a fall become less active, leading to further complications with mobility and maintaining proper physical exercise (Vellas et al, 1997). (See Chapter 7 for more information on falls and older adults.)

Impact of Social Support and Socioeconomic Status on Health Management

Older adults with sensory impairment, cognitive decline, and mobility challenges frequently rely on social support for appropriate management of medications and health. Older adults without these supports may be at an increased risk for poor management of their chronic health conditions. Additionally, socioeconomic status is an important factor to consider with health management in older adulthood. Older adults with a lower socioeconomic status are more likely to live more years with dementia compared with older adults in higher socioeconomic groups, incurring an overall higher lifetime expenditure on medication and care for their health condition (Cha et al, 2021). Individuals who have access to a variety of resources and care partner support are more likely to be on an appropriate medication management routine versus older adults without access to these services. (Refer to Promoting Best Practice 16-1 for more information regarding strategies for occupational therapy practitioners to support care partners of older adults.) This highlights an inequity in the aging process; those with financial means have the resources to care for their health conditions, whereas those without are at an increased risk for continued health decline.

PROMOTING BEST PRACTICE 16-1
Problem-Solving Training to Support Care Partners

Problem-solving training is an effective intervention to support care partners in the care partner role. For example, education and multistep strategy training to address problems improves depression among care partners of individuals post-stroke. These sessions can be conducted in person with telephone follow-up (Fields & Smallfield, 2022). Additionally, group-based intervention for care partners of individuals post-stroke improves mood and quality of life. Recommended content includes coping strategies, problem-solving skills, and education about the condition (Fields & Smallfield, 2022). Routine use of these interventions is recommended.

CASE STUDY
Occupational Profile

Lionel is an 81-year-old Black male who uses he/his pronouns. Lionel's medical history includes type 2 diabetes, peripheral artery disease (PAD), and left below-knee amputation (BKA) that occurred 4 years ago due to vascular problems. Lionel completes his ADLs without assistance, and he typically wears a prosthesis on his left lower extremity.

Lionel lives with his wife, Mary, in a one-story home in a rural area, and their two children live locally. Lionel serves as the primary caregiver for his wife, who has Alzheimer disease. He completes meal preparation, financial management, and medication management for the couple; however, he reports that keeping up with these occupations can be difficult.

Lionel was previously employed as a firefighter. He enjoys watching television and spending time with his four grandchildren, but he has given up other social activities to care for his wife. Although Lionel values his role as a husband, he reports that caring for Mary can be challenging. When he feels anxious about his role, Lionel experiences difficulty falling asleep. The couple used to walk together, but they have not done so since Lionel's amputation.

Lionel presents to his local geriatric primary care center for a well visit. During the visit, Lionel's physician identifies that it would be appropriate for him to see the center's new occupational therapist. After a brief evaluation regarding Lionel's health management and sleep routines, the occupational therapist identifies several occupational performance issues.

Identified Problem Areas Related to Health Management and Sleep
- Lionel reports difficulty managing medication.
- Lionel does not engage in regular physical activity.
- Lionel reports difficulty coping with Mary's Alzheimer disease symptoms.
- Lionel reports difficulty falling asleep.
- Lionel demonstrates poor diabetes management, such as lack of complete foot care.

Identified Strengths
- Lionel completes his ADLs without assistance.
- Lionel is experienced in donning his prosthesis during daily activities.
- Lionel lives in a one-story home, reducing the need to climb stairs.
- Lionel completes many tasks for his family, including meal preparation, financial management, and medication management.

Goals for Occupational Therapy
- Implement strategies for increasing Lionel's medication adherence
- Incorporate healthy exercise, nutrition, and sleep practices into Lionel's daily routine
- Implement appropriate coping strategies for Lionel's anxiety
- Increase Lionel's knowledge and skills regarding diabetes management

Sleep and Restoration

Sleep is a vital component of health and well-being and therefore can be considered one of the most important occupations in which humans engage (National Institutes of Health, 2017; Ramar et al, 2021; Tester & Foss, 2018; Walker, 2018). Although sleep is often considered one of the essential components of health—along with nutrition and physical activity, some researchers now consider it to be the foundation on which the others are built (Tester & Foss, 2018; Walker, 2018). AOTA (2020a) identifies sleep and rest as occupations that "...support healthy, active engagement in other occupations" (p. 32). Sleep preparation and participation are distinct from—but essential to—the management of health in older adulthood (Tester & Foss, 2018). In other words, sleep is a requirement for the management of health (Tester & Foss, 2018). The typical older adult requires 7 to 9 hours of sleep in a 24-hour period (National Institute on Aging [NIA], 2020; Ramar et al, 2021; Walker, 2018), but up to 40% to 70% of older adults may have difficulty sleeping (Gooneratne & Vitiello, 2014; Miner & Kryger, 2017; Tester & Foss, 2018). Inadequate sleep is such a significant health problem that it is recognized as a public health epidemic (CDC, 2015).

Sleep in Older Adults

Typical sleep patterns change with age, but age is not the sole cause of poor sleep (Gulia & Kumar, 2018; Loiselle et al, 2005; Vaz Fragoso & Gill, 2007). Typical sleep involves two main types of sleep: rapid eye movement (REM) sleep and nonrapid eye movement (NREM) or dream sleep. The NREM type of sleep is further divided into stages 1 through 3, with stage 3 NREM sleep being the deepest, most restorative sleep. Typical individuals sleeping 7 to 9 hours per night progress through stages 1 through 3 of NREM sleep followed by REM sleep four to five times each night (Gooneratne & Vitiello, 2014).

Compared with young adults, older adults often get sleepier earlier in the evening and wake earlier in the morning (Gulia & Kumar, 2018; Walker, 2018). Older adults have more difficulty falling asleep, sleep less deeply, and wake more frequently (Gulia & Kumar, 2018; Loiselle et al, 2005; NIA, 2020; Vaz Fragoso & Gill, 2007; Walker, 2018). Older adults average 5 to 7 hours of sleep per night, and when given the opportunity for maximum sleep capacity average 7.4 hours compared with 8.9 hours in young adults (Gooneratne & Vitiello, 2014). Additionally, time spent awake after sleep onset increases in older adults (Gooneratne & Vitiello, 2014). Because they may not get as much sleep at night as young adults, daytime napping is more common among older adults (Hereford, 2014; Walker, 2018). In addition to these objective measures of reduced sleep quality, older adults also subjectively report sleep disturbances more often than other age groups (Gooneratne & Vitiello, 2014). Furthermore, chronic health conditions, overall health status, and declining daytime activity level may be associated with aging and affect sleep quality. Therefore, occupational therapy practitioners working with older adults in a variety of settings will work with those who experience difficulties falling asleep, maintaining sleep, or getting the sleep needed for restoration.

Effects of Poor-Quality Sleep on Daytime Occupational Performance

Sleep provides the restoration needed for the performance of daytime occupations (Tester & Foss, 2018). Inadequate sleep or inconsistent sleep patterns can negatively affect the performance of daytime activity and the health of interpersonal relationships. Daytime fatigue due to poor sleep can impair safe driving; lead to decreased work productivity or an increase in errors on work tasks; strain social relationships, which can lead to isolation and loneliness; and increase risk of falling (Solet, 2019; Tester & Foss, 2018; NIH, 2017). Generally, disrupted sleep can lead to a decline in cognitive and physical function and greater use of healthcare services, including increased use of sleep medication (Chen et al,

2017; Walker, 2018). Long-term use of sleep medications has side effects of dependency, daytime drowsiness, nausea, fatigue, confusion, memory issues, and increased risk of falling (Chen et al, 2017; Walker, 2018).

The Relationship Between Sleep and Chronic Health Conditions in Older Adults

Many health conditions of aging, such as depression, anxiety, dementia, hypertension, respiratory conditions, physical disability, heart disease, diabetes, and conditions causing chronic pain, are associated with disrupted sleep (Gulia & Kumar, 2018). Those with multiple chronic health conditions get less than the recommended hours of sleep each night, have decreased quality of sleep, and experience symptoms of sleep disorders (Gulia & Kumar, 2018). Although chronic health conditions can lead to inadequate sleep, the reverse may also occur. Chronic sleep deprivation is associated with elevated risk of heart disease, stroke, and general morbidity and mortality (Gangwisch, 2014; NIH, 2017). Sleep disorders such as obstructive sleep apnea and restless leg syndrome are also more common in older adults (Gulia & Kumar, 2018).

It should be noted that there is a strong relationship between sleep and Alzheimer disease. Approximately 60% of older adults with Alzheimer disease experience sleep disorders (Walker, 2018). However, sleep deprivation also contributes to the development of Alzheimer disease (Walker, 2018). During sleep, the brain cycles through two main phases of sleep, REM sleep and NREM sleep. It is during deep NREM sleep that the brain receives a deep cleaning of cerebrospinal fluid that flushes out, among other toxins, the amyloid buildup commonly found in Alzheimer disease (Walker, 2018). Sleep deprivation, therefore, leads to increased amyloid deposits, especially in the areas of the brain responsible for NREM sleep. Without quality NREM sleep, more amyloid will accumulate. This creates a vicious cycle between poor sleep and the accumulation of the amyloid plaques common in Alzheimer disease. Adequate sleep, therefore, can delay or lower the risk of the onset of cognitive decline (Walker, 2018).

Theoretical Approaches to Successful Health Management in Older Adulthood

Theoretical knowledge guides professional reasoning. Problems are framed by theory, which drives evaluation processes and intervention decisions. One of several occupation-based models of practice such as the Kawa Model (Iwama, 2006), the Model of Human Occupation (Taylor, 2017), or the Person-Environment-Occupation-Performance Model (Baum et al, 2015) can be selected to organize professional reasoning and ensure the evaluation and intervention plan are client centered and occupation based. According to Ikiugu's framework for combining theoretical conceptual practice models in occupational therapy practice (Ikiugu et al, 2009), these occupation-based models can be combined with other complementary theoretical knowledge. Examples may include the cognitive orientation to daily occupational performance in occupational therapy (CO-OP) (Dawson et al, 2017) and the cognitive-behavioral intervention approaches. Application of these complementary theoretical approaches are highlighted in the intervention recommendations outlined next.

Occupational Therapy Assessment of Health Management and Sleep

A number of assessments can be used to measure aspects of health management and sleep. Refer to Table 16-2 for information regarding select assessment tools that might be considered. There is yet to be developed any one specific tool that captures all components of health management as discussed here. However, many assessments are available to assess the various components of health management. When used in combination, these assessments can provide a more global evaluation of the ability to manage health. Although standardized tools are recommended, informal interview or skilled observation by an occupational therapy practitioner can inform or supplement other more formal methods of data collection around health management and sleep.

In addition to the assessment methods listed in Table 16-2, it is worth noting that many software applications (apps) are available for assessment, data tracking, or monitoring of health status. Examples include apps that can track duration of physical activity, vital signs such as heart and respiration rates, blood glucose levels, medication reminders, and sleep duration and efficiency. There are also apps for tracking health information entered by the user, for example, amounts and types of food consumed, mood, or medication information. Apps can be useful in identifying trends, behaviors, habits, and routines over time, which is important for ongoing evaluation and monitoring. Computers and smartphones also serve as a primary vehicle for communicating health information with the healthcare system.

As part of the assessment process, it is also important to assess client factors, performance skills, performance patterns, and contexts that influence a person's ability to manage their own health. For example, cognitive changes may affect the ability to manage a medication routine or prepare nutritious meals. Movement-related functions such as muscle tone and endurance will influence physical activity. The living environment will influence sleep and overall wellness routines. Assessment of these factors in addition to assessment of specific components of health management are important for creating person-centered plans of care.

Occupational Therapy Interventions to Address Health Management and Sleep

A variety of evidence-based occupational therapy interventions can be utilized to address health management occupations.

TABLE 16-2 ■ Select Health Management and Sleep Assessment Tools

ASSESSMENT NAME AND CITATION	TYPE OF ASSESSMENT AND FACTORS ASSESSED	BRIEF DESCRIPTION	HOW TO OBTAIN
Social and Emotional Health Promotion and Maintenance			
Geriatric Depression Scale (Sheikh & Yesavage, 1986)	Self-report measure of depression symptoms in older adults	Participants respond yes/no to 15 items. Ten items indicate the presence of depression when answered positively, whereas five items indicate depression when answered negatively. A score greater than 5 indicates probable depression.	Available online at: https://integrationacademy.ahrq.gov/sites/default/files/2020-07/Update_Geriatric_Depression_Scale-15.pdf
UCLA three-item loneliness scale (Hughes et al, 2004)	A three-item self-report measure of loneliness: how often one feels they lack companionship, feels left out, and feels isolated from others	Each of the three items is rated on a 1 (hardly ever) to 3 (often) scale. Item scores are added so total scores range from 3 to 9. Scores of 3 to 5 indicate no loneliness, and scores of 6 to 9 indicate loneliness.	Hughes, M., E., Waite, L. J., Hawkely, L. C., & Cacioppo, J. T. (2004). A short scale for measuring loneliness in large surveys: Results from two population-based studies. *Research on Ageing, 26*(6), 655–672.
Well-being of Older People measure (WOOP) (Hackert et al, 2021)	Self-report scale that assesses well-being across nine domains: physical health, mental health, social contacts, receiving support, acceptance and resilience, feeling useful, independence, making ends meet, and living situation	Participants rate nine items on a 5-point Likert scale ranging from "bad" (1 point) to "excellent" (5 points). Higher scores indicate higher well-being.	Hackert, M., van Exel, J., & Brouwer, W. (2021). Content validation of the Well-being of Older People measure (WOOP). *Health and quality of life outcomes, 19*(1), 200. https://doi.org/10.1186/s12955-021-01834-5
Communication With the Health Care System			
eHEALS: the eHealth Literacy Scale (Norman & Skinner, 2006)	Self-report scale that assesses an individual's self-perceived F literacy	Participants rate eight items on a 5-point Likert scale ranging from "strongly agree" (1 point) to "strongly disagree" (5 points). Higher scores indicate higher eHealth literacy.	Norman, C. D., & Skinner, H. A. (2006). eHEALS: The eHealth Literacy Scale. *Journal of Medical Internet Research, 8*(4), e27. https://doi.org/10.2196/jmir.8.4.e27
Newest Vital Sign (Weiss et al, 2005)	Simulated performance-based task that assesses adult health literacy	Participants respond to six questions based on reading and interpreting a nutrition label; fewer than four correct responses indicates possibly limited health literacy.	Weiss, B. D., Mays, M. Z., Martz, W., Castro, K. M., DeWalt, D. A., Pignone, M. P., Mockbee, J., & Hale, F. A. (2005). Quick assessment of literacy in primary care: The newest vital sign. *Annals of Family Medicine, 3*(6), 514–522. https://doi.org/10.1370/afm.405
Medication Management			
Executive Function Performance Test (Baum et al, 2008)	Performance-based functional cognition assessment including medication management subtest	This is a functional cognitive assessment with four subtests: cooking, bill pay, phone use, and medication management. It involves specific guidelines for cuing.	Available free online: https://www.ot.wustl.edu/about/resources/executive-function-performance-test-efpt-308
Performance Assessment of Self-Care Skills (Rogers, 1984)	Performance-based ADLs and IADLs assessment including medication management subtest	This is a 26-item standardized assessment in which therapists can choose specific subtests relevant to the client. Two versions can be used: home and clinic. Normative data exists for Alzheimer disease and dementia.	Available free online following completion of survey: https://www.shrs.pitt.edu/ot/resources/performance-assessment-self-care-skills-pass
HOME–Rx (Somerville et al, 2019)	Performance-based medication management assessment	HOME–Rx is a medication management assessment looking at adherence to medication recommendations.	Please contact the author for assessment details.

TABLE 16-2 ■ Select Health Management and Sleep Assessment Tools—cont'd

ASSESSMENT NAME AND CITATION	TYPE OF ASSESSMENT AND FACTORS ASSESSED	BRIEF DESCRIPTION	HOW TO OBTAIN
Physical Activity and Nutrition Management			
Physical activity diary	Self-report of physical activity, including exercise and daily activities	The client completes an activity diary (physical activity log) to track physical activity, typically for a 1- to 2-week period.	There are many types of physical activity diaries. An example from the Centers for Disease Control and Prevention (CDC) is titled "My Physical Activity Diary." https://www.cdc.gov/healthyweight/pdf/physical_activity_diary_cdc.pdf
Nutrition management diary	Self-report of nutrition, including food and beverages consumed on a daily basis	The client completes a nutrition management diary to track food consumption, typically for a 1- to 2-week period.	There are varying types of nutrition management diaries. One example from the CDC is titled "My Food and Beverage Diary." https://www.cdc.gov/healthyweight/pdf/food_diary_cdc.pdf
Sleep and Rest			
Sleep diary	Self-report of daily sleep-related information such as bedtime, wake time, sleep latency, sleep interruptions, daytime naps, subjective sleep quality, substance and medication use, and exercise	Sleep diaries (also referred to as sleep logs or journals) are used to identify sleep habits and potential disruptions or factors that influence sleep quality. They are typically completed for 1 to 2 weeks at a time.	Many sleep diaries are publicly available. One example is the National Sleep Foundation Sleep Diary: https://pa-foundation.org/wp-content/uploads/NSF-Sleep-Diary.pdf
Epworth sleepiness scale (Johns, 1991, 1997)	Self-report of daytime sleepiness in eight activities: reading; watching television; sitting in public, such as in a meeting or at the theater; riding as a passenger in a vehicle; resting; talking with others; sitting quietly after lunch; and driving	Each item is scored on a scale of 0 to 3, where 0 = no dozing and 3 = high chance of dosing. Scores are totaled to determine a person's "average sleep propensity," or likeliness of daytime sleepiness ranging from normal to severe excessive daytime sleepiness.	Instructions for permission to use: https://eprovide.mapi-trust.org/instruments/epworth-sleepiness-scale
Pittsburgh Sleep Quality Index (Buysse et al, 1989)	Self-report measure of sleep quality, sleep latency, sleep duration, habitual sleep efficiency, sleep disturbances, use of medication for sleep, and daytime function over the last month	Each of the seven components is scored on a scale of 0 to 3 per instructions. Component scores are added together. A score of 5 or greater indicates poor sleep quality.	The instrument, scoring system and original article are available from the University of Pittsburgh: https://www.sleep.pitt.edu/instruments/#psqi
Health and Occupational Performance			
PROMIS Global Health	Self-report screener looking at overall health and well-being	PROMIS is a 10-question health screener measuring general, physical, mental, and social health on a 5-point scale. This screener can be completed via paper, computer, or app.	Free online: https://www.healthmeasures.net

Although these interventions have been grouped by occupation, many of these interventions benefit multiple occupations. For example, engagement in Lifestyle Redesign® or the Chronic Disease Self-Management Program may benefit both mental and physical health and addresses all categories of health management occupations (Clark et al, 2012; Lorig et al, 2019). Addressing cognition and use of cognitive approaches such as CO-OP can also improve performance and participation in all categories of health management occupations (Dawson et al, 2017). Although we have highlighted a selection of evidence-based interventions in this chapter, please note that other interventions can be useful to address health management occupations with older adult populations.

Social and Emotional Health Promotion and Maintenance

Occupational therapy interventions to address social and emotional health promotion and maintenance include Lifestyle Redesign® and Do Live Well framework.

Lifestyle Redesign®

Lifestyle Redesign® is an evidence-based intervention established by Clark and colleagues at the University of Southern California (Clark et al, 1997). This program is delivered in both group and individual formats over an extended period, and it has been modified for adults with a variety of health conditions, including hypertension, multiple sclerosis, cancer, Parkinson disease, and autism spectrum disorder. Lifestyle Redesign® enables individuals to develop, practice, and implement personalized daily routines that promote health and well-being. The program focuses on education, problem-solving, and raising self-awareness across lifestyle factors such as sleep routines, physical activity, time management, and coping strategies—all consistent with a cognitive-behavioral theoretical approach. Community-dwelling older adults who engaged in this preventative lifestyle intervention demonstrated improvements in mental well-being, including improved vitality, social function and life satisfaction, and decreased depressive symptoms (Clark et al, 2012).

Do Live Well Framework

Do Live Well is an evidence-based Canadian framework that emphasizes the impact of daily occupations on health and well-being (Moll et al, 2015). Much of the framework's supporting evidence was established through studies of older adults. The framework includes eight different dimensions of experience and five activity patterns that affect wellness outcomes. The dimensions of experience include eight categories of occupation: activating your body, mind, and senses; connecting with others; contributing to society; taking care of yourself; building security/prosperity; developing and expressing identity; developing capability and potential; and experiencing joy and pleasure consistent with cognitive-behavioral theoretical knowledge. Individuals must also experience a balance of five characteristics related to their occupational engagement; these activity patterns are engagement, meaning, balance, control/choice, and routine. The framework is particularly useful during periods of transition, such as the occupational changes experienced by older adults. Occupational therapy practitioners can use Do Live Well in their practice to promote individual reflection, community advocacy, or system-level dialogue that encourages engagement in healthful occupations and routines (Moll et al, 2015).

Symptom and Condition Management

Occupational therapy interventions to address symptom and condition management include engagement in self-management programs.

Self-Management Programs

Evidence supports the use of self-management interventions to improve occupational performance related to symptom and condition management. There is also moderate evidence that these programs support reduction in pain and increase in physical activity (Arbesman & Mosley, 2012). Self-management interventions aim to educate clients on skills needed for living with health conditions. Interventions may address goal-setting, problem-solving, and coping skills and provide opportunities for practice and mastery of these skills. These programs are consistent with a cognitive-behavioral approach and are often tailored to individuals with one or more chronic conditions. Self-management interventions can be provided in individual or group formats, and they often occur over an extended period. Although these programs may be delivered via telehealth services, several programs have found face-to-face interaction to be most effective in improving occupational performance (Jonkers et al, 2012; Lewin et al, 2013). These programs can be provided in community-based settings, and they can address goals of health promotion, maintenance, or restoration (Garvey et al, 2015). See Promoting Best Practice 16-2 for more information regarding recommendations for chronic disease self-management programs.

> ## PROMOTING BEST PRACTICE 16-2
> ### Chronic Disease Self-Management Programs
>
> Routine use of chronic disease self-management programs (CDSMPs) or modified CDSMPs is recommended to promote health management and maintenance in community-dwelling older adults with chronic conditions. These programs should include instruction in problem-solving strategies, goal-setting, and education about side effects and coping techniques (Smallfield et al, 2019).

The best-known self-management program is the Chronic Disease Self-Management Program developed by Lorig and colleagues at Stanford University (Lorig et al, 2001). This evidence-based program is a 6-week-long interactive workshop led by two professionals trained in program implementation. Participants learn skills related to problem-solving, decision-making, and action-planning across a variety of health-related topics, including self-advocacy, exercise, nutrition, and coping with the physiological and psychological effects of chronic illness, such as fatigue and pain (Lorig et al, 2019). This program has also been adapted for a Spanish-speaking population (Lorig et al, 2003).

Communication With the Health Care System

Occupational therapy interventions to address communication with the healthcare system include education and advocacy regarding health literacy.

Health Literacy Education and Advocacy

Interventions to improve health literacy can occur at the individual, community, or population level (Smith & Gutman, 2011). Occupational therapy practitioners can provide individualized education regarding health literacy topics to improve their client's understanding of health conditions and health management occupations. For example, a practitioner can educate a client on their diabetes diagnosis, break down the task of checking blood sugar, and practice this skill to ensure effective performance. At the community level, occupational therapy practitioners can develop inclusive programming that supports health literacy education and promotes healthy living regarding community-specific considerations. For example, practitioners could develop a series of educational classes and provide these classes in schools or community spaces, such as libraries or clinics. Population-level interventions strive to identify and reduce health disparities among a population. If a population has low health literacy overall, this is a health disparity. Occupational therapy practitioners can advocate for a health-literate environment within healthcare systems, engage in legislative advocacy, and implement environmental modifications and strategies that support the understanding of health information among a population (AOTA, 2020b). For example, practitioners can educate hospital systems on strategies for making their facilities more accessible and communication easier for all clients to understand.

Medication Management

Occupational therapy interventions to address medication management include use of CO-OP and the teach-back method.

Cognitive Orientation to Daily Occupations

The use of CO-OP has been found to increase health management independence among older adults with mild cognitive impairment (Saeidi et al, 2019). This cognitive strategy training approach involves setting a goal, planning to achieve the goal, actioning out the plan, and checking to understand the plan's effectiveness (Dawson et al, 2017). Individuals demonstrating difficulty in their medication management routine would complete the goal-plan-do-check process until finding a safe and effective solution to managing their medications.

Teach-Back Method

The teach-back method has been shown to increase compliance with health recommendations and self-efficacy with health management for individuals with chronic health conditions (Ha Dinh et al, 2016). Teach-back is a specific health education methodology in which the healthcare provider checks for client understanding using their own words (Talevski et al, 2020). Teach-back can ensure client understanding of their medication dosage and routines.

Physical Activity and Fall Prevention

Occupational therapy interventions to address physical activity and fall prevention include population fall-prevention initiatives, multicomponent and multifactorial training programs, and yoga, Tai chi chuan, and dance.

Population Fall-Prevention Initiatives

Population fall-prevention initiatives are implemented in a group setting and targeted toward older adults who are at risk of falling. Programs include education on controlling falls, minimizing fear of falling, reducing environmental hazards, and increasing exercise for fall prevention (National Council on Aging, 2022). Two examples of programs are A Matter of Balance and Stepping On (Elliott & Leland, 2018; Smallfield et al, 2019). These programs typically run for 7 to 8 weeks in a community setting, with 2-hour sessions.

Multicomponent and Multifactorial Fall-Prevention Training Programs

Multicomponent fall-prevention training involves a group approach toward addressing general fall-risk factors using multiple intervention strategies. Participants engage in a combination of exercises and fall-prevention education consistent with biomechanical and cognitive-behavioral theoretical approaches. Exercises involve functional activities, balance training, and strengthening. Education includes topics on environmental modifications, fall recovery, and proper hydration. Strong evidence supports the use of multicomponent programs for fall prevention (Elliott & Leland, 2018; Smallfield et al, 2019). Multifactorial fall-prevention programs use multiple intervention strategies customized to each individual. Clients frequently participate in fall-risk assessments and health screeners to provide individualized treatment. Evidence is mixed in the support of multifactorial training programs (Elliott & Leland, 2018; Smallfield et al, 2019).

Yoga, Tai Chi Chuan, and Dance

Exercise is one factor in fall prevention for older adults. Participation in yoga programs increases balance for adults and older adults with neurological conditions, including dementia. The programs were found to be most effective when combined with fall-prevention education (Green et al, 2019). Yoga also has mental health benefits and has been found to reduce anxiety, decrease depression, and improve aspects of cognition (Chugh-Gupta et al, 2013; Chobe et al, 2020). Tai chi chuan involves slow and controlled rhythmic movements with the purpose of increasing physical and mental health. Participation in Tai chi chuan increases balance, as measured on the Timed Up and Go test, and significantly reduces fear of falling in the older adult population (Hosseini et al, 2018). Participation in dance, specifically for individuals with Parkinson disease, has been found to increase balance, cognition, and fall prevention (Ventura et al, 2016).

Nutrition Management

Occupational therapy interventions to address nutrition management include education and addressing the accessibility of healthy foods.

Education and Access

While occupational therapists do not provide specific dietary recommendations, they do address the IADLs of cooking and food selection. Nutrition education can be incorporated into IADL retraining sessions to increase adherence to healthy food selection (Bailey, 2017). Due to an increase in chronic conditions in older adulthood, individuals may face barriers to reading food labels, opening containers, and food preparation. Providing education on adaptive strategies and equipment can increase participation in cooking tasks (Juckett & Robinson, 2019). Modifications to the home environment for accessibility in the kitchen can improve safety during cooking (Juckett & Robinson, 2019).

It is important to consider an individual's social and built environment, cultural factors, and access to healthy foods. Older adults are a vulnerable population at risk for food insecurity and may face environmental barriers preventing access to healthy food sources (Juckett & Robinson, 2019). Occupational therapists can connect clients with community agencies and meal delivery services to address health disparities associated with food insecurity (Mabli et al, 2015). While discussing nutrition and food preparation, the occupational therapist must demonstrate cultural humility and respect for an individual's food preferences (Song et al, 2014).

Personal Device Management

Occupational therapy interventions to address personal device management include multicomponent interventions.

Multicomponent Interventions

Personal device management includes using and caring for devices, including adaptive equipment, hearing aids, prosthetics, and sexual devices (AOTA, 2020a). Multicomponent interventions for personal device use are completed in a group or individual format. Education is provided on managing devices, with multiple sessions to provide repetition and practice (Liu et al, 2013). These interventions can increase independence and implementation of device use into daily routines. Individual training sessions with devices should include education on using the device, proper storage and cleaning, and frequency of use (Kelly et al, 2013). Older adults are more likely to use a personal device with proper education and training (Kraskowsky & Finlayson, 2001).

Sleep and Rest

Occupational therapy interventions to address sleep and rest include sleep education, cognitive-behavioral interventions, environmental modifications, and multicomponent interventions.

Sleep Education

Instruction about sleep is an effective intervention strategy as part of a multicomponent intervention based on cognitive-behavioral theoretical knowledge to enhance sleep (Lichstein et al, 2001; McCrae et al, 2007; McCurry et al, 1998). Topics may include the health benefits of sleep and maintaining a consistent sleep schedule, sleep stages, the relationship between sleep and daytime occupations, medications and sleep, substance use in relation to sleep, mind-body self-care, and strategies to enhance sleep. The use of night lights and fall prevention at night are also important topics for older adults who may have difficulty sleeping.

Cognitive-Behavioral Interventions for Sleep

Cognitive-behavioral interventions focus on bringing awareness to distorted thinking or maladaptive behaviors and the introduction of adaptive skills. Maladaptive sleep behaviors include staying up late when needing to be up early in the morning, ruminating while awake in bed, and eating heavy meals or drinking caffeinated beverages just before bed. **Sleep hygiene** is a term that is commonly used to describe the behaviors, habits, and routines that promote healthy sleep. Behaviors that contribute to improved sleep patterns include developing a consistent exercise routine and sleep/wake schedule; using a sleep log or diary; progressive muscle relaxation; meditation; limiting afternoon napping; avoiding bright light, computers, and screen time before bed; and avoiding alcohol, caffeine, and heavy evening meals. Sleep restriction, or limiting the time spent in bed, is also an important behavior, as it promotes sleep efficiency, which is the ratio of total sleep time to total time spent in bed (Sheth & Thomas, 2019). For older adults, a sleep efficiency of 80%—meaning 80% of the total time spent in bed is spent asleep—is the goal (Sheth & Thomas, 2019). Interventions using a cognitive-behavioral approach to intervention can be completed in person, over the telephone, or via computer (Brenes et al, 2012; Buysse et al, 2011; Haimov & Shatil, 2013; Kapella et al, 2011; Leland et al, 2014). These strategies can be used alone or in combination with other intervention strategies to enhance sleep among older adults. Refer to Promoting Best Practice 16-3 for single-component or multicomponent cognitive-behavioral interventions to address sleep that are supported by evidence.

> ### PROMOTING BEST PRACTICE 16-3
> #### Cognitive-Behavioral Interventions to Enhance Sleep
> Either single-component or multicomponent cognitive-behavioral interventions that include sleep hygiene, a sleep diary, sleep goals, a sleep schedule with consistent routine, and relaxation techniques are recommended for routine use with older adults with insomnia who live in the community (Smallfield et al, 2019).

Environmental Modifications

Adaptations made to the sleep environment—such as adjusting lighting, noise, external distractions, and temperature—are also important considerations (Leland et al, 2014; Sheth & Thomas, 2019). Best practices to optimize the sleep environment include ensuring a quiet, dark, cool, and safe environment. Devices should be silenced or kept out of the sleep environment to ensure a distraction-free space. Similarly, lighting is an important environmental consideration. The body's circadian rhythms are closely linked to external light. When the eyes sense darkness, the body releases the hormone melatonin, which is a signal to the body to fall asleep (Pierce & Summers, 2011; Walker, 2018). Therefore, keeping the sleep environment dark is important for falling asleep and maintaining sleep. Blue light, more than other colors of light, is linked to the suppression of melatonin levels; therefore computers, smartphones, and other electronic devices that emit high levels of blue light should be avoided a few hours before bed (Walker, 2018). Likewise, red or green shades of light should be considered for night lights, if needed. Additionally, a sleep environment with temperatures between 60 and 70 degrees Fahrenheit is optimal for quality sleep (Walker, 2018). Finally, for those who may be concerned for their safety at night, a pattern of walking through the living environment to complete a safety check of doors, windows, and other safety concerns may be one strategy for peace of mind when falling asleep.

Multicomponent Interventions to Enhance Sleep

There is strong evidence to support multicomponent interventions to enhance sleep among older adults (Leland et al, 2014; Smallfield & Lucas Molitor, 2018). The intervention components included relaxation training, physical exercise, meditation, sleep-related goal-setting, sleep hygiene education, use of a sleep journal, cognitive therapy, and problem-solving. These interventions can be delivered individually or as part of group intervention in sessions over a period ranging from 4 weeks to 6 months. Because of the strong evidence supporting the effectiveness of multicomponent interventions to enhance sleep performance, routine use of them among community-dwelling older adults is encouraged (Smallfield & Lucas Molitor, 2018). Refer to Promoting Best Practice 16-4 for recommended components to establish self-management habits and routines.

PROMOTING BEST PRACTICE 16-4
Multicomponent Intervention for Management of Chronic Conditions

A multicomponent approach that includes education, goal-setting, and problem-solving over an extended time is recommended for routine use with adults with chronic conditions to establish self-management habits and routines (Fields & Smallfield, 2022).

CASE STUDY (CONTINUED)
Intervention Plan

The occupational therapist focused on health management and sleep education to improve Lionel's occupational performance. First, she recommended that Lionel attend a local support group for spouses of individuals with Alzheimer disease to improve his ability to cope with his wife's diagnosis. Next, the therapist educated Lionel on sleep hygiene strategies, such as decreasing the amount of television he watches before bed. The occupational therapist also educated Lionel on medication management strategies, including the use of pillboxes.

When asked about foot care, Lionel reported that he cannot see the bottom of his right foot. The occupational therapist provided a telescoping mirror and educated Lionel on its use to complete daily foot checks. Lionel then demonstrated understanding of this task. He was provided educational handouts to increase retention of the information. After an hour-long session with the therapist, they planned a follow-up visit in 1 month to evaluate his progress.

Discharge Status

At Lionel's follow-up appointment, he reported that he had incorporated many of the discussed strategies into his routines. Together, Lionel and the occupational therapist problem-solved a few challenges that Lionel had identified. At the end of the appointment, the occupational therapist decided that further occupational therapy services were not needed.

Questions

1. How might decreased occupational performance affect Lionel's social and emotional health?
2. What assessments could the occupational therapist use to learn more about Lionel's health management and sleep practices?

Answers

1. Lionel is experiencing decreased occupational performance, having given up social activities, as well as exercise, due to barriers. In addition, Lionel seems to be missing previously enjoyed connectedness with his wife. Feelings of loneliness contribute to poor mental and physical health. Lack of engagement in meaningful daily occupations negatively affects quality of life, health, well-being, and life satisfaction among older adults. Lionel is also reporting difficulty sleeping. Inadequate or inconsistent sleep can impair occupational performance, lead to decreased physical and mental health, and impair one's relationships. (See Social and Emotional Health Promotion and Maintenance section and Effects of Poor-Quality Sleep on Daytime Occupational Performance section; LO 16-2.)
2. There are many assessments that may be useful to learn more about Lionel's health management and sleep practices. It may be useful to learn more about Lionel's social and emotional health through completion of a

formal questionnaire, such as the UCLA three-item loneliness scale. It may also be useful to assess Lionel's cognitive functioning, such as by completion of the Executive Function Performance Test, to ensure he can safely complete medication management for himself and his wife. Learning more about his sleep practices, such as by completion of the Pittsburgh Sleep Quality Index, may aid in identifying education and interventions to improve Lionel's sleep. Informal interview and the use of daily activity logs or diaries may provide additional information regarding Lionel's nutrition and exercise practices, along with other health management and sleep routines. (See Occupational Therapy Assessment of Health Management and Sleep section; LO 16-4.)

SUMMARY

With a growing number of older adults around the world, occupational therapy practitioners must be prepared to address health management and sleep with this population. Due to an increase in chronic health conditions and sleep disturbances in older adulthood, it is essential that occupational therapy practitioners understand their role in addressing health management and sleep from an occupation-based perspective. The definitions from the AOTA Occupational Therapy Practice Framework and ICF provide insight into overall health and well-being and can be used to better understand the different components of health management. There are several screening and assessment tools for health management and sleep that can be used in a variety of practice settings to determine an individual's current performance. Many of the screening tools can be administered by verbal report, but usage of performance-based assessments should be considered for a comprehensive understanding of functioning. This chapter highlighted the key intervention approaches and domain-specific interventions occupational therapy practitioners can use in practice while addressing health management and sleep.

Critical Thinking Questions

1. How are the occupations of health management and sleep related to each other?
2. What is occupational therapy's role in addressing health management and sleep among older adults?

REFERENCES

Alzheimer's Disease International. (2018). World Alzheimer Report 2018. Retrieved April 19, 2022 from https://www.alzint.org/resource/world-alzheimer-report-2018

American Occupational Therapy Association. (2020a). Occupational therapy practice framework: Domain and process (4th ed.). *American Journal of Occupational Therapy, 74*(Suppl. 2), 7412410010. https://doi.org/10.5014/ajot.2020.74S2001

American Occupational Therapy Association. (2020b). Occupational therapy in the promotion of health and well-being. *American Journal of Occupational Therapy, 74*(3), 7403420010p1-7403420010p14. https://doi.org/10.5014/ajot.2020.743003

Arbesman, M., & Mosley, L. J. (2012). Systematic review of occupation- and activity-based health management and maintenance interventions for community-dwelling older adults. *American Journal of Occupational Therapy, 66*(3), 277–283. https://doi.org/10.5014/ajot.2012.003327

Bailey, R. R. (2017). The Issue Is—Promoting physical activity and nutrition in people with stroke. *American Journal of Occupational Therapy, 71*(5), 7105360010p1. https://doi.org/10.5014/ajot.2017.021378

Barile, J. P., Thompson, W. W., Zack, M. M., Krahn, G. L., Horner-Johnson, W., & Bowen, S. E. (2013). Multiple chronic medical conditions and health-related quality of life in older adults, 2004–2006. *Preventing Chronic Disease, 10,* E162. https://doi.org/10.5888/pcd10.120282

Baum, C. M., Christiansen, C. H., & Bass, J. D. (2015). The Person-Environment-Occupation-Performance (PEOP) Model. In C. H. Christiansen, C. M. Baum, & J. D. Bass (Eds.) *Occupational therapy: Performance, participation, and well-being* (4th ed., pp. 49–55). SLACK Incorporated.

Baum, C. M., Connor, L. T., Morrison, T., Hahn, M., Dromerick, A. W., & Edwards, D. F. (2008) Reliability, validity, and clinical utility of the executive function performance test: A measure of executive function in a sample of people with stroke. *American Journal of Occupational Therapy, 62*(4) 446–455.

Bennett, S., & Thomas, A. J. (2014). Depression and dementia: Cause, consequence or coincidence? *Maturitas, 79*(2), 184–190. https://doi.org/10.1016/j.maturitas.2014.05.009

Bergman, B., & Rosenhall, U. (2001). Vision and hearing in old age. *Scandinavian Audiology, 30*(4), 255–263.

Brenes, G. A., Miller, M. E., Williamson, J. D., McCall, W. V., Knudson, M., & Stanley, M. A. (2012). A randomized controlled trial of telephone-delivered cognitive–behavioral therapy for late-life anxiety disorders. *American Journal of Geriatric Psychiatry, 20*(8), 707–716. https://doi.org/10.1097/JGP.0b013e31822ccd3e

Brown, J. C., Goldstein, J. E., Chan, T. L., Massof, R., & Ramulu, P.; Low Vision Research Network Study Group. (2014). Characterizing functional complaints in patients seeking outpatient low-vision services in the United States. *Ophthalmology, 121*(8), 1655–1662.e1. https://doi.org/10.1016/j.ophtha.2014.02.030

Buysse, D. J., Germain, A., & Moul, D. E. (2011). Efficacy of brief behavioral treatment for chronic insomnia in older adults. *Archives of Internal Medicine, 171*(10), 887–895. https://doi:10.1001/archinternmed.2010.535

Buysse, D. J., Reynolds, C. F., 3rd, Monk, T. H., Berman, S. R., & Kupfer, D. J. (1989). The Pittsburgh Sleep Quality Index: A new instrument for psychiatric practice and research. *Psychiatry Research, 28*(2), 193–213. https://doi.org/10.1016/0165-1781(89)90047-4

Card, A. J. (2017), Moving beyond the WHO definition of health: A new perspective for an aging world and the emerging era of value-based care. *World Medical & Health Policy, 9,* 127–137. https://doi.org/10.1002/wmh3.221

Centers for Disease Control and Prevention. (2009). *Improving health literacy for older adults: Expert panel report 2009.* U.S. Department of Health and Human Services.

Centers for Disease Control and Prevention. (2015). *Sleep and Sleep Disorders.* Retrieved April 20, 2022 from https://www.cdc.gov/sleep/index.html

Centers for Disease Control and Prevention. (2018). Summary health statistics: 2018 national health survey interview data. Retrieved January 26, 2022 from https://ftp.cdc.gov/pub/Health_Statistics/NCHS/NHIS/SHS/2018_SHS_Table_A-11.pdf

Centers for Disease Control and Prevention. (2020). *Chronic diseases and cognitive decline - a public health issue.* Centers for Disease Control and Prevention. Retrieved January 30, 2022, from https://www.cdc.gov/aging/publications/chronic-diseases-brief.html

Centers for Disease Control and Prevention. (2021). *Facts about falls.* Centers for Disease Control and Prevention. Retrieved January 30, 2022, from https://www.cdc.gov/falls/facts.html

Cha, H., Farina, M. P., & Hayward, M. D. (2021). Socioeconomic status across the life course and dementia-status life expectancy among older Americans. *SSM - population health, 15*, 100921. https://doi.org/10.1016/j.ssmph.2021.100921

Chen, T., Lee., S., & Buxton, O. M. (2017). A greater extent of insomnia symptoms and physician-recommended sleep medication use predict fall risk in community-dwelling older adults. *Sleep, 40*(11), zsx142. https://doi.org/10.1093/sleep/zsx142

Chien, W., & Lin, F. R. (2012). Prevalence of hearing aid use among older adults in the United States. *Archives of Internal Medicine, 172*(3), 292–293. https://doi.org/10.1001/archinternmed.2011.1408

Chobe, S., Chobe, M., Metri, K., Patra, S. K., & Nagaratna, R. (2020). Impact of yoga on cognition and mental health among elderly: A systematic review. *Complementary Therapies in Medicine, 52*, 102421. https://doi.org/10.1016/j.ctim.2020.102421

Chugh-Gupta, N., Baldassarre, F. G., & Vrkljan, B. H. (2013). A systematic review of yoga for state anxiety: Considerations for occupational therapy. *Canadian Journal of Occupational Therapy, 80*(3), 150–170.

Clark, F., Azen, S. P., Zemke, R., Jackson, J., Carlson, M., Mandel, D., Hay, J., Josephson, K., Cherry, B., Hessel, C., Palmer, J., & Lipson, L. (1997). Occupational therapy for independent-living older adults. A randomized controlled trial. *Journal of the American Medical Association, 278*(16), 1321–1326.

Clark, F., Jackson, J., Carlson, M., Chou, C. P., Cherry, B. J., Jordan-Marsh, M., Knight, B. G., Mandel, D., Blanchard, J., Granger, D. A., Wilcox, R. R., Lai, M. Y., White, B., Hay, J., Lam, C., Marterella, A., & Azen, S. P. (2012). Effectiveness of a lifestyle intervention in promoting the well-being of independently living older people: Results of the Well Elderly 2 Randomized Controlled Trial. *Journal of Epidemiology and Community Health, 66*(9), 782–790. http://dx.doi.org/10.1136/jech.2009.099754

Crews, J. E., Jones, G. C., & Kim, J. H. (2006). Double jeopardy: The effects of comorbid conditions among older people with vision loss. *Journal of Visual Impairment & Blindness, 100*(1_suppl), 824–848. https://doi.org/10.1177/0145482x0610001s07

Dawson, D. R., McEwen, S. E., & Polatajko, H, J. (2017). Cognitive orientation to daily occupational performance in occupational therapy: Using the CO-OP approach to enable participation across the lifespan. AOTA Press.

Elliott, S., & Leland, N. E. (2018). Occupational therapy fall prevention interventions for community-dwelling older adults: A systematic review. *The American Journal of Occupational Therapy, 72*(4), 7204190040p1–7204190040p11. https://doi.org/10.5014/ajot.2018.030494

Fields, B., & Smallfield, S. (2022). Occupational therapy practice guidelines for adults with chronic conditions. *American Journal of Occupational Therapy, 76*(2), 7602397010. https://doi.org/10.5014/ajot.2022/762001

Gangwisch, J. (2014). A review of evidence for the link between sleep duration and hypertension. *American Journal of Hypertension, 27*(10), 1235–1242. https://doi.org/10.1093/ajh/hpu071

Garvey, J., Connolly, D., Boland, F., & Smith, S. (2015). OPTIMAL, an occupational therapy led self-management support programme for people with multimorbidity in primary care: A randomized controlled trial. *BMC Family Practice, 16*(1), 1–11. https://doi.org/10.1186/s12875-015-0267-0

Gooneratne, N. S., & Vitiello, M. (2014). Sleep in older adults: Normative changes, sleep disorders, and treatment options. *Clinical Geriatric Medicine, 30*(3), 591–627. http://dx.doi.org/10.1016/j.cger.2014.04.007

Green, E., Huynh, A., Broussard, L., Zunker, B., Matthews, J., Hilton, C. L., & Aranha, K. (2019). Systematic review of yoga and balance: Effect on adults with neuromuscular impairment. *American Journal of Occupational Therapy, 73*(1), 7301205150p1–7301205150p11. https://doi.org/10.5014/ajot.2019.028944

Gulia, K. K., & Kumar, V. M. (2018). Sleep disorders in the elderly: A growing challenge. *Psychogeriatrics, 18*(3), 155–165.

Ha Dinh, T. T., Bonner, A., Clark, R., Ramsbotham, J., & Hines, S. (2016). The effectiveness of the teach-back method on adherence and self-management in health education for people with chronic disease: A systematic review. *JBI Database of Systematic Reviews and Implementation Reports, 14*(1), 210–247. https://doi.org/10.11124/jbisrir-2016-2296

Hackert, M., van Exel, J., & Brouwer, W. (2021). Content validation of the well-being of older people measure (WOOP). *Health and Quality of Life Outcomes, 19*(1), 200. https://doi.org/10.1186/s12955-021-01834-5

Haimov, I., & Shatil, E. (2013). Cognitive training improves sleep quality and cognitive function among older adults with insomnia. *PLoS One, 8*(4), e61390. https://doi.org/10.1371/journal.pone.0061390

Halaweh, H., Dahlin-Ivanoff, S., Svantesson, U., & Willén, C. (2018). Perspectives of older adults on aging well: A focus group study. *Journal of Aging Research, 2018*, 9858252. https://doi.org/10.1155/2018/9858252

Hereford, J. (2014). Sleep and rehabilitation: A guide for health professionals. Slack, Inc.

Hoffman, H. J., Dobie, R. A., Losonczy, K. G., Themann, C. L., & Flamme, G. A. (2017). Declining prevalence of hearing loss in US adults aged 20 to 69 years. *JAMA Otolaryngology–Head & Neck Surgery, 143*(3), 274. https://doi.org/10.1001/jamaoto.2016.3527

Hosseini, L., Kargozar, E., Sharifi, F., Negarandeh, R., Memari, A. H., & Navab, E. (2018). Tai Chi Chuan can improve balance and reduce fear of falling in community dwelling older adults: A randomized control trial. *Journal of Exercise Rehabilitation, 14*(6), 1024–1031. https://doi.org/10.12965/jer.1836488.244

Huber, M., Knottnerus, J. A., Green, L., van der Horst, H., Jadad, A. R., Kromhout, D., & Smid, H. (2011). How should we define health? *British Medical Journal, 343*, d4163. https://doi.org/10.1136/bmj.d4163

Hughes, M., E., Waite, L. J., Hawkely, L. C., & Cacioppo, J. T. (2004). A short scale for measuring loneliness in large surveys: Results from two population-based studies. *Research on Ageing, 26*(6), 655–672.

Ikiugu, M. N., Smallfield, S., & Condit, C. (2009). A framework for combining theoretical conceptual practice models in occupational therapy practice. *Canadian Journal of Occupational Therapy, 76*(3), 162–170. https://doi.org/10.3109/07380577.2015.1017787

Immonen, M., Haapea, M., Similä, H., Enwald, H., Keränen, N., Kangas, M., Jämsä, T., & Korpelainen, R. (2020). Association between chronic diseases and falls among a sample of older people in Finland. *BMC Geriatrics, 20*(1), 225. https://doi.org/10.1186/s12877-020-01621-9

Insel, K., Morrow, D., Brewer, B., & Figueredo, A. (2006). Executive function, working memory, and medication adherence among older adults. *Journal of Gerontology: Psychological Sciences, 61B*(2), P102–P107.

Iwama, M. (2006). The Kawa Model; Culturally Relevant Occupational Therapy. Edinburgh: Churchill Livingstone-Elsevier Press.

Johns, M. W. (1991). A new method for measuring daytime sleepiness: The Epworth sleepiness scale. *Sleep, 14*(6), 540–545.

Johns, M. W. (1997). About the ESS. Retrieved April 20, 2022 from http://epworthsleepinessscale.com/about-the-ess/

Jonkers, C. C., Lamers, F., Bosma, H., Metsemakers, J. F., & van Eijk, J. T. M. (2012). The effectiveness of a minimal psychological intervention on self-management beliefs and behaviors in depressed chronically ill elderly persons: A randomized trial. *International Psychogeriatrics, 24*(2), 288–297. https://doi.org/10.1017/S1041610211001748

Juckett, L. A., & Robinson, M. L. (2019). The occupational therapy approach to addressing food insecurity among older adults with chronic disease. *Geriatrics (Basel, Switzerland), 4*(1), 22. https://doi.org/10.3390/geriatrics4010022

Kapella, M. C., Herdegen, J. J., Perlis, M. L., Shaver, J. L., Larson, J. L., Law, J. A., & Carley, D. W. (2011). Cognitive behavioral therapy for insomnia comorbid with COPD is feasible with preliminary evidence of positive sleep and fatigue effects. *International Journal of Chronic Obstructive Pulmonary Disease, 6*, 625–635. https://doi.org/10.2147/COPD.S24858

Kelly, T. B., Tolson, D., Day, T., McColgan, G., Kroll, T., & Maclaren, W. (2013). Older people's views on what they need to successfully adjust to life with a hearing aid. *Health & Social Care in the Community, 21*(3), 293–302. https://doi.org/10.1111/hsc.12016

Kempen, G. I. J. M., Ballemans, J., Ranchor, A. V., van Rens, G. H. M. B., & Zijlstra, G. A. R. (2012). The impact of low vision on activities of daily living, symptoms of depression, feelings of anxiety and social support in community-living older adults seeking vision rehabilitation services. *Quality of Life Research, 21*(8), 1405–1411. https://doi.org/10.1007/s11136-011-0061-y

Kraskowsky, L. H., & Finlayson, M. (2001). Factors affecting older adults' use of adaptive equipment: Review of the literature. *American Journal of Occupational Therapy, 55*(3), 303–310. https://doi.org/10.5014/ajot.55.3.303

Leland, N. E., Marcione, N., Schepens Niemiec, S. L., Kelkar, K., & Fogelberg, D. (2014). What is occupational therapy's role in addressing sleep problems among older adults? *OTJR: Occupation, Participation, and Health, 34*(3), 141–149. https://doi.org/10.3928/15394492-20140513-01

Leonardi, F. (2018). The definition of health: Towards new perspectives. *International Journal of Health Services, 48*(4), 735–748. https://doi.org/10.1177/0020731418782653

Lewin, G., de San Miguel, K., Knuiman, M., Alan, J., Boldy, D., Hendrie, D., & Vandermeulen, S. (2013). A randomised controlled trial of the Home Independence Program, an Australian restorative home-care programme for older adults. *Health & Social Care in the Community, 21*(1), 69–78. https://doi.org/10.1111/j.1365-2524.2012.01088.x

Lichstein, K. L., Riedel, B. W., Wilson, N. M., Lester, K. W., & Aguillard, R. N. (2001). Relaxation and sleep compression for late-life insomnia: A placebo-controlled trial. *Journal of Consulting and Clinical Psychology, 69*(2), 227–239. https://doi.org/10.1037/0022-006X.69.2.227

Lin, F. R., Thorpe, R., Gordon-Salant, S., & Ferrucci, L. (2011). Hearing loss prevalence and risk factors among older adults in the United States. *The Journals of Gerontology. Series A, Biological Sciences and Medical Sciences, 66*(5), 582–590. https://doi.org/10.1093/gerona/glr002

Liu, C. J., Brost, M. A., Horton, V. E., Kenyon, S. B., & Mears, K. E. (2013). Occupational therapy interventions to improve performance of daily activities at home for older adults with low vision: A systematic review. *The American Journal of Occupational Therapy, 67*(3), 279–287. https://doi.org/10.5014/ajot.2013.005512

Liu, M., Hou, T., Li, Y., Sun, X., Szanton, S. L., Clemson, L., & Davidson, P. M. (2021). Fear of falling is as important as multiple previous falls in terms of limiting daily activities: A longitudinal study. *BMC Geriatrics, 21*(1), 350. https://doi.org/10.1186/s12877-021-02305-8

Loiselle, M. M., Means, M. K., & Edinger, J. D. (2005). Sleep disturbances in aging. *Advances in Cell Aging and Gerontology, 17*, 33–59. https://doi.org/10.1016/S1566-3124(04)17002-8

Lorig, K., Laurent, D., González, V., Sobel, D., Minor, M., & Gecht-Silver, M. (2019). *Living a healthy life with chronic conditions: Self-management of heart disease, arthritis, diabetes, asthma, bronchitis, emphysema and other physical and mental health conditions* (5th ed). Bull Publishing Company.

Lorig, K. R., Ritter, P. L., & González, V. M. (2003). Hispanic chronic disease self-management: A randomized community-based outcome trial. *Nursing Research, 52*(6), 361–369. https://doi.org/10.1097/00006199-200311000-00003

Lorig, K. R., Sobel, D. S., Ritter, P. L., Laurent, D., & Hobbs, M. (2001). Effect of a self-management program on patients with chronic disease. *Effective Clinical Practice 4*(6), 256–262.

Mabli, J., Redel, N., Cohen, R., Panzarella, E., Hu, M., & Carlson, B. (2015). Process Evaluation of Older Americans Act title III-C Nutrition Services Program. Retrieved from https://acl.gov/sites/default/files/programs/2017-02/NSP-Process-Evaluation-Report.pdf

McCrae, C. S., McGovern, R., Lukefahr, R., & Stripling, A. M. (2007). Research Evaluating Brief Behavioral Sleep Treatments for Rural Elderly (RESTORE): A preliminary examination of effectiveness. *American Journal of Geriatric Psychiatry, 15*, 979–982. https://doi.org/10.1097/JGP.0b013e31813547e6

McCurry, S. M., Logsdon, R. G., Vitiello, M. V., & Teri, L. (1998). Successful behavioral treatment for reported sleep problems in elderly caregivers of dementia patients: A controlled study. *Journals of Gerontology, Series B: Psychological Sciences, 53*, 122–129. https://doi.org/10.1093/geronb/53B.2.P122

McGilton, K. S., Vellani, S., Yeung, L., Chishtie, J., Commisso, E., Ploeg, J., Andrew, M. K., Ayala, A. P., Gray, M., Morgan, D., Chow, A. F., Parrott, E., Stephens, D., Hale, L., Keatings, M., Walker, J., Wodchis, W. P., Dubé, V., McElhaney, J., & Puts, M. (2018). Identifying and understanding the health and social care needs of older adults with multiple chronic conditions and their caregivers: A scoping review. *BMC Geriatrics, 18*(1), 231. https://doi.org/10.1186/s12877-018-0925-x

Miner, B., & Kryger, M. H. (2017). Sleep in the aging population. *Sleep Medicine Clinics, 12*(1), 31–38. https://doi.org/10.1016/j.jsmc.2016.10.008

Moll, S. E., Gewurtz, R. E., Krupa, T. M., Law, M. C., Larivière, N., & Levasseur, M. (2015). "Do-Live-Well": A Canadian framework for promoting occupation, health, and well-being. *Canadian Journal of Occupational Therapy, 82*, 9–23.

Monkman, H., Kushniruk, A. W., Barnett, J., Borycki, E. M., Greiner, L. E., & Sheets, D. (2017). Are health literacy and eHealth literacy the same or different? *Studies in Health Technology and Informatics, 245*, 178–182. https://doi.org/10.3233/978-1-61499-830-3-178

Monzani, D., Galeazzi, G. M., Genovese, E., Marrara, A., Martini, A. (2008). Psychological profile and social behaviour of working adults with mild or moderate hearing loss. *Acta Otorhinolaryngologica Italica, 28*(2), 61–66.

National Council on Aging. (2021a). *Can hearing loss affect mental health in older adults?* Retrieved April 20, 2022, from https://ncoa.org/article/can-hearing-loss-affect-mental-health-in-older-adults

National Council on Aging. (2021b). *Get the facts on healthy aging.* National Council on Aging. Retrieved April 20, 2022 from https://www.ncoa.org/article/get-the-facts-on-healthy-aging

National Council on Aging. (2022). *Evidence-based program: A matter of balance.* Retrieved April 4, 2022, from https://www.ncoa.org/article/evidence-based-program-a-matter-of-balance

National Institute on Aging. (2020). *A good night's sleep: Sleep and aging.* Retrieved April 20, 2022 from https://www.nia.nih.gov/health/good-nights-sleep

National Institutes of Health. (2017). *Why is sleep important?* Retrieved April 20, 2022 from https://www.nhlbi.nih.gov/node/4605

Nguyen, A. T., & Roberts, P. S. (2021). Participation in health management using patient portals: Opportunities for OT practice with the older adult population. *American Journal of Occupational Therapy, 75*(Supplement_2), 7512510223p1. https://doi.org/10.5014/ajot.2021.75S2-RP223

Norman, C. D., & Skinner, H. A. (2006). eHealth literacy: Essential skills for consumer health in a networked world. *Journal of Medical Internet Research, 8*(2), e9. https://doi.org/10.2196/jmir.8.2.e9

Osborn, R., Doty, M. M., Moulds, D., Sarnak, D. O., & Shah, A. (2017). Older Americans were sicker and faced more financial barriers to health care than counterparts in other countries. *Health Affairs (Project Hope), 36*(12), 2123–2132. https://doi.org/10.1377/hlthaff.2017.1048

Pierce, D., & Summers, K. (2011). Rest and sleep. In C. Brown & V. C. Stoffel (Eds.), *Occupational therapy in mental health: A vision for participation* (pp. 736–758). Philadelphia: F. A. Davis.

Poblador-Plou, B., Calderón-Larrañaga, A., Marta-Moreno, J., Hancco-Saavedra, J., Sicras-Mainar, A., Soljak, M., & Prados-Torres, A. (2014). Comorbidity of dementia: A cross-sectional study of primary care older patients. *BMC Psychiatry, 14*(1), 84. https://doi.org/10.1186/1471-244x-14-84

Ramar, K., Malhotra, R. K., Carden, K. A., Martin, J. L., Abbasi-Feinberg, F., Aurora, R. N., Kapur, V. K., Olson, E. J., Rosen, C. L., Rowley, J. A., Shelgikar, A. V., & Trotti, L. M. (2021). Sleep is essential to health: An American Academy of Sleep Medicine position statement. *Journal of Clinical Sleep Medicine, 17*(10), 2115–2119. https://doi.org/10.5664/jcsm.9476

Rogers, J. C. (1984). Performance Assessment of Self-Care Skills (PASS) [Database record]. PsycTESTS.

Saeidi Borujeni, M., Hosseini, S. A., Akbarfahimi, N., & Ebrahimi, E. (2019). Cognitive orientation to daily occupational performance approach in adults with neurological conditions: A scoping review. *Medical Journal of the Islamic Republic of Iran, 33*, 99. https://doi.org/10.34171/mjiri.33.99

Shankar, A., Hamer, M., McMunn, A., & Steptoe, A. (2013). Social isolation and loneliness: Relationships with cognitive function during 4 years of follow-up in the English Longitudinal Study of Ageing. *Psychosomatic Medicine, 75*(2), 161–170.

Sheikh, J. I., & Yesavage, J. A. (1986). Geriatric Depression Scale (GDS): Recent evidence and development of a shorter version. *Clinical Gerontologist: The Journal of Aging and Mental Health, 5*(1-2), 165–173. https://doi.org/10.1300/J018v05n01_09

Sheth, M., & Thomas, H. (2019). *Managing sleep deprivation in older adults: A role for Occupational Therapy*. AOTA continuing education article. Retrieved April 20, 2022 from https://www.aota.org/~/media/Corporate/Files/Publications/CE-Articles/CE-Article-March-2019-Managing-Sleep-Deprivation-Older-Adults.pdf

Smallfield, S., Elliott, S., & Leland, N. (2019). Occupational therapy practice guidelines for community dwelling older adults. Bethesda, MD: AOTA Press.

Smallfield, S., & Lucas Molitor, W. (2018). Occupational therapy interventions addressing sleep for community-dwelling older adults: A systematic review. *American Journal of Occupational Therapy, 72*(4), 7204190030. https://doi.org/10.5014/ajot.2018.031211

Smith, D. L., & Gutman, S. A. (2011). Health literacy in occupational therapy practice and research. *American Journal of Occupational Therapy, 65*(4), 367–369. https://doi.org/10.5014/ajot.2011.002139

Solet, J. M. (2019). Sleep and rest. In B. Schell, & G. Gillen, (Eds.), *Willard and Spackman's occupational therapy* (13th ed.; pp. 828–846). Wolters Kluwer/Lippincott Williams and Wilkins.

Somerville, E. K., Massey, K., Keglovits, M., Vouri, S. M., Hu, Y., Carr, D., & Stark, S. L. (2019). Scoring, clinical utility, and psychometric properties of the in-home medication management performance evaluation (HOME–Rx). *The American Journal of Occupational Therapy, 73*(2), 7302205060p1-7302205060p8.

Song, H. J., Simon, J. R., & Patel, D. U. (2014). Food preferences of older adults in senior nutrition programs. *Journal of Nutrition in Gerontology and Geriatrics, 33*(1), 55–67. https://doi.org/10.1080/21551197.2013.875502

Spuling, S. M., Wurm, S., Tesch-Römer, C., & Huxhold, O. (2015). Changing predictors of self-rated health: Disentangling age and cohort effects. *Psychology and Aging, 30*(2), 462–474. https://doi.org/10.1037/a0039111

Suchy, Y., Ziemnik, R. E., Niermeyer, M. A., & Brothers, S. L. (2020). Executive functioning interacts with complexity of daily life in predicting daily medication management among older adults. *The Clinical Neuropsychologist, 34*(4), 797–825. https://doi.org/10.1080/13854046.2019.1694702

Sumida, C. A., Vo, T. T., Van Etten, E. J., & Schmitter-Edgecombe, M. (2019). Medication management performance and associated cognitive correlates in healthy older adults and older adults with aMCI. *Archives of Clinical Neuropsychology, 34*(3), 290–300. https://doi.org/10.1093/arclin/acy038

Swanson, K. A., & Carnahan, R. M. (2007). Dementia and comorbidities: An overview of diagnosis and management. *Journal of Pharmacy Practice, 20*(4), 296–317. https://doi.org/10.1177/0897190007308594

Talevski, J., Wong Shee, A., Rasmussen, B., Kemp, G., & Beauchamp, A. (2020). Teach-back: A systematic review of implementation and impacts. *PLoS ONE, 15*(4): e0231350. https://doi.org/10.1371/journal.pone.0231350

Taylor, R. R. (2017). *Kielhofner's model of human occupation: Theory and application* (5th edition). Lippincott Williams & Wilkins.

Tester, N. J., & Foss, J. J. (2018). Sleep as an occupational need. *American Journal of Occupational Therapy, 72*, 7201347010p1-7201347010p4. https://doi.org/10.5014/ajot.2018.020651

U. S. Department of Health and Human Services. (2021). Health literacy in Healthy People 2030. Health.gov. Retrieved January 26, 2022 from https://health.gov/our-work/national-health-initiatives/healthy-people/healthy-people-2030/health-literacy-healthy-people-2030

Vaz Fragoso, C. A., & Gill, T. M. (2007). Sleep complaints in community-living older persons: A multifactorial geriatric syndrome. *Journal of the American Geriatrics Society, 55*(11), 1853–1866. https://doi.org/10.1111/j.1532-5415.2007.01399.x

Vellas, B. J., Wayne, S. J., Romero, L. J., Baumgaurten, R. N., & Garry, P. J. (1997). Fear of falling and restriction of mobility in elderly fallers. *Age and Ageing, 26*(3), 189–193. https://doi.org/10.1093/ageing/26.3.189

Ventura, M. I., Barnes, D. E., Ross, J. M., Lanni, K. E., Sigvardt, K. A., & Disbrow, E. A. (2016). A pilot study to evaluate multi-dimensional effects of dance for people with Parkinson's disease. *Contemporary Clinical Trials, 51*, 50–55. https://doi.org/10.1016/j.cct.2016.10.001

Walker, M. (2018). *Why we sleep: Unlocking the power of sleep and dreams*. Scribner.

Weiss, B. D., Mays, M. Z., Martz, W., Castro, K. M., DeWalt, D. A., Pignone, M. P., Mockbee, J., & Hale, F. A. (2005). Quick assessment of literacy in primary care: The newest vital sign. *Annals of Family Medicine, 3*(6), 514–522. https://doi.org/10.1370/afm.405

World Health Organization. (1986). *The Ottawa charter for health promotion*. Retrieved January 19, 2022 from https://www.euro.who.int/__data/assets/pdf_file/0004/129532/Ottawa_Charter.pdf

World Health Organization. (2001). *ICF: International classification of functioning, disability and health*. Geneva: World Health Organization.

World Health Organization. (2006). *Constitution of the World Health Organization* (45th ed). Retrieved January 19, 2022 from www.who.int/governance/eb/who_constitution_en.pdf

World Health Organization. (2021). *COVID-19 and the social determinants of health and health equity: Evidence brief*. World Health Organization.

CHAPTER 17

Leisure

Jenny Martínez, OTD, OTR/L, BCG, FAOTA
Monique Chabot, OTD, OTR/L, SCEM, CLIPP, CAPS
Brenda Fagan, MSDA, OTR/L

> *One thing they don't tell you about growing old—you don't feel old, you just feel like yourself. And it's true. I don't feel eighty-nine years old. I simply am eighty-nine years old.*
>
> —Betty White

LEARNING OUTCOMES

By the end of this chapter, readers will be able to:

17-1. Articulate the value of leisure to older adults.
17-2. Compare relevant theories and frameworks of reference relevant to leisure in older adults.
17-3. Summarize how environments and health conditions can affect equity in choice, availability, and engagement in leisure for older adults.
17-4. Explain older adults' participation in lifelong learning as leisure.
17-5. Select assessments relevant to occupational therapy when addressing leisure in older adults.
17-6. Create leisure interventions for older adults based on evaluation and shared goal-setting.
17-7. Understand how occupational therapy can collaborate with other professions to promote leisure in older adults.

Mini Case Study

Miss Mae is a cisgender divorced woman. She was in her late 60s when she began to experience depression. Her daughter, an avid track and field runner, took her to a fund-raising walk-and-run race. Miss Mae, as she is known to her friends, enjoyed the event so much that she began walking each day with a neighbor, then walking longer distances, and later running with a social running club. She eventually joined races around her community and is currently training for a half marathon with the help of her daughter. Miss Mae comments that she enjoys spending more time with her daughter, the social network she has built through running, and the positive changes she has noticed in her body and outlook. She hopes to continue training and racing as long as she can.

Provocative Questions

1. What are your first reactions to Miss Mae's decision to take up running as an older adult?
2. How could this activity be considered a leisure occupation?
3. What roles might occupational therapy have in supporting her ability to participate in this activity?

Longevity and an increase in life expectancy have prompted calls for a paradigm shift that normalizes aging and avoids treating old age as a problem to be fixed (Calasanti & King, 2021; Sugar, 2019). The relationship between leisure and aging is relevant to such discussions, given links between leisure and older adults' physical, psychological, social, and spiritual well-being (Nimrod & Shirira, 2014; Wang et al, 2013). Although commonly treated as a means instead of an end goal of intervention, leisure itself is a valuable treatment goal for occupational therapy treatment (Chen & Chippendale, 2018). As older adults embrace the transition from work to retirement, engagement in leisure activities also increases. Occupational therapists should consider the full role of leisure for older adults in complement with an occupational justice approach that centers on one's right to engage in personally meaningful leisure (Bundy & Du Toit, 2018).

Defining Leisure

Leisure is one's discretionary time spent in nonobligatory activities. It is free from the pressure to be productive and obligatory activities such as work, self-care, or sleep (American Occupational Therapy Association, 2020; Law et al, 2019). Leisure further requires that the client be intrinsically motivated to engage in such activities. Leisure conveys varied meanings to individuals, including what activities are categorized as such, their frequency, and their personal value to the older adult (Yoon et al, 2021a). Although leisure activities may often look like devoting time to oneself through engagement in personally meaningful activities (e.g., exercise, travel, cooking classes), leisure activities can be communal (e.g., caring for grandchildren in a multigenerational home).

Whatever form it takes, leisure has been shown to have multiple health benefits, including promoting a feeling of purposeful living and reducing loneliness (Bhattacharyya, 2022). Yet engagement in leisure activities remains unequally distributed and is limited by factors such as health and disability, socioeconomic status, political climate, and whether the older adult resides at home or in an institutional setting. Although time spent on leisure may increase after retirement, many older adults continue to work into later age, either out of choice or necessity. Further, some older adults across the globe may not be familiar with the term *leisure*, which some research suggests may be due to not experiencing a 40-hour, 5-day work system typical in Western society that promotes a separation between labor, productivity, and leisure (Yoon et al, 2021a).

Defining leisure in further detail becomes complicated, as many models exist that attempt to categorize and explain the diversity of leisure activities and the methods by which people choose and participate in these activities (Fancourt et al, 2021). Additionally, different cultures define and value leisure differently. **Leisure motivation**, or the need to be involved in leisure activities, has strong psychological and sociological underpinnings that influence a person's desire to participate in and make decisions around leisure activities. It is heavily influenced by culture, in that culture will often determine whether leisure participation is accepted and if so, if it should take on a more individualistic or collective approach (Chen & Pang, 2012).

More specifically, leisure activities can be categorized in a variety of ways (Fancourt et al, 2021). Examples of such past categorizations include:

- Mental leisure, such as reading books
- Social leisure, such as participating in a shared activity with others
- Physical leisure, such as performing home maintenance or going on a walk
- Productive leisure, such as cooking or making clothes
- Relaxed activities, such as socializing and consuming some form of media entertainment (e.g., television or music)
- Serious activities, such as goal-directed activities (e.g., sports, arts, and hobbies)
- Unclassified leisure, such as activities that do not fall into another category (e.g., thinking, resting, or studying)
- Time-out leisure activities that are a break from another task
- Achievement leisure activities, which provide challenges and a thrill

Other definitions focus on the amount of activity level required, with activities falling into categories such as active, passive, high-demand, and low-demand (Fancourt et al, 2021). Social participation is another common thread across categorizations of leisure. Regardless of the category, presence of socialization, method of completion, or overarching goal of an activity, leisure activities bring enjoyment to the person and do not involve payment.

Engagement and Leisure

Relevant to leisure in older adults is a discussion of what may characterize optimal engagement. Such engagement is accomplished when one is in a *flow*, a psychological state in which the person experiences immersion, concentration, and enjoyment from an activity (Csikszentmihalyi, 2008; Tse et al, 2022). Flow experiences remain stable from adulthood to old age, are accessible to persons across groups (e.g., gender, race/ethnicity, education), and generally enhance satisfaction with life (Tse et al, 2022). Because the experience itself is so rewarding, the person is motivated to continue participating in the activity but may find greater enjoyment when participating in social versus solitary activity (Worm & Stine-Morrow, 2021). Still, older adults may engage in a task and not be fully satisfied. For example, grandparents may provide childcare and reduce the time they spend on other personally meaningful leisure activities. This can lead to reduced satisfaction, especially for women (Ates et al, 2021).

CASE STUDY

Occupational Profile

Anay is an 83-year-old cisgender woman who lived alone and experienced a mild cerebrovascular accident (CVA) 2 months ago. She is now residing at home and receiving home health occupational therapy. Upon first meeting Anay, the occupational therapist administered the Canadian Occupational Performance Measure to learn more about her interests. Anay rated cooking for her family as the most important occupation in which she was currently dissatisfied with her performance. Upon further probing, the occupational therapist learned that at the personal or micro level, Anay was highly motivated to cook for her family. When Anay cooked big meals, she became totally caught up in timing events and creating the perfect combination of ingredients. Anay expressed that since her stroke, she still cooks, but "it's no longer the same." She has not been able to drive since her CVA and is unsure of when she will be able to get herself to the grocery store to purchase cooking ingredients. Instead, she cooks only for herself and uses mixes her friends or family have dropped off rather than beginning from scratch.

Identified Problem Areas Related to Self-Care

- Mild weakness on her left side (difficulty lifting or moving pans)
- Abnormal movements in her arm
- Decreased ability to cognitively attend to tasks

Identified Strengths Related to Self-Care

- Highly motivated to cook for her family
- Has continued to cook and adapt after her CVA
- Has insight into potential safety concerns during cooking (having something on the stove burn while she attends to something else at the sink)

Goals for Occupational Therapy

Anay will:

- Demonstrate safe management of pans during cooking with supervision

- Engage her family members in food preparation to increase socialization
- Demonstrate knowledge of options for safely obtaining groceries that do not require her to drive (e.g., delivery service, going shopping with a friend)

Theoretical Approaches

Occupational therapy recognizes the important role of leisure, its personal meaning, and the dynamic interplay of multiple factors that support or pose barriers to participation. Practitioners' approach can be informed by multiple theories, including those centered on the aging process, leisure itself, and the occupational therapy lens.

The following is a sampling of relevant theories that support occupational therapy's understanding of leisure in older adults.

Multi-Level Leisure Mechanisms Framework

Fancourt and colleagues (2021) developed a unifying framework that conceptualized multiple mechanisms by which leisure affects health. A feature of the multi-level leisure mechanisms framework (MLMF) is its understanding of leisure and health as a complex adaptive system where "all mechanisms exist symbiotically, interacting across levels and domains" (Fancourt et al, 2021, p. 333). The MLMF identifies five overarching processes (psychological, biological, social, behavioral, and health behavior processes) and more than 600 mechanisms through which leisure affects health.

These categories and mechanisms are understood to act at multiple levels:

- The micro level—includes persons or small groups
- The meso level—includes larger groups, communities, or institutions
- The macro level—including societies and cultures at large

When blended with an occupation-based lens, the MLMF can enhance understanding of how multiple layers of the environment interact with the person and leisure to affect health. The MLMF can guide occupational therapists through evaluation, goal-setting, and intervention. Figure 17-1 provides a visual representation of the MLMF's five overarching processes and corresponding selected examples of mechanisms at the micro, meso, and macro levels.

Socioemotional Selectivity Theory

Socioemotional selectivity theory proposes that people seek more emotionally satisfying and pleasurable experiences through social interactions and relationships as age increases (Carstensen et al, 1999). Prioritization is given to social activities that are emotionally satisfying. For example, older women who participated in a softball league noted social connection as a motivator to join a team and continue to play while also developing friendships off the field (Choi et al, 2018). This experience allowed players to experience the benefits of physical activity and strengthening their social networks.

Selective Optimization With Compensation Model

The selective optimization with compensation model suggests that older adults select activities that optimize their biological and psychological ability (Baltes & Baltes, 1990). For example, the ability to adapt to changing external circumstances helped older adults in Canada find ways to continue leisure involvement during the COVID-19 pandemic (Chung et al, 2021). Participants were motivated to "stay busy" to maintain their health and social connections and did so by selecting meaningful activities they could do at home, optimizing new opportunities to participate in online events, and compensating for the loss of access to community activities.

Activity Theory

The activity theory of aging explains that life satisfaction is obtained by remaining active and engaged in meaningful activities that can replace lost roles and provide support for positive self-concept (Diggs, 2008). For example, participation in team pickleball tournaments provides social interaction and potential for creating new relationships

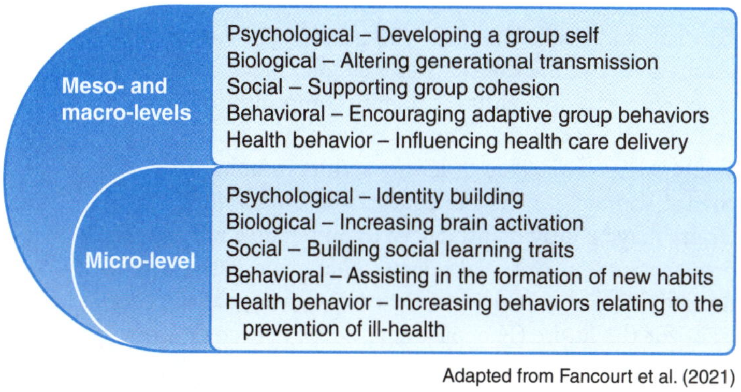

FIGURE 17-1 *Selected examples of how leisure affects health according to the multi-level leisure mechanisms framework (MLMF).*
The figure outlines selected examples of how leisure affects health according to the MLMF. This figure was adapted from original work by Fancourt et al (2021).

Meso- and macro-levels
- Psychological – Developing a group self
- Biological – Altering generational transmission
- Social – Supporting group cohesion
- Behavioral – Encouraging adaptive group behaviors
- Health behavior – Influencing health care delivery

Micro-level
- Psychological – Identity building
- Biological – Increasing brain activation
- Social – Building social learning traits
- Behavioral – Assisting in the formation of new habits
- Health behavior – Increasing behaviors relating to the prevention of ill-health

Adapted from Fancourt et al. (2021)

and may increase life satisfaction for people transitioning to retirement (Ryu et al, 2018). Older adults may replace work roles, routines, and collaboration with community activities that provide similar opportunities to maintain well-being through accountability, contribution, and social interaction.

Continuity Theory

Continuity theory states that people maintain engagement in the same activities, relationships, and behaviors they have throughout their life (Atchley, 1989). As natural aging and disability become part of daily life, people strive to continue participating in what is meaningful to them even if the activity is not exactly the same. For example, a person who loves backpacking and skiing may be unable to safely participate in those activities now. They can, however, continue to love being outside and walking in natural environments. For persons living with progressive neurocognitive disorders such as dementia, leisure can provide the added benefit of orienting the person to themselves and their identity, the physical and geographic environment, and meaningful relationships with other people (Sabat, 2018).

Life Course Theory

Life course theory considers the structural, social, and cultural contexts that contribute to the experience of aging (Elder, 1975). Socioeconomic inequality and personal role transitions contribute to differences in leisure experiences, sustainability, and leisure activity choices (Yoon et al, 2021b). Education level, social network size, and the cultural prestige of a person's last job worked influence the type of leisure a person engages in later in life. For example, leisure choices for a voluntarily retired neurosurgeon who has many social connections are more likely to include activities such as international travel or golfing at a country club, whereas a cashier at a local grocery store may engage in lower-cost and resource-intensive activities when no longer working their paid position. (Refer to Chapter 2—Theories on Aging for more information about these sociological theories.)

Impact of Environments and Health Conditions on Leisure Performance

Barriers and facilitators to engagement in leisure arise throughout the life course. For example, older adults may experience multiple shifts in family composition, romantic and sexual partnerships, the worker role, and health or disability status. The value of leisure and its meaning may also change throughout the life course. The unique meaning of leisure may be heavily influenced by an iterative relationship between cultural or social norms, others who participate in the activity, past experiences, the environment, and expectations for the future (Fancourt et al, 2021; Fenech & Collier, 2017). Such factors affect the ability, desire, and available resources to engage in leisure activities.

The Role of Environments and Contexts on Leisure Participation

Older adults' ability to engage in leisure is iterative and deeply entrenched within environments and contexts. Leisure must be considered within complex systems that include a dynamic interplay between micro, meso, and macro level contextual factors (Fancourt et al, 2021). Engagement in leisure is further influenced by multiple forces, including historical, political, economic, geographic, temporal, and interpersonal forces that affect people and communities. Leisure is affected by the environment in all of its forms (e.g., built, social, political), which significantly affects quality of life and person-level outcomes later in life (Wahl & Gerstorf, 2020).

Taken together, the result is that some older adults may face more barriers to leisure participation than others. Disability, financial resources, time availability, stress, loneliness or social isolation, and availability of high-quality programs or activities are just some factors that can pose barriers to leisure engagement. Older adults who are caregivers, or care partners, to a child, friend, or parent may also encounter barriers. (Refer to Chapter 20—Caregiving.) For example, Xu and colleagues (2022) found that caregivers of persons with dementia expressed many barriers to leisure. Such barriers included attitudes, beliefs, and available resources for the caregiver and for the person living with dementia. The loved one's needs could also be barriers, particularly when safety was a concern (e.g., a loved one who required assistance for self-care, daily activities, and supervision to avoid getting lost or hurt).

To this end, leisure may not always be accessible and freely chosen; what is leisure for one person may be considered work for another (Fenech & Collier, 2017). Such a view is congruent with occupational therapists' understanding of occupational justice and associated injustices such as *occupational deprivation,* or the "preclusion from engagement in occupations of necessity and/or meaning due to factors that stand outside of the immediate control of the individual" (Whiteford, 2000, p. 201). Occupational therapists must consider marginalization, oppression, intersectionality, personal resources, and issues of social justice as important drivers of leisure and integrate such principles into care (Son, 2018; Torregosa-Ruiz et al, 2021). Promoting Best Practice 17-1 addresses the importance of social justice topics in the context of leisure.

PROMOTING BEST PRACTICE 17-1
Leisure Participation and Social Justice

Occupational therapy considers the dynamic interplay of personal and environmental factors in leisure participation. For example, older adults' participation in leisure may be affected by disparities in social and political structures that prevent many from engaging in activities that others can access and benefit from (Pollard & Sakellariou, 2014). Such disparities may be linked to one more or more dimensions of older adults' personal and social identities (e.g., age, sex, gender identity, race/ethnicity, disability, socioeconomic status), which create overlapping and interdependent systems of discrimination or disadvantage. Occupational therapists should consider the role of marginalization, oppression, intersectionality, personal resources, and issues of social justice as important drivers of leisure (Son, 2018; Torregosa-Ruiz et al, 2021) and the delivery of occupational therapy services. Practitioners themselves must also engage in ongoing reflection and learning about their own position in society and any privileges earned as a result. Further, practitioners must help promote older adults' ability to participate in leisure via advocacy and action to transform attitudes, practice, and policy.

The Role of Disability on Leisure Participation

Engagement in leisure has been linked to improved social networks, mental health, and overall well-being, thereby demonstrating its importance for older adults (Chizari et al, 2020). Disability status and support required may limit a person's number, duration, and frequency of leisure opportunities. Further, the likelihood of experiencing a disability increases with age.

Older adults with neurocognitive disorders such as Alzheimer disease and dementia may have limited engagement in leisure activities; those who reside in institutional settings are especially at risk. For example, loneliness and depression are a concern across the spectrum of residential care, and staff may be unfamiliar with how to respond to residents' needs and neuropsychiatric symptoms (Rapaport et al, 2018; Theurer et al, 2015). Yet older adults with disabilities report increased overall health and life satisfaction in participating in activities involving social participation, indicating that this population of older adults also benefits from leisure activities (Chizari et al, 2020).

Consider the example of a resident who spends their day on passive activities and only 30 minutes once or twice a week on a valued crafting task (Causey-Upton, 2015). This resident's experience limits their participation in valued occupations, resulting in reduced quality of life. However, this experience may be markedly different for a resident in a nursing home with higher staff/resident ratios, better funding for outings or activities, and resources to match resident abilities and interests to leisure occupations.

The Impact of Isolation on Leisure Participation

Researchers have investigated leisure participation during the emergence of the COVID-19 pandemic. The COVID-19 virus was found to be highly infectious and able to spread through close contact and airborne transmission. Further, it caused worse outcomes and a higher mortality rate in high-risk groups, such as older adults (Ameis et al, 2020). Measures to reduce infection and transmission in older adults included minimizing physical contact with others and limiting activities outside of the home. Older adults were found to experience increased levels of depression, loneliness, and sedentary behavior during the pandemic, conditions exacerbated by a limited ability to use leisure as a way to cope with the stress and anxiety of isolation (Chung et al, 2021). Older adults and nursing home residents—particularly those with neurocognitive disorders—were especially vulnerable, as measures to reduce viral spread brought in-person and communal activities to a halt. Daily routines were disrupted, visitations ceased, and personnel donned necessary personal protective equipment that occluded the face and body, often disorienting residents with Alzheimer disease or dementia. Such measures exacerbated loneliness, disengagement in meaningful leisure, and connection to familiar people and surroundings.

Still, older adults also found ways to cope and thrive. Older adults across the globe benefitted from physical activity and time outdoors during the COVID-19 pandemic (Rivera-Torres et al, 2021). Although the use of technology was more likely in wealthier countries where access to modern infrastructure was more common, older adults also benefited from internet or digital technology-based leisure such as learning new skills, meditation, and attending religious ceremonies (Chung et al, 2021). Nursing home residents also engaged in creative new leisure activities, such as visitations through windows, use of online video conferencing technology, and outdoor activities.

Lifelong Learning as Leisure

Engagement in meaningful leisure occupations can facilitate the successful transition to retirement; education and volunteer leisure activities are some common activities. (Refer to Chapter 18—Work and Retirement for more information on volunteering.) Motivation plays an important role in later life learning (Chacko, 2018; Nyren et al, 2019). Learning in later life may be undertaken for a variety of purposes and can include the following:

- *Formal learning*, which is typically connected to educational systems for the purposes of gaining a formal award, qualification, credential, or other accredited outcome
- *Nonformal learning*, which involves voluntary, structured education or training outside of the institutional context and typically does not lead to a recognized qualification or credential
- *Informal learning*, which is learning that takes place through unstructured, noninstitutionalized learning activities that are related to personal interests, work, family, community, or leisure (National Seniors Productive Ageing Centre, 2010)

The reasons that older adults engage in learning are complex and multidimensional. Cognitive interest and a desire to learn are primary motivators, whether in formal, nonformal, or informal contexts (Chacko, 2018; Guo & Shan, 2019;

Illeris, 2018). Evidence suggests the following factors are also pertinent:

- Learning for its own sake
- Learning when one's circumstances are changing and new knowledge will help one deal with the new situation
- Intellectual curiosity, personal fulfillment, or growth
- Social contact or enriched social contacts
- To promote personal growth, confidence, and contributions to society
- To maintain independence and be mentally stimulated

Learning Opportunities for Older Adults Internationally

Lifelong learning as a component of positive aging has been a topic of interest since the endorsement by the Active Ageing framework by the World Health Organization in 2002 and calls for its prioritization by the United Nations Educational, Scientific and Cultural Organization (UNESCO) and the Organization for Economic Cooperation and Development (OECD) (National Seniors Productive Ageing Centre, 2010; World Health Organization, 2002). Lifelong learning has been linked to increased health, security, and psychological well-being, especially when participation in such activities is continuous (Narushima et al, 2018).

Although older adults tend to engage more in nonformal and informal learning, the number of older learners enrolled in formal classroom learning and higher education programs has been steadily increasing. For example, just over 0.3% of university students in the United States are age 65 and older (National Center for Education Statistics, 2020); these figures are only expected to rise as the number of older adults across the globe continue to grow. Such trends suggest continued and growing interest in intellectual enrichment in later life.

The availability of learning opportunities for older adults varies from country to country. Some provisions are within or supported by the formal education system. Others rely on local initiatives, and in some cases, educational programs are initiated by older adults themselves. For example, the United Kingdom provides all adults with a fully funded technical retraining and a lifelong learning loan entitlement for 4 years of post-18 education (Johnson, 2020). Still, there is a need for more research examining lifelong learning in older adults and policies that directly facilitate participation (Narushima et al, 2018).

University of the Third Age

University of the Third Age (U3A), which was founded by Professor Pierre Vellas at the Faculty of Social Sciences in Toulouse, France, in 1973, includes university courses offered in a local context. Since the early 1970s, U3As have appeared in many countries worldwide. Although courses have traditionally been humanities and social sciences courses (e.g., art, classical studies, computing, crafts, debating, drama, history, languages, literature, music, natural sciences, social sciences, and philosophy), course offerings have expanded to natural sciences and technology areas (Formosa, 2019).

The impact of U3A on a sample of persons aged 55 to 70 who attended the University Program for Older Adults (PUMA) at the Autonomous University of Madrid between 2007 and 2011 was examined by Fernández-Ballesteros and colleagues (2012). Pre–post analyses showed that even when controlling for education and age, those who participated in the PUMA demonstrated increased levels of activity, including social activity, and improved memory, and they also performed better on tests of information-seeking and general health awareness compared with the control group who did not enroll in educational courses.

Road Scholar

Road Scholar is a not-for-profit organization that provides educational travel programs for adults and older adults. Initially founded in the United States as Elderhostel, Road Scholar now offers educational programs in approximately 150 countries (Road Scholar, n.d.-a). Road Scholar also offers a Lifelong Learning Institute (LLI) Network, which provides noncredit college-level educational experiences to more than 100,000 older adults at more than 400 colleges and universities annually (Road Scholar, n.d.-b). Besides providing a variety of courses led by LLI members, host college faculty, or outside experts, these associations offer social activities such as book discussion groups, theater trips, and walking clubs. There are no prerequisite degrees and no homework assignments, examinations, or grades.

Assessments

Evaluation of leisure includes opportunities to identify and explore interests and learn about the client's routines or preferred occupations. Relevant assessments include the following:

- The **Canadian Occupational Performance Measure (COPM)** is an evidence-based outcome measure that measures performance and satisfaction in self-care, productivity, and leisure through client self-report (Law et al, 2019). The COPM may be administered with caregivers and has been translated into more than 35 languages (Law et al, 2019).
- The **Assessment of Occupational Functioning Modified Interest Checklist** collects information on client interest and participation in more than 65 leisure activities at multiple points in time (e.g., past, current, future). This assessment can be completed by the client on their own or with a therapist. Multiple versions of this assessment are available, including region-specific adaptations (e.g., United Kingdom, Ireland) and for "diverse learners/readers in a community mental health setting" (MOHO-IRM Web, 2022).
- The **Occupational Questionnaire** catalogs a client's participation in activities throughout the day. The client's

perception of competence, value, and enjoyment is rated for each occupation; listed occupations are then categorized as work, play, or leisure (MOHO-IRM Web, 2022).
- The **Patient-Reported Outcomes Measurement Information System (PROMIS®)** is a collection of person-centered outcome measures in multiple languages for children and adults. Many tools in the PROMIS® system may be relevant to leisure in older adults, such as the Ability to Participate in Social Roles and Activities scale (Cella et al, 2010).
- The **Quality of Life in Neurological Disorders (Neuro-QoL™)** system is similar to PROMIS® but has a focus on adults and children with neurological conditions (Gershon et al, 2012).
- The **World Health Organization Disability Assessment Schedule (WHODAS 2.0)** was developed by the World Health Organization to capture information of multiple domains of functioning across cultures. One domain is termed Life Activities and includes topics such as domestic responsibilities, leisure, work, and school (Üstün et al, 2010).

Applied Scenario

Oko has been newly admitted into an assisted living facility. Oko's occupational therapy evaluation begins with the COPM, where the therapist learns that Oko is dissatisfied with his ability to complete activities of daily living (ADLs) and remain engaged throughout the day. Specifically, Oko has difficulty maintaining his stability as he pulls on his pants and experiences upper extremity tremors, which make tasks such as buttoning his clothes or shaving difficult. Oko has also fallen before and is afraid of future falls and potential injury. This makes it difficult for him to engage in occupations outside of the home, such as going out for a walk and meeting friends. He feels safer being indoors and seated most of the day. Given this information, the occupational therapist administers the Occupational Questionnaire to understand more about the activities that are and have been meaningful to Oko. This information reveals a subset of activities that are intrinsically motivating to Oko and that can be incorporated as treatment goals. In this way, the occupational therapist can address Oko's current limitation in ADL performance related to weakness and fear of falling while enhancing his ability to enhance well-being through participation in valued leisure occupations.

Exemplar Interventions

A systematic review investigated occupational therapy interventions supporting social participation and leisure for community-dwelling older adults (Smallfield & Molitor, 2018). The results demonstrated strong support for education interventions and moderate evidence for self-management programs to support engagement in leisure (Smallfield & Molitor, 2018). A second systematic review investigating the effectiveness of occupational therapy interventions for leisure for older adults with low vision found few studies in this area and none addressing leisure for this specific population (Nastasi, 2022). The following are examples of interventions and approaches that target leisure and are relevant to occupational therapy.

Skills2Care

Skills2Care is an education and training program for caregivers of people with dementia living in the community. Originating at Thomas Jefferson University in the United States, Skills2Care uses many approaches to increase caregiver skill, mood, and efficacy while decreasing client need for assistance and frequency of behavioral symptoms (Gitlin et al, 2010). Although this program does not address leisure as a direct focus of intervention, one of the approaches to obtain these results is through the use of activities, such as preferred or adapted leisure activities, prior to the client completing difficult tasks. It recognizes the therapeutic power of leisure to affect behavior, mood, and independence with people with dementia.

Community Aging in Place—Advancing Better Living for Elders (CAPABLE)

Community Aging in Place—Advancing Better Living for Elders (CAPABLE) is a 4- to 5-month program created by Johns Hopkins University School of Nursing in the United States that involves an interprofessional team of occupational therapy, nursing, and home improvement professionals (Breysee et al, 2021). It has been found effective at improving independence, safety, motivation, and self-efficacy while reducing symptoms of depression (Breysse et al, 2021; Rodakowski et al, 2021). Although typically associated with home modifications and home safety, the Client-Clinician Assessment Protocol (C-CAP) is completed on the first visit. Here, goals for visits are chosen by the client and include three questions regarding social participation, leisure participation, and volunteer activities. Clients rate the difficulty of the task and its importance to them before the clinician rates their level of independence and efficiency in the task. As part of their participation in the CAPABLE program, clients can create goals around these activities, which are then addressed via home modifications, assistive devices, and brainstorming strategies.

The approach taken within the CAPABLE program is similar to coaching, a method that allows client autonomy and promotes client choice regarding goal-setting, strategy selection, and participation (Kessler et al, 2014). Coaching allows client-centered care while engaging in goal-focused problem-solving with clients. With clients who have had CVAs, the use of coaching has had a positive effect on participation and satisfaction with volunteering, recreational activities, and social participation (Kessler et al, 2014).

Lifestyle Redesign®

Lifestyle Redesign® focuses on assisting people in creating habits and routines that promote their own health and well-being. Created at the University of Southern California in the United States, Lifestyle Redesign® has had a positive impact on pain, social participation, mental health, and life satisfaction (Lund et al, 2012). Levasseur et al (2019) adapted Lifestyle Redesign® to Quebecois culture with a desire to examine its effectiveness in addressing leisure participation in French Canadians. Results showed an increase in interest and positive attitudes toward leisure across all participants as well as participation in leisure for those with disabilities. Participants also planned to participate more in familiar and unfamiliar leisure activities.

Use of Assistive Technology to Support Leisure

Despite the potential for assistive technology to support leisure participation, there is not much literature that examines the role that assistive technology can play to specifically address leisure for older adults (Klimova et al, 2018; Smallfield & Molitor, 2018). Most assistive technology research for older adults focuses on ADLs or supporting social participation to reduce social isolation, depression, and loneliness (Cruz et al, 2016; Embarak et al, 2021). More research is needed on assistive technology to support leisure participation.

There is an enduring misconception that older adults are not interested in using technology or are unable to learn how to use new technology (McLaughlin & Pak, 2020); this is simply not true. However, challenges exist regarding the adoption and use of assistive technology for leisure activities including:

- Out of pocket costs
- Risk of technology abandonment I
- Inaccessible design of technologies that do not support physiological age-related changes
- Usability concerns
- Available infrastructure
- Desire to complete tasks according to preestablished patterns and routines (Chung et al, 2021; McLaughlin & Pak, 2020; Troncone et al, 2020).

Older adults are more likely to adopt a technology if it:

- Is affordable
- Brings value to their lives
- Is a new use of an already owned device
- Is a familiar technology
- Is something being used by family and friends (Gorenko et al, 2021; Li et al, 2019).

Electronics and smart devices are highlighted as potential assistive devices, especially the use of touchscreen tablets for games, books, social media, and talking with family and friends (Embarak et al, 2021). Many older adults own a smartphone, with a large number also owning tablets and e-readers (McLaughlin & Pak, 2020). There is evidence to support virtual volunteering, virtual reality leisure activities with a gaming or sport component, and maintenance of social contact through social media and smart devices as beneficial leisure activities for mental and physical health in older adults (Jeng et al, 2020; Lachance, 2020). Smart homes are also being examined and have been found to offload many daily chores to allow for the time to participate in leisure activities (Kon et al, 2017). Promoting Best Practice 17-2 addresses the importance of addressing technology for leisure as part of occupational therapy.

PROMOTING BEST PRACTICE 17-2
Enhanced Activities of Daily Living

Given the rise in use of technology by older adults to access virtual leisure opportunities, occupational therapists should include training in *enhanced activities of daily living (EADLs)* in their practice to support older adults' abilities to access technologically-based leisure activities. Examples of EADLs include any task that involves the ability to manage technology in daily life, such as digital gaming and social networking (Rogers et al, 2020). This will assist with addressing the challenges that older adults may face with learning new technologies and different social norms stemming from the online world in leisure and lifelong learning (McLaughlin & Pak, 2020). Practitioners should be aware of resources in their community for the acquisition of needed devices and appropriate internet connectivity to ensure equal access to this form of leisure.

Interprofessional Collaboration in Evaluation and Intervention

Various professionals with whom occupational therapy practitioners may collaborate address leisure as part of their practice. Certified therapeutic recreation specialists (CTRS) use leisure and recreational activities to improve or maintain physical, cognitive, social, emotional, and spiritual abilities (American Therapeutic Recreation Association, 2022). Their work is not to be confused with recreation workers, who include the activity directors and activity assistants often found in facilities. Recreation workers are responsible for planning recreational activities for enjoyment, including group activities, programs, and events (U.S. Bureau of Labor Statistics, 2022). The activities departments of long-term care and memory care facilities support the physical and mental health of the facility's residents by organizing and facilitating activities that meet the interests and abilities of their residents. Activity directors and activity assistants are considered recreation workers who may have degrees in specific recreation activities and liberal arts or have earned certificates to work in this capacity. It is also possible that they are certified therapeutic recreation specialists or certified occupational therapy assistants who are working under the title of an activity director.

Just as occupational therapy practitioners do, other members of the care team recognize the unique value of leisure in supporting overall health and wellness, using leisure as the medium to promote physical and mental well-being. For example, practitioners can encourage clients to participate in activities of interest in long-term care or a memory care unit as run by recreation workers. Practitioners could also refer to and collaborate with a CTRS to explore new opportunities when a client has experienced a significant life-changing event that affects their typical participation in leisure activities. For instance, after a spinal cord injury, a client may find it beneficial to explore adaptive sports with both the occupational therapist and CTRS to find options and learn the sport of interest with the occupational therapist assisting in supplying pertinent information regarding the client's functional abilities and assisting in the adaptation of the sport. Additionally, recreation workers and occupational therapists can work together during group activities to adapt the activity to specific residents' needs. The occupational therapist could also incorporate the group activity into their client's individual treatment to meet treatment goals by changing the sizes of game pieces to facilitate fine motor coordination or to provide physical assistance in standing for stamina during a game.

CASE STUDY (CONTINUED)

Intervention Plan and Discharge Status

Because the occupational therapist understood that the purpose of the intervention was to enable Anay to experience leisure by gaining greater control for cooking, the therapist framed decisions in the context of leisure rather than in the context of motor control. Further, the occupational therapist collaborated with the physical therapist, who worked with Anay to facilitate more normal patterns of movement in her arm and help her move more quickly.

At the meso and macro levels, the occupational therapist and Anay identified culturally relevant recipes and foods preferred by her family. The therapist engaged Anay's grandchildren in food preparation, because Anay shared that she enjoyed cooking with them as a means to spend time together. Lastly, the occupational therapist and Anay developed a recipe book for preferred recipes using cost-conscious ingredients that she could purchase at a local grocery. They also investigated various options for safely obtaining groceries that did not require Anay to drive (e.g., delivery service, going shopping with a friend). Intervention with Anay was highly successful and took place over 6 weeks. When the occupational therapist contacted Anay by phone several weeks after the last intervention session, Anay was too busy to talk because she was involved in preparing a holiday dinner for her family.

Questions

1. How might participation in leisure affect Anay's current social, physical, and emotional health?
2. What other assessments could an occupational therapist use to better understand Anay's engagement in leisure?
3. What reasoning did the occupational therapist likely use to select the interventions described? What else would you include in Anay's plan of care?

Answers

1. Cooking has a clear social meaning to Anay. It is important to note that cooking was far more than meal preparation for eating; preparing meals for her family provided her with the most meaning. She also used cooking with her family as part of her social participation. In Anay's case, the leisure activity of cooking provided her with one of her most meaningful methods of social participation. To lose it was leading to great dissatisfaction; she did not enjoy the activity as much when it was just cooking for herself.

   Leisure activities can be used as meaningful therapeutic activities to assist in physical rehabilitation. In this case, participation in cooking provides Anay with the opportunity to practice and incorporate functional movements with her affected left upper extremity in a functional activity. Her left upper extremity strength and range of motion were also able to be worked on with multiple repetitions within the cooking task. Additionally, cooking demands many cognitive skills, such as safety awareness, insight, judgment, decision-making, multitasking, and attention. Cooking allows Anay to participate in cognitive rehabilitation in a real-world task that is also meaningful to her, thus increasing engagement and willingness to work through challenging situations within the task.

   For Anay, there are deep emotional ties to cooking for her family. She places strong meaning on this role and her ability to cook for her family in a way that she prefers, as her way to provide for them. Because of this, adaptations to cooking to allow her to continue to participate still led to dissatisfaction. Using mixes and cooking just for herself to simplify the task led her to not enjoy the activity as much. This caused less engagement in the activity and less overall health benefits from her participation due to less engagement. It is important to note that a person's emotional ties to a leisure activity and being able to complete it in a way that is satisfactory to themself both play an important role in the emotional health of a person (LO 17-1).

2. The occupational therapist may benefit from a standardized, occupation- and performance-based assessment such as the Performance Assessment of Self-care Skills or Assessment of Motor and Process Skills. Results from these assessments will provide information about Anay's abilities in the context of occupation and complement data already collected (e.g., self-report, data on factors such as strength). The Fugl-Meyer Assessment may also be useful for

capturing data about sensorimotor performance specifically in persons who have experienced stroke.

The COPM was administered and presented a view into Anay's priorities. Assessments such as the Modified Interest Checklist or PROMIS® measures may complement these results by providing further insight into her interests and multiple dimensions of what she enjoys and why. Because Anay has experienced a stroke, the Neuro-QOL™ system may be especially relevant. (LO 17-5)

3. Several types of clinical reasoning were employed by the occupational therapist to determine and deliver the described intervention plan using leisure as both a means and an outcome for Anay. Anay's difficulties with cooking related to the physical and cognitive limitations from her stroke prevented her from engaging in a personally meaningful activity that was free from the obligation to be productive, as cooking for her family had more of a social component to it versus cooking to eat. Scientific reasoning was needed to understand the impact the stroke had on Anay's performance and to decide to use a leisure activity as part of her rehabilitation plan for motor and cognitive skill return. Procedural reasoning guided the choice of assessments to better understand the stroke and its impact on Anay while also examining its impact on her leisure participation to further guide intervention choices.

Most importantly, narrative reasoning was used to understand the meaning that cooking for her family had in her life and the negative effects of her lack of participation on her social and emotional health. Although people like Anay usually will receive occupational therapy treatments that focus on biomechanical factors, such as return of her upper extremity function with a primary focus on motor control, the focus on facilitating an important leisure occupation that involved her affected skills made the intervention more meaningful, enjoyable, and effective. It also allowed her to experience her preferred leisure activity and its other benefits for her overall health and well-being through her recovery (LO 17-5).

SUMMARY

Leisure is a meaning-laden occupation and has many health benefits for older adults. Leisure is complex and includes a range of factors at the personal, group, and societal levels. Occupational therapists are well positioned to intervene at each of these levels, effecting change in persons, communities, and policies. Occupational therapists must think broadly about leisure and consider not only personal preference but also items such as cost, sociocultural factors, availability of programming, current policies, and infrastructure that supports engagement in leisure. Integration of leisure as a key component of occupational therapy assessment, treatment, and goal-setting is needed to support well-being in older adults.

Critical Thinking Questions

1. When asked about what he does in his free time, a client indicates to his occupational therapist that he has no hobbies. He describes the flow of his day as going to work, coming home, making dinner, and then enjoying the rest of the night just "sitting, doing nothing." He mentions that some call him lazy because of how he spends his nonwork time. Is this considered leisure, and if so, what classification(s) of leisure would describe his situation and why?

2. How might an occupational therapist support an older adult who has expressed interest in using their smartphone to play games and communicate with friends and family as leisure?

REFERENCES

Ameis, S. H., Lai, M. C., Mulsant, B. H., & Szatmari, P. (2020). Coping, fostering resilience, and driving care innovation for autistic people and their families during the COVID-19 pandemic and beyond. *Molecular Autism, 11*(61), 1–9. https://doi.org/10.1186/s13229-020-00365-y

American Occupational Therapy Association. (2020). Occupational therapy practice framework: Domain and process (4th ed.). *American Journal of Occupational Therapy, 74*(supplement 2), 7412410010. https://doi.org/10.5014/ajot.2020.74S2001

American Therapeutic Recreation Association. (2022). *About recreational therapy.* https://www.atra-online.com/page/AboutRecTherapy

Atchley, R. C. (1989). A continuity theory of normal aging. *Gerontologist, 29*(2), 183–190. https://doi.org/10.1093/geront/29.2.183

Ates, M., Bordone, V., & Arpino, B. (2021). Does grandparental childcare provision affect number, satisfaction and with whom leisure activities are done? *Ageing & Society,* 1–23. https://doi.org.10.1017/S0144686X2100009X

Baltes, P., & Baltes, M. (1990). Psychological perspectives on successful aging: The model of selective optimization with compensation. In P. Baltes, & M. Baltes (Eds.), Successful aging: Perspectives from the behavioral sciences (pp. 1–34). Cambridge University Press. https://doi.org/10.1017/CBO9780511665684.003

Bhattacharyya, K. K. (2022). Longevity is not an ingredient of successful aging as self-reported by community dwelling older adults: A scoping review. *Aging and Mental Health, 27*(2), 217–229. https://doi.org/10.1080/13607863.2022.2033696

Breysse, J., Dixon, S., Wilson, J., & Szanton, S. (2021). Aging gracefully in place: An evaluation of the capability of the CAPABLE approach. *Journal of Applied Gerontology, 41*(3), 718–728. https://doi.org/10.1177/07334648211042606

Bundy, A. C. & Du Toit, S. H. J. (2018). Play and leisure. In Schell, B., & Gillen, G. (Eds.), *Willard and Spackman's occupational therapy* (13th Edition), (pp. 805–827). Wolters Kluwer Health.

Calasanti, T., & King, N. (2021). Beyond successful aging 2.0: Inequalities, ageism, and the case for normalizing old ages. *The Journals of Gerontology, Series B, 76*(9), 1817–1827. https://doi.org/10.1093/geronb/gbaa037

Carstensen, L. L., Isaacowitz, D. M., & Charles, S. T. (1999). Taking time seriously. A theory of socioemotional selectivity. *Am Psychol, 54*(3), 165–181. https://doi.org/10.1037//0003-066x.54.3.165

Causey-Upton, R. (2015). A model for quality of life: Occupational justice and leisure continuity for nursing home residents. *Physical and Occupational Therapy in Geriatrics, 33*(3), 175–188. https://doi.org/10.3109/02703181.2015.1024301

Cella, D., Yount, S., Rothrock, N., Gershon, R., Cook, K., Reeve, B., Ader, D., Fries, J. F., Bruce, B., & Rose, M. (2010). The Patient-Reported Outcomes Measurement Information System (PROMIS). *Medical Care, 45*(5 Suppl 1), S3–S11. https://doi.org/10.1097/01.mlr.0000258615.42478.55

Chacko, T. (2018). Emerging pedagogies for effective adult learning: From andragogy to heutagogy. *Archives of Medicine and Health Sciences, 6*(2), 278–283. https://doi.org10.4103/amhs.amhs_141_18

Chen, M., & Pang, X. (2012). Leisure motivation: An integrative review. *Social Behavior and Personality, 40*(7), 1075–1082. https://doi.org/10.2224/sbp.2012.40.7.1075

Chen, S., & Chippendale, T. (2018). Leisure as an end, not just means, in occupational therapy intervention. *The American Journal of Occupational Therapy, 72*(4), 7204347010p1-7204347010p5. https://doi.org/10.5014/ajot.2018.028316

Chizari, H., Shooshtari, S., Duncan, K., & Menec, V. (2020). Examining the effects of participation in leisure and social activities on general health and life satisfaction of older Canadian adults with disability. *Practice in Clinical Psychology, 8*(3), 217–232. https://doi.org/10.32598/jpcp.8.3.10.713.1

Choi, W., Liechty, T., Naar, J. J., West, S., Wong, J. D., & Son, J. (2018). "We're a family and that gives me joy": Exploring interpersonal relationships in older women's softball using Socio-Emotional Selectivity Theory. *Leisure Sciences, 44*(2), 1–18. https://doi.org/10.1080/01490400.2018.1499056

Chung, W., Genoe, M. R., Tavilsup, P., Stearns, S., & Liechty, T. (2021). The ups and downs of older adults' leisure during the pandemic. *World Leisure Journal, 3*(63), 301–315. https://doi.org/10.1080/16078055.2021.1958051

Cruz, D. M. C., Emmel, M. L. G., Manzini, M. G., & Mendes, P. V. B. (2016). Assistive technology accessibility and abandonment: Challenges for occupational therapists. *The Open Journal of Occupational Therapy, 4*(1). https://doi.org/10.15453/2168-6408.116

Csikszentmihalyi, M. (2008). *Flow: The psychology of optimal experience.* Harper Perennial Modern Classics.

Diggs, J. (2008). Activity theory of aging. In S. J. D. Loue & M. Sajatovic (Eds.), *Encyclopedia of Aging and Public Health* (pp. 79–81). Springer US. https://doi.org/10.1007/978-0-387-33754-8_9

Elder Jr, G. H. (1975). Age differentiation and the life course. *Annual Review of Sociology, 1*(1), 165–190. https://doi.org/https://doi.org/10.1146/annurev.so.01.080175.001121

Embarak, F., Ismail, N. A., & Othman, S. (2021). A systematic literature review: The role of assistive technology in supporting elderly social interaction with their online community. *Journal of Ambient Intelligence and Humanized Computing, 12,* 7427–7440. https://doi.org/10.1007/s12652-020-02420-1

Fancourt, D., Aughterson, H., Finn, S., Walker, E., & Steptoe, A. (2021). How leisure activities affect health: A narrative review and multi-level theoretical framework of mechanisms of action. *Lancet Psychiatry, 8*(4), 329–339. https://doi.org/10.1016/S2215-0366(20)30384-9

Fenech, A., & Collier, L. (2017). Leisure as a route to social and occupational justice for individuals with profound levels of disability. In Sakellariou, D., & Pollard, N. (Eds.), *Occupational therapies without borders: Integrating justice with practice* (pp.123–133). Elsevier.

Fernández-Ballesteros, R., Molina, M. A., Schettini, R., & del Rey, Á. L. (2012). Promoting active aging through university programs for older adults: An evaluation study. *The Journal of Gerontopsychology and Geriatric Psychiatry, 25*(3),145–154.

Formosa, M. (2019). *The university of the third age and active ageing.* Springer.

Gershon, R. C., Shei Lai, J. Bode, R., Choi, S., Moy, C., Bleck, T., Miller, D., Peterman, A., & Cella, D. (2012). Neuro-QOL: Quality of life item banks for adults with neurological disorders: Item development and calibrations based upon clinical and general population testing. *Quality of Life Research, 21*(3), 475–486. https://doi.org/10.1007/s11136-011-9958-8

Gitlin, L. N., Jacobs, M., & Vause Earland, T. (2010). Translation of a dementia caregiver intervention for delivery in homecare as a reimbursable Medicare service: Outcomes and lessons learned. *The Gerontologist, 50*(6), 847–854. https://doi.org/10.1093/geront.gnq057

Gorenko, J. A., Moran, C., Flynn, M., Dobson, K., & Konnert, C. (2021). Social isolation and psychological distress among older adults related to COVID-19: A narrative review of remotely-delivered interventions and recommendations. *Southern Gerontological Society, 40*(1), 3–13. https://doi.org/10.1177/0733464820958550

Guo, S., & Shan, W. (2019). Adult education in China: Exploring the lifelong learning experience of older adults in Bejing. *New Directions for Adult and Continuing Education, 2019*(162), 111–124. https://doi.org/10.1002/ace.20330

Illeris, K. (2018). An overview of the history of learning theory. *European Journal of Education, 53*(1), 86–101. https://doi.org/10.1111/ejed.12265

Jeng, M. Y., Yeh, T. M., & Pai, F. Y. (2020). The continuous intention of older adult in virtual reality leisure activities: Combining sports commitment model and theory of planned behavior. *Applied Sciences, 10*(21), 7509. https://doi.org/10.3390/app10217509

Johnson, B. (2020). *PM's skills speech: 29 September 2020.* GOV.UK. https://www.gov.uk/government/speeches/pms-skills-speech-29-september-2020

Kessler, D. E., Egan, M. Y., Dubouloz, C. J., Graham, F. P., & McEwen, S. E. (2014). Occupational performance coaching for stroke survivors: A pilot randomized controlled trial protocol. *Canadian Journal of Occupational Therapy, 81*(5), 279–288. https://doi.org/10.1177/0008417414545869

Klimova, B., Valis, M., & Kuca, K. (2018). Exploring assistive technology as a potential beneficial intervention tool for people with Alzheimer's disease—a systematic review. *Neuropsychiatric Disease and Treatment, 14,* 3151–3158. https://doi.org/10.2147/NDT.S181849

Kon, B., Lam, A., & Chan, J. (2017). Evolution of smart homes for the elderly. *WWW '17 Companion: Proceedings of the 26th International Conference on World Wide Web Companion,* 1095–1101. https://doi.org/10.1145/30410221.3054928

Lachance, E. L. (2020). COVID-19 and its impact on volunteering: Moving towards virtual volunteering. *Leisure Sciences: An Interdisciplinary Journal, 43*(1-2), 104–110. https://doi.org/10.1080/01490400.2020.1773990

Law, M., Baptiste, S., Carswell, A., McColl, M. A., Polatajko, H., & Pollock, N. (2019). *COPM: Canadian Occupational Performance Measure.* COPM Inc.

Levasseur, M., Filiatrault, J., Larivière, N., Trépanier, J., Lévesque, M. H., Beaudry, M., Parisien, M., Provencher, V., Couturier, Y., Champoux, N., Corriveau, H., Carbonneau, H., & Sirois, F. (2019). Influence of Lifestyle Redesign® on health, social participation, leisure, and mobility of older French-Canadians. *The American Journal of Occupational Therapy, 73*(5), 7305205030p1-7305205030p18. https://doi.org/10.5014/ajot.2019.031732

Li, J., Ma, Q., Chan, A. H., & Man, S. S. (2019). Health monitoring through wearable technologies for older adults: Smart wearables acceptance model. *Applied Ergonomics, 75,* 162–169. https://doi.org/10.1016/j.apergo.2018.10.006

Lund, A., Michelet, M., Sandvik, L., Wyller, T., & Sveen, U. (2012). A lifestyle intervention as supplement to a physical activity programme in rehabilitation after stroke: A randomized controlled trial. *Clinical Rehabilitation, 26*(6), 502–512. https://doi.org/10.1177/0269215511429473

McLaughlin, A., & Pak, R. (2020). *Designing displays for older adults.* CRC Press: Boca Raton, LA.

MOHO-IRM Web. (2022). *MOHO assessments.* MOHO-IRM Web. https://moho-irm.uic.edu

Narushima, M., Liu, J., & Diestelkamp, N. (2018). Lifelong learning in active ageing discourse: Its conserving effect on wellbeing, health and vulnerability. *Ageing and Society, 38*(4), 651–675. https://doi.org/0.1017/S0144686X16001136

Nastasi, J. A. (2022). Occupational therapy interventions supporting leisure and social participation for older adults with low vision: A systematic review. *American Journal of Occupational Therapy, 74*(1), 740118502p1-7401185020p9. https://doi.org/10/5014/ajot2020.038521

National Center for Education Statistics. (2020). *Digest of education statistics: 2020.* National Center for Education Statistics. https://nces.ed.gov/programs/digest/d20/

National Seniors Productive Aging Centre. (2010). *Later life learning: Unlocking the potential for productive ageing.* https://library.bsl.org.au/jspui/bitstream/1/2430/1/2010%20National%20Seniors%20Report.pdf

Nimrod, G, & Shirira, A. (2014). The paradox of leisure in later life. *The Journals of Gerontology, 71*(1), 106–111. https://doi.org/10.1093/geronb/gbu143

Nyren, H., Nissinen, K., Hämäläinen, R., & De Wever, B., (2019). Lifelong learning: Formal, non-formal, and informal learning in the context of the use of problem-solving skills in technology-rich environments. *British Journal of Educational Training, 50*(4), 1759–1770. https://doi.org/10.1111/bjet.12807

Pollard, N., & Sakellariou, D. (2014). The occupational therapist as a political being. *Cadernos de Terapia Ocupacional da UFSCar, 22*(3), 643–652. https://doi.org/10.4322/cto.2014.087

Rapaport, P., Livingston, G., Hamilton, O., Turner, R., Striner, A., Robertson, S., & Cooper, C. (2018). How do care home staff understand, manage, and respond to agitation in people with dementia? A qualitative study. *BMJ Open, 8*(6), e022260. http://dx.doi.org/10.1136/bmjopen-2018-022260

Rivera-Torres, A., Mpofu, E., Keller, M. J., & Ingman, S. (2021). Older adults' mental health through leisure activities during COVID-19: A scoping review. *Gerontology and Geriatric Medicine, 7,* 23337214211036776. https://doi.org/10.1177/23337214211036776

Road Scholar. (n.d.-a). The leader in educational travel for adults since 1975. https://www.roadscholar.org/about/our-story/

Road Scholar. (n.d.-b). Welcome to the Road Scholar Lifelong Learning Institute Network. https://www.roadscholar.org/about/lifelong-learning-institutes/

Rodakowski, J., Mroz, T. M., Ciro, C., Lysack, C. L., Womack, J. L., Chippendale, T., Cutchin, M., Fritz, H., Fields, B., Niemeic Schepens, S. L., Orellano-Colon, E. M., Rotenberg, S., Toto, P. E., Lee, D., Jewell, V. D., McDonald, M. V., Arthanat, S., Somerville, E., Park, M., & Piersol, C. V. (2021). Stimulating research to enhance aging in place. *OTJR: Occupational, Participation, and Health, 41*(4), 268–274. https://doi.org/10.1177/15394492211022271

Rogers, W. A., Mitzner, T. L., & Bixter, M. T. (2020). Understanding the potential of technology to support enhanced activities of daily living (EADLs). *Gerotechnology, 19*(2), 125–137. https://doi.org/10.4017/gt.2020.19.2.005.00

Ryu, J., Yang, H., Kim, A. C. H., Kim, K. M., & Heo, J. (2018). Understanding pickleball as a new leisure pursuit among older adults. *Educational Gerontology, 44*(2–3), 128–138. https://doi.org/10.1080/03601277.2018.1424507

Sabat, S. R. (2018). *Alzheimer's disease and dementia: What everyone needs to know®.* Oxford University Press.

Smallfield, S., & Molitor, W. L. (2018). Occupational therapy interventions supporting social participation and leisure engagement for community-dwelling older adults: A systematic review. *American Journal of Occupational Therapy, 72*(4), 7204190020p1-7204190020p8. https://doi.org/10.5014/ajot.2018.030627

Son, J. S. (2018). Marginalization in leisure and health resources in a rural U.S. Town: Social justice issues related to age, race, and class. *International Journal of the Sociology of Leisure, 1,* 5–27. https://doi.org/10.1007/s41978-017-0001-7

Sugar, J. A. (2019). Introduction to aging: A positive, interdisciplinary approach. *The Gerontologist, 61*(3), 478–479. https://doi.org/10.1093/geront/gnaa211

Theurer, K., Mortenson, B., Stone, R., Suto, M., Timonen, V., & Rozanova, J. (2015). The need for a social revolution in residential care. *Journal of Aging Studies, 35,* 201–210. https://doi.org/10.1016/j.jaging.2015.08.011

Torregosa-Ruiz, M., Gutierrez, M., Alberola, S., & Tomas, J. M. (2021). Successful aging model based on personal resources, self-care, and life satisfaction. *The Journal of Psychology, 155*(7), 606–623. https://doi.org/10.1080/00223980.2021.1935676

Troncone, A., Amorese, T., Cuciniello, M., Saturno, R., Pugliese, L., Cordasco, G., Vogel, C., & Esposito, A. (2020). Advanced assistive technologies for elderly people: A psychological perspective on seniors' needs and preferences (Part A). *Acta Polytechnica Hungarica, 17*(2).

Tse, D. C., Nakamura, J., & Csikszentmihalyi, M. (2022). Flow experiences across adulthood: Preliminary findings on the continuity hypothesis. *Journal of Happiness Studies, 23*(6), 2517–2540. https://doi.org/10.1007/s10902-022-00514-5

U.S. Bureau of Labor Statistics. (2022). *Recreation workers.* https://www.bls.gov/ooh/personal-care-and-service/recreation-workers.htm

Üstün, T. B., Kostanjsek, N., Chatterji, S., & Rehm, J. (Eds.). (2010). *Measuring Health and Disability, Manual for WHO Disability Assessment Schedule: WHODAS 2.0.,* World Health Organization.

Wahl, H. W., & Gerstorf, D. (2020). Person-environment resources for aging well: Environmental docility and life space as conceptual pillars for future contextual gerontology. *The Gerontologist, 60*(3), 368–375. https://doi.org/10.1093/geront/gnaa006

Wang, H. X., Jin, Y., Hendrie, H. C., Liang, C., Yang, L., Cheng, Y., Unverzagt, F. W., Ma, F., Hall, K. S., Murrell, J. R., Li, P., Bian, J., Pei, J. J., & Gao, S. (2013). Late life leisure activities and risk of cognitive decline. *The Journals of Gerontology, 68*(2), 205–213. https://doi.org/10.1093/gerona/gls153

Whiteford, G. (2000). Occupational deprivation: Global challenge in the new millennium. *British Journal of Occupational Therapy, 63*(5), 200–204. https://doi.org/10.1177/030802260006300503

World Health Organization. (2002). *Active ageing: A policy framework.* https://apps.who.int/iris/handle/10665/67215

Worm, T., & Stine-Morrow, E. A. L. (2021). May the flow be with you: Age differences in the influence of social motives and context on the experience of activity engagement. *Journal of Adult Development, 28*(4), 265–275. https://doi.org/10.1007/s10804-021-09375-3

Xu, X. Y., Leung, D. L., Leung, A. Y. M., Kwan, R. Y. C., Lian, T. N., & Chai, A. J. (2022). "Am I entitled to take a break in caregiving?": Perceptions of leisure activities of family caregivers of loved ones with dementia in China. *Dementia (London), 21*(5), 1682–1698. https://doi.org/10.1177/14713012221093879

Yoon, H., Huber, L., & Kim, C. (2021a). Sustainable aging and leisure behaviors: Do leisure activities matter in aging well? *Sustainability, 13*(4), 1–12. https://doi.org/10.3390/su13042348

Yoon, H., Kim, E., & Kim, C. (2021b). Sociodemographic characteristics and leisure participation through the perspective of leisure inequalities in later life. *Sustainability, 13*(16), 8787. https://www.mdpi.com/2071-1050/13/16/8787

CHAPTER 18

Work and Retirement

Brent Braveman, PhD, OTR, FAOTA
Patricia Bowyer, EdD, MS, OTR, FAOTA, SFHEA

> *"It is a mistake to regard age as a downhill grade toward dissolution. The reverse is true. As one grows older, one climbs with surprising strides."*
>
> —George Sand

LEARNING OUTCOMES

By the end of this chapter, readers will be able to:

18-1. Describe patterns in changing demographics in older adults and older adult workers.
18-2. Explain models of retirement and patterns of transitioning to full retirement or part-time work in older adults.
18-3. Articulate global and cultural differences regarding work, retirement, and associated policies.
18-4. Identify special considerations for assessment of occupational performance with adults transitioning to retirement or planning or struggling with bridge employment.
18-5. Explain the focus of occupational therapy interventions with older adults transitioning to retirement.
18-6. Describe best practices for occupational therapy interprofessional collaboration, as well as evaluation and treatment of older adults who continue to work and/or are transitioning to retirement.
18-7. Describe the various types of work and volunteer occupations (i.e., named and familiar activities) typically performed by older adults.

Mini Case Study

Brian Wong has reached the age at which he planned to retire. For the past 30 years, he has been saving for his retirement. He contributed to his company's 401K and has been working with a financial advisor for the past 10 years of his employment to be sure he will have enough money to carry him through his retirement and allow him to participate in activities he has planned. Nonetheless, like many older adults, Brian worries sometimes that he may not have adequate financial resources to fully retire without some employment to supplement his retirement funds. He also wonders if he will miss aspects of working, such as having a daily routine and socializing with coworkers.

Brian plans to volunteer with a local literacy agency and the American Red Cross. He also wants to become active in his local animal rescue shelter and travel around the United States. At 68 years old, Brian is in good health and has not been placed on any medications or given any restrictions by his physician. He has been divorced for over 30 years and has no children. He has been looking forward to his retirement and intends to fully enjoy his transition to retiree and pursue many other activities.

Provocative Questions

1. Are Brian's plans sufficient to support his participation in his activities of interest in retirement?
2. What potential barriers to successful retirement might interfere with his quality of life once he retires?
3. How do Brian's plans to become involved in volunteer activities after retirement conform to emerging trends for older adults and work and retirement?

This chapter explores the topics of work, retirement, and volunteerism in older adults. In general, the term *older adults* refers to persons age 65 and older; however, it must be recognized that there is great variability in the health and functional status of persons as they age. Many older adults will continue to work well past the age of 65, either because of financial demands or because they find work rewarding and do not wish to leave the workplace. Others may choose to retire or move from full-time employment to part-time employment. Adults of all ages may be involved in volunteer activities in their communities and volunteerism can vary from a few hours per year to 20 or more hours per week. Occupational therapy practitioners can play an important role in helping older adults continue to work or return to work, to transition to fulfilling retirement, and/or to integrate a volunteer role into their lives.

Defining Older Workers and Retirement

The landscape of the labor force is changing as life span increases. In this section, the older adult workforce is described, followed by a discussion of how health conditions may impact one's options for retirement or ability to retire.

Culture and Demographics

The number of baby boomers (those born between 1946 and 1964) in the United States who have reached or who are approaching age 65 has rapidly increased. By 2024, baby boomers will have reached ages 60 to 78. Some plan to continue working even after receiving Social Security benefits. Participation in work among older adults has been on the increase since 1996 (U.S. Bureau of Labor and Statistics, 2021). The percentage of individuals in the workforce age 65 to 74 years is projected to be 30.2% in 2026 compared with 17.5% in 1996. The percentage of individuals in the workforce age 75 years or older is projected to be 10.8% in 2026 compared with 4.7% in 1996. Individuals choose to work longer for various reasons: life expectancy has increased; they are healthier or better educated; and changes to employee retirement plans and Social Security incentivize continued work.

As baby boomers move into their 60s and 70s, they face the dilemma of retiring or choosing to work beyond the traditional retirement target of age 65. This dilemma is more pronounced for women, as a gender pension gap exists not only in the United States but in most retirement income systems around the world (Ali et al, 2021). Additionally, the COVID-19 pandemic had a significant impact on baby boomers' retirement plans, accelerating retirement for some and delaying it for others (Gurchiek, 2021). According to the Pew Research Center, the leading edge of the baby boomer generation reached age 62 (the age at which U.S. workers can claim partial Social Security) in 2008. Between 2008 and 2019, the retired population age 55 or older grew by about 1 million retirees per year (Pew Research Center, 2021). As this group reaches retirement age, there may be grave shortages in the number of younger workers available to fill the void. For this and other reasons, the number of older workers will likely increase, and these workers will comprise a larger percentage of the total workforce.

In 2014, the American Association of Retired Persons (AARP) estimated that 7 of 10 aging adults planned to continue some form of work during "retirement" and that only 13% planned to fully retire. According to the U.S. Bureau of Labor Statistics, "Among people aged 75 and older, the labor force is expected to grow by 96.5% over the next decade" (U.S. Bureau of Labor Statistics, 2021, para 1). The impact of these changes on the U.S. economy and the resulting ramifications for workers and employers may be dramatic. The patterns of work for older workers can vary a great deal and have changed over time. During the 1970s and 1980s, there was an increased trend for early retirement among men due to employer incentives and access to employer-sponsored pensions and healthcare. Participation of women in the labor force increased during that time. This downward trend among men began to reverse in the 1990s (Mulvey, 2011). Since 1990, there have been reversals in trends between part-time employment and full-time employment in older workers. Between 1990 and 1995, choices were trending toward part-time rather than full-time employment or retirement, but the trend reversed after 1995 (U.S. Bureau of Labor Statistics, 2008). Between 1995 and 2014, the percentage of older adults working full-time increased from 43% to over 60% (National Institute for Occupational Safety and Health, 2015). The specific factors driving these changes are not clear, but economic conditions, unemployment, and the resulting level of opportunity to find full-time work may be responsible. Older workers were negatively affected by the significant economic recession in 2008 including lost jobs and reduced value of retirement investments. Older adults were also significantly affected by the COVID-19 pandemic although the financial context in which they are making employment decisions is significantly different from the 2008 recession. During the earlier recession there was a steep decline in financial assets forcing some older workers to remain in the labor market. However, overall household wealth has risen since the onset of the pandemic and has supported an exit from the workforce for some older adults (Fry, 2021).

It is important to employers and society to keep older workers engaged to maintain their knowledge base, facilitate the transfer of experience, and maintain the volume of active workers. Commonly cited (Columbia University Mailman School of Public Health, 2019) benefits of including older workers in the workforce include:

1. Older workers are skilled and experienced.
2. They stay in jobs longer and take fewer days off.
3. They have a strong work ethic.
4. They retain a business's knowledge and networks.
5. They play a critical role in training the next generation of workers.

As changes in workers and the workforce emerge, therapy practitioners must understand the various ways that both work and retirement can be conceptualized and the shifts that have occurred in both concepts over time. Work as paid employment can mean very different things to different people and can range from boring or repetitive part-time work sought only to bring a wage to support oneself to a career that can span decades or most of one's adult life and is approached with passion and commitment. This is not to suggest that part-time work cannot be meaningful or also approached with passion and commitment. Work can bring great meaning and significantly influence a person's identity, or it can lack meaning and add little to a person's identity or even affect it negatively. The meaning and interpretation of work across one's youth and middle age will influence how one experiences a transition to working or retirement in older age. From an occupational therapy perspective, work can also include unpaid volunteer work or unpaid duties that one performs to contribute to raising a family or managing a home or family business.

Older workers are employed in all industry types, categories, and occupations, though working later in life is not always a possibility for those with a history of physically demanding work. Older workers tend to have higher incomes and more education than their peers who are no longer in the formal workforce. In 2019, about one in six older workers (16%) were in management, about one in eight (12%) were in sales, and another one in eight (12%) provided administrative support (Jacobsen et al, 2020). Older workers have as much chance or more to be laid off than younger workers, and they often face more difficulties regaining employment after losing a job.

Impact of Health Conditions on Work and Retirement

Despite a growing body of literature on the importance of health for employment, there is limited consensus on how to objectively measure the impact of health on employment (Blundell et al, 2021). Health itself is a broad concept and is influenced by physical, psychological, social, emotional, and environmental factors, all of which can influence one's desire or ability to work. Health is a core individual resource which affects individuals' work ability and the likelihood of a longer working life (Ilmarinen, 2011). Sousa-Ribeiro and colleagues state that, "Poor health has consistently been associated with early retirement while good health status is one of the strongest predictors of late retirement preferences and decisions" (2021, p. 4).

Among older workers, physical and cognitive capacities vary as much as health status. Many older adults experience health and vitality far into older adulthood. Yet there are also those who experience significant health issues in late middle adulthood and may present as "frail elderly" while still in their 60s. Research on physical and cognitive capacities in older adults' shows that these adults are often able to compensate for slow declines in abilities. Older workers may miss more time off if they are injured, but they are less likely to have severe work injuries or injuries leading to fatality and are more likely to return to work postinjury than are younger workers. Aerobic activity with mechanical paced work may be lower, but reports of fatigue during these activities are less common (Crawford et al, 2010; Centers for Disease Control and Prevention [CDC], 2021). The slower ability to learn new material, especially when faced with rapid presentation of information, is compensated for by stronger abilities to problem-solve and to supplement learning with knowledge gained from experience.

Older workers may experience declines in health, physical strength, endurance, balance, and thermal tolerance (e.g., working in hot or cold environments) (Crawford et al, 2010). Reaction time also may be slowed but is offset by the tendency for more-experienced workers to work with caution and a focus on accuracy. Strong social support may ward off problems of emotional fatigue, and deficits in vision or hearing may be compensated for through environmental adaptations including glasses, lighting, hearing aids, or protection from noise. Finally, caregiving can be a challenge for older workers, which may also stress their health status and lead them to decrease work efforts because of their responsibility for caring for a parent, child, spouse, or friend (Principi et al, 2018). Twenty percent of caregivers are women and are over age 65 (CDC, 2021). The factors identified that may influence older workers to remain in the workforce are summarized in Box 18-1: Factors That Influence Older Workers to Remain in the Workforce.

CASE STUDY

Occupational Profile

Maria Alvarez, a 71-year-old woman, widowed 9 years ago, has a good social support network, many interests, and a variety of plans for what she will do in retirement. She has been thoughtful about planning for retirement to ensure that she had adequate resources. As she approached her retirement date, she began to volunteer with a literacy group and fully enjoys it. She has plans to travel with friends from her church over the next year. While she is active and participating, or planning to participate in, activities she has looked forward to in her retirement, she also has some concerns about being able to age in place. There are stairs to enter her home, all bedrooms and bathrooms with showers and bathtubs are on the second floor, and her washer and dryer are in the basement of her home. She realizes that to age in place she must make structural adjustments to the main living level in her home. She also worries about transportation. Because she lives alone in a rural area, she finds it important to be able to drive and maintain her vehicle. Although her family does live near her, most are 1 to 2 hours away and work, are in school, or have the responsibility of raising young children. Therefore, it would not necessarily be easy for them to take her where she needs and wants to go, such as the grocery store or church activities. She worries about maintaining her independence and not feeling like she is a burden to others. She recognizes that she will need to address all these issues before they require her to move from her home or to essentially become isolated and unable to easily move about her community. She also has realized that there are expenses associated with successfully aging in place that she had not considered or discussed in her financial planning. She has begun to rethink moving to full retirement and wonders if she should choose a phased retirement and continue to work part-time.

Because of her concerns, Maria began to gather information about the areas that could affect her ability to age

> **BOX 18-1 Factors That Influence Older Workers to Remain in the Workforce**
>
> - Age increases for Social Security eligibility (Yoe, 2019).
> - Increased life expectancy and Improved health in older age (AARP International, 2022)
> - Uncertainty in economic climate, continued need for income and/or health insurance (Simons, 2020; AARP, 2014)
> - Continued enjoyment and social and psychological fulfillment linked to identity (AARP, 2014)
> - Employer incentives and sponsored benefits are less common, yet working increases available annuity payouts or influences social security payments (Mulvey, 2011; AARP, 2014).
> - To stay physically and mentally active and prevent cognitive decline (CDC, 2021)

in place. She mentioned to a friend the structural issues with her home, and her friend had the same concerns when she retired 5 years earlier. The friend mentioned that she had been put in contact with an occupational therapist with skills in home modification. Maria obtained the occupational therapist's contact information and arranged an appointment.

Identified Problem Areas Related to Work and Retirement

Concerned about driving and maintaining her vehicle since she resides in a rural area

Identified Strengths Related to Work and Retirement

- Has a strong social support network
- Has varied interests and plans for retirement such as travel
- Is planning ahead for aging in place and retirement
- Proactively reached out to an occupational therapist for support

Goals for Occupational Therapy

- Identify driving and community mobility needs.
- Provide education on aging in place, universal design, and environmental modifications.
- Identify strategies for Maria to maintain or enhance her ability to engage in her daily activities, volunteer activities, or travel plans.

Models of Retirement and Transition to Retirement

Opportunities for employment and the forms that employment may take will vary for older adults and may include everything from traditional work schedules to flexible or incentivized programs. Calvo et al (2018) reported that retirement has shifted from the notion of retiring from full-time employment at age 65 to a destandardized and stratification of retirement sequence. They found that when and the ways in which individuals retire have become highly flexible. This change in how retirement is viewed and experienced is linked to improved health status, increased life expectancy, and less physically demanding jobs (Sargent et al, 2013; Zhou, 2022). Retirement is viewed differently by employers and employees. Employers are concerned with cost and consistency in services, while employees are concerned with being financially stable, finding meaning in retirement, and their own or family members' health status and access to health insurance if retiring before age 65 (Halama et al, 2021; Eagers et al, 2019; Heisler & Bandow, 2018).

Options include **phased retirement,** in which employees stay with the same employer while gradually reducing work hours and effort (Cahill & Quinn, 2020). Phased retirement can provide a more satisfying path to retirement for older workers and can be beneficial for the employer by preserving the institutional knowledge that enhances productivity (AARP, 2018; Cahill & Quinn, 2020). There are three factors that contribute to the decision to retire: the state, employer, and employee. There is a phase leading up to retirement that is noted as "work-ending." This is the transition between full-time work and retirement (Phillipson et al, 2019). Work-ending approaches can include job sharing, reduced work schedules, and rehiring retirees on a part-time or temporary basis (including hiring them as contractors or consultants on an ad hoc basis rather than replacing them with permanent employees) (Grødem & Kitterød, 2021; Phillipson et al, 2019). In Japan, for example, phased retirement is provided as an incentive to higher performers. The result is that the process of retiring often occurs over several years.

Changing jobs and moving to part-time employment is also common as a transition to retirement and is referred to as **bridge employment.** This approach bridges the time between leaving a career and full retirement, providing a gradual transition for some and needed supplemental income for others (AARP, 2018; Cahill & Quinn, 2020; Grødem & Kitterød, 2021). Less common transitions include starting a private business or a new career on a part-time or full-time basis and "unretirement" after several years of retirement (AARP, 2018; Cahill & Quinn, 2020).

To some extent, retirement is a concept driven by industrialized nations and heavily influenced by views on aging. Kornadt et al (2022, p. 3) note that "Even though aging can be considered a biological process, it does not happen in a vacuum, and is shaped by societal and cultural contexts and might also vary according to these contexts, which then translates into the views that people have of their own and others' aging." Socioecological variables influence perceptions of when a person can or has to stop working. "As such, it is an institutionalized age barrier, implying that after a certain age, people do not have the abilities, resources or obligations to further contribute to the workforce" (Rothermund & Kornadt, 2015, p. 126). In nonindustrialized nations, older adults may continue to actively contribute to multigenerational families through activities such as farming, agriculture, or multigenerational childcare and retirement is not a commonly recognized transition.

Theoretical Approaches to the Retirement Process

As suggested by the examples of transitions from one form of employment to another, retirement can be conceptualized as a process as well as a specific life stage. One conceptualization of the transition includes the *life course approach,* focusing on the loss of a key life role (the worker role). The life course approach examines how transitions are contextually embedded in the normal and anticipated course of life events, and the context in which the transition occurs affects adjustment and satisfaction (Komp-Leukkunen, 2020). A similar concept is *life-span development,* in which development is conceptualized as extending across the entire life span, and we do not necessarily reach a plateau or decline as we age. According to a life-span development approach, developmental events (e.g., transition to retirement) emerge at various points in the life span. Development is also multidimensional and multidirectional. Development is multidimensional because it cannot be described by a single criterion, such as increases or decreases in a behavior. Development is also multidirectional because there is no single, normal path that it must or should take. In other words, healthy developmental outcomes are achieved in a wide variety of ways. Healthy development also involves both gains and losses (Baltes, 1987; CDC, 2022). Atchley & Barusch (2004) presented a model of the retirement process that outlines the common stages experienced. Their model is shown in Box 18-2: Atchley's Stages of Retirement.

This model highlights variations in the process of adjustment to retirement as a new state and the level of satisfaction achieved by retirees. Van Solinge & Henkens (2008) differentiated between adjustment and satisfaction in the following way. Adjustment includes the ways of coping with the transition and the cognitive and behavioral efforts to manage the process and adjust to a new life stage. Satisfaction is the level of happiness with the process and new life stage and is influenced by live events. Van Solinge and Henkens further noted that often the level of individual happiness is relatively stable over time and only temporarily affected by the transition to retirement followed by a return to the individual's "normal" level of happiness. Key factors that influence satisfaction include access to key resources including financial resources, the individual's health status, and their relationship status.

Some persons experience retirement as primarily a loss, and this may be intensified in those who lack other defined roles such as family member, hobbyist, religious participant, or volunteer (Kleiber & Linde, 2014; Fadila & Alam, 2016).

BOX 18-2 Atchley's Stages of Retirement

1. Preretirement—planning for retirement and for the process of leaving the workplace.
2. Retirement—approaches to retirement can vary from focusing on rest and relaxation to focusing on travel, hobbies, or new adventures.
3. Disenchantment—a period of questioning that may be marked by a sense of loss
4. Reorientation—period of readjustment to form a retirement lifestyle that is more satisfying.
5. Retirement routine—establishing a comfortable and meaningful routine.
6. Termination of retirement—the end of retirement when an individual may no longer be able to live independently.

Source: Atchley, R. C., & Barusch, A. S. (2004). *Social forces and aging: An introduction to social gerontology* (10th ed.). Belmont, CA: Wadsworth/Thomson.

Such a perception of loss can also be accompanied by the loss of valued personal identity and role-related activities, such as socialization with coworkers or work-related travel (Fadila & Alam, 2016; Kleiber & Linde, 2014).

Successful adaptation to retirement can be facilitated through the adoption of alternative roles that fill the void and are extensions of previous worker roles, via volunteer work or through maintaining contact with previous work environment (Fadila & Alam, 2016). Continuing to practice work-related skills helps to maintain a sense of self, sustain productivity, and preserve social relationships; however, this can vary based on cultural groups. This is consistent with the "active aging" paradigm, which is the process of "optimizing opportunities for health, participation and security in order to enhance quality of life as people age" (Principi et al, p. 57, 2018; Wiseman & Whiteford, 2009; World Health Organization, 2002). Fadila & Alam (2016) noted that engagement in leisure and volunteer work is likely to increase satisfaction in retirement through maintenance of identity in alternative productive roles. Their findings were consistent with Continuity Theory as cited in Wiseman and Whiteford (2009). Continuity theory suggests that those who link past experience to current identity experience fewer negative effects of retirement, even though they no longer experience all of the same rewards (e.g., a salary). Therefore, adaptation is facilitated by maintaining a link between preretirement and postretirement life.

Barriers to Successful Continued Employment Faced by Older Workers

Although we are living longer and largely healthier lives, individuals who work into older age continue to face barriers. Yeung et al (2021) noted that fewer job opportunities exist for older workers, and participation in training for work decreases in this group. Older workers may face discrimination in hiring, promotion, and work assignment. In 2017, AARP found that two out of three workers age 45 to 74 years said they had seen or experienced age discrimination. Fifty percent of older workers were concerned that ageism could affect job prospects (AARP, 2021). These barriers and discrimination may be driven by common stereotypes about older workers, including that they are less creative, show less initiative, and may have difficulty learning new tasks (Kumar & Suresh, 2018; Yeung et al, 2021).

A Global Lens

There are great variations from country to country and culture to culture in how work and retirement are perceived and experienced. Here are a few examples:

- In some Westernized countries, retirement is viewed as the choice and responsibility of the individual, whereas other countries have a mandatory age for retirement (e.g., China, Japan) or fund retirement through state pension plans (European Union [EU] countries) (Yeung et al, 2021; Fabian et al, 2021; Che & Li, 2018).
- In EU countries, early retirement incentives allow individuals to retire in their 50s and 60s (Yeung et al, 2021).
- In cultures where homes settings are multigenerational, retirement issues are very different than in cultures in which individuals live alone or with a nuclear family (Martinez-Carter, 2015).
- In countries that hold the older generation in high esteem (e.g., Japan, China, Latin America), elders frequently retire to care for the younger family members (grandchildren/nieces/nephews) while their children assume the worker role and support all members of the family (Martinez-Carter, 2015).
- Japan and Korea have the age of retirement close to 70 for men despite a normal retirement age of 60 (Organisation for Economic Co-operation and Development [OECD], 2021).
- On average, men in Denmark, Iceland, Ireland, Portugal, and Switzerland are still in the workforce at age 65.
- In Austria, Belgium, France, Hungary, Luxembourg, and the Slovak Republic, men leave the workforce by age 60 (OECD, 2021).
- In general, women retire around 1 to 2 years earlier than men (OECD, 2021).

Roles of older workers (or retirees) from non-Westernized countries are quite different from those of older workers in Westernized countries. In some instances, parents move out of the home and the grandparents assume the child-rearing duties altogether while their children work to support the entire family. In Japan, however, there has been a slight shift in grandparents' traditional roles because of the decreased birth rate and the move of employment from rural areas to the larger cities, requiring parents to live far from the older members of a family. China addressed the issue of employment being geographically further from the multigenerational family members by enacting a law that requires the younger generation to care for and visit the older members of families or face jail time and/or a fine (Martinez-Carter, 2015; Pew Research Center, 2009). It is also important to recognize that with increased immigration, immigrants from non-Westernized countries may move to the United States and bring their cultures and perspectives on work and retirement with them.

Previously in many Westernized nations, multiple generations lived in one home. However, as nations became industrialized, there was a shift from this living arrangement. Also, in many Western countries, the older generation is not held in high esteem, which is quite different from Eastern and Latin American cultures. In the latter cultures, the older generation is viewed as knowledgeable and wise, and the collective family is more important than the individual. From its inception, the United States has valued the individual and the idea of self-sufficiency. As the nation moved from one that was agriculturally based to one that is industrialized (and now knowledge-based), there was a shift from being family oriented (Street & Parham, 2002; Vaucular, 2015) to being oriented toward the individual. Therefore, each person's occupational transition is envisioned and patterned very differently (Jonsson, 2010).

The person, context, and culture all shape how an individual's occupational transition is envisioned (Figure 18-1: Occupational Transition to a Retirement Pattern) and lived.

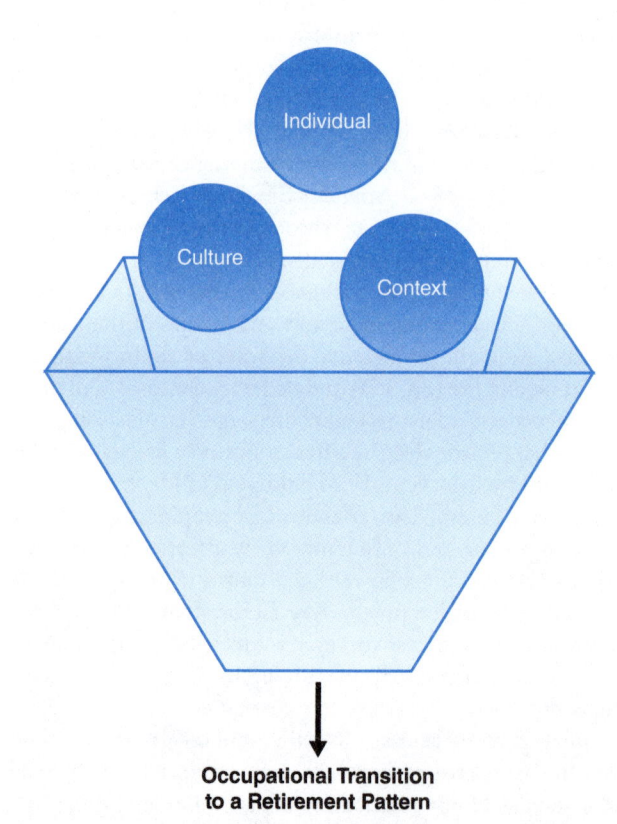

FIGURE 18-1 Occupational Transition to Retirement Pattern.

One aspect of the occupational transition does not override another; rather, each one interacts to guide life leading up to the transition, what is experienced while going through the transition, and ultimately the retirement pattern and postretirement life.

Generational and Cultural Perspectives on Work and Retirement

Generational cohort differences in groups such as the baby boomers and Generation X (those born between 1965 and 1984) are of great interest and can be a challenge for employers. Differences in these generations include different conceptualizations of work and loyalty to employers as well as differences in the need and desire for social approval; such differences are likely to result in different views of retirement (Prund, 2021). It has been suggested that general work ethic and work centrality (degree of importance that work holds at a given point in time) decreased from the baby boomers to the Generation Xers (Prund, 2021). Workers from Generation X, and from Generation Y (born between the mid-1980s and 1994) may be more likely to hold multiple jobs. Generation Y seeks approval and aligns with company values, while Generation Z (born between 1995 and 2015) is more comfortable with technology and change jobs frequently (Prund, 2021). Generation Xers are independent, like to have barriers removed, and seek work–life balance. Understanding and appreciating the generational perspectives on work and retirement will aid rehabilitation professionals to more accurately assess individual clients and remain client-centered in intervention. Another difference in views on retirement between the generations is the impact of the pandemic on when to retire and how to prepare for it. Generation Xers and Millennials (born in the 1980s to mid-1990s) are the most pessimistic about retirement (Doonan & Kenneally, 2021). Reasons for this pessimism include that they are the first generations who are less likely to have access to traditional pensions and who must rely on do-it-yourself 401K plans for their retirements. They also have faced much higher debt from college education, and personal saving may be more difficult (Doonan, 2021). Across generations, all indicate that they will delay retirement from what was originally planned (Doonan & Kenneally, 2021).

Another factor that influences retirement is culture. Within some cultures, an individual's retirement is an end goal from a lifetime of work (Principi et al, 2018). For others, it is not desirable, and for others, it is not financially feasible (Principi et al, 2018). Furthermore, the notion of retirement is influenced by whether a person lives in an industrialized Western nation or a developing nation where fewer resources and less social support may be available. Because of the decline in younger workers, many companies and governmental agencies are finding it difficult to fill open positions with qualified personnel. In some cultures, there is a set retirement age (e.g., Scandinavian countries, Italy) and forced retirement that does not allow individuals to work beyond a certain age. In each case, culture affects an individual's retirement and work life (OECD, 2019; Zhou, 2022).

Legislative and Policy Issues Around the World

A wide range of legislative and policy issues can influence the older adult worker both in the United States and internationally. Policies can vary greatly depending on cultural values regarding employment and the involvement of older persons in the workforce and in society. For example, in Germany, labor market and pension reforms have improved work incentives for older workers. These included (1) reducing maximum entitlement periods for unemployment from 32 months to 18 months; (2) enactment of regional employment pacts that have worked to raise awareness of the benefits of working later in life; and (3) increasing the age of retirement, which will reach 67 by 2029 (PricewaterhouseCoopers, LLP, 2018).

Many other countries are enacting policies and programs to promote successful employment in older adults. Descriptions of such efforts can be found at the OECD website. Individual reports are included for 67 countries with an analysis of the labor participation of older workers, current policies, and recommendations for future changes for policy is included. For example, the report for the United Kingdom notes that the employment rate of older workers is high in the United Kingdom (in 2016, 51.9% for older workers age 50 to 74, compared with the European Union average of 45.4%) (OECD, 2018). Policies cited to promote longer working lives included:

- Raising the statutory age of retirement
- Facilitating phased retirement
- Better combining of pensions (or partial pensions) and work income
- Rewarding longer careers

Kaskutas and Hildebrand (2013) provided a list of historically important policies related to employment of the older worker in the United States. These policies include, among others:

- The Ticket to Work & Work Incentive Improvement Act
- The Americans with Disabilities Act (ADA)
- The Rehabilitation Act
- Workers' Compensation legislation
- Social Security Disability Insurance
- The Family and Medical Leave Act
- Long-term disability insurance
- The Age Discrimination Employment Act
- Title VII of the Civil Rights Act

Occupational therapy practitioners working with older adults must become familiar with laws and policies that might help keep the worker on the job. Understanding and applying these policies can be complex, and practitioners should not underestimate the effort that is required to understand and apply the policies effectively. For example, older adult workers may be covered under the ADA but not simply because of their age. The Job Accommodation Network notes that "aging, by itself, is not an impairment, but a person who has a medical condition (such as hearing loss, osteoporosis, or arthritis) often associated with age has an impairment on the basis of the medical condition" (2022, para 4). Understanding when reasonable accommodation may and may not be required under the ADA can be complex and may require an in-depth understanding of the law. Practitioners who wish to provide services to older workers on a routine basis will benefit from specific training on the ADA and other legislation and policies.

Assessments

The occupational therapy process as described in the fourth edition of the "Occupational Therapy Practice Framework: Domain and Process" includes the steps of (1) evaluation including development of an occupational profile and the analysis of occupational performance; (2) intervention including development of the intervention plan, intervention implementation and intervention review; and (3) targeting of outcomes including determinants of success (American Occupational Therapy Association [AOTA], 2020). The aging process and its impact on work and retirement may also be viewed through the lens of the International Classification of Functioning (ICF) and its primary components of (1) health condition, (2) body functioning and structures, (3) activities, (4) participation, (5) environmental factors, and (6) personal factors (WIPP, 2020).

The occupational therapy process can be applied to adults who are transitioning to retirement, planning or struggling with bridge employment, or who have retired and are experiencing occupational dysfunction or dissatisfaction with their daily routines and daily life. Developing the occupational profile includes typical assessment and data gathering about a person's home and social world as well as administration of any assessments related to occupational identity or performance and in particular the person's identity, interests, and competence as a worker.

Special Considerations in Assessment

Assessments of vision, hearing, memory, and cognitive processing may be indicated if any potential deficits are noted. Assessments such as the Worker Role Interview (WRI) will contribute information to an assessment of the psychosocial factors that affect work performance (Braveman et al, 2005). The Work Environment and Impact Scale (WEIS) assesses workplace conditions that have an impact on the worker (Moore-Corner et al, 1998). Both the WRI and the WEIS are assessments based on the Model of Human Occupation and supplement the typical assessment of occupational performance that would include assessment of activities of daily living, instrumental activities of daily living, and other areas of occupation. Other assessments may be used depending on the setting and parameters, such as the amount of time available with a client and reimbursement. These assessments include the Occupational Performance History Interview (Version II), the NIH Activity Record, the Model of Human Occupation Screening Tool, or functional capacity evaluations (Gerber & Furst, 1992; Kielhofner et al, 2004; Parkinson et al, & Forsyth, 2006).

Exemplar Interventions

Interventions may occur in a range of settings including traditional rehabilitation settings as well as the home or community settings. Payment for work-related services may be a limiting factor in settings where service provision depends mainly on third-party payers such as Medicare, Medicaid, or private insurance, which traditionally do not pay for work or leisure focused interventions. Like any other worker, older workers may be covered by workers' compensation if injuries are sustained on the job, and occupational therapy practitioners may provide services to injured workers to help them return to work. Client-centered intervention planning requires that the occupational therapist involve the client in the process of establishing short- and long-term goals. Although occupational therapists are experts in the occupational therapy process, we must never forget that our clients are experts in their daily lives. Through assessment of occupational performance in all relevant areas of occupation, occupational therapists can help identify potential gaps between the client's goals (e.g., returning to full-time work) and the client's abilities, given functional limitations or deficits. Occupational therapy practitioners are also experts in assessing the physical, social, cultural, and legal environments in which the client will work. Client outcomes of the occupational therapy process can be varied and may include (a) successful return to paid employment or (b) transition from work to other productive roles including leisure and volunteer participation. See Promoting Best Practice 18-1 for an example of an occupation-based retirement program for first responders.

PROMOTING BEST PRACTICE 18-1
First Responder Retirement Transition Program

"Retire Well©" is an occupation-oriented, evidence-based, retirement transition program developed for first responders and their families. The program focuses on personal health, identity, and family cohesiveness through a multimodal approach. Twelve modules may be offered in a flexible format and were designed to include:

Preretirement	Postretirement
Stress management	Physical wellness
Family transition	Emotional wellness
Emotional detachment	Social wellness
Work plan	Occupational wellness
	Spiritual wellness
	Identity
	Generativity

Research in support of the program demonstrated a need for the program to be culturally sensitive, family centered, and peer-support driven, using a trauma-informed approach (Syrotiak, 2021).

Ergonomic and Assistive Technologies

Occupational therapy may use ergonomic strategies to assist the older worker. **Ergonomics** is the study of humans, objects, or machines and the interactions among them (Maltchev, 2012). Ergonomic approaches include examining body mechanics and posture while seated or performing work-related tasks such as reaching, bending, twisting, or lifting. Both static and repetitive tasks are examined, as is the fit of the human body in the environment (e.g., anthropometrics). Environmental considerations including noise, vibration, lighting, and contract stress are also part of ergonomic assessment and interventions.

The impact of the environment has previously been mentioned, but assessment of the physical demands of a job including the type, frequency, and duration of tasks can be included in ergonomic approaches to modifying the environment. Assessment of the effects of the environment may occur through simple observation or utilization of specific assessments, such as the Rapid Entire Body Assessment, the Revised NIOSH Lifting Equation, the Rapid Upper Limb Assessment, or the Strain Index (Innes, 2012). The University of Washington provides the following definition and explanation of universal design:

> Universal design is the process of creating products that are accessible to people with a wide range of abilities, disabilities, and other characteristics. Universally designed products accommodate individual preferences and abilities; communicate necessary information effectively (regardless of ambient conditions or the user's sensory abilities); and can be approached, reached, manipulated, and used regardless of the individual's body size, posture, or mobility. Application of universal design principles minimizes the need for assistive technology, results in products compatible with assistive technology, and makes products more usable by everyone, not just people with disabilities (University of Washington, 2021, What is Universal Design? para 1).

Universal design includes a set of strategies related to accessibility for all individuals. Such design can support older workers—and all workers—in the workplace.

Technology and the Environment

Gupta & Sabata (2010) identified the following aspects of technology related to the environment to aid with promotion of performance including the workplace: communication devices, special tools and furnishings, lighting, contrasts, visual/auditory cues, alarms and reminders, and presentation of information in alternative formats. Despite stereotypical assumptions about older adults and technology, such as the "digital divide," recent research shows that older adults express more positive attitudes about the use of technology than negative attitudes (Cotten, 2021; Mitzner et al, 2010). The term *gerontechnology* refers to "designing technology and environment for independent living and social participation of older persons in good health, comfort, and safety" (International Society for Gerontechnology, 2022).

Interventions related to work, return to work, and work transitions are often addressed by an intraprofessional team. Occupational therapists, physical therapists, rehabilitation counselors, social workers, and case managers can play a role in assisting the older adult to continue to work or transition to retirement. These services may be accessed in traditional healthcare settings, such as rehabilitation hospitals, but may also be accessed in senior settings, independent living centers, vocational rehabilitation systems operated by city or state governments, and community-based nonprofit organizations. The focus of intervention in support of the older worker or support of the older adult to transition to retirement will depend on the values, interests, and needs of the individual. Services are not routinely available or offered to all older adults and the individual, family members, or members of the care team may need to be strong advocates to help older adults receive necessary services.

Interprofessional Colleagues

In addition to occupational therapy practitioners, other types of professionals may assist older adults with issues related to work and retirement. These include physical therapists, rehabilitation counselors, social workers, and case managers.

Physical therapists are experts in movement and mobility. They work with people of all ages and in a variety of settings. Physical therapists and physical therapy assistants help people recover from injuries including work related injuries, manage chronic disease, and adopt health behaviors. Physical therapists must now enter the profession with a clinical doctorate, and physical therapist assistants must obtain an associate's degree. Both physical therapists and physical therapist assistants are licensed in all 50 states in the United States. Some of the services provided by physical therapists include:

- Diagnosing conditions and impairments related to movement and mobility
- Recommending equipment and assistive devices to aid with mobility
- Assessing physical and functional capacity for work
- Developing home exercise programs to promote improved strength, flexibility, balance, endurance, and mobility

Rehabilitation counselors help people with emotional and physical disabilities live independently. They work with clients to overcome or manage the personal, social, and professional effects of disabilities on employment or independent living (U.S. Bureau of Labor Statistics, 2022a). Rehabilitation counselors typically have a master's degree and certification, and licensure is required in some states. Rehabilitation counselors may have contact with older adults in independent living centers, rehabilitation agencies, and private practice. Some of the services provided by rehabilitation counselors include:

- Helping clients adjust to their disability through individual and group counseling
- Evaluating clients' abilities, interests, experience, skills, health, and education
- Arranging for clients to obtain services, such as medical care or career training
- Helping employers understand the needs and abilities of people with disabilities, as well as laws and resources that affect people with disabilities
- Locating resources, such as wheelchairs or computer programs, that help clients live and work more independently
- Advocating for the rights of people with disabilities to live in the community and work in the job of their choice

Social workers help people solve and cope with problems in their everyday lives, and some diagnose and treat mental, behavioral, and emotional issues. Social workers might come into contact with older adults in hospitals, independent living centers, community-based agencies, human service agencies, and rehabilitation centers. Most social workers have master's degrees and are licensed in the state in which they work (U.S. Bureau of Labor Statistics, 2022b). Some of the services provided by social workers include the following:

- Assessing clients' needs, situations, strengths, and support networks to determine their goals
- Helping clients adjust to changes and challenges in their lives, such as illness, divorce, or unemployment
- Researching and referring clients to community resources, such as food stamps, childcare, and healthcare
- Helping clients work with government agencies to apply for and receive benefits, such as Medicare
- Advocating for and helping clients get resources that would improve their well-being

Case managers work collaboratively with clients to provide "assessment, planning, facilitation, care coordination, evaluation, and advocacy for options and services to meet an individual's and family's comprehensive health needs through communication and available resources to promote quality, cost-effective outcomes" (Case Management Society of America, 2021). Case managers might come into contact with older adults in hospitals, independent living centers, community-based agencies, human service agencies, and rehabilitation centers. Case managers can have a variety of backgrounds including nursing, gerontology, and allied health professions and typically are educated at the bachelor's or master's level. Some of the services provided by case managers include:

- Assessing clients' most urgent needs, appraising the situation, and listening to the clients' concerns
- Performing an in-depth mental or physical health analysis of the client
- Developing a detailed plan of action to meet these needs, set goals, and find necessary resources to meet the goals
- Consulting with other external agencies to provide support services and resources

Staying in touch with clients to ensure the services were beneficial and that their needs are still met after pointing clients in the right direction for services.

Volunteerism and Leisure

As previously noted, the adoption of significant and meaningful volunteer and leisure occupations can facilitate the successful transition to retirement as they provide continued opportunities for socialization, promote cognitive engagement, promote mobility and fitness, and provide meaning and a source of identity. The rate of volunteerism in the United States has remained stable over the past two decades, with an estimated 30%, or 77.9 million people, reporting volunteering for an organization or association in 2019 (AmeriCorps, 2021). Although globally, it is estimated that 70% of volunteerism does not occur in the framework of organizations but rather exists informally or happens spontaneously among people in their communities. AmeriCorps estimates that the annual economic value of volunteerism in the U.S. is $147 billion (AmeriCorps, 2021).

Volunteer activities, like employment, can range from part-time or intermittent involvement to full-time or short-term, intensive experiences. Braveman (2012) described that while many volunteers routinely contribute a few hours a week, others participate in long-distance volunteering, including volunteer vacations and travel for a week to several weeks to a distant location. Organizations such as the Sierra Club (www.sierraclub.org) and others run programs in which participants may team up with local organizations or persons such as forest service rangers to restore wilderness areas, maintain trails, clean up trash and campsites, and remove nonnative plants (Sierra Club, 2022).

As you saw in Chapter 17, play and leisure activities also have a critical role in the transition to retirement. Leisure is defined in the Occupational Therapy Practice Framework as "nonobligatory activity that is intrinsically motivated and engaged in during discretionary time, that is, time not committed to obligatory occupations such as work, self-care or sleep" (AOTA, 2020, p. 47). Primeau (1996) further delineated the types of leisure activities by identifying four categories including (a) leisure as discretionary time, (b) leisure as context, (c) leisure as activity or observable behavior, and (d) leisure as disposition or experience. The benefits of leisure for the individual are wide ranging including the development of skills, personal independence and growth, socialization, developing a sense of competency, promotion of a sense of identity, and the potential to clarify personal values and priorities (National Center on Physical Activity and Disability, 2013). Leisure occupations are discussed in greater detail in Chapter 17; it is important to recognize that leisure activities can be important in ensuring a satisfying retirement.

Further, Braveman (2012) described how volunteer and leisure activities can be used with adolescents, adults, and older adults to promote participation in general but also to develop general skills, such as work habits to promote success in employment. Volunteer and leisure experiences also provide a low-risk opportunity for individuals to explore their abilities, capacities, and limitations such as fatigue, their tolerance for activity, and the application of prior skills. For older adults who may wish to transition to new areas of employment, volunteering may provide exposure to work activities to more accurately gauge interest as well as an opportunity to gain practical experience. Occupational therapy and physical therapy practitioners can benefit from using volunteer and leisure occupations to (1) assess capacity and efficacy; (2) explore values, interests and motivations; (3) develop habits and routines; (4) develop work skills and gain experience; and (5) reestablish social connections.

CASE STUDY (CONTINUED)

Intervention Plan and Discharge Status

After meeting with the occupational therapist, Maria became less concerned about aging in place as the occupational therapist provided information on universal design and environmental modifications. The occupational therapist was also able to direct Maria to another occupational therapist who was skilled in assessing driving and community mobility needs. The occupational therapist also consulted with a physical therapist skilled in working with older adults. The physical therapist determined that a physical capacity evaluation would be helpful to help Maria identify strategies for maintaining or enhancing her ability to maintain the endurance and strength needed for her daily activities, volunteer activities, and travel plans. Finally, she consulted with a financial planner again to assess whether she had adequate resources to make the types of changes to her home that would support her living there safely as she ages. After the consultation, Maria decided to alter her plans and to look for part-time work to provide her with a financial buffer for emergencies. In making this choice, she realized that it might provide an opportunity to make new friends and to remain more socially connected. With the support of occupational therapy, physical therapy, and a financial counselor to address Maria's concerns, aging in place now seems possible.

Questions

1. How did Maria prepare for retirement?
2. Why might it be important to Maria to age in place?
3. What kinds of activities or occupations do you think are most important to continue into retirement?

Answers

1. She made plans to engage in volunteer activities, travel with friends and plan ahead for possible changes to allow her to age in place as she changes physically and cognitively. She assessed her financial resources and was flexible in choosing a retirement plan that supported her goals and would meet financial demands.
2. She is familiar with her surroundings and is connected to the community in which she lives. Remaining in her home and continuing to be socially connected is likely to bolster her physical, psychological, and emotional well-being.
3. This will be dependent on each individual as to what is important to them and what they want to be able to do and achieve in retirement.

SUMMARY

This chapter explored the topics of work, volunteerism, and retirement. Large numbers of baby boomers, or those persons born between the end of World War II (1946) and 1964, are moving into their 60s and 70s. The patterns of work for these aging workers can vary a great deal and have changed over time. Full-time retirement at age 65 is no longer an option for some workers, and others are making different choices about how to approach work and retirement as older adults. Models of retirement and transitions to retirement were explored, including a life course approach, and Atchley's Stages of Retirement. Retirement planning, the context of work, and individual resources were discussed as they relate to influences on retirement adjustment and satisfaction. Generational and cultural perspectives on work and retirement were explored, and different patterns were described. Finally, the perspectives and roles of occupational therapy and physical therapy on work and retirement were described, and the potential roles for occupational therapy and physical therapy practitioners were presented.

Critical Thinking Questions

1. What are the various ways that older adults choose to approach work and retirement? How does part-time work fit and what factors influence these decisions?
2. Explain how a "life course approach" and "life-span approach" can help us to understand how retirement transitions are interpreted as healthy development.
3. Explain how leisure and volunteerism can be used to guide older adults in assessing abilities and capacities for involvement in employment and other activities as part of transition from full-time employment to retirement or part-time work.

REFERENCES

Ali, A., Knox, D., & Sonsino, Y. (2021, September 27). *How to fix the gender pension gap*. https://www.weforum.org/agenda/2021/09/how-to-fix-the-gender-pension-gap

American Association of Retired Persons. (2014, January). *Staying ahead of the curve 2013: The AARP Work and Career Study: Older workers in an uneasy job market*. https://www.aarp.org/content/dam/aarp/research/surveys_statistics/general/2014/Staying-Ahead-of-the-Curve-2013-The-Work-and-Career-Study-AARP-res-gen.pdf

American Association of Retired Persons. (2017, February 20). *10 Things you should know about age discrimination*. https://www.aarp.org/work/age-discrimination/facts-in-the-workplace

American Association of Retired Persons. (2018, August 28). *Many workers want a phased retirement but don't get it*. https://www.aarp.org/retirement/planning-for-retirement/info-2018/workers-want-phased-retirement.html

American Association of Retired Persons. (2021, January 11). *Ageism could hurt job prospects, say job-insecure older workers*. https://www.aarp.org/research/topics/economics/info-2021/ageism-job-security-older-workers.html

American Association of Retired Persons International. (2022). *What does increasing life expectancy mean for the future of work?* https://www.aarpinternational.org/initiatives/future-of-work/megatrends/longevity

American Occupational Therapy Association. (2020). The occupational therapy framework: Domain and process—fourth edition. *The American Journal of Occupational Therapy*, 74(Suppl. 2), 7412410010p1–7412410010p87. https://doi.org/10.5014/ajot.2020.74S2001

AmeriCorps. (2021, December). *Key findings from the 2019 Current Population Survey: Civic engagement and volunteering supplement*. https://americorps.gov/sites/default/files/document/2019%20CPS%20CEV%20findings%20report%20CLEAN_10Dec2021_508.pdf

Atchley, R. C., & Barusch, A. S. (2004) *Social forces and aging: An introduction to social gerontology* (10th ed.). Wadsworth Publishing, Belmont.

Baltes, P. (1987). Theoretical propositions of life-span developmental psychology: On the dynamics between growth and decline. *Developmental Psychology*, 23(5), 611–626. https://doi.org/10.1037/0012-1649.23.5.611

Blundell, R., Britton, J., Dias, M. C., & French, E. (2021). The impact of health on labor supply near retirement. *Journal of Human Resources*, 1217-9240R4. https://doi.org/10.3368/jhr.58.3.1217-9240R4

Braveman, B. (2012). Volunteerism and play: Alternative paths to work participation. In B. Braveman & J. J. Page (Eds.), *Work: Promoting participation & productivity through occupational therapy* (pp. 221–224). F.A. Davis.

Braveman, B., Robson, M., Velozo, C., Kielhofner, G., Fisher, G. S., Forsyth, K., & Kerschbaum, J. (2005). *The worker role interview* (version 10). Model of Human Occupation Clearinghouse: Department of Occupational Therapy.

Cahill, K. E., & Quinn, J. F. (2020). The importance of gradual retirement in America today. *Public Policy & Aging Report*, 30(3), 107–112. https://doi.org/10.1093/ppar/praa013

Calvo, E., Madero-Cabib, I., & Staudinger, U. M. (2018). Retirement sequences of older Americans: Moderately destandardized and highly stratified across gender, class, and race. *The Gerontologist*, 58(6), 1166–1176. https://doi.org/10.1093/geront/gnx052

Case Management Society of America. (2021). *What is a case manager?* https://cmsa.org/who-we-are/what-is-a-case-manager

Centers for Disease Control and Prevention. (2021). *Caregiving among women*. https://www.cdc.gov/aging/data/infographic/2018/female-caregiving.html

Centers for Disease Control and Prevention. (2022). *Productive aging and work*. The National Institute for Occupational Safety and Health (NIOSH). https://www.cdc.gov/niosh/topics/productiveaging/dataandstatistics.html

Che, Y., & Li, X. (2018). Retirement and health: Evidence from China. *China Economic Review*, 49, 84–95. https://doi.org/10.1016/j.chieco.2018.01.005

Columbia University Mailman School of Public Health. (2019). *The advantages of older workers*. https://www.publichealth.columbia.edu/research/age-smart-employer/advantages-older-workers

Cotten, S. R. (2021). Technologies and aging: Understanding use, impact and future needs. *Handbook of Aging and the Social Sciences* (pp. 373–392). Academic Press.

Crawford, J. O., Graveling, R. A., Cowie, H. A., & Dixon, K. (2010). The health safety and health promotion needs of older workers. *Occupational Medicine*, 60, 184–192. https://doi.org/10.1093/occmed/kqq028

Doonan, D. (2021, July 31). *High retirement anxiety for Millennials and Generation X*. https://www.forbes.com/sites/dandoonan/2021/07/30/high-retirement-anxiety-for-millennials-and-generation-x/?sh=2de50aab6535

Doonan, D., & Kenneally, K. (2021, July). *Generational views on retirement in the United States*. National Institute on Retirement Security. https://www.nirsonline.org/wp-content/uploads/2021/07/Generations-Issue-Brief-F4.pdf

Eagers, J., Franklin, R. C., Broome, K., & Yau, M. K. (2019). The experiences of work: Retirees' perspectives and the relationship to the role of occupational therapy in the work-to-retirement transition process. *Work*, 64(2), 341–354. https://doi.org/10.3233/WOR-192996

Fabian, N., Homanen, M., Pedersen, N., & Slebos, M. (2021, July 1). *Private retirement systems and sustainability: Insights from Australia, the UK, and the US*. Scholarly Commons. https://repository.upenn.edu/prc_papers/709

Fadila, D. E. S., & Alam, R. R. (2016). Factors affecting adjustment to retirement among retirees' elderly persons. *Journal of Nursing Education and Practice*, 6(8), 112–122. https://doi.org/10.5430/jnep.v6n8p112

Fry, R. (2021, November 4). *Amid the pandemic, a rising share of older U.S. adults are now retired*. Pew Research Center. https://www.pewresearch.org/fact-tank/2021/11/04/amid-the-pandemic-a-rising-share-of-older-u-s-adults-are-now-retired/#:~:text=As%20of%20the%20third%20quarter,of%20those%20adults%20were%20retired

Gerber, L. H., & Furst, G. P. (1992). Validation of the NIH activity record. A quantitative measure of life activities. *Arthritis & Rheumatism*, 5(2), 81–86. https://doi.org/10.1002/art.1790050206

Grødem, A. S., & Kitterød, R. H. (2021). Older workers imagining retirement: The collapse of agency, or freedom at last? *Ageing & Society*, 42(10), 2304–2322. https://doi.org/10.1017/S0144686X20002044

Gupta, J., & Sabata, D. (2010). Maximizing occupational performance of older workers: Applying the person-environment-occupation model. *OT Practice*, 15(7), CE-1–CE-7.

Gurchiek, K. (2021, June 28). *Employers face hiring challenge as Boomers retire in record numbers*. https://www.shrm.org/resourcesandtools/hr-topics/talent-acquisition/pages/employers-face-hiring-challenge-as-boomers-retire-in-record-numbers.aspx

Halama, P., Záhorcová, L., & Škrobáková, Ž. (2021). Meaning making in retirement transition: A qualitative inquiry into Slovak retirees. *International Journal of Qualitative Studies on Health and Well-being*, 16(1), 1985414. https://doi.org/10.1080/17482631.2021.1985414

Heisler, W., & Bandow, D. (2018). Retaining and engaging older workers: A solution to worker shortages in the U.S. *Business Horizons*, 61(3), 421–430. https://doi.org/10.1016/j.bushor.2018.01.008

Ilmarinen, J. (2011). An essay on longer working life; S 2011:05; Statens Offentliga Utredningar; Pensionsåldersutredningen.

Innes, E. (2012). Assessing and modifying the workplace. In B. Braveman & J. J. Page (Eds.), *Work: Promoting participation & productivity through occupational therapy* (pp. 325–345). F.A. Davis.

International Society for Gerontechnology. (2022). *International Society for Gerontechnology homepage*. https://www.gerontechnology.org

Jacobsen, G., Feder, J. & Radley, D. C. (2020, October 6). *COVID-19's impact on older workers: Employment, income and Medicare spending*. The Commonwealth Fund. https://www.commonwealthfund.org/publications/issue-briefs/2020/oct/covid-19-impact-older-workers-employment-income-medicare

Job Accommodation Network. (2022). *Accommodating an aging workforce*. https://askjan.org/articles/Accommodating-an-Aging-Workforce.cfm?csSearch=3937033_1

Jonsson, H. (2010). Occupational transitions: Work to retirement. In C. H. Christiansen & E. A. Townsend (Eds.), *Introduction to occupation: The art and science of living* (2nd ed., pp. 211–230). Pearson.

Kaskutas, V., & Hildebrand, M. (2013, April). *Aging workers: Work and industry special interest section business meeting, aging farmers* [Conference presentation]. AOTA Annual Conference, San Diego, CA, United States.

Kielhofner, G., Mallison, T., Crawford, C., Novak, M., Rigby, M., Henry, A., & Walens, D. (2004). *The Occupational Performance History Interview-II (OPHI-II)*. The Model of Human Occupation Clearinghouse, Department of Occupational Therapy, College of Applied Health Sciences, UIC University of Illinois at Chicago. https://moho-irm.uic.edu/productDetails.aspx?aid=31

Kleiber, D. A., & Linde, B. D. (2014). The case for leisure education in preparation for the retirement transition. *Journal of Park and Recreation Administration, 32*(1), 110–127.

Komp-Leukkunen, K. (2020). What life-course research can contribute to futures studies. *Futures, 124*, 102651. https://doi.org/10.1016/j.futures.2020.102651

Kornadt, A.E., de Paula Couto, C., & Rothermund, K. (2022). Views on aging—Current trends and future directions for cross-cultural research. *Online Readings in Psychology and Culture, 6*(2). https://doi.org/10.9707/2307-0919.1176

Kumar, D., & Suresh, B. H. (2018). Workforce diversity and its impact on employee performance. *International Journal of Management Studies. 4*(1), 48. doi:10.18843/ijms/v5i4(1)/07

Maltchev, K. (2012). Preventing injuries in the workplace: Ergonomics. In B. Braveman & J. J. Page (Eds.), *Work: Promoting participation & productivity through occupational therapy* (pp. 304–324). F. A. Davis.

Martinez-Carter, K. (2015, January 10). How the elderly are treated around the world. *The Week*. https://theweek.com/articles/462230/how-elderly-are-treated-around-world

Mitzner, T. L., Boron, J. B., & Sharit, J. (2010). Older adults talk technology: Technology usage and attitudes. *Computers in Health Behavior, 26*, 1710–1721. https://dx.doi.org/10.1016/j.chb.2010.06.020

Moore-Corner, R. A., Kielhofner, G., & Olson, L. (1998). *A user's guide to Work Environment Impact Scale (WEIS), version 2.0* (2.0 ed.). The Model of Human Occupation Clearinghouse, Department of Occupational Therapy, College of Applied Health Sciences, UIC University of Illinois at Chicago. https://moho-irm.uic.edu/productDetails.aspx?aid=12

Mulvey, J. (2011, January 5). *Older unemployed workers following the recent economic recession*. https://www.everycrsreport.com/files/20110105_R41557_efe59ef8297f3bfcd82f06c59371895f9f5a1384.pdf

National Center on Physical Activity and Disability. (2013). *Discover leisure education*. https://www.nchpad.org/discoverleisure/leisure.html

National Institute for Occupational Safety and Health. (2015). *Productive aging and work*. https://www.cdc.gov/niosh/topics/productiveaging/dataandstatistics.html

Organisation for Economic Co-operation and Development. (2018). *OECD science, technology and innovation outlook 2018: Adapting to technological and societal disruption*. OECD Publishing. https://doi.org/10.1787/sti_in_outlook-2018-en

Organisation for Economic Co-operation and Development. (2019). *OECD skills outlook 2019: Thriving in a digital world*. OECD Publishing. https://doi.org/10.1787/df80bc12-en

OECD. (2021). *OECD Skills Outlook 2021: Learning for Life*, OECD Publishing, Paris, https://doi.org/10.1787/0ae365b4-en

Parkinson, S., Forsyth, K., & Kielhofner, G. (2006). *The Model of Human Occupation Screening Tool (MOHOST)*. The Model of Human Occupation Clearinghouse, Department of Occupational Therapy, College of Applied Health Sciences, UIC University of Illinois at Chicago. https://moho-irm.uic.edu/productDetails.aspx?aid=4

Pew Research Center. (2009). *Growing old in America: Expectations vs. reality*. https://www.pewresearch.org/social-trends/2009/06/29/growing-old-in-america-expectations-vs-reality

Phillipson, C., Shepherd, S., Robinson, M., & Vickerstaff, S. (2019). Uncertain futures: Organisational influences on the transition from work to retirement. *Social Policy and Society: A Journal of the Social Policy Association, 18*(3), 335–350. https://doi.org/10.1017/S1474746418000180

PricewaterhouseCoopers. (2018, June). *PwC Golden Age index: Unlocking a potential $3.5 trillion prize from longer working lives*. https://www.pwc.co.uk/economic-services/golden-age/golden-age-index-2018-final-sanitised.pdf

Primeau, L. A. (1996). Work and leisure: Transcending the dichotomy. *American Journal of Occupational Therapy, 50*(7), 569–577. https://dx.doi.org/10.5014/ajot.50.7.569

Principi, A., Santini, S., Socci, M., Smeaton, D., Cahill, K. E., Vegeris, S., & Barnes, H. (2018). Retirement plans and active ageing: Perspectives in three countries. *Ageing and Society, 38*(1), 56–82. https://doi.org/10.1017/S0144686X16000866

Prund, C. (2021). It is time to realize generations matter on the labour market. Interesting facts about generations in the workplace. *Revista Economica. 73*(1), 88–100.

Rothermund, K., & Kornadt, A. E. (2015). Views on aging: Domain-specific approaches and implications for developmental regulation. *Annual Review of Gerontology and Geriatrics, 35*(1), 121–144.

Sargent, L. D., Lee, M. D., Martin, B., & Zikic, J. (2013). Reinventing retirement: New pathways, new arrangements, new meanings. *Human Relations, 66*(1), 3–21. https://doi.org/10.1177/0018726712465658

Sierra Club. (2022). *Volunteer connection*. https://clubvolunteer.org

Simons, S. (2020). *Seniors are working longer—out of choice and necessity* [Radio broadcast]. NPR. https://www.npr.org/local/305/2020/01/07/794209698/seniors-are-working-longer-out-of-choice-and-necessity

Sousa-Ribeiro, M., Bernhard-Oettel, C., Sverke, M., & Westerlund, H. (2021). Health- and age-related workplace factors as predictors of preferred, expected, and actual retirement timing: Findings from a Swedish cohort study. *International Journal of Environmental Research and Public Health. 18*(5), 2746. https://doi.org/10.3390/ijerph18052746

Street, D., & Parham, L. (2002). *Status of older people: Modernization*. https://www.encyclopedia.com/education/encyclopedias-almanacs-transcripts-and-maps/status-older-people-modernization

Syrotiak, B. T. (2021). *The development of a community-based occupational therapy retirement transition program for first responders and their families*. [Doctoral dissertation, Texas Woman's University]. Repository @ TWU. https://twu-ir.tdl.org/handle/11274/13258

University of Washington. (2021). What is universal design? https://www.washington.edu/doit/what-universal-design-0

U.S. Bureau of Labor Statistics. (2008). *BLS spotlight on statistics: Older workers*. https://www.bls.gov/spotlight/2008/older_workers/pdf/older_workers_bls_spotlight.pdf

U.S. Bureau of Labor Statistics. (2021, November 4). *Number of people 75 and older in the labor force is expected to grow by 96.5 percent by 2030*. https://www.bls.gov/opub/ted/2021/number-of-people-75-and-older-in-the-labor-force-is-expected-to-grow-96-5-percent-by-2030.htm

U.S. Bureau of Labor Statistics. (2022a). *Occupational outlook handbook: Rehabilitation counselors*. https://www.bls.gov/ooh/community-and-social-service/rehabilitation-counselors.htm

U.S. Bureau of Labor Statistics. (2022b). *Occupational outlook handbook: Social workers*. https://www.bls.gov/ooh/community-and-social-service/social-workers.htm

van Solinge, H., & Henkens, K. (2008). Adjustment to and satisfaction with retirement: Two of a kind? *Psychology and Aging, 23*, 422–434. https://doi.org/10.1037/0882-7974.23.2.422

Vaucular, C. (2015, July 11). *The status of older people in modern times*. https://blog.oup.com/2015/07/status-older-people-modern-times

Wiseman, L., & Whiteford, G. (2009). Understanding occupational transitions: A study of older rural men's retirement experiences. *Journal of Occupational Science, 16*(2), 104–109. https://doi.org/10.1080/14427591.2009.9686649

WIPP. (2020). *Active healthy aging in the context of the ICF-Model*. https://www.wipp-online.eu/en/active-healthy-aging-in-the-context-of-the-icf-model

World Health Organization. (2002). *Active ageing: A policy framework*. https://apps.who.int/iris/handle/10665/67215

Yeung, D. Y., Zhou, X., & Chong, S. (2021). Perceived age discrimination in the workplace: The mediating roles of job resources and demands. *Journal of Managerial Psychology, 36*(6), 505–519. https://doi.org/10.1108/JMP-04-2020-0185

Yoe, J. (2019, July). Why are older people working longer? *Monthly Labor Review*. https://www.bls.gov/opub/mlr/2019/beyond-bls/why-are-older-people-working-longer.htm

Zhou, Y. (2022, April). Comparison of pension financial systems between China and Japan. In *2022 International Conference on Social Sciences and Humanities and Arts (SSHA 2022)* (pp. 411–416). Atlantis Press. https://www.atlantis-press.com/proceedings/ssha-22/125972506

CHAPTER 19

Community Mobility and Driving

Kendra Heatwole Shank, PhD, OTR/L, CAPS

"Our transportation decisions determine much more than where roads or bridges or tunnels or rail lines will be built. They determine the connections and barriers that people will encounter in their daily lives, and thus how hard or easy it will be for people to get where they need and want to go."

—Elijah Cummings

LEARNING OUTCOMES

By the end of this chapter, readers will be able to:

19-1. Relate the occupation of driving to community mobility and participation using the language of the International Classification of Functioning, Disability and Health (ICF).
19-2. Connect age-related physiological and disease-related changes with associated driving difficulties experienced by some older adults.
19-3. Understand the continuum of care, certification programs, and members of the interprofessional team for driving and community mobility.
19-4. Appraise the utility of clinical assessments used in driving rehabilitation programs for older drivers.
19-5. Evaluate the availability and effectiveness of various driving and community mobility interventions for older drivers.
19-6. Explain the psychosocial implications of driving cessation for the older adult.
19-7. Identify alternative methods of community mobility recommended for the older adult.

Mini Case Study

Mrs. Florence Vasquez is a 72-year-old woman who is experiencing vision changes and peripheral neuropathy secondary to her chronic diabetes condition. These changes have limited her ability to drive. Specifically, she reports some fuzziness in her vision and says that it is increasingly difficult to see at a distance, such as reading upcoming signs, and while driving at dusk or in the dark. She has also noticed that occasional numbness in her feet makes using and switching pedals more difficult, causing a few "close calls" when attempting to use the brakes. Mrs. Vasquez primarily drives short distances around her town to complete the household errands and go to medical appointments for herself and her husband, who no longer drives. She also drives to visit friends' homes, to take classes for seniors at a local university, and to attend Catholic Mass services. Occasionally, she drives a friend on an errand or volunteers delivering meals for a church outreach group. Mrs. Vasquez is accustomed to driving almost daily during a typical week but has cut out some of the evening activities due to her vision, and she feels worried that she might not pass her upcoming driver's license renewal.

Provocative Questions
1. Based on this overview of Mrs. Vasquez's current patterns of engaging in the community, what areas of occupational engagement would be most influenced if she is unable to drive?
2. What suggestions might you have for facilitating continued engagement in meaningful occupations, and participation in her roles as a spouse, friend, and volunteer?

The ability to engage in activities and occupations out of the home is necessary to meet many of the demands of daily life, allowing individuals to get food and supplies, address health needs, socialize and interact, and fulfill family and worker roles. For older adults, community participation is important for a range of reasons and becomes particularly relevant for individuals who want to age in place and remain in their own home as they age. Further, well-being while aging in place is closely associated with the ability to complete these instrumental activities out of the home, which requires the ability to move about in the community (Padiero et al, 2022).

This chapter will examine the role of community mobility in facilitating participation while aging in place, the meaning of driving for older adults, and the capacities and challenges related to driving in later life. Evaluation of driving and interventions to support driving are presented, along with the implications of driving cessation. Finally, mobility alternatives are discussed, highlighting the role of occupational therapy practitioners to enhance community mobility and participation for older adults.

Defining Community Mobility Including Driving as an Occupation

Community mobility is "planning and moving around in the community using public or private transportation, such as driving, walking, bicycling, or accessing and riding in buses, taxi cabs, ride shares, or other transportation systems" (American Occupational Therapy Association [AOTA], 2020, p. 31). The actual experience of being mobile in the community is influenced by the goals and abilities of the individual, such as where someone desires to go, whether they are responsible for providing transportation for others, their physical or cognitive changes, and their sense of familiarity and competence. Mobility experiences are also shaped by the multidimensional nature of the community itself. For example, the nature and extent of travel through a community are shaped by the built environment, such as the size of roadways, density of buildings, distance of housing from retail locations, and access to mobility options such as rideshare services (Stephens et al, 2019).

Community Mobility Options

Community mobility can therefore be thought of as an example of the "activity" at the center of the World Health Organization's (WHO's) Classification of Functioning (2001) as depicted in Figure 19-1. It is shaped by environmental factors and personal factors as just described and can also be directly related to participation or involvement in life contexts. In this broad view, community mobility is what enables older adults to participate in carrying out many instrumental activities such as shopping, banking, and leisure. Community mobility enables people to attend employment, volunteer, family, or religious commitments at specific times and in designated places. Participation via community mobility is also deeply social, because being out of the home and interacting with others fosters a sense of connectedness and belonging and combats isolation and loneliness. (See Chapter 1 for more information about the WHO-ICF.)

Limitations to mobility can profoundly affect well-being for older adults, because community mobility is central to functioning and health and directly enables participation. Losses and barriers cannot always be easily compensated for; solutions like a grocery delivery service or a paratransit ride do not enable the same social participation or ability to be at specific locations that are meaningful. There are also complex environmental factors beyond the individual that affect community mobility, including neighborhood economic status, available services and resources, and community safety. Supporting community mobility for older adults, therefore, requires a broad knowledge base, collaboration with a team, and advocacy by the occupational therapy practitioner.

Driving as an Occupation

Although there are generally multiple options for moving about in the community, driving is the preferred mode of transportation for many older adults (Luiu et al, 2017). In the United States, approximately 84% of adults over the age of 65 have a driver's license and the ability to drive a personal vehicle (Federal Highway Administration [FHWA], 2022). Therefore, when considering ways that community mobility is linked with meaningful engagement in occupations for older adults, driving is often central to how many older adults want to or need to get around.

Driving is an instrumental activity of daily living for many people who ascribe meaning to it based on personal and cultural values. Driving has practical value as a means of transportation to and from a destination and as a signifier of independence (Luiu et al, 2017). Driving has additional value and meaning as an occupational enabler (Stav, 2015). Box 19-1 provides one example of how driving affects independence.

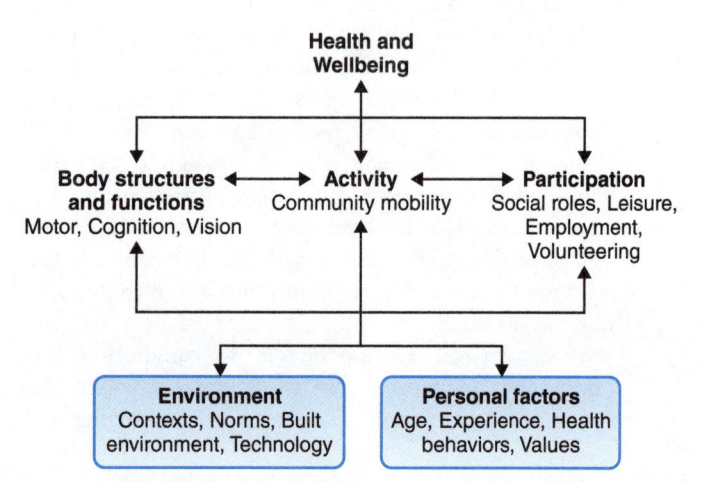

FIGURE 19-1 Community mobility facilitating participation. *(Adapted from International Classification of Functioning, Disability and Health: Short Version from the World Health Organization.)*

BOX 19-1 Driving and Community Design

A comparison of transportation patterns between the United States (Bureau of Transportation Statistics, 2021) and several countries in Europe (Organization for Economic Co-Operation and Development, 2022) shows that in the last decade (2011–2019), Americans drove approximately twice as many miles on the road. In fact, the United States is one of the busiest countries in terms of road traffic, with nearly 284 million vehicles in operation as of 2021, and more than 228.7 million drivers held a valid driver's license as of 2019 (Carlier/Statista, 2022).

This is due in part to how U.S. development and land use practices shaped the landscape of towns and cities (Weiner, 2016), where driving from a residential location (neighborhood) to a business or retail district is necessary in day-to-day life in most communities. The heavy reliance on personal cars for community mobility in the United States also reflects a cultural value of independence and autonomy across the life course, with older adults reporting that driving contributes to a feeling of being whole and provides access to the world around them and that the absence of driving—whether in the short term or permanently—feels like being imprisoned (Jones et al, 2018).

Driving and Client Factors

The occupation of driving is complex and requires skills, processing of multiple sensory stimuli simultaneously, and coordination of complex cognitive and physical tasks (Simons-Morton & Ehsani, 2016). Processing of relevant stimuli leads to the identification of objects and events and a perception of their relationships in space to one another and the overall environment. Integration of this information with past experiences provides meaning and context in relation to driving. Cues may prompt learned responses, which may result in the habitual performance of that behavior. For example, when one drives to work daily on a familiar route, the process of driving becomes routine and automatic. At the same time, higher-level processing skills are necessary to learn new skills or deal with situations that are not routine, like driving an unfamiliar car, navigating to a new destination, or responding to unexpected traffic conditions.

Central to engagement in driving are client factors, which consist of values, beliefs, and spirituality; body functions; and body structures. Individuals' interests and values guide the recognition of mobility as an important area of engagement. In addition to values, body functions such as mental functions (attention, memory, and visuospatial perception), sensory functions (vision), and neuromusculoskeletal and movement-related functions allow the individual to act in complex and coordinated ways. The body structures that support these functions include the eye, ear, and related structures along with structures related to movement.

People draw on their client factors in observable ways of acting called performance skills. Performance skills include motor and process skills and allow for the ability to operate a vehicle safely, sequence vehicle operations, interpret objects and instructions within the environment, and respond to environmental stimuli. Certain contexts, such as size of the vehicle, terrain, or traffic patterns, may affect the extent to which specific performance skills are required. Performance occurs in specific ways that develop over time and are shaped by sociocultural contexts called performance patterns. Performance patterns associated with driving can include *habits* (putting on a seat belt or using a turn signal), route and destination *routines* (taking the same route to volunteer at the hospital; going to the same grocery store each week), and *role* performance (a woman who completes the household grocery shopping for herself and her husband). Not all performance patterns are positive, and some can be negative habits (speeding), involve unsafe or limiting routines (avoiding driving in large areas of town), or burdensome roles (continuing to drive grandchildren despite impaired vision).

Client factors, performance skills, and performance patterns are activated and enacted through the environmental contexts of a community. Cultural contexts may be a special consideration, as they are imposed by family, society, and one's culture. For example, in the United States, driving is valued and viewed as a symbol of independence. In some cultures, men are the primary drivers and women are the passengers. Using public transportation may have culturally symbolic (positive or negative) meanings and may take the form of buses, taxis, motorbikes, rickshaws, or a hired car (Fig. 19-2).

Although some physical environmental features, such as roadways, parking lots, and street signage, have obvious implications for driving and getting around the community,

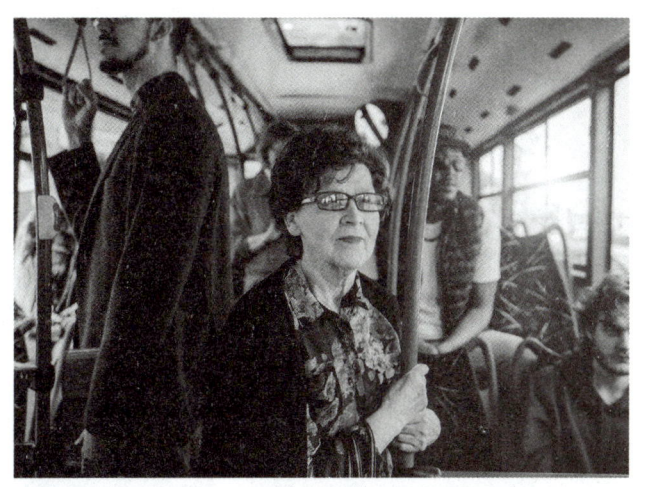

FIGURE 19-2 Perceptions of public transportation vary among older adults. *(Drazen_/E +/Getty Images.)*

there are many more aspects of an environment to consider, including:

- Culturally influenced value of driving in the community
- Products and technology integrated inside and outside of the car
- Services, systems, and policies such as qualification criteria or licensure laws
- Informal social networks that support alternative methods of driving
- Attitudes about public transportation, safety, and driving cessation

There is a significant body of literature about the environmental—and specifically neighborhood—context that influences mobility and well-being in older adulthood (Padiero et al, 2022; Stephens et al, 2019). The relationships among communities and the participation of the people who comprise a community are multidimensional and unfolding over time (Heatwole Shank & Cutchin, 2016), and effective interventions to support mobility should include context as a key consideration.

Driving and Technology

Technology is a rapidly changing aspect of the environmental context of driving. In-vehicle technology such as navigation systems, back-up cameras, blind-spot warning, and lane departure systems (Band & Perel, 2007) aim to increase the safety and decrease personal barriers to driving (Fig. 19-3). The American Automobile Association (AAA) examined the prevalence and attitudes toward these technologies and found that more than half of the older adults surveyed had at least one type of in-vehicle technology in their primary vehicles, and on average they had two such technologies (Eby et al, 2018). Although 70% of those interviewed felt that the technology made them safer drivers, these technologies were also more commonly available to males and older adults with higher incomes (Zanier et al, 2019). Furthermore, simply having access to technology that is intended to improve driving safety and performance does not mean that older drivers will adopt technology as part of their habitual driving behavior (Dickerson, 2019). Driving is a complex occupation, and the technologies intended to be solutions to safety concerns can pose increased complexity for some older drivers. The application of technology to enhance safety, compensate for driver error, and improve driving behaviors is an area of rapid growth and development.

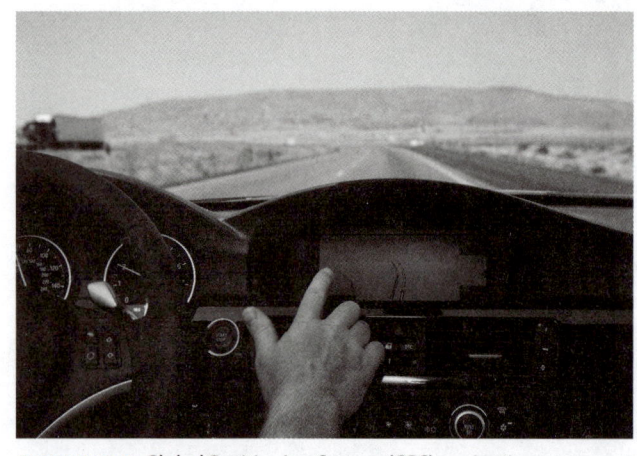

FIGURE 19-3 Global Positioning System (GPS) navigation. *(jhorrocks/E+/Getty Images.)*

CASE STUDY

Occupational Profile

Mr. Albert Smith, age 80, occasionally forgets where the keys are or what day it is. One day, Mr. Smith drives his daughter and his wife to the grocery store. During the ride, Mrs. Smith directs her husband while he is driving because he has difficulty remembering the route to take. Mr. Smith's daughter is concerned, so she makes an appointment with her father's physician to assess his cognitive skills. She tells the physician that her father has recently forgotten to turn off the stove, forgets to take his medications, rarely knows what the date is, and occasionally asks for directions to what should be familiar places. Mr. Smith has never had an accident or ticket and feels he is a safe driver. After a career as an engineer, Mr. Smith has found active pursuits like racquetball at the senior center and hiking in local parks to be most enjoyable. He drives alone to the post office, hardware store, and to a local restaurant to "meet the boys" for breakfast. He and his wife go to the grocery store and pharmacy; he takes her to the beauty parlor and to church—"Not at night, mind you"—and avoids "downtown." He reluctantly agrees to come in for an occupational therapy driving evaluation.

Identified Problem Areas and Strengths

The occupational therapist completes several types of assessments. At the end of the testing, the occupational therapist notes that Mr. Smith has some mild arthritis, which slows his walking, but he otherwise does well physically. He is independent in all his self-care. He has less than ideal vision but is within the parameters set by the state driving licensing agency, and he appears to have some mild cognitive changes. When using the Montreal Cognitive Assessment (MoCA), the occupational therapist noted difficulty with visuospatial trail-making tasks and short-term recall tasks.

Goals for Occupational Therapy

From Mr. Smith's perspective, he is faced with the prospect of not driving and loss of independence. He is also concerned about the implications for his wife, who does not have a license due to her own poor vision and physical frailty, and he fears she will be completely isolated at home if he cannot take her out and about. After the evaluation, goals set for Mr. Smith include introducing some cognitive supports, identifying alternative mobility options, and initiating family conversation about voluntary driving restrictions.

Impact of Health Conditions on Community Mobility and Driving

There is no single metric of driving safety (Souman et al, 2021), but drivers of every age rely on performance and capability to decrease risk for injury and fatality for themselves and other drivers. **Driving safety** and **driving performance** are two main indicators used in driving research. Safety involves avoidance of such adverse driving events as motor vehicle crashes, whereas performance refers to driver behavior when operating a motor vehicle. Physical driving behavior measures usually include speed, braking, lane keeping, and visual scanning. Driving performance is measured by ratings given by a trained evaluator who rides in the vehicle and uses a standardized scale. There is a complex relationship between changes associated with older age, decreasing performance over time, and risky driving behaviors (Toups et al, 2022). Some age-related changes and common medical conditions can directly affect a driver's performance skills, thus compromising driving safety as presented in Box 19-2. Section two describes other age-related changes—both typical and associated with disease processes—that may be related to changes in driving for the older driver. Several common age- and condition-related impacts are described next.

Visual Functions and Driving Performance and Safety

Changes in visual functions that are associated with driving include impairments in visual acuity, contrast sensitivity, visual field, and visual processing speed; these are most commonly experienced by older adults with cataracts, glaucoma, and macular degeneration (National Highway Traffic Safety Administration, n.d.). Grundler and Strasburger (2020) concluded that visual acuity alone is not an appropriate method for assessing fitness to drive, whereas other researchers have demonstrated that dynamic visual acuity, mimicking real-world driving conditions, is a useful predictor of impaired driving performance (Hwang et al, 2020). Contrast sensitivity is another visual function required for recognizing road signs, obstacles, and pedestrians while driving. Because contrast sensitivity may be impaired due to many of the common age-related conditions listed below, screening is particularly relevant for the older driver (Spreng et al, 2018). Research consistently indicates a relationship between impaired acuity, decreased contrast sensitivity, and reduced driving performance (Ortiz-Peregrina et al, 2020).

In terms of field of vision changes, it is generally believed that visual field impairment may elevate crash risk. Field of vision impairment is particularly associated with at-fault collisions for attempted left turns and an overall history of increased motor vehicle accidents among older adults (Swain et al, 2021). The National Highway Traffic Safety Administration (NHTSA) (n.d.) recommends that older adults with changes in their peripheral vision and processing speed seek specialized assessment by a driving rehabilitation professional.

Cognitive Functions and Driving Performance and Safety

Cognitive function has been shown to directly predict measures of driving performance (Staplin et al, 2019). Both on-road and simulated driving assessments showed that older adults with a diagnosed dementia demonstrated impaired skill and capacity (Fraade-Blanar et al, 2018), and fitness to drive is severely impaired as the dementia progresses (Toepper & Falkenstein, 2019). According to NHTSA (n.d.), dementia can reduce older driver performance and increase driving errors that lead to vehicle crashes. Problematic behaviors include becoming lost in familiar places, incorrect turning, impaired signaling, decreased comprehension of traffic signs, and lane deviation (Staplin et al, 2019). However, experts suggest that the diagnosis of Alzheimer disease alone is not sufficient to cause the immediate withdrawal of driving privileges. Not only is there a possibility of misdiagnosis, particularly in the early stages of dementia, but driving performance in the milder stages of Alzheimer disease may still be acceptable.

Although some research shows that individuals diagnosed with dementia have lower motor vehicle crash rates (e.g., Fraade-Blaner et al, 2018), this may be due to self-limiting or family intervention to reduce driving following a dementia diagnosis. In general, there is strong international consensus that individuals with moderate to severe dementia should not drive (Chee et al, 2017; Rapoport et al, 2018). Instead, these individuals should be referred for further testing when risk factors for unsafe driving exist (Rapoport et al, 2018). Physicians should refer clients with very mild and mild dementia for a driver performance evaluation by a certified examiner and reassessment every 6 months—or more often if families report concern or dementia is

---

BOX 19-2 Motor Vehicle Crashes and Fatalities

Fatal crash rates increase starting at age 70 to 74 and are highest among drivers older than 84. This increased rate of fatalities is due in part to increased susceptibility to injury and complications, rather than increased risk for crashes (Cicchino, 2015). In a recent analysis, Cox and Cicchino (2021) found that over the last several decades, fatal crashes have declined in all categories, but the greatest declines have been for those age 70 and older. However, there is still evidence that changes in cognition, such as those associated with mild cognitive impairment or Alzheimer disease, have the most pronounced and negative impact on driving performance (Toups et al, 2022). Despite the downward trend, fatal crash rates per miles traveled rise after age 70 and peak in drivers age 85 and older (American Association of Retired Persons, 2022).

rapidly progressing. In summary, moderate to severe dementia is incompatible with driving. Those with very mild to mild dementia may be safe to drive; however, individual functional assessments of driving skills should be done to determine driving safety. Reassessment is required based on the progression of dementia.

Other Medical Conditions Affecting Driving Performance and Safety

There are several conditions that can substantially affect an older adult's driving performance and safety. Parkinson disease is characterized by cognitive and perceptual changes, bradykinesia, and other motoric impacts that can lead to an increased risk for motor vehicle crashes. Ranchet and colleagues (2020) conducted a systematic review of driving behaviors of individuals with Parkinson disease, finding that during on-road assessment, there were higher fail rates and problems with the use of signals and pedals, maintaining lane position, adapting speed to traffic flow, and left turns. Although there is not a consensus, Lloyd and colleagues' (2020) recent retrospective analysis suggested that a battery of assessments to address multiple types of driving performance and capacity has the best predictive power. Drivers with mild motor disability may be fit to drive but should have a baseline comprehensive driving evaluation performed, consider having annual driving evaluations, begin planning for driving cessation, develop a plan for use of alternative transportation, and talk with family about driving retirement. Those with severe motor impairment, severe disease, and multiple risk factors, such as decreased information processing and impaired contrast sensitivity, should stop driving and seek consultative services to address transportation issues.

Diabetes, the most common chronic disease worldwide, has several safety implications for driving (Keten, 2021). Drivers with diabetes are subject to additional questions and restrictions for licensing in multiple countries (e.g., American Diabetes Association, 2014; Bédard et al, 2010), with individuals who use insulin to manage the disease having a higher risk for motor vehicle crashes due to hypoglycemic episodes while driving (Almigbal et al, 2018). Other symptoms of long-term or poorly managed diabetes that can affect driving performance and safety include diabetic retinopathy (Bro & Anderson, 2022) and peripheral neuropathy (Perazzolo et al, 2020). For older adults with diabetes, education by healthcare professionals can have a critical role in teaching strategies to maximize safety while driving (Keten, 2021).

Finally, musculoskeletal conditions such as arthritis can affect driving. Osteoarthritis and rheumatoid arthritis can make joints swollen and stiff, which can limit the movement of the shoulders, hands, head, and neck. In a recent review, Zhou and colleagues (2021) found that older adults with rheumatoid arthritis had an increased risk for motor vehicle crashes and had higher self-reported driving difficulty, rates of driving cessation, and need for driving adaptations. Functional implications of arthritis related to driving are limited ability to operate the primary controls of the vehicle, such as the foot pedals, steering wheel, ignition, gear selector, safety belt, and other controls that require reaching, strength, or leverage. Fortunately, multiple environmental adaptations can compensate for these musculoskeletal limitations (Cammarata et al, 2020), which are outlined next.

Occupational Therapy, Driving, and the Continuum of Care

The aging process and age-associated conditions described earlier may lead to declines in any of the client factor and performance skill areas. Performance patterns can also change or contract over time, and contextual factors of a community are constantly shifting. Because these various factors that can influence driving are interdependent, dysfunction that exists in one client factor or skill area may influence the demands placed on other skill areas. Furthermore, changes in driving ability that cause an individual or their family to seek input from a healthcare professional may be precipitous, such as acute changes in vision or motor skills after a stroke, or may be a gradual process, such as peripheral sensation and night vision. Occupational therapy practitioners also consider older adults' community mobility and driving performance across the care continuum. Recommendations or initial evaluations may be made as part of hospital discharge planning. Screening at a CarFit event (AOTA, 2022) or via other off-road assessments may occur as part of a community-based programming (Collins, 2020). Occupational therapists offer other community-based intervention and prevention programs (Mulry, 2018) and may have additional credentials, outlined later, for conducting specialized on-road assessments and interventions (Sanchez et al, 2016). They may also partner with individuals and families in postacute and rehabilitation settings and offer recommendations about mobility alternatives and driving cessation. Ultimately, the occupational therapist must be cognizant of the individual's client factors, contexts, and performance patterns in a wide array of settings and situations. Therefore, clinical evaluation of driving ability requires the occupational therapist to be aware of potential dysfunction that may exist in any of these areas.

Specialized Practice and the Interprofessional Team

NHTSA, the American Medical Association, and the American Geriatric Society have identified occupational therapy as the principal healthcare discipline to address driving (American Geriatrics Society & Pomidor, 2019).

Because of the complexities of diagnosis, equipment, policies, stakeholder involvement, and high risk to the client and the public, driving rehabilitation is not considered entry-level practice. Efforts to distinguish practitioners who specialize in driving rehabilitation from generalists have resulted in two certification programs.

Driving Rehabilitation Specialists

The Association for Driver Rehabilitation Specialists (ADED), an interprofessional organization, enacted the first certification program in 1995 (ADED, n.d.). The program designates individuals as certified driver rehabilitation specialists (CDRS). The CDRS credential identifies health care providers, driver educators and instructors, and equipment dealers who have met the certification requirements to plan, develop, coordinate, and implement driver rehabilitation services for individuals with disabilities (ADED, n.d.).

Certificate in Driving and Community Mobility

Driving certification is available to occupational therapists and occupational therapy assistants. It designates individuals as earning a Specialty Certificate in Driving and Community Mobility and awards a credential of SCDCM or, for occupational therapy assistants, SCADCM (AOTA, n.d.). The SCDCM or SCADCM is an application- and examination-based certification program involving professional development activities grounded in the American Occupational Therapy Association's standards of continuing competence (AOTA, 2015). Both the CDRS and the SCDCM/SCADCM certifications require hours of direct contact and continuing education; this is to ensure up-to-date and focused knowledge, skills, and experience that add credibility when working with other team members and state agencies.

Occupational Therapy Process and Collaboration

Occupational therapy practitioners are part of an interprofessional team in driving and community mobility. Areas of change in body structures, client factors, performance skills, and performance patterns should be assessed. Formalized assessment of each skill area can be accomplished by an interprofessional team including a neuropsychologist, ophthalmologist, physiatrist, and occupational therapist and can determine whether an individual has sufficient function in any given skill area to drive. Each professional focuses on the skills or functional areas aligned with their expertise. For occupational therapy practitioners in general practice, clinical reasoning skills support evaluation of the ability to drive or travel in the community safely. When a concern for performance or safety is present, a referral to a driving rehabilitation specialist should follow. See Promoting Best Practice 19-1 for more information about occupational therapy in driving and community mobility.

PROMOTING BEST PRACTICE BOX 19-1
The Occupational Therapy Process related to Driving and Community Mobility

Guidelines follow the occupational therapy process for evaluation of and intervention in driving (AOTA, 2020) and include conducting a multidimensional assessment; identifying objectives; and designing interventions that involve the family, consider external factors, and adhere to ethical considerations to promote the safety of the public (AOTA, 2016).

Five intervention approaches appropriate for occupational therapists working in this practice area are:

- **Health promotion:** Advocate for transportation system development, provide trainings and community education, conduct CarFit screenings, and consult with developers and vehicle manufacturers to improve features and adaptability.
- **Remediation and restoration:** Provide skills training; teach cognitive or scanning strategies; and offer caregiver education, public transportation training, and specialized driver rehabilitation.
- **Maintenance:** Promote wellness and regular screenings and develop walking and biking infrastructure.
- **Compensation and adaptation:** Recommend environmental modifications, recommend changes in routes and travel times, and recommend and train in the use of adaptive equipment and after-market vehicle modifications.
- **Prevention:** Consult on proposed policies and legislation, advocate for safety policies, and provide educational programming to reduce risk of injury.

All intervention approaches require regular reassessment of goals and progress to inform ongoing services, collaboration, and next steps (AOTA, 2016).

Assessment of Driving

The types of assessments an occupational therapy practitioner will conduct to evaluate **fitness to drive** range according to the setting. In most cases, evaluation begins with a driving history, interview, and driving performance, with additional cognitive or driving-specific screenings in a clinic setting. Evaluation via on-road assessment may be conducted by a practitioner with advanced specialization. Although these evaluations used alone or in combination can evaluate critical skills used for safe driving, there is no single tool that is the best for determining fitness to drive (Dickerson et al, 2014).

Medical and Driving History and Performance Patterns

Clinical assessments generally start with a medical and driving history, which may consist of a questionnaire or be part of the initial occupational profile interview. Medical information should include any diagnosed medical conditions, including psychological diagnoses, that could have implications for driving safety, including those already discussed. The examiner should inquire about prescription medications currently being taken by the individual to determine whether any might make driving hazardous. The driving history should also include basic information about the individual's driving record. In addition to a person's years of driving experience and any formal driver's education, this will generally focus on the previous 3- to 5-year period and should include driving patterns along with on-road incidents, crashes, or moving violations. An occupational profile also should be gathered to determine the client's interest and needs related to driving and other occupational engagement that is dependent on driving. Destinations to which the individual drives on a regular basis should be identified, along with driving conditions that are of particular concern.

Another key objective is to determine the level of insight the person has into their limitations and the effects of those limitations on driving performance. Particular attention should be paid to whether the individual self-regulates their driving in any way (e.g., they avoid expressways, rush-hour traffic, left-hand turns, or unfamiliar areas). Complete reliance on the older driver's self-perception of driving ability may not be a reliable way to verify whether problems will manifest themselves in driving ability. Without awareness of potential risks, it is difficult for the older adult to correct or compensate for problems identified later in the evaluation. If the client consents, obtaining input from family members may help clarify these issues. Even the seemingly innocuous observation that the client needs assistance in filling out the questionnaire and medical forms can be an indicator of visual or cognitive deficits.

Types of Assessment and Screening

Following the medical and driving history interview, the subsequent assessments should be informed by the practitioner's clinical reasoning related to the specific concerns and underlying conditions of the older adult.

Cognitive and Perceptual Screening

The objective of the cognitive-perceptual screening process is to determine the potential presence of impaired mental functions, such as attention and memory, that may potentially affect driving ability. Although there are multiple ways of assessing the cognitive and executive functioning skills that are necessary for driving, no single test or combination of tests can predict with certainty whether the degree of dysfunction measured will adversely affect driving ability.

Specific tests used as part of a clinical driving assessment vary but may include global cognitive screenings such as the MoCA, which includes an abbreviated "trails" task, short-term recall, visuospatial tasks, and speed of processing tasks. Although the MoCA has been found to have a significant association with the useful field of view assessment, it does not independently have strong predictive validity for on-road performance (Kwok et al, 2015). The Trail Making Test Parts A and B is a well-known cognitive assessment that is normed by age and measures visual search and sequencing, speed of information processing, and divided attention (Selander et al, 2020). The Trail Making Test identifies at-risk drivers if they complete the measure with slowed processing speed (Duncanson et al, 2018). When an individual takes longer than 2 minutes or cannot complete the test, the individual is at significant risk for being unfit to drive. One recent study by Barco and colleagues (2020) suggested that some common clinic-based tests such as the Traffic Sign Naming Test, which assesses recognition and naming accuracy and speed, and the Written Exam for Driving Decisions, which is a pen-and-paper assessment of driving knowledge, were found to have fair predictive ability of standardized on-road assessments. These are recommended only in combination with other performance measures (Barco et al, 2020).

One assessment that has consistently shown to be predictive of driving performance and crashes is the useful field of view test, which was designed to assess the size of the test-taker's useful field of view, or the visual processing speed. Processing speed scores that indicated a reduction of 40% or more in the useful field of view indicated cognitive performance concerns. The useful field of view test, which is now computer based, has two decades of evidence and has been revised and refined over time (Wood & Owsley, 2014). Psychometric tests have been found in various combinations to correlate with driving ability. It should be noted that even with the extensive evidence, the occupational therapist or driving rehabilitation specialist employs them only as screening tools. Any indications of cognitive deficits should be reported to the referring physician or a referral should be made for follow-up with an appropriate medical doctor.

Vision Screening

The objective of vision and perception screening should be to determine the possible presence of impaired visual functions that may affect driving ability. It is not diagnostic in nature, because there is strong evidence that visual acuity has little or no relationship to driving performance (Grundler & Strasburger, 2020). At a minimum, distant visual acuity, visual fields, contrast, and oculomotor control should be screened. The ability to renew one's driver's license does not represent proof of adequate vision for safe driving, as standards and training of licensing staff vary widely. The International Academy of Low Vision Specialists (2020) recommends that a measurement of 20/40 distant acuity or better should be the standard for unrestricted driving and that acuity measurements worse than 20/40 should be individually considered. Peripheral field recommendations state that 120 degrees horizontally and 40 degrees vertically should be the minimum standard, with peripheral fields less than this left to individual consideration.

Contrast sensitivity is the measure of the ability of the visual system to distinguish various shades of gray or shades of colors. Lighting conditions and the visual backdrop for the driver change continually. Even the color of other vehicles can have some impact on the ability of drivers to see them efficiently. Persons with cataracts, glaucoma, optic neuritis, or other diseases affecting the cornea, lens, or retina of the eye may have increased difficulty with poor lighting conditions, even when they test well for acuity clinically. Contrast sensitivity testing is conducted using a vision chart similar to a Snellen chart, with the color of the text in decreasing shades of gray. There are various handheld charts that can address contrast, such as the LEA Low Contrast Flip Chart. There are currently no standardized limitations for driving with reduced contrast, but there is evidence that impaired contrast sensitivity related to the normal process of aging is linked to increased crash risk (Ortiz-Peregrina et al, 2020; Owsley et al, 2020; Swain et al, 2021). Impaired contrast sensitivity can be a symptom of eye diseases, such as cataracts and glaucoma. Sometimes the client may be unaware of these conditions, so the clinician should refer the client to their eye specialist for follow-up.

Neuromusculoskeletal Assessment

The objective of conducting physical or motor assessments is to determine whether there are impairments in the neuromusculoskeletal functions and motor performance skills needed to safely drive a vehicle. These assessments generally focus on functional mobility, posture, coordination, strength, flexibility, and energy in relation to driving. Factors to consider are the client's ability to travel to and from the vehicle; whether the client uses an assistive device for mobility, such as a wheelchair, walker, or cane; and whether they need assistance from another person to travel to the vehicle.

Some assessments, such as the Rapid Pace Walk (Marottoli, 1994), have been found to have moderate evidence linking poor performance to decreased fitness to drive (Classen et al, 2011; Edwards et al, 2010). Other commonly used measures include manual muscle testing and range of motion testing (such as cervical rotation or shoulder flexion). Overall, research offers limited evidence for assessment of physical abilities or skills as predictors of driving performance. The observation of motor skills can inform what the therapist can expect during the behind-the-wheel (BTW) assessment. More information is available in Promoting Best Practice 19-2.

PROMOTING BEST PRACTICE BOX 19-2
Assessing Fitness to Drive

There is general agreement that practitioners are best able to evaluate fitness to drive in an off-road setting when they employ a battery of tests. Selection of these assessments should include tools that address as many skill areas as possible (Zellner et al, 2021). In a systematic review of research about screening and assessment tools for driving fitness, a clear finding was that even when a range of types of tools were frequently used, the gold standard for assessing driving performance and safety was a BTW assessment (Dickerson et al, 2014). This type of assessment process is resource intensive and may have limited availability in some regions. Clinicians in general practice should use the outcomes of screening tools and assessment batteries with strong psychometric properties to identify older adults who are at risk for unsafe driving and need more specialized or BTW evaluation (Dickerson et al, 2014).

Special Considerations in Assessment

Occupational therapists have many tools at their disposal when assessing an older adult's fitness to drive. The use of driving simulators and on-road assessments are discussed next.

Driving Simulator Assessments

Using driving simulators to assess fitness to drive is an emerging area. Simulator-based driving evaluation was shown to be correlated with Trail Making Test Parts A and B, and simulator-determined demerits were significantly associated with later on-road evaluations (Bédard et al, 2010). Other research has demonstrated that simulated and on-road driving assessments detect similar errors (Shectman et al, 2009), indicating relative validity. Because driving simulation is more resource efficient for evaluation than on-road assessment and has application to many ages and populations, the design and use of driving simulators needs significant additional research (Classen & Brooks, 2014; Caffo et al, 2020). At this time, there is a consensus that driving simulators should not be the sole evaluation of fitness to drive but could be a valuable tool as part of an assessment battery.

On-Road Assessments

The gold standard for assessing fitness to drive is an on-road assessment, sometimes called a behind-the-wheel (BTW) assessment, which is the primary evaluation specialists use when determining fitness to drive (Dickerson, 2013). During a BTW assessment, the evaluator should observe how the client's vision affects their driving ability. Visual field deficits in upper or lower quadrants can be screened via confrontation testing or by acknowledgment of stimuli presented by a laser pointer. Functionally, the evaluator should observe how well the client identifies relevant information in the periphery, including incorporation of cervical rotation to check blind spots while changing lanes. There are several structured on-road driving assessment protocols with evidence to support their discriminant validity, such as DriveSafe and DriveAware (Kay et al, 2009) or Performance Analysis of Driving Ability (P-Drive) (Patomella & Bundy, 2015), which was designed for occupational therapists without advanced training. Sawada and colleagues (2019) reviewed the reliability and validity of 21 international on-road driving protocols and found strong support for multiple tools, including P-Drive. They conclude that selecting the best tool for BTW assessment should also consider the older adult and the context of evaluation.

Exemplar Interventions to Support Driving

There are a variety of types of interventions for driving and community mobility. Generally, occupational therapy practitioners will adopt a remedial or compensatory approach (AOTA, 2016). Remediation includes cognitive or motor retraining, skills training, and specialized driving rehabilitation services. Compensation could include prescription of and training in adaptive driving equipment, recommendation of vehicle modifications, and alternative mobility plans. The evidence to support these interventions is mixed.

Interventions for Functional Mobility and Pain

For clients experiencing musculoskeletal pain or impairment, the general practice occupational therapist should consider compensatory interventions including positioning for entry and exit of the vehicle, positioning for unobstructed vision, orthotics and footwear appropriate for using the pedals, and adaptive equipment such as a seat belt pull or HandyBar. An occupational therapy specialist may explore hands-only driving adaptations, modified entrance and exit options, more significant position solutions, or the addition of supplemental mirrors (AOTA, 2022; Cammarata et al, 2020). The goal of such interventions is to improve the "fit" of the client (driver) with the physical features of the car and musculoskeletal task demands.

Interventions for Cognition and Perception

For clients experiencing cognitive or perceptual change that impairs driving and mobility, the general practice occupational therapist may design interventions that are remedial in nature. It is important to consider any underlying conditions when evaluating the strength of evidence for various interventions. For example, retraining via driving simulator has potential utility for improving driving skills for individuals with Parkinson disease (Devos et al, 2016) and certain types of neurological events (Mazer et al, 2015). In a systematic review of driving interventions targeted to improve driving performance for older adults with cognitive impairments, Spargo and colleagues (2021) found evidence to support the use of simulation interventions with improvements in use of turn signal, checking the blind spot, following distance, and braking behavior. Classroom vision sessions for this population also showed some positive impact on dynamic vision (Shimada et al, 2019). For older adults with mild cognitive impairment, a compensatory approach may also be indicated, such as the introduction of and training on audio and visual Global Positioning System (GPS) device use (Yi et al, 2015). Overall, Spargo and colleagues (2021) conclude that there is low strength of evidence existing for these interventions.

Perceptual interventions may also entail skill-building via a visual retraining program. In general, useful field of view interventions that use a computerized visual attention analyzer appear to have a positive effect on a BTW assessment (Ball et al, 2010). In commissioned systematic reviews of these interventions, the NHTSA concluded that across multiple types of interventions and age groups, there was mixed evidence for visual scanning training administered by generalist occupational therapists (Staplin et al, 2022) (Lococo & Staplin, 2018).

Vehicle Modification and Technology Interventions

Interventions involving vehicle modifications or the introduction of technology tend to be compensatory in nature. Whereas a generalist occupational therapist may recommend basic adaptive equipment, other low- and high-tech services are introduced by a CDRS or occupational therapist with SCDCM. These modifications include altered hand controls, accelerator pedal revision or extension, alternate steering devices like a spinner knob, or more advanced changes to the effort required for driving or braking systems. Technology-related interventions may include recommendations for specific original equipment installed by the manufacturer, such as lane-change alerting and rearview camera. More commonly, after-market technology modifications such as navigation systems, push-button start, and additional convex or multifaceted mirrors may be evaluated for specific clients in combination with on-road driving rehabilitation interventions.

On-Road Driving Rehabilitation Interventions

BTW interventions are conducted only by driving rehabilitation specialists. Although they are resource intensive, these interventions have the highest level of evidence from randomized control trials (e.g., Bassingthwaighte et al, 2020). Common methods used during on-road interventions include graded driving, practicing specific maneuvers, and using a modified vehicle or equipment (Unsworth et al, 2021). This specialized service may include teaching compensatory strategies and skills, and the therapist will likely generate documentation about fitness to drive in relation to these modifications or recommendations (Lane et al, 2014).

Driving Cessation

Given the occupation-enabling status of driving, the ability to access and be mobile in the community has significant implications for the health and well-being of older adults (Satariano et al, 2012). Although driving a personal vehicle is often the preferred method of transportation, older adults outlive their driving days by 11 years for women and 6 years for men (Dickerson et al, 2019). This inability to drive—whether because of a change in physical ability, cognition, or a combination of social and situational factors—can have profound and pervasive repercussions.

Implications of Driving Cessation

The need to stop driving is a difficult transition for older drivers. Losing the ability to drive oneself limits opportunities to move around in the community, which in turn negatively affects quality of life. In a 2-year cohort study, Pellichero and colleagues (2021) reported that 71% of the older drivers who ceased driving in the study period experienced declines in out-of-home occupations. Specifically, driving cessation is strongly associated with a reduction in formal employment, volunteering, and leisure (Curl et al, 2013). Driving cessation has other negative consequences, including isolation, loss of autonomy, depression, and decline in health (Chihuri et al, 2016).

Driving cessation is strongly associated with an increased risk of being socially isolated in older age (Qin et al, 2019). This is likely due to a decrease in a person's social network, thereby increasing both isolation and loneliness; an increase in depression is a particularly notable negative health outcome of driving cessation (Chihuri et al, 2016). Chihuri and colleagues noted that, in addition, driving cessation results in decline in health and function in most spheres and increases the risk of nursing home placement. In general, "life-space mobility"—the area in which one moves in daily life—is associated with quality of life, and driving cessation limits this mobility (Rantakokko et al, 2016).

The psychosocial impacts of driving cessation are wide ranging, and it is important that therapists, family members, and the individuals themselves to be aware that although age-related performance changes may lead to a decision to curtail driving, there are likely secondary losses. In this transition, additional support should be focused on alternative ways to be mobile in the community (discussed later), options for mental and social stimulation, the maintenance of community-based roles and relationships, and the ability to be physically active and engaged in meaningful activities (Pellichero et al, 2021).

Initiating the Decision to Alter or Stop Driving

The decision to stop driving has emotional and practical consequences (Chihuri et al, 2016). There may be differences in those consequences depending on the sources of the decision. In instances when older adults decide for themselves to cease driving, they may feel empowered as they initiated the transition for safety reasons. These older adults also have the opportunity to explore alternate transportation options and experiment with their use before fully relying on them for community mobility. In addition, older adults who make the choice themselves are able to slowly transition from driving over a period of time to become accustomed to the new services. On the other hand, older adults who must stop driving because they are not medically fit to drive have very different experiences. The transition is abrupt and immediate with no opportunity to consider the implications for accessing the community and desired occupations. They may feel frustrated or anxious at the prospect of using transportation systems that they never learned how to navigate. The result of these unsupported transitions can include decreased community mobility with detrimental health outcomes.

However, anticipating and planning for driving reduction or cessation leads to better outcomes when it is possible. In a longitudinal study of more than 1,000 older adults, Pellichero and colleagues (2021) found that participants who did plan for driving cessation at baseline were more likely to expect a better quality of life in the event of driving cessation and to use public transportation at follow-up despite their older age and poorer health. For those who do alter and reduce their own driving over a period of time, there are several common strategies used to increase feelings of safety and competence while reducing a sense of risk. Individuals may choose to only drive at particular times of day (Heatwole Shank, 2016). They may also avoid certain roadways, intersections, or parts of town that are particularly challenging; limit the distance they travel; or limit their own low-light driving (Molnar et al, 2018). Others rely on a co-pilot, such as a spouse, for navigational and sign-reading assistance (Ang et al, 2020). A growing number of drivers use after-market adaptations and in-vehicle technology to enhance their own driving.

These efforts are often characterized by trial and error without professional input. However, prevention and education programs do exist. For example, a pilot community-based program designed by occupational therapists provided information on the skills needed to drive, community resources, and adaptive equipment (Collins, 2020). Unfortunately, this type of education and planning is not common. Relatively few older adults had driving safety conversations with their family or physicians, and there is a significant need for supporting older adults with risk assessment and driving cessation planning to maintain community mobility (Betz et al, 2019). Conversations about driving can be difficult. More information about the role of the physician in the interprofessional team is found in Box 19-3.

Betz and colleagues (2016) synthesized older adults' own perspectives about driving communication with their health care providers, which include:

- Driving discussions are emotionally charged, and psychosocial impacts need to be acknowledged.
- The context in which conversations are initiated should be considered.
- Providers are trusted authority figures, so recommendations carry weight.
- Communication should occur over a period of time rather than suddenly.
- Older adults desire control and to have self-determination in decisions about driving.

> **BOX 19-3 Role of the Physician in Driving Cessation**
>
> As part of a network of driving support and medical care related to driving, the physician's role varies. In some states, there are mandatory physician reporting laws around cognition and vision. However, in a large retrospective analysis of national crash-related hospitalization, Agimi and colleagues (2018) found no preventive effect of mandatory physician reporting requirements and suggest that such legal requirements may unnecessarily impinge on older adults' autonomy. Beyond mandatory reporting, the role of the physician and other primary healthcare providers generally includes education, regular conversation and counseling, and planning with older adults and their family members. Using data from the AAA Longitudinal Research on Aging Drivers (LongROAD) cohort study, Betz and colleagues (2019) evaluated the frequency and nature of driving cessation conversations among family and physicians to identify patterns in this primary care. Of the 2,990 drivers age 65 to 79 years who were surveyed, 14% reported discussing driving safety with family, and only 5.5% had discussions with a primary care physician. Men with graduate education reported more frequent conversations with family, and older adults with advanced education across the board were almost twice as likely to speak to their physicians (Betz et al, 2019).

Family Involvement in Driving Decisions

Although only about one-third of older adults wish for their family members to make the decision about driving cessation for them, older adults in the United States report relying on family members for information about driving risks more frequently than their physicians (Lum et al, 2015). Family members and care partners often find the issue of driving cessation to be a difficult topic to discuss with a loved one, especially if the reason the family member needs to stop driving is related to impaired cognition. Several resources have been developed to support family members in identifying when an older adult is having difficulty driving, initiating the discussion, and assisting with the transition from driving. The Hartford worked in collaboration with the MIT AgeLab to develop a comprehensive resource for just these circumstances. The resulting book, titled *We Need to Talk ... Family Conversations With Older Drivers*, includes strategies for who should approach the older driver, the best times for the conversation, preparing for the conversation, implications when the driver has dementia, and driving behavior warning signs (The Hartford & MIT AgeLab, 2012). These kinds of tools can help ease the conversation, as both the older adult and the family gain concrete data about the driver's safety.

The identification of older adults who need to transition from driving and discussing the concerns are typically just the beginning of the journey for these older adults and their families. Transition from driving often means the end of freedom and spontaneity to travel throughout the community. New barriers now exist for older adults who want or need to travel to the grocery store, the doctor's office, a friend's home, a leisure activity, the beauty salon, or to a volunteer location. In addition, the older adult who just ceased driving may have been a source of community mobility for friends, neighbors, a spouse, or grandchildren. Driving cessation of one person may ultimately limit the community mobility of several individuals and thus may have far-reaching effects. It is important to work with the older adult and their family members to assist with filling the gaps with other modes of mobility when identifying community destinations that are frequented along with the frequency of travel and duration of trips. More information about such discussions is found in Promoting Best Practice 19-3.

> ### PROMOTING BEST PRACTICE BOX 19-3
> **Driving Cessation Conversations**
>
> Mental and physical changes that occur may make safe driving more difficult. These changes may be acute but commonly occur over a period of months or years. Driving cessation conversations should:
>
> - Empower older adults to plan ahead, consider social and engagement impacts and alternatives, and alter or reduce their driving accordingly.
> - Involve regular conversations with healthcare providers (Ammerman, 2021), with integration of assessments and individualized considerations.
> - Trigger a reassessment and focused conversation related to any change in condition, with referrals to specialists if indicated.
> - Support older adults' autonomy and self-determination and involve family members in preparation and decision-making conversations.

Mobility Alternatives to Driving

Community mobility is strongly related to maintaining social participation, decreasing loneliness, and the ability to carry out a range of occupations for older adults all around the globe (Papageorgiou et al, 2016) and should be addressed as part of any holistic intervention. Community mobility is not a specialized area of practice. Whereas driving interventions focus on the individual, community mobility is multidimensional and spans individual, community, and systems-level considerations (Di Stefano et al, 2012). Occupational therapists addressing community mobility should broadly consider their role in providing services, developing programs, engaging in education and advocacy efforts, and collaborating with a wide interdisciplinary network.

Mobility Options Beyond Driving

When an older adult needs to transition from driving to nondriving status, they need strategies and resources that will allow them to continue to meet community mobility needs.

Mobility challenges and solutions are shaped by both personal and environmental factors (Schultz-Krohn et al, 2021), so solutions will be highly variable based on the individual and the community in which they live. For example, some older adults may live near family or friends who can provide informal transportation support. Those living in urban settings are more likely to have access to public transportation routes, paratransit options (Fig. 19-4), or ride-share services—some of which are tailored for use by older adults (for example, GoGoGrandparent.com; SilverRide.com; Lively.com; UberHealth.com). Older adults living in rural settings may be more vulnerable to social isolation when they can no longer drive, and communities that are economically disadvantaged may also have fewer mobility options. In these situations, in addition to advocating for the creation of community services, the occupational therapist must be creative in identifying options and strategies. In addition to public transportation and paratransit, an older adult may establish a range of mobility supports including private drivers (e.g., professionals, college students), ride- and cost-sharing arrangements with peers, walking, and point-to-point transportation offered by some grocery stores, medical centers, religious organizations, or community centers. Cost, access, convenience, and physical requirements may all be factors in evaluating which would be most helpful to specific individuals.

It is also important to note that for many older adults, alternative transportation options are not preferred (Schultz-Krohn et al, 2021). These options may pose additional challenges—both cognitive (e.g., looking up routes, scheduling rides, and arranging dates and times in advance) and physical (e.g., transferring into a large vehicle, stepping into a bus, and walking to a pick-up location)—that must also be addressed by the occupational therapy practitioner. Optimally, a program should exist in all communities to help the older adult explore alternatives, develop new skills, and plan for the successful use of alternative community mobility options. This type of client-centered and community-based practice will help ensure the safety of the older adult and facilitate successful participation in meaningful occupations within the community.

Envisioning Community Mobility Services and Solutions

When the World Health Organization (2007) developed its plan for promoting "age-friendly cities" around the world, transportation become one of the eight primary areas for assessment and development. Specifically, the plan and associated guidebook highlight the need for community-specific initiatives to create transportation solutions that are available and adapted to the needs of older adults to support well-being and participation. Transportation is also a key indicator in the Decade of Healthy Ageing agenda of the World Health Assembly (2020) as it relates to meeting personal needs through mobility and the ability to engage in and contribute to civic life. To meet the community mobility needs of a globally aging population, community- and system-level initiatives will be necessary.

One successful program that exists in multiple cities around the United States is the Independent Transportation Network (ITN America; http://www.itnamerica.org). The comprehensive program is partially supported by local businesses allowing riders to use vouchers to travel to community partner businesses and receive a discount on purchases made in these establishments. The INT America exists in 10 states (ITN America, n.d.). Another example is the National Volunteer Transportation Center (https://ctaa.org/national-volunteer-transportation-center/), which promotes and supports volunteer transportation, shared vehicle use, and ride-sharing initiatives. Created in 2014, this national organization serves as an information hub and maintains a database of volunteer transportation in all 50 states.

Advocacy and Education

Healthcare professionals play a critical role in ensuring the development of supportive environments. Both social and physical environments have an impact on community mobility and social participation (Gardner, 2014). Amenity diversity (e.g., availability of parks, food, service, and recreational and leisure services and facilities) is associated with enhanced mobility (Rosso et al, 2013). In contrast, environments that have been allowed to deteriorate can interfere with mobility. Occupational therapists must advocate for supportive environments and collaborate with urban planners, architects, and policymakers in the design and development of enabling communities. Further, educating transportation providers, social service agencies, and local businesses is critical in creating a network supportive of community mobility.

Therapeutic services targeted at the community or population level have been repeatedly identified as a critical need, role for occupational therapy advocacy, and area requiring research (Dickerson et al, 2019).

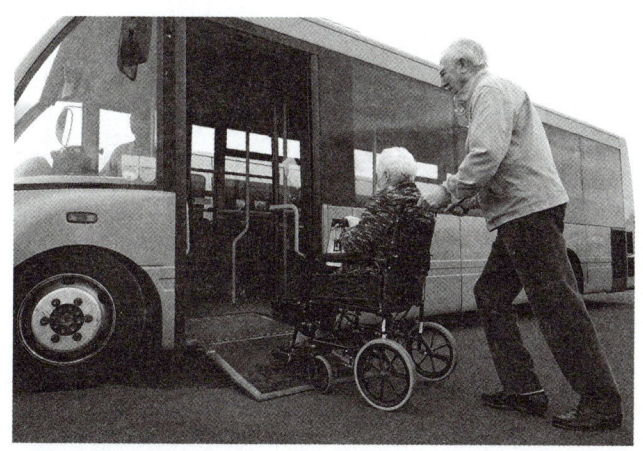

FIGURE 19-4 Using adapted and paratransit mobility options. *(SolStock/E +/Getty Images.)*

The systemic and infrastructure changes can have far-reaching benefits beyond an individual client, including services such as:

- Environmental assessment for accessibility of buses, trains, bus stops, subway stations, crosswalks, sidewalks, and public commerce areas
- Consultation with automobile manufacturers to include seating height, seating planes of movement, and handles to enhance transfers in and out of automobiles for passengers
- Vehicle modifications or inclusion of modifications for new transit vehicle purchases such as kneeling buses, convertible seating on buses, wheelchair tie-downs, and ramps
- Assistance with development of paratransit eligibility guidelines and evaluation protocols
- Facilitation of interagency collaboration for mutually beneficial transport of older adults (e.g., senior housing, local businesses, and cultural arts venues)

CASE STUDY (CONTINUED)

Intervention Plan

The occupational therapist consulted with Mr. Smith about his morning routine to establish a regular location for taking medication each morning and involved his daughter in creating and maintaining a "departure station" by the front door with a calendar of activities and his keys. The occupational therapist worked with Mr. Smith to evaluate each destination and trip he commonly took in relation to distance, time of day, and speed of the roads. For trips that were farther from home, involved dawn or dusk driving or high-speed roadways, the occupational therapist shared information about alternatives such as the senior center bus and a paratransit application for his wife, who qualifies and can use the service for medical, pharmacy, and grocery trips. They also explored informal ride options for getting to church (a 15-minute drive) and early-morning breakfast meetings with friends. Finally, the occupational therapist educated Mr. Smith and his family members about driving cessation, regular evaluation, and the potential for future referral to a driving specialist in the area.

Discharge Status

After several weeks, Mr. Smith demonstrated consistent use of cognitive strategies for taking his medicine. His daughter bought him an electronic tab for his keychain to assist with locating his keys when needed. Mrs. Smith's paratransit application was accepted, so Mr. Smith only drove her to the hairdresser down the street, the post office, and the hardware store. He signed up for the bus run by the Department of Aging to get to programs at the senior center, and a friend picked him up for breakfast socializing. At this time, a fellow church member is going to give them a ride to and from church but was unsure about the long-term commitment, so the daughter plans to follow up with church leadership to assess other options. The family unit also broached conversations about driving cessation, and Mr. Smith agreed to reassessment every 6 months going forward.

Questions

1. What are some of the client factors Mr. Smith is experiencing that would indicate a need for occupational therapy evaluation?
2. Because Mr. Smith's cognitive changes are one of the primary concerns affecting his driving performance, what might the occupational therapist intervention include using a remediation approach? What about using a compensation or adaptation approach?
3. If Mr. Smith decides that driving himself and his wife is no longer safe, what alternative mobility options might exist for Mr. Smith and his wife in their community?

Answers

1. Mr. Smith is experiencing mild musculoskeletal changes associated with arthritis; his mental (cognitive) functions also have notable impairment in short-term memory, executive function and safety decisions, and visuospatial/geographical orientation.
2. In a remediation approach, the therapist may carry out cognitive retraining related to driving and community mobility such as road sign instruction, train a client in safe and effective use of a public transportation option, or remediate perceptual skills like visual scanning. A compensation or adaptation approach would involve provision and training in adaptive equipment, suggesting changes or limitations to certain types of routes or travel times, or recommendation of vehicle modification to ease access or use features.
3. If Mr. Smith decides to no longer drive, he and his wife may be able to use a combination of formal mobility options (e.g., paratransit, public transport, agency services, and shuttles) and informal mobility options, such as getting rides from friends, fellow churchgoers, and their daughter.

SUMMARY

Driving is an important occupation and symbol of freedom and independence. Difficulties in driving may arise due to physiological and disease-related changes or changes in context that alter a person's ability to drive safely. Assessing driving performance is necessary to help determine whether the driver will be safe on the road. Understanding the role of community mobility in the individual's daily life will also inform potential areas for assessment, intervention, and adaptation. When a BTW assessment is necessary to help identify skill-area deficiencies and to provide future recommendations, a certified driving specialist offers advanced skills and knowledge about modifications. Psychosocial implications should always be considered as families and professionals collaborate with older adults to determine the best course for driving restriction or cessation. Ultimately, the practitioner must consider the balance between independence and safety for the client and other road users. Beyond driving, community mobility is an important enabling occupation because it fosters access to instrumental, social, and physical occupations beyond the home. Having viable community mobility and transportation alternatives will become increasingly important as the population ages and individuals seek options for getting around without depending on their personal vehicles. Occupational therapy practitioners have a critical role to play in informing the scope, nature, and accessibility of community mobility services and resources to support well-being and continued participation for all older adults in the community.

Critical Thinking Questions

1. How is community mobility related to participation in later life and engagement in out-of-home occupations?
2. What types of mobility interventions would be most appropriate for a cognitively typical older adult wanting to improve their driving performance?
3. How might driving cessation have differing effects for individuals who live in urban, suburban, and rural settings?

REFERENCES

Agimi, Y., Albert, S. M., Youk, A. O., Documet, P. I., & Steiner, C. A. (2018). Mandatory physician reporting of at-risk drivers: The older driver example. *The Gerontologist, 58*(3), 578–587. https://doi.org/10.1093/geront/gnw209

Almigbal, T. H., Alfaifi, A. A., Aleid, M. A., Billah, B., Alramadan, M. J., Sheshah, E., AlMogbel, T. A., Aldekhayel, G. A., & Batais, M. A. (2018). Safe driving practices and factors associated with motor-vehicle collisions among people with insulin-treated diabetes mellitus: Results from the diabetes and driving (DAD) study. *Journal of Safety Research, 65,* 83–88. https://doi.org/10.1016/j.jsr.2018.03.003

American Association of Retired Persons. (2022). *We need to talk.* Retrieved from https://www.aarp.org/auto/driver-safety/we-need-to-talk/?intcmp=AE-CAR-HEA-EOA2

American Diabetes Association. (2014). Diabetes and driving. *Diabetes Care, 37* (Supplement_1), S97–S103. https://doi.org/10.2337/dc14-S097

American Geriatrics Society, & Pomidor, A. (Eds.). (2019). *Clinician's guide to assessing and counseling older drivers* (4th ed., Report No. DOT HS 812 228). Washington, DC: National Highway Traffic Safety Administration.

American Occupational Therapy Association (AOTA). (n.d.). *Specialty Certified Practitioners.* https://www.aota.org/career/advanced-certification-program/specialty-certified-practitioners

American Occupational Therapy Association (AOTA). (2015). AOTA standards for continuing competence. *American Journal of Occupational Therapy, 69*(Suppl. 3), 479–481. https://doi.org/10.5014/ajot.2015.696S16

American Occupational Therapy Association (AOTA). (2016). Driving and community mobility. *American Journal of Occupational Therapy, 70*(Suppl. 2), 7012410050. http://dx.doi.org/10.5014/ajot.2016.706S04

American Occupational Therapy Association (AOTA). (2020). Occupational therapy practice framework: Domain and process (4th ed.). *American Journal of Occupational Therapy, 74*(Supplement_2), 7412410010p1–7412410010p87. https://doi.org/10.5014/ajot.2020.74S2001

American Occupational Therapy Association (AOTA). (2022). *Carfit.* Retrieved from https://www.aota.org/practice/practice-settings/driving-community-mobility/carfit

Ammerman, B. A. (2021). Older adults and driving cessation: Knowing when and how to approach the conversation. *Advances in Family Practice Nursing, 3,* 1–13. https://doi.org/10.1016/j.yfpn.2021.02.003

Ang, B. H., Oxley, J. A., Chen, W. S., Yap, M. K., Song, K. P., & Lee, S. W. (2020). The influence of spouses and their driving roles in self-regulation: A qualitative exploration of driving reduction and cessation practices among married older adults. *PLOS ONE, 15*(5), e0232795. https://doi.org/10.1371/journal.pone.0232795

Association for Driving Rehabilitation Specialists (ADED). (n.d.). *Certified Driving Rehabilitation Specialist.* https://www.aded.net/page/210

Ball, K., Edwards, J. D., Ross, L. A., & McGwin, G., Jr. (2010). Cognitive training decreases motor vehicle collision involvement of older drivers. *Journal of the American Geriatrics Society, 58,* 2107–2113. http://dx.doi.org/10.1111/j.1532-5415.2010.03138.x

Band, D., & Perel, M. (2007, Nov/Dec). Senior mobility series: New vehicle technologies may help older drivers. U.S. Department of Transportation, Federal Highway Administration. Issue No: Vol. 71 No. 3 Publication Number: FHWA-HRT-08-001. Retrieved from https://highways.dot.gov/public-roads/novdec-2007/senior-mobility-series-article-8-new-vehicle-technologies-may-help-older

Barco, P. P., Wallendorf, M., Rutkoski, K., Dolan, K., Rakus, D., Johnson, A., & Carr, D. B. (2020). Validity and reliability of the Traffic Sign Naming Test (TSNT) and Written Exam for Driving Decisions (WEDD) as measures of fitness to drive among older adults. *The American Journal of Occupational Therapy, 74*(3), 7403205090p1–7403205090p10. https://doi.org/10.5014/ajot.2020.034389

Bassingthwaighte, L., Griffin, J., Fleming, J., & Gustafsson, L. (2020). Evaluating the effectiveness of on-road driving remediation following acquired brain injury: A wait-list feasibility study with follow-up. *Australian Occupational Therapy Journal, 68*(2), 124–134. https://doi.org/10.1111/1440-1630.12694

Bédard, M., Parkkari, M., Weaver, B., Riendeau, J., & Dahlquist, M. (2010). Assessment of driving performance using a simulator protocol: Validity and reproducibility. *American Journal of Occupational Therapy, 64*(2), 336–340. https://doi.org/10.5014/ajot.64.2.336

Betz, M. E., Scott, K., Jones, J., & Diguiseppi, C. (2016). "Are you still driving?" Metasynthesis of patient preferences for communication with health care providers. *Traffic Injury Prevention, 17*(4), 367–373. https://doi.org/10.1080/15389588.2015.1101078

Betz, M. E., Villavicencio, L., Kandasamy, D., Kelley-Baker, T., Kim, W., DiGuiseppi, C., Mielenz, T. J., Eby, D. W., Molnar, L. J., Hill, L., Strogatz, D., Carr, D. B., & Li, G. (2019). Physician and family discussions about driving safety: Findings from the LongROAD study. *The Journal of the American Board of Family Medicine, 32*(4), 607–613. https://doi.org/10.3122/jabfm.2019.04.180326

Bro, T., & Andersson, J. (2022). The effects of visual-field loss from panretinal photocoagulation of proliferative diabetic retinopathy on performance in a driving simulator. *Eye (London), 37,* 103–108. https://doi.org/10.1038/s41433-021-01832-3

Bureau of Transportation Statistics. (2021). U.S. Passenger-Miles. Retrieved from https://www.bts.gov/content/us-passenger-miles

Caffò, A. O., Tinella, L., Lopez, A., Spano, G., Massaro, Y., Lisi, A., Stasolla, F., Catanesi, R., Nardulli, F., Grattagliano, I., & Bosco, A. (2020). The drives for driving simulation: A scientometric analysis and a selective review of reviews on simulated driving research. *Frontiers in Psychology, 11*, 917. https://doi.org/10.3389/fpsyg.2020.00917

Cammarata, M., Sangrar, R., Harris, J. E., Richardson, J., & Vrkljan, B. (2020). A scoping review of environmental factors that impact driving with arthritis: Considerations for occupational therapy. *Occupational Therapy In Health Care, 34*(3), 202–229. https://doi.org/10.1080/07380577.2020.1719451

Carlier/Statista. (2022, January). Road accidents in the United States—statistics & facts. Transportation & logistics, vehicles & road traffic. Retrieved from https://www.statista.com/topics/3708/road-accidents-in-the-us/#topicHeader__wrapper

Chee, J. N., Rapoport, M. J., Molnar, F., Herrmann, N., O'Neill, D., Marottoli, R., Mitchell, S., Tant, M., Dow, J., Ayotte, D., Lanctôt, K. L., McFadden, R., Taylor, J. P., Donaghy, P. C., Olsen, K., Classen, S., Elzohairy, Y., & Carr, D. B. (2017). Update on the risk of motor vehicle collision or driving impairment with dementia: A collaborative international systematic review and meta-analysis. *The American Journal of Geriatric Psychiatry, 25*(12), 1376–1390. https://doi.org/10.1016/j.jagp.2017.05.007

Chihuri, S., Mielenz, T. J., DiMaggio, C. J., DiGuiseppi, C., Jones, V., & Li, G. (2016). Driving cessation and health outcomes in older adults. *Journal of the American Geriatrics Society, 64*, 332–341. https://doi.org/10.1111/jgs.13931

Cicchino, J. (2015). Why have fatality rates among older drivers declined? The relative contributions of changes in survivability and crash involvement. *Accident, Analysis and Prevention, 83*, 67–73. https://doi.org/10.1016/j.aap.2015.06.012

Classen, S., & Brooks, J. (2014). Driving simulators for occupational therapy screening, assessment, and intervention. *Occupational Therapy in Health Care, 28*(2), 154–162. https://doi.org/10.3109/07380577.2014.901590

Classen, S., Witter, D. P., Lanford, D. N., Okun, M. S., Rodriguez, R. L., Romrell, J., Malaty, I., & Fernandez, H. H. (2011). Usefulness of screening tools for predicting driving performance in people with Parkinson's disease. *The American Journal of Occupational Therapy, 65*(5), 579–588. http://dx.doi.org/10.5014/ajot.2011.001073

Collins, M. E. (2020). The impact of driving education on preparedness for driving cessation. *The American Journal of Occupational Therapy, 74*(4_Supplement_1), 7411505168p1-7411505168p1. https://doi.org/10.5014/ajot.2020.74s1-po5607

Cox, A. E., & Cicchino, J. B. (2021). Continued trends in older driver crash involvement rates in the United States: Data through 2017–2018. *Journal of Safety Research, 77*, 288–295. https://doi.org/10.1016/j.jsr.2021.03.013

Curl, A. L., Stowe, J. D., Cooney, T. M., & Proulx, C. M. (2013). Giving up the keys: How driving cessation affects engagement in later life. *Gerontologist, 54*, 423–433. https://doi.10.1093/geront/gnt037

Devos, H., Morgan, J. C., Onyeamaechi, A., Bogle, C. A., Holton, K., Kruse, J., Sasser, S., & Akinwuntan, A. E. (2016). Use of a driving simulator to improve on-road driving performance and cognition in persons with Parkinson's disease: A pilot study. *Australian Occupational Therapy Journal, 63*(6), 408–414. https://doi.org/10.1111/1440-1630.12263

Di Stefano, M., Stuckey, R., & Lovell, R. (2012). Promotion of safe community mobility: Challenges and opportunities for occupational therapy practice. *Australian Occupational Therapy Journal, 59*, 98–102. https://doi.org/10.1111/j.1440-1630.2011.00993.x

Dickerson, A. E. (2013). Driving assessment tools used by driver rehabilitation specialists: Survey of use and implications for practice. *American Journal of Occupational Therapy, 67*, 564–573. http://dx.doi.org/10.5014/ajot.2013.007823

Dickerson, A. E. (2019). Evidence to support the older adults' driving and community mobility through the use of GPS. *American Journal of Occupational Therapy, 73*(4_Supplement_1), 7311515328p1. https://doi.org/10.5014/ajot.2019.73S1-PO3020

Dickerson, A. E., Meuel, D. B., Ridenour, C. D., & Cooper, K. (2014). Assessment tools predicting fitness to drive in older adults: A systematic review. *American Journal of Occupational Therapy, 68*, 670–680. http://dx.doi.org/10.5014/ajot.2014.011833

Dickerson, A. E., Molnar, L. J., Bédard, M., Eby, D. W., Berg-Weger, M., Choi, M., Grigg, J., Horowitz, A., Meuser, T., Myers, A., O'Connor, M., & Silverstein, N. M. (2019). Transportation and aging: An updated research agenda to advance safe mobility among older adults transitioning from driving to nondriving. *The Gerontologist, 59*, 215–221. https://www.doi.org/10.1093/geront/gnx120

Duncanson, H., Hollis, A. M., & O'Connor, M. G. (2018). Errors versus speed on the Trail Making Test: Relevance to driving performance. *Accident Analysis & Prevention, 113*, 125–130. https://doi.org/10.1016/j.aap.2018.01.004

Eby, D. W., Molnar, L. J., Zakrajsek, J. S., Ryan, L. H., Zanier, N., Louis, R. M. S., Stanciu, S. C., LeBlanc, D., Kostyniuk, L. P., Smith, J., Yung, R., Nyquist, L., DiGuiseppi, C., Li, G., Mielenz, T. J., Strogatz, D., & LongROAD Research Team. (2018). Prevalence, attitudes, and knowledge of in-vehicle technologies and vehicle adaptations among older drivers. *Accident Analysis & Prevention, 113*, 54–62. https://doi.org/10.1016/j.aap.2018.01.022

Edwards, J. D., Bart, E., O'Connor, M. L., & Cissell, G. (2010). Ten years down the road: Predictors of driving cessation. *The Gerontologist, 50*(3), 393–399. http://dx.doi.org/10.1093/geront/gnp127

Federal Highway Administration. (2022, January). *Highway statistics 2020*. https://www.fhwa.dot.gov/policyinformation/statistics/2020/dl20.cfm#foot1

Fraade-Blanar, L. A., Hansen, R. N., Chan, K. C., Sears, J. M., Thompson, H. J., Crane, P. K., & Ebel, B. E. (2018). Diagnosed dementia and the risk of motor vehicle crash among older drivers. *Accident Analysis & Prevention, 113*, 47–53. https://doi.org/10.1016/j.aap.2017.12.021

Gardner, P. (2014). The role of social engagement and identity in community mobility among older adults aging in place. *Disability and Rehabilitation, 36*(15), 1249–1257. https://doi.org/10.3109/09638288.2013.837970

Grundler, W., & Strasburger, H. (2020). Visual attention outperforms visual-perceptual parameters required by law as an indicator of on-road driving performance. *PLOS ONE, 15*(8), e0236147. https://doi.org/10.1371/journal.pone.0236147

Hartford, & MIT AgeLab. (2012). *We need to talk ... family conversations with older drivers*. Retrieved from http://www.thehartford.com/sites/thehartford/files/we-need-to-talk-2012.pdf

Heatwole Shank, K. (2016). What makes a community age-friendly? Conceptualizing community livability through mapping. *International Journal of Aging and Society, 7*(1), 61–76. https://doi.org/10.18848/2160-1909/CGP/v07i01/61-76

Heatwole Shank, K., & Cutchin, M. P. (2016). Processes of developing 'community livability' in older age. *Journal of Aging Studies, 39*, 66–72. https://doi.org/10.1016/j.jaging.2016.11.001

Hwang, S., Kim, S., & Lee, D. (2020). Driving performance evaluation correlated to age and visual acuities based on VR technologies. *Journal of Advanced Transportation, 2020*, 1–11. https://doi.org/10.1155/2020/5898762

International Academy of Low Vision Specialists. (2020). *DMV state driving laws*. https://ialvs.com/dmv-driving-laws/

ITNAmerica. (n.d.). *ITN affiliated communities*. Retrieved from http://www.itnamerica.org/find-your-affiliate

Jones, V. C., Johnson, R. M., Rebok, G. W., Roth, K. B., Gielen, A., Molnar, L. J., Pitts, S., DiGuiseppi, C., Hill, L., Strogatz, D., Mielenz, T., Eby, D. W., & Li, G. (2018). Use of alternative sources of transportation among older adult drivers. *Journal of Transport & Health, 10*, 284–289. https://doi.org/10.1016/j.jth.2018.07.001

Kay, L. G., Bundy, A. C., & Clemson, L. M. (2009). Predicting fitness to drive in people with cognitive impairments by using DriveSafe and DriveAware. *Archives of Physical Medicine and Rehabilitation, 90*(9), 1514–1522. https://doi.org/10.1016/j.apmr.2009.03.011

Keten, A. (2021). Diabetes and driving safety. *Accident Analysis & Prevention, 149*, 105854. https://doi.org/10.1016/j.aap.2020.105854

Kwok, J. C. W., Gélinas, I., Benoit, D., & Chilingaryan, G. (2015). Predictive validity of the Montreal Cognitive Assessment (MoCA) as a screening tool for on-road driving performance. *British Journal of Occupational Therapy, 78*(2), 100–108. https://doi.org/10.1177/0308022614562399

Lane, A., Green, E., Dickerson, A., Davis, E. S., Rolland, B., & Stohler, J. (2014). Driver rehabilitation programs: Defining program models, services and expertise. *Occupational Therapy in Health Care, 28*(2), 177–187. https://doi.org/10.3109/07380577.2014.903582

Lloyd, K., Gaunt, D., Haunton, V., Skelly, R., Mann, H., Ben-Shlomo, Y., & Henderson, E. J. (2020). Driving in Parkinson's disease: A retrospective study of driving and mobility assessments. *Age and Ageing, 49*(6), 1097–1101. https://doi.org/10.1093/ageing/afaa098

Lococo, K. H., & Staplin, L. (2018, April). *Visual scanning training for older drivers: A literature review* (Report No. DOT HS 812 514). Washington, DC: National Highway Traffic Safety Administration.

Luiu, C., Tight, M., & Burrow, M. (2017). The unmet travel needs of the older population: A review of the literature. *Transport Reviews, 37*(4), 488–506. https://doi.org/10.1080/01441647.2016.1252447

Lum, H. D., Brown, J. B., Juarez-Colunga, E., & Betz, M. E. (2015). Physician involvement in life transition planning: A survey of community-dwelling older adults. *BMC Family Practice, 16*, 1–8. https://doi.org/10.1186/s12875-015-0311-0

Marottoli, R. A. (1994). Predictors of automobile crashes and moving violations among elderly drivers. *Annals of Internal Medicine, 121*(11), 842. https://doi.org/10.7326/0003-4819-121-11-199412010-00003

Mazer, B., Gélinas, I., Duquette, J., Vanier, M., Rainville, C., & Chilingaryan, G. (2015). A randomized clinical trial to determine effectiveness of driving simulator retraining on the driving performance of clients with neurological impairment. *British Journal of Occupational Therapy, 78*(6), 369–376. https://doi.org/10.1177/0308022614562401

Molnar, L. J., Eby, D. W., Bogard, S. E., LeBlanc, D. J., & Zakrajsek, J. S. (2018). Using naturalistic driving data to better understand the driving exposure and patterns of older drivers. *Traffic Injury Prevention, 19*(sup1), S83–S88. https://doi.org/10.1080/15389588.2017.1379601

Mulry, C. M. (2018). Facilitating the participation of older adults using an occupation-based community mobility program: A mixed methods study. *The American Journal of Occupational Therapy, 72*(4_Supplement_1), 7211515248p1-7211515248p1. https://doi.org/10.5014/ajot.2018.72s1-po4028

National Highway Traffic Safety Administration (NHTSA). (n.d.). *Older drivers.* https://www.nhtsa.gov/road-safety/older-drivers#2346

Organization for Economic Co-Operation and Development. (2022). Passenger transport. Retrieved from https://data.oecd.org/transport/passenger-transport.htm

Ortiz-Peregrina, S., Ortiz, C., Casares-López, M., Castro-Torres, J. J., Jiménez del Barco, L., & Anera, R. G. (2020). Impact of age-related vision changes on driving. *International Journal of Environmental Research and Public Health, 17*(20), 7416. https://doi.org/10.3390/ijerph17207416

Owsley, C., Swain, T., Liu, R., McGwin, G., & Kwon, M. Y. (2020). Association of photopic and mesopic contrast sensitivity in older drivers with risk of motor vehicle collision using naturalistic driving data. *BMC Ophthalmology, 20*(1), 1–8. https://doi.org/10.1186/s12886-020-1331-7

Padiero, M., San Jose, J., Amado, C., Sousa, L., Oliveira, C., Esteves, A., & McGarrigle, J. (2022). Neighborhood attributes and well-being among older adults in urban areas: A mixed-methods systematic review. *Research on Aging, 44*, 351–368. https://doi.10.1177/0164027521999980

Papageorgiou, N., Marquis, R., Dare, J., & Batten, R. (2016). Occupational therapy and occupational participation in community dwelling older adults: A review of the evidence. *Physical and Occupational Therapy in Geriatrics, 34*, 21–42. https://doi.org/10.5014/ajot.2012.003327

Patomella, A. H., & Bundy, A. (2015). P-Drive: Implementing an assessment of on-road driving in clinical settings and investigating its internal and predictive validity. *The American Journal of Occupational Therapy, 69*(4), 6904290010. https://doi.org/10.5014/ajot.2015.015131

Pellichero, A., Lafont, S., Paire-Ficout, L., Fabrigoule, C., & Chavoix, C. (2021). Barriers and facilitators to social participation after driving cessation among older adults: A cohort study. *Annals of Physical and Rehabilitation Medicine, 64*(2), 101373. https://doi.org/10.1016/j.rehab.2020.03.003

Perazzolo, M., Reeves, N. D., Bowling, F. L., Boulton, A. J., Raffi, M., & Marple-Horvat, D. E. (2020). Altered accelerator pedal control in a driving simulator in people with diabetic peripheral neuropathy. *Diabetic Medicine, 37*(2), 335–342. https://doi.org/10.1111/dme.13957

Qin, W., Xiang, X., & Taylor, H. O. (2019). Driving cessation and social isolation in older adults. *Innovation in Aging, 32*(9), 962–971. https://doi.org/10.1093/geroni/igz038.3048

Ranchet, M., Devos, H., & Uc, E. Y. (2020). Driving in Parkinson disease. *Clinics in Geriatric Medicine, 36*(1), 141–148. https://doi.org/10.1016/j.cger.2019.09.007

Rantakokko, M., Portegijs, E., Viljanen, A., Iwarsson, S., Kauppinen, M., & Rantanen, T. (2016). Changes in life-space mobility and quality of life among community-dwelling older people: A 2-year follow-up study. *Quality of Life Research, 25*, 1189–1197. https://doi.org/10.1007/s11136-015-1137-x

Rapoport, M. J., Chee, J. N., Carr, D. B., Molnar, F., Naglie, G., Dow, J., Marottoli, R., Mitchell, S., Tant, M., Herrmann, N., Lanctôt, K. L., Taylor, J., Donaghy, P. C., Classen, S., & O'Neill, D. (2018). An international approach to enhancing a national guideline on driving and dementia. *Current Psychiatry Reports, 20*(3), 16. https://doi.org/10.1007/s11920-018-0879-x

Rosso, A. L., Grubesic, T. H., Auchincloss, A. H., Tabb, L. P., & Michael, Y. L. (2013). Neighborhood amenities and mobility in older adults. *American Journal of Epidemiology, 178*(5), 761–769. https://doi.org/10.1093/aje/kwt032

Sanchez, M., Schultz-Krohn, W., Pham, A., Bermudez, M., & David, N. (2016). Roles of occupational therapists in driving rehabilitation programs. *American Journal of Occupational Therapy, 70*(4), 7011505118p1. https://doi.org/10.5014/ajot.2016.70S1-PO2043

Satariano, W. A., Guralnik, J. M., Jackson, R. J., Marottoli, R. A., Phelan, E. A., & Prohaska, T. R. (2012). Mobility and aging: New directions for public health action. *American Journal of Public Health, 102*, 1508–1515. http://dx.doi.org/10.2105/AJPH.2011.300631

Sawada, T., Tomori, K., Hamana, H., Ohno, K., Seike, Y., Igari, Y., & Fujita, Y. (2019). Reliability and validity of on-road driving tests in vulnerable adults: A systematic review. *International Journal of Rehabilitation Research, 42*(4), 289.

Schultz-Krohn, W., Chan, E., Bothman, A., Bullard, L., Chambers, N., Colvin, D., & Chiao-Ju, F. (2021). Driving behaviors and community mobility of older adults living independently. *American Journal of Occupational Therapy, 75*(suppl_2), 7512505136p1. https://doi.org/10.5014/ajot.2021.75S2-RP136

Selander, H., Wressle, E., & Samuelsson, K. (2020). Cognitive prerequisites for fitness to drive: Norm values for the TMT, UFOV and NorSDSA tests, *Scandinavian Journal of Occupational Therapy, 27*:3, 231–239. https://doi.org/10.1080/11038128.2019.1614214

Shechtman, O., Classen, S., Awadzi, K. D., & Mann, W. (2009). Comparison of driving errors between on-the-road and simulated driving assessment: A validation study. *Traffic Injury Prevention, 10*(4), 379–385. https://doi.org/10.1080/15389580902894989

Shimada, H., Hotta, R., Makizako, H., Doi, T., Tsutsumimoto, K., Nakakubo, S., & Makino, K. (2019). Effects of driving skill training on safe driving in older adults with mild cognitive impairment. *Gerontology, 65*, 90–97. https://doi.org/10.1159/000487759

Simons-Morton, B., & Ehsani, J. (2016). Learning to drive safely: Reasonable expectations and future directions for the learner period. *Safety, 2*(4), 20. https://doi.org/10.3390/safety2040020

Souman, J., Adjenughwure, K., Van Dam, E., Van Weperen, M., & Tejada, A. (2021). *Quantification of safe driving.* TNO. https://publications.tno.nl/publication/34639060/3JlniP/TNO-2021-R12632.pdf

Spargo, C., Laver, K., Berndt, A., Adey-Wakeling, Z., & George, S. (2021). Occupational therapy interventions to improve driving performance in older people with mild cognitive impairment or early stage dementia: A systematic review. *American Journal of Occupational Therapy, 75*, 7505205070. https://doi.org/10.5014/ajot.2021.042820

Spreng, L., Favrat, B., Borruat, F., & Vaucher, P. (2018). Cross-sectional study assessing the addition of contrast sensitivity to visual acuity when testing for fitness to drive. *BMJ Open, 8*(1), e018546. http://dx.doi.org/10.1136/bmjopen-2017-018546

Staplin, L., Lococo, K., Mastromatto, T., Gish, K. W., Golembiewski, G., & Sifrit, K. J. (2019, January). *Mild cognitive impairment and driving performance* (Report No. DOT HS 812 577). Washington, DC: National Highway Traffic Safety Administration.

Staplin, L., Lococo, K. H., Crompton, C., Mastromatto, T., Quinones, T., & Sifrit, K. J. (2022, May). *Visual scanning training for older drivers Traffic Tech Technology Transfer Series.* Report No. DOT HS 813 296). National Highway Traffic Safety Administration.

Stav, W. B. (2015). *Occupational therapy practice guidelines for driving and community mobility for older adults* (2nd ed.). Bethesda, MD: AOTA.

Stephens, C., Szabo, A., Allen, J., & Alpass, F. (2019). Livable environments and the quality of life of older people: An ecological perspective. *The Gerontologist, 59,* 675–685. https://doi.org/10.1093/geront/gny043

Swain, T. A., McGwin, G., Antin, J. F., Wood, J. M., & Owsley, C. (2021). Left turns by older drivers with vision impairment: A naturalistic driving study. *Innovation in Aging, 5*(3), igab026. https://doi.org/10.1093/geroni/igab026

Toepper, M., & Falkenstein, M. (2019). Driving fitness in different forms of dementia: An update. *Journal of the American Geriatrics Society, 67*(10), 2186–2192. https://doi.org/10.1111/jgs.16077

Toups, R., Chirles, T. J., Ehsani, J. P., Michael, J. P., Bernstein, J. P., Calamia, M., Parsons, T. D., Carr, D. B., & Keller, J. N. (2022). Driving performance in older adults: Current measures, findings, and implications for roadway safety. *Innovation in Aging, 6*(1), igab051. https://doi.org/10.1093/geroni/igab051

Unsworth, C. A., Baker, A., Morton-Kehle, D., & Darzins, S. (2021). Survey of occupational therapy driver assessors' rehabilitation interventions with older drivers. *OTJR: Occupation, Participation and Health, 42*(2), 115–126. https://doi.org/10.1177/15394492211050634

Weiner, E. (2016). *Urban transportation planning in the United States: History, policy and practice,* 5th ed. Silver Springs, MD: Springer.

Wood, J., & Owsley, C. (2014). Gerontology viewpoint: Useful field of view test. *Gerontology, 60,* 315–318. https://doi.org/10.1159/000356753

World Health Assembly, 73. (2020). Decade of healthy ageing: The global strategy and action plan on ageing and health 2016–2020: Towards a world in which everyone can live a long and healthy life: Report by the Director-General. World Health Organization. https://apps.who.int/iris/handle/10665/355618

World Health Organization. (2001). International classification of function, disability and health. WHO: Geneva, Switzerland.

World Health Organization. (2007). Global age-friendly cities: A guide. World Health Organization. https://apps.who.int/iris/handle/10665/43755

Yi, J., Lee, H. C. Y., Parsons, R., & Falkner, T. (2015). The effect of the global positioning system of the driving performance of people with mild Alzheimer's disease. *Gerontology, 61,* 79–88. https://doi.org/10.1159/000365922

Zanier, N., Molnar, L. J., Eby, D. W., Kostyniuk, L. P., Zakrajsek, J. S., Ryan, L. H., St Louis, R. M., Stanciu, S. C., LeBlanc, D. J., Smith, J., Yung, R., Nyquist, L. V., DiGuiseppi, C., Li, G., Mielenz, T. J., Strogatz, D., & LongROAD Research Team. (2019). Improving safe mobility: An assessment of vehicles and technologies among a large cohort of older drivers. *Occupational Therapy in Health Care, 33*(1), 1–21. https://doi.org/10.1080/07380577.2018.1528653

Zellner, L., Herpich, F., Brieber, D., Herle, M., Zwanzger, P., & Brunnauer, A. (2021). Protocol for the conceptualization and evaluation of a screening-tool for fitness-to-drive assessment in older people with cognitive impairment. *PLoS One, 16*(9), e0256262. https://doi.org/10.1371/journal.pone.0256262

Zhou, D. J., Mikuls, T. R., Schmidt, C., England, B. R., Bergman, D. A., Rizzo, M., Merickel, J., & Michaud, K. (2021). Driving ability and safety in rheumatoid arthritis: A systematic review. *Arthritis Care & Research, 73*(4), 489–497. https://doi.org/10.1002/acr.24137

CHAPTER 20

Caregiving

Beth Fields, PhD, OTR/L, BCG ■ Chloe Muntefering, MS, OTR

> *"Caregiving is about enduring. It requires presence, openness, listening, doing, and cherishing of people and memories."*
>
> —Arthur Kleinman

LEARNING OUTCOMES

By the end of this chapter, readers will be able to:

20-1. Describe the trends and rise in caregiving for older adults.
20-2. Discuss the effects of caregiving on both the older adult and the caregiver.
20-3. Identify the levels of prevention that can be applied toward caregiving.
20-4. Explain current policies that support unpaid caregivers.
20-5. Formulate considerations for identifying and assessing caregivers.
20-6. Recognize exemplar interventions that can be used to support caregivers.

Mini Case Study

Darla is a 76-year-old woman with Alzheimer disease who lives with her wife, Gabriela. The couple have no children and have a limited social network due to being estranged from many members of their families who do not agree with same-sex marriage. Recently, Darla has started wandering from the couple's home during Gabriela's daily nap. Darla's balance has become increasingly impaired, requiring additional assistance with transfers when toileting and bathing. Gabriela experiences significant pain due to her rheumatoid arthritis, and attempting to assist her wife with transfers has increased her pain and made her feel unsafe. She recounts that her pain was once so bad that she had to leave Darla on the toilet for an hour before a neighbor could come assist them. Gabriela is independent in her own self-care tasks but recognizes that she does not have the physical ability to assist with supporting Darla's self-care needs. Gabriela recognizes that she needs help caring for Darla but has postponed seeking additional support because of fear of discrimination or mistreatment for being in a same-sex marriage.

Provocative Questions
1. What unique challenges does the case study of Gabriela and Darla highlight for LGBTQIA+ families?
2. How is this care situation impacting both Gabriela and Darla's health?

As adults age, they experience changes to their cardiovascular system, bones, joints and muscles, and memory and thinking skills, among others. These changes increase the risk of injury or onset of a condition or disease that affects the activities in which they can participate. While not all older adults will need care as a result of these changes, many will. Of those requiring care, some may require unpaid care from family members, friends, neighbors, or other support person designated by the older adult care recipient—herein referred to as **family caregivers.** Although some prefer the terms "care partner" or "informal caregiver," we are using the term family caregiver to align with published guidance (Stall et al, 2019). Given the suddenness of an injury or gradual onset of a condition or disease, caregiving responsibilities can vary greatly depending on the needs of the older adult. Family caregivers feel the push and pull of providing caregiving responsibilities on their own health and quality of life. As such, there is an opportunity for policymakers, healthcare providers, researchers, and educators to develop and implement solutions that better support family caregivers to fulfill their responsibilities, thereby improving their health and quality of life as well as those they care for. This chapter sheds light on the research, policy, and practice considerations for supporting family caregivers of older adults. This includes a discussion of assessments and interventions aimed at increasing recognition and support of family caregivers.

Prevalence and Trends Affecting Family Caregiving

Today there are an estimated 41.8 million family caregivers of care recipients age 50 years and older, up from the 34.2 million estimate in 2015 (AARP & National Alliance for Caregiving, 2020). In the United States alone, such care has an economic value of more than

$264 billion (White et al, 2021). The rising prevalence of family caregivers of older adults may be due to several social and demographic trends (The National Academies of Sciences, Engineering, and Medicine, 2016). The number of baby boomers (individuals who were born between 1946 and 1964) turning 65 years old. Older adults are living longer because of advances in medicine and technology. Family size continues to decline as divorce and childlessness rates increase. Healthcare systems are experiencing workforce shortages. States are expanding their home-based and community-based services. These reasons and more help explain why the lion's share of care often falls on family caregivers.

Demographics and Contextual Characteristics of Family Caregivers

"Caregiving remains an activity that occurs among all generations, racial/ethnic groups, income or educational levels, family types, gender identities, and sexual orientations" (AARP & National Alliance for Caregiving, 2020, p. 10). A 2020 report on caregiving in the United States revealed that family caregivers are about 50 years old (35%), identify as female (61%), are non-Hispanic white (61%), and help older adult care recipients who have an average age of 69 years old and identify as female (61%). Eighty-nine percent of family caregivers provide care to a relative, including parent/parent-in-law (50%), spouse/partner (12%), grandparent/grandparent-in-law (8%), sibling/sibling-in-law (7%), adult child (6%), or other relative (6%). Even children under the age of 18 assume the role of family caregiver, with about 3.4 million children helping older adults' complete daily tasks.

Seventy-six percent of family caregivers either live with or within 20 minutes of the older adult care recipient. Compared with white family caregivers, Asian American (51%), Hispanic (48%), and African American (45%) family caregivers are more likely to report living with the care recipient. Many care partners help older adults because of a long-term physical condition (63%) or memory problem (32%). Moreover, a greater number of family caregivers are helping older adults with multiple conditions. "This increasing comorbidity of conditions that require care suggests that not only are more American adults taking on the role of unpaid caregiver, but they are doing so for recipients who may have increasingly complex medical or support needs" (AARP & National Alliance for Caregiving, 2020, p. 26). The duration of care depends on the older adult care recipient's conditions. On average, the duration of caregiving is 4.5 years, but a greater proportion of family caregivers are helping older adults for 5 years or more, especially those with long-term physical conditions.

Family Caregiving Responsibilities

Level of Care Differences

Family caregivers' responsibilities across the continuum of care (e.g., healthcare settings that an older adult may experience and transition through over time) can vary greatly. The level of family caregiver involvement, duration of caregiving, and degree of control is dictated by the level of care the older adult requires (Table 20-1) (MacNaull, 2015). For example, family caregivers of older adults with chronic conditions that are predictable, like Alzheimer disease, may start by providing occasional daily care, such as management of finances and scheduling healthcare appointments. However, as the disease worsens over time, the older adult will require more intense caregiving, spanning the course of several years. Family caregivers in this situation are likely to help older adults transition to assisted living and/or skilled nursing facilities while also retaining many caregiving responsibilities (e.g., managing finances and healthcare appointments). Alternatively, some family caregivers will more abruptly step into caregiving roles. For instance, older adults are at an increased risk of falling and fracturing their hip, thus needing episodic care. This unpredictable injury often requires moderate to intense involvement of family caregivers over a span of weeks to months. Family caregivers in this situation are likely to help older adults follow their hip precautions, complete appropriate exercises, and modify their home environment to optimize safety and independence. Family caregivers may also help older adults with the following responsibilities at any given level of care: locate and coordinate services from health and human service agencies (e.g., Meals on Wheels, inhome aides), do housework, assist with complex medical and nursing tasks (e.g., tube feedings, medication monitoring), complete paperwork (e.g., advance directives, insurance plans), drive to appointments, provide companionship and emotional support, and communicate and negotiate care decisions with other family members. Each condition that the older adult encounters give rise to unique needs and challenges that the family caregiver must address across the continuum of care (Schulz & Tompkins, 2010).

Gender Differences

Gender differences in experiences and responsibilities are important issues for aging families (Xiong et al, 2020). Over their life span, women tend to experience more personal disability and need more personal assistance than their male counterparts (AARP, & National Alliance for Caregiving, 2020; Bueno & Chase, 2023). They are also more likely to be the sole caregivers for spouses, grandchildren, and other family members and less likely to hire assistants to help with these tasks. Although role flexibility has increased in the United States, women still experience considerable role strain and conflict as they juggle responsibilities as employees, parents, and caregivers for their own parents. Remarkably, while social relationships and support men during middle age, women experience significantly more social support and connection in later life (Fischer & Beresford, 2015). As women's roles continue to evolve, it will be important to continue the process of identifying emerging concerns.

TABLE 20-1 ■ Caregiver Involvement in Levels of Care

	OCCASIONAL DAILY CARE	EPISODIC CARE	CONTINUOUS/ LONG-TERM CARE	PALLIATIVE/END-OF-LIFE CARE	RECUPERATIVE CARE	HOME CARE
Caregiver involvement	Moderate to intense	Moderate to intense	Moderate to intense	Intense	Moderate to intense	Moderate to intense
Duration	Long-term May span years	Short- to midterm May span days, weeks, months	Mid- to long-term May span months, years	Unpredictable Typically 3 to 6 weeks but could last months, years	Short- to long-term May span days to years depending on condition	Short- to long-term May span days to years depending on condition
Degree of control	High and predictable Easy to plan in advance for changes to work and life responsibilities	Limited and unpredictable Impossible to plan for in advance	Mid to high Periods of high control can be disrupted with periods of midlevel control	None	None to high Depends on condition (e.g., pulled muscle vs. hip replacement after an unexpected fall)	High and predictable Easy to plan in advance for changes to work and life responsibilities
Example(s)	Groceries, yardwork, transport	Treatment-related care (e.g., appointment in response to arthritis flare-up)	Chronic and/or progressive illness or disability (e.g., Parkinson disease, Alzheimer disease)	Care in hospital, palliative care facility, community or home environments	Recovery after surgery, pneumonia, stroke	Supporting independent living (e.g., support service coordination, safety and security assistance)

Reprinted with permission from The Vanier Institute of the Family; MacNaull, 2015.

Cultural Differences

Cultural and ethnic backgrounds also affect family dynamics and expectations (Fabius et al, 2020). For example, the norm in the United States is to have nuclear families live together, with older adults living elsewhere, sometimes even at considerable distance (McMurphy, 2020). In contrast, in Mayan villages in Highland Guatemala, extended families live together in homes that are expanded to accommodate multiple generations. Older adults in these settings assist with childcare and household tasks for as long as they are physically able to do so. When they become unable to contribute, their adult children and grandchildren provide the care they need.

The belief that many Asian cultures revere older adults is accurate historically (Shea et al, 2020). Family networks are associated with psychological well-being for Chinese older adults (Mao & Han, 2018). This sense of well-being is improved in situations where there are intergenerational transfers of resources and support (Antonucci et al, 2015; Samanta et al, 2015), emphasizing the importance for older adults of being able to do for others. Current social trends have altered family dynamics, requiring adaptation on the part of each generation (Cantor, 2019). For example, in 2000, Japan introduced a long-term care insurance system rendering long-term care a right for older adults, regardless of family readiness or finances (Tsutsui et al, 2013). Analysis of this movement indicates a decreased sense of "filial obligation, or perceived norms of children's duties toward their aging parents" (Tsutsui et al, 2013, p. 797). In Scandinavia, by contrast, the existence of a social welfare system has reduced the extent to which family members may feel responsible for caring for family members (Calvó-Perxas et al, 2021). Given these cultural variations, it is critical to explore the norms of the older adult receiving support from caregivers.

Family Structure Differences

Not every older adult has a **nuclear family** (family unit that comprises a mother, father, and dependent children) structure. LGBTQIA+ older adults are less likely than others to have children and more likely to be single (Salerno et al, 2020). Additionally, individuals may be estranged from their biological family if they have not been accepted for their sexual orientation. Therefore, when in need of caregiving, LGBTQIA+ older adults may rely more on **families of choice,** which might comprise fictive kin, friends, partners, and ex-partners (Stewart & Kent, 2017). These differences highlight the importance of not making assumptions about the composition of an older adult's family. See Chapter 5: Identity, Sexuality, and Relationships for more information.

A concern for older adults who receive care from these nontraditional support sources is that most families of choice are not automatically granted legal recognition. For this reason, it is important for LGBTQIA+ older adults and their caregivers to sign basic legal documents that dictate rights for care decisions and treatment preferences (Family Caregiver Alliance, 2015). A common concern facing LGBTQIA+ caregivers is workplace leave for caregiving. The federal Family and Medical Leave Act of 1993 (FMLA) requires that most companies provide its workers a minimum of 12 weeks unpaid leave to care for sick family members. Many employers have nondiscrimination policies that extend these same benefits to LGBTQIA+ partnerships (Family Caregiver Alliance, 2015). However, many companies do not have such policies, which makes caring for a loved one much more challenging to navigate. Refer to Promoting Best Practice 20-1.

PROMOTING BEST PRACTICE 20-1
Evaluating Patient and Family Needs

When working with an older adult and their caregiver, evaluation should include holistically minded questions through the occupational profile that give insight into the patient's and caregiver's unique occupational experiences (American Occupational Therapy Association, 2021). Questions should address factors including culture, identity, societal expectations, and lived experience. Each of these occupational profile factors can affect the adult and caregiver's occupational engagement and interactions with each other. For example, the occupational therapist could ask questions about what caregiving looks like specifically in this family unit based on some of these individual factors.

CASE STUDY
Occupational Profile

Susan is an 85-year-old widowed woman who recently moved in with her daughter, Emily, and her family after a stroke that left Susan struggling to maintain her typical daily activities. Both Emily and her husband work full-time and coordinate the busy extracurricular schedules of their high school sons. Susan is often home alone during the day and mostly sits on the couch watching television in fear of falling while the family is gone. Emily has tried to create an environment in their home that is safe for Susan to navigate with her affected gait after the stroke but admits that she is not quite sure what elements of their home need to be changed. The whole family has worked hard to collectively assist Susan with some of the activities that have become more difficult for her. Despite the family's best efforts, Emily often feels uncertain and confused about how to best support her mother as she transitions into the role as her mother's caregiver. Emily feels exhausted trying to maintain her typical commitments at work and as a mother while trying to navigate a new role as her mother's caregiver.

Identified Problem Areas Related to Caregiving

- Susan has greatly limited her activity during the day due to fear of falling.
- Emily is unsure of what changes can be made in her home to increase her mother's safety.
- Emily is confused about how to best support her mother and navigate her role change from daughter to caregiver.
- Emily feels exhausted from managing her work, family life, and caregiving roles.

Identified Strengths

- Susan has a supportive daughter who assists with her care.
- Emily has tried to create a safe environment for Susan.
- Emily has a supportive husband who helps with many home-related tasks.

Goals for Occupational Therapy

- Educate Emily about resources available to help family caregivers.
- Facilitate Susan's ability to participate in valued occupations in a safe manner.
- Increase safety and reduce fall risks in Susan's environment.

Impact of Family Caregiving: A Public Health Issue

Caregiving has consequences for the caregiver as well as the older adult (Hoffman et al, 2012; Lee et al, 2015). The complexity and plurality of caregiving puts family caregivers at increased risk of physical and psychosocial morbidity. From a nationally representative survey, Schulz et al (2018) found that "nearly half of all caregivers report emotional difficulty in caring for their loved one, and one fifth report financial and physical difficulty in providing care" (p. S-41). Moreover, the restrictions enacted to protect older adults and other vulnerable populations from contracting COVID-19 have not only disrupted but amplified the family caregiving experience. Family caregivers have reported limited social and physical interactions, reduced services and supports, and increased caregiving responsibilities (Irani et al, 2021; Lightfoot et al, 2021). As a result of these changes, caregivers of older adults have reported more physical (18.7%), emotional (48.5%), and financial (14.5%) difficulties surrounding caregiving (Makaroun et al, 2021). Considering the growing number of individuals assuming caregiving responsibilities and the associated negative outcomes, family caregiving should be recognized as a public health issue much like smoking cessation, obesity prevention, and cancer surveillance. More than twice as many adults in the United States will serve as caregivers by the end of 2020 as there are adults who have ever been diagnosed with cancer. To be more precise, within the past 12 months, 53 million American adults have provided care to an adult or a child with special needs, while 23.3 million adults have received a cancer diagnosis at any time in their lives (Rosalynn Carter Institute for Caregivers, 2020, p. 8).

Levels of Prevention in Caregiving

By applying the prevention pyramid framework (Fig. 20-1), family caregiving can be better understood and recognized as a public health issue. This framework aims to "prevent [caregiving] problems occurring in the first place by targeting policies and interventions at the known risk indicators of the problem, quickly identifying and responding to problems if they do occur and minimizing the long-term effects of the problems" (World Health Organization, 2006, as cited in Australian Government, 2014).

The primary tier of the pyramid is focused on raising awareness about caregiving on a large scale. Strategies may include awareness campaigns and caregiving courses in public education. The goal of the secondary tier of the pyramid is to provide family caregivers appropriate interventions to alleviate some injury, condition, or stressors. Interventions may include a dementia caregiving support group or caregiver training on safe patient handling. The tertiary tier of the pyramid is focused on helping those caregivers in "peak crisis" who may be either suffering acutely, needing some sort of complex intervention, or requiring more assistance managing long-term health conditions. These interventions can include surgeries, antidepressants, and cognitive behavioral therapies. Understanding and recognizing caregiving through this framework is critical, not only because of the growing evidence demonstrating negative health and quality of life outcomes of family caregivers but also because these outcomes can frequently affect older adults and healthcare systems.

Example

An adult daughter helps her mother living with dementia complete both activities of daily living (ADLs) and instrumental activities of daily living (IADLs). The daughter is the only nearby relative to provide this level of care and cannot financially afford to pay for inhome support services. The daughter has served in this caregiving role for 2 years and has been struggling with depression. Unfortunately, the daughter has not been taking good care of herself and is currently experiencing a depressive episode. As a result, her mother is left alone at home and is very confused. The mother walks outside to look for her daughter and trips and falls on a curb. Luckily, a neighbor notices the accident and finds a way to calm her down before taking her to the emergency room. Once there, the neighbor calls the daughter, who immediately breaks down over the phone, casting blame on herself, thereby worsening her depression.

This case illuminates the need to "build resiliency and create a more supportive infrastructure to serve family caregivers as their caregiving experience grows more intense" (Rosalynn Carter Institute for Caregivers, 2020, p. 9). Occupational therapy's role in supporting the wellness of caregivers is addressed later in this chapter in the section on Occupational Therapy's Role in Integrating Caregivers in Care.

Policies to Support Family Caregivers

Fields and colleagues (2021) put forth guidance on the value that occupational therapists can have in supporting unpaid caregivers. This guidance is consistent with federal and state policies that have demonstrated the need to better support caregivers.

Over the past three decades, several federal- and state-level policies have been mandated in response to the need to better support family caregivers of older adults. These policies include the Older Americans Act (OAA) Reauthorization Act of 2016 (Pub. L. 114-144), the National Family Caregiver Support Program (NFCSP; Administration for Community Living, 2023), Medicare benefits, the Family Medical Leave Modernization Act (H.R. 2589 and S. 1185, 2021), the VA Maintaining Internal Systems and Strengthening Integrated Outside Networks (VA MISSION) Act

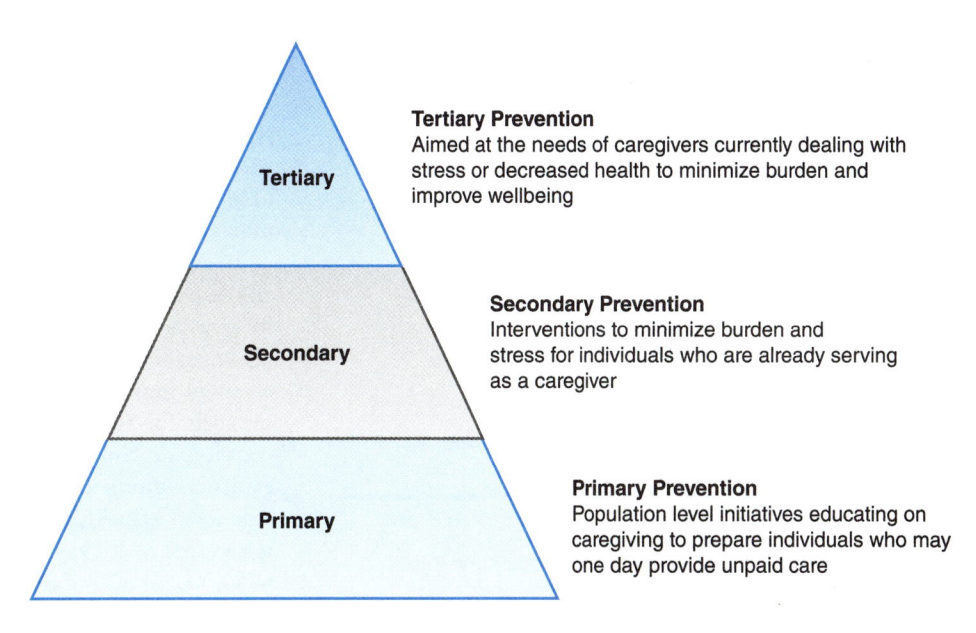

Tertiary Prevention
Aimed at the needs of caregivers currently dealing with stress or decreased health to minimize burden and improve wellbeing

Secondary Prevention
Interventions to minimize burden and stress for individuals who are already serving as a caregiver

Primary Prevention
Population level initiatives educating on caregiving to prepare individuals who may one day provide unpaid care

FIGURE 20-1 Prevention pyramid.

of 2018 (Pub. L. 115-182), and the Recognize, Assist, Include, Support, and Engage (RAISE) Family Caregivers Act (2021; Pub. L. 115-119). Table 20-2 contains supplemental information on caregiving policies at the federal and state levels.

Originally enacted in 1965, the OAA was passed to support a range of community- and home-based services to help older adults age in place. This national policy provides infrastructure for state and local agencies to implement evidence-based programs to meet the needs of older adults and their families. When the OAA was reauthorized and expanded in 2000, the NFCSP was established to better support family caregivers as well as grandparent and older kin caregivers who have minor children. "States and tribes are allocated proportional grants to work in partnership with Area Agencies on Aging and local service providers in order to provide a flexible base of caregiver services" (Bangerter et al, 2019, p. 63), including **respite care.** In addition to the programs offered through the OAA, most older adults are eligible for Medicare, a federal health insurance program that covers hospital care, outpatient services, medical equipment, and prescription drugs. The Centers for Medicare & Medicaid Services (CMS, 2020) recently expanded reimbursement for home health and telehealth services to include caregivers of beneficiaries.

The U.S. Department of Veterans Affairs enacted a program of comprehensive assistance for family caregivers of veterans injured in the line of duty after September 11, 2001, under the Caregivers and Veterans Omnibus Health Services Act of 2010 (Pub. L. 111-163). In 2018, the VA MISSION Act authorized a multiyear phase-in expansion of these services, which includes monthly stipends, mental health counseling, and enhanced respite, to caregivers of eligible veterans from other eras (U.S. Department of Veterans Affairs, 2020).

FMLA (Pub. L. 103-3) supports family caregivers by permitting full-time employed Americans to receive 12 weeks of job-protected, unpaid leave to care for a sick family member, bond with a new child, or manage a personal illness. The caveat of FMLA is that employees must work for a large company (50 or more employees) for 12 months or longer to qualify. One third of states have bolstered provisions of FMLA through more inclusive definitions of family, lower employer-size requirements, and enhanced flexibility of sick leave policies. Eight states (New York, California, New Jersey, Washington, Massachusetts, Rhode Island, Oregon, and Connecticut) have approved paid family medical leave. Another state-level initiative is the Caregiver Advise, Record, Enable (CARE) Act, model legislation that supports the integration of caregivers into hospital discharge planning to prepare them for performing care-related procedures at home (AARP, 2014, 2019). As of March 2019, the CARE Act had been adopted in 40 states (AARP, 2019).

Most recently, the RAISE Family Caregivers Act required the U.S. Secretary of Health and Human Services to convene an advisory council in 2019 to develop recommendations to systematically include, assess, and address family caregivers' needs, problems, and strengths in the care planning process. (This section reproduced from Fields et al, 2021, with permission from American Occupational Therapy Association.)

In 2021, the RAISE Family Caregiving Advisory Council released its first report to Congress describing five priority areas: (1) awareness of and outreach to family caregivers; (2) engagement of family caregivers as partners in healthcare and long-term services and supports; (3) services and supports for family caregivers; (4) financial and workplace security for family caregivers; and (5) research, data, and evidence-informed practices (RAISE Family Caregiving Advisory Council, 2021). The Credit for Caring Act (S. 1443, introduced in 2019) would allow caregivers "a tax credit of up to $3,000 for 30% of the cost of long-term care expenses that

TABLE 20-2 Supplemental Information on Caregiving Policies

FEDERAL POLICY

National Family Caregiver Support Program (2000)	Five core services include information services, access assistance, respite care, counseling, and training.
Medicare (1982)	Families can qualify to receive medical equipment, homemaker services, short-term respite care, and grief and loss counseling.
Medicare Hospice Benefits (2019) Part A and terminally ill	Families can establish a care plan with a hospice provider who then delivers the needed assistance for individuals to remain at home with their families.
Coverage for Telehealth (2018)	CMS expanded Medicare reimbursement for some services to include patient and caregiver-centered health risk assessments, advance care planning, and chronic care management to be delivered by telehealth.
Home Health Provisions (2018)	CMS implemented a new final rule for home health agencies to meet to be reimbursed by Medicare. The rule includes including, assessing, and educating caregivers of home health beneficiaries.

STATE POLICY

Caregiver Advise, Record, Enable Act[†]	43 states
Family and Medical Leave Act Expansions*	
Lower employer size	8 states
Definition expansion	14 states
Flexible sick leave	16 states
Caregiver tax credit	1 state, 10 other states considering a bill in 2019

Sources: National Academies of Sciences, Engineering, and Medicine (2016) and Aufill, Burgdorf, & Wolff (2019). [†]AARP. *National partnership. Reproduced from Fields et al, 2021, with permission of American Occupational Therapy Association.

exceed $2,000 in a taxable year" to support a spouse or other dependent relative with care needs. Moreover, in the 2021 tax year, the Child and Dependent Care Credit was initiated. Here, individuals can claim a portion of up to $8,000 in caregiving costs (IRS, 2022). While the policy landscape evolves, healthcare systems, providers, researchers, and educators can show leadership in establishing standards for integrating family caregivers in geriatric healthcare services.

Occupational Therapy's Role in Integrating Caregivers in Care

Caregiving is of particular importance for occupational therapy because it is most often a new occupation that families must learn to manage. Thoughtful assistance by the occupational therapist can reduce the stress that may be a hallmark of this occupation (de Oliveria et al, 2019) and can improve satisfaction and well-being of both the older adult and the caregiver. It is not a given that caregiving will result in stress (Geng et al, 2018), and thoughtful support from an occupational therapist in structuring caregiving can help minimize difficulties inherent in the role. In addition, an occupational therapist can help caregivers realistically examine their own emotional and instrumental resources for providing care in alternative living arrangements. This **caregiver-centered care** approach "respects and meaningfully involves the care receiver's family in the planning and delivery of supportive services" (Parmar et al, 2021) while also recognizing and addressing the needs and preferences of the family in care. To embrace a caregiver-centered care approach, occupational therapy providers can turn to a competency framework to better understand who family caregivers are, why they need support, and how best to supply this support (c.f. Caregiver Centered Care at https://www.caregivercare.ca/competency-framework). For example, through the Caregiver-Centered Care training program website, providers can earn a certificate focused on six competency domains: (1) recognizing the caregiver role, (2) communicating with family caregivers, (3) partnering with family caregivers, (4) fostering resilience in family caregivers, (5) navigating the health and social systems and accessing resources, and (6) enhancing the culture and context of care (Parmar et al, 2021). These competencies provide healthcare providers a foundation for understanding how to effectively integrate family caregivers as partners in care.

Integrating family caregivers into geriatric healthcare services will require attention to identification. Across healthcare systems and settings, providers need to offer older adults the opportunity to identify one or more family caregivers in their electronic medical record (Feinberg, 2014; National Alliance for Caregiving, 2021). Of note, it is common for older adults to not identify a family caregiver, and there are few guidelines or standards for helping older adults make decisions about family caregiver identification. This is problematic because identification helps acknowledge the responsibilities that family caregivers may assume. Once identified, there needs to be a discussion surrounding whether one or more family caregivers are willing and able to provide needed care to the older adult. Information gleaned from this conversation will shed light on the older adult's social support network and context. If a family caregiver is not willing or able to provide the needed care, then providers must make referrals to essential services and supports to help older adults maintain or improve their safety, independence, health, and quality of life.

Alternatively, providers should screen family caregivers to identify their unmet caregiving needs as well as any concerns regarding their health and well-being. The validated and standardized Caregiver Hospital Assessment Tool applies a sequential screening and referral pathway that efficiently identifies caregivers and their preferences for inclusion in the patient's hospital care and tailors referrals to address their stated preferences and unmet needs (Carbery et al, 2021; Fields et al, 2021). Other assessments that can be used in nonhospital settings to help determine how to support the caregiver include the Caregiver Strain Index, Global Health Scale, and Zarit Burden Scale (Camicia et al, 2022; Mosquera et al, 2016). Occupational therapists can also assess for signs of caregiver burnout and fatigue that may necessitate intervention. Some of the most common signs of caregiver burnout include feeling overwhelmed, frequently being tired, abnormal sleep, weight fluctuations, irritability, depression, loss of interest in activities, substance abuse, and headaches or bodily pain (American Medical Association, 2018). Utilizing both formal and informal assessments will allow therapists to better address the needs of caregivers.

Depending on family caregivers' responses to a screening tool, providers may choose to complete a more comprehensive assessment. Three practical elements that providers should consider when determining whether an assessment should be used with a population group, such as family caregivers, include whether the assessment is (1) a sensible estimate of the family caregivers' experiences and needs; (2) available, accurate, and precise for a given clinical setting; and (3) likely to affect management and planning of care to help the family caregiver (Straus et al, 2011). A comprehensive list of available family caregiver assessments, including health and well-being measures, can be found on the Family Caregiver Alliance website (c.f. https://www.carealliance.ie/userfiles/file/SelCGAssmtMeas_ResInv_FINAL_12_10_12.pdf).

The caregiver assessment framework from the National Center on Caregiving at Family Caregiving Alliance offers healthcare systems, providers, researchers, and educators areas to consider when assessing family caregivers (National Consensus Development Conference, 2006). This framework consists of several domains that represent a multidimensional approach to assessment: context; caregiver's perception of health and functional status of care recipient; caregiver values and preferences; well-being of the caregiver; skills, abilities, and knowledge to provide care to care recipient; and potential resources that the caregiver could use.

Together, these domains represent the complexities, dynamic nature, and influence of the broad range of assistance family caregivers provide to older adults who have unique characteristics, conditions, and comorbidities. Ultimately, the information gleaned from identifying and assessing family caregivers can be used to guide the selection of acceptable and effective caregiving interventions.

Exemplar Interventions

There is a large body of intervention research aimed at improving family caregiver outcomes, particularly for those providing care to older adults with Alzheimer disease and related dementias (ADRD), cancer, or stroke (The National Academies of Sciences, Engineering, and Medicine, 2016). One evidence-based, best practice, caregiving program designed to improve the quality of life and skills of family caregivers of persons living with ADRD is Skills$_2$Care (Gitlin et al, 2005). This program is delivered by certified occupational therapists and involves tailoring strategies to meet the distinct needs and environments of family caregivers. These strategies focus on teaching caregivers how to manage the everyday challenges of dementia, including communication, behaviors, home safety, and stress. Skills$_2$Care certification requirements are available through The Dementia Collaborative and are approved by the American Occupational Therapy Association for continuing-education units (The Dementia Collaborative LLC, 2022). Additionally, two treatment protocols, Reducing Disability in Alzheimer's Disease and STAR-Community Consultants, have been shown to improve care and quality of life for individuals with Alzheimer disease and reduce behavioral problems, making caregiving both easier and more rewarding (Teri et al, 2012). Each program is designed to train caregivers to improve their interactions and develop problem-solving strategies. Both have been tested using randomized, controlled studies. For more information on top dementia caregiving programs, visit the Best Practice Caregiving database (https://bpc.caregiver.org/#home). See the Promoting Best Practice 20-2 for guidance on best practice for supporting caregivers of adults with chronic conditions.

PROMOTING BEST PRACTICE 20-2
Caregivers of Persons With Chronic Conditions

> A systematic review by Rouch et al (2021) examined interventions that specifically support caregivers of adults with chronic conditions. The study found that emphasizing the problem-solving and coping skills of the caregiver were found to improve depression and quality of life. The review also found that self-management education and hands-on training led to improvements in a caregiver's sense of burden.

Family caregivers can also provide extensive care to older adults with cancer. A systematic review located and described 49 cancer-caregiving interventions (Applebaum & Breitbart, 2013). Common approaches to intervention include problem-solving/skill building, family and supportive therapy, cognitive behavioral therapy, and existential therapy. Most interventions produced favorable outcomes, such as reduced depression and anxiety and improved caregiving skills. A promising initiative that builds on the systematic review findings is the Caregivers Clinic at Memorial Sloan Kettering Cancer Center in New York City. This clinic provides a number of in person and virtual services to support caregivers as they navigate their loved one's cancer journey (c.f. https://www.mskcc.org/experience/caregivers-support/caregiver-counseling-services). Although the literature is less extensive than ADRD and cancer caregiving, interventions to support family caregivers of older adult stroke survivors are emerging and demonstrating effectiveness. One exemplar is the London Stroke Carers Training Course (LSCTC), which lasts three to five sessions (30 to 45 minutes each) and involves providing family caregivers with structured information on symptom management, goal setting, care coordination, and safe patient handling (e.g., transfers and mobility). Results from studies of the LSCTC have revealed increased quality of life and function and reduced institutionalization among older adult stroke survivors and enhanced emotional health and participation in social activities and reduced burden among caregivers (Forster et al, 2013; Kalra et al, 2004). There are several themes among family caregiving interventions. Specifically, interventions tend to use a multimodal approach involving related components (e.g., support groups, problem-solving training, coping skills training and management, and disease-related education), target similar caregiver outcomes (e.g., burden, depression, anxiety, quality of life), and offer telehealth delivery modes in combination with in-person sessions. Refer to Promoting Best Practice 20-3 for strategies to enhance caregiver health and wellness.

PROMOTING BEST PRACTICE 20-3
Improving Health and Wellness of Family Caregivers

> A study by Terranccciano et al (2020) examined the effectiveness of the Powerful Tool for Caregivers (PCT) program on burden, depressive symptoms, and self-confidence of family caregivers of older adults living with dementia. The pragmatic, two-arm, randomized controlled trial revealed that the 6-week manualized PCT program improved caregiver outcomes. Visit the PCT program website for more information (https://www.powerfultoolsforcaregivers.org).

While there is increasing public attention on developing and testing family caregiving interventions, many of these interventions have failed to move from research settings to everyday healthcare services and programs. Several existing system-level barriers may help explain this slow uptake (National Alliance for Caregiving, 2021; Schulz et al, 2018). There are few standards and associated regulatory systems to motivate providers to integrate family caregivers in service provision. To address this barrier, practice guidelines must be systematically developed to inform providers' decisions about what to assess and how to address family caregivers' physical, social, financial, and emotional needs. Another barrier is the lack of accessible Current Procedural Terminology (CPT) or Healthcare Common Procedure Coding System codes for including, assessing, and supporting family caregivers in specialty practices, hospitals, primary care, and long-term care settings. To address this barrier, health systems should create specialty and setting-specific CPT overview guides focused directly on caregiving. These guides could not only help increase reimbursement rates and ensure that family caregivers are integrated into care planning and coordination but also decrease risk of medical billing and coding errors. There is also a paucity of professional competencies and accreditation standards for licensure that focus on how to practice person- and family-centered geriatric care. To address this barrier, educational programs must train the future workforce to embody an approach to care "that is centered in collaborative partnerships among individuals, their defined family, and providers" (National Quality Forum, 2014). Elements of person- and family-centered care that should be incorporated in curricula include respecting, assessing, honoring, and addressing the needs, values, and preferences of both older adults and their families.

CASE STUDY (CONTINUED)

Intervention Plan and Discharge Status

During Susan's first appointment with her home health occupational therapist, Emily shares her concerns and uncertainty with the therapist. The occupational therapist acknowledges Emily's feelings and recommends that she look into Powerful Tools for Caregivers, national classes for caregivers that emphasize how to take care of yourself while caring for a loved one. Additionally, after learning from the Canadian Occupational Performance Measure and the occupational profile that Susan wants to return to gardening, the therapist walked through the home environment and yard with the family to identify trip hazards and barriers to accessibility for Susan. Collectively, they identified that the most difficult aspect of accessing the raised garden beds in the backyard were the steps that Susan had to descend to access the garden. Modeling intervention from CAPABLE research aimed at promoting aging in place, the therapist contacted a handyperson who worked with the family to install a ramp to exit the house into the backyard (c.f. https://nursing.jhu.edu/faculty_research/research/projects/capable/).

At discharge from occupational therapy services, Emily notes how empowered and capable she now feels caring for her mother after taking the Powerful Tools for Caregivers course. Susan shares that she is starting to finally feel like herself again, now that she is safely able to move about the home to engage in her desired occupations, including gardening. Emily comments that she feels less stress and guilt, knowing her mother is safe and engaged in activities that she enjoys throughout the day.

Questions

1. What methods of assessment might have helped to determine Emily's needs as the caregiver?
2. Understanding some of the patient/family priorities from the case study, what types of goals would be appropriate to include in the plan of care?
3. What additional interventions might be considered to meet Emily and Susan's needs?

Answers

1. Screening Emily for some of the common signs of caregiver burnout and fatigue would be helpful in determining how future interventions could equally support her as the caregiver. Additionally, the occupational therapist could have used a formal assessment like the Caregiver Strain Index, Global Health Scale, or the Zarit Burden Scale. **(LO 20-5)**
2. From this case study, we can determine that Susan is experiencing occupational deprivation and Emily is likely dealing with some degree of caregiver burnout. Therefore, goals should address improving Susan's access to and safe participation in meaningful daily activities, while also aiming to help Emily improve her self-efficacy, problem-solving, and stress management with caregiving tasks. **(LO 20-5; 20-6)**
3. An additional intervention that could be considered in this case study would be the London Stroke Carers Training Course which provides training to caregivers of adults who have suffered a stroke. This intervention could be helpful for Emily in improving her self-efficacy as Susan's caregiver. **(LO 20-6)**

SUMMARY

This chapter provided an overview of the prevalence and demographic trends affecting family caregiving, levels of care, and caregiving responsibilities and an analysis of policies and practices focused on family caregiving. Occupational therapy has much to offer throughout the care continuum to support family caregivers of older adults. By systematically identifying, assessing, and addressing the unmet needs of caregivers, the profession has the capability to make a profound difference in this growing public health concern.

Critical Thinking Questions

1. What resources and tools can support caregivers to care for their family members and friends?

2. How might the level of caregiver involvement, duration of caregiving, and degree of control affect the needs of the caregiver?
3. How can caregiving affect the health of the caregiver?

REFERENCES

AARP. (2014). *State law to help family caregivers*. https://www.aarp.org/politics-society/advocacy/caregiving-advocacy/info-2014/aarp-creates-model-state-bill.html

AARP. (2019, March). *The CARE Act implementation: Progress and promise*. https://www.aarp.org/content/dam/aarp/ppi/2019/03/the-care-act-implementation-progress-and-promise.pdf

AARP, & National Alliance for Caregiving. (2020 May). *Caregiving in the U.S.* https://www.aarp.org/content/dam/aarp/ppi/2020/05/full-report-caregiving-in-the-united-states.doi.10.26419-2Fppi.00103.001.pdf

Administration for Community Living (2023). National family caregiver support system. https://acl.gov/programs/support-caregivers/national-family-caregiver-support-program

American Medical Association. (2018). *Caring for the caregiver: A guide for physicians*. https://www.ama-assn.org/media/23686/download

American Occupational Therapy Association. (2021). Occupational therapy scope of practice. *American Journal of Occupational Therapy, 75*(Suppl. 3), 7513410030. https://doi.org/10.5014/ajot.2021.75S3005

Antonucci, T. C., Ajrouch, K. J., & Abdulrahim, S. (2015). Social relations in Lebanon: Convoys across the live course. *The Gerontologist, 55*(5), 825–835. https://doi.org/10.1093/geront/gnt209

Applebaum, A. J., & Breitbart, W. (2013). Care for the cancer caregiver: A systematic review. *Palliative & Supportive Care, 11*(3), 231–252. https://doi.org/10.1017/S1478951512000594

Aufill, J., Burgdorf, J., & Wolff, J. (2019). In support of family caregivers: A snapshot of five states. Millbank Memorial Fund. https://digirepo.nlm.nih.gov/master/borndig/101755068/MMF_Caregiver_Report_6.19.pdf

Australian Government. (2014, December). *Defining the public health model for the child welfare services context*. https://aifs.gov.au/cfca/publications/defining-public-health-model-child-welfare-services-context

Bangerter, L. R., Fadel, M., Riffin, C., & Splaine, M. (2019). The Older Americans Act and family caregiving: Perspectives from federal and state levels. *Public Policy and Aging Report, 29, 62–66*. https://doi.org/10.1093/ppar/prz006

Bueno, M. V., & Chase, J.-A. D. (2023). Gender differences in adverse psychosocial outcomes among family caregivers: A systematic review. *Western Journal of Nursing Research, 45*(1), 78–92. https://doi.org/10.1177/01939459221099672

Calvó-Perxas, L., Vilalta-Franch, J., Litwin, H., Mira, P., & Garre-Olmo, J. (2021). A longitudinal study on public policy and the health of in-house caregivers in Europe. *Health Policy, 125*(4), 436–441. https://doi.org/10.1016/j.healthpol.2021.02.001

Camicia, M., Lutz, B. J., Stram, D., Tucker, L. Y., Ray, C., & Theodore, B. R. (2022). Improving caregiver health through systematic assessment and a tailored plan of care. *Western Journal of Nursing Research, 44*(3), 307–318. https://doi.org/10.1177/01939459211045432

Cantor, M. H. (2019). Families and caregiving in an aging society. In *Families and aging* (pp. 135–144). Routledge.

Carbery, M., Schulz, R., Rodakowski, J., Terhorst, L., & Fields, B. (2021). Evaluating the appropriateness and feasibility of the Care Partner Hospital Assessment Tool (CHAT). *International Journal of Environmental Research and Public Health, 18*(24), 13355. https://doi.org/10.3390/ijerph182413355

Centers for Medicare & Medicaid Services. (2020). *Caregiver partners*. https://www.cms.gov/Outreach-and-Education/Outreach/Partnerships/Caregiver

de Oliveira, A. M., Radanovic, M., Homem de Mello, P. C., Buchain, P. C., Dias Vizzotto, A., Harder, J., Stella, F., Piersol, C. V., Gitlin, L. N., & Forlenza, O. V. (2019). An intervention to reduce neuropsychiatric symptoms and caregiver burden in dementia: Preliminary results from a randomized trial of the tailored activity program–outpatient version. *International Journal of Geriatric Psychiatry, 34*(9), 1301–1307. https://doi.org/10.1002/gps.4958

Fabius, C. D., Wolff, J. L., & Kasper, J. D. (2020). Race differences in characteristics and experiences of black and white caregivers of older Americans. *The Gerontologist, 60*(7), 1244–1253. https://doi.org/10.1093/geront/gnaa042

Family Caregiver Alliance. (2015). *Special concerns of LGBTQIA+ caregivers*. https://www.caregiver.org/resource/special-concerns-lgbt-caregivers

Feinberg, L. F. (2014). Moving toward person- and family-centered care. *Public Policy & Aging Report, 24*(3), 97–101. https://doi.org/10.1093/ppar/pru027

Fields, B., Rodakowski, J., Jewell, V. D., Arthanat, S., Park, M., Piersol, C. V., Schepens Niemiec, S. L., Womack, J., & Mroz, T. M. (2021). Unpaid caregiving and aging in place in the United States: Advancing the value of occupational therapy. *American Journal of Occupational Therapy, 75*(5), 7505347010. https://doi.org/10.5014/ajot.2021.044735

Fields, B., Schulz, R., Terhorst, L., Carbery, M., & Rodakowski, J. (2021). The development and content validation of the Care Partner Hospital Assessment Tool. *Nursing Reports, 11*(3), 522–529. https://doi.org/10.3390/nursrep11030049

Fischer, C. S., & Beresford, L. (2015). Changes in support networks in late middle age: The extension of gender and educational differences. *Journals of Gerontology, Series B: Psychological and Social Sciences, 70*(1), 123–131. https://doi.org/10.1093/geronb/gbu057

Forster, A., Dickerson, J., Young, J., Patel, A., Kalra, L., Nixon, J., Smithard, D., Knapp, M., Holloway, I., Anwar, S., & Farrin, A. (2013). A structured training programme for caregivers of inpatients after stroke (TRACS): A cluster randomised controlled trial and cost-effectiveness analysis. *The Lancet, 382*(9910), 2069–2076. https://doi.org/10.1016/S0140-6736(13)61603-7

Geng, H.-M., Chuang, D.-M., Yang, F., Yang, Y., Liu, W.-M., Liu, L.-H., & Tian, H.-M. (2018). Prevalence and determinants of depression in caregivers of cancer patients: A systematic review and meta-analysis. *Medicine, 97*(39), e11863. https://doi.org/10.1097/MD.0000000000011863

Gitlin, L. N., Hauck, W. W., Dennis, M. P., & Winter, L. (2005). Maintenance of effects of the home environmental skill-building program for family caregivers and individuals with Alzheimer's disease and related disorders. *The Journals of Gerontology: Series A, 60*(3), 368–374. https://doi.org/10.1093/gerona/60.3.368

Hoffman, G. J., Lee, J., & Mendez-Luck, C. A. (2012). Health behaviors among baby boomer informal caregivers. *The Gerontologist, 52*(2), 219–230. https://doi.org/10.1093/geront/gns003

Irani, E., Niyomyart, A., & Hickman, R. L. (2021). Family caregivers' experiences and changes in caregiving tasks during the COVID-19 pandemic. *Clinical Nursing Research, 30*(7), 1088–1097. https://doi.org/10.1177/10547738211014211

IRS. (2022, March 8). *Topic No. 602 child and dependent care credit*. https://www.irs.gov/taxtopics/tc602

Kalra, L., Evans, A., Perez, I., Melbourn, A., Patel, A., Knapp, M., & Donaldson, N. (2004). Training carers of stroke patients: Randomised controlled trial. *BMJ, 328*(7448), 1099. https://doi.org/10.1136/bmj.328.7448.1099

Lee, Y., Tang, F., Kim, K. H., & Albert, S. M. (2015). The vicious cycle of parental caregiving and financial well-being: A longitudinal study of women. *The Journals of Gerontology: Series B, 70*(3), 425–431. https://doi.org/10.1093/geronb/gbu001

Lightfoot, E., Yun, H., Moone, R., Otis, J., Suleiman, K., Turck, K., & Kutzler, C. (2021). Changes to family caregiving of older adults and adults with disabilities during COVID-19. *Gerontology and Geriatric Medicine, 7*, 1–8. https://doi.org/10.1177/23337214211002404

MacNaull, S. (2015, October 20). *Caring enough to flex, flexing enough to care*. The Vanier Institute of the Family. https://vanierinstitute.ca/caring-enough-to-flex-flexing-enough-to-care

Makaroun, L. K., Beach, S., Rosen, T., & Rosland, A.-M. (2021). Changes in elder abuse risk factors reported by caregivers of older adults during the COVID-19 pandemic. *Journal of the American Geriatrics Society, 69*(3), 602–603. https://doi.org/10.1111/jgs.17009

Mao, X., & Han, W.-J. (2018). Living arrangements and older adults' psychological well_being and life satisfaction in China: Does social support matter? *Family Relations, 67*(4), 567–584. https://doi.org/10.1111/fare.12326

McMurphy, L. (2020). It takes a village: Alternatives to the nuclear family and how the traditional model fails us. [Unpublished thesis]. Texas State University.

Mosquera, I., Vergara, I., Larrañaga, I., Machón, M., Del Rio, M., & Calderón, C. (2016). Measuring the impact of informal elderly caregiving: A systematic review of tools. *Quality of Life Research, 25*(5), 1059–1092. https://doi.org/10.1007/s11136-015-1159-4

National Academies of Sciences, Engineering, and Medicine. Families Caring for an Aging America; Report; The National Academies Press: Washington, DC, USA, 2016.

National Alliance for Caregiving. (2021, November). *Caring for the caregiver: Incentivizing medical providers to include caregivers as part of the treatment team.* https://www.caregiving.org/wp-content/uploads/2021/11/NAC_CaringForCaregiver_Paper_v2highres.pdf

National Consensus Development Conference. (2006, April). *Caregiver assessment: Principles, guidelines and strategies for change.* Vol. 1. Family Caregiver Alliance. https://www.caregiver.org/uploads/legacy/pdfs/v1_consensus.pdf

National Quality Forum. (2014, August 15). Priority setting for healthcare performance measurement: Addressing performance measure gaps in person-centered care and outcomes. https://www.qualityforum.org/Projects/n-r/Prioritizing_Measures/Care_Coordination/Final_Report.aspx

Parmar, J., Bremault-Phillips, S., Duggleby, W., Holroyd-Leduc, J., & Margriet Pot, A. (2021). Caregiver-centered care competency framework. https://uploads-ssl.webflow.com/60105a5edd88603ee79d7bda/60f5f3667195a43e406af109_202107%2017%20Caregiver%20Centered%20CAreCompetency%20Framework%20updated.pdf

RAISE Family Caregiving Advisory Council. (2021, September 22). *Recognize, Assist, Include, Support, & Engage (RAISE) Family Caregivers Act: Initial report to Congress.* Administration for Community Living, U.S. Department of Health and Human Services. https://acl.gov/sites/default/files/RAISE-InitialReportToCongress2021_Final.pdf

Rosalynn Carter Institute for Caregivers. (2020). *Recalibrating for caregivers: Recognizing the public health challenge.* (2020). Rosalynn Carter Institute for Caregivers. https://www.rosalynncarter.org/wp-content/uploads/2020/10/RCI_Recalibrating-for-Caregivers_2020.pdf

Rouch, S. A., Fields, B. E., Alibrahim, H. A., Rodakowski, J., & Leland, N. E. (2021). Evidence for the effectiveness of interventions for caregivers of people with chronic conditions: A systematic review. *American Journal of Occupational Therapy, 75*(4), 7504190030. https://doi.org/10.5014/ajot.2021.042838

Salerno, J. P., Williams, N. D., & Gattamorta, K. A. (2020). LGBTQ populations: Psychologically vulnerable communities in the COVID-19 pandemic. *Psychological Trauma: Theory, Research, Practice, and Policy, 12*(S1), S239–S242. https://doi.org/10.1037/tra0000837

Samanta, T., Chen, F., & Vanneman, R. (2015). Living arrangements and health of older adults in India. *Journal of Gerontology: Series B. Psychological Sciences and Social Sciences, 70*(6), 937–947. https://doi.org/10.1093/geronb/gbu164

Schulz, R., Beach, S. R., Friedman, E. M., Martsolf, G. R., Rodakowski, J., & James, A. E. (2018). Changing structures and processes to support family caregivers of seriously ill patients. *Journal of Palliative Medicine, 21*(S2), S-36–S-42. https://doi.org/10.1089/jpm.2017.0437

Schulz, R., & Tompkins, C. (2010). Informal caregivers in the United States: Prevalence, caregiver characteristics, and ability to provide care. In *The role of human factors in home health care: Workshop summary.* National Academies Press. https://www.nap.edu/read/12927/chapter/10

Shea, J., Moore, K., & Zhang, H. (2020). Contemporary trends in and future directions for aging and caregiving in East Asian societies. In *Beyond Filial Piety: Rethinking aging and caregiving in contemporary East Asian societies* (Vol. 6, pp. 359).

Stall, N. M., Campbell, A., Reddy, M., & Rochon, P. A. (2019). Words matter: The language of family caregiving. *Journal of the American Geriatrics Society, 67*(10), 2008–2010. https://doi.org/10.1111/jgs.15988

Stewart, D. B., & Kent, A. (2017). Caregiving in the LGBT community. https://www.sageusa.org/wp-content/uploads/2018/05/sageusa-successful-lgbt-caregiving-education-guide-longterm-care.pdf

Straus, S., Glasziou, P., Richardson, S., & Haynes, B. (2011). *Evidence-based medicine: How to practice and teach it* (4th ed.). Churchill Livingstone: Elsevier.

Teri, L., McKenzie, G., Logsdon, R. G., McCurry, S. M., Bollin, S., Mead, J., & Menne, H. (2012). Translation of two evidence-based programs for training families to improve care of persons with dementia. *The Gerontologist, 52*(4), 452–459. https://doi.org/10.1093/geront/gnr132

Terracciano, A., Artese, A., Yeh, J., Edgerton, L., Granville, L., Aschwanden, D., Luchetti, M., Glueckauf, R. L., Stephan, Y., Sutin, A. R., & Katz, P. (2020). Effectiveness of powerful tools for caregivers on caregiver burden and on care recipient behavioral and psychological symptoms of dementia: A randomized controlled trial. *Journal of the American Medical Directors Association, 21*(8), 1121–1127.e1. https://doi.org/10.1016/j.jamda.2019.11.011

The Dementia Collaborative LLC. (2022). *Skills2Care certification for occupational therapists.* https://www.dementiacollaborative.com/pages/skills2care-certification

The National Academies of Sciences, Engineering, and Medicine. (2016). *Families caring for an aging America.* National Academies Press. https://www.ncbi.nlm.nih.gov/books/NBK396401/

Tsutsui, T., Muramatsu, N., & Higashino, S. (2013). Changes in perceived filial obligation norms among coresident family caregivers in Japan. *The Gerontologist, 54*(5), 797–807. https://doi.org/10.1093/geront/gnt093

U.S. Department of Veterans Affairs. (2020). *VA caregiver support program.* https://www.caregiver.va.gov

White, D., DeAntonio, D., Ryan, B., & Colyar, M. (2021, November 8). *The economic impact of caregiving.* https://www.bcbs.com/the-health-of-america/reports/the-economic-impact-of-caregiving

Xiong, C., Biscardi, M., Astell, A., Nalder, E., Cameron, J. I., Mihailidis, A., & Colantonio, A. (2020). Sex and gender differences in caregiving burden experienced by family caregivers of persons with dementia: A systematic review. *PLoS One, 15*(4), e0231848. https://doi.org/10.1371/journal.pone.0231848

PART IV

The Context of Service Delivery

This section dives into the continuum of care contexts where older adults may receive healthcare services. Before embarking on the continuum however, it is important to understand the nuances of evaluation and assessment for the older adult. The remaining chapters are structured on the basis of healthcare systems that, in an ideal world, would provide care transitions as needed to maintain a person's highest level of function. Please note that the use of the terms "client," "patient," or "resident" is intentionally different in each chapter, reflective of the unique care contexts. Readers will follow case studies from Part II to integrate understanding of treatment contexts to the conditions formerly discussed.

A substantial challenge for individuals needing care and the institutions that provide that care is the unfortunate lack of coordination among those systems. Gaps remain and can cause significant hardship to individuals and their families. Even when the transition is relatively smooth, movement from one system to another requires the transfer of information, which may or may not happen effectively, separate evaluation to conform to system regulations, expensive transport that may not be covered by any source of funding, and adjustment by the individual—often in a weakened and confused state—to a new environment and new carers. Such transitions can result in complications and excessive stress for the individual. Single-payer systems, such as those in Canada and the United Kingdom, can provide more predictable and sustained care based on guaranteed payment for specific kinds of intervention.

The rise of chronic noncommunicable conditions, such as diabetes, heart disease, and cancers, will have social and economic costs to healthcare. Options for community-based, home, congregate, and institutional care will continue to expand (International Federation on Aging, 2018). Aging in place and "living well" in the community may be optimal choices for some but may be out of reach for those with catastrophic health challenges.

Meaningful occupation is necessary to life in all contexts. Occupational therapists play a critical role in addressing wellness and quality of life throughout the care continuum. While reading the chapters that follow, reflect on how advocacy for clients and expansion of services are important roles for occupational therapists. Identify how occupational therapy evaluation and occupation-based interventions can be designed to help individuals remain functional and satisfied with their quality of life. It is inevitable that those who live long enough will need help.

The last chapter forecasts change in aging care, including climate change, social trends, healthcare innovations, and emerging technologies. Futurist interventions have implications for both family and professional caregiving. Occupational therapists, with their holistic understanding of individuals and community, are well positioned as leaders in the healtchcare of older adults.

International Federation on Ageing. (2018). *Global health and aging.* https://ifa.ngo/publication/health/global-health-and-aging

CHAPTER 21

Special Concerns Around Evaluation of the Older Adult

Camille Ko, OTD, OTR, CBIS ■ Christine E. Haines, MBA, PhD, OTR/L

"I wasn't sure what to expect when I went to occupational therapy for the first time. During my first evaluation, the occupational therapist built an environment that made me feel hope to be able to use my arm again. I was inspired to work to meet my own objectives and get back to doing the things I enjoy most."

—Allen M. Vietnam Veteran

LEARNING OUTCOMES

By the end of this chapter, readers will be able to:

21-1. Differentiate among the various purposes and types of assessments and evaluations.
21-2. Determine the different special and ethical considerations of assessment tools when evaluating the occupational and functional performance of older adults.
21-3. Apply different theoretical models when evaluating functional and occupational performance for older adults.
21-4. Distinguish key areas of functional and occupational performance that should be assessed in older adults.
21-5. Analyze factors that affect the functional and occupational performance of older adults and need to be considered during assessment.

Mini Case Study

Ms. Annette Altman is a 68-year-old woman with a medical history of hypertension, obesity, and osteoarthritis in her cervical spine, hands, and left knee. She had a cortisone injection in her left knee that provided temporary relief of her symptoms. Ms. Altman has four adult children and lives alone in an urban townhouse. She has recently retired, having worked as a personal support worker for 25 years and, more recently, as an educational assistant in an elementary school. When asked about her current level of physical function, she reported having difficulty traversing the stairs and crouching and kneeling due to her knee pain. She is experiencing shortness of breath with exertion, which makes walking distances difficult for her. She also describes pain in her hands that affects her ability to do many of her daily chores and activities. Ms. Altman was asked by the occupational therapist working with her to identify important activities that she is unable to do or is having difficulty with due to her health. She listed five activities: (1) walking in the park and on local trails with her family, (2) using her hands to perform fine motor activities for dressing herself or for hobbies (knitting and crocheting), (3) bowling, (4) water exercise, and (5) gardening.

Provocative Questions
1. How would the occupational therapiest proceed to conduct a functional assessment with Ms. Altman based on the information presented?
2. What assessment considerations need to be made based on Ms. Altman's history?

This chapter discusses assessing and evaluating functional and occupational performance in older adults and why they need to be assessed, how to evaluate older adults' performance, conceptual frameworks to guide assessment, priority areas that often require evaluation, and specific issues to consider when evaluating older adults. This information will assist occupational therapists with completing an ethical and thorough evaluation of older adults to create the most appropriate plan of care for their clients.

Evaluating Functional and Occupational Performance

Completing a comprehensive evaluation of functional and occupational performance of older adults is integral to guiding occupational therapy services. According to the American Occupational Therapy Association's (2021)

Standard of Practice for Occupational Therapy, "evaluation requires synthesis of all data obtained, analytic interpretation of that data, reflective clinical reasoning, and consideration of occupational performance and contextual factors" (p. 2). Evaluation occurs throughout various points in the rehabilitation process, depending on the needs of the client. Some of the specific purposes for evaluation of older adults include detecting impairments with occupational performance, gathering a description of client status, predicting functional outcomes, justifying needs for ongoing services, providing required documentation, and monitoring change or goal achievement. A critical component of the evaluation process involves assessment, which refers to specific instruments, tools, and interactions used during the evaluation process to better understand a client's occupational profile, performance factors, performance skills, performance patterns, activity demands, and contexts (Kramer & Grampurohit, 2020). To complete a thorough evaluation of functional and occupational performance, clinicians need to understand the difference between the two terms.

Defining Functional and Occupational Performance

Functional performance and occupational performance are often used interchangeably in occupational therapy; however, there is a distinction between the two. **Functional performance** is used more generally across healthcare disciplines and understood as observable elements of action that include purpose and skill and result from an interaction of a person's health conditions and their context (American Occupational Therapy Association [AOTA], 2020). **Occupational performance** involves "the accomplishment of the selected occupation resulting from the dynamic transaction among the client, their contexts, and the occupation" (AOTA, 2020 p. 80).

Understanding the difference between functional performance and occupational performance is important when selecting instruments to evaluate a person's functional or occupational performance. For example, the Canadian Occupational Performance Measure (COPM; Law et al, 2014) is often used to assess a person's satisfaction with and performance of various occupations, while the Assessment of Motor and Praxis Skills and the Functional Autonomy Measurement System have demonstrated good validity in measuring functional performance of older adults (Wales et al, 2016).

Importance of Evaluating Functional and Occupational Performance

Functional and occupational performance are often evaluated in older adults because changes in functioning are common. As people grow older, changes in health status and an increasing prevalence of chronic diseases, such as cardiovascular disease, arthritis, Parkinson disease, and dementia may lead to increasing difficulties in performing the daily activities of self-care, household maintenance, community activities, voluntary or work pursuits, and recreation and leisure activities. The Federal Interagency Forum on Aging-Related Statistics (2020) found that approximately 46% of women and 31% of men over the age of 65 had difficulty performing activities of daily living (ADLs) or instrumental activities of daily living (IADLs) or were in a long-term care facility. The proportion of older adults with these difficulties increases with age, with reports that 70% of people age 85 or older had difficulties performing ADLs or IADLs compared with 30% of people age 65 to 74. In Canada, approximately 38% of people age 65 or older report limitations in their daily activities due to a long-term condition or health-related problem (Statistics Canada, 2017).

These changes in independence can lead to decreased quality of life, dependence on others, and poor physical and mental health (Motamed-Jahromi & Kaveh, 2020). The process of disablement is dynamic and involves varying functional states, such as changes in functional mobility, ADL, and IADL. The onset of disability can be slow and progressive, which often occurs with chronic disease, or sudden and acute as occurs following a catastrophic medical event (Fong, 2019). It is important for occupational therapists to be involved in the evaluation and intervention of older adults to promote independence during these dynamic transitions and to increase functional performance affected by chronic conditions.

Purposes and Types of Assessment and Evaluation

An important aspect of evaluation involves choosing appropriate assessments based on the purpose of the evaluation. Assessments can be used for multiple purposes depending on the needs of the evaluation. The first step of an evaluation frequently involves the screening process. The screening process involves reviewing available data, administering screening instruments, and observing clients. Screening tools can be a quick and straightforward method to detect potential impairments in functional and occupational performance to determine whether a formal assessment is recommended (Kramer & Grampurohit, 2020). It is important that screening evaluations are easy to do, are quick to perform, and accurately identify those who require further evaluation for intervention. Examples of screening tools include the Montreal Cognitive Assessment (MoCA; Nasreddine et al., 2005), Functional Activities Questionnaire (Fillenbaum, 1985), the Rapid Geriatric Assessment (Little, 2017), and the Berg Balance Scale (Berg et al, 1992).

Assessments used for descriptive purposes provide information on a person's current functional status, strengths, difficulties, and/or circumstances (Laver-Fawcett & Cox, 2021). **Descriptive assessments** can be used to identify issues that merit intervention; determine specific problems in the areas of impairment, activity limitation, and participation restriction; and help determine the need for therapeutic services. For example, the Functional Behavioral Profile provides a method to describe a person's capabilities with engaging in activities, social interaction, and problem-solving for adults with dementia or stroke (Baum et al, 1993). Using this information, the practitioner can decide whether there are difficulties in these different areas and whether intervention is warranted. The Assessment of Motor and Process Skills (AMPS; Fisher, 1995) is another descriptive assessment that allows the practitioner to observe the client completing meaningful activities to gather information on what might be affecting their performance with the activity.

A critical component of evaluation of older adults is detecting impairments in functional and occupational performance. Once these impairments are identified, practitioners are better able to determine how these difficulties are impacting quality of life, justify occupational therapy services, and provide appropriate therapy interventions. **Discriminative assessment** tools allow the practitioner to identify difficulties in performance by comparing a person's level of dysfunction in relation to expectations of performance of other healthy people of that age (Laver-Fawcett & Cox, 2021). Discriminative assessments are especially important in an aging population, in which some cognitive, sensory, and physical changes naturally occur due to the process of aging. For instance, a discriminative assessment can be used to distinguish whether cognitive changes are due to expected changes with aging or a pathological condition such as dementia. The Weekly Calendar Planning Activity (WCPA) is an example of a discriminative assessment that helps identify impairments with functional cognition using normative data (Toglia, 2015).

Assessments used for prediction support the occupational therapist's ability to predict outcomes for older adults based on their patterns of needs and strengths. Therapists can use the data gathered from these **predictive assessments** along with other information gleaned from the evaluation to further support the prediction of functional outcomes. Examples include the Cognitive Performance Test (Burns, et al, 1994) and the Timed Up and Go (TUG; Podsiadlo & Richardson, 1991). The Cognitive Performance Test has been used to predict functional capacity in a range of daily activities of older adults with cognitive impairment and to predict harm outcomes in older adults after hospital discharge (Douglas et al, 2013). The TUG is frequently used to determine older adults' risk for falls.

A common use for **evaluative assessments** is to evaluate outcomes or changes in persons after they receive rehabilitation services. Items included in this type of evaluative measure are those that can be demonstrated to be responsive to change in individuals when change occurs. Examples include the Continuity Assessment Record and Evaluation (CARE; Gage et al, 2012) and the COPM. The CARE is used to measure the overall performance in daily living skills through the need for assistance, providing an indicator of functional ability, and is used to evaluate the effectiveness of rehabilitation services. As mentioned previously, the COPM was designed as an evaluative tool to measure clients' self-perception of change in occupational performance and satisfaction with performance after occupational therapy intervention.

Special Considerations for Choosing Assessment Tools

During the evaluation process, practitioners use their clinical and professional reasoning skills to choose appropriate screening tools and assessments to develop an occupational profile and analyze occupational performance. One consideration when choosing an assessment is whether to use a top-down, bottom-up, or mixed approach. Top-down assessments take a global view of the person and focus on the client's participation in their living contexts and occupations to distinguish what is important to them. Some examples of top-down assessments include the COPM and AMPS. Bottom-up assessments focus on small, separate components of a person's occupational performance or skills, concentrating on the body structures and impairments of the client. These types of assessment include the Box and Block Test, which assesses upper extremity function (Mathiowetz et al, 1985). These assessments target body structures and functions related to impairments. Top-down approaches align better with evaluating occupational performance in clients, but using a mixture of both bottom-up and top-down approaches can provide a better picture of the client's overall performance in their daily routines (Goverover et al, 2020).

When using an assessment, practitioners need to be aware of the administering procedures and psychometric properties of the assessment. **Standardized assessments** have published procedures for administering and scoring, along with psychometric studies to support the use of the assessment. See Table 21-1 to learn more about three types of standardized assessments. Psychometric properties include reliability and validity, which support the quality, generalizability, and accuracy of the assessment's results. Validity determines whether the assessment measures what it is intended to measure, and reliability demonstrates whether there is consistency between scores. Strong psychometric properties facilitate accurate evaluation and intervention planning. Table 21-2 describes some of the more common types of validity and reliability. Standardized assessments are considered best practice when completing evaluations, but nonstandardized assessments are frequently used during the evaluation process to gather information. **Nonstandardized assessments** include interviews, observations, and performance testing in which there are no set procedures for administration and/or scoring (Kramer & Grampurohit, 2020). An example might be a practitioner interviewing a client to deepen understanding of a client's occupational profile. Practitioners need to be aware of the type of administration the

TABLE 21-1 ■ Different Types of Standardized Assessments

TYPE OF ASSESSMENT	DEFINITION	EXAMPLE ASSESSMENT
Normative	Compares data obtained against a sample of the general population	The Weekly Calendar Planning Activity scores can be compared with normative data for healthy youth and adults age 16 to 94 to assess for executive functioning impairments.
Criterion-referenced	Measures how well a person performs against specific criteria	The Kohlman Evaluation of Living Skills examines 17 basic living skills. Based on the score, a clinician can make recommendations on whether the client will require assistance in the home.
Ipsative	Compares the person against themselves in the same area over time	The Canadian Occupational Performance Measure has scores that are based on the client's subjective reports. The scores are compared during retesting to see if the client perceives that they have improved in the areas chosen.

Adapted from Kramer, P., & Grampurohit, N. (Eds.) (2020). *Hinojosa and Kramer's evaluation in occupational therapy* (Fifth ed.). American Occupational Therapy Association.

TABLE 21-2 ■ Psychometric Property Definitions

PSYCHOMETRIC PROPERTY	DEFINITION
Test-retest reliability	The consistency of a measure over time. If you repeat the assessment, will you get the same results?
Interrater reliability	The consistency of results between different raters. Will two different raters consistently arrive at the same score?
Internal consistency reliability	The consistency between the test items themselves to measure a concept or skill. Do the various sections of this assessment correlate with each other?
Construct validity	The coherence of an assessment with existing knowledge of the concept. Is there evidence that this assessment has a relationship with a theory of the concept being measured?
Content validity	The extent to which an assessment examines all aspects of the measured concept. Does this assessment measure all portions of the concept?
Criterion validity	The degree to which the data measured correlates with other valid measures of the same concept. Does the score on this assessment compare to other assessments measuring the same concept?
Predictive validity	The ability of the assessment to predict future outcomes or abilities. Can I predict an outcome based on the scores from this assessment?

Adapted from Ahmed, I., & Ishtiaq, S. (2021). Reliability and validity: Importance in medical research. *Journal of the Pakistan Medical Association, 71*(10), 2401–2406.

assessments require and how that can influence the results. For instance, clients might not report any difficulties with ADLs during an interview-based assessment but might demonstrate difficulties when completing an observation-based assessment.

Ethical Considerations for Evaluating Older Adults

Occupational therapy practitioners need to be aware of the different ethical implications of evaluating older adults. Practitioners should safely complete the evaluation by respecting the client's rights and not doing any harm to the client. This involves clinicians competently practicing administration of the assessment tools and recognizing if specific assessments require certification or credentialing to complete, as do the MoCA and the AMPS. Older adults may have impairments affecting activity tolerance and cognition, affecting what assessments the practitioner selects. Assessments that require a significant amount of time and effort may not be appropriate for some older adults who easily fatigue. Practitioners should consider the environment where the evaluation takes place and the method of administration when working with adults with cognitive impairments. For instance, a busy environment may be overwhelming for some adults or might not be the most appropriate when discussing intimate health changes. Assessments with multiple-step instructions might be difficult to follow for people with cognitive difficulties. Care needs to be taken to determine whether the cognitive load of the assessment is affecting the performance being evaluated and how cognition factors into the assessment scoring.

Choosing assessment tools with limited biases provides the most accurate depiction of the older adult's current status. Practitioners need to recognize possible biases in assessments including racial/ethnic, gender, informant, and socioeconomic biases. Practitioners can use multiple assessment tools to help limit bias during the evaluation. Many older adults that practitioners interact with may be from cultures with which they are unfamiliar. Finding assessment tools in a person's preferred language and using the best available interpreters can help ensure an accurate occupational profile is completed. Practitioners can strive to practice cultural humility to provide more unbiased care in which they focus on learning rather than knowing, recognizing the individuality of clients, and reflecting on power differences in healthcare (Agner, 2020). See Chapter 4 for more discussion of the impact of culture in working with older adults.

Being aware of the specific populations for whom the assessment tool was created can guide the practitioner to choose the most appropriate assessments. The results of an evaluation may not be valid if the client does not match the intended population for the assessment tools. The interpretation of the assessment tools should be concise, accurate, and written in an approach that is directed toward helping a client versus labeling the client in a way that is harmful. For example, the Occupational Therapy Driver Off-Road Assessment battery assesses multiple performance skills related to driving. How the client scores on this assessment might affect their recommendations for returning to driving, an important aspect of community mobility (Unsworth et al, 2011). Clinicians should be familiar with interpreting the tests to ensure that accurate results are made for the safety and independence of the client.

CASE STUDY

Occupational Profile and Background

Mr. Patrick is an 80-year-old man who lives alone in a single-story home with two steps into the home and a flight of 12 steps to the basement laundry and workroom. He and his spouse divorced about 35 years ago. He has two adult children, whom he seldom sees. Mr. Patrick has a history of addiction to alcohol; he reports that he is not drinking more than one beer per day now. He smokes about two packs of cigarettes per day. He was fired from his job in his early 60s and did not find work after that. He sometimes feels out of breath when ascending the basement stairs, and sometimes after bathing. He watches sports and old television shows for leisure. Mr. Patrick states that he was in a bowling league at one time and enjoyed spending evenings at the bowling alley and bar visiting with the regular customers.

He is a patient of a local primary care community health center, where the care team is concerned that he may be experiencing some early cognitive changes. He has missed three previous appointments at the clinic with his physician, the dietitian, and the foot care clinic, stating that he had no record of them. Mr. Patrick's medical history includes osteoarthritis, hypertension, type 2 diabetes, and depression.

Models Underpinning Assessment

Theoretical models provide a specific description of how a process or system works. They define scope and practice and guide the occupational therapy process. Conceptual frameworks can provide guidance to help a therapist integrate findings across several functional areas into one overall picture of the client's abilities. The World Health Organization's (World Health Organization, 2001) framework, the International Classification of Functioning, Disability and Health (ICF), is the most widely used model for assessing disability in the world (World Health Organization, 2001). The purpose of the ICF is to provide a standardized way to collect and analyze health/disability data worldwide. The ICF integrates medical and social models to evaluate outcomes of functional performance at the activity or participation level. It has allowed for increased use of assessment tools worldwide and has led to a general acceptance of an interactive biopsychosocial model in the global medical community (Lundälv et al, 2015; Mitra & Shakespeare, 2019).

The ICF has been criticized for being overly "medicalized" and falling behind in addressing a more current understanding of disability (Lundälv et al, 2015; Mitra & Shakespeare, 2019). It has also been criticized for being too person centered and understating the importance of context and the environment in assessment of a person's functioning (Cozzi et al, 2021; Mitra & Shakespeare, 2019). It is important to consider all aspects of a person's life experiences and contexts as well as how these factors influence and are influenced by each other during occupational therapy assessment. The environment and personal contexts can act as resources that enhance or deplete the outcome of the functional and occupational performance evaluation and need to be assessed separately using standardized assessments so they can be incorporated into an overall analysis of the client's functional and occupational performance.

The Occupational Therapy Practice Framework: Doman and Process (4th ed.; AOTA, 2020) is a conceptual framework from AOTA that helps to fill in gaps from the ICF for occupational therapists. For example, the Practice Framework identifies context as one of the domains in occupational therapy practice that should be evaluated in combination with occupations, performance patterns, client factors, and performance skills to determine a person's occupational identity, well-being, health, and participation in life. Both the ICF and the Practice Framework are described in more detail in Chapter 3.

Within the context of clinical practice, occupational therapists enter into partnerships with their clients. Client-centered practice occurs when a partnership is developed between the client and the therapist, allowing for empowerment of the client to engage in functional performance to meet their occupational roles in various contexts (Sumison, 2000). Using a client-centered approach during the evaluation process will make the occupational therapy process more effective.

Other theoretical models exist in occupational therapy to further guide the occupational therapy evaluation process and provide the basis for standardized assessments used in practice. For example, the COPM is based on the Canadian Model of Occupational Performance and Engagement (CMOP-E) and is the most widely used assessment tool in the world (COPM, 2021; Polatajko et al, 2007). The Model of Human Occupations (MOHO) explains human occupation through volition, habituation, performance capacity, and environmental context (Taylor, 2017). There are more available assessments based on MOHO than any other occupational therapy theory. It is important that occupational therapists base their theoretical approach to practice on evidence-based practice, context of services, as well as their own personal knowledge, skills, and preferences.

What to Assess When Focusing on Function in Older Adults

As people age, their roles and the type of activities in which they participate often change. People may not engage in paid work as they get older and instead may engage in productive roles through volunteering. Due to reductions in time spent in paid roles, the amount of available leisure time usually increases with age. Therefore, occupational therapy practitioners need to consider leisure activities as being potentially significant to the client. ADLs are often a focus of functional performance evaluation in older adults. Self-care should not be used to the exclusion of evaluation in other areas of function, including IADLs, functional and community mobility, productivity, and leisure. Functional mobility underlies many areas of performance and may be key to planning interventions to help clients meet their goals. All of these functional performance areas can be important, and together they help form the balance of activities in which people participate. The following section discusses some of the priority areas practitioners use for assessing functional and occupational performance in older adults including assessing ADLs and IADLs, functional mobility, upper-extremity function, cognition, social participation, and leisure.

ADLs and IADLs

Changes in independence in basic and instrumental ADL may occur as people age. Typically, IADL present challenges before personal care activities. Thus, some assessments are designed to demonstrate the progression of change within various instrumental and personal ADLs. The ADL Staircase, for example, includes both IADL and ADL items; IADL items were added to personal ADL items in the assessment originally formulated by Katz (Jakobsson, 2008). At times there can be gaps between observed capabilities and actual execution of daily activities when assessing ADLs and IADLs. For instance, a client may have the capability to complete household management activities but hires someone to clean their home since they would rather spend more time on leisure activities. It is important for practitioners to consider whether they want to evaluate the ability or capacity of the older adult, or whether they want to evaluate the actual usual tasks undertaken (Brick et al, 2020; Fig. 21-1).

Several systematic reviews have identified some of the more clinically relevant and valid measures used for assessing ADLs and IADLs for older adults (Pashmdarfard & Azad, 2020; Roedl et al, 2016; Wales et al, 2016). The Functional

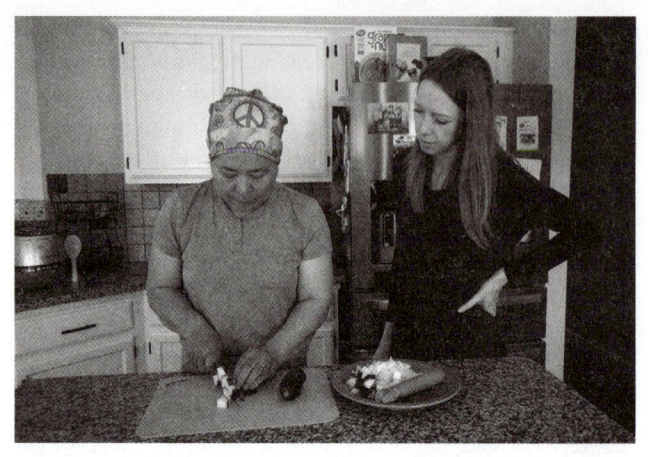

FIGURE 21-1 Assessing meal preparation in the home environment.

Autonomy Measurement Scale (Hebert et al, 1988) includes items addressing ADLs, mobility, and IADLs, as well as communication and mental functions. There are also numerous assessments that focus exclusively on personal ADLs, such as the Barthel Index (Mahoney & Barthel, 1965), the Melville Nelson Self-Care Assessment (Nelson et al, 2002), and the Katz Index of Independence in Activities in Daily Living (Katz et al, 1970). Assessments that specifically examine IADLs include the Lawton IADL scale (Lawton & Brody, 1969) and the Frenchay Activities Index (FAI; Holbrook & Skilbeck, 1983).

As with the selection of any assessment, choosing an appropriate measure of ADL or IADL function in clinical practice relies on the purpose of the assessment and review of available instruments. Evaluation of ADLs and IADLs can provide useful clinical information about an older adult's current status and the impact that a condition or set of conditions is having on their ability to manage day-to-day activities. The Kohlman Evaluation of Living Skills is a measure of IADLs that may help identify older adults' abilities to manage independently and safely in the community (Burnett et al, 2009). A new scale, the i-ADL-CDI, was created using items from the Katz Index and the Lawton Scale combined with a focus on the ICF to assess functional performance with IADLs and ADLs to help with diagnosing mild cognitive impairment and Alzheimer's disease (Cornelis et al, 2017). An important aspect of evaluating ADL and IADL involves examining the environments in which these essential activities occur. The Safety Assessment of Function and Environment for Rehabilitation Health Outcome Measurement and Evaluation Version 3 (SAFER-HOME) is a valid and reliable assessment of a client's ability to safely carry out their occupations in their home and can be used as an outcome measure to assess effectiveness of occupational therapy interventions in the home (Chiu et al, 2011).

Functional Mobility

Functional mobility involves a person's ability to move from one place to another during the performance of everyday activities including bed mobility, functional ambulation, transfers, and wheelchair mobility (AOTA, 2021). Functional mobility is linked to an older adult's ability to promote social relations, maintain independence with daily activities, avoid social exclusion, and conduct activities in society (Cuignet et al, 2020). When assessing functional mobility, a practitioner should use specific assessments concerning balance and fall risk. Falls among older adults occur at an estimated rate of up to 85%. When an older adult has concerns about falling, it can lead to avoidance of physical activity and social participation, increased depression, a decline in physical and mental performance, decreased independence with daily activities, and decreased quality of life. These concerns can also indicate impairments with functional mobility performance. The Activities-specific Balance Confidence (ABC) Scale is an example of an assessment that examines a person's concern of falling (Wang et al, 2021). Some examples of measures that assess balance in older adults include the Berg Balance Scale and the TUG.

Functional ambulation and reduced walking speed in older adults can be used as a predictor of future functional decline (Shimada et al, 2022). The Six-Minute Walk Test is an easy-to-administer assessment that examines the walking speed and endurance in older adults while comparing it to normative data (Butland et al, 1982). The Tinetti Performance Oriented Mobility Assessment is a performance-based assessment that has items that analyze the functional ambulation and balance of clients (Tinetti, 1986). An important aspect of evaluating functional mobility includes assessing a person's independence with transfers and mobility with aids. The Elderly Mobility Scale examines transfers, bed mobility, functional gait, and balance by evaluating seven functional ADLs (Smith, 1994). The Charité Mobility Index is a new assessment tool that monitors a client's ability to complete transfers, positioning, and locomotion with assistive devices as needed (Liebl et al, 2016).

Upper-Extremity Function

As people age, upper-extremity function declines due to a combination of deterioration in muscle and bone mass, muscle fiber size, and composition. Likewise, slowing of peripheral nerve conduction, central nervous system changes, and even psychosocial stress can decrease motor activity in bilateral upper extremities of older adults (Kim & Won, 2019; Roman-Liu & Tokarski, 2021; Tournadre et al, 2019). These changes cause diminished response time, coordination, and speed of movement of the upper extremities that affect independent and safe performance of occupations. Thus, assessment of upper-extremity function can contribute needed information to a rehabilitation assessment designed to assess and address functional performance. Functional activity in a person's natural context is considered the most reliable assessment and outcome of occupational and functional performance. However, there are limited direct, objective, and accurate measurements of upper-extremity function available for use in the natural context. Therefore, occupational therapists are provided with few options when assessing upper-extremity function in older adults.

Grip strength, measured with a dynamometer, is a common assessment and often used as a proxy for overall muscle strength. Norms for community-dwelling older adults have been published based on a sample of 360 older adults in Quebec (Desrosiers et al, 1995) and a sample of 224 older adults in Texas (Jansen, 2008). The link between grip strength and successful completion of daily functional activities is not always clear, and interpretation of grip strength assessment can be challenging for therapists in clinical contexts.

Other assessments of upper-extremity function include tests of motor coordination, such as the Finger–Nose Test (Gagnon et al, 2004); finger dexterity with pegboard tests, such as the nine-hole pegboard (Son et al, 2012) or the Purdue pegboard (Desrosiers et al, 1995; Tiffin & Asher, 1948) and assessments of manual dexterity through tests such as the Box and Block Test. Performance-based assessments such as the Jebsen-Taylor Hand Function Test (Jebsen et al, 1969) and self-report questionnaires like the Late-Life Function and Disability Instrument (Haley et al, 2002) should also be considered by occupational therapists assessing upper-extremity function in older adults.

Some assessments are designed to assess upper-extremity function for people with particular conditions or diseases. For example, some upper-extremity functional assessments have been used primarily for people after stroke or with other neurological conditions, for example, the Wolf Motor Function Test (Wolf et al, 2001). These may be more clinically useful to therapists in practice, particularly if the population served has a high proportion with a particular condition, such as stroke or Parkinson disease.

Cognition

The evaluation of an older adult's functional status may need to take into consideration the person's cognitive status as the risk of cognitive impairment increases with age. Assessing physical and cognitive impairments together provides a more in-depth risk assessment for impairments with occupational performance than assessing either factor alone (Aliberti et al, 2019). Limitations in functional abilities do not necessarily mean that the older adult has concomitant cognitive impairment. In situations where an older adult does not have a diagnosis related to cognitive impairment but is demonstrating cognitive difficulties, it may be useful for a therapist to administer a cognitive screening assessment, such as the MoCA or Mini-Mental Status Examination (Folstein et al, 1975; Nasreddine et al, 2005). In situations in which cognitive performance is significantly affecting performance, a more comprehensive cognitive assessment may be warranted.

People with mild cognitive impairment may have difficulties completing activities, such as IADLs, that have higher cognitive demands, such as banking or managing medications.

There are several performance-based assessment tools that evaluate different components of cognition that can help distinguish these mild cognitive impairments. The Rivermead Behavioural Memory Test is an assessment tool that examines how an older adult's memory might be affecting their functional capacity for independent living (Wilson et al, 1989). The WCPA examines a client's cognitive strategies and executive functioning skills by the client completing a weekly calendar while following specific rules and instructions (Toglia, 2015). The Executive Function Performance Test (EFPT) evaluates components of higher-level cognitive skills, asking clients to complete four everyday tasks (cooking, medication intake, bill payment, and telephone use) (Baum et al, 2008). An alternative form of the EFPT was created using internet-based tasks for bill payment and the telephone use (Rand et al, 2018).

For older adults diagnosed with cognitive impairments such as dementia, the impairment may affect the ability to manage functional activities. The Allen Cognitive Level Screen-5 is a screening tool that can be used with older adults and provides a quick estimate of a client's individual learning and problem-solving abilities after performing three visual motor tasks (Allen et al, 2007). Assessments such as the Cognitive Performance Test (Burns et al, 1994) are designed to assess cognitive status in people with dementia or other diagnoses linked to cognitive impairment. The Loewenstein Occupational Therapy Assessment Geriatric Version (LOTCA-G) is a cognitive battery created specifically for older adults with neurological impairments that assesses cognitive skills related to everyday function including orientation, memory, visual perceptual skills, praxis, visuomotor organization, and thinking operations (Katz et al, 1995). A dynamic version of the LOTCA-G (DLOTCA–G) has been created to provide clinicians an opportunity to estimate an older adult's potential for learning or receptiveness to instruction to guide the practitioner's intervention planning. (Katz et al, 2012). See Promoting Best Practice 21-1 for more information on dynamic assessments.

PROMOTING BEST PRACTICE 21-1
Using Dynamic Assessment

Dynamic assessment involves objectively measuring the degree of change that occurs in response to strategies, feedback, cues, or task conditions that are used during testing. Dynamic assessment focuses on individual changes rather than on comparison to typical performance or normative data. Using this information, practitioners can then assess the client's learning potential and ability to use strategies. The clinician can use different mediation techniques to cue the client during the assessment to assist the client with getting the correct answer. The mediation process is graded from general to more specific cues and feedback. The DLOTCA–G uses this mediation strategy and allows the practitioner to determine the most appropriate remediation techniques to use with the client (Katz et al, 2012).

Another option for dynamic assessment involves the test-teach-retest approach. In this approach, training is completed between a static pretest and posttest to determine the level and magnitude of change after training. One of the most effective methods of training involves education over strategy use. The practitioner can then observe whether the client uses the strategies discussed during the training during the posttest (Toglia & Cermak, 2009). The WCPA manual provides in-depth information on how to complete the assessment with the test-teach-retest approach (Toglia, 2015).

Social Participation and Leisure

Social participation and leisure activities are important aspects for practitioners to examine when evaluating functional and occupational performance of older adults. Some studies have indicated that limited social participation for older adults can be a larger indicator of mortality than well-established risk factors such as smoking and obesity (Turcotte et al, 2018). Currently, there are limited assessments specifically for older adults for social participation and leisure. The Activity Card Sort, 2nd edition measures an older adult's participation in IADLs, social activities, and leisure activities. This assessment tool also indicates the person's current level of engagement with the activities and whether they have discontinued the activity (Baum & Edwards, 2008). The Physical Activity Scale for the Elderly is a brief survey that assesses an older adult's participation in household, occupational, and leisure activities in the past week including volunteer work (Washburn et al, 1993). Examples of assessments that address leisure and social participation that are not specifically for older adults include the COPM and the Interest Checklist (Klyczek et al, 1997). The Interest Checklist provides an extensive list of leisure activities the practitioner can use to gather information on a person's past and present interests.

Specific Issues Related to Evaluation of Functional Performance

Regardless of the area of focus for any assessment of functional performance, therapists must always consider how the assessment findings might be influenced by circumstances beyond the specific area of assessment. For example, if an older adult is experiencing depression, it may be difficult for the person to participate actively in any physical performance testing. Other factors to consider include the older adult's education, literacy, and health literacy levels, especially if pen-and-paper assessments are being administered, as well as sensory changes, fatigue, and other concerns. Many of the factors that have potential effects on functional assessment results are highlighted next and discussed in greater detail in other chapters in this book.

Sensory Changes With Aging

Sensory loss occurs as a part of usual aging and includes changes in vision (e.g., presbyopia), hearing, and touch, all of which can influence functional performance. When evaluating functional performance, it is important to consider that changes in the sensory systems may contribute to difficulties with performance. For tests that have norms for comparison, the normative sample should include a group of older adults, so that the usual aging changes present in the normative sample are similar to those present in the older adult client group. It is also useful to set up the evaluation environment in such a way as to limit the extent to which sensory changes cause difficulties in the performance of the evaluative items, within the constraints of standardized administration. When evaluating older adults, it is useful to ensure the following:

- Adequate lighting
- Large print and contrasting background for written materials
- Minimal background noise
- Clear verbal communication and sight of the assessor's face
- Use of any prescribed aids (e.g., glasses, hearing aid)

For additional information regarding adaptations for sensory issues, refer to Chapter 10.

Fatigue

Older adults who experience fatigue associated with mobility or ADL often report a lack of energy, changes in cognitive processing, a need for increased sleep, depression, and decreased physical activity. Fatigue is a self-perceived concept, but manifests as an older person's lack of participation in physical functioning activities, such as walking or ADLs. As a result, a client experiencing fatigue may struggle to participate in assessments of mobility, cognition, ADLs, and upper-extremity function. Fatigue occurs when metabolic demands exceed energy resources and increases with aging and in the presence of chronic conditions, especially those associated with inflammation. Older adults with greater disability likely expend greater energy on tasks than those without or with lesser disability (Knoop et al, 2021). Some examples of assessment tools that examine multiple areas of fatigue include the Fatigue Severity Scale (Krupp et al, 1989) and the Multidimensional Fatigue Inventory (Smets et al, 1995). In clinical practice, if an older adult reports fatigue that is interfering with occupational performance, therapists may want to explore more in-depth assessments of fatigue to better understand and develop interventions to address this area.

Education

In clinical practice, it is important for therapists to consider the educational and literacy (including health literacy) levels of the older adult being assessed. If the evaluation requires any type of written language or numeric work, it is important to ensure that the older adult can read and understand the materials. The Short Assessment of Health Literacy—Spanish and English is a 2- to 3-minute screening tool that clinicians can use to screen English- and Spanish-speaking clients for low health literacy (Lee et al, 2010). Although some assessments consider the education level in scoring (e.g., the MoCA), others may require consideration by the clinician in interpreting scores.

Caregiver Support

Family members often take on roles as informal caregivers to ensure that older adults living in community settings are monitored and supported in activities with which they may have difficulty, including personal care and functional mobility. Commonly, family caregivers aid with transportation and community-based instrumental activities such as shopping and managing finances. The extent of caregiver support being provided is not often incorporated into the scoring of performance. For some instruments, especially ones measuring ADL, the amount of assistance or supervision required may be part of the scoring. For example, in the Functional Autonomy Measurement System (Hebert et al, 1988), consideration is given to whether a client has support and resources available to compensate for any functional impairments. Other measures, such as the Continuity Assessment Record and Evaluation (Gage et al, 2012), are scored based on the type and amount of support required to complete the task. However, whether the support is provided by paid or unpaid caregivers is not considered in the scoring.

Some older adults may become caregivers for their family members and loved ones. There are currently limited robust assessments for evaluating the needs of caregivers and how best to support them, but researchers are looking to create new tools to address this need. The Dementia Carer Assessment of Support Needs Tool is an assessment tool based on the ICF model that helps identify a caregiver's support needs when caring for a person with dementia (Clemmensen et al, 2021). Regardless of the considerations of caregiver or family supports in the administration or scoring of functional assessments, therapists will frequently consider caregiver supports in planning interventions. Refer to Chapter 20 for more information on caregiver support and caregiving.

> ### CASE STUDY (CONTINUED)
>
> #### Occupational Therapy Assessment
>
> The physician has referred Mr. Patrick to see the occupational therapist that provides services through the community health center. The occupational therapist conducted a battery of functional performance assessments, beginning with the Patient-Specific Function Scale (PSFS; Stratford et al, 1995). Mr. Patrick identifies the following activities as being affected by his health condition:
>
> 1. Walking outside the house for adequate distance: Mr. Patrick has had a recent bout of pneumonia and fell the first time he walked outside after recovery

from pneumonia. He can walk independently about three houses down from his own to get to the community mailbox. He wants to be able to walk to the corner store for food.

2. **Bathing:** Mr. Patrick reports that he showers about twice weekly. He has no safety devices in his bathroom. He states that he is independent but a bit shaky getting in and out of the bathtub when he showers. He sits down on the side of the tub to dry his lower extremities but reports difficulty ensuring that his feet are dry. He knows he should inspect his feet regularly because of his diabetes, but he is not able to do this easily.

3. **Dressing:** Mr. Patrick reports difficulty donning his socks and therefore wears shoes or slippers without socks on most days.

4. **Bowling:** Mr. Patrick believes that there is a weekly seniors' league that he would like to join.

The occupational therapist must take this occupational profile and PSFS data further and complete the assessment of Mr. Patrick to develop goals and an intervention plan.

Questions

1. Which areas of functional and occupational performance would you want to assess? Which assessment tools would you select? Justify your response.

2. You have been asked to consult on whether Mr. Patrick is safe to remain at home. Given Mr. Patrick's ADL challenges, how will you assess his performance to decide?

3. What other issues might affect the evaluation of Mr. Patrick's functional performance and why?

Answers

1. Some of the major functional and occupational performance areas to measure would include ADLs, leisure, functional cognition, and functional mobility. He reports difficulty with donning socks and drying his feet after bathing, which can be dangerous for someone with diabetes. Practitioners can use the Melville Nelson Self-Care Assessment to gather more information on his ADLs, especially bathing and dressing. For leisure, the Physical Scale for the Elderly would be a good choice to use because it has questions about bowling and mobility with leisure activities, which Mr. Patrick reports are important areas to address for him. It is stated in the case study that Mr. Patrick has been missing appointments and his physician is concerned about him having cognitive impairments, so it would be good to screen for cognition by using the Montreal Cognitive Assessment or the Mini-Mental Status Examination. If needed, more cognitive assessments, such as the WCPA or the Executive Functioning Performance Test would be beneficial to examine his cognitive abilities with completing ADLs and IADLs. Because Mr. Patrick reported falling, it would be prudent to assess his balance and functional mobility with the Tinetti Performance Oriented Mobility Assessment. The Six-Minute Walk Test could be used with assessing functional mobility, especially since he would like to be able to walk to the corner store.

2. The Kohlman Evaluation of Living Skills is specifically for assessing ADLs, IADLs, safety, and leisure to assist with determining whether someone can live independently and would be a good choice to use. A practitioner could also observe how he currently attempts to examine his feet to determine whether there are any strategies that could be used such as using a mirror to help with that aspect. Using the Melville Nelville scale to assess ADLs, the therapist could determine whether there were any adaptive equipment options to help Mr. Patrick be able to be more independent since he mentions he does not have any adaptive equipment in his bathroom. The SAFER-Home Version 3 would be beneficial to use to assess his safety while engaging in home-related activities.

3. In his medical history, it mentions that Mr. Patrick has a history of depression. This could affect his results during testing due to its effect on a person's physical and cognitive abilities. The possible cognitive impairments might impact the assessment tools used during the evaluation. The therapist should ensure that Mr. Patrick is able to follow directions and that there are limited distractions. The fact that he has diabetes is also something to consider during the evaluation because it can impact sensation in the hands and feet, and if he is having difficulty with donning socks and inspecting his feet, this could lead to more health complications. He might have decreased grip strength and dexterity in his hands, which may be affecting his independence in ADLs and IADsL. He had a recent fall, so a practitioner could assess his fear of falling using the Activities-based Confidence Scale to determine whether he has any fear of falling. There is some correlation between fear of falling and participation in daily activities and increased depression.

SUMMARY

Functional and occupational performance are critical areas of assessment for occupational therapists when working with older adults. Functional assessment can be completed for multiple purposes: screening, description, discrimination, prediction, and/or outcome evaluation; selection of the best measure is determined by the purpose of the assessment, measurement properties, and pragmatics of the assessment. Ideally, assessment of functional and occupational performance should be conducted within a conceptual framework, such as the ICF, that can help a therapist select measures and interpret findings. Although there are many areas of functional performance that can be assessed, priority areas often include functional mobility, upper-extremity function, ADLs and IADLs, cognition, social participation, and leisure. In any assessment of function, the therapist needs to consider factors that may affect results, such as sensory changes, education, fatigue, and caregiver supports. In turn, interpretation of findings and recommendations for interventions emerge from well-considered evaluations of functional performance.

Critical Thinking Questions

1. Inpatient rehabilitation requires comprehensive yet efficient assessments of function to be completed. On a geriatric rehabilitation unit, which areas and what types of assessment would be most important for an occupational therapist to complete? How could a clinician set up the environment to increase the accuracy of the results when assessing older adults in inpatient rehabilitation?

2. A home-health occupational therapist is scheduled to complete an evaluation for an older adult that is an immigrant from South America. Their primary language is Spanish, but the occupational therapist only speaks English and is not familiar with the person's native culture. What are some considerations that the occupational therapist should take when completing the evaluation process?

REFERENCES

Agner, J. (2020). Moving from cultural competence to cultural humility in occupational therapy: A paradigm shift. *The American Journal of Occupational Therapy, 74*(4), 7404347010–7404347010p7. https://doi.org/10.5014/ajot.2020.038067

Ahmed, I., & Ishtiaq, S. (2021). Reliability and validity: Importance in medical research. *Journal of the Pakistan Medical Association, 71*(10), 2401–2406. doi: 10.47391/JPMA.06-861

Aliberti, M. J. R., Cenzer, I. S., Smith, A. K., Lee, S. J., Yaffe, K., & Covinsky, K. E. (2019). Assessing risk for adverse outcomes in older adults: The need to include both physical frailty and cognition. *Journal of the American Geriatrics Society, 67*(3), 477–483. https://doi.org/10.1111/jgs.15683

Allen, C. K., Austin, S. L., David, S. K., Earhart, C. A., McCraith, D. B., & Riska-Williams, L. (2007). *Manual for the Allen Cognitive Level Screen-5 (ACLS-5) and Large Allen Cognitive Level Screen-5 (ACLS-5).* ACLS and LACLS Committee.

American Occupational Therapy Association. (2020). *Occupational therapy practice framework: Domain and process* (4th ed.) American Occupational Therapy Association.

American Occupational Therapy Association. (2021). Standards of practice for occupational therapy. *American Journal of Occupational Therapy, 75*(Suppl. 3), 7513410050. https://doi.org/10.5014/ajot.2021.75S3004

Baum, C., Edwards, D., & Morrow-Howell, N. (1993). Identification and measurement of productive behaviors in senile dementia of the Alzheimer's type. *The Gerontologist, 33*(3), 403–408. https://doi.org/10.1093/geront/33.3.403

Baum, C. M., Connor, L. T., Morrison, T., Hahn, M., Dromerick, A. W., & Edwards, D. F. (2008). Reliability, validity, and clinical utility of the Executive Function Performance Test: A measure of executive function in a sample of people with stroke. *The American Journal of Occupational Therapy, 62*(4), 446–455. https://doi.org/10.5014/ajot.62.4.446

Baum, C. M., & Edwards, D. (2008). *Activity Card Sort, 2nd edition (ACS-2). Test manual.* AOTA Press.

Berg, K. O., Wood-Dauphinee, S. L., Williams, J. I., & Maki, B. (1992). Measuring balance in the elderly: Validation of an instrument. *Canadian Journal of Public Health, 83*(Suppl. 2), S7–S11.

Brick, R., Lyons, K. D., Rodakowski, J., & Skidmore, E. (2020). A need to activate lasting engagement. *The American Journal of Occupational Therapy, 74*(5), 7405347010p1–7405347010p5. https://doi.org/10.5014/ajot.2020.039339

Burnett, J., Dyer, C. B., & Naik, A. D. (2009). Convergent validation of the Kohlman Evaluation of Living Skills as a screening tool of older adults' ability to live safely and independently in the community. *Archives of Physical Medicine and Rehabilitation, 90*(11), 1948–1952. https://doi.org/10.1016/j.apmr.2009.05.021

Burns, T., Mortimer, J. A., & Merchak, P. (1994). Cognitive Performance Test: A new approach to functional assessment in Alzheimer's disease. *Journal of Geriatric Psychiatry and Neurology, 7*(1), 46–54.

Butland, R. J., Pang, J., Gross, E. R., Woodcock, A. A., & Geddes, D. M. (1982). Two-, six-, and 12-minute walking tests in respiratory disease. *British Medical Journal (Clinical Research Ed.), 284*(6329), 1607–1608. https://doi.org/10.1136/bmj.284.6329.1607

Canadian Occupational Performance Measure. (2021, April 21). *About the COPM.* https://www.thecopm.ca/about

Chiu, T., Oliver, R., Ascott, P., Choo, L., Davis, T., Gara, A., Goldsilver, P., McWhirter, M., & Letts, L. (2011). *SAFER-HOME manual: Safety Assessment of Function and the Environment for Rehabilitation. Health Outcome Measurement and Evaluation* (4th ed.). VHA Home Healthcare.

Clemmensen, T. H., Kristensen, H. K., Andersen-Ranberg, K., & Lauridsen, H. H. (2021). Development and field-testing of the Dementia Carer Assessment of Support Needs Tool (DeCANT). *International Psychogeriatrics, 33*(4), 405–417. https://doi.org/10.1017/S1041610220001714

Cornelis, E., Gorus, E., Beyer, I., Bautmans, I., & De Vriendt, P. (2017). Early diagnosis of mild cognitive impairment and mild dementia through basic and instrumental activities of daily living: Development of a new evaluation tool. *PLoS Medicine, 14*(3), e1002250. https://doi.org/10.1371/journal.pmed.1002250

Cozzi, S., Martinuzzi, A., & Della Mea, V. (2021). Ontological modeling of the International Classification of Functioning, Disabilities and Health (ICF): Activities and participation and environmental factors components. *BMC Medical Informatics and Decision Making, 21*(1), 367. https://doi.org/10.1186/s12911-021-01729-x

Cuignet, T., Perchoux, C., Caruso, G., Klein, O., Klein, S., Chaix, B., Kestens, Y., & Gerber, P. (2020). Mobility among older adults: Deconstructing the effects of motility and movement on wellbeing. *Urban Studies, 57*(2), 383–401. https://doi.org/10.1177/0042098019852033

Desrosiers, J., Hebert, R., Bravo, G., & Dutil, E. (1995) The Purdue Pegboard Test: Normative data for people aged 60 and over. *Disability and Rehabilitation, 17*(5), 217–224. https://doi.org/10.3109/09638289509166638

Douglas, A. M., Letts, L. J., Richardson, J. A., & Eva, K. W. (2013). Validity of predischarge measures for predicting time to harm in older adults. *Canadian Journal of Occupational Therapy, 80*(1), 19–27. https://doi.org/10.1177/0008417412473577

Federal Interagency Forum on Aging-Related Statistics. (2020, September). *Older Americans 2020: Key indicators of well-being.* U.S. Government

Printing Office. https://agingstats.gov/docs/LatestReport/OA20_508_10142020.pdf

Fillenbaum, G. G. (1985). Screening the elderly: A brief instrumental activities of daily living measure. *Journal of the American Geriatrics Society, 33*(10), 698–706. https://doi.org/10.1111/j.1532-5415.1985.tb01779.x

Fisher, A. G. (1995). *Assessment of motor and process skills*. Third Star Press.

Folstein, M. F., Folstein, S. E., & McHugh, P. R. (1975). "Mini-mental state": A practical method for grading the cognitive state of patients for the clinician. *Journal of Psychiatric Research, 12*(3), 189–198. https://doi.org/10.1016/0022-3956(75)90026-6

Fong, J. H. (2019). Disability incidence and functional decline among older adults with major chronic diseases. *BMC Geriatrics, 19*(323). https://doi.org/10.1186/s12877-019-1348-z

Gage, B., Constantine, R., Aggarwal, J., Morley, M., Kurlantzick, V., Bernard, S., Munevar, D., Garrity, M., Smith, L., Barch, D., Deutsch, A., Mallinson, T., & Ehrlich-Jones, L. (2012). The development and testing of the Continuity Assessment Record and Evaluation (CARE) Item Set, volume 1 of 3. https://hsrc.himmelfarb.gwu.edu/smhs_crl_facpubs/104

Gagnon, C., Mathieu, J., & Desrosiers, J. (2004). Standardized Finger-Nose Test validity for coordination assessment in an ataxic disorder. *Canadian Journal of Neurological Science, 31*(4), 484–489. https://doi.org/10.1017/S031716710000367X

Goverover, Y., Toglia, J., & DeLuca, J. (2020). The weekly calendar planning activity in multiple sclerosis: A top-down assessment of executive functions. *Neuropsychological Rehabilitation, 30*(7), 1372–1387. https://doi.org/10.1080/09602011.2019.1584573

Haley, S. M., Jette, A. M., Coster, W. J., Kooyoomjian, J. T., Levenson, S., Heeren, T., & Ashba, J. (2002). Late Life Function and Disability Instrument: II. Development and evaluation of the function component. *The Journals of Gerontology. Series A, Biological sciences and medical sciences, 57*(4), M217–M222. https://doi.org/10.1093/gerona/57.4.m217

Hebert, R., Carrier, R., & Bilodeau, A. (1988). The Functional Autonomy Measurement System (SMAF): Description and validation of an instrument for the measurement of handicaps. *Age and Ageing, 17*, 293–302. https://doi.org/10.1093/ageing/17.5.293

Holbrook, M., & Skilbeck, C. E. (1983). An activities index for use with stroke patients. *Age and Ageing, 12*(2), 166–170. https://doi.org/10.1093/ageing/12.2.166

Jakobsson, U. (2008). The ADL-staircase: Further validation. *International Journal of Rehabilitation Research, 31*, 85–88. https://doi.org/10.1097/MRR.0b013e3282f45166

Jansen, C. W., Niebuhr, B. R., Coussirat, D. J., Hawthorne, D., Moreno, L., & Phillip, M. (2008). Hand force of men and women over 65 years of age as measured by maximum pinch and grip force. *Journal of aging and physical activity, 16*(1), 24–41. https://doi.org/10.1123/japa.16.1.24

Jebsen, R. H., Taylor, N., Trieschmann, R. B., Trotter, M. J., & Howard, L. A. (1969). An objective and standardized test of hand function. *Archives of Physical Medicine and Rehabilitation, 50*(6), 311–319.

Katz, N., Averbuch, S., & Bar-Haim Erez, A. (2012). Dynamic Lowenstein Occupational Therapy Cognitive Assessment-Geriatric Version (DLOTCA-G): Assessing change in cognitive performance. *The American Journal of Occupational Therapy, 66*(3), 311–319. https://doi.org/10.5014/ajot.2012.002485

Katz, N., Elazar, B., & Itzkovich, M. (1995). Construct validity of a geriatric version of the Loewenstein Occupational Therapy Cognitive Assessment (LOTCA) Battery. *Physical & Occupational Therapy in Geriatrics, 13*(3), 31–46. https://doi.org/10.1080/J148v13n03_03

Katz, S., Downs, T. D., Cash, H. R., & Grotz, R. C. (1970). Progress in development of the index of ADL. *The Gerontologist, 10*, 20–30. https://doi.org/10.1093/geront/10.1_Part_1.20

Kim, M., & Won, C. W. (2019). Sarcopenia is associated with cognitive impairment mainly due to slow gait speed: Results from the Korean Frailty and Aging Cohort Study (KFACS). *International Journal of Environmental Research and Public Health, 16*(9), 1491. https://doi.org/10.3390/ijerph16091491

Klyczek, J. P., Bauer-Yox, N., & Fiedler, R. C. (1997). The interest checklist: A factor analysis. *The American Journal of Occupational Therapy, 51*(10), 815–823. https://doi.org/10.5014/ajot.51.10.815

Knoop, V., Cloots, B., Costenoble, A., Debain, A., Vella Azzopardi, R., Vermeiren, S., Jansen, B., Scafoglieri, A., Bautmans, I., Bautmans, I., & Gerontopole Brussels Study group. (2021). Fatigue and the prediction of negative health outcomes: A systematic review with meta-analysis. *Ageing Research Reviews, 67*, 101261. https://doi.org/10.1016/j.arr.2021.101261

Kramer, P., & Grampurohit, N. (Eds.) (2020). *Hinojosa and Kramer's evaluation in occupational therapy* (5th ed.). American Occupational Therapy Association.

Krupp, L. B., LaRocca, N. G., Muir-Nash, J., & Steinberg, A. D. (1989). The Fatigue Severity Scale: Application to patients with multiple sclerosis and systemic lupus erythematosus. *Archives of Neurology (Chicago), 46*(10), 1121–1123. https://doi.org/10.1001/archneur.1989.00520460115022

Laver-Fawcett, A. L., & Cox, D. L. (2021). *Principles of assessment and outcome measurement for allied health professionals: Practice, research and development*. Wiley-Blackwell.

Law, M., Baptiste, S., Carswell, A., McColl, M. A., Polatajko, H., & Pollock, N. (2014). *The Canadian occupational performance measure* (5th ed.). Canadian Association of Occupational Therapists.

Lawton, M. P., & Brody, E. M. (1969). Assessment of older people: Self-maintaining and instrumental activities of daily living. *The Gerontologist, 9*, 179–186. https://doi.org/10.1093/geront/9.3_part_1.179

Lee, S. D., Stucky, B. D., Lee, J. Y., Rozier, R. G., & Bender, D. E. (2010). Short assessment of health literacy-Spanish and English: A comparable test of health literacy for Spanish and English speakers. *Health Services Research, 45*(4), 1105–1120. https://doi.org/10.1111/j.1475-6773.2010.01119.x

Liebl, M. E., Elmer, N., Schroeder, I., Schwedtke, C., Baack, A., & Reisshauer, A. (2016). Introduction of the Charité Mobility Index (CHARMI) – A novel clinical mobility assessment for acute care rehabilitation. *PloS One, 11*(12), e0169010. https://doi.org/10.1371/journal.pone.0169010

Little, M. O. (2017). The rapid geriatric assessment: A quick screen for geriatric syndromes. *Missouri Medicine, 114*(2), 101–104.

Lundälv, J., Törnbom, M., Larsson, P. O., & Sunnerhagen, K. S. (2015). Awareness and the arguments for and against the International Classification of Functioning, Disability and Health among representatives of disability organisations. *International Journal of Environmental Research and Public Health, 12*(3), 3293–3300. https://doi.org/10.3390/ijerph120303293

Mahoney, S. I., & Barthel, D. W. (1965). Functional evaluation: The Barthel Index. *Maryland State Medical Journal, 14*, 61–65.

Mathiowetz, V., Volland, G., Kashman, N., & Weber, K. (1985). Adult norms for the Box and Block Test of Manual Dexterity. *The American Journal of Occupational Therapy, 39*(6), 386–391. https://doi.org/10.5014/ajot.39.6.386

Mitra, S., & Shakespeare, T. (2019). Remodeling the ICF. *Disability and Health Journal, 12*(3), 337–339. https://doi.org/10.1016/j.dhjo.2019.01.008

Motamed-Jahromi, M., & Kaveh, M. H. (2020). Effective interventions on improving elderly's independence in activity of daily living: A systematic review and logic model. *Frontiers in Public Health, 8*, 516151. https://doi.org/10.3389/fpubh.2020.516151

Nasreddine, Z. S., Phillips, N. A., Bédirian, V., Charbonneau, S., Whitehead, V., Collin, I., Cummings, J. L., & Chertkow, H. (2005). The Montreal Cognitive Assessment, MoCA: A brief screening tool for mild cognitive impairment. *Journal of the American Geriatrics Society, 53*(4), 695–699. https://doi.org/10.1111/j.1532-5415.2005.53221.x

Nelson, D. L., Melville, L. L., Wilkerson, J. D., Magness, R. A., Grech, J. L., & Rosenberg, J. A. (2002). Interrater reliability, concurrent validity, responsiveness and predictive validity of the Melville-Nelson Self-Care Assessment. *The American Journal of Occupational Therapy, 56*(1), 51–59. https://doi.org/10.5014/ajot.56.1.51

Pashmdarfard, M., & Azad, A. (2020). Assessment tools to evaluate activities of daily living (ADL) and instrumental activities of daily living

(IADL) in older adults: A systematic review. *Medical Journal of the Islamic Republic of Iran, 34*(1), 224–239. https://doi.org/10.47176/mjiri.34.33

Podsiadlo, D., & Richardson, S. (1991). The timed "up and go": A test of basic functional mobility. *Journal of the American Geriatrics Society, 39*(2), 142–148. https://doi.org/10.1111/j.1532-5415.1991.tb01616.x

Polatajko, H. J., Townsend, E. A. & Craik, J. (2007). Canadian Model of Occupational Performance and Engagement (CMOP-E). In E. A. Townsend & H. J. Polatajko, (Eds.) *Enabling occupation II: Advancing an occupational therapy vision of health, well-being, & justice through occupation* (pp. 22–23). Canadian Association of Occupational Therapists.

Powell, L. E., & Myers, A. M. (1995). The Activities-specific Balance Confidence (ABC) scale. *The Journals of Gerontology. Series A, Biological Sciences and Medical Sciences, 50A*(1), M28–M34. https://doi.org/10.1093/gerona/50A.1.M28

Rand, D., Lee Ben-Haim, K., Malka, R., & Portnoy, S. (2018). Development of internet-based tasks for the Executive Function Performance Test. *The American Journal of Occupational Therapy, 72*(2), 7202205060p1-7202205060p7. https://doi.org/10.5014/ajot.2018.023598

Roedl, K. J., Wilson, L. S., & Fine, J. (2016). A systematic review and comparison of functional assessments of community-dwelling elderly patients. *Journal of the American Association of Nurse Practitioners, 28*(3), 160–169. https://doi.org/10.1002/2327-6924.12273

Roman-Liu, D., & Tokarski, T. (2021). Age-related differences in bimanual coordination performance. *International Journal of Occupational Safety and Ergonomics, 27*(2), 620–632. https://doi.org/10.1080/10803548.2020.1759296

Shimada, H., Doi, T., Lee, S., Tsutsumimoto, K., Bae, S., Makino, K., Nakakubo, S., & Arai, H. (2022). Identification of disability risk in addition to slow walking speed in older adults. *Gerontology, 68*(6), 625–634. https://doi.org/10.1159/000516966

Smets, E. M., Garssen, B., Bonke, B., & De Haes, J. C. (1995). The Multidimensional Fatigue Inventory (MFI) psychometric qualities of an instrument to assess fatigue. *Journal of Psychosomatic Research, 39*(3), 315–325. https://doi.org/10.1016/0022-3999(94)00125-O

Smith, R. (1994). Validation and reliability of the Elderly Mobility Scale. *Physiotherapy, 80*(11), 744–747. https://doi.org/10.1016/S0031-9406(10)60612-8

Statistics Canada. (2017). *Disability rate for both sexes in Canada by age groups* [Infographic]. https://www150.statcan.gc.ca/n1/pub/71-607-x/71-607-x2019035-eng.htm#data

Stratford, P., Gill, C., Westaway, M., & Binkley, J. (1995). Assessing disability and change on individual patients: A report of a patient specific measure. *Physiotherapy Canada, 47*(4), 258–263. https://doi.org/10.3138/ptc.47.4.258

Son, S. M., Dwon, J. W., Nam, S. H., Lee, N. K., Kim, K., & Kim, C. S. (2012). Adverse effects of motor-related symptoms on the ipsilateral upper limb according to long-term cane usage. *Neurorehabilitation, 31*(2), 137–141. https://doi.org/10.3233/NRE-2012-0782

Sumsion, T. (2000). A revised occupational therapy definition of client-centred practice. *British Journal of Occupational Therapy, 63*, 304–309. http://doi.org.10.1177/030802260006300702

Taylor, R. R. (2017). Kielhofner's Model of Human Occupation: Theory and Application, 5th ed. Wolters Kluwer.

Tiffin, J., & Asher, E. J. (1948). The Purdue pegboard; norms and studies of reliability and validity. *The Journal of Applied Psychology, 32*(3), 234–247. https://doi.org/10.1037/h0061266

Tinetti, M. E. (1986). Performance-oriented assessment of mobility problems in elderly patients. *Journal of the American Geriatrics Society, 34*(2), 119–126. https://doi.org/10.1111/j.1532-5415.1986.tb05480.x

Toglia, J. (2015). *Weekly Calendar Planning Activity (WCPA): A performance test for executive function*. American Occupational Therapy Association Press.

Toglia, J., & Cermak, S. A. (2009). Dynamic assessment and prediction of learning potential in clients with unilateral neglect. *The American Journal of Occupational Therapy, 63*(5), 569–579. https://doi.org/10.5014/ajot.63.5.569

Tournadre, A., Vial, G., Capel, F., Soubrier, M., & Boirie, Y. (2019). Sarcopenia. *Joint Bone Spine, 86*(3), 309–314. https://doi.org/10.1016/j.jbspin.2018.08.001

Turcotte, P., Carrier, A., Roy, V., & Levasseur, M. (2018). Occupational therapists' contributions to fostering older adults' social participation: A scoping review. *British Journal of Occupational Therapy, 81*(8), 427–449. https://doi.org/10.1177/0308022617752067

Unsworth, C. A., Baker, A., Taitz, C., Chan, S. P., Pallant, J. F., Russell, K. J., & Odell, M. (2011). *OT-DORA: Occupational therapy driving off-road assessment*. AOTA Press.

Wales, K., Clemson, L., Lannin, N., & Cameron, I. (2016). Functional assessments used by occupational therapists with older adults at risk of activity and participation limitations: A systematic review. *PLOS One, 11*(2), e0147980. https://doi.org/10.1371/journal.pone.0147980

Wang, C., Patriquin, M., Vaziri, A., & Najafi, B. (2021). Mobility performance in community-dwelling older adults: Potential digital biomarkers of concern about falling. *Gerontology, 67*(3), 365–373. https://doi.org/10.1159/000512977

Washburn, R. A., Smith, K. W., Jette, A. M., & Janney, C. A. (1993). The Physical Activity Scale for the Elderly (PASE): Development and evaluation. *Journal of Clinical Epidemiology, 46*(2), 153–162. https://doi.org/10.1016/0895-4356(93)90053-4

Wilson, B., Cockburn, J., Baddeley, A., & Hiorns, R. (1989). The development and validation of a test battery for detecting and monitoring everyday memory problems. *Journal of Clinical and Experimental Neuropsychology, 11*(6), 855–870. https://doi.org/10.1080/01688638908400940

Wolf, S. L., Catlin, P. A., Ellis, M., Archer, A. L., Morgan, B., & Piacentino, A. (2001). Assessing Wolf motor function test as outcome measure for research in patients after stroke. *Stroke, 32*(7), 1635–1639. https://doi.org/10.1161/01.str.32.7.1635

World Health Organization (2001). International classification of functioning, disability and health (ICF). Geneva: Author.

CHAPTER 22

Wellness and Community-Based Services

Kristin Bray Jones, MS, OTD, OTR/L
Jeanine Stancanelli, OTD, OTR/L, MPH
Noralyn D. Pickens, PhD, OT, FAOTA

"To keep the body in good health is a duty, otherwise we shall not be able to keep our mind strong and clear."

— *Buddha*

LEARNING OUTCOMES

By the end of this chapter, readers will be able to:

22-1. Appraise wellness services to support older adults' engagement in occupation.
22-2. Determine the value of different community-based services to older adults.
22-3. Discuss the role of interprofessional community agency partners.
22-4. Articulate how older adults with health issues gain value from community participation.
22-5. Create interventions to address older adult health and wellness needs.
22-6. Document wellness and community-based services to support service reimbursement.
22-7. Advocate for occupation-based community programming.

Mini Case Study

Fred is a 75-year-old man who is a resident of a senior living community in a first-ring suburb of a midsized city. He has a history of type 2 diabetes, congestive heart failure (CHF), hypertension, and neuropathy. He has been widowed for 5 years and moved to the senior community 2 years ago. Fred feels that he used to have more control over his various health conditions, especially when his wife was able to help him with health management. She used to be his main source of transportation around the community, as he was having difficulty driving due to the neuropathy in his hands and feet. She also played a vital role in helping Fred with various instrumental activities of daily living (IADLs) and took care of the household chores that required larger amounts of energy. Fred recalls fondly that once they both retired, he enjoyed spending time with her in the kitchen while she showed him how to prepare healthier meals in order to prevent exacerbation of his conditions. Fred feels that his wife was his greatest accountability to practice health and wellness. After she passed away, he felt lost and ill-equipped to manage his chronic health needs. He notes how he slowed down physically since his wife passed away, as he had decreased motivation to participate in his favorite activities due to low energy. He remained in their home by himself for a few years before he made the tough decision to move into a community living environment and sell their house.

Provocative Questions

1. What community resources would be relevant to supporting Fred's health and wellness?
2. What theoretical models would support your intervention approaches?
3. What interventions would target Fred's medical, social, and emotional needs?

Globally, there is increasing interest in health and well-being to promote healthy aging for older adults (Wilson et al, 2021). This chapter defines health and wellness; relevant factors that support positive health and wellness outcomes, including environmental influences; evidence-based programs that support health and wellness; and roles and emerging opportunities for occupational therapy practitioners on interprofessional and interdisciplinary teams. Many older adults are choosing to age in place; thus, the focus of healthcare is moving toward community-based practice. For therapists who wish to serve the healthy older adult population, it is essential that they have familiarity with both disciplinary and interdisciplinary concepts of health promotion, wellness, community practice, and research. This chapter will discuss wellness service in the context of community-based services. Topics include how occupational therapists partner with community service providers to address the health, wellness, and social needs of older adults. Additionally, there is discussion of how services are reimbursed and how to advocate for occupation-centered programming in the community.

Community-Based Wellness Services

Wellness in Older Adults

The Global Wellness Institute (GWI) defines **wellness** as the active pursuit of activities, choices, and lifestyles that lead to a state of holistic health (GWI, n.d.). There are various models of wellness, but most include interconnected dimensions that coordinate to support the active process of wellness. For example, in its model of wellness, the International Council on Active Aging (ICAA) identifies seven dimensions of wellness: emotional, environmental, intellectual, physical, social, spiritual, and vocational (ICAA, n.d.). The goal of wellness is the state of holistic health, which means that wellness is focused on the prevention of disease and promotion of lifestyles that support the health of the entire person.

Although related, health and well-being are different from wellness. For decades, the World Health Organization (WHO) has defined **health** as "a state of complete physical, mental and social well-being and not merely the absence of disease or infirmity" (WHO, 2023, para 1). Further, the WHO defines well-being as "a positive state experienced by individuals and societies. Similar to health, it is a resource for daily life and is determined by social, economic, and environmental conditions" (WHO, 2021, p. 10). The American Occupational Therapy Association (AOTA) expands the definition of well-being to include a person's satisfaction with their participation in occupations (AOTA, 2020a). Thus, both health and well-being describe states of being that humans experience. Unlike a state of being, wellness is an active process of choosing opportunities that ultimately promote both health and well-being. For a graphical representation of the relationship between wellness, health, and well-being, see Figure 22-1.

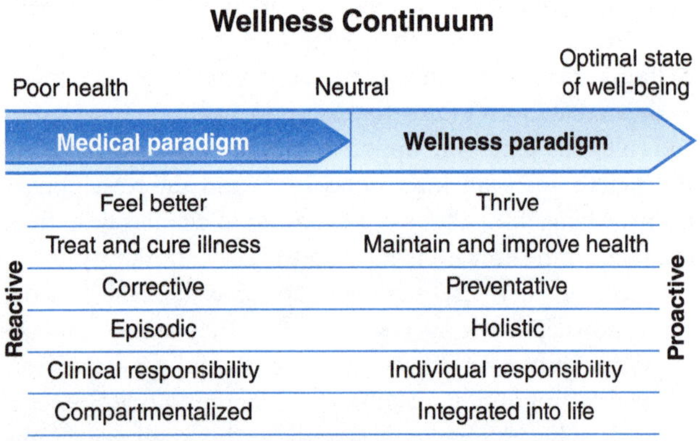

Wellness Continuum

Poor health	Neutral	Optimal state of well-being
Medical paradigm		Wellness paradigm
Feel better		Thrive
Treat and cure illness		Maintain and improve health
Corrective		Preventative
Episodic		Holistic
Clinical responsibility		Individual responsibility
Compartmentalized		Integrated into life

Reactive ← → Proactive

Source: Global Wellness Institute, adapted from Dr. Jack Travis

*The continuum concept is adapted from Dr. Jack Travis' Illness-Wellness Continuum. Travis is one of the pioneers of the modern wellness movement in the late 1970s.

Note: with permission from https://globalwellnessinstitute.org/what-is-wellness/

FIGURE 22-1 Wellness to Well-being Continuum. *(Reproduced with permission from https://globalwellnessinstitute.org/what-is-wellness/)*

Healthy Aging

The concept of healthy aging applies the process of wellness to older adults. The WHO defines healthy aging as "the process of developing and maintaining the functional ability that enables wellbeing in older age" (WHO, 2020, p. xv). Functional ability is multifaceted and includes meeting one's basic needs: learning, growing, and making decisions; being mobile; building and maintaining relationships; and contributing to society (WHO, 2020). In occupational therapy-specific terms, healthy aging is the ability of older adults to engage in occupations to which they attach value (Clemson, 2022). Thus, older adults who engage in healthy aging are actively pursuing occupational engagement and participation to promote their health and well-being.

Community-Based Wellness Services

Community-based wellness programs are designed to support healthy aging by helping older adults access necessary supports and services. A major focus of community-based wellness programs is keeping older adults living safely and independently in their homes and communities (Government of Canada, 2023). Community-based wellness programs are supported to varying degrees by national and local governments and include programs such as chronic condition management, health education, nutritional support, physical and social activities, and home safety support.

Community-based wellness services take place in a variety of community settings. Community settings include township-run senior centers, adult day centers, and Programs for All-Inclusive Care for the Elderly (PACE) centers. Each of these centers will be explained in more detail later. Other community settings that offer wellness services for older adults include local community centers, private community centers (e.g., Jewish Community Centers, YMCAs), houses of worship, universities, and fitness gyms.

With the COVID-19 pandemic, an older adult's home became a common setting for engaging in community-based wellness services. Due to the closure of many community settings, wellness services were offered through virtual, online platforms (e.g., videoconference applications, phone calls) (National Council on Aging [NCOA], 2023). As community settings reopened after the pandemic, many wellness services continued to provide online options for older adults still needing to quarantine. Thus, it is common for an older adult to choose to engage in virtual community-based services in their own home.

Senior Centers

Senior centers are the most common setting for community-based wellness services. Identified by the U.S. Older Americans Act as a community focal point, more than 10,000 senior centers serve more than one million older adults daily in the United States (NCOA, 2022). The typical participant is a 75-year-old white woman who lives alone. Compared with her peers, she is likely to have lower income but enjoys better health, greater life satisfaction, and more social contacts. She usually visits the center one to three times weekly for about 3 hours per visit (NCOA, 2022). This profile of the typical U.S. senior center participant suggests that senior centers in the United Sates may not be adequately including all persons who may benefit from wellness services, including persons of color and persons younger or older than age 70 (Kadowaki & Mahmood, 2018). There are opportunities to design programs to increase inclusion and diversity within senior centers (Pardasani & Berkman, 2021), such as ensuring senior centers have programming to welcome older adults who are monolingual non-English speakers (Lavalley, 2023) or members of LGBTQIA+ communities (Marmo et al, 2021). (See Promoting Best Practice 22-1 and 22-2 on initiatives focused on wellness in LGBTQIA+ communities and Indigenous Americans.) Outside of the United States, many countries, including Canada, Chile, China, Poland, and South Korea, use the senior center model as a method for engaging community-dwelling older adults in activities to promote wellness (Glasinovic et al, 2022; Kadowaki & Mahmood, 2018; Kim & Seo, 2022; Liu et al, 2017; Ogonowska-Slodownick et al, 2022).

PROMOTING BEST PRACTICE 22-1
LGBTQ+ Aging

SAGE is the oldest and largest organization in the United States dedicated to improving the lives of lesbian, gay, bisexual, transgender, queer, and questioning (LGBTQ+) older adults. This award-winning agency was founded in 1978 in New York City, where it continues to be headquartered, and has expanded nationwide. It provides a variety of services and programs, including social services, employment assistance, caregiver support, health and wellness, lifelong education, and arts and culture. Moreover, SAGE facilitates the National Resource Center on LGBTQ+ Aging and the Global LGBTQ+ Aging Network.

PROMOTING BEST PRACTICE 22-2
Indigenous Americans

For older adults in indigenous communities, culturally safe health and wellness programs are perceived as more appropriate and beneficial (Quigley et al, 2022). The National Indian Council on Aging (NICOA) developed NICOA Compass: A Guide to Native Wellness (NICOA, 2023), a resource for culturally informed health and wellness services for older adults in indigenous communities. These wellness services are tailored to indigenous cultures and focus on wellness interventions such as nutrition, fall prevention, brain health, home modification, and healthy aging. NICOA Compass also provides guidance for tribal leaders on how to fit the available services into their communities. (See https://nicoacompass.org/ for more information.)

Senior centers are a hub for a wide variety of community-based programs. The core of many senior center programs is congregate meals (e.g., nutritional meals provided in group settings). The Older Americans Act, which authorizes funding to many senior centers, mandates that the funded services target older adults with economic and social needs (Uivari et al, 2019). Congregate meals address both needs. Additional programs include those focusing on health and fitness, recreation, education, volunteering, and social services (NCOA, 2022). Education programs may include classes on technology, languages, or leisure activities. Recreation programming may include group field trips or excursions. Social service programing may include counseling, information and referral, employment services, legal assistance, friendly visiting, telephone reassurance, transportation, health screening, and outreach. More details on congregate meals and examples of wellness programs provided at senior centers will be discussed later in this chapter.

Senior centers are a social hub for older adults. For many older adults, they provide opportunities for socialization, which results in a sense of connectedness and psychological well-being (Kim & Seo, 2022; Pardasani & Berkman, 2021). In addition to socialization being a byproduct of senior center participation, social bonds are also a predictor of senior center engagement. Having friends at the senior center increases a person's probability of engaging in congregate meals, field trips, fitness classes, games, arts and crafts, and volunteer programs (Keyes et al, 2022).

Despite being a focal point of community-based wellness services and socialization, participation at senior centers has been declining for many years in the United States (Pardasani, 2019). The stigma of ageism may dissuade some older adults from participating (Pardasani & Berkman, 2021). For example, younger older adults have the perception that senior centers are for the very old, thus decreasing their interest in participating in senior centers (Kadowaki & Mahmood, 2018). Decreased involvement may also be due to health problems and lack of transportation (Pardasani, 2019). Older adults may also feel that they are too busy with their current social or leisure activities or that they do not need or want socialization. Lastly, the hours of operation (which are generally morning to late afternoon) may not be conducive to the schedules of working older adults (Pardasani & Berkman, 2021). See Box 22-1 for innovations that are transforming senior centers into more inviting destinations.

Adult Day Centers

Adult day centers are settings for health and wellness services for older adults who need supervised care during the day but do not require institutionalized 24-hour care (as found in nursing homes or long-term care settings). Adult day centers may prevent some older adults from being institutionalized (HelpGuide.org 2023). There are approximately 4,127 adult day centers in the United States, serving 237,400 participants (National Center for Health Statistics, 2022). In the United States, approximately 60% of adult day services are paid for through national and state Medicaid funds, with

> **BOX 22-1** **Senior Center Innovations**
>
> Innovations of the traditional senior center are on the rise. Vivalon, a senior services organization in Marin County, California, is combining affordable senior housing with a state-of-the-art senior center. This combination ensures that older adults are living in an environment that supports social connection, healthy aging, and wellness services with affordable housing (https://www.healthyagingcampus.org/).
>
> Wallis Annenberg GenSpace (https://www.annenberggenspace.org/) is a reimagination of the typical senior center. GenSpace creators were inspired by describing life as the development of new stages instead of focusing on ages and aging and designed a space that reflects growth instead of decline.

approximately 45% of adult day services being for-profit ventures (Rome et al, 2020). An adult care center has an average capacity of approximately 65 participants and an average daily attendance of 42 (Rome et al, 2020). Adult day centers operate during typical business hours 5 days a week, with some programs offering services in the evenings and on weekends (HelpGuide.org, 2023). The typical adult day center participant is a nonwhite female over 65 years of age with Medicaid benefits who needs assistance with bathing, dressing, and walking, with greater than one chronic condition (National Center for Health Statistics, 2018). Outside of the United States, many countries, including Australia, Canada, Iran, Netherlands, and Portugal, use adult day centers to provide supervised care to older adults with chronic conditions (Australian Health Directory, n.d.; Carlsson et al, 2022; Hedayati et al, 2019; HelpGuide.org, 2023).

Adult day centers offer different types of programming, depending on the older adult participants. The typical services offered in most senior day centers include socialization activities, meals and snacks, personal care assistance, physical and mental activities, and transportation to and from the center. Approximately 50% of centers offer occupational, physical, or speech therapy, with 80% staffing a nursing professional. Typically, centers will offer cognitive stimulation or memory-training programs. Most centers also offer services to support caregivers, which may include educational programs, caregiver support groups, and individual counseling (National Adult Day Services Association, 2023).

To guide programming, U.S. adult day centers focus on one or more of the following service models:

- Medical/health: emphasizing rehabilitative and health services as well as social activities
- Social: emphasizing recreation, meals, and some health-related services
- Specialized: targeting interventions and services for older adults with specific problems such as dementia or developmental disabilities

PACE Centers

PACE centers are comprehensive, full-service healthcare and social service programs in which all care is coordinated, organized, and delivered by the program (Centers for Medicare & Medicaid Services, n.d.). PACE centers house these programs. Older adults registered in a PACE program receive primary and specialized medical care to support their health, wellness, and healthy aging in the community. In addition to medical care, PACE services may include occupational and physical therapy, nutrition, recreational and socialization activities, and coordination of home care and transportation. PACE programs receive fixed monthly payments from Medicare, Medicaid, and private payers (for program participants who are not dually eligible). Each PACE program pools the funds and then delivers care to individuals according to an individual's needs. One of the benefits of involvement in a central health care program like PACE is less duplication or unnecessary services. Additionally, because community services are generally more cost effective, the organization is motivated to provide services in the community, which is typically the preference for most older adults.

Contexts of Community-Based Wellness Services

Context is a concept that describes the environmental and personal factors that affect a person's engagement and performance of occupations (AOTA, 2020b). Environmental factors encompass the physical, social, and attitudinal circumstances of a person's life. Personal factors are unique elements of a person (e.g., age, habits, cultural identification) exclusive of any health condition. Thus, how an older adult engages in community wellness programs will be affected by physical, social, and attitudinal factors of the program and their own personal factors. Occupational therapists should understand and consider both environmental and personal factors and discuss them with their older adult clients before referring to wellness programs. This consideration will ensure that the wellness services an occupational therapy practitioner suggests for the client will be a good fit for the client and enable the client to take advantage of the program's benefits.

Though not an exhaustive list, these are some of the key contexts and questions to consider when working with older adult clients:

- Human-made or natural environments: Are the environments in which the wellness services take place acceptable to the older adult? Are they concerned about getting to the location or moving within the location? For example, is the older adult comfortable engaging in wellness services taking place on the grass in a local park?
- Virtual environments: Do the wellness services rely on virtual technology or applications like smartphones or teleconferencing applications? Does the older adult have the necessary technology? Is the older adult comfortable with using the needed applications?
- Relationships: Are the wellness services in a group or individual setting? Often wellness services have a socialization

component; thus many services occur in group settings. Does the older adult have the interest and skills to be with people they may not know? Does the older adult want to attend with a friend?
- Attitudes: There are wellness services that are geared toward groups with shared cultural values or norms. Is the older adult comfortable with those cultural values or norms? For example, is the older adult comfortable engaging in wellness services taking place in a house of worship?

Service Utilization

Service Barriers

Service barriers inhibit an older adult's use of or access to community-based wellness programs. Research suggests there are four levels of service barriers (Biegel et al, 1995; Lopez et al, 2021; Sicolnofi et al, 2019; Stephan et al, 2018):

- System-level barriers are political, economic, and social forces that influence policy development. System-level barriers can include availability of government funding for services, complex or rigid regulations for accessing services, services concentrated in urban or high-income locations, disjointed coordination between in-patient and community-based services, and lack of communication of available services to older adults who need them.
- Agency-level barriers are structures, staffing, funding, and procedures within organizations that affect service delivery to older adults. Agency-level barriers include difficulty recruiting and retaining service providers, large and unmanageable caseloads, lack of coordination of agency services, and service providers with decreased knowledge or competency.
- Social-level barriers are social determinants of health that affect service delivery to older adults. Social-level barriers include internet and phone connectivity, transportation options and availability, and belonging to underserved or under resourced groups. For example, Black Americans with multiple sclerosis have been less likely to receive community-based services than their white counterparts (Fabius et al, 2018). Older adults belonging to LGBTQIA+ communities struggle to have equal access to community-based services (AARP, 2020).
- Individual-level barriers are personal attitudes toward or behaviors around service delivery for older adults. Individual-level barriers include a person's perception that community-based services are "welfare" or "charity," discomfort with group recreational activities because of shyness or fear of strangers, the belief that they do not need help, the belief that help should only come from family, and lack of personal advocate or key contact person to navigate care needs. In addition, having no friends to engage in community-based services is also a barrier (Keyes et al, 2022).

Connecting Older Adults With Services

Most communities have a variety of services for older adults. Unfortunately, as discussed earlier, a common barrier to services is a lack of knowledge of what services exist and how to access the existing services. Many countries have identified this barrier and created initiatives to address it. These initiatives entail designing methods to link older adults and their caregivers with the knowledge of and access to existent services. In 2003, the U.S. Administration on Aging (AOA) and the Centers for Medicare & Medicaid Services launched the Aging and Disability Resource Center (ADRC) initiative to help states develop a system of "one-stop shop" programs at the community level. ADRCs are designed to offer people of all ages and all abilities information, assistance, and access, particularly around the maze of fragmented long-term care options, so that they can make informed service decisions. Older Americans Act legislation in 2006 required the establishment of ADRCs in all states. Now, most states have designated area agencies on aging as the lead organization for local ADRC development, partnering with other agencies to carry out ADRC functions. The AOA hosts a website where adults can find an ADRC near their home (AOA, n.d.). Similar to ADRCs in the United States, communities in Finland have developed staffed service markets, which are central places for older adults and their carers to get help and advice (Finland Ministry of Foreign Affairs, n.d.). In Canada, anyone looking for services for older adults can call a country-wide helpline by dialing 211 (CORE Canada, 2022). For a list of ways older adults can connect with services, see Table 22-1.

CASE STUDY

Mr. Uzoma Otieno from chapter 9 in the context of community-based care

Presenting Situation

In Chapter 9, you were introduced to Uzoma Otieno. You will recall he is a married 63-year-old African American male with cardiovascular dysfunction. His health has discouraged him somewhat, and his primary care nurse practitioner would like him to engage in more regular social and physical activity.

Occupational Profile

Mr. and Mrs. Otieno had a local contractor make minor modifications to their bathroom, including adding grab bars at the toilet and shower stall. They also added a small shower bench that can be folded aside when not needed. After cardio-rehab, Mr. Otieno continued with daily walks around his block, but with seasonal winter weather coming on soon, is worried about falling on the sidewalk. One of his neighbors and a close friend recently moved to be closer to his children, leaving a void in daily conversational routine. Mrs. Otieno has tried to follow the hospital nutritionist's recommendations for meal preparation but finds the menus dull.

Assessment

An occupational therapist contracts with their local senior center and is asked by the director to meet with Mr. and Mrs. Otieno. The occupational therapist completes an occupational profile on them as a couple, with specific focus on Mr. Otieno's recent cardiovascular history.

Questions

1. What model would support the occupational therapist's approach to Mr. Otieno's care?
2. What additional information would the occupational therapist want to gather to develop an intervention plan?

Answers

1. The Health Belief Model would be useful in assessing and developing a plan to address Mr. and Mrs. Otieno's actions in making healthy changes to their lifestyles, including meals and exercise. By addressing their perceptions of the importance of health interventions, barriers to change, and the value of the interventions, the occupational therapist can target education and activities of health promotion. [LO 22-5; Models to guide intervention section]
2. The occupational therapist will want to know more about the Otienos' former meal planning and how their cultural identity influences their food choices. The occupational therapist will use this information to locate a trained dietitian who would help them develop culturally tailored medical menus. The occupational therapist will want to know about the Otienos' interests in different activities, possibly performing an interest checklist. Additionally, the occupational therapist will want to explore if Mr. Otieno is interested in partnering with the center's fitness center coordinator to help develop an individual or group exercise program. [LO 22-2, 22-5; Interprofessional partners and Intervention sections]

Role of Occupational Therapy and Interprofessional Partners

Occupational Therapy as Direct Care

Within communities, occupational therapists offer direct care wellness services to older adults. Direct care means that occupational therapists provide wellness services through personal contact either in person or virtually. Globally, occupational therapists who provide community-based wellness services work for a variety of different entities. It is common for occupational therapists providing community-based wellness services to work in private practice because private practice is inherently community based. Alternatively, occupational therapists may work for community-based health centers (e.g., mental health centers, senior health centers), local wellness organizations, healthy aging organizations, primary care clinics (see Chapter 23), or medical centers that run health initiatives within a community (e.g., healthy aging clinics, breast cancer survivor groups) (Healthy Aging Association, n.d.; Lee et al, 2022; Petruseviciene et al, 2018; Scaffa, 2020). Occupational therapists may supervise occupational therapy students in community-based wellness programs for local older adults in on-campus clinics run through occupational therapy education programs (Patch, 2023).

Occupational therapists providing direct wellness care to older adults will emphasize sustaining and enhancing occupational performance and participation in the performance areas that are most valued by the client. Occupational therapists can undertake the kind of comprehensive review of occupational performance that identifies areas of current or potential functional problems and can assist in developing strategies for sustaining performance for the longest possible period.

Some general guiding principles for occupational therapy wellness interventions include:

- Evaluation of home and community safety and identification of services or resources to support occupational performance and enable older adults to remain in the community if they desire

TABLE 22-1 Connecting Older Adults and Their Carers to Community-Based Wellness Services

RESOURCE	DESCRIPTION
Case managers	Professional case manager assigned to an older adult's case who is responsible for coordinating access to and funding of needed services. Case managers may be a variety of professionals, including nurses and occupational therapists.
Service markets (e.g., aging and disability resource centers)	Resource centers that are usually run by local area aging agencies. These are "one-stop shops" that inform older adults and their carers about the availability and accessibility of wellness services.
Senior centers	Provide lists of services available and often staffed with someone to answer questions.
Community education programs	Lectures, workshops, demonstrations, and fairs highlighting available services are hosted by local health and social service organizations, communities, universities, and local media outlets.
Information phone lines or websites	Dedicated phone lines or websites that provide older adults and their carers with information about available services.

- Education on performing occupations safely, adapting them as needed for the older adult to maintain self-care activities and other valuable occupations in their home and community if they desire, including home modifications, which are discussed in Chapter 15
- Introduction or identification of new meaningful occupations when their capacity is reduced or diminished
- Development or enhancement of socialization and leisure interests

Community-based occupational therapists may also help older adults navigate the array of older-adult-focused services. Service coordination can be a particular challenge in community settings. There is a wide array of available services, but older adults are frequently confused by the lack of coordination. There are overlapping services with similar missions, and many older adults are unfamiliar with some or all of the services. Occupational therapists, in addition to other healthcare professionals, can work as case managers to help older adults identify and coordinate the most valuable services for them given their interests and occupational strengths and limitations. Some older adults may benefit from a referral to a social worker, often through the local area agency on aging (Elliott, 2019).

Occupational Therapy as Indirect Care

Occupational therapists support community-based wellness for older adults through indirect care. Indirect care means that an occupational therapist may design or plan wellness programs but not directly administer the program to clients themselves. Rather, other professionals or support workers would administer the occupational therapy-designed wellness program. As population health grows as a focus area of occupational therapy services, addressing function in community has become a greater priority within the profession (Domholdt et al, 2020). For example, an occupational therapist may collaborate with a local aging agency to develop fall prevention programs (Elliott, 2019) or design life skills groups for intergenerational residential homes (Grohman et al, 2022). On a larger scale, occupational therapists may work in administrative roles (e.g., wellness director) at large healthcare organizations or aging agencies and be responsible for wide-reaching wellness programs or initiatives.

Indirect care also includes caregiver training. Occupational therapists are uniquely qualified to train caregivers to safely and therapeutically support an older adult's occupational performance. The training can be individual, one-on-one training, or occupational therapists may run large corporate training programs (e.g., https://www.hscaregivertraining.com). Occupational therapists are qualified to engage in community-level wellness programming. The World Federation of Occupational Therapists (WFOT, 2019) supports occupational therapists' provision of services to whole communities, focusing on eliminating barriers to community-level health, participation, and well-being. In the United States, the American Alliance of Museums has a creative aging initiative that addresses ageism through changing museum operations, including programming and accessibility (2023). Globally, the United Nations Decade of Healthy Ageing (2022) supports the initiative of age-ready cities in which cities become more adaptive and inclusive to the needs and contributions of their aging citizens. For both of these initiatives, occupational therapists may serve as leaders to identify, advocate for, and address the wellness needs of older adults through the development of building infrastructure and community-wide programming.

Interprofessional Partners

Community-based wellness services may be offered through various organizations and administered by different professionals. Occupational therapists working in the community need to understand the different services and the professionals who organize them. They will use this knowledge to build professional relationships that allow for partnerships and will ultimately facilitate efficient referrals for their older adult clients.

Professionals with whom occupational therapists may connect include:

- Administrators are the coordinators and directors of facilities like senior centers or senior day centers or community associations. They may also serve as a preliminary contact for referrals.
- Community workers may work at senior centers, adult day centers, or other community associations and administer wellness programs.
- Medical professionals, such as physicians, nurses, nutritionists and dietitians, and exercise or personal trainers manage older adults' chronic conditions, providing medical interventions and education as needed.
- Case managers assist with the arrangement and coordination of services for an older adult. They can coordinate a transition from hospitalization back home and communication between different medical professionals and caregivers and navigate insurance funding, to name a few.
- Social workers may coordinate services and act as a case manager and may be licensed to provide therapy services.

Specific Issues for Promoting Wellness of Older Adults in Community-Based Settings

Occupational therapists working with community-dwelling older adults need to be aware of unique factors that affect their health and wellness. Several of the factors reviewed here include social determinants of health and the social and community context.

Social Determinants of Health

Social determinants of health can provide insight into factors that may be supports or barriers to promoting wellness in older adults. These factors include economic stability, education access and quality, healthcare access and quality, neighborhood and built environment, and social and community context (U.S. Department of Health and Human Services, 2020). This section identifies specific aspects of social determinants of health that occupational therapists should pay particular attention to when working in community-based services. Refer to Chapter 1 for an in-depth description of social determinants of health.

Economic Stability

An older adult's economic stability affects their access to wellness and wellness services. Though usually discounted, many community-based wellness programs are fee based. Limited income may affect the amount or frequency with which an older adult engages in their preferred wellness programs. Limited income may affect their ability to pay for a wide variety of wellness supports, including nutritious food, transportation, and home modifications. Overall limited income is a barrier to occupational engagement for community-living older adults (Koh et al, 2022).

Access to Built Environments

The home environment may include a variety of assets or barriers to health and wellness for older adults. Functional limitations inherent with advanced age may lead to accessibility issues within the home (Norin et al, 2021). Solving these issues is important, because having an accessible home supports occupational performance in older adults (Nielsen et al, 2019). Refer to Chapter 15 for in-depth information on home modifications to improve accessibility.

A study of 326 community dwelling residents by Vitorino and colleagues (2019) identified access to information as an important aspect of the physical environment. Smart-home technology and information communications technologies have been developed to support aging in place and safety in the home. These technologies show potential to support health, wellness, social engagement, and daily functioning at home as one ages in place (Orlofsky & Wozniak, 2022). (See Chapter 29 for more information about advances in smart-home technologies.)

Accessibility to community buildings and outdoor spaces provides older adults with opportunities to engage in wellness options outside of their homes. Neighborhood terrain like hills, cobblestones, or uneven sidewalks can make venturing out of the house risky for some older adults. Likewise, community buildings with narrow or dark hallways, lack of places to sit, or stairs can make older adults avoid buildings in their community. Unless accessibility issues are identified and addressed, older adults who feel they are at risk of injury may eliminate some or all trips outside of the home, which could lead to decreased social participation (Townsend et al, 2021).

Loneliness and Social Isolation

Healthy aging involves the ability to build and maintain relationships with other people (WHO, 2020). The ability to maintain social connectedness as one ages can be especially challenging due to the death of friends and family and the onset of health issues. Conversely, social isolation and loneliness have been found to have a negative association with health (e.g., cardiac conditions) and well-being (Ferreira et al, 2021; Wilson et al, 2021). Social isolation may also result in greater reliance on and cost of health services (Shaw et al, 2017; Wilson et al, 2021.

Health Factors

An older adult's health can have a significant impact on their wellness. As a reminder, wellness is connected to health but is defined as active pursuit of activities, choices, and lifestyles that lead to a state of holistic health. This section explores specific health factors that can affect an older adult's pursuit of wellness.

Nutrition and Hydration

Nutrition and hydration are health factors that affect wellness in older adults. Age-related changes in senses may lead to changes in ability to taste and smell food, resulting in a reduced appetite and related reduction in food consumption. There are also age-related changes in the gastrointestinal system and dentation that may affect one's desire to eat (Calder et al, 2018). Older adults also experience reduced thirst in response to dehydration (Begg, 2017), which may be why they are less likely to meet water intake recommendations (Hooper, 2016). These changes can result in malnutrition and dehydration, which can affect normal growth and development, preservation of health, healing, and recovery from illness. In addition, dehydration is associated with decreased attention and cognitive processing speed in older female adults (Bethancourt et al, 2020). The Academy of Nutrition and Dietetics (www.eatright.org) has nutrition, hydration, and healthy eating recommendations for a variety of populations, including older adults. See Chapter 7 for more information about nutrition and hydration.

Cognitive Reserve

Cognitive reserve is a health factor that affects wellness in older adults. Cognitive reserve describes the brain's ability to optimize performance by recruiting brain networks or using alternative cognitive strategies to cope with brain dysfunctions, thereby compensating for neural loss (Alvares Pereira et al, 2022). Both innate factors and life experiences can affect cognitive reserve and the brain's ability to compensate.

Cognitive reserve is integral to support independent or community-based living. Conversely, declining cognition is a barrier to occupational engagement for older adults (Koh et al, 2022). The Lancet Commission found that cognitive decline could be prevented or delayed through reduction of modifiable risk factors (Alvares Pereira et al, 2022). For example, engagement in occupational and leisure activities, especially those associated with social interaction, appears to have a protective effect on cognitive decline (Alvares Pereira et al, 2022). For more information on cognition in older adults, see Chapter 13.

Physical Activity

Physical activity promotes positive health and wellness outcomes for older adults. Physical activity, which encompasses exercise and occupational engagement, has been shown to lower older adults' risk for cardiovascular diseases, diabetes mellitus, some cancers, weight gain, falls, depression, and cognitive decline (Calatayud et al, 2022; Collins et al, 2021). In addition to the health benefits, the wellness benefits of engaging in occupations include social connectedness (Collins et al, 2021) and productivity (Thoma et al, 2021). Results from a systematic review of 83 studies found reduced activities of daily living (ADLs) and IADLs could be predicted by low muscle mass and strength, decreased grip strength, and physical performance—all of which support the need to remain active as one ages (Wilson et al, 2021; Wang et al, 2020). Older adults who engage in a variety of physical activities are more likely to achieve recommended levels for aerobic, strengthening, flexibility, and endurance exercise.

Chronic Conditions

Chronic conditions can affect an older adult's wellness because they influence how an older adult interacts with their home and community environments. For example, an older adult with a condition that affects energy levels (e.g., CHF, rheumatoid arthritis), may find that their regular attendance to photography classes at the senior center is affected on days when their energy is low, or an older adult with diabetes and peripheral neuropathy may find that they are no longer able to make hot, nutritious meals safely. Chronic conditions are discussed extensively in Chapters 8, 10, and 11.

Psychosocial Factors

Self-Efficacy

A sense of self-efficacy, or perceived control, is associated with health and wellness among older adults. Self-efficacy is the belief that one can organize and execute courses of action needed to achieve a desired goal or to succeed at desired undertakings. Higher levels of self-efficacy positively influence health status, which in turn enables effective self-management behaviors (Peters et al, 2019). Older adults who have perceived control over their circumstances report their health as better and their lives as more satisfying. Perceived control is also associated with lower rates of hospitalization and reduced mortality (Peters et al, 2019). Reduced self-efficacy is a barrier to community-dwelling older adults' occupational engagement (Koh et al, 2022).

Resilience

Resilience, or the way one bounces back in response to adversity, is associated with wellness in older adults. The ability to successfully adapt to adversity is an important factor in aging well (Fullen et al, 2018; Ho et al, 2022). The concept of resilience has been studied in older adults of diverse backgrounds. These studies have shown a connection between resilience and quality of life (QOL), coping skills, and a reduction in chronic illness (Fullen et al, 2018). Furthermore, an older person's level of resilience has an inverse relationship to loneliness and depression (Ho et al, 2022). Resilience is related to self-esteem and may positively influence the way older adults cope with the challenges of aging (Calder et al, 2018).

Adaptation

The ability to adapt to life's challenges, particularly with regard to aging, affects an older adults' level of wellness. Adaptation is the internal processes a person follows to achieve relative mastery over occupational challenges (Schkade & Schultz, 1992). When describing the experience of adapting to occupational challenges related to aging, older adults describe the importance of accepting and making the best out of changes that occur within bodies, social structures, or environments. Adaptation may also require an older adult to adjust their standards of what is or is not acceptable and change their behaviors to accommodate for the adjusted standards (van Leeuwen et al, 2019).

Intervention

Occupational therapy has long-standing involvement in promoting health and wellness for older adults. Practice, education, policy, and research initiatives provide support for occupational therapy's contributions to positive aging. The WFOT website (www.wfot.org) has position papers supporting practice health promotion and wellness with the older adult. AOTA also identifies health and wellness intervention as a practice area that is within occupational therapists' scope of practice (AOTA, 2020a). This section will first discuss models that guide occupational therapy interventions, followed by program development, and lastly, examples of community-based wellness interventions implemented by occupational therapists.

Models to Guide Interventions

Holistic wellness models integrate multiple dimensions that contribute to wellness. Dimensions vary with different wellness models, but most models include these six dimensions: physical, mental, emotional, spiritual, social, and environmental (GWI, n.d.). Studies by Fullen and colleagues (2018) and Strout and colleagues (2016) support the use of wellness models for their usefulness in encouraging patient engagement in decision-making and compliance.

The Do-Live-Now Framework

The Do-Live-Now framework was developed in Canada by an occupational therapist to facilitate health promotion (Kim et al, 2022). The focus of this framework is on occupation. The concept of the framework is "what you do everyday matters" (p. 418), thereby increasing self-efficacy for the older adult and promoting individual autonomy. The framework has four main constructs: dimensions of experience, activity patterns, social and personal forces, and health and wellness outcomes, and it can be used with individual, group, or community programs. Kim and colleagues found that occupational therapists who had completed training in the Do-Live-Now framework valued its usefulness in supporting occupation-based practice.

The Health Belief Model

The Health Belief Model was developed to help understand the reason people fail to engage in beneficial health behaviors (Kalu et al, 2019). It has been widely used in the field of public health to encourage engagement in positive health behaviors. The Health Belief Model is a reliable model for occupational therapists to use to guide in the creation and implementation of health promotion programs for older adults. The Health Belief Model has four main constructs: perceived susceptibility, perceived severity, perceived barriers, and perceived benefit (Yazdanpanah et al, 2019). Perceived susceptibility refers to the individual's perception that they are susceptible to the problem, whereas perceived severity refers to the individual's perception of how serious the impact of the condition may be. When developing a program using this model, it is important to address the perceived barriers that may limit the individual's ability to engage in the behavior. The last stage is the individual's perception that the perceived benefits of adopting the new health behavior outweigh the cost of not adopting the new behavior.

The Preventative Correction Proactive Model

The Preventative Correction Proactive Model considers the proactive actions older adults take to adapt to age-related changes and stressors to promote successful aging and QOL (Torregrosa-Ruiz et al, 2021). The Preventative Correction Proactive model considers external resources such as financial resources and social support available to the older adult and internal characteristics (e.g., self-esteem, coping strategies, and optimism) and the ability to adapt behaviorally through the adoption of health-promotion behaviors and proactive management of illness. The interplay of these dynamics enables the older adult to cope and adapt to life stressors and changes that come with aging and experience QOL.

The Theory of Occupational Adaptation

The theory of occupational adaptation (OA) (Schkade & Schultz, 1992) is an occupational therapy-specific model that fits well with wellness promotion. OA conceptualizes the internal normative processes persons follow to achieve relative mastery over the occupational challenges that stem from a person's occupational roles (Schkade & Schultz, 1992). As discussed in this chapter and throughout the text, older adults encounter occupational challenges due to the multifaceted process of aging; they are faced with incorporating new occupations to manage chronic conditions or adapting known occupations to accommodate for changes due to aging. Regardless of the cause or type of challenge, OA provides a framework that occupational therapists can use to facilitate an older adult's experience of relative mastery over the challenges (Johansson & Björklund, 2016; Palma-Candia et al, 2019).

Program Development

Before creating wellness interventions or wellness programs, it is necessary to fully understand the needs of the community and the existing resources. Completing a needs assessment assists in fully understanding the scope of the health issue and identifying the focus of the occupational therapy intervention. A needs assessment is often completed with a community partner that can provide access to the target population and can involve collaboration of an interprofessional team. Molema and colleagues (2019) identified several conditions that may lead to successful program implementation. These include determining funding in advance, developing a program specific to the target population and supported by evidence, and good communication between stakeholders and the interprofessional team.

Development of strong community partnerships is foundational to running a successful community-based program. Aligning with community partners enables access to the population of interest and sharing of resources (Calder et al, 2018). The process of cultivating relationships can take time, but it is vital to success. Knowledge and understanding of the available resources and services available in your location or region is necessary to support best practice for the community-based older adult.

Health Promotion, Management, and Maintenance Interventions

Occupational therapy intervention focused on health promotion, management, and maintenance skills has been shown to improve occupational performance and QOL for older adults. A systematic review conducted by Berger and colleagues (2018) reviewed 36 studies on the effectiveness of health promotion interventions within the scope of occupational therapy practice. Studies reviewed looked at occupational performance, QOL, or healthcare utilization and used performance outcome measures such as basic ADLs and IADLs, leisure and social participation, and social activity questions. Interventions included standard and modified Stanford Chronic Disease Self-Management Programs, group interventions other than the Stanford Chronic Disease Self-Management Programs, individual interventions, and combined group and individual interventions. Strong evidence was found for the use of group health promotion interventions in improving occupational performance for older adults.

Chronic Condition Management

Occupational therapists can provide interventions to help older adults live with their chronic conditions. Occupational therapists can do this by educating older adults to engage in self-management activities (Berger et al, 2018; Leland et al, 2017). Occupational therapy interventions focused on chronic condition maintenance skills have been shown to improve occupational performance and QOL for older adults (Berger et al, 2018). There are also community-based Chronic Disease Self-Management Programs (cdc.gov, 2020). These programs are held in the community (e.g., senior centers, churches) and typically are taught by one healthcare provider and one non-healthcare provider who has a chronic condition. For more information, see Chapter 16.

Health Education, Health Coaching, and Health Promotion

Health education, occupational performance/health coaching, and health promotion are related programs that are designed to develop the health behaviors that support health and wellness for older adults. They are the predominant intervention approaches for healthy aging. A brief summary of their similarities and differences is included here.

Health education uses a variety of approaches to improve health outcomes and maintain health and wellness. The Joint Committee on Health Education and Promotion Terminology has adopted the definition of health education as "any combination of evidence-based/evidence-informed practices are used to provide equitable opportunities for the acquisition of knowledge, attitudes, and skills that are needed to adapt, adopt, and maintain healthy behaviors" (Videto & Dennis, 2021, p. 11). Occupational therapists may collaborate with health educators in the development and implementation of health-promotion interventions. Additionally, there are specialty certifications in health education, such as a Certified Health Education Specialist that an occupational therapist may wish to pursue.

Health coaching may have similar goals to health education, but the process is quite different. Health coaching partners with people through behavioral, individualized, evidence-based support to help manage chronic health conditions (Vanderbilt University Medical Center, 2023). Coaching may be used to promote self-care behaviors and achieve outcomes promoting health (Ahmadizadeh et al, 2023; Kessler et al, 2018). Occupational performance coaching is a technique of coaching that guides a person along the decision-making process and encourages self-direction and autonomy in the adoption of health behaviors (Ahmadizadeh et al, 2023; Kessler et al, 2018). Occupational therapists are well prepared to engage in occupational performance coaching to promote healthy aging.

Health promotion is a central intervention strategy in public health. In 2019, the United Nations identified the need to prioritize health promotion and disease prevention, health education, and health literacy as key factors in the global initiative for improved health behaviors. Health promotion is defined as "the process of enabling people to increase control over, and to improve their health. It not only embraces actions directed at strengthening the skills and capabilities of individuals, but also action directed toward changing social, environmental and economic determinants of health so as to optimize their positive impact on public and personal health. Health promotion is the process of enabling people, individually and collectively, to increase control over the determinants of health and thereby improve their health" (WHO, 2021, p. 4). This definition of health promotion emphasizes the importance of motivating people to establish health and wellness goals as a means to engage in their life passions. Three strategies for health promotion have been identified by the Ottawa Charter (WHO, 2021): advocacy for health, enabling individuals to maximize their health, and mediating the varied interests in society to improve the overall health of individuals and communities.

Lifestyle Redesign

Lifestyle Redesign intervention emerged from the landmark study by Clark and colleagues (1997) that compared the outcomes of an occupational therapy preventive intervention for older adults living in the community to a social activities program led by nonprofessionals to a group that received no intervention. The older adults who received the occupational therapy program demonstrated greater gains in physical and social functioning, mental health, and life satisfaction, with gains maintained 6 months after the intervention. The outcomes for the social activities group were similar to those who received no treatment at all (Clark et al, 1997, 2001). Lifestyle Redesign intervention focuses on educating older adults about the importance of occupation to enhance physical, mental, emotional, social, and spiritual health and on preparing older adults to be reflective about their occupational choices. The combination of knowledge of the health benefits of occupation and the skills to be reflective enables the person to "construct daily routines in a manner that would optimize their health and psychosocial wellbeing" and to participate in a process of lifestyle redesign (Jackson et al, 1998, p. 329).

Lifestyle Redesign programs continue to be implemented worldwide and adjusted to meet different cultural groups. In

Canada, the program was adapted to ensure cultural relevance for French Canadian older adults and was found to improve older adults' health and well-being (Levasseur et al, 2022). Similarly, a program adapted for Israelis was also found to be effective in improving occupational performance and QOL for those older adults (Maeir et al, 2021).

Cognitive Activities

Interventions that are focused on stimulating cognition can help delay cognitive decline and improve psychological health. Interventions can focus on specific cognitive activities like learning a language or reading complex material (Thoma et al, 2021) or on building active and enriching lifestyles. Active lifestyles that are intellectually stimulating and enriching appear to support cognitive and psychological health. The benefits of an enriching lifestyle program are based on evidence from several areas of cognitive research: cognitive-training studies, multimodal lifestyle interventions, and aerobic exercise or physical activity (Calatayud et al, 2022; Calder et al, 2018). Lifelong participation in mentally stimulating activities may promote neural connectivity as one ages, and participation in occupations that are more cognitively challenging led to lower cognitive decline in retirement (Calatayud et al, 2022).

A randomized control trial conducted in Spain analyzed the impact of an individualized cognitive stimulation program's effectiveness when developed based on the individual's preexisting cognitive levels compared with a standard cognitive stimulation program (Calatayud et al, 2022). Two hundred and eighty-eight older adults participated in the 10-week study with follow up at 6 months and 1 year. Results showed that the individualized cognitive stimulation program was effective at maintaining normal cognitive functioning and delaying cognitive decline in the older adult. The combination of "maintaining the normal cognitive function as long as possible as well as delaying the cognitive decline when this has started is an indicator of successful aging" (p. 78) and may be due to the cognitive reserve capacity (Calatayud et al, 2022).

Social Activities

A key component of most community-based wellness activities is socialization. Because social isolation and loneliness have a negative association with health (Ferreira et al, 2021; Shaw et al, 2017) and well-being (Wilson et al, 2021), creating opportunities for socialization is a key factor in promoting wellness for older adults. Wellness programs that promote socialization cover a wide range of interests and are only limited by the occupational therapist's creativity. See Table 22-2 and Promoting Best Practice 22-3 for some innovative ways to promote socialization.

PROMOTING BEST PRACTICE 22-3
EngAGED

EngAGED: The National Resource Center for Engaging Older Adults' mission is to increase social engagement of older adults by helping organizations and communities provide social engagement opportunities for older adults. EngAGED identifies trends and best practices for social engagement and develops implementation resources. EngAGED is administered by USAging and funded by the U.S. Administration on Aging. https://www.engagingolderadults.org

Physical Activity

Governmental, nonprofit, and health organizations promote physical activity as an important strategy for maintaining health and wellness in the older adult years. Physical activity includes the performance of occupations and exercise. Occupations and exercises that require moderate to high intensity may be used as part of an active lifestyle to achieve the recommended physical activity levels and physical health that support cardiovascular health and a reduced risk of cognitive decline (Alvares Pereira et al, 2022). Physical activity, such as engaging in planned or structured exercise (e.g., workouts, leisure, walking, and daily life occupations), has been cited as a predictor of QOL for older adults (Kuo et al, 2022).

TABLE 22-2 ■ Innovative Socialization Programs

PROGRAM	DESCRIPTION
Telephone Connections	Provide regular phone calls to homebound older adults (NCOA, 2023).
Intergenerational Connections	Coordinate connections between young and older generations. For example, older adults engage in creative activities with orphaned children (Government of Canada) or teenagers visiting blind and visually impaired older adults (NCOA, 2023).
Pet Connections	Facilitate pet adoption for older adults. Pet rescue organizations can match mature dogs with older adults (Anderson et al, 2015).
Security Connections	Facilitate contact between older adults and local police officers. Older adults in Sangam Vihar in South Delhi, India, met local police and were given cards with phone numbers, and police stations created a registry with the older adults so they would be recognized if they called (WHO, n.d.-b).

Evidence for Exercise

According to the Centers for Disease Control and Prevention (CDC, 2023), 150 minutes per week of moderate-intensity exercise (walking briskly is an example) is sufficient in terms of physical and mental health and well-being. That exercise can be done in small increments. Even 10 minutes at a time has been shown to reduce risk of disease and cognitive decline. Exercise can also provide opportunities for social engagement, which may, in turn, encourage continued participation in exercise. There is strong evidence that even moderate engagement in physical activity promotes health for older adults (Gahimer & Bates, 2021).

The MedlinePlus information page on exercise for seniors (2023) lists among the health benefits:

- Exercise may prevent or delay onset of many diseases and conditions.
- Physical fitness is associated with lower likelihood of developing dementia.
- Exercise helps ease arthritis pain and stiffness.
- Exercise helps to manage stress and improve mood.
- Physical activity guidelines (CDC, 2023) are summarized in Table 22-3.

Fitness Programs

Physical activity programs are generally community based and are offered through small groups, media campaigns, and online resources. A variety of physical activity options are generally available for older adults to support the different needs and perspectives regarding physical activity. Individual fitness routines, fitness programs at community organizations, online fitness programs, and/or rehabilitation fitness programs provide older adults with the necessary supports to follow national guidelines. Options are important because individuals and communities may have different preferences regarding physical activities. Occupational therapy practitioners have had a long-standing involvement in fitness programs for special populations. Tai chi (Wu et al, 2020) and yoga (Waldman-Levi et al, 2020; Green et al, 2019) are examples of fitness programs that may be extended to meet the needs of older adults with goals of positive aging, as seen in Figure 22-2.

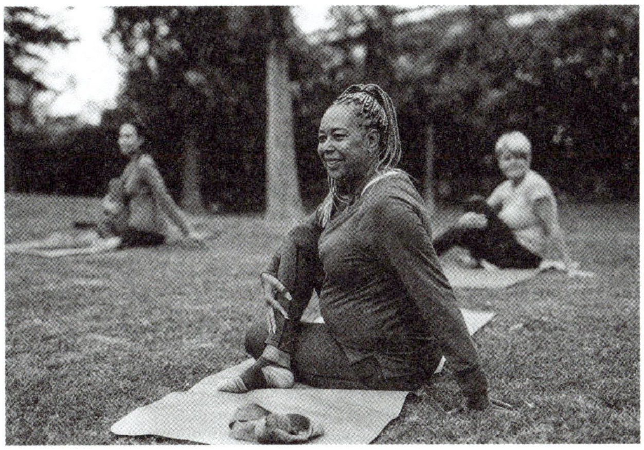

FIGURE 22-2 Women engaged in yoga fitness activity. *(Sabrina Bracher/iStock/Getty Images Plus/Getty Images.)*

Active Living and Staying-Active Programs

Active living and staying-active programs have been shown to be effective for promoting physical, psychological, and cognitive health. These programs emphasize engagement in a variety of activities beyond physical exercise, including work and volunteering, social interaction, and creative activities, to maintain involvement in daily life. The WHO's work on the United Nation's Decade of Healthy Ageing (n.d.-a) includes key proposals for age-friendly environments, combating ageism, integrative care, and long-term care. Many policy areas are aligned with occupational therapy domains of concern. For example, active aging requires barrier-free environments, options for activities, training for informal caregivers, and community mobility systems that meet the needs of an older adult population.

Maintaining an active lifestyle through the aging process has been shown to support healthy aging. A pilot study by Kuo and colleagues (2022) employed a physically active lifestyle modification program based on the Lifestyle Redesign program. The study's aim was to increase physical activity in daily routines of Taiwanese older adults. Study results showed improvements in the older adults' health, physical activity, and social engagement.

Nutritional Intervention

Nutritional intervention focuses on providing seniors with nutritious meals or the availability of nutritious food supplies. These interventions can include meal delivery, transportation to grocery stores or farmers markets, and congregate meals. Registered dietitians are skilled in addressing meal planning for medical conditions. Occupational therapists can also promote nutrition through occupations such as gardening, meal planning, and cooking.

Congregate Meal Programs

Congregate meal programs provide nutritious meals in an accessible group setting. The core of most U.S. senior center

---

TABLE 22-3 ■ Exercise Guidelines for Older Adults

Recommended Exercise for Adults Age 65 and Older (CDC, 2023)
At least 150 minutes a week (for example, 30 minutes a day, 5 days a week) *of moderate-intensity activity* such as brisk walking. OR 75 minutes a week of *vigorous-intensity activity* such as hiking, jogging, or running
At least 2 days a week of activities that *strengthen muscles*
Plus activities to *improve balance,* such as standing on one foot

programing is congregate meals. The Older Americans Act, which authorizes funding to many senior centers, mandates that the funded services target older adults with economic and social needs (Uivari et al, 2019). Congregate meals address both of these needs. Most congregate meals have no set fees, but small donations may be encouraged. In addition to providing nutrition and socialization opportunities, benefits include a variety of meals and greater food security (Stone, 2023).

Documentation, Payment Systems, and Reimbursement

Documentation of wellness services is dependent on the service context. In providing services through medically oriented community services, occupational therapists may be required to document and bill through Medicare or Medicaid (see also Chapter 23 on Primary Care). Documentation in community services may include writing reports for community agencies, providing educational materials for organizations and individual clients, or summaries of program outcomes. Measuring the outcomes of programs through regular program evaluation will support grant applications and city or county budget requests.

In the United States, occupational therapy services for health promotion and wellness programs are through Medicare, insurance plans, grant funds, private pay, or in-kind programs offered by not-for-profit organizations. As part of the Affordable Care Act, Medicare studied outcomes of adults who took part in wellness programs that focused on (1) physical activity, nutrition, and obesity; (2) falls prevention; (3) chronic disease management; and (4) mental health. After 6 months of study, participants improved most in self-reported physical activity and mental health. The program demonstrated low program costs with high return in value. Studies like this will continue to provide evidence for Medicare to reimburse health-promotion services (Centers for Medicare & Medicaid Services, 2017).

Universal health coverage in countries such as Canada and the United Kingdom provides funding for essential services such as health-promotion and prevention services (WHO, 2022). In the Netherlands, a care group (a term for part of the care system) is provided with a fixed amount of money per client from the health insurer. These funds may be used to support prevention programing to support healthy lifestyles including physical activity and diet modifications (Molema et al, 2019).

Advocacy for Community-Based Wellness Services

In the United States, occupational therapy would benefit from advocacy efforts to support reimbursement of occupational therapy for health-promotion and wellness services. Grant funds are needed to support advocacy efforts and to generate evidence supporting the role of occupational therapy in health promotion and wellness to benefit older adults. Federal and state government agencies and private organizations can provide information about grant funding opportunities (c.f. https://www.grants.gov). Advocating for community services at the local level includes promoting neighborhood senior centers and related services for meals, social participation, and wellness and health services. Advocacy also includes ensuring all older adults are aware of and have access to these services. Occupational therapists can take roles in community leadership, on city and town boards, and in community advocacy organizations using their occupational lens in support of their older adult clients.

CASE STUDY (CONTINUED)

Intervention and Disposition

Mr. and Mrs. Otieno met with a registered dietitian who helped them create meal plans that both satisfied the medical requirements for his cardiovascular health and had the flavors and textures they both appreciated. Demonstrating her belief in the value of the meal planning, Mrs. Otieno later became a go-to resource at the senior center, providing "cooking lessons" to some of the women there. Mr. Otieno worked with the fitness coordinator to learn how to safely use the center's fitness equipment and works out three times a week. He continues to prefer to work out alone, though he prefers to work out when he knows a few of the other men will also be there. He continues to be concerned about winter weather hazards and misses getting out more in the community.

Questions

1. What additional programming could Mr. Otieno benefit from to support his health and wellness?
2. What can the occupational therapist do to advocate for more wellness programming in Mr. Otieno's community?

Answers

1. The occupational therapist could invite Mr. and Mrs. Otieno to participate in a lifestyle redesign program offered at the senior center to help them explore social outlets, transportation options, and other wellness activities. [LO 22-5; Intervention section]
2. The occupational therapist can partner with senior center participants to bring in local community leaders who can help the participants inform the leaders of their community's needs and help the older adults become part of the local board membership. [LO 22-7; Advocacy section]

SUMMARY

Occupational therapy, with its holistic nature and through the power of occupation, has much to offer in supporting older adults' health and wellness. Interventions focusing on lifestyle balance, fitness, nutrition, and social needs are but some of the evidence-supported activities available. By addressing social determinants of health and health conditions through community-based services, occupational therapists can support productive and meaningful lives of older adults. Occupational therapists have many opportunities to grow their practice in both traditional and nontraditional service contexts.

Critical Thinking Questions

1. How do the different roles an occupational therapist may employ influence their collaboration with interprofessional partners in community-based care?
2. How would an occupational therapist engage older adults as a health coach?

REFERENCES

AARP. (2020). Maintaining dignity: Understanding and responding to the challenges facing older LGBT Americans. https://doi.org/10.26419/res.00217.006

Ahmadizadeh, Z., Shanbehzadeh, S., Kessler, D., Taghavi, S., Khaleghparast, S., & Akbarfahimi, M. (2023). Occupational performance coaching for adults with heart failure: Randomized controlled trial protocol. *Canadian Journal of Occupational Therapy*, 90(1),15–24. doi: 10.1177/00084174221130167

Alvares Pereira, G., Silva Nunes, M. V., Alzola, P., & Contador, I. (2022). Cognitive reserve and brain maintenance in aging and dementia: An integrative review. *Applied Neuropsychology: Adult*, 29(6), 1615–1625. doi: 10.1080/23279095.2021.1872079

American Alliance of Museums. (2023). Museums and creative aging. https://www.aam-us.org/programs/museums-creative-aging/

American Occupational Therapy Association. (2020a). Occupational therapy in the promotion of health and well-being. *American Journal of Occupational Therapy*, 74(3), 7403420010p1–7403420010p14. https://doi.org/10.5014/ajot.2020.743003

American Occupational Therapy Association. (2020b). Occupational therapy practice framework: Domain and process (4th ed.). *American Journal of Occupational Therapy*, 74(Suppl. 2), 7412410010. https://doi.org/10.5014/ajot.2020.74S2001

Anderson, K. A., Lord, L., K., Hill, L. N., & McCune, S. (2015). Fostering the human-animal bond for older adults: Challenges and opportunities. *Activities, Adaptation & Aging*, 39(1), 32–42, doi: 10.1080/01924788.2015.994447

Australian Health Directory. (n.d.). Aged care—day centers. https://www.healthdirectory.com.au/Aged_care/Day_centres/search

Begg, D. P. (2017). Disturbances of thirst and fluid balance associated with aging. *Physiology & behavior*, 178, 28–34. https://doi.org/10.1016/j.physbeh.2017.03.003

Berger, S., Escher, A., Mengle, E., & Sullivan, N. (2018). Effectiveness of health promotion, management, and maintenance interventions within the scope of occupational therapy for community-dwelling older adults: A systematic review. *American Journal of Occupational Therapy*, 72(4), 7204190010p1–7204190010p10. https://doi.org/10.5014/ajot.2018.030346

Bethancourt, H. J., Kenney, W. L., Almeida, D. M., & Rosinger, A. Y. (2020). Cognitive performance in relation to hydration status and water intake among older adults, NHANES 2011–2014. *European Journal of Nutrition* 59(7), 3133–3148. https://doi.org/10.1007/s00394-019-02152-9

Biegel, D. E., Tracy, E. M., & Song, L. Y. (1995). Barriers to social network interventions with persons with severe and persistent mental illness: A survey of mental health case managers. *Community Mental Health Journal*, 31(4), 335–349.

Calatayud, E., Jiménez-Sánchez, C., Calvo, S., Brandín-de la Cruz, N., Herrero, P., & Gómez-Soria, I. (2022). Effectiveness of cognitive stimulation personalized by the preexisting cognitive level in older adults: A randomized clinical trial. *Topics in Geriatric Rehabilitation*. 38, 73–80. doi: 10.1097/TGR.0000000000000345

Calder, P. C., Carding S. R., Christopher, G., Kuh, D., Langley-Evans, S. C., & McNulty, H. (2018). A holistic approach to healthy ageing: How can people live longer, healthier lives? *Journal of Human Nutrition & Dietetics*, 31, 439–450. https://doi.org/10.1111/jhn.12566

Carlsson, H., Pijpers. R., & Van Melik, R. (2022) Day-care centres for older migrants: Spaces to translate practices in the care landscape. *Social & Cultural Geography*, 23(2), 250–269, doi: 10.1080/14649365.2020.1723135

Centers for Disease Control & Prevention. (2020). Self-management education workshops. https://www.cdc.gov/arthritis/interventions/self_manage.htm

Centers for Disease Control & Prevention. (2023). How much physical activity do older adults need? https://www.cdc.gov/physicalactivity/basics/older_adults/index.htm#:~:text=Adults%20aged%2065%20and%20older,of%20activities%20that%20strengthen%20muscles.

Centers for Medicare & Medicaid Services. (n.d.). Programs for All-Inclusive Care for the Elderly (PACE). https://www.medicare.gov/sign-up-change-plans/different-types-of-medicare-health-plans/pace

Centers for Medicare & Medicaid Services. (2017). Wellness prospective evaluation report on 6-month follow-up survey outcomes and estimated operational costs. https://downloads.cms.gov/files/cmmi/community-basedwellnessrrevention-sixthmnthoutcomes-operationalcostrpt.pdf

Clark, F., Azen, S. P., Zemke, R., Jackson, J., Carlson, M., Mandel, D., Hay, J., Josepheson, K., Cherry, B., Hessel, C., Palmer, J., & Lipson, L. (1997). Occupational therapy for independent-living older adults: A randomized controlled trial. *JAMA*, 278(16):1321–1326. doi:10.1001/jama.1997.03550160041036

Clark, F., Azen, S. P., Carlson, M., Mandel, D., LaBree, L., Hay, J., Zemke, R., Jackson, J. & Lipson, L. (2001). Embedding health-promoting changes into the daily lives of independent-living older adults: Long-term follow-up of occupational therapy intervention. The Journals of Gerontology Series B: Psychological Sciences and Social Sciences, 56(1), 60–63. DOI: 10.1093/geronb/56.1.p60

Clemson, L. (2022). Relevance, resilience, and ageism: A bright future for occupational therapy and healthy ageing, Sylvia Docker Lecture 2021. *Australian Occupational Therapy Journal*, 69(1), 3–14. https://doi.org/10.1111/1440-1630.12783

Collins, K., Layne, K., Schooley, M., Chase, L., & Faradj-Bakht, S. (2021). Fitness in the Park: An interprofessional community-based partnership for older adults. *Topics in Geriatric Rehabilitation*, 37(3), 186–190. doi: 10.1097/TGR.0000000000000327

CORE Canada. (2022). Health aging CORE. https://healthyagingcore.ca/

Domholdt, E., Cooper, S. K., & Kleinhoff, R. J. (2020). Population health content in entry-level occupational therapy programs. *American Journal of Occupational Therapy*, 74(3), 7403205160p1–7403205160p9. doi: https://doi.org/10.5014/ajot.2020.036392

Elliott, S. J. (2019). Collaborating with an aging agency to promote healthy aging. *SIS Quarterly Practice Connections*, 4(1), 23–25. https://www.aota.org/publications/sis-quarterly/productive-aging-sis/pasis-2-19

Fabius, C. D., Thomas, K. S., Zhang, T., Ogarek, J., & Shireman, T. (2018). Racial disparities in Medicaid home and community-based service utilization and expenditures among persons with multiple sclerosis. *BMC*

Health Services Research, 18, 773. https://doi.org/10.1186/s12913-018-3584-x

Ferreira, G., Walters, A., & Anderson, H. (2021). Social isolation and its impact on the geriatric community. *Topics in Geriatric Rehabilitation. 37*(3). 191–197. doi: 10.1097/TGR.000000000000031

Finland Ministry of Foreign Affairs. (n.d.). Enabling active aging in Finland. https://finland.fi/life-society/enabling-active-ageing-in-finland/

Fullen, M, Richardson, V., & Haag-Granello, D. (2018). Comparing successful aging, resilience, and holistic wellness as predictors of the good life. *Educational Gerontology, 44*(7) 459–468 https://doi.org/10.1080/03601277.2018.1501230

Gahimer, J. E., & Bates, F. (2021). A toolbox for implementing community-based physical activity programs for older adults and adults with disabilities. *Topics in Geriatric Rehabilitation 37*(3), 134–144. doi: 10.1097/TGR.0000000000000323

Glasinovic, A., Rodríguez, C., Martín, P. S., González, D., Guzmán, R., Ureta, M. D. P., Pérez I., Feferholtz Y., & Valenzuela, M. T. (2022). Efectividad a mediano plazo de un programa multidimensional en personas mayores en centros diurnos en Chile [Effectiveness of a multidimensional therapeutic program for aged people attending senior centers]. *Revista Medica de Chile. 150*(1), 23–32. doi: 10.4067/S0034-98872022000100023

Global Wellness Institute. (n.d.). *What is Wellness?* https://globalwellnessinstitute.org/what-is-wellness/

Government of Canada. (2023). Core community support to age in community. https://www.canada.ca/en/employment-social-development/corporate/seniors/forum/core-community-supports.html

Grants.gov. (n.d.). Search grants. https://www.grants.gov/web/grants/search-grants.html?keywords = health%20promotion

Green, E., Huynh, A., Broussard, L., Zunker, B., Matthews, J., Hilton, C. L., & Aranha, K. (2019). Systematic review of yoga and balance: Effect on adults with neuromuscular impairment. *American Journal of Occupational Therapy, 73,* 7301205150p1-7301205150p11. https://doi.org/10.5014/ajot.2019.028944

Grohman, S., Hiestand, W., Park, A., & Green, V. (2022). Community-based practice to increase holistic care. *OT Practice, 27*(11) 12–15. https://www.aota.org/publications/ot-practice/ot-practice-issues/2022/community-based-practice-holistic-care

Healthy Aging Association. (n.d.) Dignity at home: Fall prevention program. https://www.healthyagingassociation.org/dignity-at-home.html

Hedayati, M., Sum, S., Hosseini, S. R., Faramarzi, M., & Pourhadi, S. (2019). Investigating the effect of physical games on the memory and attention of the elderly in adult day-care centers in Babol and Amol. *Clinical Interventions in Aging, 14,* 859–869, doi: 10.2147/CIA.S196148

HelpGuide.org (2023). Adult day care services. https://www.helpguide.org/articles/senior-housing/adult-day-care-services.htm

Ho, V., Li, X., & Smith, G. (2022). An exploratory study to assess the impact of a chair-based dance intervention among older people with depressive symptoms in residential care. *Topics in Geriatric Rehabilitation, 38*(2), 131–139 doi: 10.1097/TGR.0000000000000354

Hooper, L. (2016). Why, oh why, are so many older adults not drinking enough fluid? *Journal of the Academy of Nutrition & Dietetics. 116*(5): 774–778. https://doi.org/10.1016/j.jand.2016.01.006

International Council on Active Aging. (n.d.). *What is Wellness?* https://www.icaa.cc/business/Wellness-model-.htm

Jackson, J., Carlson, M., Mandel, D., Zemke, R., & Clark, F. (1998). Occupation in lifestyle redesign: The well elderly study occupational therapy program. *American Journal of Occupational Therapy, 52*(5), 326–336. doi: https://doi.org/10.5014/ajot.52.5.326

Johansson, A., & Björklund, A. (2016). The impact of occupational therapy and lifestyle interventions on older persons' health, well-being, and occupational adaptation, *Scandinavian Journal of Occupational Therapy, 23*(3), 207–219, doi: 10.3109/11038128.2015.1093544

Kadowaki, L., & Mahmood, A. (2018). Senior centres in Canada and the United States: A scoping review. *Canadian Journal on Aging/La Revue canadienne du vieillissement 37*(4), 420–441. https://www.muse.jhu.edu/article/708690

Kalu, M., Maximos, M., Sengiad, S., & Dal Bello-Haas, V. (2019). The role of rehabilitation professionals in care transitions for older adults: A scoping review. *Physical & Occupational Therapy In Geriatrics, 37*(4), 1–28. doi.org/10.1080/02703181.2019.1621418

Kessler, D., Egan, M. Y., Dubouloz, C. J., McEwen, S., & Graham, F. P. (2018). Occupational performance coaching for stroke survivors (OPC-Stroke): Understanding of mechanisms of actions. *British Journal of Occupational Therapy. 81*(6):326–337. doi:10.1177/0308022618756001

Keyes, L., Li, Q., Collins, B., & Rivera-Torres, S. (2022). Senior center service utilization: Do social ties affect participation patterns? *Journal of Applied Gerontology, 41*(2), 526–533. https://doi-org.ezp.twu.edu/10.1177/0733464820975905

Kim, H. K., & Seo, J. H. (2022). Effect of health status, depression, gerotranscendence, self-efficacy, and social support on healthy aging in the older adults with chronic diseases. *International Journal of Environmental Research & Public Health, 19*(13), 7930. doi.org/10.3390/ijerph19137930

Kim, S., Larivière, N., Bayer, I., Gewurtz, R., & Letts, L. (2022). Occupational therapists' application of the Do-Live-Well framework: A Canadian health promotion approach. *Canadian Journal of Occupational Therapy, 89*(4):417–426. doi: 10.1177/00084174221117717

Koh, W. Q., Chia, Y. L., Ng, W., Lim, F. Y. Q., & Cheung, T. W. C. (2022). Patterns of occupational engagement among community-dwelling older adults in Singapore: An exploratory mixed method study. *British Journal of Occupational Therapy. 85*(1):68–77. doi: 10.1177/03080226211008048

Kuo, C., Shyu, H., Park, D., Tsai, P., & Li, Y. (2022). Effects of a physically active lifestyle modification (PALM) program for independent Taiwanese older adults: A mixed-methods pilot study. *Topics in Geriatric Rehabilitation, 38*(2), 149–157. doi: https://doi.org/10.1097/TGR.0000000000000356

Lavalley, R. (2023). Occupation's role in inclusion of Spanish-speaking older adults in a senior center. *OTJR: Occupational Therapy Journal of Research. 43*(1):74–80. doi:10.1177/15394492221093311

Lee, J. J., Martínez, J., & Schepens Niemiec, S. L. (2022). Building the health of communities: A partnership between occupational therapy and *promotores de salud. SIS Quarterly Practice Connections, 7*(1), 12–14. https://www.aota.org/publications/sis-quarterly/home-community-health-sis/hchsis-2-22

Leland, N. E., Fogelberg, D. J., Halle, A. D., & Mroz, T. M. (2017). Health policy perspectives: Occupational therapy and management of multiple chronic conditions in the context of health care reform. *American Journal of Occupational Therapy, 71*(1), 7101090010p1-7101090010p6. doi.org/10.5014/ajot.2017.711001

Levasseur, M., Lévesque, M. H., Lacasse-Bédard, J., Larivière, N., Filiatrault, J., Provencher, V., & Corriveau, H. (2022). Feasibility of Lifestyle Redesign® for community-dwelling older adults with and without disabilities: Results from an exploratory descriptive qualitative clinical research design. *Australian Occupational Therapy Journal, 69*(5):514–535. doi: 10.1111/1440-1630.12807

Liu H., Eggleston K. N., & Min Y. A. N. (2017). Village senior centres and the living arrangements of older people in rural China: Considerations of health, land, migration and intergenerational support. *Ageing & Society, 37*(10), 2044–2073. doi 10.1017/S0144686X16000714

Lopez, A. M., Lam K., & Thota, R. (2021). Barriers and facilitators to telemedicine: Can you hear me now? *American Society of Clinical Oncology Educational Book, 41,* 25–36. doi: 10.1200/EDBK_320827

Maeir, T., Beit-Yosef, A., Wechsler, T., Safra, Y., Zilbershlag, Y., Katz, N., & Gilboa, Y. (2021). The feasibility and efficacy of an Israeli Lifestyle Redesign®–based program for well older adults: A pilot study. *OTJR: Occupation, Participation and Health, 41*(1), 47–55. doi: 10.1177/1539449220928141

Marmo, S., Pardasani, M., & Vincent, D. (2021). Senior centers and LGBTQ participants: Engaging older adults virtually in a pandemic. *Journal of Gerontological Social Work, 64*(8), 864–884. doi: 10.1080/01634372.2021.1937431

MedlinePlus. (2023). Benefits of exercise. Retrieved via www at: https://medlineplus.gov/benefitsofexercise.html on January 30, 2023.

Molema, C. C. M., Wendel-Vos, G. C. W., Ter Schegget, S., Schuit, A. J., & van de Goor, L. A. M. (2019). Perceived barriers and facilitators of the implementation of a combined lifestyle intervention with a financial incentive for chronically ill patients. *BMC Family Practice, 18*(1), 137. doi: 10.1186/s12875-019-1025-5

National Adult Day Services. (2023). About day services. https://www.nadsa.org/about/about-adult-day-services/

National Center for Health Statistics. (2018). Adult day services center participant characteristics: United States, 2018. https://www.cdc.gov/nchs/products/databriefs/db411.htm

National Center for Health Statistics. (2022). Adult day services centers. https://www.cdc.gov/nchs/fastats/adsc.htm

National Council on Aging. (2022, July 19). Get the facts on senior centers. https://ncoa.org/article/get-the-facts-on-senior-centers

National Council on Aging. (2023). Senior centers reaching the hard to reach. https://www.ncoa.org/article/senior-centers-reach-the-hard-to-reach

National Council on Aging. (2023, Feb, 28). Tracking health promotion guidance during COVID-19. https://www.ncoa.org/article/tracking-health-promotion-program-guidance-during-covid-19

National Indian Council on Aging. (2023). NICOA compass: A guide to native wellness. https://nicoacompass.org/

Nielsen, T. L., Andersen, N. T., Petersen, K. S., Polatajko, H., & Nielsen, C. (2019). Intensive client centred occupational therapy in the home improves older adults' occupational performance. Results from a Danish randomized controlled trial. *Scandinavian Journal of Occupational Therapy, 26* (5): 325–342. doi: 10.1080/11038128.2018.1424236

Norin, L., Slaug, B., Haak, M., & Iwarsson, S. (2021). Housing adaptations and housing accessibility problems among older adults with longstanding spinal cord injury. *British Journal of Occupational Therapy, 84*(12), 765–774. doi:10.1177/0308022620979516

Ogonowska-Slodownik, A., Morgulec-Adamowicz, N., Geigle, P. R., Kalbarczyk, M., & Kosmol, A. (2022). Objective and self-reported assessment of physical activity of women over 60 years old. *Ageing International, 47*, 307–320. doi: 10.1007/s12126-021-09423-z

Orlofsky, S., & Wozniak, K. (2022). Older adults' experiences using Alexa. *Geriatric Nursing, 48*, 247–257. https://doi.org/10.1016/j.gerinurse.2022.09.017

Palma-Candia, O., Hueso-Montoro, C., Martí-García, C., Fernández-Alcántara, M., Campos-Calderón, C., & Montoya- Juárez, R. (2019). Understanding the occupational adaptation process and well-being of older adults in Magallanes (Chile): A qualitative study. *International Journal of Environmental Research and Public Health, 16*(19), 3640. https://doi.org/10.3390/ijerph16193640

Pardasani, M. (2019). Senior centers: If you build will they come? *Educational Gerontology, 45*(2), 120–133, doi: 10.1080/03601277.2019.1583407

Pardasani, M., & Berkman, C. (2021). New York City senior centers: Who participates and why? *Journal of Applied Gerontology 40*(9): 073346482091730 doi: 10.1177/0733464820917304

Patch. (2023, Feb. 14). Dominican University launches 2023 wellness program for seniors. https://patch.com/california/sanrafael/dominican-university-launches-wellness-program-seniors

Peters, M., Potter, C. M., Kelly, L., & Fitzpatrick, R. (2019). Self-efficacy and health-related quality of life: A cross-sectional study of primary care patients with multi-morbidity. *Health Quality of Life Outcomes 17,* 37. https://doi.org/10.1186/s12955-019-1103-3

Petruseviciene, D., Surmaitiene, D., Baltaduoniene, D., & Lendraitiene, E. (2018). Effect of community-based occupational therapy on health-related quality of life and engagement in meaningful activities of women with breast cancer. *Occupational Therapy International, 2018,* 6798697. https://doi.org/10.1155/2018/6798697

Quigley, R., Russell, S. G., Larkins, S., Taylor, S., Sagigi, B., Strivens, E., & Redman-MacLaren, M. (2022). Aging well for indigenous peoples: A scoping review. *Frontiers in Public Health, 10,* 780898. doi: https://doi.org/10.3389/fpubh.2022.780898

Rome, V., Lendon, J. P., & Harris-Kojetin, L. (2020). Differences in characteristics of adult day services centers, by level of medical service provision. National Center for Health Statistics. *Vital and health statistics. Series 3, Analytical and Epidemiological Studies; no. 45;DHHS publication; no. 2020–1428.* https://stacks.cdc.gov/view/cdc/96032

Scaffa, M. E. (2020). Enhancing the health and well-being of veterans through community-based occupational therapy services. *SIS Quarterly Practice Connections, 5*(4), 17–19. https://www.aota.org/publications/sis-quarterly/home-community-health-sis/hchsis-11–20

Schkade, J., & Schultz, S. (1992). Occupational adaptation: Toward a holistic approach for contemporary practice, Part 1. *American Journal of Occupational Therapy, 46*(9), 829–837. doi 10.5014/ajot.46.9.829

Shaw, J. G., Farid, M., Noel-Miller, C., Joseph, N., Houser, A., Asch, S. M., Bhattacharya, J., Flowers, L. (2017). Social isolation and Medicare spending: Among older adults, objective social isolation increases expenditures while loneliness does not. *Journal of Aging Health. 29*(7): 1119–1143. doi: 10.1177/0898264317703559

Siconolfi, D., Shih, R. A., Friedman, E. M., Kotzias, V. I., Ahluwalia, S. C., Phillips, J. L., & Saliba, D. (2019). Rural-urban disparities in access to home- and community-based services and supports: Stakeholder perspectives from 14 states. *Journal of the American Medical Directors Association, 20*(4), 503–508.e1. https://doi.org/10.1016/j.jamda.2019.01.120

Stephan, A., Bieber, A., Hopper, L., Joyce, R., Irving, K., Zanetti, O., Portlani, E., Kepperskhoek, L., Verhey, F., de Vugh, M., Wolfs, C., Eriksen, S., Rosvik, J., Marques, M. J., Goncalves-Pereira, M., Sjolund, B-M., Jelley, H., Woods, B., & Meyer, G. (2018). Barriers and facilitators to the access to and use of formal dementia care: Findings of a focus group study with people with dementia, informal carers and health and social care professionals in eight European countries. *BMC Geriatrics, 18,* 131. https://doi.org/10.1186/s12877-018-0816-1

Stone, K. (2023, Feb 9). What is a congregate meal? How do they benefit older adults? National Council on Aging. https://ncoa.org/article/what-is-a-congregate-meal-how-do-they-benefit-older-adults

Strout, K. A., David, D. J., Dyer, E. J., Gray, R. C., Robnett, R. H., & Howard, E. P. (2016). Behavioral interventions in six dimensions of wellness that protect the cognitive health of community-dwelling older adults: A systematic review. *Journal of the American Geriatrics Society, 64*(5), 944–958. doi:10.1111/jgs.14129

Thoma, M., Kleineidam, L., Forstmeier, S., Maercker, A., Weyerer, S., Eisele, M., van den Bussche, H., König, H., Röhr, S., Stein, J., Wiese, B., Pentzek, M., Bickel1, H., Maier, W., Scherer, M., Riedel-Heller, S., & Wagner, M. (2021). Associations and correlates of general versus specific successful ageing components. *European Journal of Ageing, 18,* 549–563. https://doi.org/10.1007/s10433-020-00593-4

Torregrosa-Ruiz, M., Gutiérrez, M., Alberola, S., & Tomás, J. M. (2021). A successful aging model based on personal resources, self-care, and life satisfaction. *The Journal of Psychology, 155*(7), 606–623. doi: 10.1080/00223980.2021.1935676

Townsend, B. G., Chen J. T. H., & Wuthrich, V. M. (2021). Barriers and facilitators to social participation in older adults: A systematic literature review. *Clinical Gerontologist, 44*(4), 359–380, doi: 10.1080/07317115.2020.1863890

Uivari, K., Fox-Grage, W., Houser, A., Dean, O., & Feinberg, L. F. (2019, Feb. 4). Older Americans Act. https://www.aarp.org/ppi/info-2019/older-americans-act.html#:~:text=In%20fiscal%20year%202019%2C%20OAA,blog%20series%20on%20the%20OAA

United Nations. (2022). Decade of healthy ageing. https://www.decadeofhealthyageing.org/

U.S. Administration on Aging. (n.d.). Eldercare locator. https://eldercare.acl.gov/Public/Index.aspx

U.S. Department of Health and Human Services. (2020). *Social determinants of health.* Social Determinants of Health—Healthy People 2030. https://health.gov/healthypeople/objectives-and-data/social-determinants-health

van Leeuwen, K. M., van Loon, M. S., van Nes, F. A., Bosmans, J. E., De Vet, H. C., Ket, J. C., Widdershoven, G. A. M., & Ostelo, R. W. (2019). What does quality of life mean to older adults? A thematic synthesis. *PloS one, 14*(3), e0213263. doi 10.1371/journal.pone.0213263

Vanderbilt University Medical Center. (2023). What is health coaching? https://www.vumc.org/health-coaching/what-health-coaching

Videto, D., & Dennis, D. (2021). Report of the 2020 Joint Committee on Health Education and Promotion Terminology. *The Health Educator, 53*(1), 4-21.

Vitorino, L., Low, G., & Lucchetti, G. (2019). Is the physical environment associated with spiritual and religious coping in older age? Evidence from Brazil. *Journal of Religion and Health 58*, 1648–1660. doi.org/10.1007/s10943-019-00796-9

Waldman-Levi, A., Bar-Haim Erez, A., Katz, N., & Stancanelli, J. (2020). Emotional functioning and sense of hope as contributors to healthy aging. *OTJR: Occupation, Participation and Health, 40*(4):253–260. doi: 10.1177/1539449220920728

Wang, D. X. M, Yao, J., Zirek, Y., Reijnierse, E. M., & Maier, A. B. (2020). Muscle mass, strength, and physical performance predicting activities of daily living: A meta-analysis. *Journal of Cachexia Sarcopenia Muscle, 11*(1), 3–25. doi: 10.1002/jcsm.12502

Wilson, L., Gilusto, E., & Hansen, S. (2021). A 4 prong approach to foster health aging in older adults. *The Journal of Family Practice, 70* (8), 376–385. doi: 10.12788/jfp.0276

World Federation of Occupational Therapists. (2019). WFOT Position Paper on Community-Based Practice: https://www.wfot.org/resources/occupational-therapy-and-community-centred-practice

World Health Organization. (n.d.-a). Decade of healthy ageing. https://www.decadeofhealthyageing.org/platform-guide-to-knowledge

World Health Organization. (n.d.-b). Age-friend world. Contact programme with local police. https://extranet.who.int/agefriendlyworld/afp/contact-programme-with-local-police/

World Health Organization. (2020). Decade of healthy ageing: Baseline report. World Health Organization. https://apps.who.int/iris/handle/10665/338677

World Health Organization. (2021). Health promotion glossary of terms 2021. Geneva:.Licence: CC BY-NC-SA 3.0. ISBN 978-92-4-003834-9

World Health Organization. (2022). Universal health coverage. Retrieved via the www from www.who.int/news-room/fact-sheets/detail/universal-health-coverage-(uhc). Retrieved on 2/9/23.

World Health Organization. (2023). Constitution. https://www.who.int/about/governance/constitution

Wu, S. Y. F., Brown, T., & Yu, M. L. (2020). Older adults' psychosocial responses to a fear of falling: A scoping review to inform occupational therapy practice. *Occupational Therapy in Mental Health, 36(*3), 207–243, doi: 10.1080/0164212X.2020.1735977

Yazdanpanah, Y., Saleh Moghadam, A. R., Mazlom, S. R., Haji Ali Beigloo, R., & Mohajer, S. (2019). Effect of an educational program based on health belief model on medication adherence in elderly patients with hypertension. *Evidence Based Care, 9*(1), 52–62. doi: 10.22038/ebcj.2019.35215.1895

CHAPTER 23

Primary Care Services

Lydia Royeen, PhD, OTR/L

> *"I'd say [an occupational therapist is a] consultant ... an expert of function, which is really important for older adults, to have [a] team member who really is an expert on function and activities of daily living."*
>
> —Geriatric Service Provider

LEARNING OUTCOMES

By the end of this chapter, readers will be able to:

23-1. Articulate the differences between primary care and primary healthcare.
23-2. Discuss potential approaches and models to primary care access.
23-3. Explain the roles of occupational therapists and members of the interprofessional team working in a primary care setting.
23-4. Identify complications and concerns of patients in primary care.
23-5. Identify important areas for assessment and intervention, within primary care settings, for occupational therapists.
23-6. Discuss the importance of documentation for reimbursement.
23-7. Create a plan for advocacy for an occupational therapy practitioner in the primary care setting.

Mini Case Study

Mrs. Dottie Brown is a 75-year-old woman who lives alone in community-funded housing. Mrs. Brown's partner passed away more than a year ago. She has few social supports and a limited pension, which is her only source of income. She uses public transportation or walks to access services in the community. For health care, she goes to a primary care clinic. This clinic, with 15,000 patients, employs one full-time equivalent occupational therapist where a referral is required from the provider to perform an evaluation. The role of the occupational therapist typically includes being a generalist, focusing on function, leading self-management classes, consulting with the other health care providers, and using direct practice and consultation models of care. Today the occupational therapist will be seeing Mrs. Brown for an initial assessment as part of their direct service time.

According to the physician's note in the electronic medical record (EMR), Mrs. Brown has type 2 diabetes and chronic bilateral leg pain. The pain limits her mobility, activities of daily living (ADLs), and instrumental activities of daily living (IADLs), and it is preventing her from leaving her apartment. Numbness in her extremities makes fine motor tasks difficult and creates a fear of falling. Mrs. Brown reported a decreased appetite and weight loss at her last appointment.

Provocative Questions

1. How will the occupational therapist collaborate with Mrs. Brown to develop goals and a treatment plan?
2. What intervention approaches might the occupational therapist use with Mrs. Brown?
3. What health care professionals may be effective team members as part of an interprofessional approach to improve Mrs. Brown's function?

Occupational therapists working in the primary care setting are considered to be practicing in an innovative setting. New research emerges every year about occupational therapy services in the primary care setting, which helps further inform practice and program implementation. This chapter discusses primary care and primary health care from a broad perspective, including different models of care and conceptual health care models. The chapter explores the multiple roles occupational therapists can have when working in the primary care setting followed by specific issues occupational therapists should consider when working with older adults. Assessment and intervention exemplars relevant for occupational therapists currently working in primary care or interested in starting a practice in primary care are discussed, as are relevant documentation models and ways to advocate for this emerging practice area. The term "patient" will be used in this chapter, consistent with the primary care medical model.

Primary Care and Primary Health Care

Primary care and primary health care are terms that have distinct meanings but are often used interchangeably (Halle et al, 2018). Primary care is the entry point, or first contact, to the health care system and provides care over time. Primary health care is a health care approach to individuals and communities using a health promotion and health equity lens (Rayner et al, 2018). The World Health Organization and United Nations Children's Fund's (UNICEF) (2020) definitions further clarify the two concepts:

Primary Health Care "A whole-of-society approach to health that aims to maximize the level and distribution of health and well-being through three components: (a) primary care and essential public health functions as the core of integrated health services; (b) multisectoral policy and action; and (c) empowered people and communities" (p. XIII).

Primary Care: "A key process in the health system that supports first-contact, accessible, continued, comprehensive and coordinated patient-focused care" (p. XIII).

Occupational therapists working in primary care have been trying to expand the existing models of primary care to include occupational therapy services (Halle et al, 2018).

Successful primary care programming includes the following shared values:

- Person and family centered
- Continuous care
- Comprehensive and equitable
- Team-based and collaborative
- Coordinated and integrated
- Accessible
- High-value

(AOTA], 2020a; Patient-Centered Primary Care Collaborative, 2019, p. 9.)

These values align with occupational therapy core values and complement one another well during the evaluation service delivery process (AOTA, 2020a).

Integrating Rehabilitation Professionals and Services in Primary Care

The integration of rehabilitation professionals, including occupational therapists, in primary care is complex and depends on a variety of factors, including type of primary care setting, populations served, and reimbursement. Two important considerations when occupational therapists integrate into the primary care setting are model of care and type of service delivery. Models of care are dependent on location; these are specific settings where an occupational therapist can work with the primary health care team. Types of service delivery are approaches occupational therapists use in a variety of primary health care settings. These service delivery approaches are not exclusive to the delivery of services for older adults; however, they are important to consider in the context of delivering occupational therapy services within primary care for the assessment and management of function with this age group. These models and service delivery approaches involve a patient-centered care approach and the management of a large number of patients with a variety of conditions, including multimorbidity.

Models of Care

Models of care include primary care practice settings where occupational therapists can practice alongside the primary care team; these models are dependent on the type of primary care setting and include clinic-based, patient-centered medical home (PCMH), and Federally Qualified Health Centers (FQHCs). A common model of rehabilitation integration into primary care is clinic-based care, in which the occupational therapist is colocated with providers and other members of the health care team. The different professions deliver care in their usual scope of practice, which is typically condition (diagnosis) based. Koverman and colleagues (2017) described a successful program implementation using this model, wherein an occupational therapist worked alongside primary care providers (e.g., physicians, physician assistants, nurse practitioners) within their geriatric primary care clinic (Koverman et al, 2017).

A PCMH is a setting where medical treatment is coordinated by a primary care physician and ensures that patients receive the care they need in a patient-friendly manner (American Academy of Family Physicians, 2023). A team-based approach, where different interprofessional team members (including occupational therapists) provide services to the patients, is emphasized in a PCMH (Halle et al, 2018). However, there is no legislation that states which allied health professions are included as part of a PCMH, and occupational therapy is not a guaranteed service (Pape & Muir, 2019).

FQHCs provide primary care services to underserved populations and receive funding from the Health Resources and Services Administration (HRSA) (2018). FQHCs provide comprehensive care that may include preventative, dental, and/or mental health services. Including occupational therapy in an FQHC has the potential to improve the health of this population, and like a PCMH, occupational therapy is not a guaranteed service (Halle et al, 2018).

Types of Service Delivery

The different types of occupational therapy service delivery include outreach services, community-based rehabilitation, self-management programs, and telehealth. Outreach services are usually delivered from a clinic or academic medical institution base and may include a mobile team or satellite services to provide care for hard-to-reach populations. Community-based rehabilitation can be used to address issues of equity and inclusiveness by creating a partnership with the community to increase the capacity and autonomy to manage community health issues (Groote, 2019).

Self-management programs involve education and support provided by occupational therapists to patients to increase their confidence and skill in managing their own conditions. Mirza and colleagues (2020) demonstrated the value of a self-management intervention approach in leading an occupation-focused intervention for older adults who have chronic disease with the intent of maintaining functional independence. The intervention, Integrated Primary Care and Occupational Therapy for Aging and Chronic Disease Treatment to Preserve Independence and Functioning (IPROACTIF), occurred weekly for 6 weeks. Results demonstrated an extreme satisfaction with services provided by the occupational therapists who had support from primary care team members including physicians and nurses (Mirza et al, 2020). The participants had improved scores in patient activation, goal-setting, and physical and mental domains (Mirza et al, 2020). The occupational self-assessment was also used as an outcome measure with improved participant scores after the intervention.

The Integration of Technology to Maximize Service Delivery

The onset of the COVID-19 pandemic brought an increase in use of telehealth services for primary care practices, including practices that serve older adult populations (Doraiswamy et al, 2021). **Telehealth** is defined by the World Federation of Occupational Therapists (WFOT) (2014) as "the use of information and communication technologies (ICT) to deliver health-related services when the provider and client are in different physical locations" (p. 37). The terms *telehealth*, telemedicine, telerehabilitation, and telepractice may be used interchangeably (WFOT, 2014). Telehealth use in geriatric clinics is cost effective, increases savings on transportation for patients, improves wait times, and reduces acute hospitalization rates (Murphy et al, 2020). Telehealth also allows patients to obtain medical treatment and care while self-isolating and decreases risk of exposure to COVID-19 (Monaghesh & Hajizadeh, 2020). Telehealth has also been found to be beneficial for caregivers of older adults, specifically allowing caregivers to have increased access to care and perceived relationship building (Raj et al, 2022). Barriers to an older adult patient's participation in telehealth are hearing loss and lack of knowledge with technology (Murphy et al, 2020).

Telehealth and occupational therapy services for the older adult population should be a consideration for occupational therapists. Use of telehealth services increased during the pandemic lockdowns in 2020 and 2021 and continued to be part of service delivery for occupational therapy services post COVID-19 lockdown. However, the future of reimbursement is unknown at the time of this writing (Sanchez-Guarnido et al, 2021). Occupational therapists can provide services in a consultative model wherein they perform a one-time consult (e.g., a home safety evaluation) or provide interventions over a period of time (e.g., to monitor progress of a home safety evaluation) (AOTA, 2018).

A case report by Sclarsky and Kumar (2021) identified positive outcomes administering occupational therapy services to an older adult via telehealth. Occupational therapy practitioners are ultimately responsible to abide by the same ethical considerations when providing telehealth services as when providing services face to face and must comply with state and national governing bodies' jurisdictional, institutional, and professional regulations when applicable (AOTA, 2018; WFOT, 2014). In addition, reimbursement consideration and ethical billing practice are the responsibility of the occupational therapist, as policies from governmental regulation agencies are evolving post pandemic. Overall telehealth is another service delivery model that should be considered to be used by occupational therapists who are practicing with older adult patients and their caregivers.

CASE STUDY

Ms. Jaramillo from Chapter 8 in the context of a primary care setting

Presenting Situation

Review the case study in Metabolic Conditions (see Chapter 8). The occupational therapist is seeing Ms. Jaramillo in the geriatric primary care office for her annual visit, approximately 6 months after her last visit. Ms. Jaramillo is accompanied by her husband, Mr. Jaramillo, who also has an appointment.

Ms. Jaramillo is still working as a cashier, and the pain in her back and hips increased from a 3/10 to a 5/10. She is the primary caregiver for her husband, whose Parkinson disease is progressing, resulting in him needing more assistance with ADLs and IADLs. Her 44-year-old daughter assists with taking care of her father and grocery shopping twice a week. Ms. Jaramillo has not seen or played bridge with her church friends for a year. Ms. Jaramillo uses a cane intermittently.

Ms. Jaramillo is seen at 9:05 by the primary care provider, Dr. Ruiz. Ms. Jaramillo says everything is fine and she is doing well. Upon further examination, Dr. Ruiz learns that Ms. Jaramillo is having increased pain, including in her wrist, is more stressed caring for her husband while working full time, and often misses meals due to stress. In addition, Ms. Jaramillo had a recent fall in the shower. At the end of the visit, Ms. Jaramillo breaks down and cries because she feels overwhelmed. Dr. Ruiz asks the occupational therapist to evaluate and treat Ms. Jaramillo in a different examination room while Dr. Ruiz sees Mr. Jaramillo.

Theoretical Frameworks and Approaches

The beginning of the chapter introduced primary care and primary healthcare. It is important to understand access to health services along with these concepts. It is also important for occupational therapists to understand how and why individuals access and use health services, as this information can be used to identify health service needs and opportunities for program and service development. For example, if an occupational therapist understands the barriers to accessing primary healthcare, they can help identify strategies to overcome these barriers.

A Conceptual Framework for Access to Healthcare

Historically, access to healthcare has been defined as having physical access to a service or provider (Levesque et al, 2013). Levesque and colleagues created a conceptual framework that examined access to healthcare as an opportunity for the individual to be able to appropriately navigate the process of identifying healthcare needs, including scheduling appointments, and using healthcare services appropriately. (See Fig. 23-1 for a visual graphic demonstrating the healthcare process.)

Using the Levesque framework, individuals are able to find and locate primary care services and receive those healthcare services.

Five dimensions of accessibility are:

1. Approachability: Individuals who have health needs are obtaining appropriate healthcare information regarding services that are available and have an impact on their health.
2. Acceptability: The healthcare services are appropriate from a cultural and social point of view for the individual seeking healthcare.
3. Availability and accommodation: The healthcare team and physical space are accessible from a physical standpoint and able to be reached in a timely manner.
4. Affordability: The individual seeking healthcare can afford the services and has time to use the healthcare services appropriately.
5. Appropriateness: The healthcare services are appropriate for the individual seeking care, and the care is given in a timely manner.

Access to healthcare is a multiprong concept and is complex in nature. These dimensions are interrelated and affect one another as an individual enters and accesses the healthcare system.

Conceptual Framework in Clinical Practice

Using Levesque's five dimensions of healthcare, Kurpas and colleagues examined access to healthcare in Poland for older adult patients with frailty, their providers, and caregivers (Kurpas et al, 2018). Study participants found the services approachable but the healthcare system complex. Transparency of services—for example, a written list of therapy services and locations—supported navigating the healthcare system. A potential solution to help patients and caregivers navigate the complex healthcare system is the introduction of a liaison, a patient navigator, which will be discussed in a later section. The participants accepted the healthcare services rendered as they were culturally relevant, and the participants identified they wanted additional psychological services for the frail patients and caregivers (Kurpas et al, 2018).

Availability and accommodation were barriers to healthcare access for the participants. They believed physiotherapy and rehabilitation to be beneficial, but the availability of those services was limited (Kurpas et al, 2018). In addition, patients and providers had concerns about the appropriateness of services, especially for individuals with complex medical conditions. All patients from the study identified frustration with the affordability and inequity of care (Kurpas et al, 2018). The implications of this study can inform occupational therapists as part of the primary care services assisting frail older adults and their caregivers through advocacy efforts.

McIntyre and Chow (2020) also examined access to primary healthcare services and found that patients often had to wait more than 1 day for a primary care appointment, as opposed to being scheduled the same day. Waiting for services as a barrier demonstrated a lack of approachability, acceptability, and availability of care. The five dimensions of access are important considerations to address when the occupational therapist completes evaluations and provides interventions to older adult patients within the primary healthcare setting.

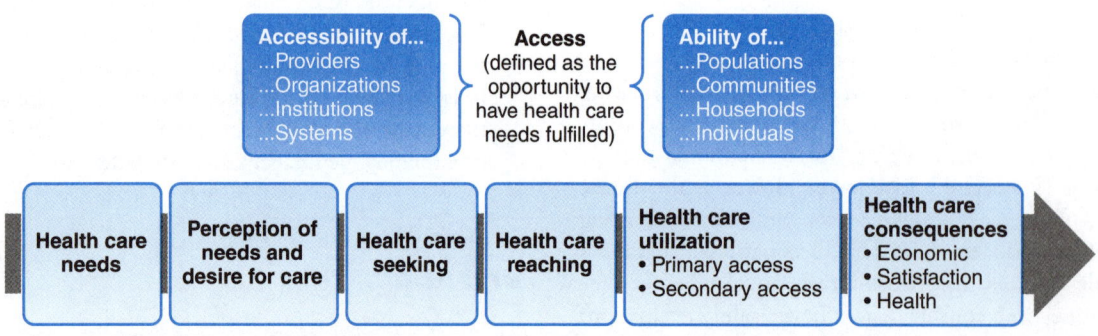

FIGURE 23-1 A definition of access to healthcare. *(Reprinted with permission from Jean-Frederic Levesque.)*

Occupational Therapy Approach and Primary Healthcare

Occupational therapy practice in primary healthcare in underserved populations will now be explored, as the concepts are applicable when working with older adults and to the five dimensions of access as described earlier. Sit and colleagues (2022) completed a scoping review of occupational therapy practice in underserved primary healthcare settings.

Their results found five approaches:

1. Patient-centered approach for goal setting and intervention
2. Team collaboration that may include interprofessional or interdisciplinary collaboration
3. Holistic focus approach was used by the therapist to understand client factors and used a health promotion approach
4. Inclusion of program outcome and standardized program evaluation measures
5. Innovative service delivery to improve access to services

It is important to understand access to healthcare from the perspective of the older adult. The occupational therapist can contribute to a team-based approach to identify barriers to access and to help the use of healthcare resources in the primary healthcare setting.

The Expanded Chronic Care Model

Older adults are at an increased risk of chronic diseases, including dementia, heart disease, type 2 diabetes, arthritis, and cancer (CDC, 2022). Occupational therapists in primary care have the opportunity to implement interventions using a chronic disease management approach to service the needs of the older adult population (AOTA, 2022). It is important for occupational therapists to understand how older adults access primary care services, but it is also important to know how to implement chronic disease management in this setting.

The **Chronic Care Model** (CCM) is an example of an approach to improve chronic disease management (Barr et al, 2003) and includes four components: (1) self-management support, (2) delivery system design, (3) decision support, and (4) clinical information systems. Quality improvement teams in primary care that focused their attention on the CCM had a positive effect on the care of patients with diabetes, including decreased levels of HbA_{1c} and decreased rates of smoking (Barr et al, 2003). Primary care providers are incentivized through reimbursement to use the CCM to help patients navigate the healthcare system (Reddy et al, 2020). There was an increased use of chronic care management codes between 2015 and 2018 with Medicare patients who have chronic conditions (Reddy et al, 2020). Coordinated care for individuals with chronic conditions is becoming prioritized and supports occupational therapy integration into the primary care team.

The Expanded Chronic Care Model (ECCM) (Fig. 23-2) was proposed in an effort to broaden the CCM through the integration of population health promotion with the prevention and management of chronic disease (Barr et al, 2003).

The ECCM supports the intrinsic role social determinants of health have in influencing individual, community, and population health and demonstrates clear associations between healthcare systems and the community (Barr et al, 2003). Table 23-1 describes components of the ECCM (Barr et al, 2003).

The ECCM comprises two sections. The two ovals in Figure 23-2 represent the community and the health system (Barr et al, 2003; p. 77). These two sectors have a porous line between them to represent the flow of ideas, resources, and people between the community and the healthcare system (Barr et al, 2003; p. 77). The four circles of self-management support, decision support, delivery system design, and information systems are placed on this line to reflect the integration and impact of these areas on the community and the health system (Barr et al, 2003). The proposed outcomes of the ECCM, which include individual, community, and population health outcomes, are reflected in the rectangle flanked by the two ovals at the bottom of model (Barr et al, 2003). This component of the model represents improved outcomes as a product of the prepared proactive practice team and the informed activated patient (Barr et al, 2003). Achieving these outcomes requires positive and productive interactions and relationships among individual community members, healthcare professionals, organizations, and community groups (Barr et al, 2003).

The ECCM and the Healthcare Professional

Occupational therapists in primary care need to consider how the services they provide align and integrate with self-management support, decision support, delivery system design, and information systems. Occupational therapists need to think broadly to identify how links with community organizations and resources that focus on both social services and health services may facilitate the delivery of care and how to maximize available resources to assist patients in reaching their rehabilitation goals. Patient navigation is an example of how occupational therapists can use the ECCM to guide the functional assessment of older adults in primary care.

Patient Navigation

The integrated care model is more comprehensive than discharge planning post-hospitalization; it is an approach to providing communication among different health entities to assist older adults who have complex needs (Kokorelias et al, 2022). A patient navigator uses an integrated care approach that stems from the ECCM and can be used for the older adult population. The ideal patient navigator should be easily accessible, have good communication skills, and have a flexible personality to meet the needs of their patients (Kokorelias et al, 2022). **Patient navigation** embraces the concept of interaction between the community, which can

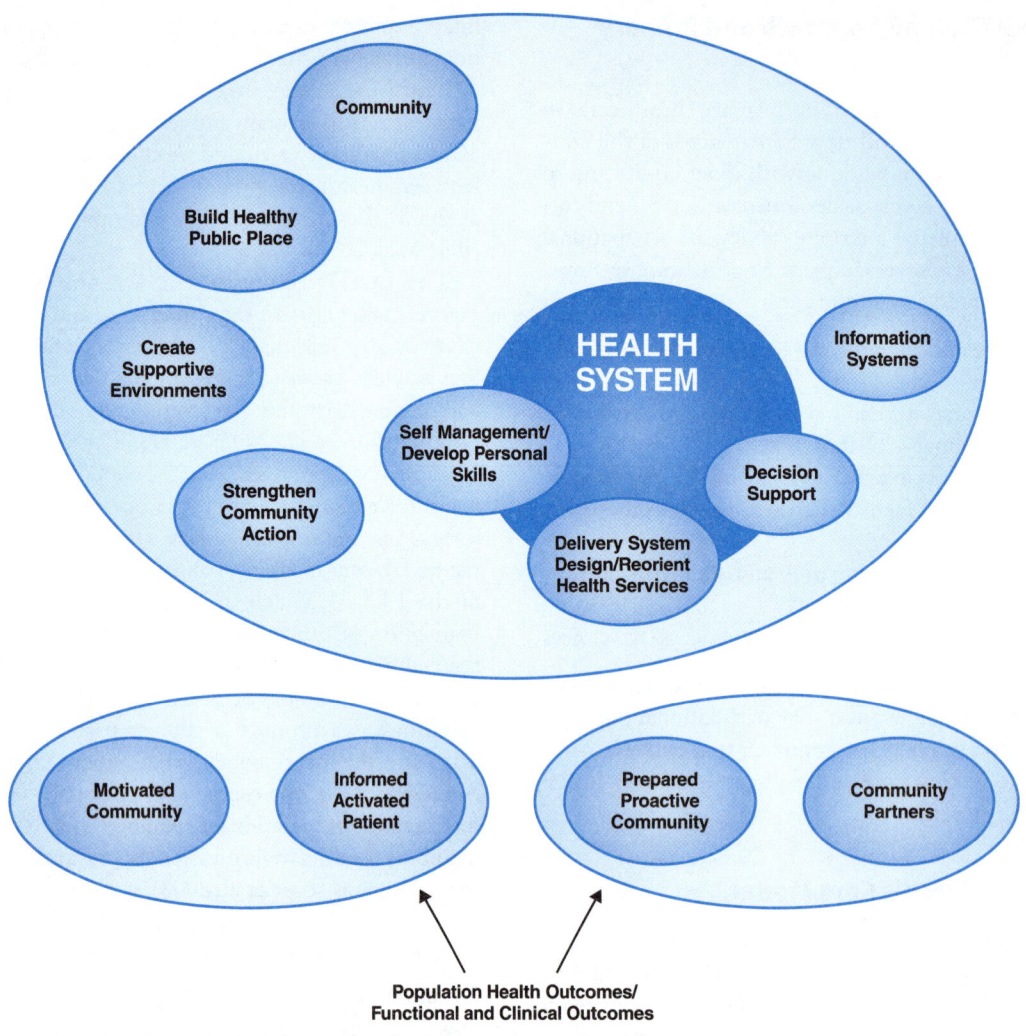

FIGURE 23-2 The Expanded Chronic Care Model. *(From Barr et al, 2003.)*

include an individual and their family, and the healthcare system (Kokorelias et al, 2022). For successful patient navigation, occupational therapists need to maintain a current inventory of available community resources that can be used to help older adults identify and access services (Kokorelias et al, 2022). As part of self-management principles, occupational therapists help older adults select and follow up with resources that the older adult perceives to be of value to their functional status.

Roles for Interprofessional Partners

Role of Occupational Therapy

Occupational therapists have many roles when working in primary care settings, and as research emerges, the roles continue to evolve and become more complex (AOTA, 2020a). The roles of the occupational therapist are dependent on the needs of the population and specialization of the primary care practice. Occupational therapy roles are multilayered and can evolve over time, especially as the primary care practice gains a better understanding of the services offered by an occupational therapist.

Personality characteristics are an important feature of the occupational therapist entering the primary care clinic. Koverman and colleagues (2017) identified the five-personality trait theory as a contributing factor to a successful program implementation: extroversion, agreeableness, conscientiousness, emotional stability, and openness to experience. Another identified contributing factor to successful program implementation was the adaptability of the occupational therapist. Occupational therapists adapt their approach depending on the particular provider's personality to increase the number of referrals and help establish rapport (Koverman et al, 2017).

A unique contribution of occupational therapy within a primary care team is a focus on the assessment and management of function as it relates to ADLs that are meaningful to the patient (AOTA, 2020a; 2020b). Occupational therapists are skilled in evaluating and providing interventions to enable the patient to participate in meaningful occupations, thereby increasing their function (AOTA, 2020a). Occupational therapists examine an individual holistically and

TABLE 23-1 ■ The Components of the Expanded Chronic Care Model

COMPONENTS OF THE EXPANDED CHRONIC CARE MODEL		EXAMPLES
Self-management/develop personal skills	Enhancing skills and capacities for personal health and wellness	■ Smoking prevention and cessation programs ■ Seniors walking programs
Decision support	Integration of strategies for facilitating the community's abilities to stay healthy	■ Development of health promotion and prevention best practice guidelines
Delivery system design/reorient health services	Expansion of mandate to support individuals and communities in a more holistic way	■ Advocacy on behalf of (and with) vulnerable populations ■ Emphasis on quality improvement of health and quality-of-life outcomes, not just clinical outcomes
Information systems	Creation of broadly based information systems to include community data beyond the healthcare system	■ Use of broad community needs assessments that take into account: ■ Smoking bylaws ■ Walking trails ■ Reductions in the price of whole wheat flour
Create supportive environments	Generating living and employment conditions that are safe, stimulating, satisfying, and enjoyable	■ Maintaining older people in their homes for as long as possible ■ Working toward the development of well-lit streets and bicycle paths
Strengthen community action	Working with community groups to set priorities and achieve goals that enhance the health of the community	■ Supporting the community in addressing the need for safe, affordable housing

From Barr et al (2003).

provide well-rounded interventions to help promote meaningful participation in occupations (AOTA, 2020b; Sit et al, 2022). It is important to educate primary care team members, including all members of the interprofessional team, on occupational therapy interventions in relation to function. For example, the medical assistant may historically educate the patient on medication management; however, the occupational therapist can evaluate and provide interventions that are patient specific to foster successful medication management. An occupational therapist may perform a cognitive screen and identify whether the patient has memory deficits and recommend the patient set an alarm when they are supposed to take medication to help promote medication compliance.

The roles of occupational therapists working in primary care will now be described. As occupational therapists integrate and establish themselves as part of the primary care team, their roles may expand and change. It is important for the occupational therapist to periodically reflect on their roles on the team and update their practice evaluations and interventions appropriately.

Generalist

An occupational therapist may work as a generalist in the primary care setting, as they are well equipped to work with a variety of diagnoses and with populations across the life span (AOTA, 2020a; Dahl-Papolizio et al, 2017; Koverman et al, 2017). Occupational therapists have a broad educational background, and the type of referral they see may differ from patient to patient (Royeen, 2020). Older adults may have a wide array of health conditions and concerns; the occupational therapist may need to implement a variety of interventions with a focus that may range from rehabilitation to health promotion and prevention of disease.

Consultant

As a consultant, the occupational therapist evaluates the patient, identifies interventions, and makes appropriate program recommendations as needed (Dahl-Papolizio et al, 2017). The occupational therapist may perform an evaluation or screening but not provide direct patient care services within the primary care setting due to reimbursement or time limitations (AOTA, 2020). For example, an occupational therapist may work at a PCMH and complete a screening to identify whether follow-up services are appropriate to refer the patient to outpatient or home healthcare (AOTA, 2020a). In addition, the occupational therapist may participate in team meetings, plan of care meetings, and other interprofessional aspects of care (AOTA, 2020a). The opening quote in this chapter is from a geriatric provider describing the role of the occupational therapist in their office. That occupational therapist serves as a consultant with a specific focus on function and is an example of the value an occupational therapist contributes to the primary care team.

Interprofessional Partners

There is potential for several different healthcare professionals to work in the primary care setting, including a medical doctor, nurse practitioner, osteopathic doctor, physician assistant, medical assistant, social worker, case manager, psychologist, occupational therapist, physical therapist, speech-language therapist, nutritionist, orthotist, geneticist, and pharmacist. The specific members of the primary care team will depend on the type of clinic and volume of patients seen. Team-based care is an aim in healthcare reform that involves healthcare professionals working together in the primary care setting to provide patient care (Vogt & Vogt, 2017).

The definition of team-based care is:

> The provision of health services to individuals, families, and/or their communities by at least two health providers who work collaboratively with patients and their caregivers—to the extent preferred by each patient—to accomplish shared goals within and across settings to achieve coordinated, high-quality care (Mitchell et al, 2012, p. 5).

Team-based care can also be referred to as "collaborative, team-based, interdisciplinary, multidisciplinary, multiprofessional, and interprofessional" (Vogt & Vogt, 2017, p. 26). The ultimate goal of team-based care is to provide the best services to patients through a collaborative patient-centered approach.

Integration of Occupational Therapy Within the Primary Care Team

Occupational therapists must understand the roles of the interprofessional team in their primary care setting for team performance. Mitchell and colleagues (2012) describe the importance of establishing clear roles: "There are clear expectations for each team member's functions, responsibilities, and accountabilities, which optimize the team's efficiency and often make it possible for the team to take advantage of the division of labor, thereby accomplishing more than the sum of its parts" (p. 9).

Integration of occupational therapy within the primary care team often requires education of team members, providers, residents, students, and other patient care providers about the occupational therapy scope of practice (Royeen, 2020). Designated space within the team charting room provides opportunities to consult with other team members on specific topics, conference on individual cases, provide advice and clinical expertise, provide assistance with assessments of patients, and review special assessments or interventions. Advocacy efforts are critical to integrating into the primary care team (Royeen, 2020).

In a pilot program, an occupational therapist adopted an "intrusionary occupational therapy" approach when starting programming in a geriatric primary care clinic (Koverman et al, 2017). Intrusionary occupational therapy is an approach that involves entering the office with confidence and assertiveness to take initiative to provide occupational therapy services to the patients while collaborating with the provider; the occupational therapist is also respectful and cognizant of not overstepping boundaries (Muir, 2014). In the pilot program, the occupational therapist came prepared with equipment and handouts that could be used for interventions. The occupational therapist was well prepared to evaluate and treat patients in front of the providers (Koverman et al, 2017).

Specific Issues for Working With Older Adults

Patient-Centeredness in Primary Care

A combination of factors necessitates healthcare delivery system reforms. Common factors across the globe include unsustainable public and private healthcare spending growth, increased prevalence of chronic health conditions, and a rising demand for healthcare services due to the aging population. Occupational therapy's focus on health promotion and disease prevention with a collaborative team-based approach supports the ideal of primary care and occupational therapy working together toward holistic and patient-centered care that can help overcome these challenges (AOTA 2020a; Halle et al, 2018; Sit et al, 2022). Patient-centered care ensures the patient's values help guide the decision-making process (Agency for Healthcare Research and Quality, 2022).

The following are important considerations from a clinical standpoint when working as an occupational therapist with the older adult population in the primary healthcare setting.

Chronic Conditions

Occupational therapists are skilled in working with individuals who have chronic conditions (AOTA, 2020a). Occupational therapists are skilled in function, as previously identified, by examining roles, routines, and habits of individuals (AOTA, 2020a; 2020b). This skill is also valuable when evaluating and providing interventions for patients who have chronic conditions (AOTA, 2020a; Leland et al, 2017). Occupational therapists can contribute to a team-based approach when evaluating and treating individuals with chronic conditions to help foster positive changes in their disease management. A self-management agenda has been adopted as a solution to address the rise in chronic health conditions and aging population, and occupational therapists can contribute to self-care management interventions (AOTA, 2020a). Occupational therapists are increasingly integrating the chronic disease management approach into their practice (Kearney et al, 2021).

Multimorbidity

Multimorbidity is the presence of two or more chronic conditions (Zheng et al, 2021). Modern medicine has increased life expectancy, and as a result, the number of older adults living with multimorbidity is increasing in the United States (Zheng et al, 2021). It is estimated that 81% of Americans age 65 years and older have multimorbidity (Buttorff et al,

2017). Multimorbidity is rising not only in the United States but also in other parts of the world (Zheng et al, 2021). Multimorbidity can have a negative impact on an individual's functioning and increase their risk of death and disability (CDC, 2022).

Behavioral Health

Occupational therapists working in primary care may play an important role in addressing the behavioral health of older adults. Occupational therapists are skilled in evaluating and providing patient-centered interventions to the person from a holistic perspective. Occupational therapists may provide interventions related to life stressors or change of health circumstances (AOTA, 2020a; Dahl-Popolizio et al, 2017).

Assessment and Intervention Exemplars

Standardized assessments help support program outcomes through documentation and reimbursement, monitor progress over time, and promote advocacy efforts (Sit et al, 2022). Performance-based evaluation measures are important to implement, as using a functional assessment demonstrates occupational therapy's unique contribution to the primary care team. Older adult patients and family members may be receptive to occupational therapy interventions more readily if occupational deficits are identified through performance-based measures.

Functional Assessment

Researchers have advocated that function should be assessed as a primary health outcome for older adults in primary care settings (Nicosia et al, 2020). Functional status is central to maintaining independence. The relationship between a person's physical function and overall health status will inform the healthcare team in assessing functional status and improving care for older adults.

Occupational therapists can work as part of a team-based approach to perform frailty evaluations to further establish and identify the patient's functioning level. Frailty with regard to geriatric medicine is "older adults at an increased risk for future poor clinical outcomes such as development of disabilities, dementia, falls, hospitalizations, institutionalization, or increased mortality" (Van Kan et al, 2010, p. 275). Components of frailty that can be assessed by the primary care team, including the occupational therapist, include gait speed, hand grip strength, fatigue, weight loss and low energy expenditure, cognition, and disability (Van Kan et al, 2010). Evidence on gait speed shows that it can be used as a measure of mobility disability and health status, as changes in gait or walking speed are predictive of the onset of further disability and dependency (Schaber, 2019). In addition, Bohannon (2019) identified grip strength is an adequate predictive biomarker for outcomes such as generalized strength and function, bone mineral density, fractures, falls, nutritional status, disease status, cognition, depression, sleep, and mortality.

The following assessments focus on ADL and IADL evaluation that can be used independently in the primary care setting or as part of a holistic frailty assessment. The Barthel Index for ADLs is a standardized assessment and measures functional independence by examining ADLs and mobility on level surfaces and stairs (Mahoney & Barthel, 1965). The Lawton Instrumental Activities of Daily Living Scale examines older adults' ability to complete tasks such as using the telephone, shopping, food preparation, housekeeping, laundry, transportation, medication management, and financial management and takes approximately 10 to 15 minutes to administer (Graf 2006; Lawton & Brody 1969). Assessments of the patient's functional performance in ADLs and IADLs are imperative to foster successful participation in ADLs and IADLs in the home environment. (For more information on ADLs and IADLs, refer to Chapters 14 and 15 respectively; for more comprehensive information about frailty, refer to Chapter 7.)

Depression, driving, and caregiver education are additional considerations when assessing function. The occupational therapist assesses the patient for depression to identify functional deficits. If the patient has depression, the occupational therapist can collaborate with the case manager or social worker to identify additional supports the patient may need for healthy aging in place. (For more information on depression, refer to Chapter 13.) Driving screening and safety is another identified area of expertise for occupational therapists practicing with older adults in primary care (AOTA, 2020a). Driving is an important IADL that should not be overlooked, as there are great safety concerns with driving. (See also Chapter 19.) Often family will be present in the primary care setting. This is an opportunity for the occupational therapist to engage in caregiver education and training as appropriate (AOTA, 2020a). (See also Chapter 20.)

Cognition

When working with the older adult population, it is imperative the occupational therapist consider whether cognition could be contributing to occupational disruption. The Montreal Cognitive Assessment (MOCA) is a comprehensive assessment that evaluates for mild cognitive impairment and requires approximately 10 minutes to administer (Nasreddine et al, 2005). The MOCA can help guide the occupational therapist as to what types of supports are needed for the patient from an IADL perspective, including bill payment, medication management, and driving. If cognitive deficits are noted, the occupational therapist may need to collaborate with the case manager or social worker to identify additional supports the patient may need for healthy aging in place. (For more information regarding cognitive evaluation, please refer to Chapter 13.)

Lifestyle Interventions

Occupational therapists working in primary care settings are in a central position to understand an older adult's concept of health and health-related goals because they are in contact with patients over a course of months or years, potentially as often as the provider is. Occupational therapists who practice in primary care settings should address modifiable risk factors associated with lifestyle, such as smoking, sleep, stress, depression, exercise, and activity levels. Many of these issues can be raised during the patient interview and discussion of the presenting problem, which may be sustained or worsened by these risk factors.

An intervention styled after the Lifestyle Redesign® program was offered to community-dwelling older adults with and without disabilities (Levasseur et al, 2022). The primary components of Lifestyle Redesign® are identifying and implementing realistic goals and changes in activity, developing strategies to overcome identified barriers, and encouraging changes in daily routines to promote participation in meaningful activities (Clark et al, 2015). All participants lived at home and were split into two groups: one without disabilities (n = 10) and another group with mild to moderate physical or cognitive disability (n = 7). The intervention program consisted of 12 modules based on the Well-Elderly Study that included occupation, health and aging, and transportation (Clark et al, 2015). Overall, the lifestyle redesign intervention was beneficial to both groups (Levasseur et al, 2022).

Occupational therapists addressing lifestyle redesign interventions with older adults need to be able to interact effectively with individuals while respecting the individual's values and priorities. Health coaching and motivational interviewing (MI) are two approaches that may be useful to address lifestyle issues with patients in primary care.

Health Coaching and Motivational Interviewing

Health Coaching

Health coaching encourages patients to change their behaviors by examining choices and barriers to facilitate positive changes and improve their health (Kivela et al, 2014). Health coaching is founded on several well-established schools of behavior change: self-efficacy (Bandura, 1997), the transtheoretical model (Prochaska & Velicer, 1997), and MI (Miller & Rollnick, 2013). Health coaching is an established method used to support patient self-management to sustain behavior change and associated health-related outcomes to help individuals achieve their goals (Long et al, 2019).

Collaborative care in the clinical encounter between the therapist and the older adult can be enhanced by using an approach that considers the patient's clinical needs, priorities, and values. A guide to how this approach can be implemented is outlined by O'Connor et al (2008). (See Figure 23-3.)

Motivational Interviewing

MI is a collaborative goal-oriented style of communication used to strengthen an individual's intrinsic motivation by exploring their reason for change. The clinician uses an accepting and compassionate approach to help to effectively elicit change in the patient's thought processes (Miller & Rollnick, 2013). It is important for the clinician using MI to engage with the patient as an equal and not as an authority (Prescott, 2020). MI is complex in nature, and the occupational therapist may require further education to implement it effectively in practice (Prescott, 2020).

Primary Clinician's Role
To diagnose the patient's clinical needs, discuss options, screen for decisional and implementation difficulties, and refer to coach as needed

Goal
Informed decision making based on clinical priorities and patient's priorities and values

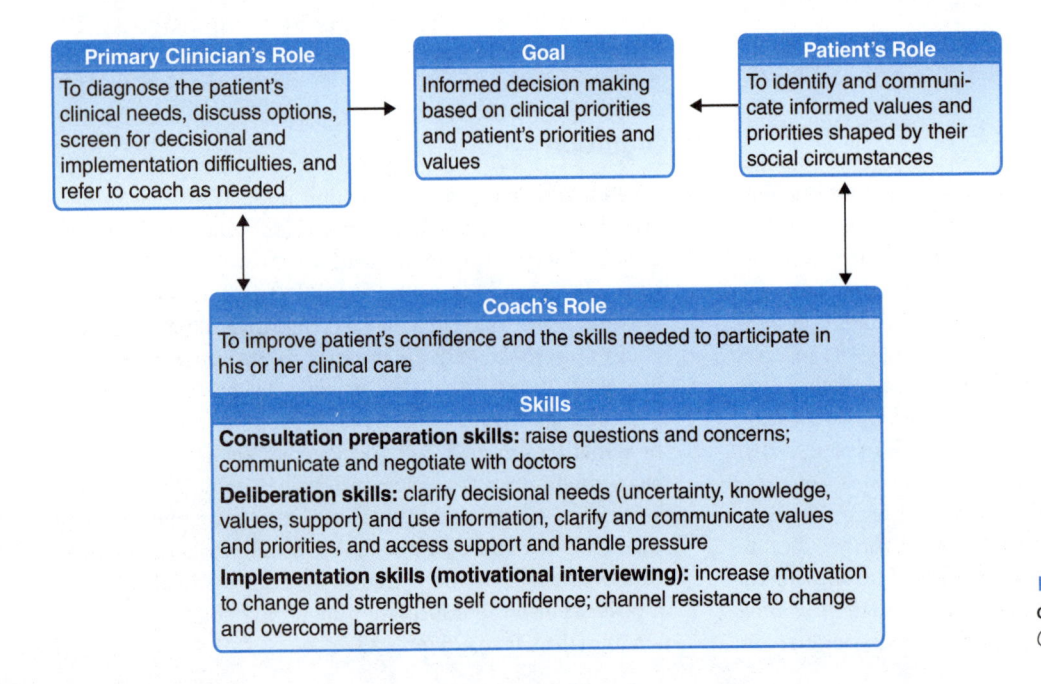

Patient's Role
To identify and communicate informed values and priorities shaped by their social circumstances

Coach's Role
To improve patient's confidence and the skills needed to participate in his or her clinical care

Skills
Consultation preparation skills: raise questions and concerns; communicate and negotiate with doctors
Deliberation skills: clarify decisional needs (uncertainty, knowledge, values, support) and use information, clarify and communicate values and priorities, and access support and handle pressure
Implementation skills (motivational interviewing): increase motivation to change and strengthen self confidence; channel resistance to change and overcome barriers

FIGURE 23-3 A coach's role in collaborative management. *(From O'Connor et al, 2008.)*

Research studies support the use of MI when working with older adults with various conditions. Poudel and colleagues (2020) completed a study on the effects of MI on adults age 58 to 79 years old with heart failure. The systematic review found an improvement in self-care behaviors, exercise capacity, quality of life, prevention of hospital admissions, and behavioral health. Harvey and colleagues (2018) conducted a randomized control pilot study on frail older adults age 65+ living in sheltered housing in Ireland. The intervention groups completed three 40-minute, face-to-face MI sessions with a physiotherapist. The sessions helped to reduce fall risk and improve lower extremity strength in both intervention groups (Harvey et al, 2018). In summary, occupational therapists working in primary care may use MI as an approach and communication style when working with older adults.

Behavioral Health Intervention Approach

Occupational therapists can contribute to a team-based approach by addressing the behavioral health aspects of a patient. Acceptance and commitment therapy (ACT) is a mindfulness-based approach occupational therapists can use in the behavioral health settings, as well as primary care settings. Promoting Best Practice 23-1 describes ACT in more detail and provides a case example reviewed in the literature.

PROMOTING BEST PRACTICE 23-1
Acceptance and Commitment Therapy (ACT)

In a case study described by Koverman and colleagues (2017), an occupational therapist was evaluating a 72-year-old patient with a diagnosis of hypertension, cerebral vascular accident, and depression in a geriatric primary care setting. During the evaluation, the occupational therapist noted the patient's deficits included visual loss related to glaucoma, decreased balance, memory loss, and noncompliance with outpatient physical therapy (Koverman et al, 2017). The interventions focused on ADLs and family education to support IADLs (Koverman et al, 2017). The occupational therapist also attempted to educate the patient on visual compensatory techniques, but the patient was reluctant (Koverman et al, 2017). Therefore, the occupational therapist, who had experience working in behavioral health, used an ACT approach and encouraged the patient to accept the visual deficits, as this would give her an increased sense of independence if she was willing to implement the visual compensatory strategies (Koverman et al, 2017). ACT is a mindfulness-based concept and is composed of six core principles: defusion, acceptance, contact with the present moment, observation of self, values, and committed action (Harris & Hayes, 2009). The overarching goal of ACT is for patients to move toward self-acceptance through compassion toward themselves related to uncontrollable conditions or events that occur in the patient's life. In addition, the patient will strive toward committed action to achieve the type of meaningful life they would like to live (Harris & Hayes, 2009).

The patient was receptive to the conversation, and the occupational therapist also informed the provider of the ACT-based intervention that occurred (Koverman et al, 2017).

Chronic Disease Self-Care Management

Chronic disease self-care management is beneficial when addressing individuals with chronic conditions (Kearney et al, 2021). Self-management occurs when an individual is able to manage their symptoms, treatments, and lifestyle changes while collaborating effectively with family, community, and healthcare professionals. It is important for occupational therapists to be aware of their patients' cultural beliefs surrounding their particular health condition(s) (Richard & Shea, 2011). Self-management can include managing symptoms, medication management, goal-setting, problem-solving, promoting behavior change, effective communication, emotional regulation, adjustment, lifestyle modification to develop new habits and routines, and IADL participation (Kearney et al, 2021).

Evidence-based occupational therapy–led self-care interventions with individuals who have chronic conditions is growing. OPTIMAL, an occupational therapy–led self-management support program, is designed to address the challenges in a primary care setting of living with multiple chronic conditions (Garvey et al, 2015). The OPTIMAL intervention, a 6-week community-based program that focused on problems associated with managing multimorbidity, consisted of weekly group meetings in local community health centers; peer support; goal-setting and prioritization based on patient preferences; and occupational therapy interventions, including:

- Self-management
- Fatigue and energy management
- Managing stress and anxiety
- Maintaining mental health and well-being
- Keeping physically active
- Healthy eating
- Managing medications
- Effective communication strategies

A significant improvement in frequency of activity participation, perceptions of activity performance and satisfaction, self-efficacy, independence in daily activities, and quality of life was found. Additionally, the intervention group had significantly higher levels of goal achievement after the intervention (Garvey et al, 2015). This intervention approach was used again in Ireland for adults who have multimorbidity (Gillespie et al, 2022). The intervention was beneficial in increasing quality-adjusted life years and beneficial from a cost-effectiveness perspective, which has potential to address overall healthcare expenditure (Gillespie et al, 2022).

A randomized controlled trial conducted by Garrison and colleagues (2020) recruited adults age 18 and older who had hypertension and/or type 2 diabetes. The intervention group received the Integrative Medication Self-Management

Intervention to improve medication adherence. The results found both the control and experimental groups improved medication adherence and HbA$_{1c}$ scores, but occupational therapy had a unique effect on the intervention group and warrants further study (Garrison et al, 2020).

A Lifestyle Redesign® randomized control trial was conducted with individuals age 18 to 75 years old, English- or Spanish-speaking, with diabetes and an HbA$_{1c}$ above 9.0% (Pyatak et al, 2020). The intervention focused on providing Lifestyle Redesign® occupational therapy (LR-OT) diabetes management as part of an interdisciplinary team at a primary care clinic (Pyatak et al, 2020). Results suggested that the LR-OT group had beneficial changes in HbA$_{1c}$, diabetes self-care and health status (Pyatak et al, 2020). A Lifestyle Redesign® randomized control trial was conducted on French Canadian community-dwelling older adults age 65 to 90 years old (Levasseur et al, 2019). The study included participants with and without a disability. The results found that participants in LR-OT had beneficial changes to mental health, leisure interest, social participation, and mobility. This research supports the use of a health promotion approach when working with older adults with and without chronic conditions.

Documentation, Payment Systems, and Reimbursement

Documentation within the EMR in primary care is similar to other practice areas. Occupational therapists must document services rendered in a way that supports reimbursement. Because this is an emerging area of practice in the United States, reimbursement may be denied, so advocacy is important. This can occur with thorough documentation, which may be required for successful reimbursement. The occupational therapist should use standardized assessments and document the rationale and results of the standardized assessments. Documentation can be used as a tool to monitor progress over time and as a way to advocate for occupational therapy services for patients. Occupational therapists documenting in a patient's EMR can have positive effects for the patient and primary care practice, and positively impact the interprofessional team (Koverman et al, 2017).

The primary care service delivery model may determine which reimbursement model the primary care practice and/or occupational therapist are using (AOTA, 2020a). Therapists seeking reimbursement must comply with their code of ethics along with regulatory boards on state and national levels (AOTA, 2020c; Koverman et al, 2017). Occupational therapists need to understand how to bill for their services to ensure payment and to sustain their practice in primary care offices. There are two primary reimbursement models: fee-for-service and value-based payment. Fee-for-service reimbursement is similar to occupational therapy billing in outpatient care. Fee-for-service occurs when the occupational therapist bills for occupational therapy services rendered in the primary care setting using the appropriate CPT codes. Koverman and colleagues (2017) described a successful program of fee-for-service billing in a geriatric primary care setting, wherein the occupational therapy practitioner bills for services provided in the geriatric clinic. Dahl-Papolizio and colleagues (2017) completed a study on billing occupational therapy services in primary care and developed a business case scenario where an occupational therapist billed for services during a simulated day working in the primary care office. Examples of CPT billing codes were provided, and potential revenue was found that offset the costs of an occupational therapist working in the primary care practice (Dahl-Poplizio et al, 2017).

Value-based payment is another common reimbursement model in the United States (AOTA, 2020a). Value-based payment is reimbursed by quality of care compared with quantity of care in fee-for-service payment (AOTA, 2020a). An example of a value-based payment system is the Veterans Affairs Home Based Primary Care model, in which an occupational therapist is part of an interprofessional team that provides primary healthcare services in veterans' homes (AOTA, 2020a; U.S. Department of Veterans Affairs, 2020). There are other reimbursement models identified by occupational therapists working in primary care. Table 23-2 describes different types of reimbursement models found by 11 occupational therapists practicing in the United States in 2019 (Royeen, 2020). Faculty practice, grant-funded practices, and student-run clinics are models of practice with their own respective reimbursement models. A consideration for these models is the sustainability aspect of programming; they may only last for a certain length of time if they are grant dependent or have limited hours based on a faculty member's availability.

International Reimbursement and Models

Reimbursement models for occupational therapists working in primary care vary by country (Bolt et al, 2019). In Canada, occupational therapists can work as part of a family health team in which the occupational therapists focus on function as part of an interprofessional team that includes providers, nurses, social worker nurses, and potentially other healthcare team members (Donnelly et al, 2014) and are paid as part of the overall service. A survey of the Council of Occupational Therapists for European Countries conducted by Bolt and colleagues (2019) found the most common payment source for occupational therapists working in primary care was health insurance, followed by self-pay, and "payment systems of the municipality and other (government, general taxation, public system and private providers)" (Bolt et al, 2019, p. 4).

Advocacy for Patients and Services

The practice of occupational therapists working in primary care has progressed and evolved over the past decade. Primary care is now included in the educational curriculum for entry-level practice for both occupational therapists and

TABLE 23-2 ■ Reimbursement Models for Occupational Therapy Practitioners in Primary Care (Royeen, 2020)

REIMBURSEMENT MODELS

Billing for Services: Billing for services. Including Medicare and non-Medicare patients. Non-Medicare patients have had some denials, but through advocacy (speaking with insurance company), reimbursement does occur after the bill has been denied intermittently. Also includes Veterans Affairs services.

Faculty Practice: Occupational therapy services are not billed; services are provided as part of a faculty practice.

Grant Funding: Funding for occupational therapy services in a primary or specialty clinic is from a grant.

Student-Run Clinic: OTD students completing research within a primary care or specialty care clinic, not reimbursed for services.

Reprinted with permission from Lydia Royeen.

---

occupational therapy assistants. Occupational therapists are beginning to conduct research and have an increased presence in primary care settings. The progression of this emerging area of practice came through advocacy of occupational therapy services and advocating to provide the best care to patients by offering access to occupational therapy services.

To advocate for this practice area for both the progression of the profession and to provide the best care to patients, occupational therapists can:

- Join state or territory and national organizations that work to support occupational therapy in the primary care setting. These organizations help to advance this practice area by providing comprehensive information and resources to practitioners and advocating through legislature. In addition, occupational therapists in primary care can connect and network through these organizations.
- Participate at local and national conferences for occupational therapists and related professions and share their unique perspective of primary care practice and research through publications, poster sessions, blogs, or magazines.
- Educate primary care providers and appropriate team members about the occupational therapy interventions provided to patients (Koverman et al, 2017). Use standardized assessments to create measurable processes and outcomes when practicing in primary care.
- Provide a brief oral explanation of their services in the primary care setting to a variety of stakeholders, including primary care team members, patients, and caregivers. The explanation may need to be tailored to a specific setting, but it should not limit the occupational therapy practitioner to a narrow scope of practice.
- Educate all students and residents through 1:1 communication or by conducting in-services on occupational therapy's role across the continuum of care, including the primary care setting.

CASE STUDY (CONTINUED)

Intervention in the Context of a Primary Care Setting

Dr. Ruiz completes a "warm handoff" with the occupational therapist, Nancy. The warm handoff includes Dr. Ruiz introducing Nancy to Ms. Jaramillo and explaining that Nancy will help Ms. Jaramillo with overall functioning. Nancy takes Ms. Jaramillo into the adjacent examination room and introduces herself. Nancy completes an occupational profile and gathers the information identified earlier by completing an occupational profile. Nancy identifies several areas of concern: back and hip pain, caregiver burden, falls, meal planning/nutrition, and self-care management, as Ms. Jaramillo has hypertension and prediabetes and often forgets to take her medication.

Nancy needs to prioritize her time with Ms. Jaramillo and takes the following steps.

1. Nancy has Ms. Jaramillo complete the Geriatric Depression Scale (GDS), which Ms. Jaramillo completes in 7 minutes. After Ms. Jaramillo is finished, she shares she has had a loss of interest in things she used to enjoy and has trouble sleeping due to repetitive stressful thoughts. Ms. Jaramillo feels overwhelmed taking care of her husband while working full time.

2. Nancy educates Ms. Jaramillo on fall-prevention interventions, especially bathroom safety. Nancy recommends a tub/shower bench, as Ms. Jaramillo has a tub/shower combination. Ms. Jaramillo has finite resources, so Nancy gives her a list of durable medical equipment (DME) organizations that have donated equipment she could obtain free or at a reduced cost. (Ms. Jaramillo's insurance does not cover bathroom DME.)

3. Nancy has Ms. Jaramillo complete a medication management activity, and Ms. Jaramillo demonstrates no difficulty. Nancy also completes the MOCA, and Ms. Jaramillo scores a 29/30, only missing one of the words for delayed recall. Ms. Jaramillo states she doesn't feel like she has any difficulties with her memory. Nancy determines Ms. Jaramillo misses medication because she doesn't prioritize herself. Therefore, Nancy discusses different medication-adherence strategies, self-care management strategies, and goal-planning with regard to medication adherence.

4. Nancy educates Ms. Jaramillo on adaptive techniques for ADLs and IADLs while following body mechanics due to her hip and back pain. Nancy is able to issue a reacher and long-handled bath sponge to Ms. Jaramillo.

5. Nancy educates Ms. Jaramillo on caregiver burden and the importance of identifying and participating

in activities that are important to her. They discuss available support that could potentially decrease caregiver burden, including talking to the social worker about respite services and asking their daughter about coming three times a week.

When Nancy is finished completing her evaluation and follow-up interventions, Nancy, Dr. Ruiz, and Ms. Jaramillo meet in the original examination room. Mr. Jaramillo is also present with the permission of Ms. Jaramillo.

Nancy discusses the following recommendations with Dr. Ruiz and Ms. Jaramillo:

1. See a counselor, psychologist, or psychiatrist for possible depression, as she scored a 13/15 on the GDS, which is indicative of depression. In addition, she has caregiver burnout and avoidant behaviors that are concerning to Nancy.
2. Obtain a shower chair to prevent future falls in the bathroom and implement fall-prevention techniques that were taught in the therapy session in day-to-day life.
3. Improve medication management through the use of strategies identified in the occupational therapy session.
4. Outpatient physical therapy to address her back and hip pain
5. Addressing possible respite services with the social worker to assist with Mr. Jaramillo's caretaking
6. Seeing a nutritionist to assist with meal planning
7. Continue occupational therapy in the primary care setting to address self-care management, medication adherence, meal planning, mindfulness education to address potential depression, leisure exploration, and follow up on ADL/IADL performance and fall-prevention techniques.

Dr. Ruiz agrees with Nancy's recommendations and puts in the appropriate orders. Dr. Ruiz will see Ms. Jaramillo again in 12 weeks. Nancy asks Ms. Jarmillo to schedule at least four follow-up appointments to address their plan of care. Nancy will update Dr. Ruiz on the occupational therapy sessions as appropriate over the next month. If Ms. Jaramillo continues to have difficulty with medication adherence, Dr. Ruiz will be notified and may schedule an appointment sooner.

Questions

1. What issues might Nancy expect to address in reimbursement?
2. What other occupation-centered assessment and intervention can be used in the primary care setting to address Ms. Jaramillo's priorities?
3. What interprofessional interventions would you expect to be part of the care plan?
4. What components need to come together for the ideal discharge (e.g., psychological, physical, relational)?

Answers

1. This is a colocated model, in which the occupational therapist provides services within the primary care office alongside the provider. Ideally, the provider can perform a warm handoff, in which the provider introduces the occupational therapist and the overall purpose of the occupational therapy evaluation alongside the occupational therapist. This would most likely be a fee-for-service model, as the occupational therapist would bill for an occupational therapy evaluation and any relevant treatment CPT codes. The process of setting up billing could be a potential issue, and these processes need to be set up and confirmed with the billing department before the evaluation. In addition, the provider must place an occupational therapy referral in the EMR before the occupational therapy evaluation. The patient will have to pay for equipment out of pocket if it is not covered by insurance.
2. In addition to obtaining the occupational profile, the occupational therapy practitioner can complete the Barthel Index of ADLs, the Lawton Instrumental Activities of Daily Living Scale, and the Canadian Occupational Performance Measure to help identify the client's priority areas and establish overall functioning.

    Interventions related to fall-prevention education are imperative for the client; a tub/bench may prevent future injuries. Educating the client on adaptive ADL and IADL techniques is also beneficial. Ms. Jaramillo can use the reacher she was issued for item retrieval from the floor and distal reaching to don her underwear and pants. Self-care management for multimorbidity is also a special consideration for older adults and appropriate with Ms. Jaramillo.
3. Collaboration with several interprofessional team members would be beneficial for Ms. Jaramillo during or after her primary care visit. Ms. Jaramillo will follow up with a counselor, psychologist, or psychiatrist to address her suspected depression and caregiver burnout. She will follow up with a physical therapist in the outpatient setting to address her hip/back pain. Dr. Ruiz will follow up with Ms. Jaramillo regarding her laboratory values and to ensure she is following up with the services at her next scheduled visit. The social worker will help connect Ms. Jaramillo with respite services so she can have caregiver relief. The outpatient nutritionist will assist with educating Ms. Jaramillo on how to meal plan and the importance of it. The occupational therapist will follow up

with Ms. Jaramillo on her plan of care and act as a patient navigator. If an unexpected issue arises, she can contact Dr. Ruiz immediately.

4. Discharge in this sense is the promotion of healthy aging in place. Ms. Jaramillo needs psychological, physical, and social supports for healthy aging in place. Psychological support would address her GDS score and ideally prevent further behavioral health symptoms that would negatively affect her function. Physical supports would help decrease her fall risk (e.g., use of cane, DME recommendation of tub/bench, follow-up occupational therapy/physical therapy in outpatient) and improve performance of ADLs and IADLS (e.g., medication management). Social supports would help address her caregiver burnout and depression, provide meal assistance, and potentially enable her to return to playing bridge with her friends.

SUMMARY

Occupational therapists working with a primary care team have a unique role in assessing and addressing older adult function. As the population ages and the prevalence of chronic conditions rises, occupational therapists, with their educational background, knowledge, and skills, are well poised to play key roles in maximizing the functional independence of older adults. Occupational therapists strive to promote participation in valued occupations for patients in the primary care setting. Occupational therapists can take on a variety of roles in the primary care setting that may evolve as the primary care team members become more aware of the value occupational therapy can bring to the multidisciplinary team and expands. By identifying measurable outcomes and using them in clinical practice, occupational therapists can establish the value of occupational therapy practice in primary care settings to external stakeholders. Telehealth and technology can also be considered when treating older adults as part of a primary care practice. Occupational therapy practitioners have the potential to bring great value to the primary care team to ultimately best serve the patients' needs.

Critical Thinking Questions

1. If you were an occupational therapist in a primary care practice of 17,000 older adult patients, why would you advocate monitoring changes in function to the director? How would you measure patient improvement? [LO 23-7]

2. Why is the occupational therapist's role in the primary care setting complex, and how does it evolve over time? [LO 23-3]

REFERENCES

Agency for Healthcare Research and Quality. (2022, December). *Six domains of healthcare quality*. Department of Health and Human Services. https://www.ahrq.gov/talkingquality/measures/six-domains.html

American Academy of Family Physicians. (2023). *Medical home*. https://www.aafp.org/about/policies/all/medical-home.html

American Occupational Therapy Association. (2018). AOTA position paper: Telehealth in occupational therapy. *American Journal of Occupational Therapy, 72*(Supplement_2), 7212410059p1-7212410059p18. https://doi.org/10.5014/ajot.2020.74S3001

American Occupational Therapy Association. (2020a). Role of occupational therapy in primary care. *American Journal of Occupational Therapy, 74*(Suppl. 3), 7413410040p1-7413410040p16. https://doi.org/10.5014/ajot.2020.74S3001

American Occupational Therapy Association. (2020b). Occupational therapy practice framework: Domain and process (4th ed.). *American Journal of Occupational Therapy, 74*(Suppl. 2), S1–S87.

American Occupational Therapy Association. (2020c). AOTA 2020 occupational therapy code of ethics. *American Journal of Occupational Therapy, 74*(Supplement_3), 7413410005p1-7413410005p13. https://doi.org/10.5014/ajot.2020.74S3006

American Occupational Therapy Association. (2022). Occupational therapy's role in chronic conditions. *American Journal of Occupational Therapy, 76*(Supplement_3), 7613410220. https://doi.org/10.5014/ajot.2022.76S3003

Bandura, A. (1997). *Self-efficacy: The exercise of control*. New York, NY: W. H. Freeman.

Barr, V. J., Robinson, S., Marin-Link, B., Underhill, L., Dotts, A., Ravensdale, D., & Salavaris, S. (2003). The expanded chronic care model: An integration of concepts and strategies from population health promotion and the chronic care model. *Hospital Quarterly, 7*, 73–82.

Bohannon, R. W. (2019). Grip strength: An indispensable biomarker for older adults. *Clinical Interventions in Aging, 14*, 1681–1691. https://doi.org/10.2147/cia.s194543

Bolt, M., Ikking, T., Baaijen, R., & Saenger, S. (2019). Occupational therapy and primary care. *Primary Health Care Research & Development, 20*, e27. https://doi.org/10.1017/s1463423618000452

Buttorff, C., Ruder, T., & Bauman M. (2017). *Multiple chronic conditions in the United States*. Santa Monica (CA): RAND Corporation. https://www.rand.org/content/dam/rand/pubs/tools/TL200/TL221/RAND_TL221.pdf?%3E

Centers for Disease Control and Prevention. (2022). *Promoting health in older adults*. National Center for Chronic Disease Prevention and Health Promotion (NCCDPHP). https://www.cdc.gov/chronicdisease/resources/publications/factsheets/promoting-health-for-older-adults.htm

Clark, F., Blanchard, J., Sleight, A., Cogan, A., Florindez, L., Gleason, S., & Vigen, C. (2015). *Lifestyle Redesign®: The intervention tested in the USC well elderly studies (2nd ed.)*. American Occupational Therapy Association Press.

Dahl-Popolizio, S., Rogers, O., Muir, S. L., Carroll, J., & Manson, L. (2017). Interprofessional primary care: The value of occupational therapy. *The Open Journal of Occupational Therapy, 5*(3). https://doi.org/10.15453/2168-6408.1363

Donnelly, C. A., Brenchley, C., Crawford, C., & Letts, L. (2014). The emerging role of occupational therapy in primary care. *Canadian Journal of Occupational Therapy, 81*, 51–61. doi: 10.1177/0008417414520683

Doraiswamy, S., Jithesh, A., Mamtani, R., Abraham, A., & Cheema, S. (2021). Telehealth use in geriatrics care during the COVID-19 pandemic—a scoping review and evidence synthesis. *International Journal of Environmental Research and Public Health, 18*(4), 1755. https://doi.org/10.3390/ijerph18041755

Garrison, T., Schwartz, J., & Moore, E. (2020). Effect of occupational therapy in promoting medication adherence in primary care: A randomized control trial. *The American Journal of Occupational Therapy, 73*(3), 7703205040. https://doi.org/10.5014/ajot.2020.74s1-po5403

Garvey, J., Connolly, D., Boland, F., & Smith, S. M. (2015). OPTIMAL. An occupational therapy led self-management support programme for people with multimorbidity in primary care: A randomized controlled trial. *BMC Family Practice, 12,* 59–68. doi: 10.1186/s12875-015-267-0

Gillespie, P., Hobbins, A., O'Toole, L., Connolly, D., Boland, F., & Smith, S. (2022). Cost-effectiveness of an occupational therapy-led self-care management support programme for multimorbidity in primary care. *Family Practice, 39,* 826–833. doi.org/10.1093/fampra/cmac006

Graf, C. (2006). Functional decline in hospitalized older adults. *The American Journal of Nursing, 106*(1), 58–68. https://doi.org/10.1097/00000446-200601000-00032

Groote, W. (2019). Concept changes and standardized tools in *community-based* rehabilitation. *Physical Medicine and Rehabilitation Clinics of North America, 30*(4), 709–721. doi: 10.1016/j.pmr.2019.07.013

Halle, A., Mroz, T., Fogelberg, D., & Leland, N. (2018). Occupational therapy and primary care: Updates and trends. *American Journal of Occupational Therapy, 72*(3), 7203090010p1-7203090010p6. https://doi.org/10.5014/ajot.2018.723001

Harris, R., & Hayes, S. C. (2009). *Act made simple: A quick-start guide to Act basics and beyond*. New Harbinger Publications Inc.

Harvey, J., Chastin, S., & Skelton, D. (2018). Breaking sedentary behaviour has the potential to increase/maintain function in frail older adults. *Journal of Frailty Sarcopenia Falls, 3*(1), 26–31. doi: 10.22540/JFSF-03-026

Health Resources & Services Administration [HRSA]. (2018, May). *Federally qualified health centers.* https://www.hrsa.gov/opa/eligibility-and-registration/health-centers/fqhc/index.html

Kearney, P., Watford, P., & Sutton, K. (2021). *Self-management interventions for people with diabetes.* [Critically Appraised Topic.] American Occupational Therapy Association.

Kivela, K., Elo, S., Kyngas, H., & Kaarianen, M. (2014). The effects of health coaching on adult patients with chronic diseases: A systematic review. *Patient Education and Counseling, 97*(2), 147–157. doi: 10.1016/j.pec.2014.07.026

Kokorelias, K., DasGupta, T., & Hitzig, S. L. (2022). Designing the ideal patient navigation program for older adults with complex needs: A qualitative exploration of the preferences of key informants. *Journal of Applied Gerontology: The Official Journal of the Southern Gerontological Society, 41*(4), 1002–1010. https://doi.org/10.1177/07334648211059056

Koverman, B., Royeen, L., & Stoykov, M. (2017). Occupational therapy in primary care: Structures and processes that support integration. *The Open Journal of Occupational Therapy, 5*(3). https://doi.org/10.15453/2168-6408.1376

Kurpas, D., Gwyther, H., Szwamel, K., Shaw, R., D'Avanzo, B., Holland, C., & Bujnowska-Fedak, M. M., (2018). Patient-centred access to health care: A framework analysis of the care interface for frail older adults. *BMC Geriatrics, 18,* 273. https://doi.org/10.1186/s12877-018-0960-7

Lawton, M. P., & Brody, E. M. (1969). Assessment of older people: Self-maintaining and instrumental activities of daily living. *The Gerontologist, 9*(3 Part 1), 179–186. https://doi.org/10.1093/geront/9.3_part_1.179

Leland, N. E., Fogelberg, D. J., Halle, A. D., & Mroz, T. M. (2017). Occupational therapy and management of multiple chronic conditions in the context of health care reform. *American Journal of Occupational Therapy, 71,* 7101090010p1-7101090010p6. https://doi.org/10.5014/ajot.2017.711001

Levasseur, M., Filiatrault, J., Larivier, N., Trepanier, J., Levesque, M. H., Beaudry, M., Parisien, M., Provencher, V., Couturier, Y., Champoux, N., Corriveau, H., Carbonneau, H., & Sirois, F. (2019). Influence of Lifestyle Redesign® on health, social participation, leisure, and mobility of older French-Canadians. *American Journal of Occupational Therapy, 73*(5), 7305205030p1-7305205030p18. https://doi.org/10.5014/ajot.2019.031732

Levasseur, M., Levesque, M. H., Lacasse-Bedard, J., Lariviere, N., Filiatrault, J., Provencher, V., & Cornveau, H. (2022). Feasibility of Lifestyle Redesign® for community-dwelling older adults with and without disabilities: Results from an exploratory descriptive qualitative clinical research design. *Australian Occupational Therapy Journal, 69*(5), 514–535. doi: 10.1111/1440-1630.12807

Levesque, J. F., Harris, M., & Russel, G. (2013). Patient-centred access to healthcare: Conceptualizing access at the interface of health systems and populations. *International Journal for Equity in Health, 12*(18). https://doi.org/10.1186/1475-9276-12-18

Long, H., Howells, K., Peteres, S., & Blakemore, A. (2019). Does health coaching improve health-related quality of life and reduce hospital admissions in people with chronic obstructive pulmonary disease? A systematic review and meta-analysis. *British Journal of Health Psychology, 24*(3), 515–546. https://doi.org/10.1111/bjhp.12366

Mahoney, F. I., & Barthel, D. W. (1965). Functional evaluation: The Barthel Index. *Maryland State Medical Journal, 14,* 61–65.

McIntyre, D., & Chow, C. (2020). Waiting time as an indicator for health services under strain; a narrative review. *Inquire, 57,* 1–15. doi: 10.1177/0046958020910305

Miller W. R., & Rollnick S. (2013). *Motivational interviewing: Helping people change.* 3rd ed. New York: The Guilford Press.

Mitchell, P., Wynia, M., Golden, R., McNellis, B., Okun, S., Webb, C. E., Rohrbach, V., & Von Kohorn, I. (2012). *Core principles & values of effective team-based health care* [Discussion paper]. Institute of Medicine, Washington, DC. https://doi.org/10.31478/201210c

Mirza, M., Gecht-Silver, M., Keating, E., Krischer, A., Kim, H., & Kottorp, A. (2020). Feasibility and preliminary efficacy of an occupational therapy intervention for older adults with chronic conditions in a primary care clinic. *The American Journal of Occupational Therapy, 74*(5), 7405205030p1-7405205030p13. https://doi.org/10.5014/ajot.2020.039842

Monaghesh, E., & Hajizadeh, A. (2020). The role of telehealth during COVID-19 outbreak: A systematic review based on current evidence. *BMC public health, 20*(1), 1193. https://doi.org/10.1186/s12889-020-09301-4

Muir, S. (2014, April 3-6). *OT as primary care: Health care systems change* [Conference session]. American Occupational Therapy Association 94th Annual Conference & Expo, Baltimore, MD, United States. https://www.aota.org/~/media/Corporate/Files/Practice/OT-as-Primary-Care.PDF

Murphy, R. P., Dennehy, K. A., Costello, M. M., Murphy, E. P., Judge, C. S., O'Donnell, M. J., & Canavan, M. D. (2020). Virtual geriatric clinics and the COVID-19 catalyst: A rapid review. *Age and Ageing, 49*(6), 907–914. https://doi.org/10.1093/ageing/afaa191

Nasreddine, Z. S., Phillips, N. A., Bédirian, V. Ã., Charbonneau, S., Whitehead, V., Collin, I., Cummings, J. L., & Chertkow, H. (2005). The Montreal Cognitive Assessment, MOCA: A brief screening tool for mild cognitive impairment. *Journal of the American Geriatrics Society, 53*(4), 695–699. https://doi.org/10.1111/j.1532-5415.2005.53221.x

Nicosia, F., Spar, M., Neumann, A., Silvestrini, M., Barrientos, M., & Brown, R. (2020). "The more they know, the better care they can give": Patient perspectives on measuring functional status in primary care. *Journal of General Internal Medicine. 35*(10), 2947–2954. doi: 10.1007/s11606-020-06075-8

O'Connor, A.M., Stacey, D., & Légaré, F. (2008). Coaching to support patients in making decisions. *BMJ, 336,* 228–229. doi: 10.1136/bmj.39435.643275.BE

Pape, S. B., & Muir, S. (2019). Primary care occupational therapy: How can we get there? Remaining challenges in patient-centered medical homes. *The American Journal of Occupational Therapy, 73*(5), 7305090010p1-7305090010p6. https://doi.org/10.5014/ajot.2019.037200

Patient-Centered Primary Care Collaborative. (2019). Investing in primary care: A state-level analysis. https://www.pcpcc.org/sites/default/files/resources/pcmh_evidence_report_2019.pdf

Poudel, N., Kavookjian, J., & Scalese, M. J. (2020). Motivational interviewing as a strategy to impact outcomes in heart failure patients: A systematic review. *The Patient-Patient-Centered Outcomes Research,* 13, 43–55. https://doi.org/10.1007/s40271-019-00387-6

Prescott, D. (2020). Motivational interviewing: As easy as it looks? *Current Psychiatry Reports, 22*(7), 35. https://doi.org/10.1007/s11920-020-01158-z

Prochaska, J. O., & Velicer, W. F. (1997). The transtheoretical model for behavior change. *American Journal of Health Promotion, 12,* 38–48.

Pyatak, E., King, M., Vigen, C. L. P., Salazar, E., Diaz, J., Schepens Niemiec, S. L., Blanchard, J., Jordan, K., Banerjee, J., & Shukla, J. (2020).

Addressing diabetes in primary care: Hybrid effectiveness-implementation study of lifestyle redesign occupational therapy. *American Journal of Occupational Therapy, 73*(5), 7305185020p1-7305185020p12. https://doi.org/10.5014/ajot.2019.037317

Raj, M., Iott, B., Anthony, D., & Platt, J. (2022). Family caregivers' experiences with telehealth during COVID-19: Insights from Michigan. *The Annals of Family Medicine, 20*(1), 69–71. https://doi.org/10.1370/afm.2760

Rayner, J., Muldoon, L., Bayoumi, I., McMurchy, D., Mulligan, K., & Tharao, W. (2018). Delivering primary health care as envisioned: A model of health and well-being guiding community-governed primary care organizations. *Journal of Integrated Care, 26*(3), 231–241. https://doi.org/10.1108/JICA-02-2018-0014

Reddy, A., Marcotte, L., Zhou, L., Fihn, S., & Liao, J. (2020). Use of chronic care management among primary care clinicians. *The Annals of Family Medicine, 18*(5), 455–457; doi: https://doi.org/10.1370/afm.2573

Richard, A. A., & Shea, K. (2011). Delineation of self-care and associated concepts. *Journal of Nursing Scholarship, 43*(3), 255–264. https://doi.org/10.1111/j.1547-5069.2011.01404.x

Royeen, L. (2020). Occupational therapy as part of a team-based approach in primary care settings. [Doctoral Dissertation 3563, Western Michigan University.] https://scholarworks.wmich.edu/dissertations/3563

Sanchez-Guarnido, A. J., Dominguez-Macias, E., Garrido-Cervera, J. A., Gonzalez-Casares, R., Mari-Boned, S., & Represa-Martinez, Å. (2021). Occupational therapy in mental health via telehealth during the COVID-19 pandemic. *International Journal of Environmental Research and Public Health, 18*(13), 1–10. doi: 10.3390/ijerph18137138

Schaber, P. (2019). Neurocognitive disorders (dementia). In C. Brown, V. C. Stoffel, & J. P. Munoz (Eds.), *Occupational therapy in mental health* (2nd ed., pp. 250–263). Philadelphia, PA: F. A. Davis Company.

Sclarsky, H., & Kumar, P. (2021). Community-based primary care management for an older adult with COVID-19: A case report. *The American Journal of Occupational Therapy, 75*(Supplement_1). https://doi.org/10.5014/ajot.2021.049220

Sit, W., Wheeler, C., & Pickens, N. (2022). Occupational therapy in primary health care for underserved populations: A scoping review. *Occupational Therapy in Health Care, 30*, 1–24. https://doi.org/10.1080/07380577.2022.2081752

U.S. Department of Veterans Affairs. (2020). Home based primary care. https://www.va.gov/GERIATRICS/pages/Home_Based_Primary_Care.asp

Van Kan, G. A., Rolland, Y., Houles, M., Gillette-Guyonnet, S., Soto, M., & Vellas, B. (2010). The assessment of frailty in older adults. *Clinics in Geriatric Medicine, 26*(2), 275–286. https://doi.org/10.1016/j.cger.2010.02.002

Vogt, H. B., & Vogt, J. J. (2017). Foundations, core principles, values, and necessary competencies of interprofessional team-based health care. *South Dakota Medicine: The Journal of the South Dakota State Medical Association*, 25–28.

World Federation of Occupational Therapists (WFOT). (2014). World Federation of Occupational Therapists' position statement on Telehealth. *International Journal of Telerehabilitation, 6*(1). doi: 10.5195/ijt.2014.6153

World Health Organization & United Nations Children's Fund (UNICEF). (2020). *Operational framework for primary health care: transforming vision into action.* Retrieved from https://www.who.int/publications/i/item/9789240017832

Zheng, D. D., Loewenstein, D. A., Christ, S. L., Feaster, D. J., Lam, B. L., McCollister, K. E., Curiel-Cid, R. E., & Lee, D. J. (2021). Multimorbidity patterns and their relationship to mortality in the US older adult population. *PLoS One, 16*(1), e0245053. doi: 10.1371/journal.pone.0245053

CHAPTER 24

Acute Care Services

Kelly S. Casey, OTD, OTR/L, BCPR, ATP, CPAM

> *"I was terrified when I woke up in the ICU with a tube down my throat and my arms tied down. I didn't believe it when they told me I had a massive stroke. I was devastated at the thought of never holding my granddaughters again, or singing in church. You believed in me, you pushed me, you showed me what was possible, even when I was so sick. You were just as excited as I was when I moved my arm again! It was the simple things like brushing my teeth. You gave me hope for so much more."*
>
> — A 74-year-old woman admitted to the ICU with a large right middle cerebral artery cerebrovascular accident

LEARNING OUTCOMES

By the end of this chapter, readers will be able to:

24-1. Distinguish between healthcare provided in the acute care and intensive care settings.
24-2. Explain the occupational therapist's role in delivering integrated care in the acute care setting.
24-3. Explain how an occupational therapy assessment is conducted in the acute care setting, including the psychosocial impact of the setting.
24-4. Assess common comorbidities older adults often present with while in the hospital.
24-5. Implement interventions for the hospitalized older adult beginning with discharge planning and addressing the patient's care in the hospital and in the future.
24-6. Discuss how acute care services are documented and reimbursed in the United States and the occupational therapist's role in ensuring payment.
24-7. Support the role of occupational therapists in advocating for patients and occupational therapy services.

Mini Case Study

Robert Iglesias, 78 years old, was struck by a car while walking in a parking lot carrying groceries to his car. His wife, who uses a walker, and 10-year-old grandson were with him but were unharmed. He was admitted to the surgical intensive care unit (ICU), with status post-open reduction external fixation of the right tibia, and right subdural hematoma.

Provocative Questions

1. What additional medical information or precautions would you want to know before completing Robert's occupational therapy evaluation?
2. What information would you assume and verify about Robert's prior level of function based on the information you have?
3. At the start of your evaluation, Robert is not responding to your questions. His eyes open briefly then close. What should you do to assess further?

Acute care is the level of care in a hospital setting after a sudden illness, injury, or surgical recovery. Within the acute care setting, older patients are often faced with a devastating new condition or progression of a diagnosis that leaves them feeling fearful and uncertain about their ability to engage in life as they knew it. The acute care hospital setting is fast paced. The focus is on medical management and stabilization in order to progress the older adult to the next level of care, be it rehabilitation or home. Acute care occupational therapists have the unique opportunity to provide support to the patient and their caregivers, prevent further debilitation or disability, and promote a return to normal functioning in everyday tasks and meaningful occupations. Engagement in early mobility and activity is key for older adults' recovery. Occupational therapists in acute care provide hope and support at an often desperate, life-changing time for many older patients.

The Acute Care and ICU Setting

Acute care is a level of healthcare in which a patient is treated for an often brief but severe episode of illness, for conditions that are the result of disease or trauma, and during recovery from surgery. Acute care is generally provided in a hospital by a variety of clinical personnel using technical equipment, pharmaceuticals, and medical supplies. The **ICU** is a department of a hospital in which patients who are critically ill are kept under constant observation. Specialized medical and nursing staff provide critical care and enhanced constant medical monitoring for organ support to sustain life. While in the ICU, best practice includes limiting sedation and encouraging early engagement in activity (Herling et al, 2018). While reducing sedation, patients sometimes need temporary restraints to prevent them from accidental self-harm by pulling out critical life-sustaining lines or airways. Providing the least-restrictive environment by limiting and removing restraints as soon as possible is encouraged to promote recovery. Healthcare provision in acute care and the ICU is fast-paced due to the rapidly changing medical complexity of patients. Patients in acute care often have many lines (e.g., peripheral IV line giving them fluids), drains (e.g., Foley catheter or postsurgical drain) and airways (e.g., nasal cannula, high-flow nasal cannula, ventilator). Patients are often recovering from major injury, surgery, or illness progression. The focus in acute care and the ICU is medical recovery. Early rehabilitation begins in the ICU and acute care settings.

Role of the Occupational Therapist and Interprofessional Partners

Hospitals rely on clinical outcomes to analyze their performance including healthcare spending and quality of care. One clinical outcome is readmission rates, or how often a patient is readmitted to the hospital post discharge. Acute care occupational therapy services decrease hospital readmission rates. A large landmark study highlighted the importance of occupational therapy in the acute care hospital setting (Rogers et al, 2017). In this study, Medicare patients with cardiopulmonary diagnoses were examined. The final sample consisted of 2,761 hospitals for the heart failure analysis, 2,818 hospitals for the pneumonia analysis, and 1,595 hospitals for the acute myocardial infarction analysis. After examining 19 different spending categories, occupational therapy was the only category examined to significantly lower readmissions. Higher spending on occupational therapy demonstrated a statistically significant association with lower readmission rates for all three medical conditions. Occupational therapy is in a critical position to recognize self-care and functional deficits leading to readmissions and can recommend alternative discharge plans. Occupational therapy addresses deficits during the hospital stay and reduces readmissions.

Role of Occupational Therapy in Acute Care

The goal of occupational therapy in acute care is to evaluate, treat, and set a discharge plan early in treatment, with the hopes of successful transition out of the hospital to home or the patient's prior living situation. For patients who are deemed medically stable but still not able to function safely at home, the acute care occupational therapist will help progress them toward a more supportive discharge location such as inpatient rehab. Occupational therapists help patients engage in functional tasks while they are early in the healing and recovery process. Occupational therapists problem-solve, and monitor vitals, medications, and overall changes in physical, cognitive, and psychosocial presentation of older adult patients. Advancing the patient through the medical crisis to the next level of care, such as returning to home or transitioning to inpatient rehabilitation or long-term care, is a primary goal of occupational therapy in the acute care hospital setting.

Interprofessional Integrated Care

Integrated care is key in the rapidly changing, medically complex, acute care setting. Incorporating other disciplines' goals and treatment plan strategies can reinforce recovery and cut down on confusion for patients and loved ones. For example, integrating communication strategies is important for patients recovering from injury or illness. Patients find themselves in the hospital as a result of either a new injury or illness or by the worsening progression of a medical condition. Many times, patients wake up in an unfamiliar environment, attached to lines, drains, or airways. It is critical that each professional who enters the room does so with the utmost healing energy, with the greatest awareness of that patient's medical condition at that time. This can be done by being overtly aware of the care that other professionals are providing to that patient. Utilizing this information within each discipline's interactions is considered interprofessional care.

Interprofessional care is "care provided by a team of healthcare professionals with overlapping expertise and an appreciation for the unique contribution of other team members, working as partners in achieving a common goal" (Donovan et al, 2018, p. 980). This term emphasizes the provision of care by a team with sufficient familiarity and mutual trust in the roles of other team members. In the acute care context, care is provided across disciplinary lines, and, to some extent, roles become shared. Examples include:

Common goals: Interprofessional care can be seen in the example of a patient needing to use a letter board for communication during functional tasks. The speech-language pathologist could be focused on the patient using proper language, word finding, and appropriate back-and-forth accurate responses. The occupational therapist could be focusing on functional communication by using the letter board with index finger isolation while reaching and pointing in preparation for social participation. The occupational therapist and the speech-language pathologist both are using the intervention of the letter board, both are addressing goals that lead to the patient being able to communicate.

Clear, consistent communication: Acute care communication includes written documentation as well as real-time communication via in-person huddles, or messaging via paging system or chat. One example of interprofessional communication is the physical therapist sending a quick message via paging system or instant messenger updating the occupational therapist on strategies that worked for sitting balance during the physical therapy session that day. The occupational therapist could then incorporate strategies such as encouraging anterior pelvic tilt while sitting at the edge of the bed preparing for activities of daily living (ADLs). Another example of interprofessional care is the occupational therapist reviewing the communication strategies the speech-language pathologist has integrated into their care or the dietary restrictions such as thickened liquids with small sips and 1:1 supervision. The occupational therapist can then integrate these goals into a self-feeding session by encouraging reach grasp of the cup using a hemiparetic upper extremity, while supporting the elbow (providing proximal support or stabilization of the arm) and bringing hand to mouth.

Collaboration: The interprofessional team extends beyond the rehabilitation professions of physical therapy, occupational therapy, and speech-language pathology. Occupational therapists collaborate closely with the medical team including the providers, such as physicians, nurse practitioners, and physician assistants. Occupational therapists often look to these medical providers to enter orders for care, such as appropriate occupational therapy consultations, activity orders, or specifics related to the patient's medical case. The providers on the medical team also outline the medical course, diagnosis, prognosis, medications, procedures, and plan of care. All of this can be helpful when the occupational therapist is determining the best therapeutic plan of care, goals, and discharge plan for the patient. Occupational therapists will interact with and rely on many medical professionals during the patient's hospital course.

- *Social workers and case managers* are professionals who work closely with occupational therapists in the acute care hospital setting. Social workers and case managers often have interrelated functions, including assessing the patient's progress with therapy; determining insurance coverage (which is essential for rehabilitation planning); setting up home equipment needs, resources, and supports at home; and helping patients complete applications for insurance or financial assistance.
- *Respiratory therapists* will collaborate on ventilation or airway changes or progression and suctioning needs.
- *Pharmacists* will share medication changes and goals for transitioning to different medications, such as for pain control or anticoagulation. This information will help occupational therapists know medication dosage and timing as well as which laboratory test values to monitor.
- *Rehabilitation aides or rehabilitation technicians* assist therapists by setting up therapy sessions, bringing equipment to the hospital room, transporting patients to the acute care therapy gyms, and assisting with transfers during therapy sessions, supporting the patient during ADLs, and providing reassurance to patients who may be in pain or anxious. Aides within the hospital are key to keeping the day-to-day running.
- *Nursing aides* assist with changing bed linens, performing ADLs and transfers to the bathroom and chair, and performing additional tasks as directed by nursing staff. Often, the occupational therapist communicates with nursing aides to guide recommendations and equipment for feeding or demonstrate safe toilet transfers.
- *Nurses:* Nurses are the most important professionals the occupational therapist will interact with in the acute care setting. Occupational therapists touch base and communicate with nurses early and often when providing occupational therapy interventions within the hospital. Communication occurs in many forms, written via paging systems, electronic documentation in note writing, computer-secure chat features, phone calls, and face-to-face communication. The occupational therapist should speak to the nurse before the session and ask targeted questions related to a patient's care. After reviewing the chart, the occupational therapist needs to elicit information that informs their treatment session plan.

Scenario

"I am from occupational therapy and am planning on treating Mr. Smith this morning by sitting him at the edge of the bed and helping him perform oral care. I read in the chart that he was taken off the ventilator and was changed to high-flow nasal cannula (HFNC) last night. I saw he had some sedatives during ventilator weaning. Has he been awake and alert this morning and tolerating the HFNC? How has his oxygen saturation been?" This provides clear information to the nurse of what the session will entail and gives the occupational therapist the information to grade the session. For instance, if the patient has not been tolerating HFNC well and has been desaturating to 85% and is not able to recover, sitting him at the edge of the bed may not be a recommended goal for the session at this time.

Communication in the Hospital Setting

When providing patient-centered care, it is important to listen to the needs and wishes of the older adult. Being patient centered also means ensuring that the patient understands the questions being asked and the information being given. (Ekdahl et al, 2010). It is essential that occupational therapists communicate directly with the patient first, then reach out to caregivers and other supporters. Providing information and education in a manner that is clear and easy to understand meets the needs of the patient and family. Awareness of the health literacy level of the patient and their caregivers, or the degree to which they are able to understand the information to inform health-related decisions, can guide the level of information given during the hospital stay. Education can include repetition, respectful and age-appropriate tone and complexity, avoiding unnecessary medical jargon, sharing real-life examples of rehabilitation strategies and recommendations, as well as printed education handouts or photos of recommended equipment for home. Not all patients of advanced age need information to be simplified. Many patients simply prefer repetition to ensure they are understanding the information correctly. For example, a 98-year-old retired biology professor, admitted for hip replacement due to avascular necrosis of the femoral head, who still consults for medical firms, likely has a better understanding of medical terminology, or a higher health literacy, than a patient having limited experience with the healthcare system and who may need more simplified yet accurate information presented in several ways.

Ensuring therapists are allowing every opportunity for the older adult patient to be engaged in decision-making is key. Patients have described healthcare as representing an institution of power and thus feeling powerless when admitted (Bláhová et al, 2021). A scoping review found seven key areas for improvement identified by older patients, including care in emergency departments, dignity, nutritional care, satisfaction of patients' needs, pain, respect and decision-making, and spiritual needs (Bláhová et al, 2021). The patients reported feeling lonely, fearful, and neglected, like passive recipients of care instead of active participants in decision-making and daily tasks. Occupational therapy in the acute care setting can highlight the capabilities and strengths of older patients. Occupational therapists can provide strategies and/or equipment, such as propping an elbow on a pillow and using built-up foam and a scoop plate so the patient can engage in self-feeding instead of waiting to be fed by a staff person. Other simple methods to help reinforce dignity around toileting include demonstrating to the nurse how a patient safely transfers via stand pivot to a bedside commode when the patient has expressed self-retention, pain, and embarrassment with being told to use a bedpan. If the patient is not able to fully stand, consider using mobility technology that can assist with a partial stand pivot while supporting the patient safely to a drop-arm bedside commode. Encourage the patient to assist with hygiene using wipes for energy conservation and ensure the patient remains as covered as possible with a gown across their back, curtains pulled, blinds drawn closed, and visitors escorted to the hallway. Refer to Promoting Best Practice 24-1.

PROMOTING BEST PRACTICE 24-1
Theoretical Foundation for Occupational Therapy in the Acute Care Setting

Occupational performance is the outcome of the transaction between the person, environment, and occupation (Weeks, 2016). While several theoretical models support the role of occupational therapy in the acute care setting, consider the Person-Environment-Occupation (PEO) model for a patient in the ICU or acute hospital setting. Personal factors could include critical illness, fatigue, weakness, pain, anxiety, delirium, shortness of breath, loss of roles (e.g., primary income earner, childcare provider, writer, etc.). Consider the environment in the ICU or acute hospital room. Various kinds of medical equipment could be beeping or making humming noises, or the room could be dark or lit by very bright overhead lights. Issues such as sensory deprivation or sensory overload leading to habituation could be occurring when no one else is in the room. The patient could suffer from impaired sleep–wake cycles, at times being awoke during the night for medication administration or vitals checks, leading to sleeping during the day. The ripple effect includes the inability to participate in therapy or actively engage in ADLs or social conversations, which could impact cognitive and physical functioning.

Consider the occupation. Is it meaningful? Typically, self-care is the first area of occupation addressed, while other areas of occupation such as instrumental activities of daily living (IADLs), productivity, and leisure activities are often overlooked in the ICU and hospital setting (Weeks, 2016). With any area of occupation, the occupational therapist in the hospital setting must modify the task to meet the needs of the patient while encouraging active engagement and the just-right challenge. Use of the PEO model in acute care hospital settings could help guide therapists to recognize that a person's environment has a direct effect on how they perform an occupation. In a study of older people's experiences of acute care hospitalization, Cheah and Presnell (2011) found that the occupations of older people lacked meaning in the hospital environment and that hospitalization was a stressful experience. The use of the model as a framework could help therapists move beyond considering the ability to manage ADLs (Maclean et al, 2012). The PEO model is consistent with treatment planning in acute care, as human behavior and occupational performance cannot be separated from contextual influence.

Occupational Therapy Evaluation in the Acute Care Hospital Setting

The occupational therapy evaluation consists of obtaining a complete occupational profile. This is done through chart review, speaking with the patient's nurse or other team members, speaking with the patient directly, as well as speaking with family members or caregivers (as recognized in the medical record). Speaking directly to the patient allows the patient to be an active participant in their occupational therapy evaluation so that they can provide key information to help determine prior level of function, goals for therapy, and considerations for determining the best discharge recommendations. Additional information can be gleaned during this interview process including screening for possible cognitive impairments or other sensory impairments such as vision or hearing. If the patient is providing inaccurate home set up information or unable to recall certain details of prior level of functioning, a further cognitive screen or assessment should be considered. Older adult patients may present with visual, hearing, speaking, and self-feeding impairments that are not new, but a result of having glasses, hearing aids, or dentures removed during an emergency room admission or before a scheduled procedure or surgery (refer to Chapter 21, Evaluation of the Older Adult).

CASE STUDY

Solveig from Chapter 7 in the context of an acute care setting

Presenting Situation and Assessment

It was 5 p.m. and Solveig was just waking up on the evening of her third day in the medical ICU. As you may recall from Chapter 7, Special Concerns in Care and Prevention, Solveig's daughter Mariane found her at home, confused after falling. Solveig has fallen several times recently, lost a significant amount of weight, has difficulty with medication management, and has tooth pain, poor vision, and urinary incontinence. "We have to get to Bible study, it starts at 5:30. We are going to be late!" Solveig panicked and quickly looked around the room. She tried but was unable to move her arms. Her wrists had straps tying her to the bed. Bilateral wrist restraints had been placed on Solveig during the night because she was delirious and trying to pull out her Foley catheter and her arterial and peripheral IV lines. Solveig had been admitted to the medical ICU straight from the emergency room. Solveig was hallucinating, a common symptom of delirium. Her sleep–wake cycle was off, compounding her delirium and fear. She was dehydrated and septic from a severe urinary tract infection (UTI). The medical team had placed a peripheral IV to provide hydration, an arterial line to accurately and consistently monitor her blood pressure, and a Foley catheter.

Occupational therapy was ordered by the medical team to assess functional ADLs, functional mobility, vision, and cognition. The Confusion Assessment Method for the ICU (CAM-ICU) delirium screen was administered, and the results confirmed Solveig was CAM-ICU positive, or positive for delirium. The occupational therapist asked Solveig to repeat orientation facts three times to encourage encoding and wrote these details on the white board in large print where Solveig could read them from her bed or chair in the room. Mariane brought in several photographs that the team used for reorientation. Advocating for the least restrictive environment and encouraging active patient engagement, the occupational therapist spoke with the providers about removing the restraints as soon as it was deemed safe. The occupational therapist encouraged nursing to challenge Solveig to stay awake and engaged during the day, keeping the blinds open and lights on, and cognitively stimulating her by asking her questions and having her problem-solve simple tasks such as oral care.

Assess Common Comorbidities Often Seen in Hospitalized Older Adults

Geriatric syndromes are multifactorial conditions prevalent in older adults. Geriatric syndromes develop when an individual experiences accumulated impairments in multiple systems that compromise their compensatory ability. Patients with geriatric syndromes are at higher risk for adverse outcomes and functional decline, both during the hospitalization as well as after discharge (Buurman et al, 2011; van Seben et al, 2019). Older hospitalized adults are also at higher risk for being readmitted to the hospital, institutionalization, and death compared their younger counterparts (Buurman et al, 2011; Wang et al, 2014). Geriatric syndromes include cognitive impairment, depressive symptoms, apathy, pain, malnutrition, incontinence, dizziness, fatigue, functional impairment, mobility impairment, fear of falling, and fall risk. Geriatric syndromes such as fatigue, functional impairment, apathy, mobility impairment, and fear of falling (van Seben et al, 2019) are highly prevalent among hospitalized older adults. Older adults who present with any of these geriatric syndromes often experience further deterioration during their hospitalization, as well as continued impairment well past discharge from the hospital (van Seben et al, 2019). It is essential that these syndromes are acknowledged during the occupational therapy evaluation, treated throughout their hospital stay, and proactively planned for to ensure good patient care after hospital discharge.

Hospital-associated deconditioning (HAD) leads to reduced functional performance after an acute hospitalization. Risk factors for HAD include age, nutritional status, mobility, and preadmission functional status, as well as cognitive impairment and depression (Chen et al, 2022). When considering the older adult who is admitted to the hospital, these risk factors are even higher. Up to 40% of older adults experience **delirium** (an acute change in cognition and a disturbance of consciousness, usually resulting from an underlying medical condition) or functional decline, both of which are associated with longer lengths of stay and higher readmission rates (Booth et al, 2019; Hoyer et al, 2014).

HAD is a strong risk factor for mortality, readmission, and institutionalization in the years after the initial hospitalization (Hoyer et al, 2014; van Rijn et al, 2016). For patients admitted to an acute inpatient rehabilitation facility, functional status near the time of discharge from an acute care hospital is strongly associated with acute care readmission, particularly for medical patients with greater functional impairments. Reducing functional status decline during acute care hospitalization may be an important strategy to lower readmissions (Hoyer et al, 2014). Researchers examined community-dwelling older adults 6 months after hospital discharge and found that 43% needed help with medication management, 24% were unable to walk a quarter of a mile, and 45% were unable to return to driving (Dharmarajan et al, 2020). During an acute hospital admission, older adults spend approximately 83% of their time in bed and 12% of their time in a chair (Falvey et al, 2015; Hartley et al, 2018). The physiological effects of bedrest include muscle loss; impaired proprioception and sensation, postural control, and joint coordination; and loss of balance. HAD and frailty are very closely related affecting similar body systems (musculoskeletal, respiratory, urinary), daily functions (sleep–wake cycle, mobility), and cognitive functioning (Chen et al, 2022). One study found that enhanced inpatient programs, including rehabilitation services in acute care, reduced the risk of declining ADL performance by 4% at discharge, reduced institutionalization (nursing home residence) by 8% at 1 month postdischarge, and reduced mortality by 23% (Smith et al, 2020).

Intervention Exemplars

Acute care occupational therapy interventions start with planning for discharge. Knowing the planned disposition after acute care informs the priorities of the therapist. Interventions are specific to the patient's care at the hospital (early mobility and activity, fall prevention, pain management, spirituality) and to future care needs (e.g., skin integrity, assistive technology). Sensory and cognitive abilities are considered in care plans and addressed where needed.

Discharge Planning as Intervention

A primary role of the occupational therapist in the acute care setting is to progress the patient to the next level of care, be it a rehabilitation program or home. Key factors in decision-making around disposition include the older adult's prior level of function, home setup, support at home, including physical assistance (e.g., help standing to get out of the shower and cognitive assistance (e.g., paying bills, taking medications, meal preparation). Additionally, the occupational therapist may recommend specialists posthospital discharge, such as optometry, neuro-ophthalmology, low-vision occupational therapy, vision therapy, or a therapeutic driving assessment. Interventions addressing early mobility and activity, fall prevention, pain management, splinting, vision, and cognition lay the foundation for the safest disposition post hospital discharge. When the medical team has determined that a patient who is recommended for inpatient rehabilitation by therapy is now "medically stable for discharge," the occupational therapist will often provide an additional therapy session and clear documentation to reinforce the need for inpatient rehabilitation after discharge. Having an updated therapy note is often a requirement of insurance.

Early Mobility and Early Activity

Older patients within the ICU are at a great risk of developing and having long-term implications due to **ICU-acquired weakness (ICUAW)** (Rahman et al, 2014). ICUAW is characterized by significant muscle loss, weakness, and even paralysis. Patients with ICUAW have poor outcomes that can have short- and long-lasting effects on overall functional ability and independence as well as increased mortality. The impaired ability to engage in meaningful occupation can be devastating. Older patients often present with reduced muscle mass and a lower level of functional independence than younger patients and are at an even higher risk of decreased strength, impaired function, medical complications, and increased mortality (Rahman et al, 2014). A contributor to ICUAW is critical illness polyneuropathy and myopathy (CIPNM). This muscle-wasting syndrome has implications for both skeletal muscle as well as peripheral nerves. Immobility and disuse atrophy can lead to loss of lean muscle mass and weakness. Older patients often present with lower amounts of lean body mass or lean muscle and decreased strength, which increases the risk of even further muscle atrophy when ill and in the acute care hospital or ICU (Dalton et al, 2012). The accelerated loss of lean muscle mass, decreased muscle function, and decreased strength define sarcopenia (Cruz-Jentoft & Sayer, 2019). The risk of sarcopenia increases with age, affecting as many as 30% of adults over 60 years of age, and 50% of those older than 80 years (Marcus et al, 2012). Sarcopenia is associated with increased adverse outcomes including falls, functional decline, frailty, and mortality. Lean muscle loss can be exacerbated in older patients facing other medical conditions such as sepsis, trauma, surgical recovery, and cancer. Poor nutrition and age are predictors of CIPNM and ICUAW (Schweickert & Hall, 2007). Additional factors compounding muscle loss and CIPNM include hyperglycemia related to diabetes and stress as well as acute respiratory distress syndrome (ARDS) (Dalton et al, 2012; Rahman et al, 2014). Older patients have a higher prevalence of both hyperglycemia and ARDS than younger hospitalized patients. Due to all of these factors, older patients are at a higher risk of ICUAW, leading to poor short- and long-term outcomes, including weakness and decreased ability to engage in meaningful occupations, and increased risk of mortality.

Early mobility is a systematic approach to encouraging patients to be out of bed and engaging in early movement as soon as they are deemed medically stable. Early mobilization can occur within 24 hours into the admission on the acute care hospital units as well as in the ICU. Early mobility is safe and feasible in older adults, even in the oldest categorized populations (>90 years old) (Goldfarb et al, 2021). Early mobilization can improve muscle strength and physical function, prevent disability, decrease rates of deep vein thrombosis, pressure sores, and delirium, and reduce intensive care and hospital length of stay (Castro-Avila et al, 2015). Early mobility is also associated with more older patients being able to discharge to home than to a rehabilitation or long-term care facility. "Bedrest is bad" is a campaign to combat hospital immobility (American Physical Therapy Association, 2019). It clearly articulates that patients lying in bed is not optimal to recovery. Patients should be awake and engaged in physical and cognitive activities, such as performing a stand pivot to a bedside commode instead of using a bedpan for toileting or sitting on the edge of the bed to brush their teeth themselves. When the occupational therapist is addressing early mobility, the goal is to help the patient return to engagement in meaningful activities, not just standing or walking. It is important for the occupational therapist to know how the patient moved around before their admission, if the patient used a device to navigate around their home and, if so, what kind of device they used and where and when they used the device. This information helps the occupational therapist set the goals and interventions for therapy.

Early mobility and early activity are at the forefront of evidence-based practice for therapy in the acute hospital setting. The occupational therapist promotes early mobility through early active engagement in functional activity, such as inbed self-grooming activities (Fig. 24-1). For example, the occupational therapist encourages a patient, while supported in bed, to actively reach for items on the tray table and use bilateral hands at midline to open the toothpaste and apply it to the toothbrush. The patient then flexes their elbow to bring their hand to mouth for brushing and continues the task while holding the arm up. An additional benefit in this example is the cognitive stimulation that occurs by encouraging the patient to plan, select, and complete the task. Deconditioned older adults can also benefit from the occupational therapist addressing activity pacing, which includes energy conservation, work simplification, and grading tasks to meet the patient's needs (Timmer et al, 2020). Patients can be taught active self-management, such as balancing activity and rest, prioritizing activity, delegating activity when needed, and modifying the task to encourage successful engagement in meaningful activities. These strategies can further promote early activity in the hospital setting and hopeful return to prior level of functioning.

Fall Prevention in the Hospital

Falls in older adults are unfortunately very common; approximately one in three older adults report falls (Lakatos et al, 2009). Of those older adults who fall, 20% to 30% sustain moderate to severe injury and 10% do so on multiple occasions (Lakatos et al, 2009; Vaishya & Vaish, 2020). Recurrent falls in older adults result in significant injury, such as a fracture or head injury, as well as increased morbidity and mortality. (Refer to Chapter 7, Special Concerns in Care and Prevention.) Older adults with a history of falls have increased anxiety and fear surrounding the risk of falling. This can affect therapy in the acute care and ICU settings, as occupational therapists often encourage early mobility and activity. Active listening, patience, and reassurance, as well

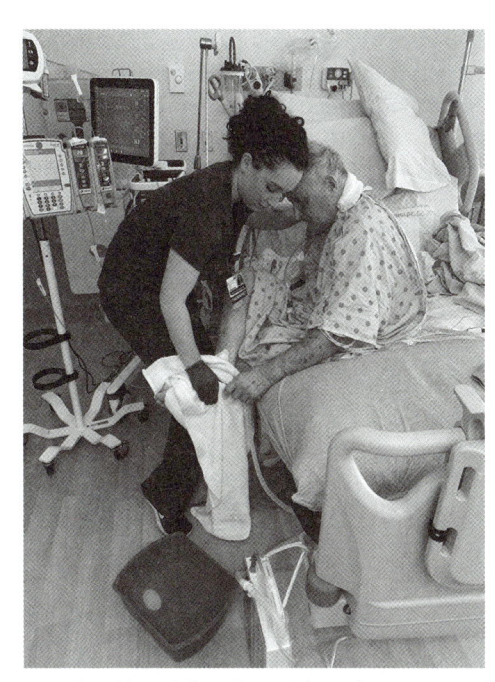

FIGURE 24-1 An older adult patient with tracheostomy on the ventilator sitting at the edge of the bed washing and drying his feet. The occupational therapist is assisting with lower body bathing, upright posture, improving breath support and trunk control and endurance. *(Courtesy of The Johns Hopkins Health System Corporation, with permission.)*

as physical assistance, durable medical equipment, and safe patient handling equipment may help the older adult feel more comfortable attempting to get out of bed in the hospital setting.

In acute care settings, interprofessional teams engage fall prevention programs that involve evaluating fall risk, safe monitoring of hospitalized patients, fall prevention products, and fall prevention interventions. Addressing fall prevention in the acute hospital setting is an ongoing initiative that is prioritized across many healthcare facilities. Most falls in the hospital setting occur in patients over 70 years of age (Lakatos et al, 2009). Older adults who fall while in the hospital setting have a hospital length of stay three times as long as those who do not fall. Many patients who fall in the hospital setting are not able to be discharged home and instead are discharged to a rehabilitation or skilled nursing facility. A significant number of patients who fall in the hospital are experiencing at least some level of delirium. While not completely eliminating fall risk, hospitals that embrace a fall prevention program addressing delirium and other risk factors can help to identify and prevent falls, specifically in the vulnerable older adult population.

Pain Management

Pain is often debilitating and not well managed for older adults in the hospital. It is important to not only document the presence of pain but to note specifics, such as location, onset (acute versus chronic), precipitating factors, alleviating factors, and time, dose, and type of medication. Pain management for hospitalized older adults is often inadequate, especially for those who cannot communicate (Bláhová et al, 2021). (See Promoting Best Practice 24-2 for intervention strategies.)

PROMOTING BEST PRACTICE 24-2
Pain Management

- Repositioning
  - Pillow under the knees to alleviate back pain
  - Rolled towel or sheet beside the head for neck pain due to weak neck muscles
  - Adjusting the bed controls, both head of bed and foot of bed
  - Elevating arms or legs on pillows
- Making recommendations for specialty supports
  - Consider consulting wound care specialists
  - Airflow mattresses
  - Air waffle cushion when in chair
  - Custom crosshatched foam cushion when in chair
- Splinting
  - Soft off-loading boots to float heels and a wedge or kickstand to prevent external hip rotation
  - Soft palm hand splints with finger separators to prevent pain due to increased tone and to protect skin of palm
- Cold or heat packs
  - Used appropriately considering cause of pain, skin integrity
    - Cold often recommended instead of heat near a postoperative incision to decrease inflammation
- Consulting
  - Providers such as physician, nursing
  - Pharmacology
  - Wound care nursing
  - Pain resource team

Skin and Joint Protection

Occupational therapists specialize in orthotics and splinting with the purpose of skin protection and prevention of pressure wounds; prevention of joint contractures or furthering joint contractures; maintaining range of motion (ROM); allowing for healing after wound, injury, or surgery; increasing functional use of weakened limbs; and pain management. As occupational therapists are assessing the patient's motor skills and ROM, they also assess the effect of impaired ROM, weakness, skin integrity, and contracture on functional tasks. Before measuring ROM and manual muscle testing (MMT) with older adults, it is important to be aware of any predisposed conditions or surgeries. When testing ROM and MMT, it is important to avoid excessive force on the joint as older adults are often weaker than their younger counterparts in the hospital (Hunter et al, 1998). However, some older adults are in excellent shape and can withstand heavy resistance during MMT. Strength testing of older adults varies with the individual patient.

It is important to weigh the possible complications of splinting, such as increased pain or skin breakdown, with the proposed benefit, such as contracture management (Riley, 2001). This is especially important with older adults and overall considerations of quality of life. For example, consider a patient who presents with right-sided weakness and increased finger flexor tone and ankle plantar flexor tone after a left middle cerebral artery cerebral vascular accident. The initial plan may be to fit the patient with a resting hand splint and a multipodus boot to be worn 4 hours on and off during the day and continuously at night. When the therapist checks adherence with the plan, the patient reports not sleeping through the night due to the pain in their right hand and ankle as well as impaired ability to attempt to use their right hand or walk during the day when wearing the splints. The aggressive splinting goal of increased ROM must be balanced with pain management, splinting tolerance, sleep quality, and the ability to engage in functional activities. One proposed solution for this case may be to wear the right resting hand splint and right boot on and off every 2 hours during the day when not engaged in functional tasks. At night, the strategy would be to position the right hand with fingers extended on a rolled towel and pillows, as well as positioning pillows at the foot of the bed to encourage dorsiflexion. This would accommodate the need for contracture prevention and skin protection balanced with good sleep quality, pain management, and increased engagement in functional activities.

Loss of muscle mass and bone density exponentially impact the aging population and lead to a higher risk of falls and factures (Padilla Colón et al, 2018). Occupational therapists work closely with other professionals, such as wound care (nursing and physical therapy) and orthopedic providers, who write orders including precautions such as weight-bearing and ROM, as well as the specific angle that they want a joint splinted (e.g., 30 degrees of elbow flexion). An example is an older adult patient who was non-weightbearing on their left leg after total hip arthroplasty or replacement. The patient would not be able to place their foot on the ground at all during transfers. Clinical problem-solving would lead to possible recommendations of a walker and drop-arm bedside commode for lateral stand pivot transfers for toileting. That same patient may also present with "foot drop," or weakness in the ankle dorsiflexors that prevents them from pulling their foot back or lifting the ball of their foot up. This can lead to plantar flexion contractors, or the foot being stuck in a pointed toe position. The occupational therapist might proactively issue a positioning boot (e.g., multipodus or soft off-loading boot). These boots support the position of the ankle in neutral which is 0 degrees dorsiflexion (appears to be at a right angle), and "floats" the heel to enhance blood circulation vital to healing by eliminating friction or pressure on the back of the foot. This is essential for preventing pressure ulcers or wounds on the heels, which can occur after just a few days of immobility in the hospital. Additionally, these boots often have a wedge or kick stand that can help support and position the entire lower leg and prevent external hip rotation (the leg rolling out or being in a "frog-leg" position). Occupational therapists can also add additional pillows lateral to the knee to prevent this from happening. Overall positioning during hospitalization is key to preventing further complications and increasing the likelihood of successful engagement in functional activities.

It is important to check skin integrity regularly when issuing, fabricating, or adjusting splints. This is especially important in older adults, who may have frail or fragile skin, more prone to bruising and skin tears. Additionally, impairments in circulation and mobility can quickly lead to pressure ulcers. Splints should be removed and skin should be checked frequently (e.g., during hygiene, functional activities, exercise, or at least every 4 hours). Any areas of redness, pain, or skin breakage should be measured using the clock method for measuring wounds. The clock method measures the wound length from head to toe (or 12:00 to 6:00) and then width (from 3:00 to 9:00). If there is redness, pain or skin breakage, splints should be removed, and nursing should be notified. In the interim, patients can be positioned using pillows and rolled towels, such as elevating arms and extending digits.

Addressing Visual Impairment

Older adults in the acute care setting often present with a higher risk of preexisting sensory limitations, such as impaired vision or hearing. Many patients may present without their usual aids, such as glasses or hearing aids. Within the fast-paced acute care setting, many areas of sensory processing can be quickly overlooked when distracted by more-obvious medical and physical impairments. Assessing vision within the hospital setting is crucial to patient safety. Visual impairments may be misconstrued as cognitive or behavioral impairments, such as the patient not making eye contact or not looking at what they are being guided to view, or could be misinterpreted as lack of attention. Assessing vision includes baseline visual impairments of which older adults are at an increased risk, such as macular degeneration, which causes blurred or central vision, or simply the need for corrective lenses or glasses that have been removed or misplaced during the hospital stay. To perform a quick, simple screening, ask if the patient wears glasses or contact lenses, and if so what type and when (e.g., bifocals, reading-only). Also ask about vision in the context of functional activity (driving, medication management, leisure activities). It is helpful to give examples instead of asking a broad-based question about vision (e.g., "Do you have blurriness when reading or black spots when using the phone?") Asking the patient to read the clock on the wall, a menu, or a name badge are simple ways to grossly screen vision. Further standardized visual assessments can be used if there is suspected visual impairment.

When in the hospital, vision can be especially affected, leading to fear, higher fall rate, impaired sleep–wake cycle, increased confusion, and delirium (LeLaurin & Shorr, 2019). To prevent falls related to visual impairment, consider the floor type and timing of floor cleaning, remove clutter, add contrast when able (such as dark-colored grip socks on a white floor), and reduce glare. Natural light is very beneficial if the hospital room has windows. Keeping the lights on and blinds open during the day and evening also helps with maintaining a proper sleep–wake cycle that may be upset during the hospital stay (LeLaurin & Shorr, 2019). The exception to that could be patients with severe photophobia, or pain with increased light, after injury, illness, or surgery. Those patients may benefit from careful use of sunglasses and verbal or physical guidance to navigate in a darkened room.

Visual impairments or the lack of visual aids such as glasses, can impact the patient's ability to use bed controls, locate the call button, see who enters the room, select items from the menu, make phone calls (using their personal cell phone or the hospital phone), and sign consent forms. Occupational therapists can engage the patient in functional tasks such as these in the acute care setting, continually reassessing the impact of their vision on function. Occupational therapists can promote proper search patterns, encourage scanning the environment, and incorporate compensatory techniques. One compensatory technique is translucent taping of a lens to accommodate for severe diplopia. Occupational therapists can also focus on remediation of specific new-onset visual impairments, such as homonymous hemianopsia, by placing items within the impaired visual field and encouraging the patient to scan to that side. Possible visual impairment, or lack of visual aids such as glasses, must be considered when assessing other areas of performance, including cognition. Being unable to read or see parts of a standardized cognitive assessment could greatly impact the patient's score. (Refer to Chapter 10, Sensory Systems.)

Addressing Cognitive Impairment

Cognitive impairment is associated with poor hospital outcomes and is common among adults admitted to acute care hospitals (Cameron et al, 2017). Of older adults presenting to the emergency room, 27% have cognitive impairment (Fogg et al, 2018). Older adults with cognitive impairment who are admitted to the hospital are more likely to have extended hospital stays, be readmitted on multiple occasions, or die (Fogg et al, 2018). Of patients 65 years or older, 40% present with a cognitive impairment during the hospital stay (Bickel et al, 2018). Cognitive impairments can be new or chronic. Some medical causes for patients presenting with confusion include abnormal laboratory test values, such as low blood glucose (hypoglycemia) or high white blood cell count (such as with sepsis) or an anoxic brain injury (for those who may have been deprived of oxygen during a medical crisis). Older adults who present with cognitive impairment demonstrate

ADL and IADL dependence at discharge (Cameron et al, 2017; Mitsutake et al, 2021). The more cognitively impaired an older adult is, the more severe the outcomes. Cognitive impairment and delirium have been linked to discharge to postacute care settings rather than home, increased risk of hospital readmission, and increased need for assistance in performing ADLs (Jackson et al, 2016). However, cognitive impairments during hospitalization are often unidentified or undiagnosed (Amini et al, 2019). Acute (new onset) and chronic (long-standing) cognitive impairments are both essential to identify during the hospital stay so that providers can promptly begin addressing functional deficits and safe discharge planning (Pritchard et al, 2019; Rogers et al, 2017). Use of a cognitive impairment screening tool is strongly recommended because cognitive impairment is associated with negative short- and long-term outcomes, including cost and persisting impairment, leading to overall impaired independence, function, and quality of life (Wilcox et al, 2021). (Refer to Chapter 13, Neurobehavioral and Cognitive Impairments.) The occupational therapist is a key healthcare provider in acute care who focuses on screening for, assessing, and treating cognitive impairment (Casey et al, 2023).

Due to the risks of unidentified cognitive impairment in the hospital setting, it is important that cognition is screened and assessed frequently. Maintaining a high level of sensitivity is important when screening a large population for cognitive impairment to be able to identify even minimal cognitive impairment. One screening tool, the AM-PAC Applied Cognitive Inpatient Short Form is a fast, reliable tool with high sensitivity (Andres et al, 2003; Activity Measure for Post-Acute Care, n.d.; Casey et al, 2023). The therapist can complete the tool based on observation of the functional performance of the patient, which is very helpful in the fast-paced environment of the acute care hospital setting. While screening for cognitive impairment is the responsibility of the interprofessional team, the occupational therapist plays a critical role. Acute care occupational therapists screen, assess, and treat cognitive impairment throughout the hospital stay. Occupational therapists may notice small changes or errors that patients may make during functional tasks, such as sequencing a grooming task or selecting the next meal from the menu. It is important to trust that gut feeling of something not being right when the patient laughs off not knowing the answer to some basic questions or diverges and starts rambling about something else instead of attending to the task at hand. The occupational therapist should document this in the medical record, including quotes, and communicate this observation to other members of the medical team. Additionally, the occupational therapist should consider completing formal standardize cognitive screens and assessments. Cognitive assessment and intervention should occur seamlessly throughout the occupational therapy process (Costigan et al, 2019). Occupational therapists in the ICU and acute care settings address delirium prevention and intervention and assess and treat a wide range of cognitive impairments.

Cognitive interventions include activities promoting orientation and executive functioning (Fig. 24-2) as well as ensuring accurate communication by incorporating assistive technology. Refer to Promoting Best Practice 24-3.

PROMOTING BEST PRACTICE 24-3
Delirium

Occupational therapists play a significant role in the identification, prevention, and treatment of delirium. Occupational therapists are viewed as the cognitive specialists focusing on delirium management, arousal, and awareness in the critical care setting (Algeo & Aitken, 2019). One screening tool for delirium is the CAM-ICU (MDCalc, n.d.). With a focus on encouraging patients to actively engage in activity and meaningful occupations, occupational therapists use a systematic approach to the analysis of occupational performance problems (Pozzi et al, 2020). In the sometimes-chaotic environments of the ICU and acute care setting, occupational therapists provide structure by encouraging the patient to engage in simple, habitual self-care tasks, such as brushing their teeth or organizing their self-care routine. By focusing on the intersection of personal, environmental, and occupational factors, occupational therapists address delirium prevention in a unique and meaningful manner.

- Personal factors include physical abilities and limitations, motor planning difficulty, lack of initiative, or cognitive impairment. Examples include:
  - A tremor in their right hand
  - Arthritis in their knees that cause them to buckle when they stand
  - Errors with bill pay and now their adult children have taken over this task to ensure accuracy
- Environmental factors include cultural, values, the role of caregiver, and the hospital setting. Examples include:
  - All one-level home setup and their toilet may be next to the sink, which they can hold to stand.
  - Culturally, it may be important to rest and allow the younger generation to complete all ADLs for them so they can heal.
- Occupational factors include routines, interests, personal choices, motivation, experiences with that occupation, as well as the challenge of task. Examples include:
  - How they complete that task at home. Likely all their oral care supplies are kept in the same location in the right side of the sink.
  - They likely use the same brand of toothpaste and may have for years.
  - Their spouse puts their socks on them every day.

By considering these factors, the occupational therapist reorients the patient and engages them in meaningful activities. By engaging the older adult patient in meaningful tasks, the occupational therapist can prevent and treat delirium in a safe and feasible manner (Pozzi et al, 2020).

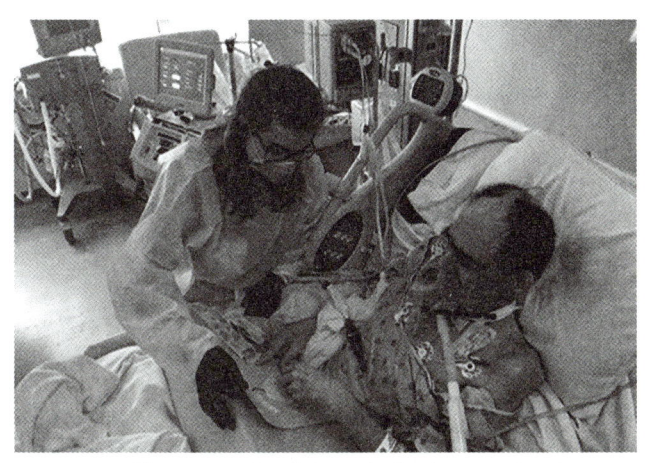

FIGURE 24-2 The occupational therapist having a patient in the ICU perform sticker by number task, using wedge pillow, encouraging sequencing, reaching, using bilateral hands at midline. This patient had previously been an artist and was actively engaged in a task for the first time since being in the hospital. *(Courtesy of The Johns Hopkins Health System Corporation, with permission.)*

Assistive Technology: Considerations for the Older Adult in the Hospital

For older adults who are hospitalized, assistive technology can serve to aid for many new or progressing impairments. High- and low-tech assistive technology options exist. Easy-to-use text-to-speech (e.g., Speech Assistant AAC) or picture-based (e.g., Small Talk Intensive Care or Proloquo2go) communication programs provide simple communication options. An eye-gaze communication system may work well for patients who are unable to speak or move their arms or hands, such as those with a higher-level spinal cord injury, amyotrophic lateral sclerosis (ALS), or an endotracheal tube on a ventilator with weakness or restraints. Older adults may already be using high-tech options that are mass marketed for user-friendly access (e.g., home surveillance systems). Some patients are more engaged in using assistive technology if they are allowed to use their own devices, such as a smartphone or tablet. Lower-tech options, such as the SPEACS program, offer communication options for use in the acute care and ICU settings. (More information on the SPEACS program can be found at https://sites.pitt.edu/~cmh1/happ/index.html.) The SPEACS program is a free program online that provides suggestions for improved patient communication, such as marker boards and markers, reader glasses, voice amplifiers, magnifying glasses, and composition paper and large grasp pens. All of these strategies for functional communication encourage social participation, such as with family video calls. Communication software creates opportunities for self-initiated communication and private conversations that do not require another person in the room. The use of assistive technology such as eye-gaze communication systems in the hospital setting has been shown to decrease frustration and improve the patient's sense of competence, adaptability, and self-esteem. Patients in the ICU using eye-gaze devices demonstrated an overall improvement in engagement in therapy and interactions with other professionals (e.g., nurses, doctors) and family members (Garry et al, 2016). Patients who are unable to speak or move, can use assistive technology to better communicate basic wants and needs, such as "I need suction" or "please move my leg" or "please call my wife." Incorporating assistive technology for patients who are unable to demonstrate verbal or written communication may also decrease the duration of delirium in these patients (Garry et al, 2016). Assistive technology should be considered for older adult patients even when lower-tech options have not worked to ensure all patients have the opportunity to engage in their care.

Addressing Spirituality in the Hospitalized Older Adult

Many older patients may experience sadness, fear, and anxiety while in the hospital setting. They may lean on their spirituality during these times. Patients and their loved ones may rely on their hope and faith during medical crises. However, many patients report that their spiritual needs are often ignored during hospitalization (Bláhová et al, 2021; Hodge & Wolosin, 2012). Medical staff may respect their patients' beliefs but lack the skills required to satisfy those needs or ability to refer to others who can support those spiritual needs within the hospital. As an acute care occupational therapist, it is important to be aware of the spiritual needs of patients, noting specific cultural and religious implications. During a hospitalization, patients and families often need spiritual support the most during critical moments, such as when making end-of-life decisions. Occupational therapists address patients' abilities to engage in meaningful activities based on their personal values, beliefs, and spirituality (American Occupational Therapists Association, 2020; McColl, 2011). In the hospital setting, such recommendations may include adaptive positioning to allow the patient to pray, such as kneeling on the floor and flexing forward with the head to the ground for prayer or grasping and holding the Bible in bed. Occupational therapists should also be aware of and respect specific times of the day or week that are sacred and not schedule other activities or therapy at those times. Additionally, occupational therapists should be aware of spiritual or cultural healing music or audio prayers and delicately discuss with the patient and family about how that auditory stimulation can be lessened in cases where the patient may be overstimulated. Finally, ensuring the patient has a safe space, if they request prayer or song during their occupational therapy session, allows them the ability to engage in an activity that can be incredibly powerful in the healing process.

Acute Care Documentation

Documentation of the patient's hospital stay often takes place within the electronic medical record (EMR). Although hospital systems have proprietary systems and regulatory requirements, documentation can be customized in many situations. Patients receive a new "episode of care" with each admission. It is important to view the current admission, as well as previous admissions, if possible, to understand if the episode involves a new, acute, or chronic diagnosis. With computers in patient rooms, everything from chart review to completing documentation and billing can take place locally and quickly. Documentation in acute care settings must provide clear and concise information as the medical case evolves. Occupational therapists in acute care settings must be able to demonstrate accurate and quick chart review skills and identify "red flags", such as a change in medical status, new deep vein thrombosis, or new-onset confusion. They must be able to quickly scan the EMR, digest the information, and identify key items that will dictate the course of action. Occupational therapists may decide to withhold evaluation or further treatment due to a new medical concern or change in status. Clearly documenting the reason for withholding care and then communicating those needs to appropriate interprofessional team members is essential. There can be significant medical risks to delayed documentation. For example, the medical team may delay extubating a patient from a ventilator if the patient had an eventful and effortful occupational therapy session, such as desaturating and struggling to breathe after sitting at the edge of the bed for ADLs. If documentation including vital signs (e.g., a significant pulse oxygen desaturation) is entered in a timely manner during or immediately after a therapy session, the medical team will be able to consider all current and relevant information when determining whether to perform a procedure as significant as removing the patient from a ventilator. Delayed documentation can also delay discharge. Social workers or case managers often are waiting for updated therapy notes to share with a potential rehabilitation facility or home care agency. Sometimes these are needed for insurance authorization or to recommend appropriate durable medical equipment (e.g., walker, bedside commode) for safety at home. These delays can deter what is called "throughput," or advancing the patient to the next level of care. Refer to Promoting Best Practice 24-4 for more information on acute care documentation.

PROMOTING BEST PRACTICE 24-4
Documenting Skilled Occupation-Centered Interventions in Acute Care

- Encouraged proper search patterns via scanning or head turns during functional tasks with moderate verbal cues
- Utilized compensatory strategies such as adaptive equipment
- Promoted energy conservation by sitting for shower
- Promoted engagement in social participation
- Encouraged bilateral hands at midline during ADLs/functional activity
- Challenged sitting balance by propping with unilateral or no upper extremity support during functional tasks/ADLs
- Encouraged reach and grasp outside of base of support in sitting edge of bed or standing sink side for ADLs
- Challenged standing balance by encouraging weight shifting
- Opened containers with bilateral hands
- Utilized hemiparetic upper extremity for stabilization
- Encouraged attention to left/right side with minimal oral or tactile cues

Payment Systems and Reimbursement for Acute Care Services (US)

Payment for occupational therapy services performed in the hospital setting varies by location. In the United States, reimbursement structures can vary by state. For instance, in the state of Maryland, occupational therapy services are covered under one charge for the overall hospital stay, which is determined by the patient's diagnosis. Older adults often have Medicare insurance coverage. The social worker and case manager can help patients apply for Medicaid or medical assistance if they do not already have insurance coverage.

Payment systems or insurance companies often require updated rehabilitation notes for approval for discharge to a rehabilitation unit, skilled nursing facility or for home care. Standardized assessments such as the American Spinal Injury Association Impairment Scale (Jha, 2018) or Coma Recovery Scale-Revised (Giacino et al, 2004) may help reinforce the need for specialty rehabilitation for patients with conditions such as spinal cord injury or traumatic brain injury. Unfortunately, one of the considerations often examined for these specialty facilities is the ability to tolerate 3 hours of intensive therapy. The payment system or insurance company may assume that the older adult has limited tolerance, making it more difficult for the older adult to be accepted to these specialty facilities. The occupational therapist can play a role in advocating for older adults and demonstrate potential recovery and progress made during the acute care stay.

Many older adults are on a fixed income, which may affect their ability to self-pay for equipment, such as a tub transfer bench or copayment for a power wheelchair. Financial status is also a factor when considering recommendations for home renovations, such as creating a roll-in shower for safer transfers. Additionally, there may be a cap on the number of inpatient rehabilitation hospital days a patient is allowed to use. If an older adult has had more than one admission or a long hospital stay, they may have difficulty being accepted into a rehabilitation facility when discharged from the hospital. The occupational therapist should have knowledge of insurance coverage to help guide the older adult. For example, the occupational therapist could advise an older adult with a progressive disease such as ALS to consider a loaner manual wheelchair and save their insurance benefit for a sophisticated power wheelchair when they may need it later, as wheelchairs are often covered only every 5 years. The occupational therapist can advocate for the older patient and save their insurance benefit for what they may likely need in the future.

Advocacy for Patients and Occupational Therapy Services

Occupational therapy is essential for hospitalized older adults, focusing on helping the patient return to engagement in meaningful activities. The older adult may struggle with a new diagnosis or sudden progression of a disease process that results in hospitalization. The occupational therapist can offer reassurance and comfort by letting the patient know they may still be able to engage in self-care tasks as well as other occupations that are meaningful, even if in an adaptive manner. Although it may be assumed that hospitalized older adults need to rest and are safer in bed, occupational therapists should advocate for early activity and empower older adults to actively participate in their healing (Wick, 2011). This process begins in the ICU or acute care setting and continues throughout the hospital stay. Patients who receive occupational therapy in acute care settings are less likely to be readmitted to the hospital (Rogers et al, 2017). Occupational therapists advocate for the provision of occupational therapy services by encouraging referrals from physicians and providers. Empowering the older adult in the hospital with hope and reassurance of functional healing after injury or illness is the end goal of occupational therapy in acute care.

> ### CASE STUDY (CONTINUED)
>
> #### Intervention in the Context of an Acute Care Setting
>
> Later in their treatment session, the occupational therapist moved the IV lines, peripheral IV pole, arterial blood pressure bag, and Foley catheter to the side of the bed near the window so that Solveig could sit on the edge of the bed and brush her teeth while getting natural light and seeing her environment to help with cognitive stimulation. The occupational therapist provided short direct cues to perform each task. "Solveig, we are going to sit up." The occupational therapist then tapped the bed near Solveig's hip providing tactile stimulation. The occupational therapist provided direct oral cues and assisted with problem-solving by providing minimal cues such as "What do you need to do first" to guide Solveig to remove the toothpaste lid. Solveig continued and terminated the task of oral care appropriately, then stated she felt dizzy. The occupational therapist observed that Solveig's blood pressure had dropped while sitting at the edge of the bed and assisted her in lying back down with the head of the bed elevated. She reapplied the restraints, turned the bed alarm on, and documented posttherapy vital signs, which showed that Solveig's blood pressure had returned to goal range. The occupational therapist left the lights on and blinds open to help Solveig reestablish a normal sleep–wake cycle.
>
> After 2 days, Solveig was transferred to the medical unit. She no longer has the arterial blood pressure line or indwelling Foley catheter but now has a Purewick external female catheter. Her cognition has improved but she is still occasionally impulsive, mostly due to urinary urgency and wanting to go to the bathroom instead of letting the Purewick collect the urine. The occupational therapist completed a standardized cognitive assessment in preparation for Solveig being medically ready for discharge. Mariane had been an active participant in therapy sessions and was hoping to have Solveig return to her home and live independently. The occupational therapist administered the Hopkins Medication Schedule (Carlson et al, 2005) to assess cognition and determine how much assistance Solveig may need with medication management at home. The occupational therapist recommended setting alarms on Solveig's phone, using a pillbox that is filled with Mariane's supervision, and reminder phone calls from Mariane. Both Solveig and Mariane agreed to the plan. After completing a medication management assessment, the occupational therapist addressed Solveig's goal of toileting in the bathroom. The occupational therapist removed the Purewick and encouraged Solveig to use her rolling walker to the bathroom to practice toileting. Solveig completed toileting in the bathroom and grooming and washing her hands while standing at the sink and then gathered her robe before she returned to the chair in the room, all with supervision.
>
> The occupational therapist discussed discharge recommendations with Solveig and Mariane and then consulted with the rest of the care team. The physical therapist recommended home physical therapy and use of the rolling walker. The speech-language pathologist stated that Solveig was able to swallow with no signs of dysphagia and recommended eating softer foods, given her tooth pain and possible dental concerns. The medical team agreed with the occupational therapist's recommendation for follow-up with home occupational therapy to address medication management, meal preparation, and ADL strategies to ensure ongoing progress at home. The occupational therapist recommended follow-up with Solveig's primary dentist as well as pelvic floor therapy should her urinary urgency continue after discharge. Low-vision occupational therapy was also recommended, as Solveig demonstrated blurred central vision, which may indicate macular degeneration. Solveig was happily discharged to her home. Her daughter stayed the first few nights with her to ensure her safety. Home occupational therapy was scheduled to begin the next day.
>
> #### Questions
> 1. What treatment options could the occupational therapist use if Solveig's cognitive impairment persists, indicating that her delirium was not a result of her UTI, dehydration, and medication errors but instead was due to a progressive cognitive decline?

2. What changes would you make to Solveig's discharge plan with this revised scenario?

Answers

1. Train Solveig in compensatory strategies such as alerts and reminders on her phone, or phone calls from family to take medications, pay bills. Have the family take over bill paying, shopping, and setting out pills in pill case daily. Discuss therapeutic driving evaluation or cessation of driving and alternate methods for transportation. Use a memory notebook, memory board, or calendar.
2. Ask if the family is able to provide full-time supervision, or supervision during ADLs and IADLs as needed. Consider placement in long-term care, such as an assisted-living facility.

SUMMARY

Older adults in the acute care hospital setting may experience fear and uncertainty about their ability to engage in life as they knew it. They may be facing a new devastating illness or injury. The fast-paced environment of the acute care hospital is focused on medical management and progressing the patient to the next level of care, such as rehabilitation or home. Acute care occupational therapists are poised to evaluate and treat the patient's abilities, the environment, and the demands of the tasks in order to guide the patient back to engagement in meaningful occupations. Occupational therapists in acute care are also quick to modify treatments and prepare for safe discharge planning. Early engagement in mobility and activity within the hospital setting helps propel recovery for older adults. Supporting older adults and their loved ones as they return to meaningful participation in life often provides hope at an initially desperate and critical time.

Critical Thinking Questions

1. What is the best approach for older adults to recover from a medical procedure in the presence of decreased activity tolerance?
2. An older patient presents with confusion or impaired cognition during their occupational therapy evaluation in the hospital. What factors should be examined as a possible cause to help guide safe discharge planning?
3. Safe discharge planning begins during the first occupational therapy session on evaluation. What details should be considered when discharge planning for the older adult to leave the acute care hospital setting?

REFERENCES

Algeo, N., & Aitken, L. M. (2019). The evolving role of occupational therapists in adult critical care in England: A mixed methods design using role theory. *Irish Journal of Occupational Therapy, 47*(2), 74–94. https://doi.org/10.1108/IJOT-04-2019-0005

American Occupational Therapists Association. (2020). Occupational therapy practice framework: Domain and process—fourth edition. *American Journal of Occupational Therapy, 74*(Suppl. 2), 7412410010p1-7412410010p87. https://doi.org/10.5014/ajot.2020.74S2001

American Physical Therapy Association. (2019, June 30). 'Bedrest is bad': New #everyBODYmoves campaign combats hospital immobility. https://www.apta.org/article/2019/07/01/bedrest-is-bad-new-every-bodymoves-campaign-is-combatting-hospital-immobility#:~:text=According%20to%20researchers%2C%20bedrest%20can,development%20of%20thromboembolic%20disease%20increases

Amini, R., Chee, K. H., Swan, J., Mendieta, M., & Williams, T. (2019). The level of cognitive impairment and likelihood of frequent hospital admissions. *Journal of Aging and Health, 31*(6), 967–988. https://doi.org/10.1177/0898264317747078

Boston University Activity Measure for Post-Acute Care. *AM-PAC Homepage.* (n.d.). Retrieved May 12, 2022, from http://am-pac.com/

Andres, P. L., Haley, S. M., & Ni, P. S. (2003). Is patient-reported function reliable for monitoring postacute outcomes? *American Journal of Physical Medicine & Rehabilitation, 82*(8), 614–621. https://doi.org/10.1097/01.PHM.0000073818.34847.F0

Bickel, H., Hendlmeier, I., Baltasar Heßler, J., Nora Junge, M., Leonhardt-Achilles, S., Weber, J., & Schäufele, M. (2018). The prevalence of dementia and cognitive impairment in hospitals. *Deutsches Ärzteblatt International, 115*(44), 733–740. https://doi.org/10.3238/arztebl.2018.0733

Bláhová, H., Bártová, A., Dostálová, V., & Holmerová, I. (2021). The needs of older patients in hospital care: A scoping review. *Aging Clinical and Experimental Research, 33*(8), 2113–2122. https://doi.org/10.1007/s40520-020-01734-6

Booth, K. A., Simmons, E. E., Viles, A. F., Gray, W. A., Kennedy, K. R., Biswal, S. H., Lowe, J. A., Xhaja, A., Kennedy, R. E., Brown, C. J., & Flood, K. L. (2019). Improving geriatric care processes on two medical-surgical acute care units: A pilot study. *Journal for Healthcare Quality, 41*(1), 23–31. https://doi.org/10.1097/JHQ.0000000000000140

Buurman, B. M., Hoogerduijn, J. G., de Haan, R. J., Abu-Hanna, A., Lagaay, A. M., Verhaar, H. J., Schuurmans, M. J., Levi, M., & de Rooij, S. E. (2011). Geriatric conditions in acutely hospitalized older patients: Prevalence and one-year survival and functional decline. *PloS One, 6*(11), e26951. https://doi.org/10.1371/journal.pone.0026951

Cameron, J., Gallagher, R., & Pressler, S. J. (2017). Detecting and managing cognitive impairment to improve engagement in heart failure self-care. *Current Heart Failure Reports, 14*(1), 13–22. https://doi.org/10.1007/s11897-017-0317-0

Carlson, M. C., Fried, L. P., Xue, Q.-L., Tekwe, C., & Brandt, J. (2005). Validation of the Hopkins Medication Schedule to identify difficulties in taking medications. *The Journals of Gerontology Series A: Biological Sciences and Medical Sciences, 60*(2), 217–223. https://doi.org/10.1093/gerona/60.2.217

Casey, K., Sim, E., Lavezza, A., Iannuzzi, K., Friedman, L. A., Hoyer, E. H., & Young, D. L. (2023). Identifying cognitive impairment in acute care hospital setting: Finding an appropriate screening tool. *American Journal of Occupational Therapy, 77*(1), 7701205010. https://doi.org/10.5014/ajot.2023.050028

Castro-Avila, A. C., Serón, P., Fan, E., Gaete, M., & Mickan, S. (2015). Effect of early rehabilitation during intensive care unit stay on functional status: Systematic review and meta-analysis. *PloS One, 10*(7), e0130722. https://doi.org/10.1371/journal.pone.0130722

Cheah, S., & Presnell, S. (2011). Older people's experiences of acute hospitalisation: An investigation of how occupations are affected. *Australian*

Occupational Therapy Journal, 58(2), 120–128. https://doi.org/10.1111/j.1440-1630.2010.00878.x

Chen, Y., Almirall-Sánchez, A., Mockler, D., Adrion, E., Domínguez-Vivero, C., & Romero-Ortuño, R. (2022). Hospital-associated deconditioning: Not only physical, but also cognitive. *International Journal of Geriatric Psychiatry, 37*(3); 1-13. https://doi.org/10.1002/gps.5687

Costigan, F. A., Duffett, M., Harris, J. E., Baptiste, S., & Kho, M. E. (2019). Occupational therapy in the ICU: A scoping review of 221 documents. *Critical Care Medicine, 47*(12), e1014–e1021. https://doi.org/10.1097/CCM.0000000000003999

Cruz-Jentoft, A. J., & Sayer, A. A. (2019). Sarcopenia. *The Lancet, 393*(10191), 2636–2646. https://doi.org/10.1016/S0140-6736(19)31138-9

Dalton, R. E., Tripathi, R. S., Abel, E. E., Kothari, D. S., Firstenberg, M. S., Stawicki, S. P., & Papadimos, T. J. (2012). Polyneuropathy and myopathy in the elderly. *HSR Proceedings in Intensive Care & Cardiovascular Anesthesia, 4*(1), 15–19.

Dharmarajan, K., Han, L., Gahbauer, E. A., Leo-Summers, L. S., & Gill, T. M. (2020). Disability and recovery after hospitalization for medical illness among community-living older persons: A prospective cohort study. *Journal of the American Geriatrics Society, 68*(3), 486–495. https://doi.org/10.1111/jgs.16350

Donovan, A. L., Aldrich, J. M., Gross, A. K., Barchas, D. M., Thornton, K. C., Schell-Chaple, H. M., Gropper, M. A., Lipshutz, A. K. M., & University of California, San Francisco Critical Care Innovations Group. (2018). Interprofessional care and teamwork in the ICU. *Critical Care Medicine, 46*(6), 980–990. https://doi.org/10.1097/CCM.0000000000003067

Ekdahl, A. W., Andersson, L., & Friedrichsen, M. (2010). "They do what they think is the best for me." Frail elderly patients' preferences for participation in their care during hospitalization. *Patient Education and Counseling, 80*(2), 233–240. https://doi.org/10.1016/j.pec.2009.10.026

Falvey, J. R., Mangione, K. K., & Stevens-Lapsley, J. E. (2015). Rethinking hospital-associated deconditioning: Proposed paradigm shift. *Physical Therapy, 95*(9), 1307–1315. https://doi.org/10.2522/ptj.20140511

Fogg, C., Griffiths, P., Meredith, P., & Bridges, J. (2018). Hospital outcomes of older people with cognitive impairment: An integrative review. *International Journal of Geriatric Psychiatry, 33*(9), 1177–1197. https://doi.org/10.1002/gps.4919

Garry, J., Casey, K., Cole, T. K., Regensburg, A., McElroy, C., Schneider, E., Efron, D., & Chi, A. (2016). A pilot study of eye-tracking devices in intensive care. *Surgery, 159*(3), 938–944. https://doi.org/10.1016/j.surg.2015.08.012

Giacino, J. T., Kalmar, K., & Whyte, J. (2004). The JFK Coma Recovery Scale-Revised: Measurement characteristics and diagnostic utility. *Archives of Physical Medicine and Rehabilitation, 85*(12), 2020–2029. https://doi.org/10.1016/j.apmr.2004.02.033

Goldfarb, M., Semsar-Kazerooni, K., Morais, J. A., & Dima, D. (2021). Early mobilization in older adults with acute cardiovascular disease. *Age and Ageing, 50*(4), 1166–1172. https://doi.org/10.1093/ageing/afaa253

Hartley, P., Keevil, V. L., Westgate, K., White, T., Brage, S., Romero-Ortuno, R., & Deaton, C. (2018). Using accelerometers to measure physical activity in older patients admitted to hospital. *Current Gerontology and Geriatrics Research, 2018*, 3280240. https://doi.org/10.1155/2018/3280240

Herling, S. F., Greve, I. E., Vasilevskis, E. E., Egerod, I., Mortensen, C. B., Møller, A. M., Svenningsen, H., & Thomsen, T. (2018). Interventions for preventing intensive care unit delirium in adults. *Cochrane Database of Systematic Reviews, 2019*(11), Article CD009783. https://doi.org/10.1002/14651858.cd009783.pub2

Hodge, D. R., & Wolosin, R. J. (2012). Addressing older adults' spiritual needs in health care settings: An analysis of inpatient hospital satisfaction data. *Journal of Social Service Research, 38*(2), 187–198. https://doi.org/10.1080/01488376.2011.640242

Hoyer, E. H., Needham, D. M., Atanelov, L., Knox, B., Friedman, M., & Brotman, D. J. (2014). Association of impaired functional status at hospital discharge and subsequent rehospitalization. *Journal of Hospital Medicine, 9*(5), 277–282. https://doi.org/10.1002/jhm.2152

Hunter, S., White, M., & Thompson, M. (1998). Techniques to evaluate elderly human muscle function: A physiological basis. *The Journals of Gerontology Series A: Biological Sciences and Medical Sciences, 53A*(3), B204–B216. https://doi.org/10.1093/gerona/53A.3.B204

Jackson, T. A., MacLullich, A. M. J., Gladman, J. R. F., Lord, J. M., & Sheehan, B. (2016). Undiagnosed long-term cognitive impairment in acutely hospitalised older medical patients with delirium: A prospective cohort study. *Age and Ageing, 45*(4), 493–499. https://doi.org/10.1093/ageing/afw064

Jha, A. (2018). ASIA impairment scale. In J. S. Kreutzer, J. DeLuca, & B. Caplan (Eds), *Encyclopedia of clinical neuropsychology* (pp. 354–356). Springer, Cham. https://doi.org/10.1007/978-3-319-57111-9_1793

Lakatos, B. E., Capasso, V., Mitchell, M. T., Kilroy, S., Lussier-Cushing, M., Sumner, L., Repper-Delisi, J., Kelleher, E. P., Delisle, L., Cruz, C. L., & Stern, T. (2009). Falls in the general hospital: Association with delirium, advanced age, and specific surgical procedures. *Psychosomatics, 50*(3), 218–226. https://doi.org/10.1176/appi.psy.50.3.218

LeLaurin, J. H. & Shorr R. I. (2019). Preventing falls in hospitalized patients: State of the science. *Clinics in Geriatric Medicine, 35*(2), 273-283. https://doi.org/10.1016/j.cger.2019.01.007

Maclean, F., Carin-Levy, G., Hunter, H., Malcolmson, L., & Locke, E., (2012). The usefulness of the person-environment-occupation model in an acute physical health care setting. *British Journal of Occupational Therapy, 75*(12), 555–562. https://doi.org/10.4276/030802212X13548955545530

Marcus, R. L., Addison, O., Dibble, L. E., Foreman, K. B., Morrell, G., & Lastayo, P. (2012). Intramuscular adipose tissue, sarcopenia, and mobility function in older individuals. *Journal of Aging Research, 2012*, Article 629637. https://doi.org/10.1155/2012/629637

McColl, M. A. (2011). *Spirituality and occupational therapy*. Canadian Association of Occupational Therapists.

MDCalc. (n.d.). *Confusion Assessment Method for the ICU (CAM-ICU)*. Retrieved July 8, 2022, from https://www.mdcalc.com/calc/1870/confusion-assessment-method-icu-cam-icu

Mitsutake, S., Ishizaki, T., Tsuchiya-Ito, R., Furuta, K., Hatakeyama, A., Sugiyama, M., Toba, K., & Ito, H. (2021). Association of cognitive impairment severity with potentially avoidable readmissions: A retrospective cohort study of 8897 older patients. *Alzheimer's & Dementia, 13*(1), e12147. https://doi.org/10.1002/dad2.12147

Padilla Colón, C. J., Molina-Vicenty, I. L., Frontera-Rodríguez, M., García-Ferré, A., Rivera, B. P., Cintrón-Vélez, G., & Frontera-Rodríguez, S. (2018). Muscle and bone mass loss in the elderly population: Advances in diagnosis and treatment. *Journal of Biomedicine, 3*, 40–49. https://doi.org/10.7150/jbm.23390

Pozzi, C., Tatzer, V. C., Álvarez, E. A., Lanzoni, A., & Graff, M. J. L. (2020). The applicability and feasibility of occupational therapy in delirium care. *European Geriatric Medicine, 11*(2), 209–216. https://doi.org/10.1007/s41999-020-00308-z

Pritchard, K. T., Fisher, G., McGee Rudnitsky, K., & Ramirez, R. D. (2019). Policy and payment changes create new opportunities for occupational therapy in acute care. *The American Journal of Occupational Therapy, 73*(2), 7302109010p1-7302109010p8. https://doi.org/10.5014/ajot.2018.732002

Rahman, A., Wilund, K., Fitschen, P. J., Jeejeebhoy, K., Agarwala, R., Drover, J. W., & Mourtzakis, M. (2014). Elderly persons with ICU-acquired weakness. *Journal of Parenteral and Enteral Nutrition, 38*(5), 567–575. https://doi.org/10.1177/0148607113502545

Riley, M. A., Lohman, H., Berger, S., Cavanaugh, M., & Coppard, B. (2001). Splinting on elders. In B. Coppard, & H. Lohman (Eds.), *Introduction to splinting: A clinical-reasoning and problem solving-approach*. (2nd edition, pp. 359–395). Mosby.

Rogers, A. T., Bai, G., Lavin, R. A., & Anderson, G. F. (2017). Higher hospital spending on occupational therapy is associated with lower readmission rates. *Medical Care Research and Review, 74*(6), 668–686. https://doi.org/10.1177/1077558716666981

Schweickert, W. D., & Hall, J. (2007). ICU-acquired weakness. *Chest, 131*(5), 1541–1549. https://doi.org/10.1378/chest.06-2065

Smith, T. O., Sreekanta, A., Walkeden, S., Penhale, B., & Hanson, S. (2020). Interventions for reducing hospital-associated deconditioning: A systematic review and meta-analysis. *Archives of Gerontology and Geriatrics, 90,* 104176. https://doi.org/10.1016/j.archger.2020.104176

Timmer, A. J., Unsworth, C. A., & Browne, M. (2020). Occupational therapy and activity pacing with hospital-associated deconditioned older adults: A randomised controlled trial. *Disability and Rehabilitation, 42*(12), 1727–1735. https://doi.org/10.1080/09638288.2018.1535630

Vaishya, R., & Vaish, A. (2020). Falls in older adults are serious. *Indian Journal of Orthopaedics, 54*(1), 69–74. https://doi.org/10.1007/s43465-019-00037-x

van Rijn, M., Buurman, B. M., MacNeil-Vroomen, J. L., Suijker, J. J., ter Riet, G., Moll van Charante, E. P., & de Rooij, S. E. (2016). Changes in the in-hospital mortality and 30-day post-discharge mortality in acutely admitted older patients: Retrospective observational study. *Age and Ageing, 45*(1), 41–47. https://doi.org/10.1093/ageing/afv165

van Seben, R., Reichardt, L. A., Aarden, J. J., van der Schaaf, M., van der Esch, M., Engelbert, R. H. H., Twisk, J. W. R., Bosch, J. A., Buurman, B. M., Kuper, I., de Jonghe, A., Leguit-Elberse, M., Kamper, A., Posthuma, N., Brendel, N., & Wold, J. (2019). The course of geriatric syndromes in acutely hospitalized older adults: The hospital-ADL study. *Journal of the American Medical Directors Association, 20*(2), 152-158.e2. https://doi.org/10.1016/j.jamda.2018.08.003

Wang, H.-H., Sheu, J.-T., Lotus Shyu, Y.-I., Chang, H.-Y., & Li, C.-L. (2014). Geriatric conditions as predictors of increased number of hospital admissions and hospital bed days over one year: Findings of a nationwide cohort of older adults from Taiwan. *Archives of Gerontology and Geriatrics, 59*(1), 169–174. https://doi.org/10.1016/j.archger.2014.02.002

Weeks, A. (2016). Integration of theory into assessment and treatment: The person-environment-occupation model in the intensive care unit. *Physical Disabilities Special Interest Section Quarterly, 1*(3), 22–24.

Wick, J. Y. (2011, January 13). Bedrest: Implications for the aging population. *Pharmacy Times, 77(1).* https://www.pharmacytimes.com/view/featurebedrest-0111

Wilcox, M. E., Girard, T. D., & Hough, C. L. (2021). Delirium and long term cognition in critically ill patients. *BMJ, 373,* n1007. https://doi.org/10.1136/bmj.n1007

CHAPTER 25

Rehabilitation Services

Cara L. Brown, PhD, OTReg(MB) ■ Vanina Dal Bello-Haas, PhD, Med, BSc(PT)

> *"In his 87th year of life, the great Michelangelo Buonarroti (1475-1564) was believed to have said, "Ancora imparo" ("Still, I am learning").*

LEARNING OUTCOMES

By the end of this chapter, readers will be able to:

25-1. Describe the different service contexts in which geriatric rehabilitation can be delivered and why geriatric rehabilitation is believed to be effective for older adults.

25-2. Identify factors that may alter the role of the scope of the occupational therapist's assessment and intervention and their role on the interprofessional team.

25-3. Create a reference resource of person-level factors that influence rehabilitation that the occupational therapist can identify during assessment and address during intervention.

25-4. Debate the role of the occupational therapist in identifying and addressing the impact of social determinants of health that may have an impact on the rehabilitation trajectory.

25-5. Identify two evidence-based interventions for older adults that can be delivered across settings and explain why they are believed to be effective.

25-6. Provide a rationale for the importance of documentation that supports transfer of patient information from one level of care to another.

25-7. Partner with interprofessional colleagues to address micro-, meso-, and macro-level constraints to accessing rehabilitation services.

Mini Case Study

Mrs. Zelda Chompsky is 76 years old and widowed and lives alone. She is described by her family as having "so much zest for life, always painting, dancing, baking, planting, and helping others in need." Mrs. Chompsky's family found her lying on the kitchen floor when they arrived one evening for a family dinner. She was not fully conscious, so they called an ambulance. At the hospital, Mrs. Chompsky was diagnosed by medical staff with left middle cerebral artery stroke and underwent surgery to reduce the swelling in her brain. Mrs. Chompsky had weakness and poor sensation in her right arm and leg, was unable to get out of bed or walk on her own, had receptive aphasia and bladder incontinence, and was more anxious and cautious than her typical self.

While in the acute care ward, Mrs. Chompsky received physical therapy, occupational therapy, and speech-language therapy for post-operative evaluation and early mobilization. After 5 days, Mrs. Chompsky was transferred from acute care to the hospital's inpatient rehabilitation unit for a 6-week stay. She received 4 hours of therapy a day from speech-language pathology, occupational and physical therapy, psychology, and social work. She also was able to access a bowel and bladder nurse and a rehabilitation physician. In the last 2 weeks of her rehabilitation stay, she and her team were focused on planning her discharge, including needed equipment and health and social services. Mrs. Chompsky hopes that although she is much slower than before, she will be able to go home to do some of the things that bring her joy and purpose, like knitting for charity and tending her plants.

Provocative Questions

1. Thinking about Mrs. Chompsky, what are some reasons that inpatient rehabilitation was the best option for her at first?
2. At what point in her rehabilitation trajectory do you think they decided that she should transition from inpatient to outpatient rehabilitation? What would be the facilitators and barriers for transitioning to outpatient rehabilitation for Mrs. Chompsky?

This chapter surveys important aspects of rehabilitation services for older adults. It starts with a brief overview of rehabilitation settings for the older adult across the healthcare continuum and includes more detail for some of the contexts not covered in other chapters, such as virtual rehabilitation. The second main topic in this chapter is specific issues for older adults in rehabilitation and includes a discussion of personal and environmental factors that can influence rehabilitation outcomes. The third main topic is interventions that apply to multiple settings that are best practice care for older adult rehabilitation, such as

comprehensive geriatric assessment (CGA) and discharge planning. Finally, this chapter touches briefly on documentation, payment systems, and reimbursement in addition to the role of occupational therapy in advocacy for older adults and services.

Rehabilitation and Service Contexts

Rehabilitation has been defined by Wade as "a person-centered process, with treatment tailored to the individual patient's needs and, importantly, personalized monitoring of changes associated with intervention, with further changes in goals and actions if needed" (2020, p. 571). This process-oriented definition is an important advancement from what the World Health Organization (WHO) (2022) describes simply as interventions. To deliver the rehabilitation process, services need to be embedded in health and social services across the entire continuum—from public and primary healthcare to specialized care in intensive care units and long-term care environments, such as nursing homes. Through a client-focused partnership, usually involving several healthcare professionals and including family and caregivers whenever possible, rehabilitation provides people with the tools they need to attain the highest possible level of independence and self-determination. Occupational therapy services play an important role in maximizing activities and tasks of daily life that have value and meaning for the older adult and in improving their overall independence and quality of life. It is important to note that the definition and description of healthcare services are limited to individuals. Rehabilitation also plays an important role in serving communities and collectives, and this approach may be desired or needed in combination with an individual approach to best serve our culturally diverse communities and collectives (Egan & Restall, 2022). This chapter will address rehabilitation at the community or collective level in only a very limited way. (See also Chapter 22.)

Rehabilitation can be carried out in a variety of settings, and the scope, types, and intensity of services provided, the type of patients served, and the overall philosophy and focus of the program offered within each setting will vary. Rehabilitation is known to be most effective when delivered using an interprofessional team and a variety of intervention approaches (Wade, 2020). Thus, occupational therapists should be a part of the health and social care team across the continuum and should be advocates for a team-based approach in all settings.

Evidence is building to support the use of rehabilitation in multiple service contexts. This includes specialty inpatient wards (e.g., stroke unit), outpatient and day hospital settings, nursing homes, and the private home (Wade, 2020). In these settings, rehabilitation uses a biopsychosocial approach to determine needs, develop goals and an associated plan to work towards the goals, and constant monitoring and adaptation of the plan. Rehabilitation aims to minimize disability occurring from acute or chronic health conditions and injuries and includes supporting individuals and collectives to restore activity limitations and participation, relearn skills, and develop self-management skills. Rehabilitation makes a particularly significant contribution to healthcare for individuals with a persistent and chronic condition causing disability (where standard medical approaches are limited in their contributions to improving quality of life) and in progressive conditions (where the individual will need to engage in a continual adaptation of processes to engage in daily life, such as with Parkinson disease). See Figure 25-1 for an evidence-based depiction of the therapy process. While this process was developed for all ages, addressing the needs of the aging population around the world is a major health priority now and for the coming decades (Heinemann et al, 2020).

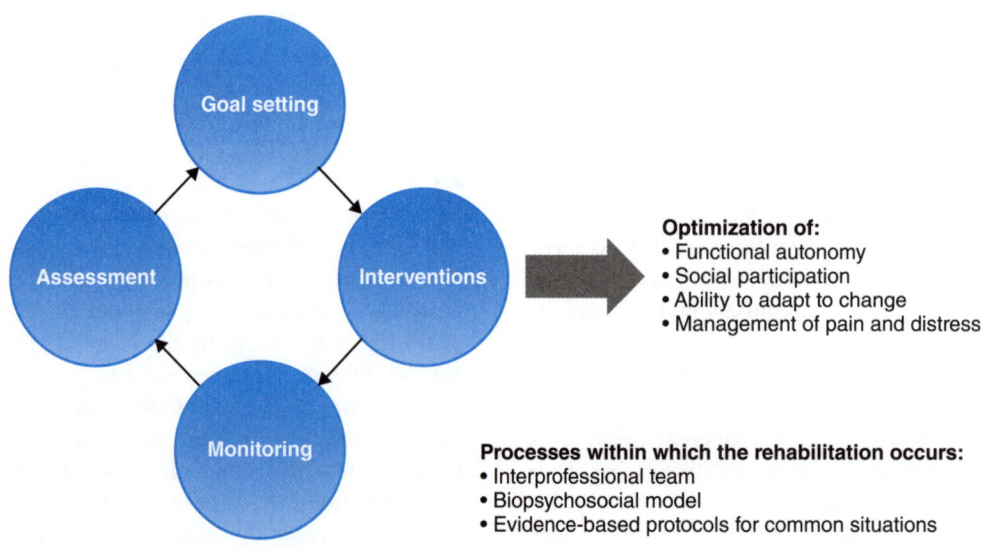

Optimization of:
- Functional autonomy
- Social participation
- Ability to adapt to change
- Management of pain and distress

Processes within which the rehabilitation occurs:
- Interprofessional team
- Biopsychosocial model
- Evidence-based protocols for common situations

FIGURE 25-1 The process of rehabilitation.

Evidence is also building in relation to the use of interprofessional teams for delivering rehabilitation to older adults for some conditions and settings. For example, mobility training is associated with improved mobility and functional status in community-dwelling older adults who meet the criteria for being frail. Also, multidisciplinary care in the hospital after hip surgery is associated with reduced mortality and need for institutional care (Handoll et al, 2021). Although positive outcomes are also seen by clinicians in non-hospital settings, more research is needed to confirm this. Evidence supporting rehabilitation approaches typically supports interventions that include care bundles rather than individual interventions (Gibson et al, 2022). There is less understanding of what specific combination of interventions and professionals is best for different types of conditions and settings. Therefore, the clinician should ensure that older adults are receiving multidisciplinary care, tailor the intervention plan to the individual, and stay up to date on the latest evidence.

Rehabilitation Settings and Services

Rehabilitation can be carried out across a continuum of settings, such as in a hospital, an outpatient clinic, in the older adult's home, or in other community settings (Box 25-1). Internationally, rehabilitation settings and programs vary widely by availability, type, level, scope, and content of care provided. One reason for this variation is overall country health funding. In many low- and middle-income countries, more than 50% of the people requiring rehabilitation do not receive rehabilitation services. In high-income countries, the variation is related to government and health system organization, financing, and priorities. Variation also occurs within countries. For example, in Canada, jurisdictional issues between the federal and provincial governments results in some First Nation communities not having access to the same adult rehabilitation services offered in other rural settings. Another example is the United States, where there is variation in spending on mental health services—with Maine spending about $362 per capita and Idaho spending only $36 per capita (American Addiction Centers, 2022).

Inpatient Rehabilitation Units

As illustrated in the mini-case study at the beginning of this chapter, many older adults become disabled by an acute health condition or illness such as a stroke, fractures, or pneumonia and require emergency hospital admission. Inpatient rehabilitation units provide the individual with the medical and therapy care that they require for recovery from illness or injury, most often following a short acute care unit stay. (See Chapter 24, Acute Care.)

Promoting Best Practice 25-1 provides a brief summary of the vast body of literature on discharge planning from an acute care setting in terms of what is best practice and where interprofessional teams' attention needs to be focused on improving hospital discharge planning processes. Inpatient rehabilitation programs are typically located within the hospital setting or in specialized rehabilitation centers. In larger centers, inpatient rehabilitation units are often specialized by health condition, an approach strongly supported by evidence for some conditions, such as stroke and hip fracture (Langhorne & Ramachandra, 2020; Moyet et al, 2018). Inpatient rehabilitation programs specialized for older adults are common in developed countries, where care is specialized by age versus condition. These geriatric rehabilitation inpatient programs are distinct units housed within community hospitals, free-standing rehabilitation hospitals, or long-term care facilities and are staffed by multidisciplinary teams specializing in the management of the medical, social, physical, psychological, and economic well-being of older adults. Finally, as mentioned earlier, in some developed countries, rehabilitation programs are stratified by both age and condition.

PROMOTING BEST PRACTICE 25-1
Discharge Planning

Discharge planning is the assessment and development of a comprehensive plan to support the older adult transitioning from one health setting to another, typically from an inpatient acute or rehabilitation setting to another setting. Research supports the use of discharge planning to promote a safe transition from the hospital back to one's home (Gonçalves-Bradley et al, 2022). Discharge planning can reduce hospital lengths of stay while also reducing hospital readmission rates. A discharge planning assessment involves predicting the social, functional, and health needs of the older adult upon discharge by exploring their previous level of function and support and comparing that to their current level of function and supports. A plan is developed to ensure safety of the older adult and that their basic daily living needs are met—for example, determining whether they require equipment like a raised toilet seat or a wheelchair for long distances or services like Meals on Wheels or home housekeeping.

Research has determined specific components of the hospital discharge intervention that are particularly important. The Re-Engineered Discharge (RED) intervention has been very widely studied and involves the following components:

- Ascertaining the need for language assistance in the discharge planning process
- Ensuring that follow-up appointments are in place prior to the older adult's discharge from hospital
- Ensuring there is a plan in place for pending tests or test results
- Ensuring all needed medical equipment is in place
- Ensuring all required services such as home healthcare are set up
- Ensuring the discharge plan is congruent with national guidelines for that health condition
- Educating the older adult on their health condition and assessing their level of understanding of their health condition
- Identifying the correct medications and developing a plan for the older adult to take them

> **BOX 25-1 Geriatric Rehabilitation**
>
> Geriatric rehabilitation is a specific model of rehabilitation for older adults that may be delivered in many setting types. It is a multidimensional approach to enhance functional "capacity, promote activity and preserve functional reserve and social participation" (p. 234) in older adults with impairment and disability (Grund et al, 2020). Geriatric rehabilitation focuses on goals that are developed in conjunction with the older adult and their circle of care. It is most often a step between acute care and home healthcare, such as an inpatient rehabilitation setting or a day hospital setting.
>
> Geriatric rehabilitation has the following principles:
>
> 1. Delivered by an interprofessional rehabilitation team that includes a physician trained in geriatric rehabilitation
> 2. Includes those with cognitive impairment, confusion, or delirium when there is rehabilitation potential
> 3. Uses a comprehensive geriatric assessment to develop the care plan
> 4. Incorporates multimorbidity needs into the care plan
> 5. Considers the time limits of the care plan
> 6. Measures progress regularly using outcome measures with a contribution and involvement from the older adult and/or their circle of care
> 7. Organizes care around neurological and orthopedic conditions when possible (van Balen et al, 2019)
>
> The principles of geriatric rehabilitation are generally the same as standard rehabilitation programs. However, the program is designed to support common age-related conditions such as pre-existing disability, cognitive impairment, and sensory loss (Achterberg et al, 2019). Geriatric rehabilitation programs generally have different expectations in relation to the quantity and intensity of daily rehabilitation, recognizing that comorbidities like lower cardiorespiratory capacity may limit the older adult's ability to meet the quantity and intensity of rehabilitation expectations in a standard rehabilitation setting. The rehabilitation team is more aware of special considerations for older adults, such as common complications like delirium or different medication regimens, and is aware of programs and services in the community specific to the needs of older adults (Achterberg et al, 2019). With this awareness, the team designs **restorative** rehabilitation goals and interventions that are intended to promote successful outcomes.
>
> Geriatric rehabilitation structures vary by country, but in most high-income countries, restoration of function may not be the primary goal of rehabilitation. Instead, goals that balance autonomy and dependency may be the best approach depending on the older adult's pre-existing and current health conditions and injuries. Some limitations and critiques of geriatric rehabilitation within the current health systems exist. One is that the admission criteria are not clear for geriatric rehabilitation compared to a standard rehabilitation program. This can result in geriatric rehabilitation being the default setting for an older adult when they would have been able to tolerate the intensity of a standard rehabilitation program. In the United States, a particular concern is that geriatric rehabilitation is making up for underfunding in other areas of rehabilitation (Achterberg et al, 2019). Since there is more insurance for geriatric rehabilitation than home care services, there is speculation that geriatric rehabilitation is a setting used for some individuals who would be able to return home without rehabilitation if supportive home care services are available (Flint et al, 2019).
>
> A survey of geriatric rehabilitation in Europe found great variation in types of rehabilitation services across countries. The most common type of geriatric rehabilitation was inpatient settings, with 14 of the 22 countries reporting that their inpatient geriatric rehabilitation also had subspecialty units, such as geriatric orthopedic rehabilitation. Eight countries did not have formal recognition for geriatric specialists. Consistent with these findings, outpatient geriatric rehabilitation centers varied in number from 1 in Romania to 200 in Finland, Sweden, and France. Even with the variation among countries, no European countries surveyed were meeting the need for geriatric rehabilitation of their overall population (Grund et al, 2020; Grund et al, 2020).

- Reviewing with the older adult what to do if a problem arises
- Teaching a written discharge plan the older adult can understand
- Reconciling medications
- Expediting the written discharge summary to the providers receiving the older adult's care post-discharge
- Providing telephone reinforcement of the discharge plan within 3 days of discharge (Popejoy et al, 2020)

Discharge planning is now more focused on continuity of care/transitional care interventions that follow the older adult from the hospital to their home setting to ensure the long-term continuity in the management of their care and to prevent related factors (such as the older adult's self-management capabilities, socioeconomic issues, and poor community resources) from prompting illness (Facchinetti et al, 2020). Further, there needs to be more focus on equity and social determinants of health in these interventions, as individual (e.g., low socioeconomic status and education level) and community (e.g., neighborhood poverty rates) factors drive up hospital readmission rates (Zhang et al, 2020). Therefore, discharge planning continues to be very important, but a focus on the whole trajectory of the transition needs to be incorporated into the care of older adults returning home from the hospital.

A **physiatrist**, a doctor who specializes in physical medicine and rehabilitation, determines who will be transferred to an inpatient rehabilitation program from the acute care setting. The physiatrist determines if the individual would benefit from the rehabilitation stay by looking at factors like capacity for recovery and ability to participate in the intensive rehabilitation process. In many settings, for older adults to be admitted to a rehabilitation unit, they must be medically stable and able to tolerate at least 3 hours of intervention a day, 5 or 6 days a week. It is common for the older adult to need to demonstrate measurable progress during the duration of the stay, and thorough documentation is essential to demonstrate the need for continued care. The older adult must continually be reassessed in the inpatient rehabilitation setting to ensure that it is the best setting for their needs (Achterberg et al, 2019). Once the older adult has reached their personal capacity for remediation and can manage at home with or without supports, they may be discharged to home. If returning home is not feasible, then transfer to a long-term care facility is a typical discharge plan. Discharge to a long-term care facility can be predicted by the presence of medical complications, lower functional status at discharge from the acute facility, and severity of impaired gait status.

Transitional Care

"Transitional care is a set of strategies and services offered to improve care transitions, and aspects of safe and timely passage of patients between levels of healthcare and across care settings and are time limited to these situations" (Morkisch et al, 2020, p. 2). Transitional care models vary, with some programs being inpatient programs and others spanning care delivery across settings from acute care to a community setting. Delivery models for community-based transitional care include outpatient transitional care clinics and mobile interdisciplinary care teams that provide most of the care in the older adult's home. Transitional care has an objective of reducing readmission rates to acute care, a common challenge in healthcare for older adults.

In the United States, skilled nursing facilities (SNFs), subacute units, or transitional care units are the most commonly described transitional care settings. The difference between transitional care and subacute care is not particularly clear. Some health organizations have subacute care units that are designed to offer a setting that is less hectic than acute care and where adults who need more time or rehabilitation for recovery can stay until they are ready for discharge to home, which can range from a few days to a few weeks.

Skilled Nursing Facilities

"Skilled care is nursing and therapy care that can only be safely and effectively performed by, or under the supervision of, professionals or technical personnel. It's healthcare given when you need skilled nursing or skilled therapy to treat, manage, and observe your condition, and evaluate your care." (U.S. Centers for Medicare and Medicaid Services, n.d.a., "What it is"). The care needs of individuals admitted to SNFs vary considerably due to factors such as a lack of standardized evaluation processes, lack of a clear primary decision-maker for selection of patients for SNF, characteristics of the older adult (older, more likely to have dementia than in home health or inpatient rehabilitation), and the pressure to clear acute care hospital beds (AOTA & APTA, 2021; Burke et al, 2017). Therefore, the rehabilitation team needs to be able to adapt rehabilitation approaches and plans for each individual. (For more information about rehabilitation in SNFs, see Chapter 27.)

Outpatient and Ambulatory Care

Outpatient rehabilitation is for people who are recovering from an acute event, can live at home, and need specific rehabilitation services. Like inpatient rehabilitation, services are typically organized by health condition, but outpatient services tailored to the older adult may also be an option. A thorough assessment of the older adult's abilities and needs may help in determining the correct outpatient setting. For example, for older adults with few comorbidities, intact cognitive status, and a condition that may benefit from a specialist approach (e.g., spinal cord injury), a setting specific for that condition may be the best. On the other hand, conditions more common in older adults (e.g., heart failure), that require moderate-intensity rehabilitation and tailoring to potential cognitive impairment, a geriatric outpatient program may be more efficacious.

These outpatient services can be provided in various settings, including hospitals, free-standing clinics, or private practices. In the United States, comprehensive outpatient rehabilitation facilities (CORFs) offer a variety of rehabilitation services to Medicare beneficiaries in one location. CORFs need to include in their services, at minimum, a physician, physical therapy, and psychological or counseling services and may also include occupational therapy, speech-language pathology, and/or respiratory therapy, among others (U.S. Centers for Medicare and Medicaid Services, n.d.b.).

Recent evidence supports the use of outpatient occupational therapy and physical therapy for older adults with various health conditions. A randomized controlled trial found that older adults with cancer improved activity expectations and self-efficacy (as measured by the Possibilities for Activity Scale) with outpatient rehabilitation (Pergolotti et al, 2019). There is also evidence that outpatient rehabilitation can improve performance of activities of daily living (ADLs) following hip fracture (Freitas et al, 2021) and reduce mortality post hip fracture (Pan et al, 2018). However, an interesting finding in the Pan study (2018) was that the rehabilitation group had an increased risk of rehospitalization, potentially due to acquiring an infection, as many of the rehospitalizations were due to pneumonia (Pan et al, 2018). This raises an interesting consideration for designing rehabilitation facilities and the potential benefits of home-based rehabilitation.

Day-Care Services

Day-care programs vary in their objectives. Some may be time limited and focus on transitional care after an acute care stay, whereas others may be long-term programs that aim to enhance the quality of life and support older adults to remain in their own home as long as possible. This means that some programs may have a more medical focus and others a more social focus. Most day-care programs provide transportation to the care site, a meal while the older adult is on site, and recreational and social activity programs. More medically focused programs will also include physician monitoring and/or rehabilitative care. In the United States, day-care service models include day hospital, **maintenance model** programs, and social programs (Bakerjian, 2020).

The day hospital model was first developed in the United Kingdom and is now common in the United Kingdom, the United States, and Canada. This model emphasizes rehabilitation or skilled care for people recovering from an acute condition. These programs are usually time limited (e.g., 6 weeks to 6 months). In the United States, Medicare does not reimburse for day-care services. Funds generally come from the Older Americans Act, Medicaid waiver programs, long-term care insurance, and private funds. Some centers use donated funds to subsidize transportation and a sliding-fee scale to match aid with the patient's financial need.

Adult day-care (a U.S. term) programs offer maintenance and social models. They provide an alternative to institutionalization for newly or chronically disabled adults who cannot stay alone during the day but who do not need 24-hour inpatient care. These programs are designed to promote maximum independence, and older adults usually attend on a scheduled basis. Services may include nursing, counseling, social services, restorative services, medical and healthcare monitoring, medication administration, well-balanced meals, transportation to and from the facility, exercise programs, field trips, and recreational activities along with occupational, physical, and speech therapy. In the United States, such programs may serve individuals with physical limitations and individuals with cognitive impairments (Maffioletti et al, 2019). (See Chapter 22 for more on day program services.)

Telerehabilitation

The COVID-19 pandemic that began in March 2020 stimulated an increase in the offering of tele- and virtual rehabilitation options. **Telerehabilitation,** according to van den Bergh et al (2021), includes three categories:

1. Teleconsultation, comprising coaching or consultation sessions via information and communication technology (ICT) such as telephone and videoconferencing
2. Telemonitoring, comprising data collection via a remote monitoring tool, such as a wearable device or app, to inform healthcare providers in treatment provision
3. Teletreatment, which includes direct delivery of various therapies remotely using ICT devices

Telehealth is the provision of healthcare remotely by means of a variety of telecommunication tools, including telephones, mobile wireless devices, and computers. While this a fairly new means of providing care, evidence is building on the use of this rehabilitation approach with older adults. Telerehabilitation has many potential benefits, including increased access to rehabilitation for people living in rural and remote settings, prevention of unnecessary delays in care, and improved collaboration and coordination of care. There is also evidence that it is as effective as in-person rehabilitation, although older adults are less likely to choose telerehabilitation care (Hayes, 2020). It is thought that the lack of uptake of telerehabilitation is a combination of older adults' and therapists' attitudes and beliefs. Older adults may feel hesitant to try a new model of rehabilitation, and therapists express concerns with patient safety, lack of physical contact, developing rapport, and issues relating to lack of technical support (Hayes, 2020). However, once they have tried telerehabilitation, older adults tend to be satisfied with the service, particularly with the convenience. Furthermore, telerehabilitation is preferable for some caregivers. Ariza-Vega and colleagues (2021) compared those who received telerehabilitation and those who received in-home rehabilitation and found that the caregivers in the telerehabilitation group expressed less stress and anxiety.

Velayati and colleagues (2020) found that methods of telerehabilitation delivery ranged from a virtual reality–based system delivered via the internet to a multicomponent intervention that included weekly telerehabilitation sessions, telemonitoring, and phone calls. Health conditions addressed included stroke, post knee replacement, chronic obstructive pulmonary disease, post-stroke, and congestive heart failure. There are no reported differences between the use of telerehabilitation and traditional rehabilitation for improvement of physical function, including hand function and balance for the older adults in these studies who had intact cognitive status (Velayati et al, 2020). Some conditions, such as certain musculoskeletal conditions and stroke, require a hands-on assessment, but in these cases, there is evidence that telerehabilitation can be an effective adjunct to in-person treatment (Hayes, 2020). More research is needed to determine for which populations telerehabilitation versus in-person care is the most appropriate intervention; for example, in the case of multimorbidity, different levels of function and different levels of cognitive capacity.

CASE STUDY

Mr. George from Chapter 12 in the context of a rehabilitation setting

Presenting Situation

To consider in- and outpatient rehabilitation contexts, we will revisit the case study from Chapter 12 of Mr. George who has Parkinson disease and also broke his wrist in a fall. After reviewing this case study, consider the multiple settings of care Mr. George has experienced until now and may experience in the future considering his progressive condition. When Mr. George broke his wrist and had difficulty with function due to his wrist in combination with his Parkinson disease symptoms, he had a home visit from an occupational therapist to assess his safety in the home. He was provided with equipment, and his home care services were temporarily increased as a result of this assessment. When it was time for Mr. George's cast to come off, he was seen by an occupational therapist in a hospital outpatient department for an assessment of his hand function.

Role of Occupational Therapy and Interprofessional Partners

The role of the occupational therapist will vary based on factors that are both patient centered and setting dependent:

- Extent of patient's injury across different body function domains (e.g., physical, cognitive, emotional)
- Severity of patient's condition
- Setting of care
- Interprofessional team members in the setting

When an individual presents with one focal issue, such as a fracture of the upper extremity, the occupational therapist tends to focus on that issue. The occupational therapist will stay attuned to cues from the older adult and screen for other issues (e.g., cognitive) as needed but will focus the assessment and intervention on the focal issue. For someone presenting with a chronic condition that tends to affect multiple domains, the therapist may take a broader approach to assessment, looking at cognitive, emotional, and physical abilities, and developing a priority list of interventions. If the occupational therapist works in a setting where there are older adults with more minor issues or early disease onset, the therapist may be able to provide more preventative care (Whyman, 2022).

For many professions, there is some blurring of role. For example, dependent on state or regional licensure, occupational therapists and physical therapists are both able to assess for and provide intervention and prescriptions for walking aids. Occupational therapists and social workers are both able to provide supportive counseling. Thus, the types of members on the team and the typical issues of the older adults that the team services often will influence the specific team roles. Developing role clarity and negotiating roles to provide the most effective and efficient care is an important part of working on a team, and time should be dedicated to this, rather than seeing it as an "extra." Occupational therapists who are not working in a team will need to consider what other services or professionals the older adults they are serving would benefit from and make referrals to other needed professionals (Canadian Interprofessional Health Collaborative, 2010).

Interprofessional Partners

The most important member of the rehabilitation team is the older adult. Rehabilitation is maximized when there is a comprehensive and holistic approach, with input from family, friends, and other supports and a variety of skilled professionals.

The health-care professionals who make up the rehabilitation team for an older adult vary greatly depending on the care setting and the needs of the older adult but typically include a **geriatrician** (a physician who specializes in geriatric medicine) or a physiatrist (a physician who specializes in physical medicine and rehabilitation), rehabilitation nurses and/or a geriatric nurse practitioner, a social worker, a physical therapist, an occupational therapist, a speech-language pathologist, a dietitian, and support personnel. Other health professionals, such as psychologists, audiologists, recreational therapists, respiratory therapists, and pharmacists, are also frequently part of a team that may evaluate and manage care for the older adult (Nordström et al, 2018). In some countries, team members can have specialized skills or specialist certification. For example, in the United Kingdom, there is a diploma in geriatric medicine program for regulated health professionals such as physicians and occupational therapists. In the United States, occupational therapists may be board certified in gerontology.

Teams need to be aware that the presence of an interprofessional team does not guarantee better quality care. In fact, a team that does not work well together can lead to inefficiency, fragmented care, and confusion for the older adult receiving care. Teams should ensure that they have common goals and philosophy, as the team members need to work with a shared set of values (Singh et al, 2018). Teams also need to recognize how group dynamics are at play in their work and engage in an evaluative process to continually improve their ability to work together cooperatively. The Interprofessional Collaborative Relationship-Building Model outlines the stages of interprofessional relationships and how these relationships can be facilitated to support effective teamwork (Wener et al, 2022). Working on improving teamwork and interprofessional relationships and communication is a core function of teams, is required to promote quality care, and needs to be given the time and energy it requires (Singh et al, 2018).

Specific Issues for Working With Older Adults

While not all older adults who require rehabilitation will have complex health and social needs, many do because of a variety of personal and environmental factors related to aging and society. It is important that these personal and environmental factors are considered during the assessment and intervention plan development process to best meet the needs of the older adult. It is a role of the occupational therapist to identify and, where applicable, support the modification of these factors through intervention or referrals to improve rehabilitation outcomes.

Personal Factors

Physiological Age

Chronological age is not always a reflection of physiological age, as everyone ages at a different physiological pace.

A great deal of heterogeneity and variability exists in the overall presentation and functional limitations in older adults, secondary to differences in decline in the physiological systems, such as cognitive, neuromuscular (e.g., strength), cardiovascular, sensory (e.g., vision), and other physical functions and the number and extent of health conditions, impairments, and limitations. (See Part II, Aging: Body Structures, Body Functions.) Therefore, an individual's rehabilitation potential or program should not be developed based on their chronological age, as it may be misleading in relation to their physiological capacity (Soto-Perez-de-Celis et al, 2018).

Frailty

Frailty is a medical condition of reduced function and health in older adults and is predictive of mortality and health service use (Canadian Frailty Network, 2021–2022). It is often related to loss of physiological reserve, but many factors are considered in combination to determine an older adult's frailty status, including physical, cognitive, social, and behavioral impairments and issues. The most common and medically accepted features of frailty include slowed muscle speed, such as slow gait, muscular weakness, fatigue, and low activity levels. Other factors include few social supports, cognitive decline, multiple medications, and low mood. Regardless of the reason for the rehabilitation admission, factors related to frailty need to be included in the rehabilitation plan to ensure rehabilitation success. For example, even if the condition is neurological, general strengthening may be required, and the rehabilitation program may need to increase gradually to account for the need for muscular and endurance gains for the older adult to participate fully in the rehabilitation program (Wang et al, 2020). The plan may also need to include improving social and health supports to address social and cognitive issues.

Motivation

Numerous theories of motivation try to explain why people behave as they do, what sustains and directs a person's attention, and what arouses and instigates behavior, gives direction or purposes to behavior, allows behavior to persist, or leads a person to choose or prefer a particular behavior (Cole & Tufano, 2020). Motivation should not be confused with adherence, which is the extent to which an older adult follows a healthcare professional's advice or recommendations. It is important to remember that motivation is associated with mood and mood disorders and that lack of motivation is a cue for clinicians to screen for mood or make a referral for a screen. Because rehabilitation is often being provided in the context of a traumatic incident and significantly affects day-to-day life and relationships, medical intervention for mood may help support the individual's transitional time in rehabilitation and improve individual outcomes (Grahek et al, 2019).

A common way to address motivation in rehabilitation is to involve the older adult and their circle of care in the development of rehabilitation goals. Goal-setting is a complex intervention. Challenges can include unrealistic expectations on the part of the older adult receiving rehabilitation, which in turn creates conflict between the older adult and the occupational therapist. Another challenge includes the older adult being unclear on the purpose of the goal-setting process (Knutti et al, 2022). However, therapists should invest time and energy in developing skills in collaborative goal-setting, as it has been shown to improve outcomes related to physical ability, mood, quality of life, occupational performance and satisfaction, rehabilitation satisfaction, and self-efficacy (Yun & Choi, 2019).

Depression and Grief

In the older adult undergoing rehabilitation, depression, loss, and grief are common; can influence motivation; and need to be considered in the context of therapy. Depression is associated with diminished coping mechanisms that can negatively affect outcomes of rehabilitation. Depression often goes unrecognized in the older adult because of ageism and the overlapping of depression and dementia symptoms, such as somatic complaints (pain, constipation, dyspnea), apathy, and decreased memory or concentration (Stanetić et al, 2020). With their knowledge of both mental illness and physical illness, occupational therapists can play an important role in the identification and treatment of depression for adults undergoing rehabilitation regardless of the primary reason for the rehabilitation.

Dementia and Cognitive Impairment

In many countries, older adults with cognitive impairments often have problems with being admitted to, receiving, or being reimbursed for rehabilitation services (McGilton et al, 2012; Ankuda et al, 2020). This is most likely related to evidence that suggests the odds of successful rehabilitation outcomes in those with cognitive impairments to be lower than in those without dementia (Cameron et al, 2012). As described in Chapter 13, people with dementia are capable of learning, and rehabilitation should be considered for those in the early stages of a disorder that is causing cognitive impairment. Strategies for supporting function in individuals with cognitive impairment are discussed in Chapter 13. Although severity of cognitive impairment has been found to be related to higher mortality and less successful return to independent living, the evidence related to cognitive impairment and positive rehabilitation outcomes is equivocal. The occupational therapist can draw on applied theories to support intervention planning for older adults with dementia, such as Allen's Cognitive Levels Frame of Reference (Cole & Tufano, 2020).

Comorbidities and Pre-Existing Disability

The potential for disability increases with age, with the greatest number of disabilities affecting the very old. The WHO recognizes that although people are living longer, there is really no change in disability as one ages. The most common causes of disability in older people are chronic, non-communicable diseases, including depression, falls, diabetes, dementia, and osteoarthritis (WHO, 2017). As a result, the older adult frequently presents with multiple diagnoses or pathologies in combination with changes associated with normal aging. The interaction between conditions and normal aging may exacerbate impairments and limitations and may affect the response to some rehabilitation interventions. Please see Chapter 7 for more information about common health issues for older adults.

Environmental Factors That May Influence Rehabilitation

Immediate Social Supports

Social supports like family members and other people who support and care for the older adult are an integral part of the care team. They know the older adult and can often provide additional information about the older person's perspectives, habits, behaviors, and needs; can provide emotional and instrumental support; and can facilitate focus on the rehabilitation goals. Other older adults may be lacking in social supports and be dependent on social services to be able to maintain living in the community. This is common with aging, as the older adult's own life partner, family, and friends also develop disabilities or die as they age. About half of women who are 75 years of age and older live alone (Administration on Aging, 2021). Even those with large families who live very long lives may outlive their children, limiting their social circle of care. Chapter 20 discusses caregiving in detail.

Social Determinants of Health

The social determinants of health framework emphasizes the social, economic, cultural, and political influence of society on individual health and wellness. People's health and illness are not solely the outcome of their own individual choices. Rather, an individual's context within their community and wider society—including age, gender, race, ethnicity, education, occupation, and income—influences their socioeconomic position and thus their health (Northwood et al, 2018). In the context of rehabilitation, this can best be understood by contrasting the experience of two older adults who have just had a stroke. The first is a white middle-income woman living in an urban setting. She has a university-level education and a wide network of friends who are doctors, lawyers, and counselors. Her time to hospital at the time of her stroke was short due to a quick ambulance response and living fairly close to the specialist hospital. She was treated by primarily white individuals who had a shared language, values, and cultural understanding with her. She generally understood the instructions she was given, or if she did not, she was not afraid to ask for clarification. Her grown children spent time learning about community resources while she was in the hospital. Upon discharge, they ensured that she continued to receive outpatient therapy; some was public, but they paid for private services to fill some gaps. One of her children was able to afford to take unpaid leave from work to spend time with her in the first 2 weeks following discharge to take her to appointments and provide practical and supportive care.

The second individual is an Indigenous woman who had a stroke in her rural community. She delayed phoning the ambulance because she was afraid she couldn't afford it. Her time to hospital was more than 12 hours. Because of past trauma related to institutional settings, she feared the institutional hospital setting and was afraid to ask any questions. None of her family was able to come with her to the hospital because they needed to work and couldn't afford to travel and stay in the city. She did not understand her discharge instructions. She was discharged home to her community, where there are no rehabilitation services for adults, and where she depended on community members to help her with tasks she could not complete but had not told the rehabilitation team about, such as taking out garbage down a very long gravel driveway. Even without emphasizing the racism, ageism, and ableism present in our healthcare systems, the contrast of these two stories helps to illustrate how the social context has a large influence on rehabilitation outcomes.

It is the responsibility of the therapist to:

- Assess for and work to mitigate social factors that may impede rehabilitation recovery (e.g., ensure social needs are met rather than assuming that family or friends will do it)
- Advocate for improved services at the community level when services are inadequate
- Learn about and work to interrupt oppression, including white supremacy, racism, and ageism in daily healthcare delivery (Grenier, 2020)
- Ensure that the rehabilitation approach, including the type of assessments and the types of goals, are socially and culturally relevant to the care receiver.

Intervention Exemplars

This section outlines best practices for approaching older adult rehabilitation. It includes best practice considerations for assessment, intervention, care coordination, and continuity and addresses both individual and collective approaches to rehabilitation.

Comprehensive Geriatric Assessment

A CGA is "a multidimensional, multidisciplinary process which identifies medical, social and functional needs, and the development of an integrated/coordinated care plan to meet those needs" (Parker et al, 2018, p. 150). In the literature, CGA is also sometimes referred to as a program that provides the intervention, considering the CGA as a program rather than solely an assessment. CGA helps healthcare professionals determine and prioritize problems, develop long- and short-term plans of care, and implement rehabilitation strategies that optimize management, improve function and outcomes, prevent further deterioration, optimize living location, decrease unnecessary healthcare resources and service use, arrange long-term case management, and prolong survival of older adults.

CGA has several major measurable dimensions, usually grouped into these domains:

- Physical health (e.g., traditional history and physical examination, medical assessment, nutritional assessment, medication review, laboratory data, disease-specific severity indicators, and preventative health practices)
- Functional status (e.g., ADLs, and instrumental ADLs and other functional status, such as mobility and quality of life)
- Psychological health (mainly cognitive and affective status)
- Socioenvironmental parameters (e.g., social networks and supports, economics, and environmental safety, adequacy, and needs)

CGA has been shown to reduce death, disability, and re-institutionalization. When first introduced, CGA was revolutionary in its time for looking beyond the medical condition of the older adult and for taking a coordinated approach to the provision of multidisciplinary care. It is now considered to be the best approach to care, particularly for older adults with frailty and/or comorbidities that influence quality of life. CGA helps to re-center quality of life rather than taking a purely medical and remediation approach with the older adult. Although there is consistency in the concept of CGA, how it is delivered varies—from a screening assessment to thorough diagnostic assessment and management by a multidisciplinary team (Pilotto et al, 2017).

A CGA typically includes assessment of functional status, mobility, gait speed, cognition, mood, nutritional status, comorbidities and polypharmacy, conditions related to aging (e.g., vision and hearing loss, delirium), disease-specific rating scales (e.g., parkinsonism, dementia), goals of care, social and environmental situation (e.g., social support needs, financial concerns), and advance care planning. Typically, a core team (e.g., geriatrician, nurse, and/or social worker) will conduct the assessment, with other professions contributing as needed (e.g., occupational therapy, physical therapy, dietetics, and speech-language pathology). Then a care plan is developed based on those findings and is carried out by a multidisciplinary team.

CGA can be delivered in a variety of settings. While research on CGA has waned since 2010 (Pilotto et al, 2017), there is strong evidence that a dedicated inpatient unit for older adults using CGA is an effective intervention for reducing death, improving functional status, and addressing cognitive impairment. This approach has been found to be more effective than a geriatric consultation team that provides consultative support to older adults dispersed across different wards of mixed ages. There is also less evidence that a post-hospital CGA is effective at improving outcomes, but this may be because many of the components of CGA are now standard practice in hospital discharge-planning practices (see Box 25-1). It may be that in community, a preventative approach using home visits to conduct CGA is more effective at improving outcomes and reducing hospital admission in older adults (Pilotto et al, 2017).

Case Management

Case management is a process that comprises a variety of consecutive collaborative phases that culminates in ensuring older adults have access to available and relevant resources necessary to attain identified goals (Hudon et al, 2018). Case managers facilitate communication among healthcare providers and ensure that services are not duplicated. Case management offers a practical, one-step approach to helping older adults coordinate their care.

Key elements of the case management process include:

- Service recipient identification (screening)
- Assessment
- Stratifying risk
- Planning
- Implementation (care coordination)
- Monitoring
- Transitioning
- Evaluation

Globally, case management for older adults is a central part of rehabilitation (Alejandro, 2021). Case management assumes that people with complex health problems need assistance in using the healthcare system effectively and efficiently. Older adults often use multiple healthcare providers and require varied social services to help them live independently. During the course of rehabilitation, many older adults will require services from several healthcare professionals. To ensure that the correct interventions are applied in the correct order and that complications, delays, and duplications are avoided, many decisions will have to be coordinated. This means that decisions must be made in full awareness of many other older adult care issues, such as preferences, post-discharge resources in the older adult's home, availability of family and caregivers, and community resources.

Case management has been found to be an effective strategy for people who have high healthcare use (e.g., frequent hospitalizations, frequent visits to general practitioner) in primary care settings. In this role, the case manager can coordinate care, advocate for services for the older adults and their family, and monitor health and social status. The positive benefits include reducing emergency room visits and improvements in health and social status. The occupational therapist—with their background in biopsychosocial approaches and a strong understanding of the influence of environmental factors on health—is well positioned to be a case manager.

Integrated Care Models

Integrated care models promote the integration of social supports and healthcare as well as different levels of healthcare (primary care, secondary care, and tertiary care). These types of models are becoming more recognized as being very important for maintaining continuity of care and supporting older adults in the community to avoid institutionalization. These models typically have a screening process to determine eligibility and focus on those older adults who require more supportive community care. Integrated models can bring together primary care supports with more specialist geriatric care and social services that are needed for supporting people with complex health and social needs (Mann et al, 2021). Practically, this is the provision of multiple services and supports to ensure that the older adult's needs are met. This can include home visits from health professionals like physicians and therapists, the provision of transportation to appointments and social settings, social programming, and flexibility in the provision of care in the home to adapt to health and functional needs (e.g., increasing and decreasing home care needs as required to prevent the need for hospitalization when the health needs can be supported at home). These models often incorporate other best practices for older adults, such as case management and CGA. One example is the Programs for All-Inclusive Care for the Elderly model found in Chapter 22.

Documentation, Payment Systems, and Reimbursement

Although rehabilitation settings are generally similar across developed countries, the payment systems, reimbursement, and documentation requirements for these settings vary widely depending on the national healthcare systems. In developed countries, there is a continuum of private/public funding systems. For example, the United States has a primarily private insurance-funded system, where 67% of the population's healthcare is covered by private insurance, and supplemental insurance for older adults and people who are disabled is funded with national and state tax revenue, leaving 8.5% of adults uninsured (Tikkanen et al, 2020a). England has a national healthcare system that provides public coverage to 100% of the population, with only 10.5% of the population buying supplemental insurance for more extensive access to the system (Tikkanen et al, 2020b). In Canada, tax revenue covers basic healthcare services for the entire population (e.g., primary care physician, hospital care), with private insurance being required for supplemental services not covered in the national healthcare system, such as dental and optometry care; 67% of the population has supplementary insurance (Tikkanen et al, 2020c). These different healthcare models drive delivery models.

Documentation

There are several purposes to documentation of the rehabilitation process. These include:

- Interprofessional communication
- Tracking rehabilitation progress
- Ensuring continuity of care (e.g., documenting the care plan, and progress can ensure that another therapist can provide care in the event the primary therapist is absent)
- Communication with other programs or institutions (e.g., review for admission by a rehabilitation program, information to support safe transfer of care to another facility)

The requirements for documentation vary between countries. To be reimbursed by Medicare and/or Medicaid in the United States, specific requirements for the features and delivery of rehabilitation must be reflected in the documentation. For example, for outpatient therapy, documentation must include a plan of care and documentation of how time is spent in therapy in 15-minute blocks (Medicare Learning Network, 2022), demonstrating the need for an interdisciplinary team. In Canada, public rehabilitation services do not have documentation requirements for reimbursement purposes, but some third-party payers (such as worker's compensation or automotive injury benefits) have specific documentation requirements for reimbursement purposes.

Documentation of the care of the older adult in an inpatient setting needs to include the older adult's previous level of function and service and support needs for goal-setting and discharge planning. This is because older adults are more likely to have pre-existing disability, but pre-existing disability should not be assumed. The rehabilitation team needs to be aware of the goals intended to support the older adult in achieving their previous functional status through the rehabilitation process. The occupational therapist should also ensure that information gleaned from the older adult's supports, such as family and friends, is documented and shared with the team. This information will assist the team in determining and planning the older adult's needed supports.

Occupational therapists working with older adults should be familiar with common conditions in older adults, such as delirium and urinary tract infections, and carefully document (as well as communicate verbally) any changes in behavior or cognition or daily fluctuations in physical status to support the team in identifying and treating these conditions (Seematter-Bagnoud & Büla, 2018). The practitioner should also consider the type of information they are sharing with the older adult and their circle of care. Typically, chart documentation is not accessible physically, and even if the older adult and family get access to the chart, it may not be helpful from a health literacy perspective. The therapist should work to understand how the older adult would best like to receive information about their care plan and share this information in a way that works best for the older adult to ensure that they understand and consent to the care plan.

Payment Systems and Reimbursement

United States

In the United States, the Affordable Care Act requires that private health insurance plans cover rehabilitation services and devices as one of ten essential healthcare services. The details of this coverage are determined at the state level. Medicare is a major component of rehabilitation funding for older adults, potentially in combination with Medicaid for older adults with low income. Medicare is the federal health insurance program for people who are age 65 or older. Medicare Part A is the basic program and covers inpatient hospital service, hospice and home healthcare. It is free for individuals who have paid in to social security for at least 10 years. Medicare Part B is medical insurance that covers services and supplies not covered by Medicare Part A. It requires a monthly premium from the user. Inpatient rehabilitation services are covered by Medicare Part A if it is determined necessary by a doctor. There is deductible that needs to be paid by the user. Medicare Part B pays for 80% of outpatient rehabilitation services, and the user pays 20% and a deductible. For outpatient services, Medicaid may be able to address the 20% user fees (U.S. Centers for Medicare and Medicaid Services, n.d.b).

There are also regulations in the United States specific to SNFs. Prior to 2019, Medicare and Medicaid reimbursed SNFs according to the intensity of rehabilitation provided (e.g., number of minutes). However, financial incentives have shifted with new policy and reimbursement is now associated with patient characteristics and need. This policy shift was made because of a large increase in reimbursement requests for high-intensity services without an associated change in self-care capacity, but it left some concerned that it would result in fewer therapy hours and less functional gain for people in SNFs, as higher intensity rehabilitation is associated with greater functional gain (Edelman, 2021; Prusynski et al, 2021). Another critique is that the length of SNF stay is associated with eligibility for copayment, suggesting that length of stay is based on financial resources rather than need (Werner et al, 2019).

Canada

The financing of the Canadian healthcare system is driven by a universal health insurance plan first enacted in 1962. Because only some services are covered by this plan, Canada has a mixed model of care reimbursement. The Canadian universal insurance is robust in terms of hospital services. When rehabilitation is provided in a hospital, whether it be inpatient or outpatient, it is covered by the universal healthcare system. Once outside the hospital system, coverage for rehabilitation varies by service and by province, because provinces have some autonomy in how they choose to organize and deliver healthcare (Tikkanen et al, 2020c). Depending on the political climate in a province, there may be expansion or contraction of rehabilitation services. For example, in Manitoba, there were large cuts to outpatient orthopedic physical therapy provided in hospitals, which forced consumers to seek these services through private providers (CBC News, 2017). Another example is rehabilitation providers in primary care. Some provinces have invested more than others in having occupational therapists and physical therapists on primary care teams. A disadvantage of the Canadian system is that there is less expectation for documentation and tracking of quality performance of different rehabilitation programs, making it difficult to determine the impact of rehabilitation on health at the population level. An advantage is that therapists do not need to adhere to specific timelines and requirements for the rehabilitation program, which may allow for more individualized care planning and timing.

Australia

The Australian healthcare system consists of a mix of public and private providers. Australians can access one or the other or a mix of both. The public system is primarily funded with taxes and is called Medicare. Australians can access this system free for healthcare services like physician visits, hospitalization, prescribed medications, and primary healthcare. Australians have private insurance for things not covered in the public system, such as ambulance costs. People requiring rehabilitation following significant illness will be funded through the public hospital system. Further, the public system covers rehabilitation telehealth visits and extra services for older adults (e.g., rehabilitation provider costs, supplies for incontinence). Australians can also purchase additional insurance for things like private hospital care and private rehabilitation across the spectrum of care (The Department of Health and Aged Care, 2019).

Advocacy for Older Adults and Rehabilitation Service

The evidence on the benefits of rehabilitation for older adults is clear. However, like rehabilitation services generally, older adult rehabilitation is not prioritized within health systems because of competing and urgent demands from the acute care system and because of societal beliefs about the limited benefit of rehabilitation with older adults due to ageism (Heyman et al, 2020). Advocacy should be embedded in the occupational therapist's day-to-day practice (AOTA, 2022). In the Canadian Association of Occupational Therapy Profile of Practice, advocacy is a key role for occupational therapy practice (CAOT, 2012). The occupational therapist's work in advocacy can range from the micro (or individual) level to the meso (organizational) and macro (population) levels.

Micro-level advocacy is a regular part of everyday practice and involves ensuring that older adults are receiving the best care for them. For example, for an acute care occupational therapist, advocacy could include reaching out to a rehabilitation program that has declined acceptance of an older adult that you think would be a good candidate for the program. It could involve advocating for funding for equipment that would promote independence or requesting medical or other care that has not yet been identified as needed (e.g., a hearing assessment). Or it could involve pointing out ageist beliefs and attitudes that are expressed by team members about an older adult's capacity for rehabilitation.

Advocacy at a meso level might involve working with your rehabilitation program or organization to improve its accessibility for older adults, such as ensuring information is accessible for those with reduced hearing and/or vision, ensuring that there is adequate physical space and workplace culture for ensuring that caregivers are included in care. At a macro level, advocacy could involve becoming involved in your local occupational therapy association or other organization to advocate for fair and equitable rehabilitation reimbursement systems and coverage of services that are important for older adult health, such as home assessments and equipment for fall prevention.

CASE STUDY (CONTINUED)

Intervention in Context of a Rehabilitation Setting

At this time, Mr. George's difficulty with mobility and ADLs was also noted by the therapist. The occupational therapist advocated for a referral to a day hospital program that could do a more comprehensive geriatric assessment and provide multiple therapies to Mr. George a few times a week, which would also give his spouse some time to herself. It is hoped that Mr. George will see an overall improvement in function by the time this time-limited program is over, rather than needing to look at inpatient care options like an SNF stay. Mr. and Mrs. George were able to receive this comprehensive care in the United States because they were enrolled in Medicare and had private insurance. Although much of Mr. George's rehabilitation was covered by Medicare, it is very time limited and more robust for coverage of acute situations, like the wrist fracture. Some private insurance was used to extend the therapy time frames for the wrist fracture, to account for some of the additional therapy needed due to the comorbidity of Parkinson disease, and to supplement home care services.

Questions

1. Considering the different settings of therapy for Mr. George, what do you think the extent of interprofessional collaboration was in these settings?

2. What are two evidence-based interventions that would be used in this case study, and in which setting do you anticipate that intervention being used?

Answers

1. In the home healthcare setting, it is typical for there to be a home care case coordinator who consults other professionals as required. This case coordinator typically conducts a home visit and does a global assessment of function and need, typically by self-report from the older adults and supports. This individual is often a nurse, social worker, or occupational therapist. It is likely that a physical therapist would also have been involved to look at how to support improvement with mobility and maintenance of strength.

   For Mr. George's rehabilitation of the wrist, it is typical for the occupational therapist to have an extra hand therapy designation that provides them with extra skills in hand rehabilitation, particularly with designing and teaching rehabilitation exercises for home for strength and flexibility. If the case is not straightforward, the occupational therapist may refer to a physical therapist who can provide more specialized care in relation to the remediation of hand strength.

   In a day hospital setting, it is typical for an interprofessional team to work together; often this team consists of a geriatrician, nurse social worker, occupational therapist, physical therapist, and speech-language pathologist. These professionals will share their assessment findings with one another, develop a rehabilitation plan together, and meet regularly to review progress of the day hospital participants. (Role of Occupational Therapy and Interprofessional Partners, LO 25-2)

2. It is likely that the day hospital team uses a comprehensive geriatric assessment approach to ensure that a multi-domain assessment is completed and that a multi-domain intervention plan is designed and implemented.

   In the home care setting, typically a case management approach is used, with a nurse, social worker, or occupational therapist acting as a case manager or care coordinator to ensure that care is coordinated and that all the older adult's needs are met. (Intervention Exemplars, LO 25-5)

SUMMARY

Older adult care can occur in many different settings, depending on the older adult's specific care needs. Regardless of the setting in which the care is occurring, there are considerations for older adults that should be carried across all settings because of biological, environmental, and social commonalities in older adults that are best addressed by a multidisciplinary team with knowledge in older adult healthcare. To best serve older adults, occupational therapists need to be aware of best practice in terms of how service is best designed and delivered and reimbursed. Developing advocacy skills will ensure that the older adult receives the extent of rehabilitation services that they require.

Critical Thinking Questions

1. One of the roles of an occupational therapist is to help determine the best setting for an older adult's rehabilitation. Consider the settings discussed in this chapter. What personal and social characteristics would influence the setting that an occupational therapist would recommend?

2. Identify two issues for which you could do advocacy work in your community that would help older adults participate more fully in their community (macro level).

REFERENCES

Achterberg, W. P., Cameron, I. D., Bauer, J. M., & Schols, J. M. (2019). Geriatric rehabilitation—State of the art and future priorities. *Journal of the American Medical Directors Association, 20*(4), 396–398. doi: 10.1016/j.jamda.2019.02.014

Administration on Aging. (2021). *A profile of older Americans.* Retrieved from https://acl.gov/sites/default/files/Aging%20and%20Disability%20in%20America/2020ProfileOlderAmericans.Final_.pdf

Alejandro J. (2021). Considering case management practice from a global perspective. *Professional Case Management, 26*(2):99–103. doi: 10.1097/NCM.0000000000000489

American Addiction Centers. (2022). *Mental health spending by state across the US.* https://rehabs.com/explore/mental-health-spending-by-state-across-the-us/

American Occupational Therapy Association. (2022). *Everyday advocacy.* https://www.aota.org/advocacy/everyday-advocacy

American Occupational Therapy Association (AOTA) & American Physical Therapy Association (APTA). (2021). *Therapy Outcomes in Post-Acute Care Settings (TOPS) Study Chartbook.* https://www.apta.org/contentassets/c998db9173664112ae6e5c95b81eceae/tops-study-chartbook.pdf

Ankuda, C. K., Leff, B., Ritchie, C. S., Rahman, O. K., Ferreira, K. B., Bollens-Lund, E., & Ornstein, K. A. (2020). Implications of 2020 skilled home healthcare payment reform for persons with dementia. *Journal of the American Geriatric Society, 68*(10), 2303–2309. doi: 10.1111/jgs.16654

Ariza-Vega, P., Castillo-Pérez, H., Ortiz-Piña, M., Ziden, L., Palomino-Vidal, J., & Ashe, M. C. (2021). The journey of recovery: Caregivers' perspectives from a hip fracture telerehabilitation clinical trial. *Physical Therapy, 101*(3), pzaa220. https://doi.org/10.1093/ptj/pzaa220

Bakerjian, D. (2020). *Day care for older adults.* In MSD manual, professional version. https://www.msdmanuals.com/professional/geriatrics/providing-care-to-older-adults/day-care-for-older-adults

Burke, R. E., Lawrence, E., Ladebue, A., Ayele, R., Lippmann, B., Cumbler, E., Allyn, R., & Jones, J. (2017). How hospital clinicians select patients for skilled nursing facilities. *Journal of the American Geriatrics Society (JAGS), 65*(11), 2466–2472. https://doi.org/10.1111/jgs.14954

Cameron, I. D., Schaafsma, F. G., Wilson, S., Baker, W., & Buckley, S. (2012). Outcomes of rehabilitation in older people—functioning and cognition are the most important predictors: An inception cohort study. *Journal of Rehabilitation Medicine, 44*, 24–30. doi: 10.2340/16501977-0901

Canadian Association of Occupational Therapy. (2012). *Profile of practice of occupational therapists in Canada.* https://caot.ca/document/3653/2012otprofile.pdf

Canadian Frailty Network. (2021–2022). *What is frailty?* https://www.cfn-nce.ca/frailty-matters/what-is-frailty/

Canadian Interprofessional Health Collaborative. (2010). *A national interprofessional competency framework.* BC: University of British Columbia, Vancouver (2010). https://phabc.org/wp-content/uploads/2015/07/CIHC-National-Interprofessional-Competency-Framework.pdf

CBC News. (2017). *Some Manitobans will pay out-of-pocket for physiotherapy starting this Fall.* https://www.cbc.ca/news/canada/manitoba/manitoba-physiotherapy-occupational-therapy-payments-1.4200596

Cole, M., & Tufano, R. (2020). Model integration (Chapter 11). In *Applied theories in occupational therapy: A practical approach* (2nd edition). SLACK Incorporated.

Edelman, T. (2021). *CMS confirms steep decline in therapy at nursing facilities.* Center for Medicare Advocacy. https://medicareadvocacy.org/cms-confirms-steep-decline-in-therapy-at-nursing-facilities/

Egan, M., & Restall, G. (2022). *Promoting occupational participation: Collaborative relationship-focused occupational therapy: 10th Canadian occupational therapy guidelines* (M. Egan & G. Restall, Eds.). Canadian Association of Occupational Therapists.

Facchinetti, G., D'Angelo, D., Piredda, M., Petitti, T., Matarese, M., Oliveti, A., & De Marinis, M. G. (2020). Continuity of care interventions for preventing hospital readmission of older people with chronic diseases: A meta-analysis. *International Journal of Nursing Studies, 101*, 103396. https://doi.org/10.1016/j.ijnurstu.2019.103396

Flint, L. A., David, D. J., & Smith, A. K. (2019). Rehabbed to death. *The New England Journal of Medicine, 380*(5), 408–409. https://doi.org/10.1056/NEJMp1809354

Freitas, M. M, Antunes, S., Ascenso, D., & Silveira, A. (2021). Outpatient and home-based treatment: Effective settings for hip fracture rehabilitation in elderly patients. *Geriatrics (Basel), 6*(3), 83. https://doi.org/10.3390/geriatrics6030083

Gibson, E., Koh, C. L., Eames, S., Bennett, S., Scott, A. M., & Hoffmann, T. C. (2022). Occupational therapy for cognitive impairment in stroke patients. *Cochrane Library, 3*(3), CD006430. https://doi.org/10.1002/14651858.CD006430.pub3

Gonçalves-Bradley, D. C., Lannin, N. A., Clemson, L., Cameron, I. D., & Shepperd, S. (2022). Discharge planning from hospital. *Cochrane Library, 2*(2), CD000313. https://doi.org/10.1002/14651858.CD000313.pub6

Grahek, I., Shenhav, A., Musslick, S., Krebs, R. M., & Koster, E. H. W. (2019). Motivation and cognitive control in depression. *Neuroscience and Biobehavioral Reviews, 102*, 371–381. https://doi.org/10.1016/j.neubiorev.2019.04.011

Grenier, M. L. (2020). Cultural competency and the reproduction of White supremacy in occupational therapy education. *Health Education Journal, 79*(6), 633–644. https://doi-org.uml.idm.oclc.org/10.1177/0017896920902515

Grund, S., Gordon, A. L., van Balen, R., Bachmann, S., Cherubini, A., Landi, F., Stuck, A. E., Becker, C., Achterberg, W. P., Bauer, J. M., & Schols, J. M. G. A. (2020). European consensus on core principles and future priorities for geriatric rehabilitation: Consensus statement. *European Geriatric Medicine, 11*(2), 233–238. https://doi.org/10.1007/s41999-019-00274-1

Grund, S., van Wijngaarden, J. P., Gordon, A. L., Schols, J. M. G. A., & Bauer, J. M. (2020). EuGMS survey on structures of geriatric rehabilitation across Europe. *European Geriatric Medicine, 11*(2), 217–232. https://doi.org/10.1007/s41999-019-00273-2

Handoll, H. H., Cameron, I. D., Mak, J. C., Panagoda, C. E., & Finnegan, T. P. (2021). Multidisciplinary rehabilitation for older people with hip fractures. *Cochrane Database of Systematic Reviews,* (4), CD007125. https://doi.org/10.1002/14651858.CD007125.pub3

Hayes. (2020). Telerehabilitation for older adults. *Topics in Geriatric Rehabilitation, 36*(4), 205–211. https://doi.org/10.1097/TGR.0000000000000282

Heinemann, A. W., Feuerstein, M., Frontera, W. R., Gard, S. A., Kaminsky, L. A., Negrini, S., Richards, L. G., & Vallée, C. (2020). Rehabilitation is a global health priority. *Canadian Journal of Occupational Therapy, 87*(2), 89–90. doi: 10.1016/j.apmr.2019.08.468

Heyman, N., Osman, I., & Ben Natan, M. (2020). Ageist attitudes among healthcare professionals and older patients in a geriatric rehabilitation facility and their association with patients' satisfaction with care. *International Journal of Older People Nursing, 15*(2), e12307. https://doi.org/10.1111/opn.12307

Hudon, C., Chouinard, M. C., Dubois, M. F., Roberge, P., Loignon, C., Tchouaket, É., Lambert, M., Hudon, É., Diadiou, F., & Bouliane, D. (2018). Case management in primary care for frequent users of health care services: A mixed methods study. *The Annals of Family Medicine, 16*(3), 232–239. doi: 10.1370/afm.2233

Knutti, K., Björklund Carlstedt, A., Clasen, R., & Green, D. (2022). Impacts of goal setting on engagement and rehabilitation outcomes following acquired brain injury: A systematic review of reviews. *Disability and Rehabilitation, 44*(12), 2581–2590, doi: 10.1080/09638288.2020.1846796

Langhorne, P., & Ramachandra, S. (2020). Organised inpatient (stroke unit) care for stroke: Network meta-analysis. *Cochrane Database of Systematic Reviews, 4*(4), CD000197–CD000197. https://doi.org/10.1002/14651858.CD000197.pub4

Maffioletti, V., Baptista, M. A. T., Santos, R. L., Rodrigues, V. M., & Dourado, M. C. N. (2019). Effectiveness of day care in supporting family caregivers of people with dementia: A systematic review. *Dementia & Neuropsychologia, 13*(3), 268–283. https://doi.org/10.1590/1980-57642018dn13-030003

Mann, J., Thompson, F., McDermott, R., Esterman, A., & Strivens, E. (2021). Impact of an integrated community-based model of care for older people with complex conditions on hospital emergency presentations and admissions: A step-wedged cluster randomized trial. *BMC Health Services Research, 21*(1), 1–11. https://doi.org/10.1186/s12913-021-06668-x

McGilton, K. S., Davis, A., Mahomed, N., Flannery, J., Jaglal, S., Cott, C., & Rochon, E. (2012) An inpatient rehabilitation model of care targeting patients with cognitive impairment. *BMC Geriatrics, 12*, 21–21. doi: 10.1186/1471-2318-12-21

Medicare Learning Network. (2022). *Complying with outpatient rehabilitation therapy documentation requirements: MLN fact sheet.* U.S. Department of Health & Human Services (HHS). https://www.hhs.gov/guidance/sites/default/files/hhs-guidance-documents/OutptRehabTherapy_Booklet_MLN905365.pdf

Michelangelo. (n.d.) Ancora imparo (Still, I am learning). Retrieved from https://www.goodreads.com/quotes/215155-ancora-imparo-i-am-still-learning

Morkisch, N., Upegui-Arango, L. D., Cardona, M. I., van den Heuvel, D., Rimmele, M., Sieber, C. C., & Freiberger, E. (2020). Components of the transitional care model (TCM) to reduce readmission in geriatric patients: A systematic review. *BMC Geriatrics, 20*(1), 1–345. https://doi.org/10.1186/s12877-020-01747-w

Moyet, J., Deschasse, G., Marquant, B., Mertl, P., & Bloch, F. (2018). Which is the optimal orthogeriatric care model to prevent mortality of elderly subjects post hip fractures? A systematic review and meta-analysis based on current clinical practice. *International Orthopaedics, 43*(6), 1449–1454. https://doi.org/10.1007/s00264-018-3928-5

Nordström, P., Thorngren, K. G., Hommel, A., Ziden, L., & Anttila, S. (2018). Effects of geriatric team rehabilitation after hip fracture: Meta-analysis of randomized controlled trials. *Journal of the American Medical Directors Association, 19*(10), 840–845. https://doi.org/10.1016/j.jamda.2018.05.008

Northwood, M., Ploeg, J., Markle-Reid, M., & Sherifali, D. (2018). Integrative review of the social determinants of health in older adults with multimorbidity. *Journal of Advanced Nursing, 74*(1), 45–60. https://doi.org/10.1111/jan.13408

Pan, P. J., Lin, P. H., Tang, G. J., & Lan, T. Y. (2018). Comparisons of mortality and rehospitalization between hip-fractured elderly with outpatient rehabilitation and those without: A STROBE-compliant article. *Medicine (Baltimore), 97*(19), e0644–e0644. https://doi.org/10.1097/MD.0000000000010644

Parker, S. G., McCue, P., Phelps, K., McCleod, A., Arora, S., Nockels, K., Kennedy, S., Roberts, H., & Conroy, S. (2018). What is comprehensive geriatric assessment (CGA)? An umbrella review. *Age Ageing, 47*(1), 149–155. doi: 10.1093/ageing/afx166

Pergolotti, M., Deal, A. M., Williams, G. R., Bryant, A. L., McCarthy, L., Nyrop, K. A., Covington, K. R., Reeve, B. B., Basch, E., & Muss, H. B. (2019). Older adults with cancer: A randomized controlled trial of occupational and physical therapy. *Journal of the American Geriatrics Society (JAGS), 67*(5), 953–960. https://doi.org/10.1111/jgs.15930

Pilotto, A., Cella, A., Pilotto, A., Daragjati, J., Veronese, N., Musacchio, C., Mello, A. M., Logroscino, G., Padovani, A., Prete, C., & Panza, F. (2017). Three decades of comprehensive geriatric assessment: Evidence coming from different healthcare settings and specific clinical conditions. *Journal of the American Medical Directors Association, 18*(2), 192.e1–192.e11. doi: 10.1016/j.jamda.2016.11.004

Popejoy, L. L., Vogelsmeier, A. A., Wakefield, B. J., Galambos, C. M., Lewis, A. M., Huneke, D., & Mehr, D. R. (2020). Adapting project RED to skilled nursing facilities. *Clinical Nursing Research, 29*(3), 149–156. doi:10.1177/1054773818819261

Prusynski, R. A., Gustavson, A. M., Shrivastav, S. R., & Mroz, T. M. (2021). Rehabilitation intensity and patient outcomes in skilled nursing facilities in the United States: A systematic review. *Physical Therapy, 101*(3), pzaa230. https://doi.org/10.1093/ptj/pzaa230

Seematter-Bagnoud, L., & Büla, C. (2018). Brief assessments and screening for geriatric conditions in older primary care patients: A pragmatic approach. *Public Health Reviews, 39*(1), 8. https://doi.org/10.1186/s40985-018-0086-7

Singh, R., Küçükdeveci, A. A., Grabljevec, K., & Gray, A. (2018). The role of interdisciplinary teams in physical and rehabilitation medicine. *Journal of Rehabilitation Medicine, 50*(8), 673–678. https://doi.org/10.2340/16501977-2364

Soto-Perez-de-Celis, E., Li, D., Yuan, Y., Lau, Y. M., & Hurria, A. (2018). Functional versus chronological age: Geriatric assessments to guide decision making in older patients with cancer. *The Lancet Oncology, 19*(6), e305–e316. https://doi.org/10.1016/S1470-2045(18)30348-6

Stanetić, K., Petrović, V., Stanetić, B., Kević1V, S. M., & Matović, J. (2020). Screening of undiagnosed depression among elderly primary care patients: A cross-sectional study from the Republic of Srpska, Bosnia and Herzegovina. *Medicinski Glasnik, 17*(1), 1103–1120. doi:10.17392/1103-20

The Department of Health and Aged Care. (2019). *The Australian Health System.* Australian Government: Department of Health and Aged Care. https://www.health.gov.au/about-us/the-australian-health-system#:~:text=Medicare%20and%20the%20public%20hospital,cost%20of%20your%20health%20care

Tikkanen, R., Osborn, R., Mossialos, E., Djordjevic, A., & Wharton, G. A. (2020a). *International health care system profiles: The United States.* New York: NY. The Commonwealth Fund. https://www.commonwealthfund.org/international-health-policy-center/countries/united-states

Tikkanen, R., Osborn, R., Mossialos, E., Djordjevic, A., & Wharton, G. A. (2020b). *International health care system profiles: England.* New York: NY. The Commonwealth Fund. https://www.commonwealthfund.org/international-health-policy-center/countries/england

Tikkanen, R., Osborn, R., Mossialos, E., Djordjevic, A., & Wharton, G. A. (2020c). *International health care system profiles: Canada.* New York: NY. The Commonwealth Fund. https://www.commonwealthfund.org/international-health-policy-center/countries/canada

U.S. Centers for Medicare and Medicaid Services. (n.d.a.). *Skilled nursing facility (SNF) care.* https://www.medicare.gov/coverage/skilled-nursing-facility-snf-care

U.S. Centers for Medicare and Medicaid Services. (n.d.b.). *What Medicare covers.* https://www.medicare.gov/what-medicare-coversvan

van Balen, R., Gordon, A. L., Schols, J. M. G. A., Wes, Y. M., & Achterberg, W. P. (2019). What is geriatric rehabilitation and how should it be organized? A Delphi study aimed at reaching European consensus. *European Geriatric Medicine, 10*(6), 977–987. https://doi.org/10.1007/s41999-019-00244-7

van den Bergh, R., Bloem, B. R., Meinders, M. J., & Evers, L. (2021). The state of telemedicine for persons with Parkinson's disease. *Current Opinion in Neurology, 34*(4), 589–597. https://doi-org.uml.idm.oclc.org/10.1097/WCO.0000000000000953

Velayati, F., Ayatollahi, H., & Hemmat, M. (2020). A systematic review of the effectiveness of telerehabilitation interventions for therapeutic purposes in the elderly. *Methods of Information in Medicine, 59*(2-03), 104–109. https://doi.org/10.1055/s-0040-1713398

Wade, D. T. (2020). What is rehabilitation? An empirical investigation leading to an evidence-based description. *Clinical Rehabilitation, 34*(5), 571–583. https://doi.org/10.1177/0269215520905112

Wang, Z., Hu, X., & Dai, Q. (2020). Is it possible to reverse frailty in patients with chronic obstructive pulmonary disease? *Clinics (São Paulo, Brazil), 75*, e1778. https://doi.org/10.6061/clinics/2020/e1778

Wener, P., Leclair, L., Fricke, M., & Brown, C. (2022). Interprofessional collaborative relationship-building model in action in primary care: A secondary analysis. *Frontiers in Rehabilitation Sciences, 3*, 890001. https://doi.org/10.3389/fresc.2022.890001

Werner, R. M., Konetzka, R. T., Qi, M., & Coe, N. B. (2019). The impact of Medicare copayments for skilled nursing facilities on length of stay, outcomes, and costs. *Health Services Research, 54*(6), 1184–1192. https://doi.org/10.1111/1475-6773.13227

Whyman, J. (2022). Geriatric occupational therapy: Achieving quality in daily living. In Pathy's *Principles and practice of geriatric medicine* (pp. 1574–1584). John Wiley & Sons, Ltd. https://doi.org/10.1002/9781119484288.ch126

World Health Organization. (2017). *10 facts on ageing and health (Fact Sheet)*. Geneva: World Health Organization. https://www.who.int/news-room/fact-sheets/detail/10-facts-on-ageing-and-health

World Health Organization. (2022). *Rehabilitation (Fact Sheet)*. Geneva: World Health Organization. https://www.who.int/news-room/fact-sheets/detail/rehabilitation#:~:text=Rehabilitation%20is%20defined%20as%20%E2%80%9Ca,in%20interaction%20with%20their%20environment%E2%80%9D

Yun, D. W., & Choi, J. (2019). Person-centered rehabilitation care and outcomes: A systematic literature review. *International Journal of Nursing Studies, 93*, 74–83. https://doi.org/10.1016/j.ijnurstu.2019.02.012

Zhang, Y., Zhang, Y., Sholle, E., Abedian, S., Sharko, M., Turchioe, M. R., Wu, Y., & Ancker, J. S. (2020). Assessing the impact of social determinants of health on predictive models for potentially avoidable 30-day readmission or death. *PLoS ONE, 15*(6), e0235064. https://doi.org/10.1371/journal.pone.0235064

CHAPTER 26

Home Health Services

Keegan McKay, OTR, MOT, OTD

> *"What counts in life is not the mere fact that we have lived. It is what difference we have made to the lives of others that will determine the significance of the life we lead."*
>
> —Nelson Mandela

LEARNING OUTCOMES

By the end of this chapter, readers will be able to:

26-1. Analyze how the concept of home health occupational therapy services is successfully delivered in different contexts.

26-2. Evaluate the role of an occupational therapist in home health in order to determine what skills and knowledge are needed to be successful in this setting.

26-3. Compare and contrast the roles of different disciplines seen in the home health setting that create a collaborative interprofessional team.

26-4. Relate the Medicare rules and regulations that affect home health to the practice of occupational therapy in order to ensure compliant and ethical standards are met.

26-5. Synthesize information related to the assessment process in home health and to data collection and documentation requirements for reimbursement.

26-6. Synthesize information about exemplar occupational therapy interventions to address patients' occupational challenges.

26-7. Explore and design new ways to advocate for occupational therapy services in home health.

Mini Case Study

Mr. Omar Ali Bey is a 68-year-old retired postal worker who lives in a small two-story bungalow in a low-income neighborhood near the city center. The home has three bedrooms and one bathroom, all located on the second floor. He has had diabetes for 30 years and recently underwent a left, below-knee amputation secondary to his diabetes. Mr. Bey was fitted with a prosthesis, had 2 weeks of inpatient rehabilitation with occupational therapy and physical therapy, and has been discharged to his home. His wife, also 68 years old, has rheumatoid arthritis and macular degeneration and struggles to take care of herself. Their three children live within several miles of their parents but have full-time jobs and adolescent children at home. Although the family is emotionally close and supportive, the children have limited time to provide instrumental assistance.

Provocative Questions

1. What aspects of Mr. Bey's health status and living situation would qualify him for home health services?
2. What are some of the immediate areas of concern that an occupational therapist could address?
3. What skills would an occupational therapist need to successfully develop a plan of care and provide interventions that are best practices?
4. What other disciplines in an interprofessional team might be needed as part of Mr. Bey's home health plan of care?

Home health is a healthcare setting that has allowed patients to have better access to services by providing these services in the patient's own home. The setting of home health has proven to be a cost-effective and quality-measured option for patients with illness, injury, or other conditions. These conditions are often due to older age, disability, or chronic conditions and can lead to difficulties in occupational performance. As the population ages, the need for home health services grows. Practitioners of multiple disciplines work with patients in the home health setting. Occupational therapists play an essential role in the delivery of home health services, with a focus on treating a patient within the context of their home environment. Refer to Figure 26-1 for an example of a patient participating in the occupation of meal preparation in their home, one of the many activities that can be addressed in home health.

This chapter will explore the interprofessional nature of home health and will feature some of the important contributions that occupational therapy in particular makes to this setting. Additionally, because home health is so highly regulated, key concepts related to the provision of services, reimbursement, and other administrative considerations will be reviewed.

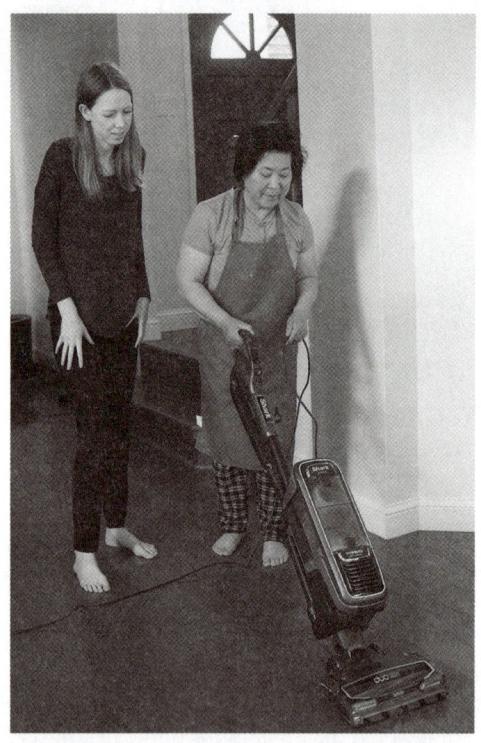

FIGURE 26-1 Observing the patient in his or her environment can provide important information about how specific occupations are accomplished.

Defining Home Health Services

Home health services is defined as the provision of a wide range of services for patients of all ages within their own home environment (Medicare.gov, 2022a). The Centers for Medicare and Medicaid Services (CMS) states that home health is a covered service consisting of part-time, medically necessary skilled care (nursing, and occupational, physical, and speech therapies) that is ordered by a physician or other certain types of providers (Medicare.gov, 2022a). These services are typically prescribed for patients experiencing an illness or injury that has resulted in the need for intervention from a variety of healthcare professionals. These conditions might include, for example, an individual with mobility issues due to a recent joint replacement surgery, a deconditioned patient returning home after a hospital stay due to pneumonia, or an older adult with difficulty managing their healthcare needs after an exacerbation of congestive heart failure. The decrease in length of stay at acute care hospitals, which was influenced by CMS and insurance companies, has created a need for continued healthcare services after acute care discharge.

There are multiple advantages for patients in the home health setting compared with an inpatient setting, such as an acute care hospital, inpatient rehabilitation facility, or skilled nursing facility. Providing care in the home is much more convenient for the patient, equally effective, and less expensive than stays in an inpatient facility (Medicare.gov, 2022a). The services described in this chapter are provided to patients who are either unable to leave the home or for whom it would be challenging to leave the home.

The types of home health services explored in this chapter include interventions not only from occupational therapists but from the other interprofessional partners. Occupational therapists are especially important in the home health setting because of their skills in activity and occupation analysis, ability to assess occupational performance of patients in their unique environments, and knowledge of home safety, fall prevention, and environmental modifications.

The Context of Home Health

Home health services can occur in a variety of different settings, depending on the patient's home situation. A patient's residence is "wherever he or she makes his or her home. This may be his or her own dwelling, an apartment, a relative's home, a home for the aged, or some other type of institution" (CMS, 2021a, §30.1.2). In this language, *institution* refers to community-based institutions, such as assisted- and independent living facilities. Hospitals, skilled nursing homes, and long-term care facilities do not qualify as a patient's residence.

There is a strong and continued desire among older adults to remain in their own homes for the long term as they age (Davis, 2021). When patients receive occupational therapy services in their private homes, they are observed in their own environment (where they may have lived for many years), allowing the occupational therapist to determine their ability to safely perform daily occupations in their typical manner. While living in community-based institutions tends to be a more-controlled environment that is supported by facility employees, a home health patient living in their private home might encounter situations out of their control that could affect their safety. For example, an older home may have been built during a time when specifications for buildings could have resulted in a less-than-ideal environment for the homeowner (e.g., narrow doorways, lack of accessibility in bathrooms, inappropriate counter heights). This requires that the occupational therapist utilize their skills to problem-solve very challenging situations, which could entail educating the patient on a safer way to complete an activity or recommending a significant change in the physical environment or structure of the building itself. Aging in place is the ideal for many patients; for others, the home environment may not always be optimal for their safety and occupational performance.

Assisted-Living Facilities

Many older adults choose to transition to an alternative long-term care option, such as an **assisted-living facility.** Beyond housing, assisted-living facility residents may receive support and healthcare services (National Health Care Association, 2023). Examples include instrumental activities of daily living (IADLs), such as meals, transportation, and medication management, and basic activities of daily living (BADLs), such as dressing, toileting, and bathing. In an assisted-living facility, employees include trained support caregivers, such as certified nurse assistants. Certified nurse assistants must complete a required number of hours of training to obtain and maintain certification and act as care staff who assist residents with BADLs, IADLs, and functional transfers. Caregivers provide the appropriate amount of assistance to residents, under the supervision of nursing staff, to meet residents' daily needs.

There is still a need for the provision of occupational therapy services under the home health benefit in an assisted-living setting. This includes the patient's desire to work on increasing independence or implementing compensatory strategies with IADLs and BADLs, improving satisfaction with occupational performance, improving quality of life, and reducing the need for caregiver assistance. Occupational therapists can work with the patient and caregivers on creating a plan of care that supports patient-centered goals and includes interventions for the patient and caregivers. While there are advantages to living in an assisted-living facility, such as accessible bathrooms and safe appliances, occupational therapists can recommend modifications to the environment to increase autonomy and safety.

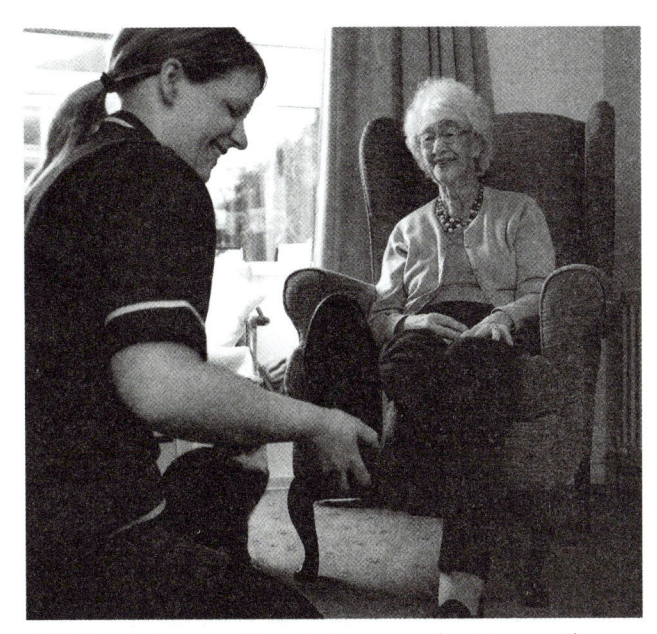

FIGURE 26-2 Home health patients may need assistance with activities of daily living when they first leave an acute care setting. *(Dean Mitchell/iStock/Getty Images.)*

CASE STUDY

Mr. Martinez from Chapter 11 in the context of home healthcare

Presenting Situation

In Chapter 11, you were introduced to Mr. Juan Martinez. As you may recall, Mr. Martinez is a 78-year-old man who sustained a right proximal femur fracture and underwent an open-reduction, internal fixation procedure. The fracture occurred when he was exiting his bathtub and his leg gave way. Mr. Martinez lives with his wife in a two-story home, which has several steps (with no railings) leading into the home. Mr. and Mrs. Martinez's bedroom and bathroom are on the second level. Before his fall and proximal femur fracture, he was independent with mobility and BADLs and IADLs, except he needed minimal assistance to get in and out of the bathtub. Some of his hobbies include gardening and playing bridge.

The Role of Occupational Therapy in Home Health

Home health services is an interesting, often complex, setting of healthcare that includes many rules and regulations that are an essential part of these services. The home health setting allows occupational therapists to use their vast knowledge of human occupation to help patients live a fulfilling life in their own home environment. When a patient first leaves an acute care setting, they may require assistance with BADLs and IADLs. Refer to Figure 26-2, which shows an occupational therapist assisting a patient with dressing. Dressing is often a high priority for patients in home health. Occupational therapists working in home health care address BADLs, IADLs, home safety, chronic health management, medication management, and family education and training (see Chapters 14, 15, and 16 for more intervention ideas). Hospice care is also often provided in the home (see Chapter 28).

Interprofessional Partners

Beyond occupational therapists, many other individuals contribute, both clinically and administratively, to the success of meeting a home health patient's needs.

Physical Therapy

Physical therapists and physical therapist assistants work closely with occupational therapists when addressing the autonomy and safety needs of a patient. An occupational therapist may be concerned with a patient's ability to safely and independently perform their IADLs, such as meal preparation. A physical therapist or physical therapy assistant might take a closer look at the patient's movement patterns and perhaps have the patient perform therapeutic exercises in a way that could ultimately help the patient use their arms when they need to perform a meal preparation task, such as using a mixing bowl (Hayhurst, 2020). The patient benefits from meaningful interventions from both occupational and physical therapy. There are times when the roles of occupational therapists and physical therapists overlap, which is why it is essential that both disciplines collaborate and discuss the patient's goals and how they can work together to meet the needs of the patient. From a reimbursement point of view, it is important to avoid duplication of services, which can be achieved through regular face-to-face, telephone, and e-mail correspondence.

For example, physical therapists and occupational therapists are trained, and it is in their scope of practice, to address safety and independence with transfers and mobility. However, the issue of duplication of services arises if both disciplines attempt to address a patient's goal of improving these activities. One solution could be to focus on each discipline's strengths. When developing the plan of care, the physical therapist might focus on a patient's ability to perform a sit-to-stand transfer, including using an assistive device safely and increasing lower-extremity strength for greater ease in standing. In addition, they could provide opportunities to practice walking on even surfaces and uneven surfaces and upgrade a walking device from a walker to a single-tip cane. On the other hand, an occupational therapist might choose to address transfers and mobility within the context of the patient's chosen occupations. This could include performing toilet transfers and bathtub/shower transfers for bathroom occupations, mobility in the yard to work on gardening activities, or mobility in the kitchen for safety with meal preparation. By working together, the physical therapist and occupational therapist can significantly accelerate the progress of a home health patient during an episode of care.

Speech Therapy

In home health, speech therapy services are provided by speech-language pathologists. The focus of their interventions varies, though speech-language pathologists often address functional communication, such as spoken language comprehension and expression, as well as swallowing difficulties (American Speech–Language–Hearing Association, n.d.). While speech-language pathologists also address cognitive deficits in their practice, information found in the Medicare Benefit Policy Manual (CMS, 2021a) does not specify the inclusion of cognitive treatment under the home health benefit. It is important for home health agencies to research and determine the local rules of cognitive treatment, though quite often cognition is not addressed by speech-language pathologists in home health due to the ambiguous verbiage in the manual. This leads to another opportunity for occupational therapists to partner with speech-language pathologists. While a speech-language pathologist might focus on communication skills, including receptive language, an occupational therapist could use occupations and activities in the home to address cognition in a functional way (e.g., problem-solving, sequencing, other higher executive functioning skills used when performing occupations in the home).

Another way in which a speech-language pathologist and occupational therapist could collaborate is that speech therapy includes treatment of swallowing disorders (dysphagia) while occupational therapy focuses on the fine motor and coordination skills needed to feed oneself at the dinner table. Together, a speech-language pathologist and an occupational therapist practitioner can help improve the independence, safety, and enjoyment of mealtimes for patients at home.

Skilled Nursing

Skilled nursing services are one of the largest parts of any home health agency. Nurses address the medical needs of their patients and are essentially the "eyes and ears" for a physician, assessing and reporting updates on a patient's medical condition. This is true of all disciplines, but in skilled nursing, often the treatments can be of a more serious nature, such as providing infusions, wound care, and injectable medications and monitoring unstable patients to ensure their safety at home (CMS, 2021a). While therapy services can be an important part of a patient's plan of care, the highest priority is to help medically stabilize a home health patient before addressing other needs.

All disciplines are required to monitor the patient's vital signs (blood pressure, temperature, respiration and heart rate) on every visit. When an occupational therapist discovers a vital sign that is out of parameters or something else of concern, they collaborate with home health nursing staff, clinical nursing managers (usually based in the home health office), and the physician's office to make sure that these urgent issues are addressed.

Social Services and Home Health Aides

Medical social services and home health aide services are considered dependent services, meaning they are covered under the home health benefit only if they are provided alongside skilled services. Medical social workers are brought in as part of the patient's plan of care when assistance is needed with finding or accessing resources (e.g., equipment, long-term living options, need for caregiver assistance). Additionally, a medical social worker might be brought in to the case if there are issues with neglect, abuse, unsafe living conditions in the patient's home, or other psychosocial issues. Medicare beneficiaries may qualify for medical social services if there is a need to resolve social or emotional problems that could affect the overall treatment plan for the patient (CMS, 2021a).

A home health aide provides personal care assistance to patients on a part-time and intermittent basis. Home health aides are typically certified nurse assistants, and it is very important that they have the required number of hours of training so as to ensure home health patients are being cared for by qualified and competent employees. The type of assistance provided includes activities such as bathing, dressing, grooming, positioning in bed, and assistance with ambulation. Typically, a home health aide will provide assistance on a temporary basis as part of the plan of care. However, if ongoing assistance will be needed with BADLs and IADLs after discharge from home health services, the interprofessional care team will collaborate and provide recommendations for a long-term solution. Discharge planning is an important consideration that begins at the start of care and continues for the duration of the episode of care. A **start of care** is the initial billable visit that is completed when home health services are initiated by a home health agency.

Administrative Staff

Professionals and paraprofessionals who work with patients in a home health agency are often called the "field staff." To complement the field staff, every home health agency must have a home office that consists of administrative staff who support the field operations. Each agency must have both an administrator and an alternative administrator, who are appointed by a governing body (CMS, 2019). These roles are an essential part of the requirements of a home health agency. The administrator is ultimately responsible for ensuring that the agency is compliant with Medicare rules and regulations. Within a typical home health agency, it is the administrator who has oversight of processes and procedures, including the clinical care, financial budgets, and any other considerations for the day-to-day functioning of the agency. You will also find clinical managers, usually registered nurses, who focus on the clinical needs of the patient and supervisory functions of field clinicians and are often responsible for facilitating quality care and outcomes. Support staff also work in a home health office to perform administrative, nonclinical tasks but often interact with patients and family members telephonically or via other routes of communication.

Home Health Agencies and Medicare

There are important ways in which Medicare rules and regulations relate to home health services. It is important to note that home health services are reimbursed by a variety of payers, including commercial insurance, Medicare advantage plans, Medicaid, private pay, and other sources. However, for the purpose of this chapter, when looking at home health services provided for older adults, the focus is on Medicare rules and regulations that affect this healthcare setting. It is important to have an understanding of which parts of Medicare fund home health services, and the policies that are required to receive and provide Medicare-certified home health services.

Home health agencies are agencies or organizations that are primarily involved in providing skilled services, including nursing and other therapeutic services, to home health patients (CMS, 2022a). They are required to adhere to the rules and regulations outlined by CMS, including maintaining clinical records on all patients. An agency must be Medicare certified to provide home health services to a Medicare recipient. This involves implementing and following Medicare requirements, which will be discussed later in this section. Home health agencies can be either: (1) public agencies, which are operated by state or local government; (2) nonprofit agencies, which are private, nongovernmental agencies; or (3) proprietary agencies, which are private, for-profit organizations (CMS, 2022a).

The Medicare program extends healthcare coverage to Americans age 65 or older, people younger than age 65 with certain disabilities, and people of all ages with other specified conditions.

There are multiple parts of Medicare that cover specific services. Below are some of these parts and how they affect home health services (CMS, 2021b).

- **Medicare Part A (Hospital Insurance)** covers costs for Medicare-certified home health services, in addition to other inpatient care services and hospice.
- **Medicare Part B (Medical Insurance)** covers costs for doctor's services, outpatient therapy services, and some specific home healthcare costs, such as durable medical equipment.
- **Medicare Part C (Managed Advantage)** is an alternative for Part A and Part B coverage and is provided through private insurance, which Medicare must approve. Part C may also include the Part D drug benefit.
- **Medicare Part D** is a stand-alone prescription drug coverage plan.

In this chapter, the discussion of home health services is specific to Medicare-certified home health that focuses on skilled nursing and therapeutic services. Although there are other organizations that use the title "home health care" when describing their services, they may be providing private duty care, sometimes called home care, such as housekeeping services, transportation, or companionship. These latter services are most often paid for privately or out-of-pocket, though some insurance plans or state-funded programs may cover some of these services. For home health services, Medicare remains the single largest payer in the United States. Although a home health agency may serve patients with a variety of payer sources, all patients must be treated under the same regulatory guidelines established by Medicare in order to participate in the Medicare program. It is critical for occupational therapists, physical therapists, and speech-language pathologists to be familiar with the guidelines because failure to meet specific criteria could result in a denial of coverage, which would be harmful to the patient.

As previously mentioned, CMS has developed regulations for both the home health agency and the beneficiary. There are generally two terms used when discussing regulatory guidelines: *conditions* and *standards*. Conditions are global in nature and are made up of standards. For example, the *condition* "Comprehensive Assessment of Patients" (Code of Federal Regulations [CFR], 2022, §484.55) consists of many *standards* that are separately surveyed and assessed. Conditions for Coverage are criteria that a beneficiary must meet to be eligible for coverage of services under Medicare. Conditions of Participation are regulatory mandates that a provider (e.g., home health agency) must comply with to participate in the Medicare program (CFR, 2022). These are minimum health and safety standards that must be measurable and continually met by the home health agency provider to remain in the Medicare programs. These conditions are, however, changed from time to time. The intent of the regulatory mandates is to ensure quality care provision and protection of the safety of the beneficiaries. Detailed knowledge of all the Conditions of Participation is beyond the scope of an entry-level occupational therapist. A discussion on some parts of these CMS regulations in consideration for practitioners working in home health appears later in this chapter.

Criteria for Medicare Reimbursement to Home Health Agencies

The Medicare Benefit Policy Manual (CMS, 2021a) states that, a home health agency must meet specific criteria to be reimbursed for the provision of home health services. The following list of criteria must be met on *all* counts by the home health agency:

1. The person to whom the services are provided is an eligible Medicare beneficiary.
2. The home health agency that is providing the services to the beneficiary has in effect a valid agreement to participate in the Medicare program.
3. The beneficiary qualifies for coverage of home health services.
4. The services for which payment is claimed are covered.
5. Medicare is the appropriate payer.
6. The services for which payment is claimed are not otherwise excluded from payment.

Criteria for Coverage of Home Health Services for Medicare Beneficiaries

To qualify for the Medicare home health benefit, a Medicare beneficiary must meet all of the following criteria:

- Be confined to the home
- Be under the care of a physician or allowed practitioner
- Be receiving services under a plan of care established and periodically reviewed by a physician or allowed practitioner
- Be in intermittent need of skilled nursing, physical therapy, speech-language pathology, or occupational therapy

For any skilled services (nursing, occupational therapy, physical therapy, speech pathology) to be covered under the home health benefit of Medicare, a beneficiary's eligibility for home health services must be established at the start of care. Although occupational therapy alone may not establish eligibility for Medicare beneficiaries, it is a covered skilled service. Once program eligibility has been determined, a beneficiary may be discharged from skilled nursing, speech-language pathology, or physical therapy, and occupational therapy may remain as the only service involved. As of January 1, 2022, occupational therapists are allowed to complete the initial visit (e.g., the start of care) along with the comprehensive assessment for home health patients under the Medicare benefit (AOTA, 2021a). Two important conditions must be met for this to occur. Occupational therapists may complete the start of care if (1) occupational therapy is on the home health plan of care, in addition to either physical therapy or speech therapy; and (2) skilled nursing services, such as the need for wound care, medication management, or monitoring medical stability, are not initially included on the plan of care.

Confined to Home

The requirement of being **confined to home** is generally referred to by practitioners as "being homebound." Medicare requires that for a beneficiary to be eligible to receive home health services, a physician or allowed practitioner must certify that the patient is confined to their home. While the beneficiary does not have to be bedridden, their condition must be such that (1) there is the inability to leave home, (2) leaving home would require a considerable and taxing effort, and/or (3) trips away from the home are for short and infrequent periods of time (Box 26-1). Health-related care is an uncontested reason for leaving the home, but Medicare has further clarified that "occasional absences from the home for nonmedical purposes; e.g., an occasional trip to the barber, a walk around the block or a drive, attendance at a family reunion, funeral, graduation, or other infrequent or unique event would not necessitate a finding that the patient is not homebound if the absences are undertaken on an infrequent basis or are of relatively short duration and do not indicate that the patient has the capacity to obtain the healthcare provided outside rather than in the home" (CMS, 2021a, §30.1.1).

Documentation of homebound status is an important part of the patient record and must include a patient report as well as a clinical observation and assessment of the

---

BOX 26-1 Criteria for "Confined to Home"

Criterion 1:
1. *The patient must either:*
   - Because of illness or injury, need the aid of supportive devices such as crutches, canes, wheelchairs, and walkers; the use of special transportation; or the assistance of another person in order to leave their place of residence
   OR
   - Have a condition such that leaving his or her home is medically contraindicated

If the patient meets one of the criterion 1 conditions, then the patient must ALSO meet both additional requirements defined in criterion 2.

Criterion 2:
- There must exist a normal inability to leave home; and
- Leaving home must require a considerable and taxing effort (CMS, 2021a).

patient's physical and mental status (CMS, 2021a). If any question should arise by the payer related to homebound status, proper and adequate documentation will establish such status.

The requirement that the patient be homebound raises some significant issues in terms of occupational therapy interventions. Occupational therapy is concerned with maximizing function and quality of life; remaining permanently homebound may not be consistent with these goals. For example, reimbursement will not be provided for interventions that are implemented outside of the home (e.g., locations around and in the community). Practitioners must think carefully about how they might assist patients in regaining functions that would allow them to participate more fully in life beyond the home while still working within the regulations of homebound status of the patient. As an example, an occupational therapist might encourage the patient to practice climbing stairs to enter or exit the home to retrieve their mail. In this scenario, the patient is performing at an optimal level and preparing for advancement from home health services (and increasing their walking distance in the home as a mechanism for increasing physical capacity that might later facilitate movement outside the home). Although this kind of movement outside the home is consistent with Medicare regulations, therapy-related trips further into the community—to the grocery store, the bank, a senior center—would make the patient ineligible for home health as they are no longer homebound.

An Approved Plan of Care

Medicare has a clear expectation that any beneficiary receiving home health services is under the active care of a physician or allowed practitioner who is qualified to sign the certification and plan of care. Allowed practitioners include nurse practitioners, clinical nurse specialists, and physician assistants (CMS, 2021a, §484.2). Allowed practitioners can certify and recertify beneficiaries for eligibility, order home health services, and establish and review the care plan in the same way that physicians can.

As part of the certification of patient eligibility for the Medicare home health benefit, a face-to-face encounter (in person or via telehealth) must have occurred where the patient was seen by certain types of practitioners for reasons related to their need for home health. This face-to-face encounter needs to occur within 90 days before the start of care of home health services or within 30 days after the start of care. This encounter must be performed either by the certifying physician or allowed practitioner, a physician or allowed practitioner that cared for the patient in the acute or postacute setting, or by an allowed nonphysician practitioner. Nonphysician practitioners include nurse practitioners, clinical nurse specialists, physician assistants, and certified nurse midwives. Due to the COVID-19 pandemic, CMS has modified its rules allowing not just physicians but other allowed practitioners to be responsible for the care of a home health patient (CMS, 2021a).

Skilled Nursing Care and Therapy Services

Skilled nursing services are covered when a patient's condition requires the skills of a nurse, such as the provision of wound care to improve a condition, maintain the patient's current condition, or prevent or slow further deterioration. If the skills of a nurse are not deemed necessary for care—usually because they can be performed by patient or caregiver—then these services would not be covered (CMS, 2021a).

For occupational therapy, physical therapy, and speech-language pathology services to be included under the home health benefit, the services being provided need to be of a certain level of complexity that demonstrates the need for a licensed therapy practitioner to oversee the treatment being provided (CMS, 2021a). These practitioners use their specialized skills, breadth of knowledge, and their judgment to monitor the safety of a patient while performing different activities and ensure the effectiveness of the treatments being provided (CMS, 2021a). In basic terms, the therapy services must be consistent with the severity of the patient's need and must be reasonable and necessary. The home health medical record must clearly reflect these principles.

Any therapy service must be reasonable and necessary to the treatment of the patient's illness or injury or to the restoration or maintenance of function that has been affected by illness or injury. The decision whether services are reasonable and necessary is the responsibility of the entity that pays the home health agency and is based on the beneficiary's plan of care, medical record, documentation, and diagnosis. Medicare policy states that while a "patient's particular medical condition is a valid factor in deciding if skilled therapy services are needed, a patient's diagnosis or prognosis should never be the sole factor in deciding that a service is or is not skilled" (CMS, 2021a, §40.2.1). See Promoting Best Practice 26-1 for an example of determining "reasonable and necessary."

PROMOTING BEST PRACTICE 26-1
Reasonable and Necessary Therapy Services

> To understand reasonable and necessary therapy services, consider two patients with the same diagnosis. Both Mrs. S and Mrs. J have returned home after hip arthroplasty. Mrs. S is married and able to dress herself and, with her husband's assistance, can bathe and manage light IADLs. Mrs. J lives alone and is unable to shower or manage IADLs and does not have any available assistance. The occupational therapy evaluation would be reviewed by the payer source to determine whether the services needed were reasonable and necessary. It would be appropriate to assume that while both patients may require the services of an occupational therapist, Mrs. J would be a candidate for a longer duration of services.

Home Health Assessment

There are specific processes in which a patient is assessed during the implementation of home health services. These include the use of Medicare-approved assessment tools to collect data on patients and the **start of care** visit with a new home health patient, which includes a comprehensive assessment.

Outcome and Assessment Information Set and Section GG

In 1999, CMS mandated that a home health agency must collect and transmit data for all adult patients (with the exception of obstetric patients) who receive skilled services reimbursed by Medicare. The instrument, the **Outcome and Assessment Information Set,** commonly referred to as OASIS (CMS, 2022b), is a group of standard data elements developed over decades of research. OASIS data are designed to allow systematic comparison of measurement of a patient's status at two time points. These time points include, but are not limited to, start of care, recertification, discharge from home health services, as well as other required events (e.g., returning home from a hospital stay). Data from OASIS assessments are collected through direct observations and interactions with the patient. Data collection can be completed only by a registered nurse, physical therapist, speech-language pathologist, or occupational therapist. A licensed practical nurse, physical or occupational therapy assistant, social worker, or aide cannot collect OASIS data.

While the data collected from the OASIS assessment affect reimbursement to the home health agency for home health services provided, the data are also reported to the government where it is analyzed and published as a "report card" for a home health agency. In this era of technology, there are a multitude of sites where a consumer, referral source, or specific discipline can assess information on how an entity or individual is rated compared with similar services. In home health, the main source is a website called Home Health Compare (Medicare.gov, 2022b). A star-rating system is published using the collected data to assist the consumer. Occupational therapy plays a vital role in the ratings; the best scores result from quality, evidenced-based best practice.

In addition to the OASIS content, clinicians are required to utilize another data collection tool, Section GG. **Section GG** measures a variety of functional activities, including ADLs and mobility/transfers, and when documented must include a prior level of function, admission performance, a discharge goal, and the discharge performance for each item being assessed. These assessment items, in addition to the OASIS assessment questions, help create a reliable picture of the patient's functional performance.

The Initial Visit and Comprehensive Assessment

CMS mandates that an initial assessment visit be performed to determine eligibility for the home health benefit and to identify the immediate needs of the patient (CFR, 2022). The initial assessment must be performed within 48 hours of referral, within 48 hours of the patient's return home, or on a physician-ordered start of care date. For patients receiving only nursing services or both nursing and therapy services, a registered nurse *must* perform the initial assessment visit. As mentioned earlier, for therapy-only cases that include occupational therapy, in addition to physical and/or speech therapy orders, an occupational therapist can complete the initial visit and perform the comprehensive assessment of the patient's medical, rehabilitation, social, and discharge planning needs (CFR, 2022).

A home health agency may choose to have a registered nurse perform all initial assessment visits, regardless of the services ordered, and some state practice acts may require this. Conversely, a therapist may not perform the initial assessment visit if nursing services are ordered at the start of care. This applies to any nursing services that may be ordered.

The comprehensive assessment of patients is a condition of participation that mandates each beneficiary must receive a patient-specific comprehensive assessment that reflects the patient's current health status accurately, supports the development of a plan of care, and justifies the beneficiary's need for skilled home health services, including homebound status and discharge needs (CFR, 2022). Furthermore, this condition mandates that the comprehensive assessment must incorporate the current OASIS data items for Medicare beneficiaries receiving skilled services. If a patient is receiving skilled services but these services are reimbursed by insurance other than Medicare, the comprehensive assessment is still required, but the collection of OASIS data is not.

Timeliness of the Comprehensive Assessment

Medicare mandates that the comprehensive assessment must be completed in a timely manner and defines this time frame as no later than 5 calendar days after the start of care (CFR, 2022). The start of care date is the first billable home health visit. The outcome and financial rationale is that the more accurate the picture of the patient, the easier it is to measure true progress and predict the necessary agency costs of care provided.

The comprehensive assessment must be updated and revised as needed but no less frequently than the last 5 days of every 60-day home health episode of care (CFR, 2022). This assessment is performed by the appropriate discipline to determine the patient's current status and justify the need for continued home health services. There are other occasions when a comprehensive assessment must be updated and revised (e.g., when a patient returns home from a hospital or inpatient stay).

The comprehensive assessment must include a review of all medications, including nonprescription drugs, that the patient is currently taking (CFR, 2022). This review is performed to identify potential adverse effects and/or drug reactions. Occupational therapists, physical therapists, and speech-language pathologists are expected to be aware of the medications a patient is taking, and documentation should reflect the monitoring of medication changes by all disciplines involved. For example, on therapy-only cases, an agency may have the clinician call the office and review the medications with a nurse over the phone to determine any significant issues. In another instance, if the clinician learns during a routine home visit that the patient is now taking a new drug, they must communicate this information as outlined in agency policy. Depending on the policy, the clinician might need to call the nursing supervisor or write an update in the medical record.

A wide array of issues may be identified during assessment that guide the plan of care (CFR, 2022). There are common elements involved in assessment but also discipline-specific considerations. Establishing a plan that addresses these concerns based on the scope of expertise of each discipline is important to ensuring that overall goals are met.

Intervention in the Context of Home

In order to work as a practitioner in home health, it is important for the therapist to utilize clinical reasoning skills, creativity, and problem-solving abilities. Quite often, when working in a patient's home, a therapist may not have the typical equipment found in a clinic setting, including exercise equipment, a fully outfitted kitchen, or an accessible bathroom with durable medical equipment. Having this equipment can often help occupational therapists to educate and train a patient in a safe, controlled environment. Working in a patient's home, on the other hand, requires the therapist to utilize what equipment is available, while working within the possible limitations of a patient's home environment. This is both an exciting opportunity to utilize occupational therapy skills, as well as a challenge that helps the novice practitioner gain autonomy and confidence as a clinician.

It is important to note that working with a patient in their own home environment also has many advantages. The opportunity to observe a patient in their natural environment versus a simulated environment has great benefits when training and educating a patient in home safety and engaging in chosen occupations. Patients often return home from a stay in an inpatient setting where they have received intensive occupational therapy services. This is an important step in the continuum of care where the focus is on preparing a patient to eventually return to their prior level of function in their chosen place of residence. When a patient does return home, the role of the occupational therapist is to first assess how safely a patient can perform their daily activities; determine whether or not assistance, equipment, or other outside considerations are required; and develop a plan that focuses on the patient's goals. Quite often, this may be to increase a patient's independence in performing their occupations, increase safety with occupational performance, and increase caregiver satisfaction by decreasing caregiver burden (Stolee et al, 2012). See Promoting Best Practice 26-2 for an example of how an occupational therapist would problem-solve through a challenging home healthcare situation.

PROMOTING BEST PRACTICE 26-2
Problem-Solving Example: Mr. Lin

The Problem: Mr. Lin is a 52-year-old man who experienced a cerebrovascular accident. He lives at home with his wife, who works remotely from her home office. Due to his stroke, Mr. Lin needs a significant amount of assistance with his BADLs. He spends most of his day in his hospital bed, which is placed in the middle of the living room due to the challenging layout of the family home. Mr. Lin's wife would very much like for her husband to enjoy a shower in their bathroom, which includes a bathtub/shower combination, and an available bathtub transfer bench. Mr. Lin has been receiving sponge baths for the past few weeks, as the bathroom does not have sufficient space for him to access it through the narrow door using his wheelchair. Because of the family's main goal of bathing in the bathtub/shower, the home health occupational therapist was tasked with determining the best way in which to achieve this goal.

The Solution: The occupational therapist began by assisting Mr. Lin with mobility by transferring to the chair to work on BADLs. Later, therapeutic activities were performed while standing to build his strength and endurance. With a continued focus on preparatory activities and within several sessions, Mr. Lin was strong enough to safely rise from his wheelchair, placed outside the bathroom door, and walk 10 feet into the bathroom and sit on the bathtub transfer bench. Assistance from the occupational therapist was required throughout the process. The patient's wife was able to observe and eventually received training on how to assist her husband. Mr. Lin received his first full shower in several weeks, and even though the process was fatiguing, he was extremely happy with the outcome. His wife, too, was very pleased that her husband had progressed from being in bed, to sitting and performing BADLs, to standing while participating in activities, to ultimately being able to walk a short distance in order to reach his long-term goal.

The example of Mr. Lin demonstrates the unique ability of an occupational therapist to problem-solve challenging situations. In this example, not only did the occupational therapist need to consider the client factors, including strength, balance, and endurance, they also had to consider both the limitations and advantages of the environment, what durable medical equipment was needed to provide safety in occupational performance, and what family training and education was needed for a long-term solution. In this example, the outcome was ideal for both the patient and his family and permanently affected his ability to perform his BADLs in a safer manner.

However, what would happen if a different outcome occurred? Continuing with the example of Mr. Lin, consider what education or recommendations could be made if Mr. Lin was unable to walk into the bathroom for his bathing needs. At this point, an occupational therapist might consider recommending alternative options, such as the need for a paid caregiver to provide an "extra pair of hands" for bathing, a plan for possible home modifications if financially feasible, or a referral to a social worker to assist the family in finding resources that may help. It is important to be aware that home health services are provided on a short-term basis, and discharge planning and implementing long-term solutions for the future are essential. Occupational therapists are an essential part of the discharge planning process, as patients often are in need of recommendations for the long term, what equipment will be needed in the future, and what would be the safest way to complete their occupations after home health services have ended. It is important for the interprofessional team of clinicians to address all aspects of their patients' lives to prepare for discharge, including both physical and psychosocial issues and any other part of that patient's daily life that might create challenges in the future.

There are many areas of concern that often arise for home health patients. The ability to perform both BADLs and IADLs is often a goal for patients in this setting, so that they may be able to return to completing the daily activities they previously enjoyed. However, there are times when any of the other areas of occupation would be appropriate to address with a patient. To summarize this section, the focus of intervention is unique to the patient but can often include (1) increasing independence with occupations, (2) increasing safety with occupational performance, or (3) training caregivers to provide a long-term solution for participation in daily activities.

When working on these considerations, an occupational therapist might examine client factors that affect occupational performance; the environment, which may require modifications or the addition of equipment; or the occupation itself and provide alternative options or ways to adapt the occupation to better match with the patient's abilities. Promoting Best Practice 26-3 includes a table of common problem areas encountered by practitioners when working with home healthcare patients. The solutions include just a few possible approaches that can be used to train and educate patients and recommendations that can be made.

PROMOTING BEST PRACTICE 26-3
Problem Areas and Solutions

Problematic Area	Possible Solutions
Bathing	■ Recommend structural modifications of shower/tub ■ Lower cost modifications such as nonskid mats or strips and installing grab bars ■ Durable medical equipment, such as shower chair or bathtub transfer bench ■ Safer techniques including using towels to avoid wet floor surfaces ■ Use of long-handled equipment, such as sponge, and use of handheld showerhead
Medication management	■ Organization of medications, including pill box ■ Assistive technology, such as pill dispensers and electronic reminders ■ Larger labels on medications from pharmacy for low vision ■ Prepackaged medication services
Functional mobility in the home	■ Practice using assistive device in the home, navigating small spaces such as bathroom ■ Use of kitchen appliances while using assistive devices (use of walker tray, walker bag, baskets) ■ Retrieving mail from mailbox safely ■ Address ability to walk around yard while gardening ■ Focus on fall prevention, including functional balance activities, modifying the environment by reducing clutter and hazards, and addressing fall recovery
Laundry	■ Using equipment, such as reacher, to move clothes between washer and dryer ■ Use of walker trays and rolling baskets to move clothes between rooms ■ Energy conservation techniques (perform tasks in sitting, taking rest breaks, performing at optimal time of day)

Documentation and Reimbursement

With rising healthcare costs and increased scrutiny by payers and the public, practitioners must be sure to properly document care. Documentation is extremely important to demonstrate continual communication, effectiveness of services provided, beneficiary response to treatment, and ongoing assessment to determine if there is any need to change the plan of care (CFR, 2022).

Through objective documentation, practitioners can demonstrate that they have implemented evidence-based treatment that drives best practice that will increasingly be required in future home health reimbursement models. It plays a key role in justifying the need for skilled therapy. In the two recognized types of home health therapy, rehabilitative and maintenance, quality documentation is essential to payment. For rehabilitative therapy, documentation supports that (1) the patient's condition has the potential to improve and (2) the expectation that improvement is attainable in a reasonable period of time. For maintenance therapy, documentation supports that the skills of a therapist are needed to maintain current function or prevent or slow further deterioration (CMS, 2021b).

Confirmation of homebound status, measurable and attainable goals, written clinical notes reflecting progress toward goals and response to treatment, timely and thorough reassessments, and comprehensive discharge summaries are minimum standards that must be met. CMS has specific policy directives that are routinely updated to reflect best practice captured within the documentation. Ultimately, the home health record must justify the need for skilled services. This justification is initiated at the evaluation and continues throughout the entirety of the therapy intervention (CFR, 2022).

Initial Evaluation

The initial evaluation serves to elicit baseline data for the practitioner to determine the patient's skilled service needs, establish measurable and attainable goals, and anticipate rehabilitation progress and serves as the foundation for subsequent documentation. The evaluation addresses both physical and mental status, and the interpretation of the acquired data serves as the justification and individualization of the occupational therapy, physical therapy, and speech-language pathology plan of care. Note that this evaluation goes beyond the OASIS to incorporate specific concerns of the individual disciplines: ability to complete self-care occupations, safe ambulation in the home and adequate physical capacity for function, and ability to communicate effectively. Objective tests and measurements should be used whenever possible and should be used consistently at various time points. Selecting the appropriate tests and measurements has two components: (1) tests and measures appropriate for the demographic clientele of the agency and (2) the practitioner's clinical judgment to determine which tests and measures are most appropriate for the patient. These requirements are consistent with occupational therapy, physical therapy, and speech-language pathology professional guidelines, which focus on the individual needs of the patient (see Chapter 21, Special Concerns Around Evaluation of the Older Adult).

Reassessment

Reassessments must be performed by a qualified practitioner from each ordered discipline at least every 30 days or earlier if it is clinically indicated by a change in the patient's functional status. An occupational therapist, physical therapist, or speech-language pathologist must provide the ordered therapy service and functionally reassess the patient. This policy is discipline neutral, which means where more than one therapy is being provided, each discipline has its own reassessment clock. This does not change the need for interprofessional communication but allows for increased ease in focusing on patient care by reducing anxiety over "exact" visit count. The 30-day "clock" begins on the evaluation date and resets with each reassessment performed.

It is important to use the same tests and measures over time to accurately document progress (or lack thereof) toward patient goals. This reassessment includes a summary of the practitioner's clinical assessment of effectiveness of current therapy and any modifications needed to the plan of care. A primary way that occupational therapists in home health demonstrate improvement is the measurement of levels of assistance in BADLs and IADLs. Although measuring levels of assistance is required, the occupational therapist must ensure that each measure is distinctly related to a functional activity with factors such as response to assistance and projected potential future gain.

In home health, each visit note must "stand-alone" and justify the skilled need. This justification occurs by properly documenting assessments, treatment and training, outcomes of interventions, patient response or change in behavior, communication among the home healthcare team, and plan for next visit. A well-written note paints a picture of the patient and allows auditors or reviewers to clearly understand the rationale for the need for skilled therapy services.

Payment Systems

All practitioners must understand the payment system in which they provide services. There are many third-party payers of home health services, but Medicare is the largest and sets the standards for all other payers in the United States. Although it is crucial for practitioners to comprehend the payment criteria for coverage of specific therapy services, it is critical to our continued success in home health to understand the global picture of the reimbursement system. Occupational therapists, physical therapists, and speech-language pathologists do not practice in a silo in the home health arena, and their actions and documentation affect the greater whole of a home health agency. Understanding the reimbursement structure for a home health agency solidifies practitioners' value and makes them vital members of the home health team.

Patient Driven Groupings Model

Past reimbursement models for home health services focused, in part, on levels of reimbursement that were affected by the number of therapy visits provided for cases that included therapy involvement. In home health, the **Patient Driven Groupings Model (PDGM)** is the reimbursement model that focuses on the *quality* of care versus the *quantity* of visits. In this model, patients are placed into payment groups based on the following criteria (AOTA, 2021b):

- Admission source (institutional versus community-based referrals)
- Episode timing
- Clinical characteristics and diagnoses (12 possible clinical groups)
- Functional impairment level, based on data from OASIS and Section GG
- Comorbidity adjustment

It is these criteria that are responsible for determining the amount of reimbursement that the home health agency receives for services provided. For all disciplines in home health, it is important to focus on each patient's unique needs to provide the best and most appropriate number of services that demonstrate good clinical outcomes. Because of this shift, it is increasingly apparent how important the use of effective assessment tools, evidence-based interventions, and a focus on the provision of excellent care have become. This continues to become even more important as initiatives continue to move toward reimbursement using value-based purchasing. In this model, agencies are reimbursed for services they have provided based on quality outcomes. In other words, reimbursement could be higher for those home health agencies who demonstrate excellent quality and functional outcomes and the reduction of any negative outcomes or inappropriate care. While this is becoming more common in some states, value-based purchasing is not yet mandatory for all Medicare-certified home health agencies in all states.

Overlap of Home Health and Outpatient Services

In the context of providing services in the home, some areas of services can overlap and/or cause confusion. Part B outpatient therapy is such an area. This is commonly seen when a beneficiary begins outpatient therapy (under Part B) from one provider while under a home health plan of care (under Part A) of another provider. In this instance, the home health agency will receive payment, and if the outpatient provider does not have a written contract or agreement with the agency, the outpatient provider will not be reimbursed, regardless of the number of services provided.

Other Sources of Payment

Although Medicare is by far the most frequent payer for home health services, there are many other options. The Veterans Health Administration and Medicaid are other federal funders (CMS, 2021b). The federal government also provides block grants to states that are used to cover specific services. A number of private insurance companies offer long-term care insurance that includes a home-health benefit. A variety of community initiatives have been implemented around the United States; these vary widely in terms of the services provided. Finally, individuals who have the resources to do so can self-pay for care.

International Home Health and Domiciliary Care

This chapter focuses on home health services that are provided within the United States. However, other countries have similar types of services, though the terminology may be different, reimbursement may come from different payers, and the actual services provided may differ.

In many countries, *domiciliary care* refers to a range of services that are provided to an individual to support them in their own home (Department of Health, n.d.). Quite often these services might be similar to that of a nonskilled home care agency in the United States, where caregivers provide assistance with dressing, bathing, household chores, meal preparation, and other tasks. However, some domiciliary programs utilize nurses and other healthcare professionals to provide medical services in the home.

In the United Kingdom, healthcare is based on a government-sponsored universal system called the National Health Service (NHS). Many services are provided free, including some types of home care services. Whether a service is provided without a cost to the patient or whether they have an out-of-pocket expense depends on multiple factors, including a financial assessment of their income and savings. The home services provided include home adaptations and equipment, such as stair handrails, grab bars, and ramps, among other items. Typically, in order for patients to receive these benefits, social services will make a referral to an occupational therapist, who performs a home assessment to determine the patient's needs. If the changes and additions made to the home amount to less than £1,000, they must be provided to the patient at no cost (NHS, 2022).

In addition, the NHS provides other benefits that some may qualify for, such as monetary allowances for personal care attendants (NHS, 2022). Also, when patients return home from the hospital, intermediate care, or reablement, focuses on helping residents return to living as independently as possible (NHS, 2022). This could involve home modifications and adaptations, as well as paid caregivers. For individuals with more serious disabilities or illnesses, the NHS might provide its continuing healthcare package, which includes healthcare services at home, personal care, and reimbursement for accommodation costs (NHS, 2022).

While many countries do have some type of home health services, reimbursement is based in part on the healthcare system of that country. As noted in the United States, the primary payer for home health services for older adults is Medicare; however, there are a variety of private payers as well. In Australia, the healthcare system includes universal healthcare (also called Medicare), but consumers have the choice of private insurance, which allows care from providers outside the public system (Australian Government, 2019). The Australian Government provides reimbursement to approved aged care providers using a "Home Care Packages Program." With these programs, services provided include assistance with household tasks, durable medical equipment, minor home modifications, and allied health services (including occupational therapy) (Australian Government, 2022).

To summarize, home health occurs in many shapes and forms across many countries and continents. Each country has its own healthcare system with its own nuances. As part of that, many healthcare systems do include a home care or domiciliary service, what would be described as nonskilled home care in the United States. However, a lot of these systems, especially those in developed countries, do include nursing services and allied health professions. One common theme is that in most countries, when occupational therapists are involved in home health, they can recommend home modifications and assess the patient within their own home environment to help the patient have a better quality of life.

Advocacy in Home Health

The home health industry has seen many changes over the past few decades. Much of the positive changes in home health have resulted from advocacy from multiple groups. AOTA was instrumental in advocating for occupational therapists to be able to perform the initial start of care for home health patients, something which has now become a reality (AOTA, 2021b). Previously, occupational therapists were unable to perform the start of care visit, until the COVID-19 pandemic began. During this time, Medicare made temporary allowances for occupational therapists to initiate the first start of care visits, but it was not until 2022 that this became a permanent change. Occupational therapists are uniquely qualified to assess a home health patient and complete a comprehensive assessment and can collaborate with other therapy disciplines to create a complete picture of the patient's needs.

Other organizations are also advocates for home care agencies and patients. For example, the National Association for Home Care & Hospice (NAHC) is the largest professional association representing the interests of chronically ill, disabled, and dying Americans of all ages and the caregivers who provide them with in home health and hospice services (NAHC, 2019). Because of their advocacy initiatives, many victories have been achieved, such as the permanent allowance of nonphysician providers to certify patients for eligibility for home health.

CASE STUDY (CONTINUED)

Intervention in the Context of Home Healthcare

After spending a few days in the acute care hospital, Mr. Martinez returned to his home, with orders for occupational therapy. These services would need to be provided under the home health benefit. The physician in the hospital has also included physical therapy in the discharge orders. The social worker at the hospital had assisted Mr. Martinez by ordering necessary equipment that had been recommended by the acute care occupational therapist.

Review and answer the following questions that pertain to Mr. Martinez, and his experience as a patient being treated by a Medicare-certified home health agency.

Questions

1a. What are the reimbursement models that affect your ability to provide care to the case study patient?

1b. What are the issues you might expect to address in reimbursement?

2. What are two or three evidence-based, occupation-centered, exemplar interventions that address the case study patient's priorities specific to the home health setting?

3. What are interprofessional interventions you would expect done?

4. What ingredients need to come **together** for the ideal discharge from home health services?

Answers

1a. It is important to note that because of Mr. Martinez's age, he would qualify for Medicare benefits. As stated, the home health agency he is being treated by is a Medicare-certified agency. The reimbursement model being used in this setting is called the PDGM. In this model, the reimbursement for services is based on multiple factors, including the admission source (e.g., Mr. Martinez's case is an "institutional" referral versus a "community-based" referral as he is transitioning from an acute care hospital), the episode timing (this is his first episode of care), clinical characteristics and diagnoses, functional impairment level (based on OASIS and Section GG data), and comorbidity adjustment. All of these factors will affect how much the agency is reimbursed for the care they provide to Mr. Martinez. In addition, the specific number of occupational therapy visits that Mr. Martinez receives will not directly correlate to how much the agency is reimbursing, as the PDGM model is based on a model of "quality" instead of "quantity".

1b. The previous model of reimbursement in home health consisted of a tiered system that increased reimbursement based on higher numbers of therapy visits (with other requirements and limitations). With the implementation of PDGM, this is no longer the case and there is a focus on the "quality" of the therapy services provided versus the number of visits (e.g., the "quantity"). It is essential that the occupational therapist considers the frequency and duration of the home health plan of care carefully. From a reimbursement point of view, the number of total occupational therapist visits should not be directly related. However, home health agencies need to provide the right number of services that will result in positive outcomes to help patients achieve their goals. Better outcomes lead to a higher-star rating for the home health agency, which shows that the services they provide are of high quality.

2. There are multiple occupation-centered interventions that could be provided for Mr. Martinez. One of the benefits of being in the home health setting is that instead of simulating occupations, mobility, and transfers, these activities can be performed in the patient's actual home using the equipment, appliances, and furniture that they will need to utilize going forward.

- Bathing is such an essential part of many people's lives. For Mr. Martinez, the case study suggested he had a bathtub/shower combination. Because of his hip surgery, getting in and out of the low surface of the bathtub might not be the best option. Utilizing a bathtub transfer bench would be ideal in this situation. This will allow Mr. Martinez to sit on a bench while performing his bathing activities, and still be able to use the shower feature of

the bathtub/shower combination from a sitting position. The occupational therapist could train Mr. Martinez in the appropriate way to transfer in and out of the shower using the bathtub transfer bench, how to use long handled adaptive equipment (such as a long-handled sponge) to compensate for his temporary difficulty in reaching forward, and train in other safe techniques for performing BADLs in a wet environment. Also, recommendations for placement of grab bars could potentially be a huge benefit to the patient. After bathing, more BADL training could be provided with a focus on lower-body dressing using adaptive equipment. This includes the use of a reacher, sock aide, and dressing stick.
- Mr. Martinez enjoys gardening in the summer. An occupational therapist could train him in adapted ways to complete this occupation. This could include recommending and helping find places to obtain a gardening stool that he could safely sit on and use long-handled equipment for digging/weeding/planting for his gardening activities. In addition, because Mr. Martinez has not yet found ways to occupy his time in the winter, the occupational therapist could assist in identifying appropriate activities that Mr. Martinez might find enjoyable and perform safely.
- Mr. Martinez enjoys playing bridge. It would be important for the occupational therapist to assess whether he is still able to perform this occupation or if his hip surgery has affected his performance in any way. While Mr. Martinez may be able to play a card game with ease, as his upper body is not significantly affected, there are other considerations, such as emotional state (whether Mr. Martinez is suffering from any change in mood or frustration because of his condition), and the physical environment when playing bridge, by considering positioning, comfort, and ways for Mr. Martinez to successfully perform this occupation while interacting with friends and family.

3. There are some noticeable areas that occupational therapy can collaborate with physical therapy when working with Mr. Martinez. There are several steps leading up to the entry of the house, and there is no railing on this staircase. While occupational therapy could provide intervention by recommending the most appropriate railings, and helping find resources for the installation of railings, the physical therapist could focus on the act of ascending and descending the stairs to better help Mr. Martinez enter and leave the house when needed for appointments and other activities. Additionally, Mr. Martinez's bedroom and bathroom are on the second floor. As he continues to heal and gain independence, and have the desire to move around the house, his ability to ascend and descend the stairs is important. While occupational therapy could be focused on all the different IADLs that Mr. Martinez could perform by being able to move around his home, once again physical therapy could focus on his mobility, safety with gait, and the ability to navigate the stairs.

4. Ultimately, in order for Mr. Martinez to be discharged from services with successful outcomes, there are several important considerations.
    - Assessing his ability to move safely around the home, enter and exit the home, go upstairs and downstairs, be able to navigate his home, and access all areas he desires to is essential. Also, the goal is essentially for Mr. Martinez to no longer be "home bound" after his plan of care has been completed, and therefore increasing the ease with which he can leave the home would be beneficial.
    - Maximizing Mr. Martinez's independence with both BADLs and IADLs would be important, as his prior level of functioning was mostly independent. This would occur by both training Mr. Martinez in safer ways of completing his BADLs and IADLs, helping restore function, and adapting the occupation, the patient, and/or the environment for maximized occupational performance.
    - Ensuring the psychosocial needs of the patient have been met. Mr. Martinez should be able to return to all previously performed occupations, including BADLs, IADLs, play and leisure activities, and social participation. This would ultimately improve his quality of life.

SUMMARY

Home health offers several significant advantages in helping older adults maximize function. Patients may manage differently in a familiar environment compared with their performance in clinical settings, and their cultural beliefs and habits can be incorporated into care. Older adults receiving rehabilitation in their home were equal or higher in function, cognition, and quality of life and reported higher satisfaction (Stolee et al, 2012). Home health has proven to be an avenue for occupational therapists to demonstrate their effect on the occupational performance of patients in their own unique environment, assessment of client factors, and use of home modifications and adaptation to ensure patients are as safe as possible in their homes. As a home health clinician, it is important to remember what a privilege it is to be a guest in a patient's home and be able to provide care that improves a patient's quality of life within their own natural environment.

Critical Thinking Questions

This chapter examined the nuances of the home health setting including the role of an occupational therapist, the collaborative nature of an interprofessional team, and best practices for assessment and intervention in home health. Additionally, it explored the regulations and requirements of a Medicare-certified home health agency, reimbursement, and documentation considerations.

1. Consider why the home health setting is so highly regulated by Medicare. Even though all rules and regulations are important, which ones would most directly affect an occupational therapist working in home health?

2. How are the focus and benefits of occupational therapy a good fit for the home health setting? What exactly does an occupational therapist bring to the table?

3. Why is it so important for occupational therapists working in home health to be aware of the reimbursement model in home health?

REFERENCES

American Occupational Therapy Association. (2021, November 5). *AOTA victory for occupational therapy: Final Medicare rule allows occupational therapists to open home health cases.* https://www.aota.org/advocacy/advocacy-news/2021/home-health-medicare

American Occupational Therapy Association. (2021, November 24). *Payment policy: Home health payment.* https://www.aota.org/practice/practice-essentials/payment-policy/home-health-pdgm

American Speech-Language-Hearing Association. (n.d.). *Getting started in home health.* https://www.asha.org/slp/healthcare/start_home

Australian Government Department of Health and Aged Care. (2019). *The Australian health system.* https://www.health.gov.au/about-us/the-australian-health-system

Australian Government Department of Health and Aged Care. (2022). *Home care packages program.* https://www.health.gov.au/initiatives-and-programs/home-care-packages-program

Centers for Medicare and Medicaid Services. (2019, January 23). *Home health agency (HHA) frequently asked questions (FAQs).* https://www.cms.gov/Medicare/Provider-Enrollment-and-Certification/SurveyCertificationGenInfo/Downloads/AdminInfo19-07-HHA.pdf

Centers for Medicare and Medicaid Services. (2021a). *Medicare benefit policy manual: Chapter 7—home health services.* https://www.cms.gov/Regulations-and-Guidance/Guidance/Manuals/Downloads/bp102c07.pdf

Centers for Medicare and Medicaid Services. (2021b). *Medicare program—general information.* https://www.cms.gov/Medicare/Medicare-General-Information/MedicareGenInfo

Centers for Medicare and Medicaid Services. (2022a). *Home health providers.* https://www.cms.gov/Medicare/Provider-Enrollment-and-Certification/CertificationandComplianc/HHAs

Centers for Medicare and Medicaid Services. (2022b). *OASIS user manuals.* http://www.cms.gov/Medicare/Quality-Initiatives-Patient-Assessment-Instruments/HomeHealthQualityInits/HHQIOASISUserManual.html

Code of Federal Regulations. (2022). *Part 484—home health services.* https://www.ecfr.gov/current/title-42/chapter-IV/subchapter-G/part-484

Davis, M. R. (2021, November 18). *Despite pandemic, percentage of older adults who want to age in place stays steady.* AARP. https://www.aarp.org/home-family/your-home/info-2021/home-and-community-preferences-survey.html

Department of Health. (n.d.). *Domiciliary care.* https://www.health-ni.gov.uk/articles/domiciliary-care

Hayhurst, C. (2020, February 1). *Good to be home: Physical therapists working in home health discuss their evolving role in the continuum of patient care.* American Physical Therapy Association. https://www.apta.org/apta-magazine/2020/02/01/good-to-be-home

Medicare.gov. (2022a). *What's home health care?* https://www.medicare.gov/what-medicare-covers/whats-home-health-care

Medicare.gov. (2022b). *Home health compare.* https://data.cms.gov/provider-data/search?theme=Home%20health%20services

National Association for Home Care and Hospice. (2019). *About NAHC.* https://nahc.org/about-nahc

National Health Care Association. (2023). Assisted living. *https://www.ahcancal.org/Assisted-Living/Pages/default.aspx*

National Health Service. (2022). *Care and support you can get for free.* https://www.nhs.uk/conditions/social-care-and-support-guide/care-services-equipment-and-care-homes/care-and-support-you-can-get-for-free

Stolee, P., Lim, S. N., Wilson, L., & Glenny, C. (2012). Inpatient versus home-based rehabilitation for older adults with musculoskeletal disorders: A systematic review. *Clinical Rehabilitation, 26*(5), 387–402. https://doi.org/10.1177/0269215511423279

CHAPTER 27

Long-Term Care Services

Patricia J. Watford, OTD, MS, OTR/L ■ Vanessa Jewell, PhD, OTR/L, FAOTA

"Caring for seniors is perhaps the greatest responsibility we have. Those who have walked before us have given so much and made possible the life we all enjoy."

—Senator John Hoeven

LEARNING OUTCOMES

By the end of this chapter, readers will be able to:

27-1. Summarize the types of residents typically found in long-term care settings today.
27-2. Appraise the occupational needs of residents in long-term care.
27-3. Evaluate the benefits of restorative care for older adults in a nursing home.
27-4. Create occupation-centered interventions that are appropriate within the long-term care context.
27-5. Analyze the application of strength-based approaches in long-term care.
27-6. Appraise critical legislation that created the modern nursing home.
27-7. Compare and contrast advocacy plans for an older adult in a long-term care setting at the person, group, and population levels.

Mini-Case Study

Miguel is a 73-year-old former electrician who retired at age 65. He had lived with his wife, Lucinda, of 51 years in a small two-story house. He was independent in all activities of daily living (ADLs) and instrumental activities of daily living (IADLs), handled all home maintenance and yard work, and played soccer once a week with a group of friends. Five weeks ago, Miguel experienced a cerebrovascular accident (CVA) that left him with right hemiplegia and expressive aphasia. He spent a week in an acute care facility and was transferred to a rehabilitation center. He made some progress over his monthlong stay in rehabilitation but was unable to return home safely due to needing a two-person assist for all transfers and increased impulsivity. Unable to afford private care in their home, Lucinda made the difficult decision to move Miguel to a long-term care facility.

Provocative Questions
1. What client and contextual factors would be most critical to consider in helping Miguel adjust to his new life in a long-term care facility?
2. In what ways may the occupational therapist need to advocate for Miguel during his stay in the long-term care facility?

As the number of older adults living in the United States continues to increase, so does the number of older adults experiencing physical or cognitive disabilities. Moreover, approximately 80% of older adults live with a chronic condition, and 68% live with two or more chronic conditions (National Council on Aging, 2023). The increased prevalence of older adults living longer with chronic conditions leads to an increased need for **long-term care services** (Sengupta et al, 2022). It is expected that as many as 70% of older adults will require a form of long-term care at some point in their lives (U.S. Department of Health and Human Services, 2020). In the United States, **long-term care services** encompass a large group of services that include assistance for personal care, healthcare, and support services. These services help with tasks such as ADLs, IADLs, health management, and other important daily care. Long-term care services are needed by individuals who require assistance due to chronic illness; a physical, cognitive, or mental disability; injury; or other health conditions (Harris-Kojetin et al, 2019). Long-term care can be provided in a variety of settings, but most frequently includes nursing homes or skilled nursing facilities (SNFs). This chapter discusses the vital role of occupational therapy to improve or maintain function and quality of life for those who need long-term care services.

Define Long-Term Care Services Context

Long-term care includes more than traditional nursing home care services (Grabowski, 2022). There is an increasing emphasis on consumer choice and preference, leading to the establishment of community, assisted-living, and home health programs. These programs have emerged to address the needs of older adults who need ongoing, relatively intensive support due to declining functional performance in their daily occupations. This chapter focuses on long-term care as provided in nursing homes or SNFs. Nursing home care is generally described in two main categories: **skilled care,** which provides high-level care after a qualifying inpatient hospital stay that can only be provided by licensed nursing or therapy staff; and **custodial care,** in which ADLs or personal needs can be reasonably and safely provided by nonlicensed caregivers (Medicare.gov, n.d.-c). Long-term care services are frequently paid for by a client's Medicare or Medicaid insurance, the military or Department of Veterans Affairs, federal or state employee health care plans, private insurance, or self-pay. However, Medicare is the largest healthcare funder for adults over the age of 65, and many private healthcare policy companies follow the rules and policies set by Medicare.

Profile of Nursing Home Residents

In 2019, only 2.4%, or 1.2 million, adults age 65 years or older lived in institutional settings. However, the percentage increases dramatically with age, ranging from 1% for persons 65 to 74 years, to 2% for persons 75 to 84 years, and 8% for persons 85+ (Administration on Aging, 2021). Most nursing home residents are female (66.6%) and do not have a spouse (Sepgupta et al, 2022). Because women have a longer life expectancy than men and generally have marital partners their own age or older, they are less likely than men to have a caregiver at home should they become disabled or unable to independently care for themselves. Additional risk factors for nursing home placement include various social determinants of health, such as low income, poor accessibility of the neighborhood and built environment, lack of access to and quality of healthcare, and poor family support. Those who experience the highest likelihood of nursing home placements are individuals with high frailty scores, functional impairments, and conditions that are likely to impose a burden on informal caregivers (Duan-Porter et al, 2019). There are significant racial disparities in nursing home admission, with particularly low rates among Hispanic (5.7%) and black (15%) populations. It is not clear whether this is due to limited access or to preference for family care and support in the home (Sengupta et al, 2022).

Nursing home residents are especially affected by chronic disease and often require assistance with their health management routines (Boscart et al, 2020). For example, 49.1% of nursing home residents live with Alzheimer's disease or other dementias (Septupta et al, 2022). Other highly prevalent chronic conditions in this population include hypertension (77%), arthritis (28%), hypertension (20%), heart disease (20%), and osteoporosis (11%).

Because the frequency of disabilities increases with age, many of those living in nursing homes require assistance with three or more ADLs. Sepgupta and colleagues (2022) found that among nursing home residents, 97% required assistance with bathing, and 98% needed help with dressing. Most of these residents experienced urinary incontinence (62%) and fecal incontinence (43%), and approximately one third had hearing or vision loss (McCreedy et al, 2018; Musa et al, 2019; Stefanacci et al, 2022). Although most nursing home residents age 65 years or older receive various forms of medical care, only 19% receive rehabilitation services, such as occupational therapy.

When an individual is unable to return to a less-restrictive environment after a hospitalization and a stay in an inpatient rehabilitation facility, a long-term care facility can become home. This is especially true for older adults with developmental or intellectual disabilities or those who require substantial care (Egan et al, 2022). These individuals may have previously lived independently or with some support from parents, other informal caregivers, or home health organizations. After admission to a long-term care facility, it is likely that an individual will experience physical, cognitive, sensory, and social changes and will need to redefine personal relationships, life roles, and self-esteem. Therefore, it is critical to support these individuals with interventions that encourage a homelike environment. Practitioners should consider an individual's health needs and health improvements without sacrificing the social environment. This might include simple measures such as giving residents choices about sleep schedules, providing access to snacks and drinks, decorating their rooms with items from home, and offering meal choices.

CASE STUDY

Tom from chapter 13 in the context of long-term care
Presenting Situation

Tom, a 73-year-old retired fireman was introduced in Chapter 13. He retired 5 years ago when diagnosed with dementia with Lewy bodies. He and his wife have been married for 45 years. His wife, Mandie, is a nurse and retired 2 years ago to take care of Tom. They have two children who live out of state. Tom was an only child and has no other family. Mandie has four siblings and is only in contact with one sister. Tom was functioning up to 2 years ago. He was driving locally, playing golf, and caring for the home while his wife worked. He showed gradual declines in memory and was able to rely on lists and reminders from his wife. With the cognitive decline, Tom required supervision for safety. His wife became his caretaker, and he became anxious if she left Tom's sight. Mandie enrolled him in Lee Silverman Voice Treatment (a Parkinson disease program designed to improve functional mobility and movement for everyday activities) classes, and Tom participated for a few months. However, the disease caused him to be paranoid during classes and often disruptive and require that his wife was in sight.

> **Question**
>
> 1. In what ways can the occupational therapist collaborate with the interprofessional team to ease the adjustment for Tom from his home to the long-term care facility?
>
> **Answer**
>
> 1. The occupational therapist would support physical therapy interventions by recommending client-centered strengthening exercises that also support his sense of self; (e.g., asking about how he maintained strength as a firefighter). Occupational therapy would work with speech-language pathology and social services to support a sense of comfort at the facility through memory boards and clear signage for way-finding. (LO 27.2; Interprofessional partners section)

Role of Occupational Therapy and Interprofessional Partners

The role of occupational therapy in long-term care, as in other settings, begins with an assessment of the client. After the assessment, the occupational therapist and the client collaboratively set goals, and then the therapist plans and implements programs for individuals or groups to promote functional independence, education and practice with adaptive equipment and in compensatory techniques, environmental modifications, falls prevention, dementia management, restraint reduction, positioning programs, or therapeutic groups for behavioral and mental health issues. Scoping reviews have indicated that occupation-based interventions are underutilized in SNFs, despite evidence of their efficacy (Durocher et al, 2022; Jewell et al, 2019). See the following section on Occupational Therapy Evaluation and Intervention Exemplars for more detailed information.

Consistent with the fourth edition of the Occupational Therapy Practice Framework: Domain and Process (OTPF-4; American Occupational Therapy Association [AOTA], 2020), occupational therapy in long-term care addresses the individual's ability to accomplish needed and desired activities. Because long-term care residents tend to have significant cognitive or physical limitations, collaboration with the family or social support system, along with the healthcare team is critical to develop an occupational therapy care plan. Specifically, practitioners should identify a resident's strengths and limitations, personal goals, and a series of strategies or interventions developed to facilitate those goals. Specific interventions depend on the nature of the condition and expectations about whether the person will return to their home environment. When developing an occupational therapy care plan for an older adult in long-term care, it is critical to consider not only their current occupations, contexts and environments, habits, routines, roles, performance skills, and client factors but also their previous life experiences. (AOTA, 2020). A comprehensive occupational profile and targeted questions about the client's life experiences will describe a person's routines, habits, values, and interests for both the present and the past. Occupational therapists should utilize the connectedness older adults have with their previous seasons of life and past relationships, as well as their physical, emotional, social, and cognitive abilities, to create a well-rounded and person-centered care plan.

Goals for occupation-centered programs in long-term care can focus on a wide variety of target areas, including promoting change in intrapersonal skills (appropriately tolerating frustration due to memory decline, developing realistic expectations of self in a new setting), promoting change in communication skills, demonstrating appropriate impulse control, actively listening; promoting change with cognitive and task performance skills (organizing their own ADL schedule, self-correcting safety errors during ADLs), promoting change in independent living skills (effectively managing increased leisure time, using appropriate safety judgment, developing a sense of emotional well-being in their new environment), and promoting maintenance or improvement of physical skills (increasing functional balance for self-care independence, ability to transfer to and from the toilet independently). Occupational therapists should consider designing intervention plans that incorporate evidence-based interventions to decrease loneliness and improve the well-being of older adults, such as pet therapy, laughter therapy, reminiscence, exercise, gardening, green visiting, green exercise, and horticulture therapy (Gagliardi & Piccinini, 2019; Quan et al, 2020). Occupation-centered therapy has as many diverse goals met through a creative intervention plan. For example, an occupational therapist could coordinate with the dietary staff to utilize cooking supplies to bake the client's favorite cookies while simultaneously addressing client factors such as safety awareness, endurance, and transporting items in the kitchen.

Interprofessional Partners

An interprofessional care team works collectively to emphasize improving or maintaining a resident's functional performance and common issues experienced by long-term care residents, such as dementia-related symptoms (van Voorden et al, 2023), depression, and decreased quality of life (Arrieta et al, 2018). Given the wide variety of needs of long-term care residents, a variety of healthcare professionals are required to meet these needs. As a result, occupational therapists creating occupation-centered programs for long-term care residents must work as part of an interprofessional team. Members of the interprofessional team must work in collaboration with one another, advocating for the rights and needs of the resident. The interprofessional team typically comprises healthcare professionals such as nurses, nursing assistants, physicians, social workers, and therapists from various disciplines, including art therapy, audiology, dietitians, music therapy, occupational therapy, physical therapy, speech-language pathology, and recreation therapy.

Occupational therapists and physical therapists typically work very closely together, often sharing a clinic, gym, or other workspaces. While occupational therapy focuses on a resident's ability to participate in meaningful and necessary occupations, physical therapy emphasizes the resident's strength and mobility required to complete those occupations. For example, a resident who sustained a CVA may need a physical therapy care plan to maintain or improve range of motion in affected extremities, strengthening, and balance. Intervention focused on these goals would support an occupational therapy intervention emphasizing the client's ability to participate in occupations such as self-care and leisure activities (Fig. 27-1). Participation in occupations requires sufficient ability to complete performance skills or modification of the occupation. Furthermore, motivation for undertaking physical exercise is often based on the desire to participate in meaningful occupations. For this reason, collaborative occupational therapy/physical therapy intervention is critical in long-term care facilities.

Occupational therapists also work closely with speech-language pathologists in nursing homes, with overlapping scopes of practices in cognition, feeding, and swallowing. However, the approaches to care are varied, as speech-language pathology focuses on issues of communication and disabilities of the upper gastrointestinal tract, whereas occupational therapy is concerned with how cognition, speech, feeding, and swallowing affect daily function and meaningful occupations of their clients. Occupational therapy, physical therapy, and speech-language pathology services complement each other in long-term care settings, and all share the goal of increasing function and providing the best outcomes for residents. For example, a client who has difficulty swallowing after sustaining a stroke may work with the speech-language pathologist to determine the appropriate thickness of liquids and foods, while the occupational therapist may fabricate an adaptive device to increase the client's ability to hold a cup and bring it to their mouth to drink without spilling.

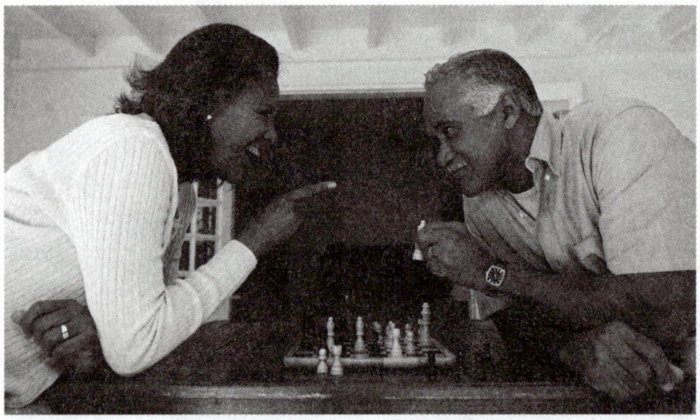

The most important, and often forgotten, member of the interprofessional team when working in long-term care, is the resident. Whereas therapists and other medical professionals are experts in their respective disciplines and specialty areas, the resident is the expert on the person. Too often, decisions are made for the resident in long-term care with little or no input from the resident on their preferences. Care that includes the emotional needs and preferences of the resident is also known as resident-centered care or person-centered care. The person-centered care model has become more prevalent and promotes the partnering of healthcare providers with the resident to deliver high-quality personalized care (Santana et al, 2017). In addition to including the resident in the interprofessional team, it is imperative to include the residents' client constellation, or social support system, whenever possible to assist in establishing goals and making informed decisions. Family members are vital to effective care and help to reduce staffing and other care costs (Barken & Lowndes, 2018). Such caregiving can be both rewarding and stressful for families. Acknowledging family contributions, providing caregiver training, and addressing potential caregiver stress can have positive benefits for residents and their caregivers. The entire interprofessional team, including the resident and the family, develops a comprehensive, personalized plan of care outlining all aspects of care delivery for the resident.

Interprofessional meetings for each resident are held at least quarterly or more frequently when a resident has an improvement or decline in medical status. The team is charged with developing a care plan that will maximize an individual's abilities and focus on successful interactions while maintaining the resident's dignity and feelings of self-worth. Effective documentation of a resident's observed behavior, response to intervention, and changes in health or function can ensure that team members are well-informed.

A successful interprofessional plan provides the highest quality care for a resident, respects the wishes of the resident and family, and allows the resident to reach their highest level of independence. Staff attitudes and communication are the most significant determinants of whether the care plan of the interprofessional team will be successful. Staff members must focus on the needs of the resident and set aside individual differences and potential competitiveness among disciplines. This may be especially challenging in an era of managed care and changes within government entitlement programs. It is critical for all providers to work cooperatively to create and maintain supportive environments and optimal programming for residents.

Many other disciplines work within the interprofessional team in the long-term care setting. For example, social services partners with other members of the interprofessional team, such as occupational therapists, to identify the

FIGURE 27-1 Chess, checkers, and other board games can be used as interventions to address concentration, fine motor skills, and social interaction. *(Stockbyte/Stockbyte/Getty Images.)*

emotional, mental, and psychosocial needs of the resident and promote services to meet those needs; dining services works with the resident to support autonomy with food choices while ensuring that adequate hydration and nutrition are achieved, and pharmacy professionals partner with the interprofessional team to review and make recommendations concerning medications for the resident (Dietitians of Canada, 2019; Sadowski et al, 2019; National Association of Social Workers, 2020). It is also important to include the contributions of nurses and nursing assistants in the long-term care setting. These individuals provide most of the direct care to residents and are considered the "cornerstone of nursing homes" (Franzosa et al, 2022, p. 905). They can provide valuable input about residents' behavior and needs based on consistent observation and can implement a variety of aspects of care identified by other disciplines. For example, a resident with dementia may require comprehensive rehabilitation services after a fall and subsequent hip fracture. The occupational therapist may collaborate with nursing to manage the timing of pain medications and overnight bed positioning to reduce pain and facilitate healing of the resident's hip, the physical therapist may provide education on strength training and range of motion to promote the resident's ability to walk from their room to the dining hall, the speech-language pathologist may complete a screening to assess cognition, social services may provide input on the resident's family support system, and the occupational therapist may provide education and training on how to complete dressing using adaptive equipment and follow their hip precautions.

Specific Issues for Working With Older Adults in Long-Term Care

Working with older adults in a long-term care setting brings with it specific needs tailored to the setting and population. This section discusses several important issues that affect the care of older adults, such as individual restorative care plans after the discontinuation of therapy services, the importance of oral care on the health of the individual, the increased risk of depression, and how the interprofessional team can address dementia.

Intensity of Rehabilitation After Hospitalization

The increase in medical conditions in older adults leads to increased hospitalizations. During those hospitalizations, older adults often experience functional deterioration of their sensorimotor and cognitive client factors (Urquiza et al, 2020). When an older adult is admitted or readmitted to long-term care after a hospitalization, occupational therapists work with client to help them return to their prior level of function or their new maximum level of function. A meta-analysis found that a posthospitalization interprofessional rehabilitation program contributed to improved functional mobility in older adults at 3 months after discharge, supporting the use of occupational therapists (Verweij et al, 2019).

An important consideration when evaluating the results of rehabilitation services in SNFs is the intensity, or number of therapy minutes, or therapy services provided per day or week. A retrospective study of older adults receiving care in SNFs found that 60 minutes per week of combined therapy, including occupational therapy, physical therapy, and speech-language pathology, was associated with a higher frequency of residents returning to the community and shorter length of SNF stay, allowing residents to return home quicker. Less than 60 minutes per week of combined therapy was associated with more hospitalizations and higher mortality rates (O'Brien & Zhang, 2018). A systematic review of rehabilitation intensity and patient outcome in SNFs in the United States concluded with moderate evidence that higher intensity therapy (more than 60 to 90 minutes per day of combined therapy) was associated with shorter length of SNF stay and higher community discharge rates (Prusynski et al, 2021).

The Value of Restorative Care

When residents have received full benefit and are no longer making functional gains during therapy, occupational therapy services may pause or terminate (AOTA, 2020). In such cases, restorative care plans can prevent or limit a resident's physical, cognitive, and functional decline. Restorative care programs, sometimes called maintenance programs, are programs "established by a therapist that consists of activities and/or mechanisms that will assist a beneficiary in maximizing or maintain the progress he or she has made during therapy or to prevent or slow further deterioration due to a disease or illness" (Centers for Medicare and Medicaid Services [CMS], 2014). Restorative care programs are usually provided by nursing assistants, preferably with specialized training in therapeutic activities. At the end of therapy services, an occupational therapist or physical therapist will develop an individualized restorative care plan and provide training to the nursing assistant on the plan so that the assistant can implement the restorative care plan. An example of a restorative care plan for an older adult being seen by an occupational therapist for a decline in functional independence due to weakness would be an upper-extremity exercise plan and scheduled functional mobility around the facility. Minimizing decline contributes to resident well-being and reduced care costs to the resident and long-term care facility.

Restorative care programs can be viewed as an ongoing, long-term approach to the maintenance and enhancement of functional abilities and thus a preventative health program rather than a short-term solution to a specific deficit. The programs should also include the development of and maintenance of social activities, as they are especially salient for long-term care residents. As of June 2006, CMS guidelines and regulations regarding activities provided to residents emphasize the need to ensure that activities match an individual resident's personal interests and needs and to enrich their maximum level of physical, mental, and psychosocial well-being. Among the many benefits linked to social activities include reduced depression symptoms, less cognitive decline, and decreased negative behaviors (Bethell et al, 2021). The occupational therapist must collaboratively work with the resident, nursing, and other rehabilitation professionals to develop a feasible and sustainable maintenance program.

Addressing Oral Hygiene

Oral hygiene is an often-overlooked element of long-term care, but it has significant implications for residents' well-being. Good dental health is vital to adequate nutrition and the ability to communicate effectively. Absence of good dental health can also increase pain and discomfort, making engagement with activities difficult. An interprofessional team of healthcare providers can enhance a resident's dental health (Ástvaldsdóttir et al, 2018). Dietitians can focus on appropriate diet and adequate hydration, speech-language pathologists can emphasize strength of oral and throat muscles, and occupational therapists can address proper positioning for feeding and oral hygiene. Occupational therapists can also address social aspects of eating, as well as managing flossing and brushing of teeth. (See Chapter 7 for more information about oral health.)

Depression

In the United States, it is estimated that 1% to 5% of older adults living in the community experience depression (Centers for Disease Control and Prevention, 2022). For long-term care residents, that number increases to 49% (Sengupta et al, 2022). Occupational therapists can provide interventions to improve a resident's depression symptoms by promoting engagement in creative occupations or activities, occupational balance and time use, skills and habit development, group and family approaches, and animal-assisted therapy (Kirsh et al, 2019).

Dementia

In 2018, an estimated 49% of long-term care residents were diagnosed with dementia (Sengupta et al, 2022). An interprofessional team may provide support to residents and their families living with effects of dementia. Innovation, creativity, and research are essential to ensure that the principles and philosophy of occupational therapy will be part of engagement for long-term care residents who have dementia (Fazio et al, 2018). (See Chapter 13 for more information about depression and dementia.)

Occupational Therapy Evaluation and Intervention Exemplars

Evaluation

As in many other settings, occupational therapy services in long-term care settings begin with an evaluation that includes the residents' occupational profile, an occupational performance analysis, and standardized assessments and screening tools (AOTA, 2020). In some circumstances, an occupational therapist may choose to complete a screen or consultation to determine whether a full occupational therapy evaluation is required. In this situation, the therapist would review the client's history, consult with the interprofessional team, and utilize standardized screening tools. After completing the screen, the practitioner may determine that a complete occupational therapy evaluation is appropriate or that occupational therapy services are not necessary (AOTA, 2020). A list of common assessment and screening tools used with older adults in long-term care can be found in Table 27-1. After completing the evaluation, the occupational therapist synthesizes the information from the occupational profile, the occupational performance analysis, assessment findings, and the residents' preferences to collaboratively develop a treatment plan with the resident. See Promoting Best Practice 27-1 for a sample occupational therapy treatment plan.

TABLE 27-1 ■ Commonly Used Assessments and Screening Tools in Long-Term Care

TYPE OF ASSESSMENT	NAME OF ASSESSMENT
ADLs/self-care	Assessment of Motor and Process Skills (AMPS) Barthel Index/Modified Barthel Index Katz Index of Independence in Activities of Daily Living (Katz ADL)
ADLs and IADLs	Kohlman Evaluation of Living Skills (KELS) Routine Task Inventory (RTI)
Balance	Berg Balance Scale (BBS) Functional Reach Test/Modified Functional Reach Test Timed Up and Go (TUG) Test
Upper-extremity function	Disabilities of the Arm, Shoulder, and Hand (DASH)/Short DASH
Cognition	Allen Cognitive Level Screen- 5 (ACLS-5) Mini-Mental State Examination (MMSE) Montreal Cognitive Assessment (MoCA)
Leisure	Activity Card Sort
Quality of life	WHO Quality of Life (WHOQOL)/WHOQOL-Bref
Depression	Beck Depression Inventory (BDI)

PROMOTING BEST PRACTICE 27-1
Sample Occupational Therapy Treatment Plans

Sample Occupational Therapy Treatment Plan

Assessment: Client is a 92-year-old female post right CVA affecting L side with resulting left-sided weakness. Client lives with sisters in two-story home and was previously independent in ADLs and IADLs, including driving, and did not use an assistive device for mobility. Client currently presents with one-sided weakness with left upper-extremity (UE) flaccid, pain, left shoulder subluxation, and impaired sequencing. Client presents with impaired ADLs and IADLs and decreased functional transfer ability, safety awareness, and functional activity tolerance. Client would benefit from skilled occupational therapy services to address these deficits and promote a safe return home at the highest level of functional ability.

Learning Barriers: None

Rehabilitation Potential: Good

Performance Deficits: Decreased independence/safety with activities of daily living; decreased independence/safety with IADLs, decreased UE passive/active assist/active range of motion, decreased UE strength; decreased gross motor skills, decreased fine motor skills, decreased standing balance/tolerance, decreased activity tolerance, decreased cognitive functioning; decreased sensory/motor skills, decreased sequencing, decreased safety wheelchair positioning, decreased safety awareness

Long-Term Goal 1: Client will be modified independent (Mod I) for feeding, grooming, UE dressing/bathing, and supervised for lower-extremity (LE) dressing/bathing, and toileting using durable medical equipment (DME) as needed to return to baseline functional abilities and prevent the need for 24-hour care.

Long-Term Goal 2: Client will be supervised during toilet and shower transfers using DME as needed to return to baseline functional abilities and prevent the need for 24-hour care.

Long-Term Goal 3: Client will be supervised when performing simple meal preparation and light cleaning tasks and Mod I for medication and money management using DME as needed to return to baseline functional abilities and prevent need for 24-hour care.

Short-Term Goal 1: Client will safely complete cognitive self-care tasks graded in levels of complexity with good accuracy and requiring only one to two verbal cues for attention, awareness, and problem-solving.

Short-Term Goal 2: Client will require minimal assistance (Min A) for LE dressing with efficient use of DME as needed while demonstrating good safety techniques.

Intervention Plan: ADL education/training, IADL education/training, therapeutic activities, sensory/motor intervention, cognitive training, resident/family education

Intervention Exemplars

Once the goals have been written and the plan of care has been established, the intervention process begins. The occupational therapy intervention process consists of three steps: (1) the intervention plan, (2) intervention implementation, and (3) intervention review. For the intervention plan, the therapist uses information gathered in the evaluation process to devise occupation-centered interventions to meet the established goals. Therapists have a variety of intervention approaches to utilize during a resident's care plan, including occupation and activities, interventions to support occupations, education and training, advocacy, group interventions, and virtual interventions. See Table 27-2 for a

TABLE 27-2 Occupational Therapy Interventions in Long-Term Care

TYPE OF INTERVENTION	EXAMPLES
Occupations and activities	• ADLs and IADLs • Games (bingo, cards, puzzles, etc.) • Book clubs • Crafts
Interventions to support occupations	• PAMs—Electrical stimulation, ultrasound, diathermy, heat, cold • Retrograde massage to reduce edema
Orthotics and prosthetics	• Fabricate and issue orthosis • Prosthetic for amputee
Assistive technology and environmental modifications	• Visual schedule • List of steps to complete an activity • Increase accessibility and safety in the facility
Wheeled mobility	• Adapted wheeled mobility to the individual client • Train in electric mobility
Self-regulation	• Create a sensory room • Work with dining staff on best environment for eating
Education and training	• Educate client on using adaptive equipment during ADLs and IADLs • Educate client on precautions after surgery • Train staff on donning and doffing a client's immobilization sling
Advocacy	• Work with client to improve food choices in the dining room • Work with client to implement a resident's board in the facility
Group interventions	• Functional groups—Learning to use a walker safely • Activity groups—Baking or cooking • Task groups—Creating a community garden • Social groups—Support, new resident
Virtual interventions	• Online support groups • Bring in a nutrition expert to virtually discuss managing diabetes

Note. *ADLs*, Activities of daily living; *IADLs*, instrumental activities of daily living; *PAMs*, physical agent modalities.
Interventions from American Occupational Therapy Association. (2020). Occupational therapy practice framework: Domain & process (4th ed.). *American Journal of Occupational Therapy, 74*(Suppl. 2), 7412410010p1–7412410010p87. www.doi.org//10.5014/ajot.2020.74S2001

list of examples of how an occupational therapist can utilize these interventions in a long-term care setting. Approaches can include creating or promoting, establishing or restoring, maintaining, modifying, and preventing declining function in occupations (AOTA, 2020). See Table 27-3 for a list of examples of how an occupational therapist can utilize these approaches in a long-term care setting.

After the occupational therapist creates the intervention plan, the therapist implements the intervention plan using purposeful and occupation-based approaches. The Occupation-Centered Intervention Assessment (OCIA) is an excellent tool, with established validity and reliability, for occupational therapists to use quickly and easily to develop and implement creative, occupation-centered interventions (Jewell et al, 2022). The OCIA promotes the use of a top-down approach with a focus on client-centered, ecologically valid, and occupationally relevant interventions. The OCIA includes three continua, each with four numeric ratings for scoring an occupational therapy intervention. The personal relevance continuum "represents the meaning and purpose, including motivation, purpose, or experience, a client holds for the intervention" or the client-centered aspects of an intervention (Jewell et al, 2022, p. 25). The contextual relevance continuum includes the client's "context and environment as they related to engagement in occupations" (p. 29), or the ecological validity of an intervention. The occupational relevance continuum examines the therapeutic modality that is provided to and with the client and closely examines if it includes an occupation as the therapeutic means, or the occupational relevance. The OCIA is shown in Figure 27-2.

TABLE 27-3 ■ Occupational Therapy Approaches in Long-Term Care

TYPES OF APPROACHES	EXAMPLES
Create, promote (health promotion)	■ Develop an energy conservation program for a client diagnosed with COPD. ■ Develop a falls prevention program for your facility.
Establish, restore (remediation, restoration)	■ Establish a sleep hygiene routine for a client who is having difficulty sleeping. ■ Work with a client to restore function to their upper-extremity after an injury.
Maintain	■ Run a group session to maintain social participation for clients with dementia. ■ Increase lighting in rooms for residents with low vision.
Modify (compensation, adaptation)	■ Rearrange a client's room to allow for safe mobility. ■ Work with the facility to provide a more accessible and safer environment for residents.
Prevent (disability prevention)	■ Develop an exercise program for a client. ■ Implement a tai chi program in the facility.

Note. COPD, Chronic obstructive pulmonary disease.
Approaches from American Occupational Therapy Association. (2020). Occupational therapy practice framework: Domain & process (4th ed.). *American Journal of Occupational Therapy, 74*(Suppl. 2), 7412410010p1-7412410010p87. www.doi.org//10.5014/ajot.2020.74S2001

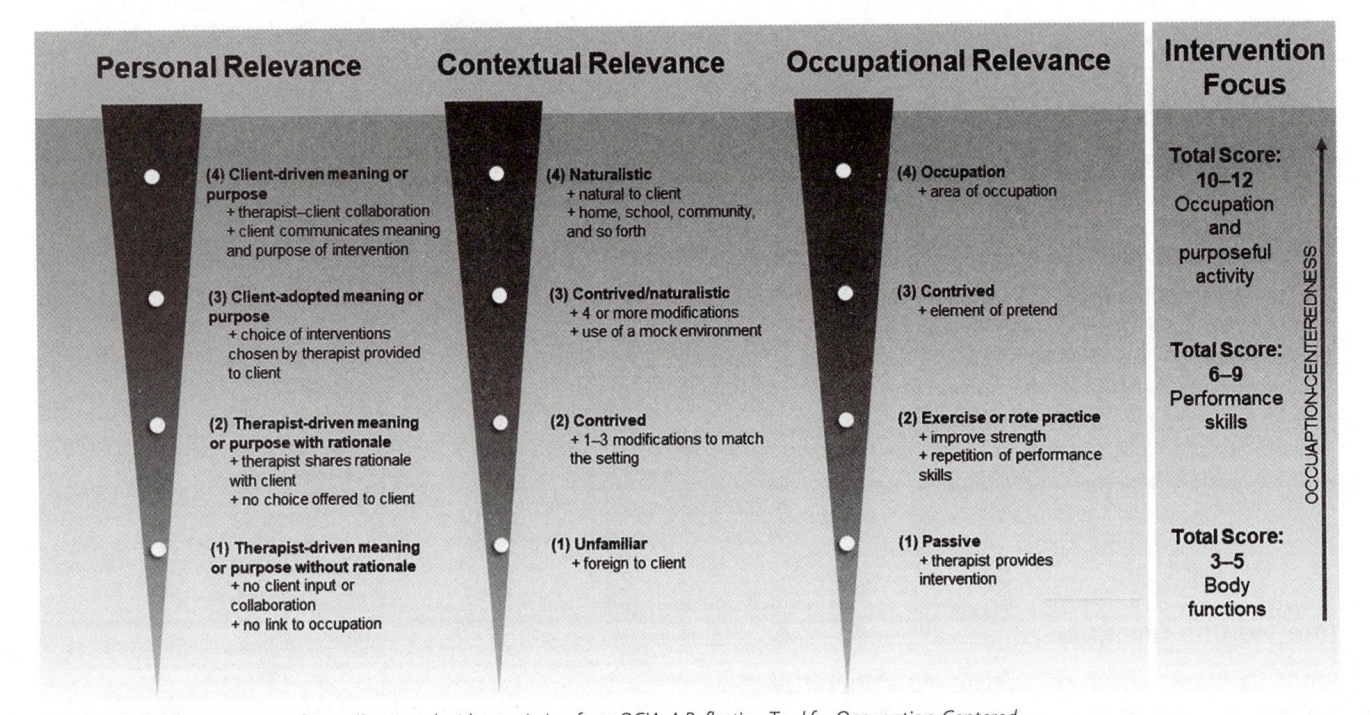

FIGURE 27-2 OCIA scoring sheet. *(Reprinted with permission from OCIA: A Reflection Tool for Occupation-Centered Practice, Appendix A: OCIA Scoring Sheet, AOTA Press.)*

An important part of intervention implementation is continuous evaluation and reevaluation of the resident's response to the intervention. The final step in the intervention process is intervention review, in which the therapist and client reevaluate and review the intervention plan and collaborate to assess progress toward goals and desired outcomes. The intervention plan may need to be modified, and the continuation or discontinuation of therapy services should be determined, along with referral to any needed services (AOTA, 2020).

Therapeutic Environments. Along with the expertise and attitude of the staff, the organization environment can support the delivery of a quality occupation-centered program (Bethell et al, 2021). Each resident has an array of previous life skills that can be incorporated into programming. It is a mistake to believe that rehabilitation can occur only within a traditional clinic setting focusing on tabletop tasks and therapy materials. Practitioners must look beyond the obvious and utilize the total living environment as an element in treatment planning. Fortunately, guidelines are shifting in this direction for overall nursing home care.

The goal of care in nursing homes is to enhance the overall well-being of the residents. An effective model for conceptualizing care, known as the Green House Model, emphasizes the environment, philosophy, and service capacity of the long-term services (Grabowski, 2022). This model emphasizes the importance of both private space and public shared space. Availability of single rooms that include familiar resident furnishings and a welcoming and supportive public environment have an important role in the residents' overall quality of life. Strong evidence supports the importance of person-centered care, a philosophy that allows residents to control and choose how they spend their time and receive their daily care. Service capacity in this setting must encompass both routine care and specialized services (The Green House Project, 2021).

These characteristics are evident in several models of care, including those being integrated into existing nursing home facilities, as well as stand-alone models of care, such as the Wellspring Program and the Eden Alternative (Fazio et al, 2018). The Green House Model, Wellspring Program, and Eden Alternative are examples of programs that focus on using the full 24-hours in a day as potential time for engagement in the various areas of occupation, such as social participation or IADLs. The Wellspring Program, developed for residents with memory loss, is designed to foster a self-regulating series of behavior-based feedback loops among the resident, staff, and family members. This approach fosters independence and spontaneity, creating activities "for the moment," meaning capturing a moment of pleasurable occupational engagement (The Well-Spring Group, 2022). The Eden Alternative attempts to redesign the experience of aging and limitations by using animals, plants, and children to transform the nursing home environment into habitats where individuals enjoy living. Staff, including everyone in contact with residents, continually ask, "What is best for the resident?" The resident always remains the central focus,

ensuring that each day reflects the natural rhythms of life and freedom of choice (The Eden Alternative, 2021).

At Menorah Park, in Beachwood, Ohio, the treatment environment includes a horticulture area; an in-house nature center; in-house pets; therapeutic and recreational swimming facilities; work trial areas in a snack shop, gift shop, or reception area; an onsite child care facility for volunteer opportunities for residents (Fig. 27-3); available technology such as environmental controls, aids for the visually impaired, internet access, and computer learning modules; vehicles for exploring and integrating into the community at large; a specific place for worship and meditation; a resident bank and beauty shop, exterior garden spaces with putting greens, and raised flower beds (Fig. 27-4); an ice cream parlor; an auditorium used for entertainment, evenings of formal dining with visiting family members, and dances; and so on (Menorah Park, 2022). Development of an engaging and homelike environment such as this requires input from a variety of team members and uniquely positions occupational therapy to take a leadership role in ensuring maximum participation of the residents in meaningful occupations while ensuring safety and providing modifications to the environment to improve access and participation in daily activities.

Improving the Dining Experience. Person-centered care can also be expanded into the dining experience to provide maximal levels of personal choice in dining options and can enhance quality of life for nursing home residents. Ideas that improve the quality of dining in long-term care include expanding menus to include easy-to-swallow food choices, food carts and self-service buffets that allow the individual to select the type and amount of food, flexible mealtimes to allow residents to eat when they are hungry rather than at prescribed times that are more convenient for the facility, and tableside service to recreate the atmosphere of a restaurant. These innovative ideas also provide opportunities for staff to notice a resident's nutrition, food choices and needs, changes in cognition or physical functioning, and social

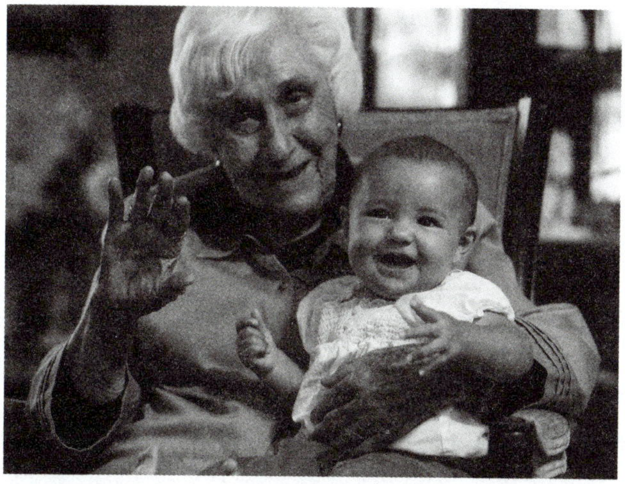

FIGURE 27-3 On-site childcare facilities in long-term care settings allow for older adults to participate in volunteer experiences. *(Monkeybusinessimages/iStock/Getty Images.)*

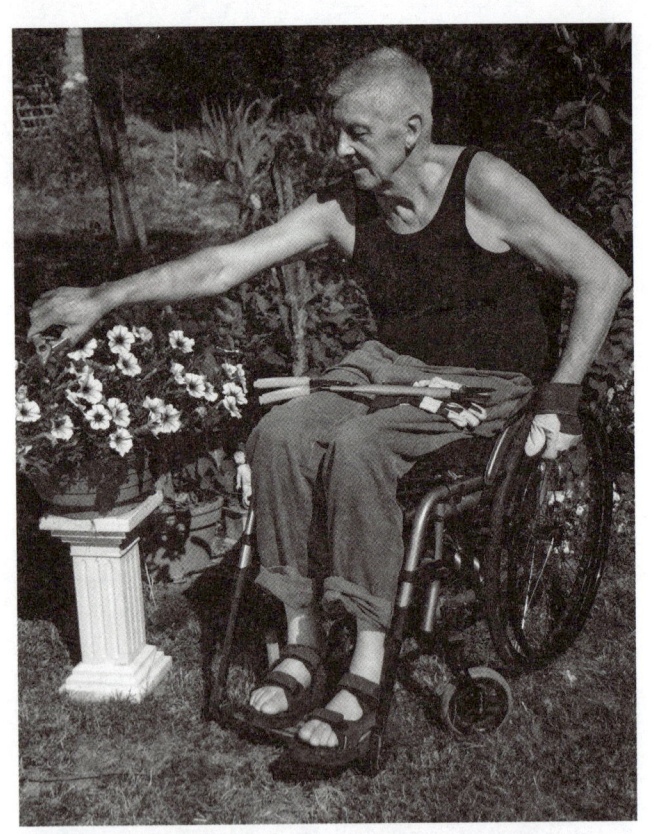

FIGURE 27-4 Raised planters. The use of assistive devices and modified environments makes outdoor gardening accessible to residents. *(Sorcerer44/iStock/Getty Images.)*

interaction (Keller et al, 2021; McLaren-Hedwards et al, 2021). An occupational therapist may work closely with a speech-language pathologist to assess and treat issues with swallowing to promote safe feeding, eating, and swallowing. The occupational therapist will assess the dining environment to ensure proper lighting and contrast of feeding tools and materials, safe positioning at the table, and that food consistencies and adaptive tools are present and utilized properly to promote feeding.

Dementia Care Exemplars. Occupational therapists can work with individuals experiencing dementia to maintain existing function, promote positive relationships and social interactions, and increase participation in meaningful and necessary occupations (AOTA, 2017). Evidence supports three therapeutic interventions to address the behavioral and psychological symptoms of dementia: (1) sensory practices (aromatherapy, massage, multisensory stimulation, and bright light therapy), (2) psychosocial practices (validation therapy, reminiscence therapy, music therapy, pet therapy, and meaningful activities), and (3) structured care protocols to address bathing and oral care. These interventions should be responsive to the preferences and experiences of each individual and client-centered to promote optimal well-being for those with dementia (Scales et al, 2018). Both bathing and oral care protocols should be developed by the occupational therapist, with input from nursing, through careful consideration of the client's personal and contextual factors.

For example, bathing protocols should be scheduled during a time that the client is the most responsive to the self-care activity, which will limit agitation and promote sleep habits. The occupational therapist can trial various sensory strategies to promote a relaxing environment during bathing, such as the use of music or aromatherapy. Evidence suggests that consistent routines, with the use of strategies to promote a person-centered self-care routine, are beneficial for residents with dementia (Gozalo et al, 2014).

Cognitive loss can affect the ability to perform ADLs and IADLs, as a resident may forget to perform necessary daily occupations such as eating, bathing, taking medicine, or attending appointments. Therapists working with residents who have memory difficulties will often provide education and training in the use of external memory aids to residents and their care staff. These memory aids can include low-tech devices such as diaries, memory books, note-taking, and lists. Interventions may also include more high-tech solutions such as Google Calendar or Outlook Calendar, smartphones, smart watches, and text reminder systems. External memory aids can be helpful in assisting residents to achieve therapeutic goals (Jones et al, 2021). Additionally, social interaction and social supports are of vital importance for individuals with dementia in long-term care settings. Organizing systems in which residents interact regularly among themselves and with loved ones can enhance a variety of outcomes. Increasing residents' social interactions may involve attending activities and communicating with family and relatives to minimize behavioral problems for residents (Arai et al, 2021). Another example includes the use of an intergenerational program. These programs bring different generations together to participate in organized combined activities. Gerritzen and colleagues reported successful intergenerational dementia programs that incorporated buddy systems, Montessori-based activities, and reminiscence programs (2020). All activities demonstrated benefits for residents with dementia and younger generations.

Originally developed as an approach for working with children, Montessori-based activities have also been used with individuals experiencing dementia in long-term care facilities (Camp, 2010; Mbakile-Mahlanza et al, 2020; Tschanz & Hammond, 2020; Wilkes et al, 2019). The Montessori method simplifies tasks, offers immediate feedback, and provides hands-on opportunities for older adults with dementia to participate in meaningful activities and connect with previous long-term memories. This approach is based on the idea that there may be a developmental progression to the loss of abilities in dementia and has been found beneficial for residents with significant and deteriorating cognitive impairments (Wilkes et al, 2019).

Outcomes of Occupational Therapy Services in Long-Term Care

The final component in the occupational therapy process is the target outcomes. An occupational therapist should administer the same standardized and non-standardized assessments during client evaluation, reevaluation, and discharge to accurately report on the resident's goal progression and completion. If the client has met all goals or chooses to no longer receive services, the client may discontinue occupational therapy services. At the end of occupational therapy services, the resident may return to their home, move to another residential facility such as assisted living, or remain in the current facility for a short period of time or as a long-term resident. Planning for discontinuation of occupational therapy services should begin during the evaluation and continue throughout the intervention process by preparing the resident, family members, and caregivers for a safe transition to the next level of care, thereby preventing readmission to a hospital or an SNF. During discharge planning, a therapist may provide education to the resident and their caregiver on the use of adaptive equipment, adaptations of occupations, environmental modifications, or helping the resident and family decide on the best setting for the transition of care. If a resident is remaining in a nursing home for an extended period, the therapist may create and implement a restorative care plan in collaboration with the client.

Documentation, Payment Systems, and Reimbursment

Occupational therapists must objectively prove to regulators and reimbursement sources that occupation-centered programs designed and implemented by skilled practitioners provide positive, objective, and sustained functional and quality of life outcomes to residents in long-term care contexts. Documentation of occupational therapy is required for long-term care facilities to receive insurance payment for therapy services, report the medically necessary service provided, document a resident's goal progression, and support the submitted therapy charges. In addition, CMS requires all occupational therapy documentation to follow state and local laws and adhere to professional guidelines. CMS also requires that therapy documentation supports the time spent with the resident, the billed Current Procedural Terminology code, and follows all Medicare regulations.

To receive Medicare or Medicaid funding for rehabilitation therapy services, the minimum required therapy documentation for each resident includes evaluation and any reevaluations, plan of care/certification of the plan of care, progress reports, treatment notes, and a discharge note. For evaluations, Medicare requires a medical diagnosis, long-term functional goals, a detailed list of the types of interventions performed, and the quantity and frequency of treatment. The care plan should be consistent with the evaluation and can be two separate documents or the same document. After the occupational therapist creates the plan of care, a physician or nurse practitioner must sign and date it. If the resident completed their first plan of care and requires additional occupational therapy services past the initial plan of care date, the therapist must complete a reevaluation. A recertification is required after 90 days, regardless of the plan of care established in the initial evaluation. Daily notes are required and should contain the date of service, all services provided, time spent on each service, changes to treatment, and observations of the patient made during treatment. Progress reports provide justification for the medical necessity of treatment and must be completed once every 10 treatment days or once during each certification interval, whichever is less. Progress notes should include an assessment of progress toward each goal, plans to continue treatments, and additional evaluation results. Treatment notes are intended by CMS to be a record of all encounters of the therapist with the patient. At a minimum, they should include the type of treatment and intervention and total treatment time. A sample clinical note can be found in Promoting Best Practice 27-2. The final documentation required by CMS is the discharge note. It is intended to be a progress note describing all treatment provided from the last progress note to the time of discharge (CMS, n.d.-b.).

PROMOTING BEST PRACTICE 27-2
Sample Clinical Note (Occupational Therapy)

Total Individual Time (Min): 75.
SUBJECTIVE: "I told myself I was going to work hard on the weekends." PAIN: No complaint of pain
OBJECTIVE: client seen for morning ADL session SELF CARE: GROOMING: Modified independent seated in w/c at sink to wash/rinse/dry face, apply deodorant and complete oral care including mouthwash, brushing teeth. Increased time to complete. Moving at a slow pace, completed mouthwash ×2. Large amount of time spent on thoroughly brushing teeth. Client completed own setup at w/c level, no assist required to open containers on this date. BATHING: Modified independent to wash/rinse/dry upper body while seated in w/c at sink. Increased time spent on thoroughness. UE DRESSING: modified independent seated to doff pullover shirt over head. MOD I to don pullover shirt/CGA to don open front jacket while seated in w/c.
ASSESSMENT: increased time to complete full ADL session due to slow pace. Significant progress demonstrated during ADL session.
INTERVENTION PLAN: continue to work toward goals

Payment Systems and Reimbursement

In the United States, Medicare and Medicaid are the primary payment systems for residents receiving care in nursing homes (CMS, n.d.-a.). Medicare covers up to 100 days of skilled nursing care and requires that the nursing home placement be preceded by a hospitalization. Medicaid is the primary source of longer-term coverage, particularly when there is no immediate precipitating medical trigger, and the care is deemed "custodial." For example, Medicaid would be more likely to pay for long-term care for an individual who has a cognitive impairment that is likely to worsen over time. Some individuals pay privately or through personal long-term care insurance; however, the cost for nursing home care averaged $260 per day for a semiprivate room in 2021 (Genworth, 2022), making it difficult for most individuals and families to cover the cost of care.

Medicare determines payment to facilities using a Prospective Payment System (PPS) (CMS, 2021b). Occupational therapists need to be aware of changes to the PPS in SNFs, as this has a tremendous effect on therapy service delivery, and such changes occur frequently. In October 2019, the Patient Driven Payment Model (PDPM) went into effect, replacing the previous payment system, Resource Utilization Groups (RUG), which had been in place since 2000. Under the RUG system, SNFs were reimbursed according to the number of therapy minutes provided to a resident for the previous week. When the resident participated in more therapy minutes in a week, the SNF reimbursement for services also increased. Now, with PDPM as the PPS for Medicare, reimbursement is determined by specific resident characteristics to determine the daily amount, or per diem, paid for each resident. The specific resident characteristics are determined by a five case-mix adjusted component and a variable per diem adjustment. The case-mix adjusted components are physical therapy, occupational therapy, speech-language pathologist, nontherapy ancillary services, and nursing (CMS, 2021a).

Payment for residents with occupational therapy and physical therapy needs is determined by the primary diagnosis for the SNF stay and the client's functional status, which will place a patient into one of 16 case-mix classification groups. CMS determined the four categories of diagnosis for the occupational therapy and physical therapy component by examining the cost for therapy services, and grouping certain clinical categories together based on similar costs. These categories include major joint replacement or spinal surgery, nonorthopedic/musculoskeletal, orthopedic surgery, acute infections, and medical management. These five categories are further divided into another four categories based on functional status, which is calculated using data from Section GG of the Minimum Data Set 3.0. Section GG contains 10 items determined by CMS to predict occupational therapy and physical therapy costs per day and consists of two bed mobility items, three transfer items, one eating item, one toileting item, one oral hygiene item, and two walking items. The speech-language pathology component utilizes a different classification system (CMS, 2021a). The final component determining reimbursement for the PDPM payment system is the variable per diem schedule. Because resource utilization for residents is higher at the beginning and decreases over the course of a length of stay, payment under PDPM slowly declines from day 21 of the stay until day 100, which is the last day of coverage of an SNF stay by Medicare (CMS, 2021a).

The PDPM allows for therapy to be broken down into three modes: individual, concurrent, and group. Individual therapy is considered by CMS to be the most appropriate mode of therapy for residents in an SNF, as it allows for specific, focused interventions that meet the individual needs of each resident. Another mode of therapy, concurrent therapy, is defined as one therapist treating two patients at the same time, with the residents not performing the same or similar activities. Group therapy, the third mode of therapy permitted by PDPM, is the concurrent treatment of two to six residents who are performing the same or similar activities by one therapist. Under PDPM, the combination of group and concurrent therapy minutes for a patient cannot exceed 25% of their total therapy minutes (CMS, 2021a).

State Regulations

In addition to the numerous federal guidelines regulating nursing homes, individual states have established their own policies (Chen et al, 2020). Among the areas that are often governed by state law are qualifications for nursing home administrators, licensing and inspection of facilities, admission rules, resident rights, programming, and a host of other factors. Differences exist in many aspects of nursing home management and programming, extending to building codes, furnishings, staffing, and programming.

International Reimbursement and Models

This chapter focuses primarily on long-term care in the United States. Because of the wide range of types of long-term care and the centrality of specific government and third-party payer regulations, it is beyond the scope of a single chapter to cover long-term care worldwide. In some countries, long-term care facilities are rare, either because economic circumstances make it impossible to afford such care or because families feel strongly about providing care themselves. In other countries, an array of long-term care options may provide alternative models worthy of consideration for implementation in the United States. For example, in Canada, older adults can receive 24-hour long-term care services through the Canada Health Transfer (Considra Care, 2022), while Latin American countries do not have an established national coverage (Scheil-Adlung, 2015). Certainly, as the population ages, options for ensuring adequate care for older adults at the end of their lives will become increasingly important worldwide.

Advocacy for Clients and Service

Occupational therapists frequently need to advocate for long-term care residents' needs and services. For example, an occupational therapist advocating at the person level may contact a resident's insurance company when a termination date for therapy services has been issued, but the resident continues to require therapy services to return home safely. At the group level, a practitioner might advocate for a meeting space for a group of residents who are interested in starting a grief support group. Advocating at the population level may include a therapist talking with facility administrators about ways to decrease inequities in care offered to underserved populations (AOTA, 2021).

The OTPF-4 lists advocacy as a type of intervention used in delivering occupational therapy services (AOTA, 2020). Practitioners not only advocate for residents directly, but they also provide support and training to residents on how to successfully advocate for themselves (self-advocacy). Self-advocacy is a powerful tool that residents can use not only in their current situation but throughout their lives in a variety of situations. Occupational therapists can advocate for residents during many occasions and contexts, including during informal conversations with coworkers in a facility, when speaking in interprofessional team meetings, when making phone calls or sending emails, or when presenting at meetings or conferences.

CASE STUDY (CONTINUED)

Intervention in the Context of a Long-Term Care Setting

Mandie tried a day care program for a few days a week to give her respite. After 2 weeks, Tom refused to go to day care, and the day care felt he was not adjusting. Tom is continuing to decline and now needs assistance with basic self-care, eating, and functional mobility. Tom is frequently confused, disoriented, and sometimes asks Mandie who she is. He acts out in his sleep at night. Mandie realizes she is no longer able to care for Tom. She has mixed feelings about moving her husband to a long-term facility but feels she must for his safety and her health. Tom moves to a long-term care facility that is only a 10-minute drive from their home. Mandie visits daily to reassure Tom of her presence and to encourage his participation in facility programming. She also helps with meals and self-care activities when she is present. Tom is less engaged with his daily living tasks and his environment than Mandie would like, and she hopes occupational therapy will be able to support his continued participation to his best ability.

Questions

1. Utilizing the OCIA to guide your thinking, what is an occupation-centered intervention the occupational therapist could provide to promote Tom's safe dining room experience and eating?
2. What factors should the occupational therapist consider when setting up a bathing/showering protocol with the nursing staff?

Answers

1. The person factors of choice of food and seating location as well as the context of the dining experience would need to be assessed for their therapeutic value. (LO 27.4, 27.8; Evaluation section and Intervention exemplar section)

2. The personal and contextual factors around the time of day that is best for the resident and providing a soothing sensory experience (e.g., smells and sounds) should be considered when setting up such a protocol. If the protocol is considered restorative, the therapist would schedule opportunities to assess the restorative care program and modify as needed. (LO 27.2, 27.3; Interprofessional partners section and Special Issues section)

SUMMARY

Occupational therapists must continue to demonstrate positive resident outcomes through the provision of skilled interventions, research, and advocacy for their residents' needs. Because older adults are living longer and with more chronic conditions, it is expected that occupational therapists will need to continue to provide complex, skilled services within the context of long-term care facilities. Long-term care residents require safety, autonomy, and excellent medical services. To meet the needs of residents and deliver services in long-term care settings, therapists must be creative and innovative when designing skilled, occupation-centered programs.

An individual's age should not be the determinant of whether a person should or should not participate and benefit from a therapeutic activities program, but will third-party payers understand the significance of quality-based activities programs for the older adult and be willing to reimburse therapists for their skills? Long-term care guidelines are increasingly focused on function and quality of life. This may well portend a renewed interest in providing truly therapeutic programs for long-term care residents. If so, the skills and knowledge of occupational therapists may become more salient to facilities seeking to comply with regulatory imperatives.

Critical Thinking Questions

1. Describe the characteristics of a typical person who utilizes long-term care services.
2. Compare and contrast single discipline intervention to interprofessional care in a nursing home setting.
3. Create three occupation-centered long-term goals for a client in an SNF.

REFERENCES

Administration on Aging. (2021, May). *2020 Profile of older Americans.* https://acl.gov/sites/default/files/Aging%20and%20Disability%20in%20America/2020ProfileOlderAmericans.Final_.pdf

American Occupational Therapy Association. (2017). *Fact sheet: Dementia and the role of occupational therapy.* https://www.aaa7.org/Portals/_AgencySite/Functional%20Fridays/AOTA%20Fact%20Sheet%20Dementia.pdf

American Occupational Therapy Association. (2020). Occupational therapy practice framework: Domain & process (4th ed.). *American Journal of Occupational Therapy, 74*(Suppl. 2), 7412410010p1-7412410010p87. https://www.doi.org//10.5014/ajot.2020.74S2001

American Occupational Therapy Association. (2021). *Everyday advocacy decision guide.* https://www.aota.org/-/media/corporate/files/advocacy/everyday-advocacy-decision-guide.pdf

Arai, A., Khaltar, A., Ozaki, T., & Katsumata, Y. (2021). Influence of social interaction on behavioral and psychological symptoms of dementia over 1 year among long-term care facility residents. *Geriatric Nursing, 42*(2), 509–516. https://doi.org/10.1016/j.gerinurse.2020.09.008

Arrieta, H., Rezola-Pardo, C., Echeverria, I., Iturburu, M., Gil, S. M., Yanguas, J. J., Irazusta, J., & Rodriguez-Larrad, A. (2018). Physical activity and fitness are associated with verbal memory, quality of life, and depression among nursing home residents: Preliminary data of a randomized controlled trial. *BMC Geriatrics, 18*(80), 1–13. https://doi.org/10.1186/s12877-018-0770-y

Ástvaldsdóttir, Á., Boström, A. M., Davidson, T., Gabre, P., Gahnberg, L., Sandborgh Englund, G., Skott, P., Ståhlnacke, K., Tranaeus, S., Wilhelmsson, H., Wårdh, I., Östlund, P., & Nilsson, M. (2018). Oral health and dental care of older persons—A systematic map of systematic reviews. *Gerodontology, 35*(4), 290–304. https://doi.org/10.1111/ger.12368

Barken, R., & Lowndes, R. (2018). Supporting family involvement in long-term residential care: Promising practices for relational care. *Qualitative Health Research, 28*(1), 60–72. https://doi.org/10.1177/1049732317730568

Bethell, J., Aelick, K., Babineau, J., Bretzlaff, M., Edwards, C., Gibson, J., Colborne, D. H., Iaboni, A., Lender, D., Schon, D., & McGilon, K. S. (2021). Social connection in long-term care homes: A scoping review of published research on the mental health impacts and potential strategies during COVID-19. *Journal of the American Medical Directors Association, 22*(2), 228–237.e25. https://doi.org/10.1016/j.jamda.2020.11.025

Boscart, V., Crutchlow, L. E., Taucar, L. S., Johnson, K., Heyer, M. Davey, M., Costa, A. P., & Heckman, G. (2020). Chronic disease management models in nursing homes: A scoping review. *BMJ Open, 10*, e032316. https://www.doi.org//10.1136/bmjopen-2019-032316

Camp, C. J. (2010). Origins of Montessori programming for dementia. *Non-Pharmacological Therapies in Dementia, 1*(2), 163–174.

Centers for Disease Control and Prevention. (2022). *Depression is not a normal part of growing older.* https://www.cdc.gov/aging/depression/index.html

Centers for Medicare and Medicaid Services. (2014, January 14). CMS manual system: Pub 100-02 Medicare Benefit Policy, transmittal 179. https://www.cms.gov/Regulations-and-Guidance/Guidance/Transmittals/Downloads/R179BP.pdf

Centers for Medicare and Medicaid Services. (2021a). *Patient driven payment model.* https://www.cms.gov/Medicare/Medicare-Fee-for-Service-Payment/SNFPPS/PDPM

Centers for Medicare and Medicaid Services. (2021b). *Prospective payment systems – general information.* https://www.cms.gov/Medicare/Medicare-Fee-for-Service-Payment/ProspMedicareFeeSvcPmtGen

Centers for Medicare and Medicaid Services. (n.d.-a.). *Nursing homes.* https://www.cms.gov/medicare/health-safety-standards/quality-safety-oversight-general-information/nursing-homes

Centers for Medicare and Medicaid Services. (n.d.-b.). *Medicare benefit policy manual. Chapter 15: section 220—coverage of outpatient rehabilitation therapy services (physical therapy, occupational therapy, and speech-language pathology services) under medical insurance.* https://www.cms.gov/Medicare/Prevention/PrevntionGenInfo/Downloads/bp102c15.pdf

Centers for Medicare and Medicaid Services. (n.d.-c.). *Custodial care vs skilled care.* https://www.cms.gov/Medicare-Medicaid-Coordination/Fraud-Prevention/Medicaid-Integrity-Education/Downloads/infograph-CustodialCarevsSkilledCare-%5BMarch-2016%5D.pdf

Chen, A. T., Ryskina, K. L., & Hye-Young, J. (2020). Long-term care, residential facilities and COVID-19: An overview of federal and state policy responses. *Journal of the American Medical Directors Association, 21*(9), 1186–1190. https://doi.org/10.1016/j.jamda.2020.07.001

Considra Care. (2022). *Senior care options in Canada.* https://www.considra-care.com/senior-care-options-in-canada/#:~:text=Long%2Dterm%20care%20(LTC),and%20other%20daily%20living%20activities

Dieticians of Canada. (2019). Best practices for nutrition, food service, and dining in long term care homes: A working paper of the Ontario LTC Action Group 2019. https://www.dietitians.ca/DietitiansOfCanada/media/Documents/Resources/2019-Best-Practices-for-Nutrition,-Food-Service-and-Dining-in-Long-Term-Care-LTC-Homes.pdf

Duan-Porter, W., Ullman, K, Rosebush, C., McKenzie, L., Ensrud, K. E., Ratner, E. Greer, N., Shippee, T. Gaughler, J., and Wilt, T. J. (2019, May). Systematic review: Risk factors and interventions to prevent or delay long-term nursing home placement for adults with impairments. VA ESP Project #09009. https://www.hsrd.research.va.gov/publications/esp/nursing-home-delay.pdf

Durocher, E., Njelesani, J., & Crosby, E. (2022). Art activities in long-term care: A scoping review. *Canadian Journal of Occupational Therapy, 89*(1), 36-43. https://doi.org/10.1177/00084174211064497

The Eden Alternative. (2021). *Well-being is a human right.* https://www.edenalt.org/

Egan, C., Mulcahy, H., & Naughton, C. (2022). Transitioning to long-term care for older adults with intellectual disabilities: A concept analysis. *Journal of Intellectual Disabilities, 26*(4), 1015–1032. https://doi.org/10.1177/17446295211041839

Fazio, S., Pace, D. P., Flinner, J., & Kallmyer, B. (2018). The fundamentals of person-centered care for individuals with dementia. *The Gerontologist, 58*(Suppl. 1), S10–S19. https://doi.org/10.1093/geront/gnx122

Fazio, S., Pace, D., Maslow, K., Zimmerman, S., & Kallmyer, B. (2018). Alzheimer's Association dementia care practice recommendations. *The Gerontologist, 58*(Suppl. 1), S1–S9. https://doi.org/10.1093/geront/gnx182

Franzosa, E., Mak, W., Burack, O. R., Hokenstad, A., Wiggins, F., Boockvar, K. S., & Reinhardt, J. P. (2022). Perspectives of certified nursing assistants and administrators on staffing the nursing home frontline during the COVID-19 pandemic. *Health Services Research, 57*(4), 905–913. https://doi.org/10.1111/1475-6773.13954

Gagliardi, C., & Piccinini, F. (2019). The use of nature-based activities for the well-being of older people: An integrative literature review. *Archives of Gerontology and Geriatrics, 83*, 315–327. https://doi.org/10.1016/j.archger.2019.05.012

Genworth. (2022). *Cost of care survey.* https://www.genworth.com/aging-and-you/finances/cost-of-care.html

Gerritzen, E. V., Hull, M. J., Verbeek, H., Smith, A. E., & De Boer, B. (2020). Successful elements of intergenerational dementia programs: A scoping review. *Journal of Intergenerational Relationships, 18*(2), 214–245. https://doi.org/10.1080/15350770.2019.1670770

Gozalo, P., Prakash, S., Qato, D. M., Sloane, P. D., & Mor, V. (2014). Effect of the bathing without a battle training intervention on bathing-associated physical and verbal outcomes in nursing home residents with dementia: A randomized crossover diffusion study. *Journal of the American Geriatrics Society, 62*(5), 797–804. https://doi.org/10.1111/jgs.12777

Grabowski, D. C. (2022). Putting the nursing and home in nursing homes. *Innovative Aging, 6*(4), 1–6. https://doi.org/10.1093/geroni/igac029

The Green House Project. (2021). *The transformation of institutional long-term and post-acute care.* https://thegreenhouseproject.org

Harris-Kojetin, L., Sengupta, M., Lendon, J. P., Rome, V., Valverde, R. & Caffrey, C. (2019). *Long-term care providers and services users in the United States: 2015-2016.* National Center for Health Statistics. Vital and health statistics. Series 3, analytical and epidemiological studies; no 43; DHHS publication; no. 2019-1427. https://stacks.cdc.gov/view/cdc/76253

Keller, H. H., Wu, S. A., Iraniparast, M., Trinca, V., & Morrison-Koechl, J. (2021). Relationship-centered mealtime training program demonstrates efficacy to improve the dining environment in long-term care. *Journal of the American Medical Directors Association, 22*(9), 1933–1938e2. https://doi.org/10.1016/j.jamda.2020.11.008

Jewell, V. D., Pickens, N., & Burns, S. (2019). Identification and effectiveness of occupational therapy interventions in skilled nursing facilities: A scoping review. *Annals of International Occupational Therapy, 2*(2), 79–90. https://doi.org/10.3928/24761222-20190218-03

Jewell, V. D., Wienkes, T. L., & Pickens, N. D. (2022). *The occupation-centered intervention assessment: A reflection tool for occupation-centered practice.* AOTA Press.

Jones, W. E., Benge, J. F., & Scullin, M. K. (2021). Preserving prospective memory in daily life: A systematic review and meta-analysis of mnemonic strategy, cognitive training, external memory aid, and combination interventions. *Neuropsychology, 35*(1), 123–140. https://doi.org/10.1037/neu0000704

Kirsh, B., Martin, L., Hultqvist, J., & Eklund, M. (2019). Occupational therapy interventions in mental health: A literature review in search of evidence. *Occupational Therapy in Mental Health, 35*(2), 109–156. https://doi.org/10.1080/0164212X.2019.1588832

Mbakile-Mahlanza, L., van der Ploeg, E. S., Buija, L., Camp, C., Walker, H., & O'Conner, D. W. (2020). A cluster randomized crossover trial of Montessori activities delivered by family carers to nursing home residents with behavioral and psychological symptoms of dementia. *International Psychogeriatric Association, 32*(3), 347–358. https://doi.org/10.1017/S1041610219001819

McCreedy, E. M., Weinstein, B. E., Chodosh, J., & Blustein, J. (2018). Hearing loss: Why does it matter for nursing homes? *Journal of the American Medical Directors Association, 19*(4), 323–327. https://doi.org/10.1016/j.jamda.2017.12.007

McLaren-Hedwards, T., D'cunha, K., Elder-Robinson, E., Smith, C., Jennings, C. March, A., & Young, A. (2021). Effect of communal dining and dining room enhancement interventions on nutrition, clinical and functional outcomes of patients in acute and sub-acute hospital, rehabilitation and aged-care settings: A systematic review. *Nutrition & Dietetics, 79*(1), 140–168. https://doi.org/10.1111/1747-0080.12650

Medicare.gov. (n.d.). *Skilled nursing facility (SNF) care.* https://www.medicare.gov/coverage/skilled-nursing-facility-snf-care

Menorah Park. (2022). *Excellence in caring.* https://www.menorahpark.org

Musa, M. K., Saga, S., Blekken, L. E., Harris, R., Goodman, C., & Norton, C. (2019). The prevalence, incidence, and correlates of fecal incontinence among older people residing in care homes: A systematic review. *Journal of the American Medical Directors Association, 20*(8), 956–962.e8. https://doi.org/10.1016/j.jamda.2019.03.033

National Association of Social Workers- Massachusetts Chapter. (2020). *Nursing home model job description.* https://www.naswma.org/page/90#:~:text=The%20nursing%20home%20social%20worker,being%20and%20quality%20of%20life

National Council on Aging. (2023, Aug 31). *The top 10 common chronic conditions in older adults.* https://www.ncoa.org/article/the-top-10-most-common-chronic-conditions-in-older-adults

O'Brien, S. R., & Zhang, N. (2018). Association between therapy intensity and discharge outcomes in aged Medicare skilled nursing facility admissions. *Archives of Physical Medicine and Rehabilitation, 99*(1), 107–115. https://doi.org/10.1016/j.apmr.2017.07.012

Prusynski, R. A., Gustavson, A. M., Shrivastav, S. R., & Mroz, T. M. (2021). Rehabilitation intensity and patient outcomes in skilled nursing facilities in the United States: A systematic review. *Physical Therapy. 101*(3), pzaa230. https://doi.org/10.1093/ptj/pzaa230

Quan, N. G., Lohma, M. C., Resceniti, N. V., & Friedman, D. B. (2020). A systematic review of interventions for loneliness among older adults living in long-term care facilities. *Aging and Mental Health, 24*(12), 1945–1955. https://doi.org/10.1080/13607863.2019.1673311

Sadowski, C. A., Charrois, T. L., Sehn, E., Chatterly, T., & Kim, S. (2019). The role and impact of the pharmacist in long-term care settings: A systematic review. *Journal of the American Pharmacists Association, 60*(3), 516–524.e2. https://doi.org/10.1016/j.japh.2019.11.014

Santana, M. J., Manalili, K., Jolley, R. J., Zelinsky, S., Quan, H., & Mingshan, L. (2017). How to practice person-centred care: A conceptual framework. *Health Expectations, 21*(2), 429–440. https://doi.org/10.1111/hex.12640

Scales, K., Zimmerman, S., & Miller, S. J. (2018). Evidence-based nonpharmacological practices to address behavioral and psychological symptoms of dementia. *The Gerontologist, 58*(Suppl. 1), S88–S102. https://doi.org/10.1093/geront/gnx167

Scheil-Adlung, X. (2015). *Extension of Social Security: Long-term care protection for older persons: A review of coverage deficits in 46 countries.* International Labour Office, Geneva. https://www.social-protection.org/gimi/RessourcePDF.action?id=53175

Sengupta, M., Lendon, J. P., Caffrey, C., Melekin, A., & Singh, P. (2022, May 1). Post-acute and long-term care providers and service users in the United States, 2017–2018. Vital and health statistics. Series 3, analytical and epidemiological studies; no. 47. https://stacks.cdc.gov/view/cdc/115346

Stefanacci, R. G., Yeaw, J., Shah, D., Newman, D. K., Kincaid, A., & Mudd, P. N. (2022). Impact of urinary incontinence related to overactive bladder on long-term care residents and facilities: A perspective from directors of nursing. *Journal of Gerontological Nursing, 48*(7), 38–46. https://doi.org/10.3928/00989134-20220606-06

Tschanz, J. T., & Hammond, A. G. (2020). A Montessori-based approach to treat behavioral and psychological symptoms in dementia. *International Psychogeriatrics, 32*(3), 303–306. https://doi.org/10.1017/S1041610220000149

Urquiza, M., Echeverria, I, Besga, A Amasene, M. Labayen, I., Rodriguez-Larrad, A., Barroso, J., Aldamiz, M., & Irazusta, J. (2020). Determinants of participation in a post-hospitalization physical exercise program for older adults. *BMC Geriatrics, 20*, 408. https://doi.org/10.1186/s12877-020-01821-3

U.S. Department of Health & Human Services. (2020). *How much care will you need?* Administration for Community Living. https://acl.gov/ltc/basic-needs/how-much-care-will-you-need#:~:text=Here%20are%20some%20statistics%20(all,supports%20in%20their%20remaining%20years

van Voorden, G., Koopmans, R. T., Smalbrugge, M., Zuidema, S. U., van den Brink, A. M., Persoon, A., Voshaar, R. & Gerritsen, D. L. (2023). Well-being, multidisciplinary work and a skillful team: Essential elements of successful treatment in severe challenging behavior in dementia. *Aging & Mental Health*, 1–8. https://doi.org/10.1080/13607863.2023.2169248

Verweij, L., van deKorput, E, Daams, J. G., ter Riet, D., Peters, R. J., Engelbert, R. H., Scholte op Reimer, W. J. M., & Buurman, B. M. (2019). Effects of postacute multidisciplinary rehabilitation including exercise in out-of-hospital settings in the aged: Systematic review and meta-analysis. *Archives of Physical Medicine and Rehabilitation, 100*(3), 530–550. https://doi.org/10.1016/j.apmr.2018.05.010

Well-Spring Group. (2022). *Well-spring solutions.* https://www.well-spring-solutions.org/services/adult-memory-care-services

Wilkes, S. E., Boyd, P. A., Bates, S. M., Cain, D. S., & Geiger, J. R. (2019). Montessori-based activities among persons with late-stage dementia: Evaluation of mental and behavioral health outcomes. *Dementia, 18*(4), 1373–1392. https://doi.org/10.1177/1471301217703242

CHAPTER 28

Hospice and Palliative Care

Karen la Cour, MSc, PhD, OT ▪ Line Lindahl-Jacobsen, PhD, MPH ▪
Marc Sampedro Pilegaard, OT, MSc, PhD

*"We exploit the uncertainty about the end of our existence
to live as if we were not to die."*

—K.E. Løgstrup

LEARNING OUTCOMES

28-1. Articulate contemporary definitions and understandings of palliative care and hospice philosophy.
28-2. Explain the role of occupational therapy as a part of hospice and palliative care services, also in relation to interprofessional partners.
28-3. Reflect on end-of-life circumstances among older adults like general ageing, functional changes, and existential challenges such as grief and bereavement.
28-4. Critically appraise programs addressing the everyday life needs of older adults facing limited life expectancy in relation to occupational therapy.
28-5. Apply knowledge about health policy and political-societal systems as they pertain to documentation, payment, and reimbursement models in hospice and palliative care services in the United States and internationally.
28-6. Advocate for clients and palliative care services, including occupational therapy interventions and implications for collaboration and clinical practice.
28-7. Critically reflect on appropriate outcomes in palliative care.

Mini Case Study

Sarah Winford is a 75-year-old woman with lung cancer that has metastasized to her liver and brain. No treatment is available. She lives in a house in the countryside with her partner, Jim. Sarah has two sons, Peter and Poul. Peter is married and has a daughter. Poul lives by himself and has had difficulties establishing a life on his own. Sarah has always been active and has many interests; however, she is increasingly burdened by breathlessness and side effects from chemotherapy, which cause pain in her fingers and toes. Sarah worries about decline and how her sons and Jim will manage when she is no longer there. The symptoms of fatigue and pain especially impinge on her daily activities, keeping her from doing even the smallest tasks and forcing her into passivity and dependency.

Provocative Questions
1. In addition to her concerns about her partner and sons, what might be significant issues for Sarah at this point in her care?
2. How might her resources to engage in occupations best be assessed and prioritized?

Hospice and palliative care concerns the services for persons with a life-limiting illness facing the end of life. The period during which hospice and palliative care may be required can last for days, weeks, months, or years and hence does not only pertain to the terminal phases and dying. The need for hospice and palliative care continues to rise due to the growth of life expectancy and increases in noncommunicable diseases (American Occupational Therapy Association [AOTA], 2023). Older adults in particular may need end-of-life hospice and palliative care as their life expectancy is affected by aging, including decreasing abilities and deterioration, and incurable diseases. Their families may need support as they strive to deal with closure, transition, grief, and bereavement. Occupational therapists can play a significant role in hospice and palliative care for older adults with life-limiting illness facing the end of life, by addressing issues related to functioning as well as pain relief, grief, and bereavement (Cooper, 2006). Hence it is necessary to have knowledge about the challenges and needs of older adults living with life-limiting illness.

This chapter introduces definitions of hospice and palliative care conceptualizations and philosophy. It describes the roles of the occupational therapist and interprofessional partners along with possible implications for the provision of occupational therapy. Furthermore, the specific issues, including challenges and needs of older adults with life-limiting illness who may benefit from hospice and palliative care services, are presented. The chapter also describes some of the challenges of grief and bereavement related to both the person facing life-limiting illness with forthcoming death and the affected relatives. To support the understanding of occupational therapy and the collaboration with interprofessional partners in hospice and palliative care, intervention exemplars are provided. Finally, the chapter presents models for documentation, payment systems, and reimbursement in the United States and internationally along with suggestions for advocacy for clients and services.

Hospice and Palliative Care

Research shows that hospice and palliative care for older adults facing the end of life is slowly developing (Eva & Morgan, 2018). One of the reasons for the slow progress is that healthcare professionals receive limited education in palliative care. Furthermore, death and dying have not, until recently, been part of a public discourse (AOTA, 2023; Stein Duker & Sleight, 2019). However, education of occupational therapists preparing for work in hospice and palliative care is limited. A study of preparedness for palliative care among six occupational therapy schools from Australia and New Zealand found that the schools reported 2 to 10 hours of palliative care–specific education and that less than 50% of clinicians recalled undergraduate education in palliative care (Meredith, 2010). Recent studies confirm occupational therapists' lack of training in the palliative care setting (Talbot-Coulombe & Guay, 2020), with special attention to areas such as grief, bereavement, loss, and achieving a good death. Talbot-Coulombe and Guay (2020) point out a need for self-reflection, exposing students to the harsh realities of end-of-life care, and providing a safe learning environment.

Because activities of daily living (ADLs) and instrumental activities of daily living (IADLs) are considered essential occupations in **end-of-life** care, implementing educational programs would teach students to explore a client's role and their interests beyond the ADLs and IADLs. Hence, education programs focusing on occupational therapists in palliative care would raise the influence of occupation and engagement during the last stages of life regardless of what abilities the client may or may not have (Chow & Pickens, 2020).

Little attention has been paid to death and dying in old age, possibly because life-limiting illnesses such as cancer attract more economic and societal support when the individual is a younger person. Evidence shows that older adults who are dying suffer unnecessarily, in part due to insufficient assessment and undertreatment of their problems, including lack of access to home care, hospice care, palliative care, and other specialist services. In response to these problems, the World Health Organization (WHO) has emphasized the care of older adults facing the end of life through two evidence-based reports to guide policies and palliative healthcare for this group of people (WHO, 2011).

Supporting older adults with life-limiting illnesses at the end of life calls for a holistic understanding of the cycle of human life. Occupational therapists need a holistic understanding to address the occupational needs of older adults at end of life with functional challenges and to alleviate pain and mourning for the individual who is dying and their family. Thus, providing occupational therapy in contexts of interdisciplinary hospice and palliative care is a highly complex healthcare service requiring specialized education. To serve people who are dying, occupational therapists must possess competencies to enable and support clients to manage meaningful occupation—that is, what people do to occupy time and bring meaning and purpose to life (World Federation of Occupational Therapists, 2012) and preserve integrity while coping with unavoidable physical insults/decline and losses, grief, and bereavement (Fig. 28-1).

Hospice as a concept derives from the Latin word *hospitum* and means a guesthouse of rest for weary travelers (MedicineNet.com, 2021). The hospice movement was founded by Dame Cicely Saunders in the early 1960s in Great Britain, where she established the St. Christopher's Hospice near London and provided palliative care for dying patients. The hospice movement constitutes the foundation for today's end-of-life care, based on the central idea that death is part of life and that the experience of dying should be meaningful. Emphasis is placed, for example, on the idea that patients should be supported in opportunities for physical and mental activity to preserve self-control and independence as much as possible. Thus, hospice is perceived as a care system provided by an interdisciplinary team in residential facilities, such as nursing homes, private and public residences, or inpatient hospice settings. Hospice care is the most comprehensive interdisciplinary care system available to patients, families, and caregivers of persons living with a life-limiting illness.

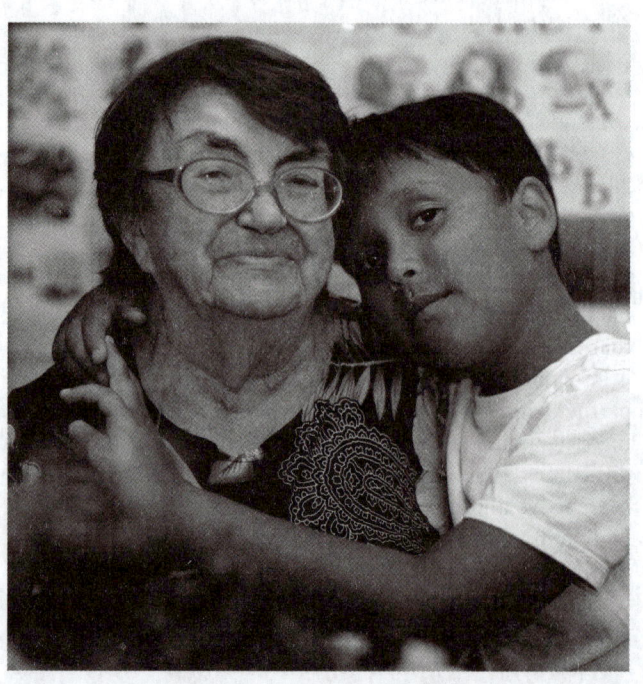

FIGURE 28-1 Occupations that promote meaning can be particularly important at the end of life. *(Danr13/iStock/Getty Images.)*

Palliative care comprises the active total care of persons with a disease unresponsive to curative treatment. Control of pain and other symptoms and support to manage physical, psychological, social, and other problems are of paramount importance. The goal of palliative care is achievement of the best quality of life for the person and their family.

According to the WHO, all patients facing the end of life are potential recipients of palliative care (Sepúlveda et al, 2002). The European Association for Palliative Care (EAPC) has proposed a definition of palliative care that complements that of the WHO and extends to the understanding of palliative care (Box 28-1). The EAPC definition specifies that palliative care is called for when curative treatment is no longer possible.

The terms "palliative" and "terminal" have been used interchangeably, and today the palliative phase is considered as a continuum starting from the time of diagnosis to the end of life and for those mourning (Fig. 28-2).

A person may receive palliative care for a variable amount of time even when death is not anticipated. For instance, an older adult with chronic obstructive pulmonary disease whose condition is not terminal may benefit from palliative care. Based on this understanding, palliative care applies not only to people in the later stages of illness but also to people in early stages and throughout their disease trajectory. Palliative care, however, becomes particularly relevant when the person's condition deteriorates and cure is no longer expected. Here, progressive deterioration and death is anticipated, and the emphasis of care moves from active treatment of the disease to comfort and control of symptoms such as pain. In such circumstances, the medical treatment that is used to treat the disease may be helpful for symptom control as part of palliative care. An example is radiotherapy, which can be used to alleviate pain (palliative treatment).

The model of total pain, described by Cicely Saunders in the early 1960s, is a central organizing concept for hospice and palliative care. It embraces the complex and multifaceted nature of pain as suffering, which can comprise physical, psychological, social, and spiritual dimensions. Total pain defines the goal of modern palliative care as relief of suffering toward the end of life using multidisciplinary approaches and technologies. Furthermore, providing palliative care requires a measure of patient compliance, including accepting the use of powerful pain-relieving medications, which are often limited in other contexts; being willing to engage in end-of-life conversations; life review; the reconciliation of troubled relationships; and the acceptance of death (Timm et al, 2021).

BOX 28-1 Definition, Aims, and Principles of Palliative Care

Definition: World Health Organization (www.who.int)

Palliative care is an approach that seeks to improve the quality of life of patients and their families who face problems associated with life-threatening illness, through the prevention and relief of suffering by means of early identification and impeccable assessment and treatment of pain and other problems, physical, psychosocial, and spiritual.

Palliative care:

- Provides relief from pain and other distressing symptoms
- Affirms life and regards dying as a normal process
- Intends neither to hasten nor postpone death
- Integrates the psychological and spiritual aspects of patient care
- Offers a support system to help patients live as actively as possible until death
- Offers a support system to help the family cope during the patient's illness and in their own bereavement
- Uses a team approach to address the needs of patients and their families, including bereavement counseling, if indicated
- Will enhance quality of life and may also positively influence the course of illness
- Is applicable early in the course of illness, in conjunction with other therapies that are intended to prolong life, such as chemotherapy or radiation therapy, and includes those investigations needed to better understand and manage distressing clinical complications

The European Association for Palliative Care (EAPC) has extended the understanding of palliative care by stating that:

"Palliative care is the active, total care of the patients whose disease is not responsive to curative treatment. Control of pain, of other symptoms, and of social, psychological and spiritual problems is paramount. Palliative care is interdisciplinary in its approach and encompasses the patient, the family and the community in its scope. In a sense, palliative care offers the most basic concept of care – that of providing for the needs of the patient wherever he or she is cared for, either at home or in the hospital. Palliative care affirms life and regards dying as a normal process; it neither hastens nor postpones death. It sets out to preserve the best possible quality of life until death." (www.eapcnet.eu)

The EAPC definition specifies that palliative care is called for when curative treatment is no longer possible. Furthermore, the EAPC emphasizes an interdisciplinary approach in the definition.

Researchers often use the terms "palliative" and "terminal" interchangeably and make fairly strict distinctions between the curative and the palliative phase. The palliative phase is instead considered as a continuum starting from the time of diagnosis (WHO, 2020b; Timm et al, 2021).

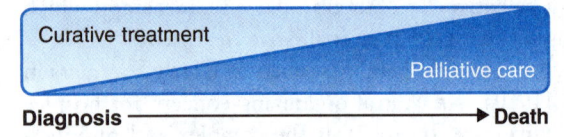

FIGURE 28-2 Previous and present understanding of palliative care.

CASE STUDY

Mrs. Spiros from Chapter 10 in the context of hospice care.

Presenting Situation
Mrs. Aleka Spiros, whom you met in Chapter 10, is now an 83-year-old woman and has been referred from a nursing facility to palliative occupational therapy at a hospice.

Occupational Profile
While completing the occupational profile before Mrs. Spiros is admitted to the hospice, the occupational therapist obtains further information. Mrs. Spiros has been living for 1 year in a nursing facility after having lived with her son and daughter-in-law, who have both been very involved throughout the disease trajectory and her continuous decline. Mrs. Spiros is from Greece and had only been in the United States for 2 years when her husband died. She speaks very little English and relies on family to communicate. Unfortunately, her son's and daughter-in-law's work schedules conflict with the ability to translate as often as needed.

Over the past year, Mrs. Spiros continued to experience pain when performing her daily activities and routines. Furthermore, she has had a noticeable weight loss and appears to be increasingly withdrawing from activity with limited engagement. Her son and daughter-in-law are quite affected and concerned by her deteriorating condition and also faced the immense challenges of pushing the nursing home for further examination.

The family reports that Mrs. Spiros often appears to be in pain when walking and changing positions (e.g., sit to stand). During the first meeting with her in the hospice facility, Mrs. Spiros demonstrates poor endurance and discomfort with movement—including reactions of possible pain and fatigue, and she needs assistance to walk and move from chair to bed and seems fearful of using her body. Mrs. Spiros and her family report she loves cooking, although she has not been participating much in cooking or any other activities since she moved from Greece. They report no concerns with cognition but state that people often think she is confused due to her language barrier.

Medical History
The review of Mrs. Spiros's medical record reveals that she has lived with peripheral vascular disease and congestive heart failure for approximately 3 years. She was referred to a skilled nursing facility after she had a fall while trying to ambulate to the bathroom in her son's home. She landed on her right side, and although she reported pain the day of the fall, there was no evidence of fracture. A recent medical examination showed that Mrs. Spiros has colon cancer that has spread to the lungs and liver. Emotionally, she is under observation for depression.

Evaluation
The occupational therapist decides to talk to Mrs. Spiros and her son and daughter-in-law and observe Mrs. Spiros performing various activities during a day in the hospice facility.

During the meeting with Mrs. Spiros and her family, the occupational therapist uses the person-centered conversation tool called the one-page profile (see Role of Occupational Therapy).

By using this tool, the occupational therapist, just like interprofessional collaborators and the family, gets an opportunity to support Mrs. Spiros's needs, which is crucial. Mrs. Spiros's one-page profile reports: (1) People find me to be helpful and social. (2) It is important for me that I can take an active part in my personal hygiene and be with my family as much as possible. (3) It is important for me that people let me try to do an activity independently, although it may take some time. I need the time to try by myself before someone offers to assist me.

The occupational therapist observes that Mrs. Spiros appears to get fatigued by walking a short distance. Likewise, she has difficulties taking a shower and putting on clothes. Furthermore, she cannot find any comfortable resting positions, and she lacks activities and opportunities for engagement within the range of what is possible for her to do.

Questions
1. Based on the presented information, what assessments would you choose to learn more about Mrs. Spiros's function?
2. What more do you need to know that would be assessed by other team members?

Answers
1. It would be important to understand factors that affect Mrs. Spiros's functioning, including how her pain influences her energy and stamina. It is also important to determine her interest and abilities in engaging in occupations of meaning. Pain scales,

such as the Wong-Baker FACES Pain Rating Scale (see Chapter 10) and the Canadian Occupational Performance Measure (COPM) are good options. (LO 28-2; Assessment section)
2. It would be important to gain nursing reports on Mrs. Spiros's functioning through the hours of the day and a physiotherapist's assessment of Mrs. Spiros's mobility. A chaplain would assess her spiritual end-of-life needs. (LO 28-2; Interprofessional partners section and Hospice and Palliative care section)

The Role of Occupational Therapy

Occupational therapists working in hospice and palliative care integrate the knowledge they have from different areas of therapy in collaboration with interprofessional partners. Palliative interventions incorporate knowledge of physical dysfunctions, psychiatry, and social functioning while maintaining the palliative focus of relief of total pain to effectively serve the needs of the person and the family.

The role of occupational therapy in palliative care delivery has evolved during the last decades. However, this evolvement varies across countries, highlighting the need for further development of occupational therapy in palliative care (Eva & Morgan, 2018). The main goal of **palliative occupational therapy** is to enable engagement in meaningful occupation despite illness or dysfunction and to maintain functions and occupational roles of daily living that the individual perceives to be important. Regarding palliative care, meaningful occupations that in particular provide relief from pain and suffering are important as the palliative focus predominates. Meaningful occupation may be related to ADLs, education, work, leisure, or social life. ADLs consist of personal ADLs (PADLs) and instrumental ADLs (IADLs). Research has shown that people with life-limiting illnesses and advanced disease experience difficulties engaging in meaningful occupations (Bendixen et al, 2014; Pilegaard et al, 2019; Wæhrens et al, 2020) and that there is an association between these difficulties and reduced quality of life (Brekke et al, 2019; Kaptain et al, 2020), highlighting the need for occupational therapy in palliative care.

Assessment

The work of the occupational therapist should be based on a thorough assessment of the person's everyday life rather than focusing on the person's diagnosis, including:

- What kinds of meaningful occupations are causing challenges (are they related to ADLs, work, education, leisure, social life)?
- What occupations does the person consider meaningful and relevant?
- What is the person's functional level (physical, psychological, social, and spiritual)?
- Which factors influence the person's ability to perform and engage in their daily occupations?
- How is the interaction with the family and what are their needs?

To clarify these factors, occupational therapists use assessment tools that are developed to provide them with the best possible knowledge of the person's activity status. This information can be used to develop goal-related interventions that can be adjusted on an ongoing basis. Occupational therapists collaborate with the person and their family and other relevant health professionals to identify goals and adjust them as necessary based on the progression of the person's illness.

Occupational therapists, like other health professionals in palliative care, may benefit from using the one-page profile. This tool is one simple sheet that focuses on what is important to the individual. The one-page profile was developed by Helen Sanderson and presents what the individual finds meaningful to them, covering the following questions: (1) What people appreciate about me; (2) What is important to me; and (3) How to support me (Helen Sanderson Associates, n.d.).

Intervention

In a European survey from 2018, the most common interventions (of European and UK occupational therapists) were provision of assistive equipment to optimize clients' independence in ADLs and assessing persons' functional capacity, positioning, postural and comfort needs, and strategies to manage occupations (Eva & Morgan, 2018). Occupational therapists also provide support and advice to carers and colleagues on resources and strategies to enable clients to manage their occupations.

A scoping review from 2019 of 74 papers dealing with occupational therapy in palliative care found the following themes: "the importance of *valued occupations* even at the end of life, an exploration of how *occupations change* over the trajectory of a terminal illness, the balance between *affirming life and preparing for death*, valued occupations might be *doing, being, becoming, or belonging* occupations and the emphasis of *a safe and supportive environment* as an essential dimension for effective palliative care" (Essential Yeh & McColl, 2019, p. 108). Together, these studies show that occupational therapy in palliative care can include a variety of interventions. In extension, the AOTA recommends that occupational therapy in palliative and hospice care addresses the areas of PADLs, IADLs, sleep/rest, leisure pursuits, and psychosocial and behavioral health (see Promoting Best Practice 28-1).

PROMOTING BEST PRACTICE 28-1
Occupational therapy in palliative and hospice care addresses these areas (AOTA, 2016, 2023).

PADLs

- *Dressing:* Use adaptive equipment, modified techniques, energy conservation principles, and proper body mechanics to minimize fatigue, overexertion, and pain (e.g., getting dressed in bed to maximize independence and safety).

- *Bathing and showering:* Use specialized or adaptive equipment to maximize safety (e.g., grab bars, shower bench) and incorporate energy-conservation principles.
- *Functional mobility:* Incorporate fall prevention strategies (e.g., remove hazards like scatter rugs, improve lighting) and foster awareness of safety issues and limitations within the environment while reinforcing confidence and capabilities. Provide optimal positioning and mobility devices to increase comfort and safety while decreasing risk for pressure sores.

IADLs

- *Meal preparation:* Incorporate energy-conservation principles and activity modifications such as using wheeled carts and reorganizing kitchen storage for easier access. Encourage a healthy diet and provide resources for nutrition management.
- *Home management:* Assess activity tolerance and body mechanics with tasks such as house cleaning or doing laundry, if appropriate. Suggest activity modifications, support systems, adaptive equipment, pacing, and energy-conservation techniques.
- *Health management:* Provide strategies on how to manage symptoms associated with fatigue, pain, anxiety, or shortness of breath during daily activities.
- *Religious or spiritual activities:* Modify activities or resources to help develop or maintain spiritual involvement, if desired (Pizzi, 2010).

Rest and Sleep

- Assess sleeping habits and the person's sleep/wake cycle and develop pre-sleep routines to facilitate longer restorative sleep periods.
- Provide relaxation techniques and positioning to increase comfort, improve ability to rest, and reduce skin breakdown from pressure.

Leisure Participation

- Identify and facilitate ways to participate in enjoyable leisure and community activities despite altered capabilities and roles through modifications and/or by exploring alternatives.
- Use relaxation techniques, coping strategies, anxiety management, time management, and activity pacing to facilitate participation in desired activities.
- Identify and facilitate ways to maintain cognitive function (e.g., memory and concentration) to participate in meaningful activities.
- Use creative and performing arts to provide a means to deal with emotional responses to living with a life-limiting disease and facilitate community engagement with end-of-life issues (Kleijberg et al, 2021; la Cour et al, 2016; Sakaguchi & Okamura, 2015).

Psychosocial/Behavioral Health

- Engage clients and their family in discussions about their feelings, fears, and anxieties. If appropriate, provide support and resources to assist in creating a client-centered, end-of-life plan and staying organized during the process (Pizzi, 2010).
- Encourage communication and family involvement to support the client's wishes and promote continued social connections (Lala & Kinsella, 2011).
- Support the role of the caregiver, including communication about realistic expectations, education on safe body mechanics and techniques during daily activities and transfers, management, and resources to decrease burnout (e.g., caregiver support group, or adult hospice day care).
- Therapeutic use of the narrative (e.g., life review, life stories, dignity therapy) may decrease depression and anxiety and promote quality of life, well-being, and a sense of meaning and purpose (Roikjær et al, 2022; Sakaguchi & Okamura, 2015; Sposato, 2016).

Using a holistic approach, occupational therapists collaborate with the palliative care team and other relevant health professionals to develop a comprehensive intervention plan that addresses the full range of problems and needs as prioritized in collaboration with the person and their family.

Evaluation of Outcomes

Occupational therapists should evaluate whether the person's goals have been achieved and whether the intervention addressed and met these goals. A person's condition can worsen rapidly, and therefore, goals often have to be short term so that they can be achieved. For example, did the intervention help the person reduce pain during particular occupations? Did the team provide appropriate support for the family? Such considerations are crucial to evaluate the effectiveness of the therapy provided and to adjust interventions as necessary. Such outcome measures typically pertain to functioning, task performance, occupational balance, and quality of life. Diaries, for example, can help occupational therapists obtain information about daily routines, which are useful for planning interventions that address the client's desired outcomes related to changes in occupational patterns and balance.

The ultimate outcome of end-of-life care is supporting or improving the person's and family's quality of life. Therefore quality-of-life measures are commonly employed as a primary outcome when testing the effectiveness of end-of-life interventions, such as palliative occupational therapy. To properly measure effects, it is pertinent to use outcome measures proximal to the given intervention, for example, ADL ability. At the same time, well-being and quality of life should not be ignored, although they can be difficult to measure.

Interprofessional Partners

As described in the beginning of this chapter, the hospice philosophy builds on holistic approaches requiring team cooperation to secure coherence and coordination of care and support. Optimally, this requires that occupational therapy is part of palliative care or at minimum that these services are delivered in close collaboration and coordination with other services. Quality of life of both client and caregivers can be improved by coordinated support (Stadelmaier et al, 2022).

Some of the challenges for collaboration with interprofessional partners may be caused by cultural barriers within systems and among healthcare professionals. Communication and coordination between partners can make cultural barriers visible and raise awareness of existing and tacit knowledge supporting possibilities for collaboration. A shared mutual understanding of care among different healthcare providers can facilitate interdisciplinary collaboration and coordination by drawing on the model of total pain. Collaboration in palliative care pertains not only to the health professions involved but equally to collaboration with clients and families. There is a growing interest among healthcare providers in involving clients in the design and planning of services to ensure specialists provide more client-centered care. Evidence is lacking, but clients reported positive outcomes (Høgsgaard, 2016; Jakobsen et al, 2021).

Specific Issues for Working With Older Adults

To understand the palliative needs for occupational therapy, it is important to understand the general palliative care needs of older adults in the last stages of life. Of deaths in high-income countries, 75% are caused by progressive advanced chronic conditions. Hence, the majority of adults in need of palliative care have chronic diseases such as cardiovascular diseases (38.5%), cancer (34%), chronic respiratory diseases (10.3%), AIDS (5.7%), and diabetes (4.6%) (WHO, 2020b). Older adults with a life-limiting illness are, in contrast to younger people, more often dealing with ongoing losses closely related to the deterioration and fragility that accompanies aging concurrent with other health conditions, comorbidity and symptoms, side effects of treatment, and problems related to body function, activity, and participation in life situations (Tang et al, 2021). Faced with progressive life-limiting illness, older adults struggle to uphold daily routines and self-defining roles (AOTA, 2023).

A report made by the Health Evidence Network for the WHO (Davies, 2004) identified unmet needs that included pain, issues for noncancer illnesses (such as heart conditions and dementia), multiple problems of aging, concerns about communication, and preferences for place of care and place of death. According to Strang and Strang (2001), palliative care problems and needs in end-of-life stages pertain to four dimensions covering physical, psychological, social, and existential areas, which are in line with the total pain model.

- *Physical dimensions* typically include control of symptoms such as pain, fatigue, and sensibility problems; problems due to functional decrease, including mobility, endurance, and body mechanics; and loss of daily routines and activities, including ADL ability, self-care, home management, and leisure.

- The most common *psychological dimensions* are issues of fear and worry, anxiety, and increased risk of depression and loss of identity and self-worth.
- *Social dimensions* pertain to, for example, loss of prior social roles and network, communication, and interaction with family members and caregivers; dealing with marginalization; and issues related to where the client can live (home/home care, hospital, nursing home, hospice, or other).
- The *existential dimension* involves life crisis and the awareness of end of life (Davies, 2004).

Problems and needs deriving from these dimensions affect quality of life in the end-of-life phase in many ways, for example, by interfering with sleep, ADLs, and social interaction. A recent cross-sectional study undertaken in Ireland and England among people with a life-limiting illness shows that clients prioritized services focusing on quality of life over services focusing on quantity of life. They valued barrier-free access to services and sufficient support for their relatives (Johnston et al, 2022).

Palliative care needs in relation to occupational therapy primarily concern levels of occupations in relation to:

- Problems and needs related to physical functioning such as pain, depression, fatigue, worry/anxiety, physical weakness, and physical inactivity (Cheville, 2001; Cheville et al, 2008; Cheville et al, 2009)
- Ability to perform and engage in meaningful occupation contributing to quality of life on a daily basis, to preserve physical and mental functions, and to maintain a sense of well-being (Lyons et al, 2002)

The needs vary widely among persons and different cultures. Older adults may wish to spend time and energy with family and friends, for example, visiting old friends or sharing memories with relatives. Some wish to prepare for death while making memory items for their loved ones, telling their personal history, or writing farewell letters. A cross-sectional study of the needs related to meaningful occupation in the home environment with 164 persons with advanced cancer showed that the problems identified primarily were within recreational activities, social activities, mobility, and domestic activities (Wæhrens et al, 2020).

Older adults with life-limiting illness prioritize maintaining a sense of control, integrity, and being connected with important others (Lala & Kinsella, 2011). In old age, as persons may lose hope for cure and prolonged life, their need and desire for meaningfulness, integrity, and dignity at the very end of life may be more important than problems related to function. For older adults in the final stages of life, there is a significant focus to connect to past, present, and future lives—not only of the life the person has been part of themselves but also the life ahead of their descendants (la Cour et al, 2005). Likewise, research has shown that older adults with life-limiting illness seek solutions to maintain meaningful occupations that contribute to joy (Bentz et al, 2022) and have a need for perspectives that brighten their moods and emotional lives (Raunkiær, 2022). Identification of needs from the perspective of the older adult and their immediate relatives in an ongoing dialogue with the health professionals is essential, as they must integrate functional dimensions of illness and functioning along with the older adult's personal meanings, coping strategies, preferences, values, motivation, and resources (Fig. 28-3).

Lindqvist and colleagues (2006) identified that for those living with conditions such as incurable cancer, bodily problems such as deterioration and impaired functionality were given meaning by patients' perceptions of living in a cyclic movement of losing and reclaiming wellness. In addition to the decline in body systems and body function, typical physical problems for older adults with life-limiting illness are pain, fatigue, nausea, and confusion along with psychological problems such as anxiety and depression. Older adults are particularly prone to experience losses that affect their capacity to carry out and engage in ADLs, social roles, and valued relationships (Wæhrens et al, 2020). Regarding the latter, it is well known that social relations are of essential importance for well-being in end of life (Fig. 28-4).

Changes in the way families live and work can leave older adults increasingly isolated and vulnerable, which in turn affects their sense of belonging within society (Davies, 2004). In addition, older adults face existential concerns because life is moving toward its end (McKechnie et al, 2007). Thus, old age and a life-limiting illness can elicit strong emotional reactions exacerbated by a discourse of death associated with fear and uncertainty.

The individual must adjust to the unpredictability of illness and fear of the future, exacerbated by increasing pain, while simultaneously struggling to maintain or regain physical strength, independence, and possibilities for meaningful occupation in the face of increasing limitations. Hence, older adults living with a life-limiting illness often commute between feelings of having control and feelings of powerlessness, between hope and fear, and between benefit and loss. In seminal research on how occupational therapists handle these apparent contradictions, Bye (1998) developed a therapeutic framework for people who are approaching end of life. The framework deals with affirming life while preparing for death. The occupational therapist handles this contradiction by rethinking processes and goals while recognizing the ambiguous orientation in life and toward death.

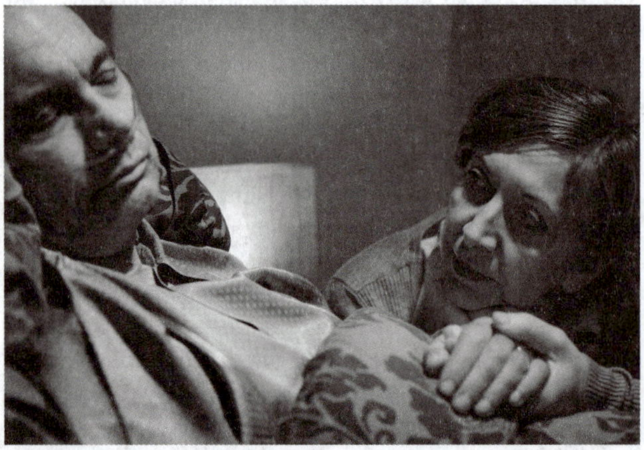

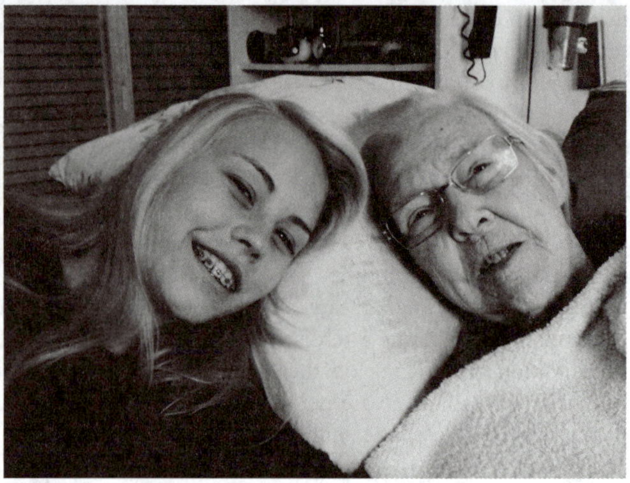

FIGURE 28-4 Family support means a great deal for older adults approaching the end of life and can form warm memories for younger individuals. *(Courtesy of Karen la Cour. Reprinted with permission.)*

FIGURE 28-3 Perspectives of the older adult and immediate relatives are important to consider. *(CandyBoxImages/iStock/Getty Images.)*

Grief and Bereavement

Grief is a common and universal reaction to a loss and can be defined as a psychological and physical reaction that may cause emotional, cognitive, behavioral, and somatic symptoms (Shear, 2015). Grief reactions after the loss of a close relative are often intense around the time of the loss, with symptoms such as longing, yearning, preoccupation with the deceased person, and sense of meaninglessness (Shear, 2015). In most individuals, the intensity of grief symptoms decreases over time as the bereaved person gradually adapts to the consequences of the loss (Shear, 2015), but grief reactions may vary in intensity and duration (Nielsen et al, 2019). Researchers Stoebe and Shut (1999) conceptualized grief and bereavement as a transactional process between loss and reestablishment without a specific goal, during which the bereaved address challenges and changes in everyday life caused by the loss.

The end of life affects both the person with life-limiting illness and the immediate family and significant others. In Western countries, women are likely to live, on average, 4 to 7 years longer than men; this means that when an older person loses a spouse or partner, more often the woman is the one left to live on (Ginter & Simko, 2013). Toward the end of life, people living with a life-limiting illness progressively deteriorate in their functional independence and ability to participate in life, often requiring increasing amounts of help and care from others in the period leading up to death.

Becoming a family caregiver of a person with life-limiting illness is a challenge. The caregiver may be confronted with the person's deterioration, loss of future plans, and uncertainties of the near future (Moon, 2016). For the family, the decline of the person can have consequences for practical matters like having to take over roles and obligations and provide more extensive support in everyday life in addition to the emotional implications, including coping with concerns, fears, and mourning for the dying process and the future. Furthermore, the disease trajectory may affect socioeconomic status, social networks, and personal resources, including quality of life (Hellbom et al, 2011; Steinvall et al, 2011). Challenges can include communication and interpersonal problems in the family, which in turn may complicate the dying trajectory (Fletcher et al, 2010; Song et al, 2011). The emotional strain caused by concerns for a partner or family member can lead to stress, depression, and psychosomatic reactions, especially when the relative is the primary support and caregiver (Ezer et al, 2011; Steinvall et al, 2011). Hence, the end-of-life phases may be a challenging time for the family. The emotional strain of living in proximity to a person with life-limiting illness can continue for extended periods, even after the loved one's death (Arnaert et al, 2010). Although hospice and palliative care services aim to meet the needs of family and relatives, many issues can influence the dying process and affect persons and their families (Arnaert et al, 2010; Ezer et al, 2011).

Along with the growing awareness of the relational consequences of end-of-life circumstances, there is an increasing need to develop ways in which occupational therapists can address relational issues, grief, and bereavement when working in hospice and palliative care to support the persons affected (Jacques & Hasselkus, 2004). Engaging in typical occupations with family members and being a part of the care process can foster a sense of normalcy that can be supported by occupational therapists (Pickens et al, 2010). For the relatives, lack of appropriate palliative care and support can be an additional burden. (See Chapter 20 – Caregiving.)

CASE STUDY (CONTINUED)

Assessments

After the meeting with the family and the observations of Mrs. Spiros, the occupational therapist plans the assessments for Mrs. Spiros to complete while her family is present to translate. Both pain and fatigue appear to be affecting her function, so it is essential to determine the location and intensity of the pain. The Wong-Baker FACES Pain Rating Scale (Wong-Baker FACES Foundation, 2020) could be useful in determining the level of pain, combined with the COPM, which the occupational therapist uses with Mrs. Spiros to measure her self-reported occupational performance and to identify the most important occupations in order to set goals as part of the occupational therapy process.

Assessment Results

Mrs. Spiros confirms that her pain is becoming significant in her lower extremities, especially with movement or when she sits for long durations. A main concern of Mrs. Spiros and her family is her decreased endurance and that she "tires so quickly." Results from the COPM interview show that showering and putting on clothes are important occupations for Mrs. Spiros. Being able to take a short walk is also important to her.

Interprofessional Communication

The occupational therapist communicates concerns regarding Mrs. Spiros's fatigue and problems taking a bath and putting on clothes during the interprofessional team meeting. Barriers to successful communication due to the language differences are also discussed, and they agree on cooperation with an interpreter. The occupational therapist collaborates with a physiotherapist to organize a treatment plan to improve Mrs. Spiros's physical function and improve her skills in walking a short distance. Finally, the team will focus on her challenges with finding resting positions.

Questions

1. How do the assessment results inform your interventions?
2. What are two or three evidence-based, occupation-centered exemplar interventions that address the case study client's priorities?
3. What assistive technologies or environmental modifications would you recommend?

Answers

1. The interventions would be guided by Mrs. Spiros's goals as set forth in the COPM and as influenced by her pain and function assessment, which will vary throughout the day. (LO 28-2; Role of Occupational Therapy section)
2. The occupational therapist would use Mrs. Spiros's meaningful occupations to integrate pain management techniques, energy conservation, and legacy activities. (LO 28-4; Intervention exemplars section)
3. Mrs. Spiros has a goal to do her own bathing as much as she is able. The occupational therapist would provide a tub-transfer slide bench and instruct the patient and care providers in the use of grab bars, tub bench, handheld shower, and wall-mounted soap dispenser (LO 28-4; Intervention exemplars section)

Intervention Exemplars

Older adults are typically characterized with multimorbidity, including advanced cancer. Worldwide, the prevalence of advanced cancer is highest among older adults. This section, therefore, presents three examples of interventions that aim to support the everyday life of people living with advanced cancer. The interventions, delivered at three different care contexts, aim to support peoples' occupations and quality of life despite living with a life-limiting illness and draw on aspects from rehabilitation and palliative care. In the following paragraphs, the three interventions are described in more detail, including how they were developed.

Hospice Day-Care Intervention

The first intervention was developed in 2013 and was a rehabilitation intervention delivered at a hospice day-care. The intervention content and structure were developed through involvement of stakeholder consultations, patient focus groups, and interviews. The day-care program was provided by an integrated multidisciplinary team and consisted of the following components:

1. Systematic assessment
2. Goal-setting
3. Review of goals
4. Care package
5. Documentation, communication, and care plans
6. Multidisciplinary clinical meetings
7. Review
8. Emergency
9. Discharge
10. Additional services

The assessment was done by senior medical and nursing staff using the National Assessment and Care Planning Framework. Based on this, goals and plans for each participant were developed in mutual collaboration between the participants and the multidisciplinary team, referred as the participant's "care package." The care package included the actual delivered interventions and were individualized and tailored to each participant's goals and needs. It could be, for instance, physical exercise and/or psychological and complementary therapies. Additional available services were also offered, such as acupuncture, art therapy, massage, relaxation group, writing therapy, nutritional therapy, and physiotherapy/hydrotherapy. During the intervention period, documentation and care plans were evaluated, and the multidisciplinary team met regularly to review the progress of each participants' goals and to discuss potential new problems arising. The medical and nursing staff also assessed the need for emergency contacts, if this was necessary during the period. Discharge was considered when outpatient specialist palliative care no longer was required. The discharge was coordinated by a nurse who, in dialog with relevant professionals in the community and a general practitioner, supported the transition from hospice to community-based palliative care. The duration of the intervention lasted about 3 months, with the possibility to extend the period. See Table 28-1 for more detailed information.

Cancer Home-Life Intervention

The second intervention was developed in 2014 and comprised an occupational therapy-based intervention delivered in the home environment (Lindahl-Jacobsen et al, 2021). The Cancer Home-Life Intervention was developed based on:

- Existing evidence of home-based intervention studies in people with cancer and other chronic illnesses
- Findings from a cross-sectional study investigating problems and needs with meaningful occupation of people with advanced cancer (Wæhrens et al, 2020)
- Occupational therapy clinical guidelines and position statements within the cancer field
- Experiences and inputs from two researchers and a panel of experts consisting of occupational therapists and people with advanced cancer (Lindahl-Jacobsen et al, 2021)

The Cancer Home-Life Intervention was provided by trained occupational therapists in the homes of people with advanced cancer (Table 28-2).

Adaptation was used as the overarching intervention approach and is a coping strategy that exists in all people. This strategy is applied when a person encounters challenges with daily life that require them to change the way they usually do things. This may include intrinsic adjustment—a process in which a person receives support to change habits and behavior to overcome challenging situations. It can also be extrinsic adjustment that encompasses changing the person's physical home environment and providing devices or tools to enhance the ability to perform occupations. The Cancer Home-Life Intervention aimed to enable meaningful occupations that the participants wanted to perform at home but had difficulties performing (e.g., engagement in leisure and ADLs). The occupational therapists and the participant collaborated to identify those occupations that were important to target in the intervention, and these occupations became the main target of the intervention. The occupational therapist provided the participants with adaptive strategies that compensated for their functional limitations and enabled them to perform their selected occupations with less difficulty. The intervention consisted of the following six components: (1) a mandatory interview to clarify problems and needs with their occupations at home; (2) prioritization of resources, energy, and tasks; (3) adaptation of occupations; (4) adaptation of posture and seating positioning; (5) provision of assistive technology; and (6) modification of the physical home environment. Component 1 was mandatory, whereas the composition of the remaining components was optional, meaning that they were tailored to each participant based on their selected meaningful occupations identified in component 1.

The participant was given instructions on and practice performing the selected adaptive strategies. The occupational therapists observed the participants while they performed their selected occupations (component 3 and component 5). In total, one to three home visits (maximum 2 hours) and one to three follow-up telephone contacts were offered. The

TABLE 28-1	Intervention Features

INTERVENTION FEATURES

Setting	Hospice
Format	Individual
Intervention period	3 months

Components

Component 1	**Assessment**	

Patients are assessed in the nurse-led clinic or medical clinic. All patients have access to the core elements of the service, which include the outpatient clinic, nurse-led clinic, the day suite, volunteer support, and relaxation groups.

Component 2 — **Goal setting**
Patients may present with aims, problems, and/or goals to be met or achieved. For some patients, these may be specific and measurable goals, for example, to walk to the bus stop. For other patients, they may be expressed as existential needs, for example, the need to feel safe. Patients may express problems or issues that they wish to address where clearly measurable goals are not appropriate or the patients may not want to engage in a goal-setting process.

Component 3 — **Review of goals**
Goals/issues/problems are reviewed with the patient at each visit to the medical or nursing clinic on an individual basis depending on the expected time it will take to achieve them.

Component 4 — **Care package**
Once goals have been agreed to, a program of services is arranged. This is referred to as the patient's "care package" and is documented on the care plan in the patient's records. Patients may only require access to the core elements of the service; however, the additional elements are offered to the patient singly or in combination on the basis of meeting their individual needs and goals.

Component 5 — **Documentation, communication, and care plans**
The assessment is recorded in the patient notes using the assessment and care planning framework documentation. A care plan is agreed to with the patient and a copy is given or sent to the patient.

Component 6 — **Multidisciplinary clinical meetings**
The clinical team meets weekly to plan and review appropriate involvement of different disciplines. At this meeting, there is case review of all new referrals and all patients who have been seen in the medical or nurse-led clinic. This meeting also provides an opportunity for individual therapists to discuss problems that have risen over the previous week.

Component 8 — **Review**
All patients have a set review date when they are seen either in the medical or nurse-led clinic. At this appointment, the clinician discusses the content, difficulties, and benefits of the care plan with the patient. The package of care is reviewed and reformulated or plans for discharge are set.

Component 9 — **Emergency**
Patients requiring emergency care are triaged by the medical or nursing staff. If appropriate, patients may be admitted to the hospice inpatient unit. If the patient has a need for acute care in hospital, then the staff will contact the patient's hospital medical team to arrange appropriate transfer.

Component 10 — **Discharge**
Discharge will be considered when outpatient specialist palliative care is no longer required. Decisions related to discharge are made with the patient and discussed in the multidisciplinary meeting.

Component 11 — **Additional services**
Physiotherapy: All patients who wish to access the gym or hydrotherapy pool are assessed by a member of the medical team before assessment by the physiotherapist. Initial assessment by the physiotherapist consists of a consultation identifying the current issues affecting physical function, and specific goals are set. The physiotherapist will develop the exercise program with the patient in this session before joining our group sessions. They are continually monitored by the physiotherapy team and gym volunteers, and programs are adapted and progressed as necessary.

Complementary therapies: Hypnotherapy may be useful in helping patients who are phobic or anxious or perhaps are experiencing sleep disturbance. Touch techniques such as aromatherapy or healing reflexology may engender a sense of well-being and reinstate the sense of touch as a pleasurable rather than invasive experience.

Psychosocial team: The psychosocial team comprises counseling staff, art therapist, chaplain, and social workers. Team members offer advocacy on a range of complex social issues, including access to care, benefits and financial problems, and legal issues—including wills, funeral arrangements, housing, and immigration. The team also offers emotional support to patients, carers, family members, and friends through sessions of varying lengths to talk through fears and anxieties, to explore emotions such as depression and low self-esteem, and to enable people to adapt to living with and surviving illness and to dying.

Table created by la Cour, Lindahl-Jakobsen, and Pilegaard.

TABLE 28-2 ■ Description of the Cancer Home-Life Intervention

INTERVENTION FEATURES	INTENSITY AND CONTENT
Setting	Participant's home
Format	Individual
Number of home visits	1–3
Intervention period	≤3 weeks
Time per visit	60–120 min
Telephone follow-up	1–3

Mandatory Component

Component 1		*Interview*
		Addressing problems with meaningful occupation, symptoms, and needs in the home environment

Optional Components

Component 2		*Prioritization of resources, energy, and occupations*
		Instructing in energy-conservation techniques, talking about time to rest during the day, and delegating activities to family members or other people, for instance, so that participants could perform and participate in their meaningful occupations
Component 3		*Adaptation of occupations*
		Instructing performance of occupations in other ways according to symptom management (e.g., by working in a seated position instead of standing, splitting tasks into actions, and reordering actions)
Component 4		*Adaptation of posture and seating positioning*
		Instructing and practicing seated positioning and ergonomics when performing occupations
Component 5		*Provision of assistive technology*
		Instructing and practicing using assistive technology when performing occupations
Component 6		*Modification of the physical home environment*
		Providing home safety and home modification

scheduling of these visits and contacts were also tailored to the participants' needs. The telephone contacts were made to support the participants' use of the selected adaptive strategies when performing their selected occupations and to resolve new problems they might face in between the home visits.

The efficacy of the Cancer Home Life-Intervention was evaluated in a full-scale randomized controlled trial (RCT). The Cancer Home-Life Intervention was delivered mostly through one home visit and one follow-up telephone call (Pilegaard et al, 2018). A process evaluation conducted alongside the RCT showed that people with advanced cancer preferred interventions that focused on their resources and contributed to enjoyment rather than interventions focusing on problems and activities they no longer could perform (la Cour et al, 2020). This indicated a need to adjust the content of the intervention to better meet the needs and preferences of people with advanced cancer.

Resource-Oriented Intervention

The third intervention example was a resource-oriented palliative rehabilitation intervention developed in 2021 for people with advanced cancer, which built on the knowledge from the Cancer Home-Life Intervention. The intervention combines rehabilitation and palliative care principles and was developed based on existing research, clinical experiences, and input from a panel of users, including people with cancer and advanced cancer and relevant healthcare professionals. The intervention aimed to support peoples' resources, enhance occupational balance, and underpin enjoyment and quality of life. The novel intervention consisted of two residential care stays with a home stay between to use the resources and tools before returning for further intervention. The person with cancer first had a 5-day stay, followed by a return home for 6 weeks with supportive contact at about 3 weeks. The person with cancer then returned for a 2-day residential care follow-up stay for intervention. The intervention was delivered by a multidisciplinary team consisting of a nurse, an occupational therapist, a physiotherapist, a medical trained artist, a mindfulness coach, and a social worker.

The resource-oriented palliative rehabilitation intervention encompassed 15 sessions provided during the 5-day stay and 2-day follow-up stay. This included workshops and engagement in physical and creative occupations. Each session had a duration of 45 to 150 minutes. Additionally, two individual conversations were offered at both stays as well as one optional session during the 2-day stay, the contents of which were determined by the participants. An optional half-way follow-up telephone contact was also offered to the participants. The intervention was primarily group-based, and all 15 sessions were mandatory. (See Table 28.3 for a resource-orientated intervention example.)

The resource-oriented palliative rehabilitation intervention is currently being evaluated in a feasibility study that will provide further knowledge that will be used to adjust the content of the intervention. The next step will be to pilot test the intervention in a community-based setting (Pilegaard et al, 2022).

Documentation, Payment Systems, and Reimbursement

It is estimated that around 40 million people worldwide are in need of palliative care each year, with 78% of them living in low- and middle-income countries. According to a WHO survey relating to noncommunicable diseases that was conducted among 194 member states in 2019, 95% of countries had a unit, branch, or department responsible for noncommunicable diseases within their ministry of health.

Funding for palliative care was available in 68% of the countries, and only 40% of the countries reported that the services reached at least half of patients in need of palliative care (WHO, 2020a).

National health systems are responsible for including palliative care for people with noncommunicable diseases and life-limiting illness, including financing national healthcare systems, strengthening and expanding human resources, and training health professionals. Early palliative care not only improves quality of life but also reduces hospitalizations and use of healthcare services. Because of the differences in healthcare systems around the world, the provision of hospice and palliative care varies among countries and within regions of each country. In many countries, for example, there is limited or no government support for palliative care. In others, however, charitable palliative care has developed and operates through non-profit organizations.

In the United States, palliative occupational therapy services may be covered under Medicare or private insurance. Charitable and religious organizations also support end-of-life care services (Hospice Foundation of America, 2022). With the Medicare hospice benefit, occupational therapy

TABLE 28-3 Description of a Resource-Oriented Intervention

INTERVENTION FEATURES				INTENSITY AND CONTENT
Setting				Residential stay
Format				Primarily group-based
Intervention provider				Multidisciplinary
Number of sessions				15 mandatory and 1 optional
Intervention period				7 days
Time per session				45 min to 2.5 hours
Telephone follow-up				1

MANDATORY SESSIONS AND FORM	DAY			TIME AND PROVIDER
Session 1 Introduction to activity, balance, and everyday life: group-based	1	This session provides an overall introduction to the intervention and the significance of occupations for people's daily life, health, and well-being. The session also provides knowledge about the importance of having appropriate occupational balance. The content consists of: • Introduction to the residential stay • Introduction to the concept of occupations (e.g., activity, health and well-being, and occupational balance)		45 min Occupational therapist
Session 2 Introduction to "Walk to get happy"— activities in nature: group-based	1	This session aims to provide the participants with knowledge about walking and physical activity as important factors to improve physical and mental health and that nature as context can increase happiness/joy and well-being. The content consists of: • Introduction to walking as an activity and the use of the nature as a source of obtaining increased energy and happiness/joy • Providing knowledge about physical activity in nature and how to prioritize this in daily life to achieve happiness/joy and well-being • Providing knowledge about how to integrate physical activity in daily life		45 min Physiotherapist

Continued

TABLE 28-3 ■ Description of a Resource-Oriented Intervention—cont'd

MANDATORY SESSIONS AND FORM	DAY		TIME AND PROVIDER
Session 3 My everyday routine and occupations: introduction to diaries: group-based	2	The session introduces the participants to diary as a method to get insight into their occupational pattern. The content consists of: ■ Introduction to diary and its usefulness ■ Discussion in pairs of their filled-out diary over 1 day of activities ■ Plenary discussion about the diaries *Material: time-geography diary method over 1-day activities*	60 min Occupational therapist
Session 4 Balancing resources, fatigue and energy—how to?: group-based, including lectures, discussions, and individual assignments	2	The session provides participants with strategies to better balance resources and energy in everyday life. They gain knowledge about: ■ Fatigue: use of breaks, occupational adaptation, and positioning ■ How to plan and prioritize activities bringing meaning and joy: introduction to energy schema and score ■ Assistive devices: guidance in application hereof *Material: energy schema and score*	60 min Nurse
Session 5 My everyday life—balance, challenges, and joys: group-based	2	The session combines the achieved knowledge from sessions 3 and 4 and provides the participants with more in-depth knowledge about ways in which to improve their occupational balance (e.g., change their occupational pattern so it includes a mix of activities regarding chores, social activities and relations, physical activities, creative activities, and general activities bringing joy). The content consists of: ■ Reflections on the participant's occupational balance—are they satisfied? ■ Using occupations to better achieve occupational balance ■ Introduction to and work with activity wheel as method to achieve activity balance *Material: The activity wheel is a circle divided around the clock illustrating which activities the participants have performed and how much time they have used on those activities. It is a visual illustration of their everyday activity balance.*	60 min Occupational therapist and nurse
Session 6 "Walk to get happy"—activities in nature: group-based	2	In this session, the participants engage in different movement and physical occupations in the form of games indoor and outdoor in the nature. The content consists of: ■ Doing physical occupations in the nature, walk and movement games ■ Doing physical occupations indoors	75 min Physiotherapist
Session 7 Life in movement: group- and individual-based	3	The session explores and starts a reflection among the participants on what contributes to a meaningful life and involves them in brainstorming ideas to implement these meaningful aspects in their daily life. The content consists of: ■ Introduction to sources of meaning ■ Individual work in which the participants choose three to five cards that symbolize important and meaningful things ■ Group discussion based on the cards ■ Ideas on how sources of meaning can be a larger part of participants' daily life *Material: Sources of Meaning Card Method*	150 min Psychologist
Session 8 Yoga: group-based	3	The session introduces the participants to yoga and breathing and relaxation exercises. The participants will obtain more knowledge about how yoga can be used to experience stress relief both physically and mentally. The content consists of: ■ Warm-up focusing on movement and breathing ■ Doing meditation and breathing exercises ■ Doing yoga exercises ■ Stress relief	90 min Physiotherapist and certify yoga instructor
Session 9 Meaningful occupation; What makes you happy?: group-based	4	The session provides knowledge of and starts a reflection among the participants about how meaningful occupations have changed during their course of life, for instance because of illness. The participants get insights into their meaningful occupations and what contributes to their joy and happiness. They will also reflect on which occupations should be part of their future daily life. The content consists of: ■ Short presentation about the meaning of occupations through phases of life ■ Participants engaging in reflective teams where they discuss and present which occupations should be part of their future narrative by using a timetable filled out before the session ■ Peer-to-peer support based on participants' narrative with new occupations *Material: timetable with the participants meaningful occupations*	60 min Occupational therapist

TABLE 28-3 ■ Description of a Resource-Oriented Intervention—cont'd

MANDATORY SESSIONS AND FORM	DAY		TIME AND PROVIDER
Session 10 Creative expression: group-based	4	This session introduces the participants to creative occupations as a means of alleviating suffering and diverting attention from illness and problems. The content consists of: ■ Doing simple mindfulness exercises in preparation for the creative activity ■ Making a collage of important aspects of their daily life	150 min Medical-trained artist and mindfulness coach
Session 11 Relaxing massage "Be good to yourself": individual-based	4	This session offers relaxing massage to provide rest, well-being, and more energy to the participants. The content consists of: ■ Relaxing massage using soft and dynamic grips	45 min Massage therapist
Session 12 Values and action plan: group-based	5	This session introduces a plan of action to implement the new strategies and meaningful occupations into the participants' daily life when returning home. They will also return to what they value and how this can be a larger part of their daily life. The content consists of: ■ Discussion of values ■ Setting goals and wishes for their daily life ■ Group discussions about the plan of action	60 min Social worker and occupational therapist
Session 13 "Developments since the previous session": group-based	6	This session follow ups on session 12 regarding how the participants have worked with and succeed with their goals and changes after the 5-day residential stay. The content consists of: ■ Group discussions about achieved goals and changes in participants' daily lives ■ How these goals and changes have affected their quality of life	60 min Social worker
Session 14 Life in movement—family, friends, and network: group- and individual-based	6	This session focuses on social relationships, particularly on belonging as an important aspect of experiencing meaning in life. The session therefore supports the participants to beware of their social network of family, friends, and other kinds of persons in their lives. The content consists of: ■ Introduction to social relationships and changes after life-threatening illness ■ Participants individually brainstorming about which persons should be in their social network and how to be closer to them in their daily lives ■ Plenum discussion of advices and actions to take to accomplish a more fruitful social network	90 min Psychologist
Session 15 Body and movement: group-based	7	In this session, the participants again engage in doing physical occupations that bring joy and happiness. The content consists of: ■ Doing physical occupations both indoors and outdoors	30–90 min Physiotherapist
Optional session	7	In this session, the content is determined by the participants.	90 min

services "may be provided for purposes of symptom control or to enable the individual to maintain activities of daily living and basic functional skills" (Centers for Medicare and Medicaid Services, 2020, Section 40.1.8).

Health policy is fundamental to developing and securing conditions of palliative care services, including support of families and caregivers (Connor & Gwyther, 2018). Despite the growing population of older people and the awareness of end-of-life challenges, studies in different countries have shown that care for dying patients is far from optimal because of lack of communication, unmitigated symptoms, inadequate pain control, unaddressed fear and spiritual needs, and patients being isolated or even left to die alone. Although occupational therapy has always been provided to the elderly population, care focused on persons with life-limiting illness has been given little attention.

Integrated care pathways, which include structured multidisciplinary care plans that detail essential steps in caring for persons with specific clinical problems, have been developed to improve care of persons who are in the last days of life (Chan et al, 2016). These care pathways aim to ensure that the most appropriate management occurs at the most appropriate time and that it is provided by the most appropriate health professionals. They can also be used to introduce clinical guidelines and systematic audits of clinical practice (Hockley et al, 2005).

In the United Kingdom, the Leadership Alliance for the Care of Dying People developed five priorities for palliative care (2014). The priorities are:

■ The possibility that a person may die within the next few days or hours should be recognized and communicated

clearly. Decisions about care should be made in accordance with the person's needs and wishes. Regular reviews and revisions should occur.
- Sensitive communication should take place at the earliest moment between staff, the dying person, and those important to them.
- Decisions regarding treatment and care should be made with the involvement of the patient and those important to them.
- People who are important to the patient should be listened to and their needs respected and addressed.
- An individual care plan, which includes food and drink, symptom control, and psychological, social and spiritual support, should be agreed, coordinated, and delivered with compassion.

These priorities put the person who is dying and their family foremost in the plan, promotes communication, and supports a multidisciplinary approach.

Another kind of policy document to ensure optimal palliative care for older adults facing end of life can be enabled through advance care planning (ACP), increasing the likelihood that person and family preferences are respected (Brown et al, 2005; Tan et al, 2013). However, the implementation of directives for ACP varies across nations and within countries (Brown et al, 2005; Malpas, 2011; Tan et al, 2013). (See Chapter 6 – Legal and Ethical Issues.)

Profession-specific policies and clinical guidelines advising palliative occupational therapy are being developed worldwide. The EAPC has defined the roles of occupational therapists, the British Pain Society has made clinical guidelines for cancer pain management supported by the Association for Palliative Medicine and the Royal College of General Practitioners, and in countries such as Denmark, clinical guidelines for occupational therapy within palliative care have been developed. The guidelines typically consist of clinical recommendations for practice based on recent research, such as concrete competencies, tasks, and education. Clinical guidelines can ensure the implementation of best practices but may also increase the risk of missing specific individual needs.

Advocacy for Clients and Service

Occupational therapists may play a vital role in hospice and palliative care by facilitating the client's occupational engagement through discernment of goals, contextual demands, and personal factors to enhance occupational performance, coping with occupational losses, and preparing for death.

Clients' perspectives are crucial when delivering optimal services like occupational therapy in hospice and palliative care. Though research regarding occupational therapy in hospice and palliative care is growing, knowledge about the persons' perspectives and experiences is required to inform the continued development of such services. Nevertheless, occupational therapy remains underused in hospice and palliative care (Chow & Pickens, 2020). A scoping review of the palliative care preferences of adults with life-limiting illnesses without possible cure found that continuing engagement in meaningful occupations is important for people receiving palliative care (von Post & Wagman, 2019). More specifically, the study identified that maintaining previous occupational patterns—feeling needed, being involved in the social environment, leaving a legacy, and living as long as you live—was of great importance to the participants (von Post & Wagman, 2019). Other studies have shown that people with life-limiting illnesses such as advanced cancer want to manage their meaningful occupations and experience enjoyment in their everyday lives (Bentz et al, 2022; Peoples et al, 2017). Furthermore, they want to prioritize spending time with their families (social activities and relations), remain mobile, and participate in community and recreative occupations to the extent possible (Peoples et al, 2017; Wæhrens et al, 2020).

The results from these studies show that occupation is of great importance to people who may need hospice and palliative care. The results also cohere with the recommendations of WHO, emphasizing that active engagement should be part of palliative care. The value of being able to perform and engage in some kind of occupation should not be underestimated; the WHO recommendations supports occupation-based palliative care services. For instance, when people are no longer able to work or conduct any of their other usual occupations, it is important to enable other possibilities for stimulating occupation for as long as people desire to engage and do something. An occupation-based approach is useful, as it includes attention to occupational needs and uses occupation as a means to address such issues.

Enabling being active is not simply about the necessity of being physically active; it also encompasses cognitive, emotional, and relational engagement. Regarding palliative care, adaptive approaches may be warranted as people with life-limiting illness are suffering from functional decline. According to Morgan and colleagues, functional decline can be based on two simplified trajectories that take place either slowly or rapidly, both trajectories representing opportunities to plan for responsive healthcare that will support clients and their relatives (Morgan et al, 2019). Although it may no longer be possible to restore functioning as it was before illness, the client may be able to maintain functioning with the use of compensatory strategies. In that regard, technology and social media could be used to enable engagement and as a means to continue being active, such as with religious practice via the internet or television (Sampedro Pilegaard et al, 2022). Being able to continue meaningful occupations and do the things a person prioritizes has been shown to affect hope, dignity, and quality of life despite life-limiting illness (Morgan et al, 2017).

Such findings call for the use of an array of occupations that require continuous adjustment and grading according to the client's needs and priorities. Occupational therapists can contribute to this by taking a highly person-centered approach with attention to what matters most for the person and by drawing on the unique skills for analyzing, using, and grading occupations as means and ends in occupation-based interventions integrated with other palliative care services.

CASE STUDY (CONTINUED)

Interventions
Based on the evaluation results and consultation with Mrs. Spiros and her family, the occupational therapist plans the intervention sessions to address Mrs. Spiros's occupational performance barriers, including fatigue, pain, and decreased endurance.

Occupation-Based Interventions
While performing the occupations, the therapist plans to implement education and training in energy conservation, breathing techniques, and general safety (e.g., taking time when changing positions) along with introduction to one or two occupations that can enable enjoyment. From the one-page profile, the occupational therapist recognizes Mrs. Spiros's social skills. This is included in the prioritization of activities, resulting in Mrs. Spiros taking a break several times during the day to be able to spend time with her family.

Meaningful Occupation
Based on the observation and the information from the COPM interview, the occupational therapist decides to address Mrs. Spiros's needs for maintaining and (if possible) improving her skills when taking a shower and putting on clothes. The occupational therapist will also collaborate with a physical therapist to work with Mrs. Spiros on taking short walks. The entire team of health professionals are informed about the intervention plan to make sure that everyone incorporates the overall plan in their approach to Mrs. Spiros.

Environmental Modification
The occupational therapist organizes a plan to maintain and increase function within the skilled nursing environment. Mrs. Spiros and the occupational therapist agree to get a bath stool to use during showering, and smaller assistive devices will be supplied to improve her dressing skills. They agree that the occupational therapist will be ready to assist Mrs. Spiros in both activities (showering and dressing) when she asks for help.

Caregiver Education Including Support to the Family
All staff interacting with Mrs. Spiros need to understand her language barrier and that she may not understand or respond to communication. The therapist organizes a list of translation services that can be used to strengthen communication when family or the interpreter is not present.

Question
1. What contextual elements from the case study's occupational therapy profile influence your treatment planning?

Answer
1. Appreciating the context of being an immigrant with a primary language other than the language spoken at the hospice would influence services, such as providing a translator, chaplaincy in her primary language, and culturally oriented interventions. The occupational therapist may have a role in advocating for the client as understood in context. (LO 28-6, 28-7; Intervention exemplar section; Advocacy section)

SUMMARY

Occupational therapy in end-of-life contexts of hospice and palliative care is a critical and complex area of practice, requiring specialized education. To best serve people who are dying and their families, occupational therapists must possess competencies to enable and support clients to engage in and find relief in meaningful occupation throughout the dying process. Best practice involves access to resources, knowledge of community services, and providing evidence-based intervention. People with life-limiting illnesses maintain a sense of purpose and participation, living while dying.

Critical Thinking Questions

1. What do you think are the most important contributions occupational therapy can provide for older adults with life-limiting illness receiving hospice or palliative care?

2. What kind of functional and existential challenges may older adults experience when facing end of life?

3. How would you decide which assessment instruments should be part of an occupational therapy intervention for older adults with life-limiting illness, and what should you be aware of?

REFERENCES

American Occupational Therapy Association. (2016). The role of occupational therapy in end-of-life care. *American Journal of Occupational Therapy, 70*(Supplement_2), 7012410075p1. https://doi.org/10.5014/ajot.2017.706s2raccreview

American Occupational Therapy Association. (2023). End-of-life care and the role of occupational therapy. *American Journal of Occupational Therapy.* https://www.aota.org/-/media/corporate/files/secure/practice/officialdocs/position/end-of-life-care-and-role-of-ot-position-statement.

American Occupational Therapy Association. (2023, in press). The role of occupational therapy in end-of-life care.

Arnaert, A., Gabos, T., Ballenas, V., & Rutledge, R. D. H. (2010). Contributions of a retreat weekend to the healing and coping of cancer patients' relatives. *Qualitative Health Research*, *20*(2), 197–208. https://doi.org/10.1177/1049732309352855

Bendixen, H. J., Ejlersen Wæhrens, E., Wilcke, J. T., & Sorensen, L. V. (2014). Self-reported quality of ADL task performance among patients with COPD exacerbations. *Scandinavian Journal of Occupational Therapy*, *21*(4), 313–320. https://doi.org/10.3109/11038128.2014.899621

Bentz, H. H., Madsen, S. H., Pilegaard, M. S., Østergaard, L. G., Brandt, Å., Offersen, S. M. H., & la Cour, K. (2022). Occupations creating joy for people living with advanced cancer: A qualitative descriptive study. *British Journal of Occupational Therapy*, *85*(3), 187–198. https://doi.org/10.1177/03080226211009419

Brekke, M. F., la Cour, K., Brandt, Å., Peoples, H., & Wæhrens, E. E. (2019). The association between ADL ability and quality of life among people with advanced cancer. *Occupational Therapy International*, *2019*, 1–10. https://doi.org/10.1155/2019/2629673

Brown, M., Grbich, C., Maddocks, I., Parker, D., Roe, P., & Willis, E. (2005). Documenting end of life decisions in residential aged care facilities in South Australia. *Australian and New Zealand Journal of Public Health*, *29*(1), 85–90. https://doi.org/10.1111/j.1467-842X.2005.tb00754.x

Bye, R. A. (1998). When clients are dying: Occupational therapists' perspectives. *Occupational Therapy Journal of Research*, *18*(1), 3–24. https://doi.org/10.1177/153944929801800101

Centers for Medicare & Medicaid Services. (2020). Coverage of Hospice Services under Hospital Insurance. In Medicare Benefit Policy Manual (rev 10437). Retrieved August 19, 2022 from: https://www.cms.gov/Regulations-and-Guidance/Guidance/Manuals/downloads/bp102c09.pdf

Chan, R. J., Webster, J., & Bowers, A. (2016). End-of-life care pathways for improving outcomes in caring for the dying. *Cochrane Database of Systematic Reviews*, Vol. 2016. https://doi.org/10.1002/14651858.CD008006.pub4

Cheville, A. (2001). Cancer rehabilitation in the new millennium rehabilitation of patients with advanced cancer. *CANCER Supplement*, *92*(4), 1039–1048. https://doi.org/10.1002/1097-0142(20010815)92:4+<1049::AID-CNCR1418>3.0.CO;2-H

Cheville, A. L., Bech, L. A., Petersen, T. L., Marks, R. S., & Gamble, G. L. (2009). The detection and treatment of cancer-related functional problems in an outpatient setting. *Supportive Care in Cancer*, *17*(1), 61–67. https://doi.org/10.1007/s00520-008-0461-x

Cheville, A. L, Troxel, A. B, Basford, J. R., & Kornblith, A. B. (2008). Prevalence and treatment patterns of physical impairments in patients with metastatic breast cancer. *Journal of Clinical Oncology*, *26*(16), 2621–2629. https://doi.org/10.1200/JCO.2007.12.3075

Chow, J. K., & Pickens, N. D. (2020). Measuring the efficacy of occupational therapy in end-of-life care: A scoping review. *American Journal of Occupational Therapy*, *74*(1), 7401205020p1–7401205020p14. https://doi.org/10.5014/ajot.2020.033340

Connor, S. R., & Gwyther, E. (2018). The Worldwide Hospice Palliative Care Alliance. *Journal of Pain and Symptom Management*, *55*(2), S112–S116. https://doi.org/10.1016/j.jpainsymman.2017.03.020

Cooper, J. (2006). *Occupational therapy in oncology and palliative care* (2nd ed.). London: Whurr.

Davies, E. (2004). What are the palliative care needs of older people and how might they be met. *WHO Regional Office for Europe*. Retrieved from http://www.euro.who.int/document/E83747.pdf

Essential Yeh, H. H., & McColl, M. A. (2019). A model for occupation-based palliative care. *Occupational Therapy in Health Care*, *33*, 108–123. https://doi.org/10.1080/07380577.2018.1544428

Eva, G., & Morgan, D. (2018). Mapping the scope of occupational therapy practice in palliative care: A European Association for Palliative Care cross-sectional survey. *Palliative Medicine*, *32*(5), 960–968. https://doi.org/10.1177/0269216318758928

Ezer, H., Chachamovich, J. L. R., & Chachamovich, E. (2011). Do men and their wives see it the same way? Congruence within couples during the first year of prostate cancer. *Psycho-Oncology*, *20*(2), 155–164. https://doi.org/10.1002/pon.1724

Fletcher, K. A., Lewis, F. M., & Haberman, M. R. (2010). Cancer-related concerns of spouses of women with breast cancer. *Psycho-Oncology*, *19*(10), 1094–1101. https://doi.org/10.1002/pon.1665

Ginter, E., & Simko, V. (2013). Women live longer than men. *Bratislavske lekarske listy*, *114*(2), 45–49. https://doi.org/10.4149/bll_2013_011

Helen Sanderson Associates. (n.d.). Retrieved April 26, 2022 from http://helensandersonassociates.co.uk/person-centred-practice/one-page-profiles/one-page-profile-templates/

Hellbom, M., Bergelt, C., Bergenmar, M., Gijsen, B., Loge, J. H., Rautalahti, M., Smaradottir, A., & Johansen, C. (2011). Cancer rehabilitation: A Nordic and European perspective. *Acta Oncologica*, *50*, 179–186. https://doi.org/10.3109/0284186X.2010.533194

Hockley, J., Dewar, B., & Watson, J. (2005). Promoting end-of-life care in nursing homes using an "integrated care pathway for the last days of life." *Journal of Research in Nursing*, *10*(2), 135–152. https://doi.org/10.1177/174498710501000209

Høgsgaard, D. M. (2016). Tværsektoriel samarbejde og kommunikation imellem sundhedsprofessionelle når ældre patienter udskrives. *RUC*, (1-10), 1–173. Retrieved from https://ruc.dk/sites/default/files/2017-03/Afhandling-Ditte-Hoegsgaard.pdf

Hospice Foundation of America. (2022, January 19). Paying for hospice care. Retrieved August 19, 2022 from: https://hospicefoundation.org/End-of-Life-Support-and-Resources/Coping-with-Terminal-Illness/Paying-for-Care

Jacques, N. D., & Hasselkus, B. R. (2004). The nature of occupation surrounding dying and death. *OTJR Occupation, Participation and Health*, *24*, 44–53. https://doi.org/10.1177/153944920402400202

Jakobsen, F. A., Ytterhus, B., & Vik, K. (2021). Adult children's experiences of family occupations following ageing parents' functional decline. *Journal of Occupational Science*, *28*(4), 525–536. https://doi.org/10.1080/14427591.2020.1818611

Johnston, B. M., Daveson, B., Normand, C., Ryan, K., Smith, M., McQuillan, R., Higginson, I., Selman, L., Tobin, K., & BuildCARE. (2022). Preferences of older people with a life-limiting illness: Evidence from a discrete choice experiment. *Journal of Pain and Symptom Management*, *64*(2), 137–145. https://doi.org/10.1016/j.jpainsymman.2022.04.180

Kaptain, R. J., Helle, T., Patomella, A. H., Weinreich, U. M., & Kottorp, A. (2020). Association between everyday technology use, activities of daily living and health-related quality of life in chronic obstructive pulmonary disease. *International Journal of COPD*, *15*, 89–98. https://doi.org/10.2147/COPD.S229630

Kleijberg, M., Hilton, R., Ahlberg, B. M., & Tishelman, C. (2021). Play elements as mechanisms in intergenerational arts activities to support community engagement with end-of-life issues. *Healthcare*, *9*, 764. https://doi.org/10.3390/healthcare9060764

la Cour, K., Gregersen Oestergaard, L., Brandt, Å., Offersen, S. M. H., Lindahl-Jacobsen, L., Cutchin, M., & Pilegaard, M. S. (2020). Process evaluation of the Cancer Home-Life Intervention: What can we learn from it for future intervention studies? *Palliative Medicine*, *34*(10), 1425–1435. https://doi.org/10.1177/0269216320939227

la Cour, K., Josephsson, S., & Luborsky, M. (2005). Creating connections of life during life-threatening illness: Creative activity experienced by elderly people and occupational therapists. *Scandinavian Journal of Occupational Therapy*, *12*(3), 98–109. https://doi.org/10.1080/11038120510030889

la Cour, K., Ledderer, L., & Hansen, H. P. (2016). Storytelling as part of cancer rehabilitation to support cancer patients and their relatives. *Journal of Psychosocial Oncology*, *34*(6), 460–476. https://doi.org/10.1080/07347332.2016.1217964

Lala, A. P., & Kinsella, E. A. (2011). Phenomenology and the study of human occupation. *Journal of Occupational Science*, *18*(3), 195–209. https://doi.org/10.1080/14427591.2011.581629

Leadership Alliance for the Care of Dying People. (2014). One chance to get it right: Improving people's experience of care in the last few days and hours of life. https://assets.publishing.service.gov.uk/government/uploads/system/uploads/attachment_data/file/323188/One_chance_to_get_it_right.pdf

Lindahl-Jacobsen, L. E., la Cour, K., Gregersen Oestergaard, L., Sampedro Pilegaard, M., Peoples, H., & Brandt, Å. (2021). The development of the 'Cancer Home-Life Intervention': An occupational therapy-based intervention programme for people with advanced cancer living at home. *Scandinavian Journal of Occupational Therapy, 28*(7), 542–552. https://doi.org/10.1080/11038128.2020.1735514

Lindqvist, O., Widmark, A., & Rasmussen, B. H. (2006). Reclaiming wellness—Living with bodily problems, as narrated by men with advanced prostate cancer. *Cancer Nursing, 29*(4), 327–337. https://doi.org/10.1097/00002820-200607000-00012

Lyons, M., Orozovic, N., Davis, J., & Newman, J. (2002). Doing-being-becoming: Occupational experiences of persons with life-threatening illnesses. *American Journal of Occupational Therapy, 56*(3), 285–295. https://doi.org/10.5014/ajot.56.3.285

Malpas, P. J. (2011). Advance directives and older people: Ethical challenges in the promotion of advance directives in New Zealand. *Journal of Medical Ethics, 37*(5), 285–289. https://doi.org/10.1136/jme.2010.039701

McKechnie, R., Macleod, R., & Keeling, S. (2007). Facing uncertainty: The lived experience of palliative care. *Palliative and Supportive Care, 5*(4), 367–376. https://doi.org/10.1017/S1478951507000569

MedicineNet.com. (2021). Medical definition of hospice care. Retrieved January 5th from: https://www.medicinenet.com/hospice_care/definition.htm

Meredith, P. J. (2010). Has undergraduate education prepared occupational therapy students for possible practice in palliative care? *Australian Occupational Therapy Journal, 57*(4), 224–232. https://doi.org/10.1111/j.1440-1630.2009.00836.x

Moon, P. J. (2016). Anticipatory grief: A mere concept? *American Journal of Hospice and Palliative Medicine, 33*(5), 417–420. https://doi.org/10.1177/1049909115574262

Morgan, D. D., Currow, D. C., Denehy, L., & Aranda, S. A. (2017). Living actively in the face of impending death: Constantly adjusting to bodily decline at the end-of-life. *BMJ Supportive and Palliative Care, 7*(2), 179–188. https://doi.org/10.1136/bmjspcare-2014-000744

Morgan, D. D., Tieman, J. J., Allingham, S. F., Ekström, M. P., Connolly, A., & Currow, D. C. (2019). The trajectory of functional decline over the last 4 months of life in a palliative care population: A prospective, consecutive cohort study. *Palliative Medicine, 33*(6), 693–703. https://doi.org/10.1177/0269216319839024

Nielsen, M. K., Carlsen, A. H., Neergaard, M. A., Bidstrup, P. E., & Guldin, M. B. (2019). Looking beyond the mean in grief trajectories: A prospective, population-based cohort study. *Social Science and Medicine, 232*, 460–469. https://doi.org/10.1016/j.socscimed.2018.10.007

Peoples, H., Brandt, Å., Wæhrens, E. E., & la Cour, K. (2017). Managing occupations in everyday life for people with advanced cancer living at home. *Scandinavian Journal of Occupational Therapy, 24*(1), 57–64. https://doi.org/10.1080/11038128.2016.1225815

Pickens N., O'Reilly, K., & Sharp, K. (2010). Family caregiving at end of life: Dimensions of occupation. *Canadian Journal of Occupational Therapy, 77*(4), 230–236. doi: 10.2182/cjot.2010.77.4.5

Pilegaard, M. S., la Cour, K., Brandt, Å., Lozano-Lazano, M., & Oestergaard, L. G. (2019). The impact of pain, dyspnea and fatigue impact on occupational performance in people with advanced cancer. *Scandinavian Journal of Occupational Therapy, 27*(7), 507–516. https://doi.org/10.1080/11038128.2019.1690042

Pilegaard, M. S., la Cour, K., Gregersen Oestergaard, L., Johnsen, A. T., Lindahl-Jacobsen, L., Højris, I., & Brandt, Å. (2018). The 'Cancer Home-Life Intervention': A randomised controlled trial evaluating the efficacy of an occupational therapy–based intervention in people with advanced cancer. *Palliative Medicine, 32*(4), 744–756. https://doi.org/10.1177/0269216317747199

Pilegaard, M. S., Timm, H., Birkemose, H. K., Dupont, S. B., Joergensen, D. S., & la Cour, K. (2022). A resource-oriented intervention addressing balance in everyday activities and quality of life in people with advanced cancer: Protocol for a feasibility study. *Pilot and Feasibility Studies, 8*(1), 86. https://doi.org/10.1186/s40814-022-01038-8

Pizzi, M. (2010). Promoting health and well-being at the end of life through client-centered care. *Scandinavian Journal of Occupatioal Therapy, 22*, 442–449. doi:10.3109/11038128.2015.1025834

Raunkiær, M. (2022). The experiences of people with advanced cancer and professionals participating in a program with focus on rehabilitation and palliative care. *Journal of Death and Dying, 302228211058307*. https://doi.org/10.1177/00302228211058307

Roikjær, S. G., Gärtner, H. S., & Timm, H. (2022). Use of narrative methods in rehabilitation and palliative care in Scandinavian countries: A scoping review. *Scandinavian Journal of Caring Sciences, 36*(2), 346–381. https://doi.org/10.1111/scs.13050

Sakaguchi, S., & Okamura, H. (2015). Effectiveness of collage activity based on a life review in elderly cancer patients: A preliminary study. *Palliative and Supportive Care, 13*, 285–293. https://doi.org/10.1017/S1478951514000194

Sampedro Pilegaard, M., La Cour, K., Baldursdottir, F., Morgan, D., Gregersen Oestergaard, L., & Brandt, Å. (2022). Assistive devices among people living at home with advanced cancer: Use, non-use and who have unmet needs for assistive devices? *European Journal of Cancer Care, 31*(4), e13572. https://doi.org/https://doi.org/10.1111/ecc.13572

Sepúlveda, C., Marlin, A., Yoshida, T., & Ullrich, A. (2002). Palliative care: The World Health Organization's global perspective. *Journal of Pain and Symptom Management, 24*(2), 91–96. https://doi.org/10.1016/S0885-3924(02)00440-2

Shear, M. K. (2015). Clinical practice: Complicated grief. *The New England Journal of Medicine, 372*(2), 153–160. https://doi.org/10.1056/NEJMcp1315618

Song, L., Northouse, L. L., Braun, T. M., Zhang, L., Cimprich, B., Ronis, D. L., & Mood, D. W. (2011). Assessing longitudinal quality of life in prostate cancer patients and their spouses: A multilevel modeling approach. *Quality of Life Research, 20*(3), 371–381. https://doi.org/10.1007/s11136-010-9753-y

Sposato, L. (2016). Occupational therapy interventions for adults at the end of life: A systematic review of dignity therapy. *Occupational Therapy in Mental Health, 32*(4), 370–391. https://doi.org/10.1080/0164212X.2016.114693

Stadelmaier, N., Assesmat, L, Paternostre, B, Bartholome, C., Duguey-Cachet, O., & Quintard, B. (2022). Supporting family members in palliative phases of cancer: A qualitative study comparing health care professionals and non-health care professionals. *Journal of Hospice and Palliative Care, 24*(2), E18–E25. doi:10.1097/NJH0000000000000827

Stein Duker, L. I., & Sleight, A. G. (2019). Occupational therapy practice in oncology care: Results from a survey. *Nursing and Health Sciences, 21*(2), 164–170. https://doi.org/10.1111/nhs.12576

Steinvall, K., Johansson, H., & Berterö, C. (2011). Balancing a changed life situation: The lived experience from next of kin to persons with inoperable lung cancer. *American Journal of Hospice and Palliative Medicine, 28*(2), 82–89. https://doi.org/10.1177/1049909110375246

Strang, S., & Strang, P. (2001). Spiritual thoughts, coping and 'sense of coherence' in brain tumour patients and their spouses. *Palliative Medicine, 15*(2), 127–134. https://doi.org/10.1191/026921601670322085

Stroebe, M., & Schut, H. (1999). The dual process model of coping with bereavement: Rationale and description. *Death studies, 23*(3), 197–224. https://doi.org/10.1080/074811899201046

Talbot-Coulombe, C., & Guay, M. (2020). Occupational therapy training on palliative and end-of-life care: Scoping review. *British Journal of Occupational Therapy, 83*(10), 609–619. https://doi.org/10.1177/0308022620926935

Tan, H., Digby, R., Bloomer, M., Wang, Y., & O'Connor, M. (2013). End-of-life care in a rehabilitation centre for older people in Australia. *Australasian Journal on Ageing, 32*(3), 184–187. https://doi.org/10.1111/j.1741-6612.2012.00654.x

Tang, L. H., Harrison, A., Skou, S. T., & Doherty, P. (2021). To what extent are comorbidity profiles associated with referral and uptake to cardiac rehabilitation. *International Journal of Cardiology, 343*, 85–91. https://doi.org/10.1016/j.ijcard.2021.09.016

Timm, H., Thuesen, J., & Clark, D. (2021). Rehabilitation and palliative care: Histories, dialectics and challenges. *Wellcome Open Research*, 6(171), 1–19. https://doi.org/10.12688/wellcomeopenres.16979.1

von Post, H., & Wagman, P. (2019). What is important to patients in palliative care? A scoping review of the patient's perspective. *Scandinavian Journal of Occupational Therapy*, 26, 1–8. https://doi.org/10.1080/11038128.2017.1378715

Wæhrens, E. E., Brandt, Å., Peoples, H., & la Cour, K. (2020). Everyday activities when living at home with advanced cancer: A cross-sectional study. *European Journal of Cancer Care*, 29(5), e13258. https://doi.org/10.1111/ecc.13258

Wong-Baker FACES Foundation. (2020). Wong-Baker FACES® Pain Rating Scale. Retrieved with permission from http://www.WongBakerFACES.org. Originally published in *Whaley & Wong's Nursing Care of Infants and Children*.

World Federation of Occupational Therapists. (2012). About occupational therapy. Retrieved May 1, 2022, from https://wfot.org/about/about-occupational-therapy

World Health Organization. (2011). Palliative care for older people: Better practices Dunhill Medical Trust. *WHO Regional Office for Europe*.

World Health Organization. (2020a). *Assessing national capacity for the prevention and control of noncommunicable diseases: Report of the 2019 global survey*. Retrieved May 1, 2022 from https://www.who.int/publications/i/item/9789240002319

World Health Organization. (2020b). Palliative care. Retrieved May 1, 2022 from https://www.who.int/news-room/fact-sheets/detail/palliative-care

CHAPTER 29

The Future of Aging

Noralyn D. Pickens, PhD, OT, FAOTA ■ Bette Bonder, PhD, OTR, FAOTA

"It's good to take a longer view and think, what would I really like to do if I had no limitations whatsoever?"

—Laurie Anderson, artist

LEARNING OUTCOMES

29-1. Articulate the current intersection of global aging demographics and healthcare needs.
29-2. Distinguish between virtual care options for occupational therapy provision.
29-3. Articulate the interprofessional role occupational therapists have in ensuring safe patient care transitions.
29-4. Develop strategies for remote monitoring of activity and occupational performance using healthcare technologies.
29-5. Assess smart home and transportation technology for occupation-centered interventions.
29-6. Describe collaborations with and educational strategies for caregivers in using meaningful technologies to support the older adult.
29-7. Describe various approaches to framing the role of occupation-centered therapy in the future of healthcare for older adults.

Mini-Case Study

Maja Wójcik, age 82, lives in a small town in Poland. She raised her three children alone and supported her family for many years as a domestic worker after her husband died at an early age. Dosia, her youngest child, moved to the United States for work and to provide financial support for her mother back home. Maja's two older children live in towns near their mother. Maja experienced a stroke at age 72 and received brief rehabilitation, but her right upper extremity remained nonfunctional, and she used a hemi-cane for walking. Dosia was able to purchase a small apartment for her mother across the street from the town's Catholic church and regularly sent money for medication and internet service. Dosia visits her mother in Poland twice a year for 2 to 3 weeks and has support from her older siblings, though they are busy with their families and jobs. Dosia often uses video conference technologies to talk with her mother while Dosia does chores or cooks. Maja often describes the ways her visits with friends, the garden she has planted and nurtured, and the knitting projects she wants to do for her grandchildren have all become more difficult (or even impossible) since her stroke. Maja remains positive in attitude and committed to her community; however, as she ages, she is not able to get out as frequently, especially in the winter months, and has been experiencing more weakness and falls. The situation came to the attention of the occupational therapist when Dosia sought care for depression stemming from the pressure of caring for her mother from a distance.

Provocative questions
1. What technology could Maja, Dosia, and her siblings use to help communicate and monitor Maja's health and wellbeing as well as Maja's ability to live independently?
2. How could an occupational therapist provide caregiving support to Dosia and her siblings?
3. How might the therapist help Maja continue or replace some of the occupations that were important to her quality of life?

Throughout this book, a variety of environmental and contextual considerations have been discussed. The focus has been on developments that alter the experience of aging and the circumstances in which occupational therapy is provided. This chapter highlights several of these factors as they may unfold in the future, with significant potential benefits and challenges for positive aging and for the role of occupational therapy in facilitating this positive experience to the greatest extent possible.

Healthcare systems and technologies are rapidly changing to address the needs of older adults. This chapter reviews global demographic shifts, including financial and living arrangements. Emerging technologies, including health and activity monitors, smart homes and transportation, and robotics, can improve quality of life for older adults. Technology will also affect family and informal caregiving in the future. There is considerable opportunity for occupational therapy in these service and technology areas. Occupational therapists, with their occupational lens and skills in activity analysis, can make significant contributions to aging in the future.

Demographic and Societal Trends

As noted throughout the text, demographic changes have had a profound effect on older adults. Worldwide, in 2019 there were 703 million people age 65 or older, with expectations of 1.5 billion older adults by 2050. There is a tripling of people living into their 80s, something not seen in such numbers in prior generations (United Nations, 2019). Addressing long-term health issues of aging is a new phenomenon globally, as only in the past 50 years have countries experienced so many people aging into their eighth, ninth, and even 10th decades (Rudnicka et al, 2020). Japan, Italy, and Finland have the greatest proportion of older adults in their populations. In Japan, the dependency ratio is 51 people over age 65 for every 100 people age 20 to 64 (United Nations, 2019). The expectation is that by 2050, this ratio will increase to 81 older adults for every 100 adults. Some countries in South and Latin America, which have not anticipated the rapid aging of their populations that they are now experiencing, are rapidly catching up to their European counterparts (United Nations, 2019).

The "simple" act of defining aging is undergoing something of a change. The social marker of age 65 being "old" (the typical understanding in many Western cultures) is no longer consistent with changing lifestyles, including longer work lives, healthier lives, and younger adult children and grandchildren because of later childbearing. Around the world, life expectancy at age 65 is increasing; in 2015, a person age 65 could expect to live an additional 17 years and by 2050, a person age 65 can expect to live an additional 19 years (United Nations, 2019). The number of younger people is growing at a slower pace, shifting the care focus from young children to older adults.

Financial and healthcare policies are often slow to adapt to these changing demographics. A concern is the availability of care, especially as provided by informal caregivers. There is also a shortage of younger workers in every field that seems likely to persist for the foreseeable future. Not only are there fewer young people, but women's roles in society continue to evolve as more women have entered the workforce. This means rethinking the traditional expectation that women will provide informal care while ensuring that healthcare professions, such as nursing and therapy (which historically were largely female), must now attract a more varied workforce. There is a call to increase the number of well-trained healthcare providers; strengthen public health measures; develop new approaches to healthcare monitoring and delivery; improve palliative, end-of-life, and long-term care services; and remediate health disparities (Fulmer et al, 2021).

Healthy Aging

The World Health Organization (WHO) has defined healthy aging as a process of maintaining functional ability to enable wellbeing in older age (Rudnicka et al, 2020). Globally there is a focus on healthy behaviors linked to an improved aging experience. Physical activity and improved diet (Lærum-Onsager et al, 2021) have made positive effects on physical health, whereas poor hydration and limited medication adherence continue to negatively affect physical and cognitive health outcomes (Edmonds et al, 2021; Mendes et al, 2019). Older adult mental and physical health is positively affected by having a sense of purpose. A sense of purpose positively affects sleep, diet, physical activity, and the use of preventative healthcare. This is a place where occupational therapy offers great potential in supporting positive aging. An increased focus on healthful behaviors among better educated older adults is counterbalanced by increasing obesity and associated diseases (e.g., diabetes) that disproportionately affect older adults in socioeconomically disadvantaged groups. Thus, occupational therapy may need to increase its focus on these disadvantaged groups.

Living Arrangements

Living arrangements in later life may be affected by particular social trends. For example, a larger number of baby boomers are unmarried and childless compared with previous generations. Given that older adults rely heavily on family for instrumental and emotional support, this may significantly affect older adults' ability to continue to live in the community. When family networks are limited, older adults often turn to neighbors and community groups for socialization. Older adults who are childless are more likely to live in poverty and have food insecurity (Valerio et al, 2021). At the same time, many baby boomers are continuing to provide care for their parents, who are surviving into very old age, and grandchildren, as the availability of paid childcare workers has diminished. In some places, the consequences of this lack of extended family are already being seen. Recent reports indicate that younger individuals in Puerto Rico are leaving the island, resulting in a lack of care for older individuals who remain there (Matos-Moreno et al, 2022). Japan is already facing issues in providing care for older individuals whose younger family members have left rural areas for more urban settings. The consequences of China's one-child policy have left many families with no one to care for parents as they age (Chen et al, 2019).

Rural, suburban, and urban-residing older adults often have different social and health needs. Providing consistent access to mental and physical health services will demand commitment from government agencies. Addressing these concerns will require thoughtful policy and development. Efforts are already underway to experiment with new multigenerational living arrangements (Kuraoka et al, 2017). As noted in Chapters 1 and 2, housing options are more plentiful yet often not affordable for many older adults.

The COVID-19 pandemic has increased a trend away from residential care, especially nursing homes, for older adults. At the same time, the pandemic reduced access and availability for those needing support in their homes (Reinhard et al, 2022). Numerous nursing homes, especially those in disadvantaged areas, were already struggling to maintain services, and the pandemic has accelerated closures in these communities (Estrada et al, 2022). Thus, the pandemic exacerbated the problem of adequate support for older adults who have been disadvantaged throughout life.

Advocating for public policies that support aging in place and resource-rich communities is crucial for occupational therapists interested in occupational justice. The COVID-19 pandemic demonstrated how important technological competence and access was for all people, especially older adults. Occupational therapists can both provide individual technology training as part of therapy provision and advocate for equitable access for the communities they serve. Read about OATS – Older Adult Technology Services in Box 29-1 for an example of how addressing a local need grew into a national program supporting older adult social, educational, and healthcare participation.

Reemergence of Ageism

Ironically, the COVID-19 pandemic has increased societal expressions of ageism at a time when the resources provided by older adults are more needed than ever (Lytle & Levy, 2022). Older adults were disproportionately affected by the illness, something that has continued during the shift in disease from pandemic to endemic. They remain more likely to have severe illness and die compared with the younger population, leading to advice that they isolate themselves more extensively than younger individuals and a sense that the pandemic was not as serious as it might have been because it was older people who were experiencing its worst effect.

There has been an increase in negative stereotypes of older individuals (Sutter et al, 2022) that has persisted into the next phase of COVID-19. This ignores the fact that many older individuals provide substantial benefits to society, benefits that are more crucial than ever as workforce shortages affect the global economy. Older adults often work for pay, volunteer, and provide childcare that might otherwise be unavailable or unaffordable. This increased ageism has negatively affected quality of healthcare, quality of life, and positive aging (Nicklett et al, 2022). Occupational therapists can make important contributions to fighting ageist stereotypes and improving access to and quality of care for older adults through direct care as well as advocacy efforts.

Climate Change and Aging

Climate change is now acknowledged as a critical concern around the world. Changes in temperature have already led to increasing numbers and intensity of storms, drought, flooding, and forest fires, among many other serious consequences. These events have led to increased mortality and morbidity, and the effects are greatest on the most vulnerable populations (Pörtner et al, 2022). Older adults are at higher risk of malnutrition, illness, and premature mortality as a result of climate change that has already occurred, and it is likely that, for the foreseeable future, the situation will worsen.

Occupational therapy interventions need to recognize and acknowledge climate change as one of the environmental factors that may influence treatment outcomes. Ensuring that clients have adequate access to food, safe living situations, and medical care will become increasingly important until such time as action from around the world moderates climate deterioration.

Aging in the Future

While factors like climate change and pandemics worsen outcomes for older individuals, there is considerable research in healthy aging and in extending the lifespan. Scientists are already able to extend the healthy lives of simple organisms and mice by targeting cellular functions that age the structures of the body. These scientists approach aging itself as a disease to be addressed rather than addressing the individual diseases that shorten life (Powell, 2019). Biotechnology firms and academic researchers are also seeking out approaches to specific diseases, such as studying how proteins, such as the growth differentiation factor 11, target cellular rejuvenation in organs to address cancer, cardiovascular diseases, and metabolic conditions (e.g., diabetes) (Ma et al, 2021; Simoni-Nieves et al, 2019). Scientists are looking to extend not just the lifespan but the "health span—the amount of time that people spend healthy and active, with a good quality of life" (Lama, 2023, para 5). For occupational therapists, and all healthcare providers, this means a reconceptualization

---

BOX 29-1 OATS – Older Adult Technology Services

Beginning with a small group of volunteers, project OATS went to senior centers and living facilities in New York City to train older adults in virtual technologies. They developed a curriculum, now in five languages, helping address access to the best technology while embracing the call for racial justice around the country. OATS addresses connectivity and access across urban and rural communities. As of 2021, OATS was established in five U. S. states, with 87 program sites. When older adults become comfortable with technology use they are empowered in everyday decision making and networking. Products from OATS include:

- Aging connected: Exposing the Hidden Connectivity Crisis for Older Adults
- Fly Like an Eagle: Measuring Transformational Social Outcomes Among Seniors Using Technology
- Patients Accessing Technology at Home (PATH) Project

Find these reports and more information at oats.org.

OATS advocates for older adult technology access by engaging older adults as advocates. Programs like OATS are excellent resources for information, training, and self-advocacy through community involvement.

of the intersection of health and age. Many conditions may not be "conditions of the old" but rather simply healthcare conditions.

CASE STUDY: Mrs. Smythe

Occupational Profile

Harriet Smythe is a 78-year-old widow who lives in a small town in Iowa. Her husband, who had been a farmer, died 12 years ago, at which point Mrs. Smythe moved from the farm into the nearby town. She was increasingly uncomfortable with driving and felt she would be closer to help if she lived in town. Mrs. Smythe is an active and enthusiastic gardener. She belongs to four book clubs (three of them online) and communicates regularly with her former coworkers. She uses Zoom and Facebook to stay in touch with her daughter and grandchildren in New York, though she wishes they were closer and worries about them. She has numerous Facebook friends.

Mrs. Smythe retired 2 years ago from her position as bookkeeper for a local business, a job she held for 30 years. She has no pension and a very modest income from social security. She also has a small income from investments made after the sale of the farm. She now lives in a compact two-story cottage that has not been updated since 1970. The town is rapidly losing population as young people move to urban areas. In addition, only one of five health clinics remains open; the three physicians there are over age 70 and talking about retiring. A hospital 100 miles away offers weekly telehealth appointments via the health clinic.

Before her bookkeeping job, she was a stay-at-home mother for her two daughters. One daughter has moved to a city in the same state, at a distance of 300 miles from her mother. She and her husband and three children visit twice per year. Mrs. Smythe used to visit them but no longer feels comfortable making the drive. The other daughter lives in New York City, where she manages a dance troupe. This daughter never married.

Identified Problem Areas

Mrs. Smythe has lost muscle mass, which makes it difficult for her to carry groceries and other moderately heavy items. She sometimes feels unsteady on her feet. She has slightly elevated blood pressure. Joint pain has begun to limit her ability to work in the garden for sustained periods. Her home environment may need modifications to support her aging in place.

Identified Strengths

Mrs. Smythe has strong family support, a friend network, leisure pursuits, and generally good physical and mental health. She describes herself as being, on the whole, satisfied with her life, though she has concerns about the potential for worsening health in the future and about the services that are available in her town.

Goals

1. Increase strength and balance to perform valued occupations, such as gardening.
2. Demonstrate safety in driving.
3. Demonstrate safe use of simple assistive technologies to help her age in place.

Intervention Plan

1. Develop a strengthening program.
2. Recommend participation in tai chi or yoga for balance and endurance.
3. Recommend a driving evaluation by a certified driving rehabilitation specialist.
4. Evaluate digital health literacy and comfort with technologies in order to provide guidance on wearable technologies to provide Mrs. Smythe with real-time feedback on her progress as well as balance during instrumental activities of daily living (IADLs) and vital signs.

Trends in Healthcare

In addition to advances in biomedicine, trends in healthcare include shifts in how care is delivered and technology. While many of these changes have been in process for years, the COVID-19 pandemic demonstrated both efficacy and importance of virtual health and therapy visits and care provision in the home.

Telehealth and Virtual Care

Virtual care is an umbrella term for remote delivery of services including synchronous and asynchronous telehealth and remote patient monitoring (Dunning & Servat, 2022). The American Medical Association (AMA) uses the term *digitally enabled care* to describe "full and hybrid virtual care models that deliver based on medical need, appropriateness, convenience, and cost" (AMA, 2021). Older adults can be served at home through teams' and specialists' remote visits, services, and monitoring. Medical services are more frequently being performed at home (e.g., dialysis, infusions, home-based diagnostics). These services are especially helpful for people who are frail and those with advanced or chronic illnesses where community travel may be challenging or put them at risk.

Occupational therapists are increasingly using telehealth services in therapy provision. In their scoping review, Ding and colleagues (2023) found that occupational therapists were engaged with older adults via telehealth in preventative care and health maintenance, caregiver education and training, assessment and intervention of the home environment, falls and mobility, as well as cognitive retraining. Therapists were also reviewing data from activity monitors to track progress and supplement their care plan decision making. Remote data collection of health information through the use of at-home devices (from activity monitors to guardrails) can inform and be used for in-time care plan modifications and allow for virtual coaching and closer management of health and lifestyle (AMA, 2021). Ding and colleagues noted that a few studies demonstrated better therapy outcomes when treatment was provided via telehealth than in traditional settings. They suggest that the home environment, caregiver support, and activity monitoring were key factors in those successes. Telehealth can be used to monitor engagement in work, leisure, and creative occupations as well as self-care. Therapists can check in with clients to ascertain their level of social engagement, their participation in formal and informal leisure activities, and issues that may arise in work or volunteer settings. The question then is not whether to do telehealth, but how to do it, reconsidering best practices in assessment, intervention, and measurement of outcomes.

Virtual care is reliant on adequate access to the internet as well as comfort and competence with technology. There are vast areas around the globe that do not have access to the required infrastructure. Therapists need to be intentional about selecting devices and products that have an accessible, client-centered user interface, and need to modify and develop content for best practices in the virtual medium. From a health inequities and occupational justice lens, occupational therapists can support clients and communities in advocating for access to virtual care.

Facilitating Transitions and Interprofessional Practices

This text presented chapters from the perspective of different kinds of institutions or settings for care—community based, short-term rehabilitation, home health, long-term care facilities, and so on—as they are structured in the United States. It has also described systems in many other countries around the world. Although many of those other countries have some form of universal healthcare payment, none has a single, seamless system for providing care. In every country, movement among institutions and into and out of the home is typical in later life. Such fragmented care presents significant difficulties ranging from poor care to inefficient use of resources (Lynn & Montgomery, 2015). These concerns may grow as economic and societal pressure lead to reductions in numbers of care facilities.

Transitions from one facility to another are periods at which patients are at particular risk (Cadogen et al, 2016; WHO, 2016). Cadogen and colleagues (2016) gave the example of the dangers inherent in the period after discharge from the emergency department for older adults who are not admitted to the hospital. They note that this is a point in care at which medical errors and adverse effects are at heightened risk, and that the potential for subsequent repetition of medical tests that generate added costs affects availability of resources.

The World Health Organization (WHO, 2016, p. 6) advocates for evidence-based interventions to improve care transitions, including:

- Standardizing documentation and agreeing on which information should be included in referral and discharge documents
- Discharge planning with agreed-upon criteria and protocols
- Improving the quality and timeliness of discharge documentation
- Implementing effective medication reconciliation practices
- Conducting timely and appropriate patient follow-ups, including telephone calls and home visits
- Improving the effectiveness and timeliness of clinical handovers between clinicians
- Establishing primary care hotlines to hospital emergency departments
- Assigning care coordinators or case managers to people with complex needs
- Increasing the involvement of primary care physicians
- Educating and supporting patients, families, and carers

Interprofessional collaboration is critical to patient transition. There is considerable literature on the importance of medication safety and communication during patient transfers from one care environment to another. In their study of the patient's transition journey over space and time, Carayon and colleagues (2020) noted the large number of people at different locations at different times, all making decisions that affect the success of the transfer. Multiple medical record systems, scheduling, and organizational and provider priorities all affect transition. Their Systems Engineering Initiative for Patient Safety (SEIPS) 3.0 model has an ecological lens in approaching the patient within different healthcare systems, home contexts, and care services. Their suggested focus on patient safety through the SEIPS 3.0 model has improved outcomes for physical, mental, and emotional health; patient and caregiver burden; quality of provider work life; safety; and health and improved provider satisfaction and organizational performance (Carayon, 2020). It is incumbent on interprofessional care providers to recognize the challenges and develop strategies such as education for family care providers, coordination of referrals, and follow-up, which will be vital if outcomes are to be improved (Cadogan et al, 2016; WHO, 2016).

Interprofessional Collaboration

Occupational therapists work with myriad professionals. Interprofessional collaboration is critical in all healthcare delivery contexts. In transitional care, there are demonstrable positive outcomes for older adults when providers and organizations facilitate teamwork, eliminate hierarchies, and create an environment supportive of shared and bidirectional learning (Junge-Maughan et al, 2021). Occupational therapists are often a part of comprehensive geriatric assessment teams. These teams work to provide patient-centered assessment and intervention plans that promote health and often support aging in place (Ivanoff et al, 2018). It is important for each profession to have a clear understanding of the different team members' roles and areas of expertise in order to provide efficient and effective care. In a study of palliative home care, Klarare and colleagues (2019) found that mature interprofessional teams were most effective when they understood each other's roles, were flexible and able to adapt, and demonstrated mutual trust.

Team Strategies and Tools to Enhance Performance and Patient Safety (TeamSTEPPS®) 2.0 is a set of communication, leadership, and teamwork skills developed to improve patient outcomes and strengthen healthcare team function. Initially developed for institutional teams, the core concepts can be applied in any setting. See Promoting Best Practice 29-1 for the Agency on Healthcare Research and Quality TeamSTEPPS® 2.0 key principles.

PROMOTING BEST PRACTICE 29-1
TeamSTEPPS® 2.0

TeamSTEPPS® 2.0 is an evidence-based framework to optimize team performance across the healthcare delivery system.
Key Principles
Team Structure: Identification of the components of a multiteam system that must work together effectively to ensure patient safety
Communication: Structured process by which information is clearly and accurately exchanged among team members
Leadership: Ability to maximize the activities of team members by ensuring that team actions are understood, changes in information are shared, and team members have the necessary resources
Situation Monitoring: Process of actively scanning and assessing situational elements to gain information or understanding, or to maintain awareness to support team functioning
Mutual Support: Ability to anticipate and support team members' needs through accurate knowledge about their responsibilities and workload
TeamSTEPPS® 2.0 training and implementation focuses on learning and using skills in communication, leadership, situation monitoring, and mutual support to create a safe environment and provide quality care. Many occupational therapy faculty members and clinicians are trained in TeamSTEPPS. Learn more about it at https://www.ahrq.gov/teamstepps/index.html, and download the TeamSTEPPS Pocket Guide app free through online app stores.

Acute Care at Home

Home-based services and technology are already shaping the future of healthcare. European countries introduced the concept of acute care at home in the late 1990s as a means to provide comfort and reduce exposure to hospital-based infections. Now a standard practice in Europe and Australia (Zolot, 2018), it is demonstrating value in other countries, especially during and after the COVID-19 pandemic. Researchers have found that older adults receiving acute services at home, compared with hospital-based acute services, have less delirium (Isaia et al, 2009), fewer hospital or emergency department visits, fewer complications from immobility (e.g., pressure sores, mobility problems) (Levine et al, 2020), reduced mortality, and high patient and caregiver satisfaction (Caplan et al, 2012).

In the United States, the Centers for Medicare and Medicaid Services (CMS) is focusing on home and community-based services as alternatives to institutional care. During the COVID-19 pandemic, CMS's Hospitals Without Walls program provided a waiver to allow hospitals to provide services to patients at ambulatory care facilities, long-term care facilities, and homes in response to the crisis of availability of acute care hospital beds. As a result of this successful action, CMS is working with a number of hospital systems to provide acute care at home to eligible patients. These patients will receive daily virtual physician visits, therapy services, and nursing care. Some services may be provided in person; however, this program differs from home healthcare skilled services in that these patients need 24-hour (remote) monitoring (CMS, 2020). For more information, see the Acute Care Delivery at Home Tip Sheet (Administration for Strategic Preparedness and Response, Technical Resources, Assistance Center, and Information Exchange, 2021; link in reference list).

Occupational therapists have an opportunity to demonstrate the value of occupation-centered interventions for home-based acute care patients. The home context provides the natural environment to assess activities of daily living (ADLs), IADLs, and leisure performance to create patient- and family centered interventions (see also Chapters 15 and 17). For patients who have progressive or short-term cognitive impairments, performing occupations such as hair care or board games in their natural environment supports confidence and success. The Occupation Centered Intervention Assessment (OCIA; Jewell et al, 2022) is a reflective assessment tool that can assist therapists in developing interventions by addressing the occupation's contextual, occupational, and personal relevance in the home environment. For more information on the OCIA see Chapter 27.

Creative Response to Staff Shortage and Funding Issues

Much of what has been discussed in this chapter so far emphasizes best practice, as should be the case in meeting professional obligations. However, at present there are significant staffing and funding concerns that make it more difficult to ensure that best practice. For several decades there have been staffing issues in healthcare, but these have worsened significantly as the pandemic has unfolded (Harms et al, 2022). The pandemic caused considerable staff stress with associated mental health issues and burnout causing many to leave their jobs through retirement or resignation. This problem is not unique to the United States, with Europe and other areas also seeing increased vacancies (Pruszyński et al, 2022).

As Harms and colleagues (2022) note, solutions will be multifaceted, and occupational therapists, along with many of their colleagues in other health professions, will need to be creative in providing care efficiently to the greatest number of clients, and in finding ways to fund vital services. Many of the most important occupational therapy interventions do not fall under traditional insurance goals (e.g., strategies to enhance quality of life through leisure occupations), so alternate payment mechanisms must be sought.

Technology in Healthcare and Social Environments

In his 2017 Slagle lecture during the centennial celebrations of occupational therapy in the United States, Smith (2017) argued that technology has had the greatest effect on the quality of life for people with disabilities. Biotechnologies, rehabilitation technologies, and assistive technologies are a part of everyday lives. They influence how people live in their homes, relate to others, receive medical care, and engage in daily occupations, and enable older adults to engage in work, leisure, creativity, and other occupations that contribute to meaning in life. Low-tech assistive technologies are often simple devices that are ubiquitous in homes, such as magnifiers, one-handed can openers, and reachers. Occupational therapists use assistive technologies in their daily practice and are increasingly using high-tech assistive technology and artificial intelligence to support decision-making.

- **Assistive technology** is an umbrella term covering the systems and services related to the delivery of assistive products and services. Assistive technology supports independence and function, enabling people to live dignified lives and have a sense of personal well-being (WHO, 2023).
- **Artificial Intelligence (AI),** composed of software systems that make decisions that require a human-level of expertise, help to anticipate problems. AI is "a wide-ranging tool that enables people to rethink how we integrate information, analyze data, and use the resulting insights to improve decision making—and already it is transforming every walk of life" (West & Allen, 2018, para 1).

AI is contributing to medical advances, including predicting health outcomes, generating solutions, and simplifying decision-making. Technology is neither dystopian (human obsolescence and security gaps) nor utopian (a fix for overworked healthcare workers and independent living). Technology is a tool or means for occupation, not the end.

This section includes a discussion of current and future ways older adults and occupational therapists will interact with technology to enable occupational participation.

Health Monitoring

Wearables, technology that people wear on their bodies, include watches and devices with accelerometers, smart fabrics used in clothing, implantable devices, electrodes, and monitors, such as for blood glucose levels. These technologies monitor vital signs, location, and body movement, including falls, and with additional apps and settings, allow direct synchronous and asynchronous communication to care teams and/or family care providers. Monitoring biometric data can be useful for medical teams needing remote monitoring. For example, a drastic change in the number of steps taken during a time frame may indicate an injury or illness, a change in symmetry of gait or widening of step width could demonstrate orthopedic instabilities, or increased dizziness that could affect a person's ability to complete activities of daily living or to engage in meaningful occupations such as gardening, woodworking, and socializing. Wearable systems reduce costs and burden of travel for short inperson visits. For people hesitant to reach out, these data allow the medical team to initiate action and provide early intervention, yielding better outcomes (Li et al, 2019).

The stigma of wearable devices has decreased as the fashion emphasis has improved, and wearing devices to monitor health and exercise habits has become ubiquitous among athletes and the general public. For acceptability, the devices need to integrate into a person's lifestyle and align with their health and communication goals (Moore et al, 2021). Occupational therapists have a role to educate their patients and clients and to advocate for the best use of wearable technologies, considering the context of use, personal choice, perceived value and ease of use, and access to healthcare technologies.

Vital signs that can be monitored by wearable technologies include:

- Respiration
- Blood pressure
- Temperature
- Activity, mobility, and falls
- Heart rate variability
- Brain electrical activity
- Muscle activity
- Galvanic skin response
- Blood glucose

Risks to clients may include costs, privacy violations and concerns about wearing electronic devices. While wearables may allow communication with medical providers and family care providers, not everyone wants to share such information. Those older adults who use wearables tend to be more confident with technology and have healthier habits (Chandrasekaran et al, 2021).

IBM's Aging in Place and Accessibility Research laboratories are working on home environment atmospheric measurements (via carbon-dioxide and carbon-monoxide levels) to determine sleep habits, movement patterns, when and where people eat, and monitor for fall prevention. In their labs they are developing systems to help keep older adults with cognitive disabilities living in their homes and in support of family caregiving (IBM, n.d.). Occupational therapists have a role in partnering with researchers and companies to provide the occupational lens to their development projects.

ADL Monitoring Through Technology

Occupational therapists may recommend the use of technologies for remote monitoring through cameras, or devices and apps with voice activated alarms for appointments and medication reminders (Camp et al, 2021). Families and practitioners can monitor ADLs to determine assistance needs through wearable accelerometers and biometric data, as well as through environmental monitoring using video or motion sensors. In addition to wearables, bed pressure sensors can monitor time in and out of bed. Door, drawer, floor, and room sensors can monitor time in different spaces to suggest time and space needs for dressing and toileting. Toileting can be further monitored through water usage, accelerometers attached to flush mechanism and smart switches for lighting (Camp et al, 2021).

Digital Health Literacy

The successful use of any personal technology is dependent on the client's comfort with technologies and their digital health literacy. As noted in prior chapters (e.g., Chapters 1 and 16), health literacy involves the competent use of electronic technologies for accessing information. Wearables, remote monitoring, and other smart technologies necessitate sharing and accessing data via the internet. As a social determinant of health, digital health literacy will become more of a factor in widespread use of these technologies across populations (Heath, 2022).

Smart Homes

In addition to ADL supports, technologies can support IADLs and home management and leisure occupations. The smart home uses apps and devices to assist with everyday life. For safety and security technology can unlock and lock doors, facilitate automatic door openers and monitor through cameras. For comfort, technologies can open window blinds, monitor room temperatures, and turn on and dim lights. People use technology to order groceries, call family, and control televisions. Smart appliances can provide cognitive supports with digital step-by-step directions for placing foods in devices and selecting the right settings and includes sensors to avoid burning. Tips for recommending these daily—and assistive technologies—include finding simple and intuitive products, using "off-the-shelf" products that have mainstream usage for support needs, and ensuring a best fit for the older adult's needs

and desires. Occupational therapists play an important role through activity analysis and helping the older adult integrate their desired technology into their habits and routines.

As seen in Chapter 15, technologies in the home can assist aging in place and support occupational participation for the older adult and their family. Occupational therapists with a strong interest in assistive technologies may consider obtaining their assistive-technology practitioner credential to demonstrate and maintain expertise. See Box 29-2 for more information.

In implementing any technological interventions in occupational therapy, it is important to consider the client's health literacy (Bryant et al, 2022). According to research reported by Bryant and colleagues, as many as 88% of individuals in the United States lack needed health literacy skills. This means that they may not understand instructions or may not grasp the value, importance, and procedures for making effective use of health information. The problem is compounded when technology is added, given that significant numbers of older adults are not comfortable with the technologies that might improve their lives (Wang et al, 2019). Thus, therapists must consider their clients' reading comprehension if written instructions are to be provided. They must also ensure that they work closely with clients to select technologies that are acceptable to the individual and that they provide careful training to ensure the clients' comfort with the devices.

BOX 29-2 Assistive Technology Resources

Smart home-made simple website and resources: https://smarthomesmadesimple.org/

- Including a self-assessment tool—what tech people might want and need

Australian Rehabilitation & Assistive Technology Association https://www.arata.org.au/

Rehabilitation Engineering and Assistive Technology Society of North America (RESNA) https://www.resna.org/ - and https://www.resna.org/AT-Standards to access standards for technologies and activity

Australia Assistive Technology resources https://at-aust.org/home/assistive_technology/assistive_technology

Canadian Assistive Technology resources https://canasstech.com/pages/resources

U.S. Assistive Technology Resource Centers https://at3center.net/state-at-programs/

Transportation

Many older adults drive, and use public transportation, on-call transportation, and ride-hailing services (as discussed in Chapter 19), and delivery services for groceries, meals, and general products. Driverless cars, also known as automated vehicles, engage AI in using sensors to detect objects and movement to make decisions to control the vehicle. These AI systems engage with already ubiquitous GPS systems for mapping routes and locations. Driverless cars are not yet in common use, but occupational therapists should monitor progress, as these vehicles have the potential to dramatically improve quality of life for older adults when they have been adequately designed and tested.

Automated vehicles will provide options for older adults and people with disabilities who are no longer able or desire to drive. Compared with other forms of transportation, automated vehicles will allow older adults to travel at any desired time, to locations of interest, and travel with friends and companions (Faber & van Lierop, 2020). Rahman and colleagues (2019) found that older adults had positive attitudes toward perceived usefulness and acceptance, including trust in the automated vehicles' abilities, and that the more familiar the vehicles became in the social environment, the more likely acceptance would increase.

Acceptance of driverless cars also needs to take into consideration the view of the older adult as pedestrian. In their same study, Rahman and colleagues (2019) found that older adults had concerns about interaction between automated vehicles and pedestrians. As with all new technologies, access may be limited for those with limited incomes and communities with less infrastructure. Vehicle features, including size, comfort, and access also need to be considered (Rahman et al, 2019). And while vehicles may transport people from one place to another, the "last 50 feet" of safe mobility to and from the vehicle and the home or building still needs to be considered.

Robotics

Robotics, first introduced in industry and manufacturing to improve efficiencies, are now a part of the healthcare delivery system. Many health facilities have robots that transport medications and specimens and act as greeters or information providers. Robots will have a range of purposes depending on the care setting.

Care Assistance and Service Robotics

Pennsylvania State University's Rehabilitation Robotics Laboratory, including occupational therapy, has developed Lil'Flo, a socially assistive robot that is intended to interact with people with simple games and assist in measuring upper extremity motor assessment through virtual care (Johnson et al, 2019). Lil'Flo is remotely activated by healthcare providers and has the potential to be of value in telehealth and rural health settings (Sobrepera et al, 2021). As of this writing, Lil'Flo is undergoing validation studies on its ability to accurately measure vital signs.

An example of a robot tailored for the home is the Labrador Retriever personal robot (labradorsystems.com). It is essentially a moving cart with upper and lower trays that carries items and, with AI, learns to move about the house to support independent activities. Students are encouraged to explore the latest in care robotics as this is a highly dynamic field.

Social Robotics

Social robots are being developed using artificial intelligence to understand and respond to human behaviors through social cues, facial and voice recognition, and movement patterns. In the future, social robots will interact with patients and family caregivers, potentially to play games, chat, and motivate to exercise (Čaić et al, 2019). Companionship pet robots are already highly used to address anxiety for people with dementia. These robot cats and dogs are relatively inexpensive and provide comfort, companionship, and have helped reduce social isolation (Koh et al, 2021). As with other forms of technology, acceptance may be related to the value of interaction and meeting the intended needs of the older adult.

It is important to note here that relatively straightforward technologies like Zoom contribute widely to engagement in meaningful occupations. While social robots may be an additional option, older adults embraced applications like Zoom and Facetime during the pandemic. Not only do these technologies allow for social interaction, but there has been a dramatic increase in other kinds of online programs that enrich life: classes, art and craft instruction, cooking classes, virtual tours, online book clubs, discussion groups, and many other applications remain popular even after the loosening of restrictions.

Caregiving in the Future

Caregiving is an occupation for older adults through caring for partners, grandchildren, friends, and possibly adult children with special needs. Older adults also are the recipients of caregiving. Family and professional caregivers provide self-care and household support, transportation, communication and cognitive supports, mental health and social supports. Chapter 20 discussed the range and need of caregiving at length. In the future, their caregivers living in different communities may continue to experience differences in supports. Research shows that rural caregivers have more financial difficulty caring for older adults, yet have better coping strategies and skills. Rural caregivers have more community and family support as part of the fabric of the community and social expectations. In comparison, urban caregivers have better access to medical care for their loved one and for themselves (Bouldin et al, 2018).

In many areas, both rural and more populated, availability of professional healthcare personnel has become a significant issue, one that is likely to worsen in coming years (Zallman et al, 2019). The COVID-19 pandemic has increased the rate at which healthcare staff have left the field, a trend that is continuing as the pandemic shifts to a more endemic pattern. Immigration policy has exacerbated the problem because many home health support personnel have historically been drawn from immigrant populations (Fig. 29-1).

The availability of technology as described above will allow older adults to remain in place longer. Family caregivers expect to use technology to manage parents and family members with functional and health needs (Egan et al, 2022). Caregiving is also a very personal and intimate occupation. Technology as monitoring is not an answer for all caregiving needs. Occupational therapists need to be mindful of the meaning that caregiving has for older adults and their loved ones. As people live longer, there will be more families and households with multiple generations—as many as five—living together. Multigenerational homes provide rich opportunities for "meaning making" while sharing and learning household responsibilities. Another housing alternative is "skipped generation" or "grand-families," where adult grandchildren share households with grandparents (Kaufman, 2022). For young people with limited first-career incomes and grandparents desiring companionship, "grand-mates" can be an answer.

Implications for Occupational Therapy

Occupational therapists are foremost problem solvers. The foundational art of activity analysis drives professionals to determine the best practices necessary for their older adult clients to engage in meaningful occupations. Throughout this chapter, ways in which occupational therapists can advocate for their clients was discussed, including supporting access to in-person and virtual care, personal fit and purposeful use of technologies, addressing health literacy, and engagement with interprofessional teams. Occupational therapists need to be curious about their clients and families, the context in which their clients live, and about the vast array of innovative interventions becoming available. Occupational therapists can promote best practice with older adults by engaging in research such as evaluating technologies and medical devices for accessibility by older adults with disabilities. Occupational therapists have made important contributions to rehabilitation engineering and biotechnology companies because of the primacy of the human occupation lens.

Occupational therapists must advocate for full participation of older adults in society. Many of the trends and issues faced by older adults and the therapists striving to support them are systemic: insurance limitations, staffing shortages, ageism, to name just some. Occupational therapists have an obligation to advocate for individuals, but they also have an obligation to advocate through social and political activism for policies and funding that support quality of life for older adults.

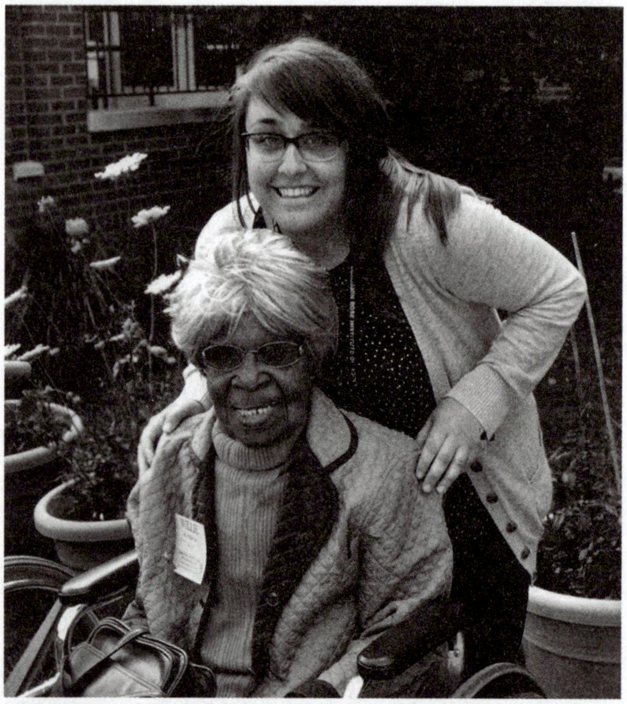

FIGURE 29-1 Availability of care providers may be an issue in the future as the proportion of the population that is older continues to increase. *(Photo courtesy of Benjamin Rose Institute, reprinted with permission.)*

CASE STUDY (CONTINUED)

Discharge Status

Mrs. Smythe actively participates in a local tai chi program with other seniors at her community senior center and performs simple yoga-like stretching activities each morning. She completed the driving evaluation, and with simple mirror adjustments and seat adaptations, she is more comfortable driving locally, though she limits her driving to daytime hours. The occupational therapist completed a home safety assessment. Mrs. Smythe and her family followed the recommendation, adding a second handrail at all stairs in and outside the home, grab bars at the bathtub, and additional lighting both in and out of the home. Mrs. Smythe is not yet sure if she wants to use a smartwatch but is considering her options.

Questions

1. What factors in Mrs. Smythe's situation reflect emerging trends in aging?
2. How could Mrs. Smythe's care plan, as determined in the above scenario, engage her daughters in her healthcare, help her age-in-place, and maintain occupations she finds most meaningful?

Answers

1. Mrs. Smythe lives in a small rural community with reduced access to regular healthcare. Her physicians are retiring with potential effect on the one remaining healthcare clinic. Telehealth services are available via a hospital. She has limited finances and no pension.

Her children live at a distance and are unable to be immediately available. (Location: Demographic and social trends; LO 29.1 and Telehealth and Virtual care; LO 29.2)

2. Should Mrs. Smythe elect to use wearable technologies, she could allow shared access to her daughters, and remote access to health providers. Smart home technologies, such as remote locking system, video doorbells, and eventually a care assist robot (such as the Labrador Retriever robot) to transport groceries, food, and leisure tools that Mrs. Smythe may need to engage in her daily occupations, would be particularly useful. Voice-activated video technologies can be used to stay in contact with family, friends, and social partners. (Location: Technology in healthcare and social environments; Caregiving in the future; LO 29.4, LO 29.5, LO 29.6)

SUMMARY

Demographic changes, including the growth of the older adult population, are driving healthcare systems to innovate models of service delivery including virtual care and acute care at home. In addition, social and healthcare technologies are rapidly growing. Assistive technology products, which were once the domain of people with rehabilitation needs, are now ubiquitous to everyday living for all people. Products that once seemed futuristic, such as automated vehicles, virtual health monitoring, and care robots, are a part of mainstream life. How people interact with technologies and how technologies become part of the habits and routines of older adults, their caregivers, and healthcare professionals are important to occupational therapists. The value of occupational therapy continues to grow. Occupational therapists were pioneers in health and assistive technology, seen as something to admire and embrace. The future promises opportunities and growth for the field of occupational therapy.

Critical Thinking Questions

1. What are ways that occupational therapists can use virtual remote monitoring for care planning?

2. How can an occupational therapist support social participation and engagement in meaningful occupation in acute care at home environments?

3. How can an occupational therapist gain expertise in finding the right technologies to support their clients' occupational participation?

REFERENCES

Administration for Strategic Preparedness and Response, Technical Resources, Assistance Center, and Information Exchange. (2021, April). *Acute care delivery at home. Tip sheet.* https://files.asprtracie.hhs.gov/documents/aspr-tracie-acute-care-delivery-at-home-tip-sheet-.pdf

Agency on Healthcare Research and Quality (n.d.) TeamSTEPPS 2.0 https://www.ahrq.gov/teamstepps/index.html

American Medical Association. (2021, May). *Return on health: Moving beyond dollars and cents in realizing the value of virtual care.* https://www.ama-assn.org/system/files/ama-return-on-health-report.pdf

Bouldin, E. D., Shaull, L., Andresen, E. M., Edwards, V. J., & McGuire, L. C. (2018). Financial and health barriers and caregiving-related difficulties among rural and urban caregivers. *The Journal of Rural Health, 34*(3), 263–274. https://doi.org/10.1111/jrh.12273

Bryant, A. M., Gee, B. M., & Gitlow, L. (2022). Health literacy and occupational therapy: A discussion on assessing and addressing limited health literacy. *The Open Journal of Occupational Therapy, 10*(4), 1–5. https://doi.org/10.15453/2168-6408.1996

Cadogan, M. P., Phillips, L. R., & Ziminski, C. E. (2016). A perfect storm: Care transitions for vulnerable older adults discharged home from the emergency department without a hospital admission. *The Gerontologist, 56*(2), 326–334. https://doi.org/10.1093/geront/gnu017

Čaić, M., Mahr, D., & Oderkerken-Schröder, G. (2019). Value of social robots in services: Social cognition perspective. *Journal of Services Marketing, 33*(4), 463–478. https://doi.org/10.1108/JSM-02-2018-0080

Camp, N., Lewis, M., Hunter, K., Johnston, J., Zecca, M., Di Nuovo, A., & Magistro, D. (2021). Technology used to recognize activities of daily living in community-dwelling older adults. *International Journal of Environmental Research and Public Health, 18*(1), 163. https://doi.org/10.3390/ijerph18010163

Caplan, G. A., Sulaiman, N. S., Mangin, D. A., Ricauda, N. A., Wilson, A. D., & Barclay, L. (2012). A meta-analysis of "hospital in the home." *Medical Journal of Australia, 197*(9), 512–519. https://doi.org/10.5694/mja12.10480

Carayon, P., Wooldridge, A., Hoonakker, P., Hundt, A. S., & Kelly, M. M. (2020). SEIPS 3.0: Human-centered design of the patient journey for patient safety. *Applied Ergonomics, 84*, 103033. https://doi.org/10.1016/j.apergo.2019.103033

Centers for Medicare and Medicaid Services. (2020, November 25). *CMS announces comprehensive strategy to enhance hospital capacity amid COVID-19 surge* [Press release]. https://www.cms.gov/newsroom/press-releases/cms-announces-comprehensive-strategy-enhance-hospital-capacity-amid-covid-19-surge

Chandrasekaran, R., Katthula, V., & Moustakas, E. (2021). Too old for technology? Use of wearable healthcare devices by older adults and their willingness to share health data with providers. *Health Informatics Journal, 27*(4). https://doi.org/10.1177/14604582211058073

Chen, R., Xu, P., Song, P., Wang, M., & He, J. (2019). China has faster pace than Japan in population aging in next 25 years. *Bioscience Trends, 13*(4), 287–291. https://doi.org/10.5582/bst.2019.01213

Ding, J., Yang, Y., Wu, X., Xiao, B., Ma, L., & Xu, Y. (2023). The telehealth program of occupational therapy among older people: An up-to-date scoping review. *Aging Clinical and Experimental Research, 35*(1), 23–40. https://doi.org/10.1007/s40520-022-02291-w

Dunning, L., & Servat, C. (2022). *Advancing tech-enabled health and home care.* Milken Institute. https://milkeninstitute.org/report/tech-enabled-health-home-care

Edmonds, C. J., Foglia, E., Booth, P., Fu, C. H. Y., & Gardner, M. (2021). Dehydration in older people: A systematic review of the effects of dehydration on health outcomes, healthcare costs and cognitive performance, *Archives of Gerontology and Geriatrics, 95*, 104380. https://doi.org/10.1016/j.archger.2021.104380

Egan, K. J., Clark, P., Deen, Z., Paputa Dutu, C., Wilson, G., McCann, L., Lennon, M., & Maguire, R. (2022). Understanding current needs and future expectations of informal caregivers for technology to support health and well-being: National survey study. *JMIR Aging, 5*(1), e15413. https://doi.org/10.2196/15413

Estrada, L. V., Levasseur, J. L., Maxim, A., Benavidez, G. A., & Pollack Porter, K. M. (2022). Structural racism, place, and COVID-19: A narrative review describing how we prepare for an endemic COVID-19 future. *Health Equity, 6*(1), 356–366. https://doi.org/10.1089/heq.2021.0190

Faber, K., & van Lierop, D. (2020). How will older adults use automated vehicles? Assessing the role of AVs in overcoming perceived mobility barriers. *Transportation Research Part A: Policy and Practice, 133*, 353–363, https://doi.org/10.1016/j.tra.2020.01.022

Fulmer, T., Reuben, D. B., Auerbach, J., Fick, D. M., Galambos, C., & Johns, K. S. (2021). Actualizing better health care for older adults. *Health Affairs 40*(2), 219–225. https://doi.org/10.1377/hlthaff.2020.01470

Harms, L., Schmidt, R. N., Dame, M., Brockman, M., & Stuart, D. (2022). Multi-faceted human capital workforce solutions and innovative staffing strategies for healthcare systems during the COVID-19 pandemic. *Journal of Business and Behavioral Sciences, 34*(1), 131–146. https://asbbs.org/files/2021-22/JBBS_34.1_Spring_2022.pdf

Heath, S. (2022, April 26). *Digital health literacy stands in the way of patient tech adoption.* Patient Engagement HIT. https://patientengagementhit.com/news/digital-health-literacy-stands-in-the-way-of-patient-tech-adoption

IBM. (n.d.). Tour the IBM "Aging in Place" environment. Retrieved October 14 2023, from https://www.ibm.com/blog/tour-the-ibm-aging-in-place-environment/

Isaia, G., Astengo, M. A., Tibaldi, V., Zanocchi, M., Bardelli, B., Obialero, R., Tizzani, A., Bo, M., Moiraghi, C., Molaschi, M., & Ricauda, N. A. (2009). Delirium in elderly home-treated patients: A prospective study with 6-month follow-up. *Age, 31*(2), 109–117. https://doi.org/10.1007/s11357-009-9086-3

Ivanoff, S. D., Duner, A., Eklunda, K., Whilhemsond, K., Lidénc, E., & Homgren E. (2018). Comprehensive geriatric assessment of frail older people: Ideals and reality. *Journal of Interprofessional Care, 32*(6), 728–734 https://doi.org/10.1080/13561820.2018.1508130

Jewell, V. L., Wienkes, T. D., & Pickens, N. (2022). *The Occupation-Centered Intervention Assessment (OCIA).* AOTA Press.

Johnson, M., Sobrepera, M. J., Kina, E., & Mendonca, R. (2019). Design of an affordable socially assistive robot for remote health and function monitoring and prognostication. *International Journal of Prognostics and Health Management, 10*(3), 1–15. https://doi.org/10.36001/ijphm.2019.v10i3.2706

Junge-Maughan, L., Moore, A., & Lipsitz, L. (2021). Key strategies for improving transitions of care collaboration: Lessons from the ECHO-care transitions program. *Journal of Interprofessional Care, 35*(4), 633–636. https://doi.org/10.1080/13561820.2020.1798900

Kaufman, J. (2022, September 30). Grand-mates: Generations sharing a special bond (and sometimes the rent). *The New York Times.* https://www.nytimes.com/2022/09/30/realestate/grandparents-grandchildren-living-together.html

Klarare, A., Hansson, J., Fossum, B., Fürst, C. J., & Lundh Hagelin, C. (2019). Team type, team maturity and team effectiveness in specialist palliative home care: An exploratory questionnaire study. *Journal of Interprofessional Care, 33*(5), 504–511. https://doi.org/10.1080/13561820.2018.1551861

Koh, W. Q., Ang, F. X. H., & Casey, D. (2021). Impacts of low-cost robotic pets for older adults and people with dementia: Scoping review. *JMIR Rehabilitation and Assistive Technologies, 8*(1), e25340. https://doi.org/10.2196/25340

Kuraoka, M., Hasebe, M., Nonaka, K., Yasunaga, M., & Fujiwara, Y. (2017). Effective community-based program for multigenerational cyclical support system. *Innovation in Aging, 1*(Suppl. 1), 1111. https://doi.org/10.1093/geroni/igx004.4069

Lærum-Onsager, E., Molin, M., Olsen, C. F., Bye, A., Debesay, J., Hillestad Hestevik, C., Bjerk, M., & Pripp, A. H. (2021). Effect of nutritional and physical exercise intervention on hospital readmission for patients aged 65 or older: A systematic review and meta-analysis of randomized controlled trials. *International Journal of Behavioral Nutrition and Physical Activity, 18*, 62. https://doi.org/10.1186/s12966-021-01123-w

Lama, D. J. (January 4, 2023). As a doctor, I see aging differently. *The New York Times.* https://www.nytimes.com/2023/01/04/opinion/anti-aging-science-longevity.html#:~:text=Knowing%20our%20patients'%20ages%20allows,grade%20its%20degree%20of%20tragedy

Levine, D. M., Ouchi, K., Blanchfield, B., Saenz, A., Burke, K., Paz, M., Diamon, K., Pu, C. T., & Schnipper, J. L. (2020). Hospital-level care at home for acutely ill adults: A randomized controlled trial. *Annals of Internal Medicine, 172*(2), 77–85. https://doi.org/10.7326/M19-0600

Li, J., Ma, Q., Chan, A. H. S., & Man, S. S. (2019). Health monitoring through wearable technologies for older adults: Smart wearables acceptance model. *Applied Ergonomics, 75*, 162–169. https://doi.org/10.1016/j.apergo.2018.10.006

Lynn, J., & Montgomery, A. (2015). Creating a comprehensive care system for frail elders in "age boom" America. *The Gerontologist, 55*(2), 278–285. https://doi.org/10.1093/geront/gnu175

Lytle, A., & Levy, S. R. (2022). Reducing ageism toward older adults and highlighting older adults as contributors during the COVID-19 pandemic. *Journal of Social Issues.* https://doi.org/10.1111/josi.12545

Ma, Y., Liu, Y., Han, F., Qiu, H., Shi, J., Huang, N., Hou, N., & Sun, X. (2021). Growth differentiation factor 11: A "rejuvenation factor" involved in regulation of age-related diseases? *Aging, 13*(8), 12258–12272. https://doi.org/10.18632/aging.202881

Matos-Moreno, A., Santos-Lozada, A. R., Mehta, N., Mendes de Leon, C. F., Lê-Scherban, F., & De Lima Friche, A. A. (2022). Migration is the driving force of rapid aging in Puerto Rico: A research brief. *Population Research and Policy Review, 41*(3), 801–810. https://doi.org/10.1007/s11113-021-09683-2

Mendes, R., Martins, S., & Fernandes, L. (2019). Adherence to medication, physical activity and diet in older adults with diabetes: Its association with cognition, anxiety and depression. *Journal of Clinical Medicine Research, 11*(8), 583–592. https://doi.org/10.14740/jocmr3894

Moore, K., O'Shea, E., Kenny, L., Barton, J., Tedesco, S., Sica, M., Crowe, C., Alamäki, A., Condell, J., Nordström, A., & Timmons, S. (2021). Older adults' experiences with using wearable devices: Qualitative systematic review and meta-synthesis. *JMIR Mhealth Uhealth, 9*(6), e23832. https://doi.org/10.2196/23832

Nicklett, E. J., Ory, M. G., Johnson, K. E., & Dwolatzky, T. (2022). COVID-19, aging, and public health. *Frontiers in Public Health, 10*, article 924591. https://doi.org/10.3389/fpubh.2022.924591

Pörtner H.-O., Roberts, D. C., Tignor, M., Poloczanska, E. S., Mintenbeck, K., Alegría, A., Craig, M., Langsdorf, S., Löschke, S., Möller, V., Okem, A., & Rama, B. (Eds.). (2022). *Climate change 2022: Impacts, adaptation, and vulnerability. Contribution of Working Group II to the sixth assessment report of the Intergovernmental Panel on Climate Change.* Cambridge University Press. https://report.ipcc.ch/ar6/wg2/IPCC_AR6_WGII_FullReport.pdf

Powell, A. (2019, March 8). Longevity and anti-aging research: "Prime-time for an impact on the globe." *Harvard Gazette.* https://news.harvard.edu/gazette/story/2019/03/anti-aging-research-prime-time-for-an-impact-on-the-globe

Pruszyński, J., Cianciara, D., Pruszyńska, I., & Włodarczyk-Pruszyńska, I. (2022). Staff shortages and inappropriate work conditions as a challenge geriatrics and contemporary healthcare service at large faces. *Journal of Education, Health and Sport, 12*(7), 136–147. https://doi.org/10.12775/JEHS.2022.12.07.014

Rahman, M. M., Shuchisnigdha, D., Strawderman, L., Burch, R., & Smith, B. (2019). How the older population perceives self-driving vehicles. *Transportation Research Part F: Traffic Psychology and Behaviour, 65*, 242–257, https://doi.org/10.1016/j.trf.2019.08.002

Reinhard, S. C., Flinn, B., & Blakeway Amero, C. (2022, April 27). COVID-19's impact on community-based long-term services and supports. *Generations, 2021.* https://generations.asaging.org/covid-19s-impact-community-based-ltss

Rudnicka, E., Napierała, P., Podfigurna, A., Męczekalski, B., Smolarczyk, R., & Grymowicz, M. (2020). The World Health Organization (WHO) approach to healthy ageing. *Maturitas, 139*, 6–11. https://doi.org/10.1016/j.maturitas.2020.05.018

Simoni-Nieves, A., Gerardo-Ramírez, M., Pedraza-Vázquez, G., Chávez-Rodríguez, L., Bucio, L., Souza, V., Miranda-Labra, R. U., Gomez-Quiroz, L. E., & Gutiérrez-Ruiz, M. C. (2019). Implications in cancer biology and metabolism. Facts and controversies. *Frontiers in Oncology, 9*, article 1039. https://doi.org/10.3389/fonc.2019.01039

Smith, R. O. (2017). Technology and occupation: Past, present, and the next 100 years of theory and practice. *American Journal of Occupational Therapy, 71*(6), 7106150010p1–7106150010p15. https://doi.org/10.5014/ajot.2017.716003

Sobrepera, M. J., Lee, V. G., & Johnson, M. J. (2021). The design of Lil'Flo, a socially assistive robot for upper extremity motor assessment and rehabilitation in the community via telepresence. *Journal of Rehabilitation and Assistive Technologies Engineering, 8*. https://doi.org/10.1177/20556683211001805

Sutter, A., Vaswani, M., Denice, P., Choi, K. H., Bouchard, J., & Esses, V. M. (2022). Ageism toward older adults during the COVID-19 pandemic: Intergenerational conflict and support. *Journal of Social Issues*. https://doi.org/10.1111/josi.12554

United Nations, Department of Economic and Social Affairs, Population Division. (2019). *World population ageing 2019: Highlights* (ST/ESA/SER.A/430). https://digitallibrary.un.org/record/3846855/files/WorldPopulationAgeing2019-Highlights.pdf

Valerio, T., Knop, B., Kreider, R. M., & He, W. (2021). *Childless older Americans: 2018.* Current Population Reports, 70-173. U.S. Census Bureau & National Institute on Aging. https://upload.wikimedia.org/wikipedia/commons/d/d0/Childless_Older_Americans_2018_P70-173.pdf

Wang, S., Bolling, K., Mao, W., Reichstadt, J., Jeste, D., Kim, H. C., & Nebeker, C. (2019). Technology to support aging in place: Older adults' perspectives. *Healthcare, 7*(2), 60. https://doi.org/10.3390/healthcare7020060

West, D. M., & Allen, J. R. (2018, April 24). *How artificial intelligence is transforming the world*. Brookings Institute Center for Technology Innovation. https://www.brookings.edu/research/how-artificial-intelligence-is-transforming-the-world

World Health Organization. (2016). *Transitions of care: Technical series on safer primary care.* https://apps.who.int/iris/bitstream/handle/10665/252272/9789241511599-eng.pdf

World Health Organization. (2023, May 15). *Assistive technology.* https://www.who.int/news-room/fact-sheets/detail/assistive-technology

Zallman, L, Finnegan, K. E., Himmelstein, D. U., Touw, S., & Woolhandler, S. (2019, June). Care for American's elderly and disabled people relies on immigrant labor. *Health Affairs, 38*(6), 919–926. https://doi.org/10.1377/hlthaff.2018.05514

Zolot, J. (2018). At-home hospital care reduces readmissions and length of stay, enhances patient satisfaction. *American Journal of Nursing, 118*(10), 13. https://doi.org/10.1097/01.NAJ.0000546363.97759.db

APPENDIX A

Answers to Critical Thinking Questions

Chapter authors have provided answers to the critical thinking questions in each chapter, along with locations of where to find the answers in the chapter, and the related chapter learning objective (LO). Many of these questions have additional answers that could be generated from class discussion, or other in-class learning activities such as evidence searches.

Chapter 1

1. A healthcare provider's negative expectations of performance and limited patience in ensuring the older adult is fully informed could lead to inability of the older adult to act on information they were given, leading to a downward spiral of poor health decisions, health, and well-being.
   (LO 1-2; LO 1-4; Subsections on Health Literacy and Attitudes)
2. Age-friendly environments: Address neighborhood safety at a community and population level; provide home safety assessment and affordable technologies.
3. Combatting ageism: Advocate for services for older adults in their care setting.
4. Integrated care: Maintain excellence in skills and best practices to provide effective therapy.
5. Long-term care: Ensure clients receive the full continuum of care through the end of life by providing occupation-centered, relevant therapy.
   (LO 1-6; Social and Occupational Justice section; subheader – UN Decade of Healthy Aging)

Chapter 2

1. The therapist would complete an occupational profile and assess the new resident's occupational history and desire for continuity in meaningful occupations. (Occupation and Home section, LO 2-7)
2. Spirituality and religion encourage both a feeling of connection and a sense of the presence of something greater than the self. A wide array of occupations reflect spirituality and support these occupations. Attending religious services, observing religious customs at home, and community with nature are examples of such occupations. (Spirituality and Religion as Contributors to Existential Meaning, LO 2-4)
3. Ability to complete self-care can contribute to perceived self-efficacy and independence. For some, these may be highly valued outcomes. Others, however, might find such activities to be routine and not particularly fulfilling. These individuals might prefer to get help with such activities and save their energy for other activities that matter more to them. (Themes of Meaning, LO 2-3)
4. As an example, holding a job for pay involves *doing* of the job content, which can satisfy the need to accomplish something useful. It involves *being* in providing a role or title that can support self-identity. It can involve *becoming*, as it allows for new challenges and increasing competence. It supports *belonging* in allowing the worker to feel like part of the team. (Occupation, Cooccupation, and Meaning section, LO 2-2)

Chapter 3

1. Numerous theories in this chapter, such as the Situational Model of Care, implement comprehensive approaches to understanding the aging process. Ideally, those that include biological/person, environmental, social, and occupational elements are most appropriate for guiding occupational therapy practice. (LO 3-1)
2. Theories provide a frame of reference or a way to guide thinking of the therapist. Many times, therapists use a combination of theories to develop client-centered care plans. An understanding of a variety of theories enables occupational therapists to have breadth and depth when selecting the most appropriate evidence-based interventions and goal planning for older adults. (LO 3-6)

Chapter 4

1. Practitioners can integrate an older adult client's culture into intervention by first taking the time to get to know the client and the client's culture. See Defining Culture to understand what culture is. Refer to Promoting Best Practice Box 4-1 for suggestions on conversation starters. Defer to the client as the expert on their culture and identity (see Clinical Implications: Using Cultural Humility to Promote Participation and Health Outcomes). Consider the unique experience of the client's intersecting spheres of their life. Be sensitive to how ageism and power imbalances may limit their participation (see Effect of Cultural Perceptions of Aging on Participation). Based on the

client's culture, think about what may be of value and interest to them. Brainstorm together on what the client would like to focus on in treatment. (LO 4-1, 4-2, 4-3, 4-5, 4-6)
2. In this chapter, Tamika considered the context of her hospice team and then worked to get buy-in by presenting the goals and the reasons behind the art lesson book during her team meeting. She focused on a common goal of providing client-centered care for Sam at the end of life and invited the team to be involved. Similarly, when providing interventions that are unique to any practice setting, consider first the context of care. What is the culture of the context and the common goals that could connect the intervention to the setting? Are there environmental systems that pose power imbalances, discriminate, and/or limit participation? Try to initiate discussions within the team, centering on the main goal of client-centered care based on the client's culture. In the end, do not be discouraged. It may take time to get support and make changes, but each conversation is a starting point. See Effect of Cultural Perceptions of Aging on Participation and Effect of Environmental Systems on Older Adult Health Outcomes. (LO 4-3, 4-4)

Chapter 5

1. Social networks are relationships between individuals, families, and groups. These networks provide social engagement and reinforce meaningful roles within a family and community. (under heading: Social Support). Instrumental support provides assistance with ADLs and IADLs; information support provides advice, problem-solving, and information; and emotional support provides love and friendship. (LO 5-1, 5-3; Social Network Types)
2. Over time, social networks become less diverse, although larger, more diverse networks are associated with positive well-being. Kin ties provide more instrumental social support, but non kin ties and friends can provide emotional support, companionship, and morale. Non kin ties are becoming more important sources of support than family relationships as family structures evolve over time. (LO 5-1, 5-3; Social Network Characteristics and Social Support)

Chapter 6

1. The occupational therapy practitioner should be aware of the dynamics of the aging population and the laws put into place to prevent ageism against older adults. The occupational therapy practitioner can advocate for the older adult in their care for specific issues. Moreover, the occupational therapy practitioner can be involved at the local, state, and national levels in professional organizations to advocate for laws and policies that recognize older adults as important members of society. (LO 6-1)
2. Ms. Parks's case constituted a true ethical dilemma between valuing her autonomy (allowing her to not report the abuse) and offering her beneficence (stopping the abuse). To evaluate this case, the occupational therapy practitioner would need to consider which principle is most important, because they cannot be upheld at the same time. In this government locality, the occupational therapy practitioner was told the laws constrained them from reporting the abuse unless Ms. Parks was willing to do so. To offer beneficence, the occupational therapy practitioner would have to report the abuse anyway and experience the potential legal and employment consequences. To offer autonomy, the occupational therapy practitioner would have to let the abuse continue, per Ms. Parks's wishes. The case does not end satisfactorily, because the occupational therapy practitioner does not know what Ms. Parks decides to do. However, the practitioner afforded Ms. Parks the autonomy she desired while providing persuasive information that there were options other than just letting the abuse continue. There is no absolutely correct answer in this scenario; the important thing is to work through the ethical problem-solving framework and arrive at a decision that the occupational therapy practitioner can live with (LO 6-6, Box 6-2).

Chapter 7

1. The main barrier facing an older adult with these special concerns is that a single issue can have a chain reaction on other multiple systems. For example, poor oral health can lead to increased risk for systemic disease and decreased ability to eat. These factors may lead to poor nutrition, frailty, and increased risk for falls, resulting in reduced participation with additional physical decline. Further complicating the client's condition, aging body structures may limit the client from recovering or adapting well. Environmental and contextual supports may help the client adapt, but additional effort, attention, and cognitive load are needed by older adult clients compared with younger persons. Providing the client with assistive technology, training a caregiver on how to maximize the client's occupational engagement, and/or instilling a routine to support occupational engagement may promote greater well-being in older adulthood. For this example, see Oral Health With Aging and Nutrition and Hydration With Aging.
2. An older adult with special concerns addressed in this chapter has inefficient and impaired body structures and functions, which negatively affect participation in activities. Any intervention plan for an older adult must include education about aging body processes

and their outcomes and how to mitigate or attenuate these effects. For example, as part of the aging process, reduced body water and loss of muscle promote fatigue, so more rest periods are needed during intervention activities to counter fatigue and prevent falls. Another example is that aging leads to inefficient renal and hydration processes, indicating the need for rehydration and toileting opportunities during intervention sessions and daily life activities. See Nutrition and Hydration With Aging and Implications for the Older Adult in Treatment: Malnutrition and Dehydration.

Chapter 8

1. The Health Belief Model may be particularly useful in this situation. It is possible that Juanita's perceptions about the benefits of and barriers to taking medications as prescribed are influencing her self-management (refer to Health Belief Model). It would be useful to have a conversation with Juanita to determine why she is not taking the medications as prescribed. Medication management is inherently complex, and other problems, such as cost, lack of symptoms, and even mistrust in pharmaceutical companies may influence Juanita's reasoning for not taking the medications as prescribed. It is necessary that the occupational therapist further explores additional factors that may be perpetuating the problem (Refer to Medication Management). Following the IMedS protocol (Promoting Best Practice 8-2) could be one approach toward solving this problem. (LO 8-3)

2. First, health events like a stroke can be a powerful motivator for health behavior change. The term *teachable moment* is often used to describe this motivation. It appears that Steve may be in the preparation or action stage of the Transtheoretical Model, meaning he is ready and beginning to make changes. People in the preparation stage believe that they can make changes to their health behaviors and work toward having a healthier lifestyle. It is important to consider that although Steve may be ready to commit to behavior change, it is possible that he could move either forward or backward, as the steps do not always occur in a linear process. It may be motivating to discuss the transtheoretical stages and how sometimes clients move back a stage but it is always possible to move forward again. The occupational therapist can support Steve's self-management by: (1) helping him create goals, (2) providing education on risk reduction, (3) supporting strategy development for engaging in healthy behaviors considering any residual effects from his stroke, and (4) providing ongoing support in helping him meet his goals in the context of everyday life (The Transtheoretical Model). (LO 8-2, 8-4)

Chapter 9

1. Acute care: Most individuals have either had an exacerbation of their cardiovascular and/or cardiopulmonary condition or an associated surgery. These individuals typically present with an overall decrease in strength, activity tolerance, and ADL performance; therefore, it is valuable to provide a remediation, restoration approach to intervention with these individuals. Inpatient rehabilitation/skilled nursing focus on interventions related to the continuation of pursed lip breathing, O_2 management, diaphragmatic breathing, and progress intervention related to ADL/IADL retraining, along with patient education related to self-management and lifestyle changes. Outpatient/community rehabilitation focuses on interventions specifically associated with patient education for self-management and empowerment, increased expansion on understanding MET levels and integration of energy conservation and work simplification, community resources, psychosocial supports, and lifestyle changes to support the intervention approaches within this setting. (See Box 9-7; LO 9-3; 9-9)

2. MET levels, pursed lip breathing, dyspnea control postures, diaphragmatic breathing, O_2 management, client education (self-management, empowerment, and lifestyle changes), ADL/IADL retraining, ECWS, and caregiver education. See interventions for older adults section. (LO 9-3; 9-9)

3. Interprofessional teams promote holistic and inclusive care for individuals within these populations. Each professional's contribution to treatment improves the quality of healthcare by shifting the focus of care from medical treatment toward promoting health and wellness with these individuals. Interprofessional collaboration also promotes patient satisfaction and improves carryover for individuals within these populations. (See interprofessional colleagues: collaboration and referrals.; LO 9-8)

Chapter 10

1. Changes in the sensory systems may affect the older adult's behaviors in many ways, including decreased participation in ADLs and IADLs due to decreased vision, hearing, taste, smell, touch, or pain. An older adult may also withdraw socially or experience decreased safety due to sensory changes. Are any changes generally more devastating than others? Why or why not? Low vision can be detrimental, because it limits driving ability and safe interaction with the physical environment. Decreased ability to hear can limit a person's social interactions and participation in social situations. (LO 10-1, 10-2, 10-3, 10-4, 10-5)

2. Sensory changes often cause decreased functional performance without intervention. An older adult may

need to increase visual contrast in their homes and/or rearrange items so they can be located more easily. Or they may have to cease some activities, such as driving, altogether due to safety concerns. Auditory changes? The older adult may choose not to participate in certain activities due to difficulty with participation. They may need to explore assistive technology options like flashing lights to draw attention to items in the home such as the phone or smoke alarms. They may also need to explore using a TTY to be able to hear the television or a conversation on their phone. Pain? They may need to modify certain activities to decrease pain or modify their schedule around pain-relieving measures like medications or periods of inactivity. (LO 10-1, 10-2, 10-3, 10-4, 10-5)

3. Regarding taste and smell, a person may be at risk for food poisoning if they do not detect that food has gone bad. Additionally, with smell, a person may not be able to detect certain hazards, such as fires or gas leaks. Changes in superficial sensations could lead to the older adult not being able to detect when something is too hot or too cold or localizing stimuli. (LO 10-3, 10-4, 10-5)

Chapter 11

1. Some of the most profound changes in the musculoskeletal system that are associated with typical aging and that we might expect to observe for Mrs. Sampson are decreased muscle strength and power, decreased skeletal muscle mass, decreased number of functional motor units, decreased percentage of type II (fast twitch) fibers, changes in postural alignment, decreased bone mass, cartilage changes, decreased elasticity of connective tissues, decreased flexibility, changes in balance and gait, decreased maximal speed of movement and initiation of motor responses, decreased proprioception, decline in the total number of muscle fibers, and increased adipose tissue. (LO 11-1, 11-2)

2. Implications of musculoskeletal system changes for occupational performance in older adults can include decreased functional mobility, decreased walking speed, poor balance, decreased joint range of motion, and an increased risk of falls that may contribute to injuries such as falls, impaired occupational performance, and loss of independence. (LO 11-3, 11-4)

3. Occupational therapy practitioners should consider the following approaches when prescribing an exercise program to an older adult. Use simple directions and gestures; ensure adequate warm-up and cool-down; take into consideration current and potential musculoskeletal problems, chronic conditions (e.g., osteoporosis), and functional limitations; institute short and graded exercise sessions but apply the overload principle; use a variety of muscle contractions; establish an exercise program with a focus on multiple components (low-impact aerobic, muscular strength, power, endurance, flexibility, and balance); monitor skin for signs of heat stress; monitor vital signs, including blood pressure, respirations, and pulse rate in response to exercise; and exercise at a rate of perceived exertion of 12 to 14 ("somewhat hard") or use the *talk test* (the older adult should be able to engage in a conversation during the exercise). (LO 11-3, 11-4, 11-5, 11-6)

Chapter 12

1. A. Feeling off-balance and at risk of falls walking on uneven ground in parks, forests, and marshes. Intervention remediative: Individualized balance program that challenges her balance that she can do several times a week between bird-watching sessions. Intervention adaptive: Use of walking stick or Nordic poles during bird watching. B. Struggling with precision in adjusting binoculars. Remediative: Individualized fine dexterity program to do a few times a week between bird-watching sessions, including practice with the binoculars in more supportive sitting position and moving toward less postural support to increase the challenge. Adaptive: See if a repair person can experiment with changing the force required to adjust the lenses. C. Cannot capture a photo in time due to slowed motor response. Intervention remediation: Reaction time exercises using her iPad that she enjoys using and skills are very transferable to her iPhone that she uses for pictures. Adaptive intervention: Acquire video equipment that would run continuously and learn how to edit video.

2. The evidence tells us that a motor learning approach is the most effective intervention, most specifically a task-oriented approach, where the intervention matches the goal of the intervention (e.g., practicing dressing in order to get better at dressing). This theory considers the complex networks of the brain that work in an integrated fashion rather than being solely driven by sensory information input. Motor response is also dependent on context, personal factors, prior learned patterns, and the nervous system's ability to suppress motor reflexes in response to sensory information. With special training, a therapist may use a motor control approach when an individual has a completely paretic limb and is unable to complete any tasks with it regardless of complexity of the task. Sensory input is used in this scenario to trigger reflexive movement that stimulates the motor system, potentially as a building block toward voluntary movement.

3. It is important to consider natural progression of the injury/disease in goal-setting. Someone in the middle stage of Parkinson disease can be encouraged to set goals that will support their participation, with maintenance rather than improvement in physical skill. An

example would be transitioning to using a ball ramp for bowling to allow for participation in the present rather than focusing exclusively on improving physical performance for bowling in the future (which may not be possible due to disease progression and hampers enjoyment of current possibilities for enhancing quality of life). In contrast, someone who has recently had a stroke can be encouraged to set goals that are cautious yet hopeful related to improving physical function, because natural improvement is typical in the natural recovery of stroke and can be enhanced with rehabilitation.

Chapter 13

1. Genetics, socioeconomics, access to healthcare, and lower education have been linked to declines in cognitive function with aging. Factors such as participation in cognitively stimulating activities, physical activity and exercise, and socialization have been linked to facilitating enhanced cognitive reserve. Interventions promoting cognitive functioning should include an environment that promotes both social and cognitively stimulating activities. Occupations must be of interest to the individual. Exercise or activity must be of interest to the client and performed almost daily, and exercise or activity is most beneficial if it engages cognitive functions (such as with dance or sports). See section on Optimizing Cognitive Functioning in Older Adults. (LO 13-2, LO 13-3)

2. Cognitive changes include slowed processing, working memory, and fluid intelligence. Other conditions include loss of hearing and changes in vision. Strategies to help adapt for these changes include speaking at a slower pace, ensuring the person hears you (can ask them to look at you), having the individual repeat what was said, encouraging depth of processing with repeating, and ensuring good light and low distraction. See each section on "Impact of ……. on older adults". (LO 13-1, 13-3, 13-8)

3. Primary cognitive symptoms of dementia include difficulties with short-term memory; attention; orientation to time, place, and person; visuospatial processing; language production and comprehension; and executive functioning. Individuals with dementia also experience difficulties performing day-to-day activities, such as handling finances, grocery shopping, participating in leisure activities and hobbies, and carrying out self-care tasks. Individuals with dementia may experience changes in their emotions and usual behaviors. Most people with even mild dementia will experience some changes in behavior. Severe changes or problematic behavioral changes lead to earlier institutionalization.

    Occupational therapy assessment and interventions must focus on promoting quality of life and participation for the client with dementia and the caregiver(s).
Exercise, sensory-based treatments, cognitive stimulation, reminiscence therapy, validation therapy (accepting the person's reality), and simulated presence (video played of loved one) are interventions found to affect behaviors. Treatments that align with the client's interest and ability contribute to the effectiveness of interventions, especially in enhancing function and reducing responsive behaviors. Interventions must also consider the needs of the caregiver(s). Skill-building education, mindfulness practices, and cognitive behavioral therapy have been shown to be effective in decreasing depression, anxiety, and stress in caregivers. LO 13-8, 13-9, 13-10 See sections Factors Impacting Functioning for Persons Living with Dementia and Occupational Therapy Interventions with Persons with Dementia. Refer to Table 13-3 on Cognitive Reserve.

Chapter 14

1. Maintaining functional performance in daily living tasks promotes self-esteem and social well-being. Older adults who maintain competence in ADL are less lonely and isolated, supporting cognitive and psychological health. (LO 14-2; Location: Importance of Self-Care for Self-Identity and Socialization)

2. The Quality of Life in Neurological Disorders (Neuro-QoL) measures are a set of standardized assessments that holistically addresses self-care among other functional activities, including the ability to participate in social roles and activities. (LO 14-5; Location: Special Considerations in Evaluation)

3. Modifications to the bathroom for safe performance of ADLs for mobility needs could include grab bars, tub or shower benches, raised toilet seats, and widened doorways. These basic environmental modifications and assistive devices support safe transfers and stability while the person is in the bathroom area. [LO 14-6; Location: Environmental modifications. Assistive devices for self-care]

Chapter 15

1. It would be important to understand the physical, environmental, and social aspects. Like many older adults, Mrs. Wilson has multiple chronic conditions, combined with a new injury. Her home is very meaningful to her but not optimal in terms of accessibility. Her social support is strong in terms of financial and emotional support, but support with performing daily tasks is currently limited due to her son's distance and daughter's health. Many older adults face these challenges with adult children living at a distance and aging and facing their own health issues. (LO 15-2: Complexities of Aging: Physical, Environmental, Social)

2. It would be important to get to know the older adult in terms of their personal and health history, their environment and their attachment to their environment, their support system, and their personal goals and priorities. The use of the Occupational Profile Interview would be helpful in terms of guiding the discussion. Once you have that discussion, using the COPM or some other way of co-developing the goals and understanding the person's priorities, you can finalize the goals. At that point, it is important to observe the client performing the activities that need to be addressed to assess the person's function in their natural environment. Further assessments need to be chosen to assess more specific IADL needs. Typically, more than one intervention will be needed to address performance. For example, if cooking is an area of concern, the occupational therapist may need to address environmental adaptation, skill training, fatigue management, grocery list development, meal planning, and so on. (LO 15-4 and 15-5: Importance of Person-Centered Care for Older Adults, Special Considerations in Assessment, COPM)

Chapter 16

1. Sleep is critical to overall health and wellness. Although sleep and health management are two distinct occupations, achieving quality sleep is essential to managing health. Conversely, managing components of health such as physical activity, nutrition, and symptoms of chronic conditions can promote healthy sleep habits. (LO 16-1; see The Relationship Between Sleep and Chronic Health Conditions in Older Adults)
2. The role of occupational therapy is distinct from other health professions in addressing health management and sleep because of the unique focus on the development of habits and routines that promote health. Occupational therapy interventions focus on active engagement in occupations that promote and maintain healthy behaviors and habits among older adults. In addition, occupational therapy intervention includes client education, problem-solving strategies, and goal-setting, which can be used to improve health management and sleep occupational performance and participation. (See Promoting Best Practice features, LO 16-1)

Chapter 17

1. The only common definition of leisure is that it brings enjoyment to the person and does not involve payment. The client enjoys not participating in any particular activity in the evening, and no payment is involved; therefore it counts as leisure. Specifically, it could be considered a passive, low-demand, unclassified leisure activity. (See Defining Leisure, LO 17-1)

2. An occupational therapist should view the smartphone as both a source of leisure and a potential assistive device for leisure. A clinician can teach the client about accessibility settings on the device to increase its ability to be used with any age-related changes, such as vision, fine motor coordination, hearing, and voice. The client can also be trained on problem-solving, care of the device, and general setup to establish patterns and routines of use. Finally, the occupational therapist can teach the client how to use the games and apps of interest to most effectively interact with their desired audience. (See "Use of Assistive Technology to Support Leisure" and Promoting Best Practice 17-2; LO 17-5)

Chapter 18

1. Whereas some older adults choose to move to full-time retirement and leave work behind, others transition to part-time employment. A wide variety of factors influence these decisions, including financial factors (e.g., can they afford to leave work altogether), health factors, and personal interests. (See "Culture and Demographics.")
2. Development is multidimensional and multidirectional. Development is multidimensional because it cannot be described by a single criterion, such as increases or decreases in a behavior. Development is also multidirectional because there is no single normal path that it must or should take. In other words, healthy developmental outcomes are achieved in a wide variety of ways. Healthy development also involves both gains and losses. (See "Theoretical Approaches to the Retirement Process.")
3. Volunteer and leisure experiences also provide a low-risk opportunity for individuals to explore their abilities, capacities, and limitations, such as fatigue, their tolerance for activity, and the application of prior skills. For older adults who may wish to transition to new areas of employment, volunteering may provide exposure to work activities to more accurately gauge interest as well as an opportunity to gain practical experience. (See "Volunteerism and Leisure.")

Chapter 19

1. Community mobility enables older adults to participate in carrying out many instrumental activities and attend employment, volunteer, family, or religious commitments. It is social in nature, because being out of the home and interacting with others fosters a sense of connectedness and belonging and combats isolation and loneliness. Limitations to mobility can negatively affect well-being for older adults, because community mobility directly enables participation. (See "Community Mobility Options," LO 19-1)

2. Interventions that focus on remediation could improve a cognitively typical older adult's driving performance. These include cognitive or motor retraining, skills training, simulation experiences, and specialized driving rehabilitation services with the addition of compensatory strategies, such as audio and visual GPS devices. (Location: "Exemplar Interventions," LO 19-5)

3. Adults living in urban settings are more likely to have access to public transportation routes, paratransit options, or ride-share services, whereas older adults living in rural settings may be more vulnerable to social isolation when they can no longer drive. (Location: "Mobility Options Beyond Driving," LO 19-6)

Chapter 20

1. There are multiple policies that can support caregivers, including those listed in Table 20-2. Other interventions and tools that can support caregivers are Skills2Care®, Powerful Tools for Caregivers, Reducing Disability in Alzheimer's Disease (RDAD), and STAR-Community Consultants (STAR-C). (Refer to Sections: Policies to Support Family Caregivers, & Exemplar Interventions, LO 20-4, 20-6)

2. The great duration, less degree of control, and increased level of caregiver involvement could all place more demands on the caregiver. Therefore, caregivers at these extreme ends of the care spectrum might be especially in need of additional support. (Refer to Section: Levels of Care and Family Caregiving Responsibilities, LO 20-2)

3. Evidence has shown that individuals providing care are at an increased risk of physical health challenges. Additionally, caregivers frequently report emotional and social challenges in relation to their caregiving responsibilities. (Refer to Section: Impact of Family Caregiving: A Public Health Issue, LO 20-1, 20-2)

Chapter 21

1. The focus of inpatient rehabilitation is on promoting the safety and independence of clients when performing ADLs and IADLs so that they can transition to living at home. Important assessment areas would include ADLs, IADLs, and functional mobility. (*What to Assess When Focusing on Function in Older Adults*). Evaluative assessments would be appropriate to use with the clients to measure progress and to provide evidence to insurance that a client is benefiting from intensive therapy. Predictive measures would be helpful to administer to determine what progress is possible during their stay and what kind of assistance clients might need once they are discharged. (*Purposes and Types of Assessment and Evaluation*). The clinician could try to create an environment that is not overwhelming for the client by limiting the number of distractions during the assessment, making sure the client is using any hearing aids or glasses when needed, speaking slowly and clearly, providing written materials that are large enough for the client to read, and using assessments with appropriate health literacy levels. (*Specific Issues Related to Evaluation of Functional Performance*, LO 21-1; LO 21-4; LO 21-5)

2. The therapist should try to eliminate biases based on language and culture when choosing assessment tools. The therapist could do this by researching more about the client's culture while practicing cultural humility and recognizing that each person is an individual. The therapist should also use the best available Spanish interpreter to provide the most accurate results during the evaluation. The therapist could look for written assessments that have Spanish translations that can be completed with help from the interpreter. Using many different types of assessment tools can help limit bias as well. (*Ethical Considerations for Evaluating Older Adults*, LO 21-2; LO 21-5)

Chapter 22

1. In a direct care role, the occupational therapist would provide hands-on services through addressing the client's performance skills, partnering with other medical professionals. Additionally, the occupational therapist may address the physical or social environment, partnering with contractors and architects, or social support organizations. Lastly, in addressing quality of life, the occupational therapist may partner with case managers, spiritual leaders, and, in all cases, with family and other important life partners. (LO 22-3; Role of OT and Interprofessional Partners section)

2. Occupational therapists could function as health coaches through their holistic background in medical conditions, social and emotional health, activity analysis, ability to appraise best evidence, and a lens of occupational adaptation to provide occupation-oriented health coaching to empower the individual to meet their health goals. Coaches guide their clients into making personally relevant and meaningful choices to improve and sustain health. (LO 22-5; Health education, health coaching, and health promotion section)

Chapter 23

1. It would be measured through regular evaluation of ADL and IADL assessments in the EMR. Important note: When working with older adults, It is important to phrase questions about ADLs/IADLs in terms of level of difficulty rather than what they need help with (Nicosia et al, 2020). (LO 23-7)

2. Roles will vary and are dependent on the primary care setting's needs and the occupational therapist's skill set. The roles may evolve over time as the providers may become more aware of occupational therapy's scope of practice. As the providers learn more about occupational therapy evaluation and intervention, they may ask for additional occupational therapy services or base programming based on occupational therapy services, for example, adding a frailty evaluation program. Occupational therapy's focus on function is an important consideration, and as the needs of the patients change, the occupational therapy interventions may as well. (LO 23-3)

Chapter 24

1. Evidence supports the engagement in early activity and mobility within the ICU and acute care hospital setting. Prevention of other sequalae of factors such as ICU-AW and delirium are additional reasons to encourage the patient to engage in early activity and mobility. "Bedrest is bad" is a campaign to combat hospital immobility. It clearly articulates that patients lying in bed is not optimal to recovery. Patients should be awake and engaged in physical and cognitive activities such as performing a stand pivot to a bedside commode instead of using a bed pan for toileting or sitting on the edge of the bed to brush their teeth themselves. (Early Mobility section, LO 24-5)
2. Obtain an accurate occupational profile to determine the patient's prior level of function. Was the patient able to successfully perform IADL tasks such as medication, financial management, and driving? Ask family members or caregivers if the patient had confusion, memory, or attention problems before coming to the hospital. Determine whether the patient has their sensory aids (glasses or hearing aids). Check the patient's medical chart for medications, including sedatives, as well as infections such as a urinary tract infection. Examining the medical course also lends to deciphering the cause of the cognitive impairment. Cognitive impairment would be expected in an older adult patient who has just had a massive right frontal subdural hematoma but not in a patient who has had a spinal fusion surgery. Checking laboratory values may also help problem solve impaired cognition such as low blood glucose (hypoglycemia) or high white blood cell count (such as with sepsis). (Discharge Planning Section and Addressing Cognitive Impairment for Older Adults in Acute Care; LO 24-4)
3. a. Is there someone at home who can provide the level of assistance needed for the older adult patient? This includes physical and cognitive assistance. For example, can the caregiver physically lift the patient from the edge of the bed to standing or be in charge of managing the medications and medication changes after a hospital admission? Does the caregiver have any limitations themselves, such as needing an assistive device to walk? Is there someone who can call and check on the patient to ensure medications are taken, meals are consumed, etc.? What is the home setup? Is it one floor, or are steps required for access to the bathroom? Do they have any equipment at home? Are there supportive resources such as loaner closets or churches to donate equipment not covered by insurance for those on a fixed income? (Discharge Planning Section, LO 24-5)
   b. Is this a progressive decline in function? Physical and/or cognitive? Should long-term care placement be considered if the family is no longer able to care for the patient? (Addressing Cognitive Impairment for Older Adults in Acute Care, LO 24-5)

Chapter 25

1. Skilled nursing facilities would be appropriate for individuals who do not yet have the physical capacity to return to their home setting, but there is potential for improvement and they may improve adequately to be supported at home by services and/or friends and family within approximately 3 months. Inpatient care can allow for more time to assess for safety to return home or to provide important health education, as well as gain strength and improve function.

   Outpatient and ambulatory care services and day care services are for older adults who can remain in their home safely and can travel to therapy. They would need to have cognitive, physical, and emotional capacity to complete activities of daily living or have enough support from friends, family, and social services to do any activities of daily living that they are not able to do themselves. They or their family would need to understand and be confident with managing any healthcare conditions that they had. Some day care services are long term, which would be helpful for someone who needs long-term monitoring and/or family or friends who require respite occasionally from the caregiving role.

   Telerehabilitation is best offered to an older adult with skills for technology or someone who can help them. The individual needs to be able to conceptualize the ideas being shared online to their own physical environment and needs to have good safety insight so they do not overextend themselves without standby physical supervision. (Rehabilitation and Service Contexts; Role of Occupational Therapy and Interprofessional Partners; LO 25-1, 25-2)
2. In most communities, transportation for older adults is problematic. Often transportation is not adequately

accessible, is expensive, or has barriers to access, such as complex scheduling. You could make sure that transportation is an issue being addressed by your local politician.

Another common community-level issue for older adults is lack of access to services because most information is now going online. How is your community making sure that older adults are aware of services they can access? What ideas could you suggest to your municipality or local library? (Advocacy section; LO 25-7)

Chapter 26

1. It is essential that an occupational therapist ensures that their patient is appropriate for home health services. An individual must meet multiple criteria to qualify for home health. These can be found under the main heading Home Health Agencies and Medicare, in the section on Criteria for Coverage of Home Health Services for Medicare Beneficiaries. As a clinician working in home health, one must ensure their patient qualifies for services by being "homebound." If a therapist is aware that a patient is leaving the home excessively and for inappropriate reasons, they are required to report this to their home health agency so that a decision can be made, in collaboration with the physician or allowed practitioner, about the homebound status of the patient. The patient must be under the care of a physician or an allowed practitioner at all times during the episode of care, as collaboration between the home health clinicians and the physician/practitioner is essential. All home health clinicians are the "eyes and ears" for the physicians/practitioners and are required to report back findings that affect the patient's plan of care. Lastly, to qualify for home health services, the patient must require the skilled services of nursing, physical therapy, or speech therapy. Occupational therapy on its own does not make a patient eligible for home health. However, if occupational therapy is working with a patient alongside one of the other disciplines mentioned, the occupational therapist can in fact continue to work with the patient even if the other discipline(s) discharge the patient from their services.

   Additionally, it is important that occupational therapists be aware of the many nuances of home health, including the rules related to the initiation of care (i.e., Start of Care), the comprehensive assessment, developing a plan of care, and communicating with the interdisciplinary team and the physician or allowed practitioner. (All this information can be found under the main heading Home Health Agencies and Medicare, LO 26-4, 26-5)

2. Occupational therapy practitioners are well suited for working in the home health setting, as the main focus is helping patients get back to performing their chosen occupations. The Context of Home Health Services explains the benefit of working with patients in their own surroundings. This allows occupational therapists to work with patients in their own natural environment versus having to simulate occupations. Occupational therapists can provide education and training in safety with ADL and IADL performance, assist in maximizing independence or providing compensatory strategies, train caregivers to assist their loved ones, and address all areas of occupation in a very effective way. The physical therapist may want to focus on gait, balance, and endurance, whereas the occupational therapist will use the improvement of these skills to increase the patient's occupational performance. For example, as a patient improves safety of walking up and down steps with the physical therapist, the occupational therapist can use this skill to assist the patient in retrieving their mail from the mailbox. (This information can be found under the main heading The Role of OT in Home Health and Intervention, LO 26-1, 26-2, 26-6)

3. Although the main focus of an occupational therapist is to provide excellent clinical care, it is also important for therapists to be aware of how services are reimbursed by Medicare so that the best possible services can be provided that are appropriate to the setting. Because home health reimbursement is not affected by the number of occupational therapy visits alone, an occupational therapist should be aware when they assess a patient that they need to develop a plan of care that meets the patient's needs and consists of a frequency and duration that will allow the patient to meet the decided-upon goals. There is a very big focus on use of evidence-based practice and providing visits that are of high quality to achieve good outcomes. Occupational therapists should be providing education (both orally and written) training patients in appropriate home exercise programs (if applicable) and preparing for discharge from the very first visit. (Information on this topic can be found under Documentation and Reimbursement, LO 26-5)

Chapter 27

1. The typical person who uses long-term care services has at least one chronic condition, needs assistance with ADLs such as bathing and dressing, is female, has no spouse, has a higher level of frailty, is White, and is incontinent of bladder. (Introduction, Profile of Nursing Home Residents, LO 27-1)

2. Single-discipline interventions such as occupational therapy and physical therapy provide care to a client from the frame of reference of one profession, but interdisciplinary care offers a more holistic approach

that encompasses the viewpoint of many disciplines working together to provide the best outcome for the client. (Role of Occupational Therapy and Interprofessional Partners, LO 27-4)
3. Answers will vary, but could include:
   1. The client will independently identify and attend three group activities in the skilled nursing facility within 2 weeks to increase participation in leisure activities and decrease social isolation.
   2. The client will complete shower routine with supervision and good safety within 1 month to increase independence with self-care.
   3. The client will participate in watering and weeding the facility's accessible garden with modified independence within 3 weeks.

      (Role of Occputional Therapy and Interprofessional Partners, Occupational Therapy Process, LO 27-5)

Chapter 28

1. Most importantly, occupational therapy can enable engagement in and alleviate barriers to participation in meaningful occupations despite imminent death. (LO 28-2)
2. Older adults facing the end of life are often burdened by deteriorating function along with grief and sorrow at having to leave loved ones behind. (LO 28-3)
3. Decisions about assessment instruments should be based on a thorough assessment of the person's everyday life and activity status, taking their individual circumstances into account. (LO 28-7)

Chapter 29

1. Occupational therapists can use accelerometer data to assess activity and movement in the home and community and sensors in the home to gain data on how long clients are in rooms and are accessing drawers, closets, and different rooms of the house. Additionally, family members may need consultation on remote monitoring video cameras or smart home technologies.

   (Found in Technology in Healthcare and Social Environments section, LO 29-4)
2. The home, as a place of meaning, provides an occupationally rich context to pursue basic ADL and leisure activities while the person is limited in function. For example, the client can engage in cognitive activities with family by playing games while sitting at edge of the bed or participate in daily home management activities through guiding and directing others, if unable to physically perform the tasks. Engagement in meaningful, person-centered occupations supports health and recovery. (Found in Acute Care at Home section, LO 29-1, 29-7)
3. Occupational therapists who want to gain expertise in assistive technologies can become assistive technology practitioners, attend technology-related conferences, and participate in service and research activities that provide direct contact with clients and technologies. Such examples are working with home modification service groups and veterans' organizations. (Found in Box 29.2 Assistive Technology Resources; Implication for Occupational Therapy section, LO 29-7)

APPENDIX B

Index of Assessments

APPENDIX B ■ Index of Assessments

NAME	FORMAT	ICF DOMAIN	PURPOSE	SOURCE	CHAPTER
Activity Card Sort (ACS)	Interview	Participation	Measures a person's participation in IADL, leisure, and social activities	Baum, C. M., & Edwards, D. (2008). *Activity Card Sort (ACS)*. St. Washington University School of Medicine. Access: https://myaota.aota.org/shop_aota/product/1247	16, 21, 27
ADL Staircase	Interview and observation	Activity	Assesses functional changes in performance in ADL and IADL over time	Jakobsson, U. (2008). The ADL-staircase: Further validation. *International Journal of Rehabilitation Research, 31*, 85–88. https://doi.org/10.1097/MRR.0b013e3282f45166	16, 21
Assessment of Occupational Functioning Modified Interest Checklist	Questionnaire	Activity; Participation	Assesses interest and participation leisure activities at multiple points in time	Kielhofner, G., & Neville, A. (1983). The modified interest checklist. *Chicago: University of Illinois.*	9, 17, 21
Barthel Index of ADL	Performance-based on observation, interview, or records	Activity	Assesses the functional status of hospital patients in ADLs	Mahoney, S. I., & Barthel, D. W. (1965). Functional evaluation: The Barthel index. *Maryland State Medical Journal, 14*, 61–65. Access: https://www.kcl.ac.uk/nmpc/assets/rehab/tools-bifunctional-evaluation-the-barthel-index.pdf	9, 16, 21, 23, 27
Beck Depression Inventory (BDI)	Questionnaire	Body Function	Screening tool for signs and symptoms of depression.	Beck, A. T., Ward, C. H., Mendelson, M., Mock, J., & Erbaugh, J. (1961). An inventory for measuring depression. *Archives of general psychiatry, 4*(6), 561–571. https://doi.org/10.1001/archpsyc.1961.01710120031004	2, 27
Berg Balance Scale	Performance-based Rating Scale	Activity	Measures older adults balance to determine risk for falling	Berg, K. O., Wood-Dauhpinee, S. L., Williams, J. I., & Maki, B. (1992). Measuring balance in the elderly: Validation of an instrument. *Canadian Journal of Public Health, 83*(Suppl. 2), S7–S11. https://pubmed.ncbi.nlm.nih.gov/1468055/ Access: https://www.sralab.org/rehabilitation-measures/berg-balance-scale	16, 21, 27
Brain Injury Visual Assessment Battery for Adults (biVABA)	Performance-based	Body Function	A collection of assessments for visual acuity, contrast sensitivity, and visual field, specifically postbrain injury	Warren, M. (n.d.). THE biVABA (Brain Injury Visual Assessment Battery for Adults). https://www.visabilities.com/bivaba.html	10
Canadian Occupational Performance Measure (COPM)	Semistructured interview	Participation	Assesses change in a client's self-perception of occupational performance over time	Law, M., Baptiste, S., Carswell, A., McColl, M. A., Polatajko, H., & Pollock, N. (2014). *The Canadian Occupational Performance Measure* (5th ed.). Canadian Association of Occupational Therapists. https://www.thecopm.ca/	1, 2, 9, 15, 16, 17, 21
Cognitive Performance Test (CPT)	Standardized graded task performance	Activity	Assesses a person's ability to complete IADL and ADL requiring working memory and executive functioning	Burns, T., Mortimer, J. A., & Merchak, P. (1994). Cognitive Performance Test: A new approach to functional assessment in Alzheimer's disease. *Journal of Geriatric Psychiatry and Neurology, 7*, 46–54. https://doi.org/10.1177/089198879400700109	2, 14, 16, 21
Cougar Home Safety Assessment (CHSA)	Questionnaire and environmental observation	Environmental Factors	Assessment of the home environment specific to safety features	Fisher, G, Burgess, B., DiMassimo, H., Florenzo, C., Hymers, B, Kuchta, K., & Natale, O. (2019) Cougar Home Safety Assessment 5.0. https://resources.finalsite.net/images/v1587754449/misericordia/ectokqd4oenv9yx8seau/chsa_50_April_11_2019.pdf	15

APPENDIX B ■ Index of Assessments 529

Assessment	Format	ICF Domain	Description	Reference	Chapter(s)
Dementia Carer Assessment Needs Tool (DeCANT)	Questionnaire	Participation	Identifies a caregiver's needs when working with clients with dementia.	Clemmensen, T. H., Kristensen, H. K., Andersen-Ranberg, K., & Lauridsen, H. H. (2021). Development and field-testing of the Dementia Carer Assessment of Support Needs Tool (DeCANT). *International Psychogeriatrics, 33*(4), 405-417. https://doi.org/10.1017/S1041610220001714	16, 21
eHEALS: The eHealth Literacy Scale	Questionnaire	Activity; Personal factors	Assesses measures consumers' combined knowledge, comfort, and perceived skills at finding, evaluating, and applying electronic health information to health problems	Norman, C. D., & Skinner, H. A. (2006). eHEALS: The eHealth Literacy Scale. *Journal of Medical Internet Research, 8*(4), e27. https://doi.org/10.2196/jmir.8.4.e27	16
Elder Maltreatment Screen and Follow-up Plan	Questionnaire	Participation	Assessment to help identify older adults at risk for abuse for action planning.	American Medical Association (2019) Elder maltreatment screen and follow-up plan. https://qpp.cms.gov/docs/QPP_quality_measure_specifications/CQM-Measures/2020_Measure_181_MIPSCQM.pdf	6
Elderly Mobility Scale (EMS)	Performance-based	Activity, Participation	Assesses a person's ability to complete transfers, their gait, and balance through functional activities of daily living	Smith, R. (1994). Validation and reliability of the Elderly Mobility Scale. *Physiotherapy, 80*(11), 744-747. https://doi.org/10.1016/S0031-9406(10)60612-8	16, 21
Falls Efficacy Scale-International (FES-I)	Questionnaire	Activity	Measures concerns about falling and fear of falling while completing daily activities.	Yardley, L., Beyer, N., Hauer, K., Kempen, G., Piot-Ziegler, C., & Todd, C. (2005). Development and initial validation of the Falls Efficacy Scale-International (FES-I). *Age and Ageing, 34*(6), 614-619. https://doi.org/10.1093/ageing/afi196	7
Functional Behavioral Profile (FBP)	Rating scale in checklist or interview format	Environmental Factors	Provides caregivers with a method of describing the impaired person's capabilities in interacting with others, solving problems, and performing tasks; for persons with dementia or stroke.	Baum, C., Edwards, D., & Morrow-Howell, N. (1993). Identification and measurement of productive behaviors in senile dementia of the Alzheimer's type. *The Gerontologist, 33*, 403–408. https://doi.org/10.1093/geront/33.3.403	16, 21
Functional Reach Test (FRT)	Performance-based	Activity	A performance-based balance screening that identifies a person's limits of stability when reaching forward	Duncan, P. W., Weiner, D. K., Chandler, J., & Studenski, S. (1990). Functional reach: a new clinical measure of balance. *Journal of Gerontology, 45*(6), M192-M197. https://doi.org/10.1093/geronj/45.6.M192	7, 27
Geriatric Depression Scale (GDS)	Questionnaire	Body Function	Screens for presence of depression	Sheikh, J. I., & Yesavage, J. A. (1986). Geriatric Depression Scale (GDS): Recent evidence and development of a shorter version. *Clinical Gerontologist: The Journal of Aging and Mental Health, 5*(1-2), 165–173. https://doi.org/10.1300/J018v05n01_09	16

Continued

APPENDIX B ■ Index of Assessments

NAME	FORMAT	ICF DOMAIN	PURPOSE	SOURCE	CHAPTER
Home Environment Assessment Protocol (HEAP)	Questionnaire and observation	Participation, Environmental Factors	An assessment specific to the home environment of caregivers and people who have dementia. Provides recommendations for home modification.	Gitlin, L. N., Schinfeld, S., Winter, L., Corcoran, M., Boyce, A. & Hauck, W. (2009). Evaluating home environments of persons with dementia: Interrater reliability and validity of the Home Environmental Assessment Protocol (HEAP). *Disability and Rehabilitation, 24*(1-3), 59-71. https://doi.org/10.1080/09638280110066325 Access: Gitlin, L., & Corcoran, M. (2005). *Occupational Therapy in Dementia Care.* Bethesda, MD: AOTA	15
Home Environment Lighting Assessment (HELA)	Questionnaire	Environmental Factors	Assessment of home lighting environments to provide intervention strategies for low vision.	Perlmutter, M. S., Bhorade, A., Gordon, M., Hollingsworth, H., Engsberg, J. E., & Baum, M. C. (2013). Home lighting assessment for clients with low vision. *American Journal of Occupational Therapy, 67,* 674–682. http://dx.doi.org/10.5014/ajot.2013.006692	10
HOME-Rx	Performance-based	Activity	Assesses medication management, through performance problems, safety concerns, and environmental barriers to guide intervention	Somerville, E., Massey, K., Keglovits, M., Vouri, S., Hu, Y. L., Carr, D., & Stark, S. (2019). Scoring, clinical utility, and psychometric properties of the in-home medication management Performance Evaluation (HOME-RX). *American Journal of Occupational Therapy, 73*(2), 7302205060p1- 7302205060p8. https://doi.org/10.5014/ajot.2019.029793	16
i-ADL-CDI	Performance-based	Activity	Assesses functional performance with IADL and ADL to help with diagnosing mild cognitive impairment and Alzheimer's disease.	Cornelis, E., Gorus, E., Beyer, I., Bautmans, I., & DeVriendt, P. (2017). Early diagnosis of mild cognitive impairment and mild dementia through basic and instrumental activities of daily living: Development of a new evaluation tool. *PLOS Medicine, 14*(3), e1002250. https://doi.org/10.1371/journal.pmed.1002250	21
In Home Occupational Performance Evaluation (I-HOPE)	Performance-based	Participation, Environmental Factors	Assesses activity participation, client's rating of performance, client's satisfaction with performance, and severity of environmental barriers in the home.	Stark, S. L., Somerville, E. K., & Morris, J. C. (2010). In home occupational performance evaluation (I-HOPE). *American Journal of Occupational Therapy, 64*(4), 580-589. https://doi.org/10.5014/ajot.2010.08065 Access: https://starklab.wustl.edu/resources/i-hope/i-hope-kit/#order	15
Independent Living Scale (ILS)	Questionnaire	Activity, Participation	Helps assess an individual's ability to achieve successful independent community living through five sub scales: memory orientation, managing money, managing home and transportation, health and safety, social adjustment.	Loeb, P.A. (1996). *The independent living scales (ILS).* San Antonio, TX: Pearson Assessment. https://www.pearsonassessments.com/store/usassessments/en/Store/Professional-Assessments/Cognition-%26-Neuro/Independent-Living-Scales/p/100000181.html	15
Interest Checklist	Questionnaire	Activity, Participation	Assesses an adult's past and present leisure interests	Klyczek, J. P., Bauer-Yox, N., & Fiedler, R. C. (1997). The Interest Checklist: A factor analysis. *The American Journal of Occupational Therapy, 51*(10), 815-823. https://doi.org/10.5014/ajot.51.10.815	16

APPENDIX B ■ Index of Assessments 531

Katz Index of Independence in Activities of Daily Living	Interview and observation	Activity	Screens for independence with ADL and type of assistance required to complete the ADL	Katz, S., Downs, T. D., Cash, H. R., & Grotz, R. C. (1970). Progress in development of the Index of ADL. *The Gerontologist, 10*, 20-30. https://doi.org/10.1093/geront/10.1_Part_1.20	16, 21, 27
Kitchen Picture Test (KPT)	Performance-based	Body Function	Assessment of practical judgment and basic cognitive problems through the use of pictures that the client describes, highlights safety problems and is tested on recall.	Mansbach, W. E., MacDougall, E. E., Clark, K. M., & Mace, R. A. (2014) Preliminary investigation of the Kitchen Picture Test (KPT): A new screening test of practical judgment for older adults. *Aging, Neuropsychology, and Cognition: A Journal on Normal and Dysfunctional Development, 21*(6), 674-692. https://doi.org/10.1080/13825585.2013.865698	15
Kohlman's Evaluation of Living Skills (KELS)	Interview and task-performance	Activity, Participation	Assesses a person's living and community skills	Burnett, J., Dyer, C. B., & Naik, A. D. (2009). Convergent validation of the Kohlman Evaluation of Living Skills as a screening tool of older adults' ability to live safely and independently in the community. *Archives of Physical Medicine and Rehabilitation, 90*, 1948–1952. https://doi.org/10.1016/j.apmr.2009.05.021	14, 15, 16, 21, 27
Lawton IADL Scale	Questionnaire	Activity, Participation	Assessment of independence in IADLs. Identifies how a person is functioning at the present time and their improvement or deterioration over time.	Lawton, M. P., & Brody, E. M. (1969). Assessment of older people: Self-maintaining and instrumental activities of daily living. *Gerontologist, 9*(3), 179-186. Access: https://www.alz.org/careplanning/downloads/lawton-iadl.pdf	15, 16, 21, 23
Loewenstein Occupational Therapy Assessment Geriatric Version (LOTCA-G)	Performance-based	Body Functions	Assesses cognitive skills related to everyday function including orientation, memory, visual perceptual skills, praxis, visuomotor organization, and thinking operations.	Katz, N., Elazar, B., & Itzkovich, M. (1995). Construct validity of a geriatric version of the Loewenstein Occupational Therapy Cognitive Assessment (LOTCA) Battery. *Physical & Occupational Therapy in Geriatrics, 13*(3), 31-46. https://doi.org/10.1080/J148v13n03_03	21
Mini Nutritional Assessment (MNA)	Questionnaire	Body Function	A screen of the nutritional status, addressing food intake, weight loss, mobility, psychological status, and either body mass index (BMI) or calf circumference.	Kaiser, M. J., Bauer, J. M., Ramsch, C., Uter, W., Guigoz, Y., Cederholm, T., Thomas, D. R., Anthony, P., Charton, K. E., Maggio, M., Tsai, A. C., Grathwohl, D., Vellas, B., & Sieber, C. C. (2009). Validation of the Mini Nutritional Assessment Short-Form (MNA®-SF): A practical tool for identification of nutritional status. *JNHA-The Journal of Nutrition, Health and Aging, 13*(9), 782-788. https://doi.org/10.1007/s12603-009-0214-7	7
Mini-Mental Status Examination (MMSE)	Performance-based questionnaire	Body Function	Screening for cognitive abilities	Folstein, M. F., Folstein, S. E., & McHugh, P. R. (1975). "Mini-mental state": A practical method for grading the cognitive state of patients for the clinician. *Journal of Psychiatric Research, 12*(3), 189-198. https://doi.org/10.1016/0022-3956(75)90026-6	2, 9, 10, 16, 27

Continued

APPENDIX B ■ Index of Assessments

NAME	FORMAT	ICF DOMAIN	PURPOSE	SOURCE	CHAPTER
Montreal Cognitive Assessment (MoCA)	Performance-based	Body Function	Screening for cognitive abilities; sensitive for mild cognitive impairment	Nasreddine, Z. S., Phillips, N. A., Bédirian, V., Charbonneau, S., Whitehead, V., Collin, I., Cummings, J. L., & Chertkow, H. (2005). The Montreal Cognitive Assessment, MoCA: A brief screening tool for mild cognitive impairment. *Journal of the American Geriatrics Society, 53*, 695–699. https://doi.org/10.1111/j.1532-5415.2005.53221.x Get certified: https://mocacognition.com/	2, 10, 16, 19, 21, 23, 27
Multi-Direction Reach Test (MDRT)	Performance-based	Body Function	Assesses a person's limits of stability when reaching in four different directions, one at a time.	Newton, R. A. (2001). Validity of the Multi-Directional Reach Test: A practical measure for limits of stability in older adults. *The Journals of Gerontology: Series A, 56*(4), 248–252. https://doi.org/10.1093/gerona/56.4.M248 Access: https://www.sralab.org/rehabilitation-measures/multidirectional-reach-test-reach-four-directions-test	7, 12
Occupation Centered Intervention Assessment (OCIA)	Questionnaire	Participation	Assessment to assist therapists in developing interventions by addressing the occupation's contextual, occupational, and personal relevance in the home environment	Jewell, V. L., Wienkes, T. D., & Pickens, N. (2022). *The Occupation-Centered Intervention Assessment (OCIA)*. AOTA Press. https://myaota.aota.org/shop_aota/product/900622U	27, 29
Physical Activity Scale for the Elderly (PASE)	Questionnaire	Activity, Participation	Assesses an adult's participation with household, occupational, and leisure activities	Washburn, R. A., Smith, K. W., Jette, A. M., & Janney, C. A. (1993). The physical activity scale for the elderly (PASE): Development and evaluation. *Journal of Clinical Epidemiology, 46*(2), 153–162. https://doi.org/10.1016/0895-4356(93)90053-4	16, 21
Rapid Geriatric Assessment (RGA)	Questionnaire and performance-based	Body Function, Activity	Screens for cognitive impairments, frailty, muscle loss, and functional mobility in older adults	Little, M. O. (2017). The Rapid Geriatric Assessment: A quick screen for geriatric syndromes. *Missouri medicine, 114*(2), 101–104. https://www.ncbi.nlm.nih.gov/pmc/articles/PMC6140035/pdf/ms114_p0101.pdf	16, 21
Safety Assessment of Function and Environment for Rehabilitation Health Outcome Measurement and Evaluation Version 3 (SAFER-HOME)	Performance-based and environmental observation	Participation, Environmental Factors	Assesses ability to safely carry out their occupations in their home and can be used as an outcome measure to assess effectiveness of occupational therapy interventions in the home.	Chiu, T., Oliver, R., Ascott, P., Choo, L., Davis, T., Gara, A., Goldsilver, P., McWhirter, M., & Letts, L. (2011). *SAFER-HOME manual: Safety Assessment of Function and the Environment for Rehabilitation. Health Outcome Measurement and Evaluation* (4th ed.). VHA Home Healthcare.	15, 21
Sit to Stand	Performance-based	Activity	Assessment of lower body strength necessary for transfers and functional mobility	Csuka, M., & McCarty, D. J. (1985). Simple method for measurement of lower extremity muscle strength. *American Journal of Medicine, 78*, 77–81. http://dx.doi.org/10.1016/0002-9343(85)90465-6. Access: https://www.sralab.org/rehabilitation-measures/five-times-sit-stand-test	11
Six-Minute Walk Test (6MWT)	Performance-based	Activity	Measures functional mobility and activity tolerance to indicate overall physical performance and functional mobility	Butland, R. J., Pang, J., Gross, E. R., Woodcock, A. A., & Geddes, D. M. (1982). Two-, six-, and 12-minute walking tests in respiratory disease. *British Medical Journal (Clinical Research Ed.), 284*(6329), 1607–1608. https://doi.org/10.1136/bmj.284.6329.1607	16, 21

APPENDIX B ■ Index of Assessments 533

Assessment	Type	Domain[a]	Description	Reference	Chapter
Sock Test for Sitting Balance	Performance-based	Activity	Assesses a person's unsupported sitting balance during ADL performance of donning a slipper sock.	Franc, I. A., Baxter, M. F., Mitchell, K., Neville, M., & Chang, P. F. (2020). Validity of the Sock Test for Sitting Balance: A Functional Sitting Balance Assessment. *OTJR: Occupation, Participation and Health*, 40(3), 159-165. https://doi.org/10.1177/1539449220905807	7
Timed Up and Go (TUG)	Performance-Based	Activity	Assesses older adults walking ability and balance	Podsiadlo, D., & Richardson, S. (1991). The timed "up and go": A test of basic functional mobility. *Journal of the American Geriatrics Society*, 39, 142–148. https://doi.org/10.1111/j.1532-5415.1991.tb01616.x	16, 21, 27
Tinetti Balance and Gait Test	Performance-Based	Body Function	Assesses standing balance and gait.	Tinetti, M. E., Williams, T. F., & Mayewski, R. (1986). Fall risk index for elderly patients based on number of chronic disabilities. *The American journal of medicine*, 80(3), 429–434. https://doi.org/10.1016/0002-9343(86)90717-5	7
Tinetti Performance Oriented Mobility Assessment (Tinetti POMA)	Performance-based	Activity	Measures fall-risk, gait, and balance	Tinetti, M. E. (1986). Performance-Oriented Assessment of Mobility Problems in elderly patients. *Journal of the American Geriatrics Society (JAGS)*, 34(2), 119-126. https://doi.org/10.1111/j.1532-5415.1986.tb05480.x	7, 16, 21
Well-being of Older People Measure (WOOP)	Questionnaire	Participation	Assessment captures a comprehensive set of well-being domains through self-report	Hackert, M., van Exel, J., & Brouwer, W. (2021). Content validation of the Well-being of Older People measure (WOOP). *Health and quality of life outcomes*, 19(1). https://doi.org/10.1186/s12955-021-01834-5	16
Westmead Home Safety Assessment (WeHSA)	Questionnaire	Participation, Environmental Factors	Assessment to identify fall hazards in the home environment.	Clemson, L., Fitzgerald, M., & Heard, R. (1999). Content validity of an assessment tool to identify home fall hazards: the Westmead Home Safety Assessment. *British Journal of Occupational Therapy*, 62(4), 171-179. https://doi.org/10.1177/030802269906200407	15

Note: [a] Domain determined through ICF taxonomy definitions https://icd.who.int/dev11/l-icf/en

GLOSSARY

Activities of daily living (ADL): Routine activities used to take care of one's own body. ADL activities identified by AOTA (2020) include bathing, showering, toileting, dressing, eating, swallowing, feeding, functional mobility, personal hygiene and grooming, and sexual activity.

Acute care: Level of health care in which a patient is treated for an often brief but severe episode of illness, for conditions that are the result of disease or trauma, and during recovery from surgery. Acute care is generally provided in a hospital by a variety of clinical personnel using technical equipment, pharmaceuticals, and medical supplies.

Advance care planning: A process of planning to meet future medical needs. This process may include advance care directives, end-of-life care wishes, and designating a health care power of attorney. A person indicates their values, goals, and preferences in regard to health care decisions in advance care directives.

Age-related macular degeneration (AMD): Retinal atrophy and scarring, along with hemorrhages in the macula, resulting in a gradual loss of the central field of vision.

Ageism: A process of systematic stereotyping or discrimination against people because of their age (Levy et al., 2020).

Ageusia: Absence of taste.

Aging in place: Aging in place is a term used to describe a person living in the residence of their choice for as long as they are able as they age. It also means that the older person has the services and things they need in their daily life so that aging in place is feasible. The goal is to maintain or improve their quality of life.

Alternating attention: The ability to direct or switch attentional resources between two or more tasks or activities.

Ambivalent: The simultaneous existence of contradictory feelings and attitudes toward the same person, object, event, or situation (American Psychological Association, n.d.a.).

Anosmia: Lack of smell.

Artificial intelligence (AI): "Artificial intelligence (AI) is a wide-ranging tool that enables people to rethink how we integrate information, analyze data, and use the resulting insights to improve decision making—and already it is transforming every walk of life." (West & Allen, 2018).

Assistive technology: An umbrella term covering the systems and services related to the delivery of assistive products and services. AT supports independence and function to live dignified lives and have a sense of personal wellbeing (WHO, 2022).

Atrial fibrillation: an irregular cardiac rhythm associated with very rapid heartbeat that can lead to blood clots forming in the heart.

Attention: The ability to focus on stimuli for the purpose of processing information.

Bradykinesia: Abnormal slowness in the execution of voluntary movements (APA, 2022).

Bridge employment: Changing jobs and moving to part-time employment is also common as a transition to retirement.

Caregiver-centered care: A collaborative working relationship between families and health care providers, with providers supporting family caregivers in their caregiving responsibilities.

Co-occupation: Occupations that can only exist when two or more individuals are part of the process.

Cognitive reserve: The amount of cognitive resources left over and available after an individual engages in a task.

Community mobility: Planning and moving around in the community using public or private transportation, such as driving, walking, bicycling, or accessing and riding in buses, taxi cabs, rideshares, or other transportation systems.

Comprehensive geriatric assessment (CGA): 'a multi-dimensional, multidisciplinary process which identifies medical, social and functional needs, and the development of an integrat-ed/co-ordinated care plan to meet those needs' (p. 150, Parker et al., 2018).

Conductive hearing loss: Block of acoustic energy that prevents the conduction of sound to the inner ear.

Confined to home: One of the Medicare requirements for a patient to receive home health services; it is a taxing and considerable effort to leave home.

Crepitus: A grating sound or sensation produced by friction between bone and cartilage or the fractured parts of a bone.

Crystallized intelligence: The accumulation of knowledge, experience, and acculturation that is highly representative of individual differences.

Cultural competency: Inferred mastery of knowledge about identified cultural groups (Hughes et al., 2020). Such knowledge, often presented in cultural competency training programs, is thought to help practitioners provide better services for members of these cultural groups; however, there is lack of evidence to substantiate whether cultural competency training programs foster better service (Lekas et al., 2020).

Cultural humility: "The ability to have a humble and other-oriented approach to others' cultures" (Rullo et al., 2022, p. 169). The practitioner recognizes the client as the expert of their own culture, commits to reflect on how personal biases may affect care provision, and acknowledges power imbalances (Bernstein & Gukasyan, 2019).

Culture: A construct composed of the shared languages, customs, beliefs, rules, arts, knowledge, and identities and memories of a group. These elements form a "collective agreement to the rules and norms that allow us to cooperate, function as a society, and live together..." (Cole, 2019, "Why Culture Matters to Sociologists" section).

Custodial care: Refers to a type a long-term care that does not include skilled rehabilitation, but instead includes any "nonmedical care that can reasonably and safely be provided by nonlicensed caregivers," such as a nursing assistant. (CMS, n.d.-c).

Cytokines: A protein made by immune and non-immune cells which also effect the immune system by either stimulating or slowing down the immune system.

Dehydration: A body state characterized by fluid usage (loss) that exceeds fluid intake; there is not enough water to carry out normal body functions such as respiration, neural conduction, gastrointestinal function, etc. This may result from emesis, sweating, or low fluid consumption. Dehydration is reversible but there is a point when it is nonreversible and death occurs.

Delirium: Acute change in cognition and a disturbance of consciousness, usually resulting from an underlying medical condition

Descriptive assessments: Assessments used to identify issues that merit intervention; to determine specific problems in the areas of impairment, activity limitation, and participation restriction; and to help determine the need for therapeutic services.

Diabetic retinopathy: Damage to the blood vessels of the retina due to diabetes.

Discriminative assessments: Assessments that provide a method for the practitioner to identify difficulties in performance by comparing a person's level of dysfunction in relation to expectations of performance of other healthy people of that age.

Disuse atrophy: Muscle atrophy that occurs with lack of physical activity.

Divided attention: The ability to allocate attentional resources to two or more tasks or activities at the same time.

Driving performance: Operating a moving motor vehicle under the categories of general and blind spot observation, indication, braking-acceleration, lane positioning, gap selection, and approach.

Driving safety: Having the physical, sensory, visual-perceptual, and cognitive skills critical for driving and safely operating a motor vehicle.

Dyslipidemia: Imbalance between lipids in the bloodstream such as cholesterol, low density lipoprotein cholesterol, triglycerides, and high density lipoprotein cholesterol.

Early mobility: A systematic approach to encouraging patients to be out of bed and engaging in early movement as soon as they are deemed medically stable.

eHealth literacy: The ability to seek, appraise and understand health information from electronic sources and apply the knowledge to solve problems related to one's health.

Elder abuse: Actions causing physical, psychological, emotional, or financial harm or neglect to an older adult. (See Box 6.1 for different forms of elder abuse).

End-of-life care: Support for people who are in the last months or years of their life. End-of-life care should help people to live as well as possible until they die. Wishes and preferences are considered and taking into account when planning the care (NHS, 2017).

Enhanced activities of daily living (EADLs): Activities related to the use and management of electronic devices in daily life, including leisure activities and technology used for daily activities of daily living.

Epigenetics: The scientific exploration of how behavioral, social, and environmental factors impact genetic expression and change.

Episodic memory: The memory of past events including the people present, date and time, location, and general recall of things said and done during the episode.

Ergonomics: The study of humans, objects, or machines and the interactions among them.

Ethical dilemma: A conflict between two (or more) ethical principles in which the practitioner must choose to honor one principle over another.

Ethical issue: A problem or concern relating to ethical principles and standards necessitating that the practitioner chooses a course of action that provides the most care or benefit and the least amount of harm to a client.

Ethical problem: A situation involving one or more issues that have ethical principles in question. Ethical problems require deliberation and evaluation in order to reach a resolution.

Evaluative assessments: Assessments that evaluate outcomes or changes in persons after they have received rehabilitation services. They include items that are responsive to change in individuals when change occurs.

Executive functioning: Refers to higher-order cognitive processes such as reasoning, decision-making, problem-solving, judgment, abstract thought, cognitive flexibility, initiation, and inhibition.

Explicit bias: Conscious attitudes and beliefs we have about people (*Explicit Bias Explained*, n.d.).

Explicit processing: Intentional, occurs with awareness, and is effortful, requiring moderate to substantial cognitive resources.

Fall: An unintentional landing of the body on a lower surface, with or without injury is a fall (e.g., floor, ground or another lower surface). Mechanical falls involve an external object or force that precipitated the fall, whereas nonmechanical falls are due to body structure and body function issues (e.g., weak muscle and brittle frail bones or pain and orthostatic hypotension).

Families of choice: Family support networks that include but are not limited to partners, friends, and other non-related or legally recognized loved ones.

Family caregiver: Includes children, partner, home caregiver, relatives, friends, or other support person designated by the older adult care recipient.

Fitness to drive: The ability to drive safely by managing complications caused by physical ability, injury, mental health condition, or medications.

Flow: A psychological state in which the person experiences enjoyment, immersion, and concentration from an activity.

Fluid intelligence: The ability to use abstract reasoning, flexibly shift one's mental set, and initiate and complete purposeful action.

Frailty: Frailty is a geriatric syndrome characterized by multisystem dysregulation and decreased physiological reserve. It is identified through a screen such as Fried's Frailty Phenotype, where a person has at least three of five outcomes: diminished strength, slowness, low physical activity, self-reported exhaustion, and unintentional weight loss (Travers et al., 2019).

Functional cognition: Described as the cognitive ability to perform basic (BADL) and instrumental activities of daily living (IADL) incorporating attention, memory, executive functions, and areas of processing.

Gender identity: One's innermost concept of self as male, female, a blend of both or neither – how individuals perceive themselves and what they call themselves. One's gender identity can be the same or different from their sex assigned at birth (Wamsley, 2021).

Geriatric syndromes: Multifactorial conditions prevalent in older adults. Geriatric syndromes are important indicators for adverse outcomes and functional decline, both during the hospitalization as well as post discharge.

Geriatrician: A physician who is specialized in care of the older adults.

Gerontology: The scholarly and scientific exploration of aging and old age.

Glaucoma: A group of diseases characterized by progressive optic nerve damage.

Grief: Grief is a common and universal reaction to a loss and can be defined as a psychological and physical reaction, which may cause emotional, cognitive, behavioral, and somatic symptoms (Shear, 2015).

Health: "A state of complete physical, mental and social well-being and not merely the absence of disease or infirmity" (WHO, 2023, para 1).

Health coaching (HC): Patient oriented and encourages patients to change their behaviors by examining choices and barriers to help facilitate positive changes to improve their health (Kivela et al., 2014).

Health coaching: Health coaching partners with people through behavioral, individualized, evidence-based support to help manage chronic health conditions (Vanderbilt University Medical Center, 2023).

Health education: "Any combination of evidence-based/evidence-informed practices are used to provide equitable opportunities for the acquisition of knowledge, attitudes, and skills that are needed to adapt, adopt, and maintain healthy behaviors" (Videto & Dennis, 2021, p. 11).

Health management: Engagement in occupations and routines related to promoting or maintaining one's health and wellness, such as physical activity, nutrition, medication management, condition management or communication with the health care system.

Health promotion: The process of enabling people, individually and collectively, to increase control over the determinants of health and thereby improve their health" (WHO, 2021, p. 4).

Heart blocks: Occur when then electrical signals from the atriums do not conduct effectively with the ventricles; there are associated with 4 types (first-degree, second-degree Wenckebach, classic second-degree, and third-degree).

Homeostatic hydration: A balanced proportion and amount of water and electrolytes that are readily available for bodily needs and processes.

Hospice: Hospice is perceived as a care system provided by an interdisciplinary team in residential facilities, such as nursing homes, private and public residences or inpatient hospice settings. Hospice care is the most comprehensive interdisciplinary care system available to patients, families, and caregivers of persons living with a life-limiting illness.

Hyperglycemia: An excess of blood glucose in the bloodstream.

Hyperinsulinemia: Excess levels of insulin in the blood relative to glucose which is higher than what is expected or normal.

Hypertrophy: The enlargement of an organ or tissue due to increased cell size.

Implicit Bias: Subconscious attitudes and beliefs we have about people (Bernstein & Gukasyan, 2019).

Implicit processing: Unintentional, occurs without awareness, and is effortless, requiring minimal cognitive resources.

Instrumental activities of daily living (IADL): Higher level living skills necessary for self-care and living in the community. IADL activities identified by AOTA (2020) include care of others, care of pets and animals, child rearing, communication management, driving and community mobility, financial management, home establishment and management, meal preparation and cleanup, religious and spiritual expression, safety and emergency maintenance, and shopping.

Intensive care unit (ICU): a department of a hospital in which patients who are dangerously ill are kept under constant observation. Specialized medical and nursing staff provide critical care and enhanced constant medical monitoring for organ support to sustain life.

Intention tremor: The trembling of a body part that arises near the conclusion of a directed, voluntary movement, such as touching a finger to one's nose (APA, 2022).

Intersectionality: The intersection of a person's identities across different spheres of life that "incorporates the vast array of cultural, structural, sociobiological, economic, and social contexts by which individuals are shaped and with which they identify" (APA, 2017, p.19).

Joint protection strategies: Self-management strategies that maintain function and prevent further degradation of a joint by modifying work strategies and movement patterns of the affected joint; often utilized by individuals with OA.

Legal blindness: (1) Visual acuity of 20/200 or less in the better eye after best possible standard correction or (2) a visual field of no greater than 20 degrees in the better eye.

Leisure: Discretionary time spent in nonobligatory activities which are free from the pressure to be productive and are intrinsically motivating.

Leisure motivation: The need to be involved in leisure activities, which is underlied by strong psychological and sociological underpinnings (e.g., cultural norms, social environment, etc.) which influence a person's desire to participate in and decisions around leisure activities.

Life course perspective: Explicitly dynamic, focusing on the life cycle in its entirety while allowing for deviations in trajectories.

Life expectancy: A mathematical construct capturing the estimate of average age at which a person from a particular population category will die and is influenced by such realities as war, poverty, and disease.

Life span: The maximum years a human body can live, around 120 years.

Long-term care services: "Long-term care involves a variety of services designed to meet a person's health or personal care needs during a short of long period of time. These services help people live as independently and safely as possible when they can no longer perform everyday activities on their own." (National Institute on Aging, 2017).

Low vision: An untreatable loss of sight that is not correctable with standard eyeglasses and interferes with the functioning of the individual.

Maintenance model: A rehabilitation program that is designed to preserve health. This could be maintain progress after intensive rehabilitation or preventing decline in function.

Meaning: "What we create for ourselves in our mind that explains experiences and, in turn, motivates us and spurs us on to create new experiences" (Polatajko, Backman, et al., 2013, p. 61).

Metabolic equivalent (MET): A concept that represents a simple procedure for associating energy expenditure with physical activities.

Micronutrient-related malnutrition: Either deficiencies or excesses of vitamins and minerals; often a result of the aging process when breakdown, absorption, and excretion is impeded (e.g., low vitamin B_{12} due to diminished stomach acid breaking it down for absorption) (WHO, 2021).

Minimum data set (MDS): "A standardized, comprehensive assessment of an adult's functional, medical, psychosocial, and cognitive status. It is commonly used in long-term care facilities and outpatient and home-based social service program for older adults." (American Psychological Association, 2011).

Moral distress: The emotional experience of psychological distress that occurs in response to an event or situation that has moral implications.

Moral injury: The cumulative experience of moral distress, resulting in a reduced capacity to manage moral distress in the future.

Narrative ethics: Consideration of the person's life story as a means of ethical decision making.

Neuroplasticity: Neural and synaptic change and/or growth following new learning, experience, or recovery from injury.

Nonstandardized assessments: Assessments that include interviews, observations, and performance testing in which there are no set procedures for administration and/or scoring.

Nuclear family: A family unit that comprises a mother, father, and dependent children.

Occupational deprivation: Prelusion from engagement in occupations of necessity and/or meaning due to factors that stand outside of the immediate control of the person.

Organizational health literacy: The degree to which organizations enable individuals to obtain, interpret, and use information to make appropriate health-related decisions.

Osteoarthritis: Degeneration of joint cartilage and the underlying bone causing pain and stiffness.

Osteoporosis: A skeletal disorder characterized by compromised bone strength, predisposing a person to increased risk of fracture.

Osteoporosis: A disease process where the bones thin and become brittle and fragile leading to fractures after experiencing very little force or rotation.

Outcome and assessment information set (OASIS): Group of standard data elements that are designed to allow systematic comparison of measurement of a patient's status at two time points.

Oxidative stress: An imbalance between the free radicals and antioxidants in the body.

Palliative care: According to the World Health Organization (WHO) palliative care is an approach that aims to improve patients' and their families' quality of life by addressing the problems they face when living a life-threatening illness, such as physical, psychosocial and spiritual aspects of life.

Palliative occupational therapy: The main goal of occupational therapy in palliative care is to enable engagement in meaningful occupation despite illness or dysfunction, and to maintain functions and occupational roles of daily living that are perceived to be important by the individual. The interventions are often using an adaptive approach.

Patient navigation: Embraces the concept of interaction between the community and the health-care system highlighted in the ECCM. For successful patient navigation, OTPs need to maintain a current inventory of available community resources that can be used to help older adults identify and access services. They also need to support an older adult, as part of self-management principles, to select and follow up with resources that they perceive to be of value to their functional status.

Patient-driven groupings model (PDGM): The reimbursement model for home health services that began on January 1, 2020. Removed the emphasis on the number (quantity) of visits and replaced it with a focus on quality of care.

Personal health literacy: "The degree to which individuals have the ability to find, understand, and use information and services to inform health-related decisions and actions for themselves and others" (U.S. DHHS, Office of Disease Prevention and Health Promotion, 2022).

Personal health literacy: An individual's ability to obtain, interpret, and use information to make appropriate decisions regarding health.

Pharmacodynamics: How a drug affects or influences the body (Ruscin & Linnebur, 2021b).

Pharmacokinetics: How the body processes a drug; includes absorption, metabolism, distribution, and elimination of a drug (Ruscin & Linnebur, 2022).

Phased retirement: Employees stay with the same employer while gradually reducing work hours and effort.

Physiatrist: A physician who specializes in rehabilitation care.

Pneumonia: An infection in the lungs that causes inflammation that can either be viral or bacterial in nature.

Pneumothorax: A collection of air or gas in the pleural cavity that results in a partially collapsed or collapsed lung.

Population health: A concept of health characterized by both objective and subjective determinants and health outcomes of a population.

Postural stability: A tendency to fall or the inability to keep oneself from falling; imbalance (Apeadu & Gupta, 2020).

Postural sway: The unconscious, small movements that happen around the body's center of gravity in order to maintain balance. It is your body's natural adaptation to changing stimuli.

Predictive assessments: Assessments that support the ability to predict functional outcomes for clients based on their patterns of needs and strengths.

Presbycusis: Age-related hearing loss; a typical degradation of the hearing sensory system associated with age.

Presbyopia: An age-related refractive error leading to difficulty clearly focusing on objects up close.

Primary care: "A key process in the health system that support first-contact, accessible, continued, comprehensive and coordinated patient-focused care (UNICEF, 2020, XIII)."

Primary health care: "A whole-of-society approach to health that aims to maximize the level and distribution of health and well-being through three components: (a) primary care and essential public health functions as the core of integrated health services; (b) multisectoral policy and action; and (c) empowered people and communities (UNICEF, 2020, XIII)."

Procedural or nondeclarative memory: A nonverbal-based memory system that stores information for motor-based skills and behaviors (i.e., muscle memory), habits, emotional associations, priming, and classical conditioning.

Pronouns: Pronouns are the words people should use when they are referring to you, but not using your name. Examples of pronouns are she/her/hers, he/him/his, and they/them/theirs (Wamsley, 2021).

Prospective memory: Enables individuals to remember future-oriented or scheduled tasks without the use of external memory aids (e.g., written note or list).

Pulmonary embolism: Occurs when a blood clot or other foreign material occludes an artery within pulmonary circulation.

Pulmonary fibrosis: Lung disease with associated scarring and damage to the lung tissue which impedes the lungs ability to work properly.

Quality of life: Satisfaction with circumstances and health, as well as concrete markers of economic and social well-being.

Reciprocity: The quality of an act, process, or relationship in which one person receives benefits from another and, in return, provides an equivalent benefit (American Psychological Association, n.d.b.).

Religious occupations: Occupations undertaken in association with formally constituted religious organizations, such as churches, mosques, or synagogues.

Residual volume: The amount of air remaining in the lungs after an individual fully exhales.

Respite care: Temporary or short-term relief from being a primary caregiver.

Resting tremor: A trembling that occurs when the affected body part is at rest (APA, 2022).

Restorative care: A "philosophy of care that emphasizes the evaluation of residents' underlying capabilities with regard to function and helping them to optimize and maintain functional abilities" often provided by nonlicensed medical staff such as a nursing assistant (Talley et al., 2015, p. S89).

Restorative: Rehabilitation that focuses on maximizing abilities.

Rigidity: Inability of the muscles to relax normally. The condition can affect any of the muscles in the body, causing sharp pain that makes it difficult to move (APA2022).

Sarcopenia: Loss of muscle mass associated with aging.

Sarcopenic obesity: A condition characterized by low muscle mass combined with high fat mass.

Section GG: A functional scoring system that is used in post-acute settings, such as home health.

Selective attention: The ability to direct attentional resources to a task or activity while simultaneously directing attentional resources to ignore distracting information.

Self-care: Taking action to support personal physical, mental, and psychological health.

Semantic memory: The knowledge of language including words, phrases, definitions, and grammar.

Senescence: Biological deterioration of cells with age.

Sensory memory: The processing of information through the vestibular, visual, auditory, and tactile systems.

Shared decision making: A process in which the client, client's family, and the health care team collaborate and share in the decision-making process on treatment and care.

Short-term memory: Can take on two forms. The first is new information reliant on sensory inputs, thought to be limited to about seven pieces of information; the second form is memories that have been stored and retrieved through cueing such as smelling an odor and recalling a feeling or conversation.

Skilled care: "Skilled care is nursing and therapy care that can only be safely and effectively performed by, or under the supervision of, professionals or technical personnel. It's health care given when you need skilled nursing or skilled therapy to treat, manage, and observe your condition, and evaluate your care" (Centers for Medicare and Medicaid Services, n.d.-c).

Sleep hygiene: Lifestyle modifications to improve sleep.

Social determinants of health: "Nonmedical factors that influence health outcomes. They are conditions in which people are born, grow, live, and age, and the wider set of forces shaping the conditions of daily life" (WHO, 2022b, para 1).

Social support: Social support is an individual's perception and reality of having the level of family, friend, neighbors, organizations, etc. needed to live and for quality of life. It can include many types of support such as emotional, informational, and tangible such as financial support, among others.

Spiritual occupations: Occupations identified as connecting individuals to a higher power.

Standardized assessments: Assessments that have published procedures for administering and scoring, along with psychometric studies to support the use of the assessment.

Start of care: The first billable home health visit when services are initiated. The initial assessment must be performed within 48 hours of referral, within 48 hours of patient's return home, or on a physician-ordered start of care date Includes the start of the comprehensive assessment.

Sternotomy: A surgical procedure that allows access to the heart and nearby organs with an incision being made vertically along the sternum.

Subjective well-being: A feeling that current circumstances are positive.

Sustained (or focused) attention: The ability to direct attentional resources to a single task or activity, such as reading a book.

Telehealth: Defined by the World Federation of Occupational Therapists (2014) as "the use of information and communication technologies (ICT) to deliver health-related services when the provider and patient are in different physical locations (p. 37)." Telehealth may also be used interchangeably with telemedicine, telerehabilitation and telepractice (WFOT, 2014).

Telerehabilitation: Provision of rehabilitative care remotely by means of a variety of telecommunication tools, including telephones, mobile wireless devices, and computers.

Urinary tract infection: An infection of any part of the urinary system—the kidneys, ureters, bladder, and urethra (Mayo Clinic, 2021a).

Virtual care: An umbrella terms for remote delivery of services including synchronous and asynchronous telehealth and remote patient monitoring (Dunning & Servat, 2022).

Wellness: The active pursuit of activities, choices and lifestyles that lead to a state of holistic health (GWI, n.d.).

Wisdom: Typically reflects knowledge gained through experience, the ability to understand what others may not, and good sense or judgment.

Working memory: Not only demands attention like short term memory, but it also requires intentional use of strategies to manipulate, store, and maintain information.

Xerosis: Dry skin.

Xerostomia: Dry mouth (Xu et al., 2018).

Index

Page numbers followed by "f" denote figures and "t" denote tables.

A

A Matter of Balance: Managing Concerns About Falls, 117
Abandonment, 86t
Abdominal adiposity, 129
Ableism, 10
Abuse. *See* Elder abuse and neglect
Acceptance and Commitment Therapy (ACT), 411
ACE inhibitors, 152b
Action tremor, 221t
Active aging, 327
Active living, 395
Activities of daily living (ADLs)
  assessment of, 156b, 271–272, 374, 409, 472t
  balance as necessary for completing, 225
  basic, 241, 247, 254, 452–454, 460
  bathroom modifications, 273, 273f
  in cardiopulmonary conditions, 159
  in cardiovascular conditions, 159
  classification of, 264
  cognitive loss effects on performance of, 476
  dementia effects on, 268
  difficulties in performing, prevalence of, 370
  dressing area modifications, 273
  in end-of-life care, 484
  enhanced, 318
  environmental modifications for, 273, 273f
  instrumental. *See* Instrumental activities of daily living (IADLs)
  interventions for, 272–274
  limitations of, prevalence of, 266–267
  musculoskeletal system functioning for, 188
  in palliative care, 487–488
  personal, 487–488
  retraining, 159, 198
  as self-care activities, 264
  skill training for, 272–273
  stroke effects on, 267
  task modifications for, 274
  technology for monitoring of, 510
  vision impairment effects on, 268
Activities-specific Balance Confidence (ABC) Scale, 375
Activity, 42
Activity analysis, 103, 512
Activity Card Sort, 376
Activity limitations, 42
Activity theory, 313–314
Activity tolerance, 156b
Acute care
  advocacy for patient in, 431
  cognitive impairment in, 427–428
  cognitive interventions in, 428, 429f
  communication in, 421–422
  definition of, 419–429
  delirium in, 428
  description of, 157b
  discharge planning, 424
  documentation of, 429–430
  early activity, 424–425
  early mobility, 424–425
  evaluation in, 422–423
  fall prevention in, 425
  home-based, 508
  in ICU setting, 419
  interprofessional integrated care, 420–421
  intervention in, 431
  joint protection, 426–427
  occupational therapists in, 419–422, 424
  occupational therapy in, 419–423
  pain management in, 425–426
  payment systems for, 430
  range of motion in, 426
  reimbursement for, 430
  skilled occupation-centered interventions in, 430
  skin protection, 426–427
  visual impairment in, 427
Acute coronary syndrome (ACS), 151
Acute respiratory distress syndrome (ARDS), 153–154, 424
Adaptation, 224, 391, 492
ADED. *See* Association for Driver Rehabilitation Specialists
A-delta fibers, 181
Adherence
  definition of, 442
  medication, 102–103, 127, 296
  motivation versus, 442
ADL Staircase, 374
Administration on Aging (AOA), 387
Adult day centers, 385–386
Adult day-care programs, 440
Advance care planning, 83, 498
Advance directives, 83, 83t
Advocacy
  acute care, 431
  community mobility, 349–350
  community-based wellness services, 396
  description of, 302–303
  home health, 462–463
  long-term care services, 478–479
  micro-level, 446
  palliative care, 498–499
  primary care, 412–413
  rehabilitation, 446–447
Affordable Care Act, 396, 446
Age Discrimination Act of 1975, 81, 81t
Age Discrimination in Employment Act (ADEA), 81, 81t
Age in place, 8, 30
Age stratification perspective, 41
Aged person, 36
Ageism
  benevolent, 54
  compassionate, 54
  COVID-19 pandemic effects on, 505
  description of, 9–10, 52–53
  digital, 54
  elder abuse and neglect, 88
  global nature of, 81
  healthcare affected by, 81–82
  laws that address, 81, 81t
  social determinants of health affected by, 80–81
  societal effects of, 81
  structural, 53–54
  surveys regarding, 80
Age-related erectile dysfunction (ARED), 71
Age-related macular degeneration (AMD), 169–170
Ageusia, 177
Aging
  active, 327
  activity theory of, 313–314
  attitudes about, 9–10
  auditory system affected by, 166t, 173–174
  biological changes associated with, 282
  body function changes associated with, 106
  bone loss associated with, 192
  brain changes associated with, 212, 243
  cancer and, 128b, 128–129
  cardiopulmonary system affected by, 148, 149t
  cardiovascular disease and, 125–128
  cardiovascular system affected by, 126b
  cognition and, 38–39, 238, 244
  cognitive processes affected by, 239t
  cognitive theories of, 243
  complexity of, 281–282
  context of, 4–7
  cultural factors that affect, 10, 52–53
  cultural perceptions of, 52–53
  dehydration and, 106
  demographic trend in, 10
  as developmental process, 36
  diabetes mellitus and, 129–130
  dietary habits affected by, 107
  ecological model of, 39, 40t
  economic influences on, 11–12
  environmental factors, 281–282
  factors that affect, 7–12, 281–282
  falls and, 112–117
  future of, 503–512
  gastrointestinal disorders and, 130
  gender factors that affect, 11–12
  genetic factors that affect, 11
  healthy, 63, 384, 504
  at home, 8
  hydration affected by, 105–109
  inflammatory markers associated with, 129
  intersectionality with, 52–53
  leisure and, 311
  medication effectiveness and adherence affected by, 102–103
  memory changes associated with, 240
  migration effects on, 9
  muscle mass affected by, 190–191
  muscle power affected by, 189, 190b
  muscle strength affected by, 189, 190b, 190f
  muscle structure affected by, 190–192, 191f
  musculoskeletal system changes, 188–195
  negative stereotypes of, 238, 505
  neuromotor system changes, 212–216
  nutrition affected by, 105–108
  olfactory sense affected by, 133, 176–177

541

oral health affected by, 104–105
pain and, 180–181
performance skill declines with, 23
personal factors that affect, 11
personality and, theories regarding, 38, 38t
physical environment effects on, 8–9
physical factors, 281–282
physiological changes associated with, 132
positive, 4, 12, 202, 264
as positive phenomenon, 9
process of, 36
psychology of, 37–38
public policy and, 10
pulmonary diseases and, 129
self-perceptions of, 82
sexuality affected by, 70–72, 71t
skin changes associated with, 179–180
sleep affected by, 135
social determinants of health and, 7f, 7–8
social factors, 281–282
sociocultural factors that affect, 9–10
socioeconomic factors that affect, 11
socioeconomic status and, 11
sociological theories of aging, 41–44, 42t
stereotypes of, 9–10
taste affected by, 166t, 176–177
temperature detection affected by, 179–180
theories of. *See* Theories of aging
trends in, 10
upper extremity movement affected by, 215
visual system changes, 166t, 167–168
Aging and Disability Resource Center (ADRC), 387
Aging in community, 30
Aging in place, 8–9, 29–30, 282, 337
Aging in Place and Accessibility Research Laboratories, 509
Aging in the right place, 40, 40t
Agrarian cultures, 5
Airways, 148
Akinesia, 221t
Allen Cognitive Level Screen-5, 376
Alternating attention, 238
Alveolar capillary wall, 149
Alzheimer disease
bipolar disorder and, 252
dementia caused by, 246, 248t
description of, 37, 39
sleep and, 299
visual impairments caused by, 171
Alzheimer disease and related dementias (ADRD), 72, 362
Alzheimer's Association, 247
Ambulatory care, 439
American Association of Retired Persons (AARP), 282, 328
American Automobile Association (AAA), 340
American Medical Association (AMA), 506
American Occupational Therapy Association (AOTA)
Code of Ethics, 80, 82–83, 90–91
home health advocacy by, 462–463
Occupational Therapy Practice Framework, 13
Practice Guidelines for Older Adults with Low Vision, 171
Standard of Practice for Occupational Therapy, 369–370
well-being as defined by, 384

American Spinal Injury Association Impairment Scale, 430
Americans with Disabilities Act (ADA), 329–330
AM-PAC Applied Cognitive Inpatient Short Form, 428
Amputation, 199–201
Amyotrophic lateral sclerosis (ALS), 217t, 232, 430
Angle-closure glaucoma (ACG), 170
Anosmia, 177
Anterior cerebral artery, 219t
Antibiotics, 154b
Antidepressants, 251
Anxiety disorders, 251
Aorta, 126b
Aortic valve replacement, 152b
Aphasia, 232
Appraisal support, 65
Apraxia, 216
Aquatic exercise, for osteoarthritis, 196
Area Agencies on Aging (AoA), 81
Aristotle, 20
Arm Activity Measure, 225
Arnadottir OT-ADL Neurobehavioral Evaluation (A-ONE), 271
Arousals from sleep, 135b
Arterial hypertension, 126
Arterial saturation, 161
Arthritis
instrumental activities of daily living affected by, 282
osteoarthritis, 195–197, 342
rheumatoid, 71, 268, 342
self-care affected by, 268
Artificial intelligence (AI), 509
Aspiration pneumonia, 232
Assessment(s). *See also specific assessment*
activities of daily living, 156b, 271–272, 374, 409
biases in, 372
descriptive, 370–371
evaluative, 371
functional mobility, 374–375
home health, 457–459
instrumental activities of daily living, 156b, 374, 409
predictive, 371
psychometric properties in, 371, 372t
theoretical models, 373–374
Assessment of Motor and Praxis Skills, 370
Assessment of Motor and Process Skills (AMPS), 13, 271, 285t, 371
Assessment of Occupational Functioning Modified Interest Checklist, 316
Assigned female at birth, 68t
Assigned male at birth, 68t
Assisted-living facilities, 452–453
Assistive listening devices (ALDs), 176, 177f
Assistive technology
definition of, 509
for home management, 287
in hospital, 429
for leisure participation, 318
low-tech, 509
resources, 510b
for retirement, 331
for self-care, 274
for work, 331

Association for Driver Rehabilitation Specialists, 343
Associative stage, of motor learning, 223
Astigmatism, 167
Ataxia, 217
Atchley's Stages of Retirement, 327, 327b
Atherosclerosis, 126
Atherosclerotic cardiovascular disease (ASCVD), 71
Atrial fibrillation, 136
Atrial systole, 147f
Attention, 238–239
Attitudes
about aging, 9–10, 12
education effects on, 10
negative, 9
positive, 9, 12
Audiogram, 173
Auditory system. *See also* Hearing; Hearing loss
age-related changes in, 166t, 173–174
pathological changes of, 175
Australia, 446
Autonomous stage, of motor learning, 223–224
Autonomy, 80, 90t

B

Baby Boomers, 5, 6t, 324, 504
Back-scratch test, 201
Balance
age-related changes in, 213–214
assessment of, 115–116, 225–227, 226t, 227b, 472t
cognitive demand and, 214b
interventions for, 228–229
physiology of, 214b
postural, 113
Ballistic stretching, 204
Barthel Index, 156b, 271, 409
Basal ganglia, 211, 215
Basic activities of daily living (BADLs), 241, 247, 254, 452–454, 460
Bathroom modifications, 273, 273f
Behavioral health
description of, 409
intervention approach, 411
in palliative care, 488
Behaviour Change Wheel, 136
Behind-the-ear (BTE) hearing aids, 176
Behind-the-wheel (BTW) assessment, 345–346
Beneficence, 80
Benevolent ageism, 54
Bereavement, 136, 490–491
Berg Balance Scale, 115
Beta blockers, 152b
Biases
cultural perceptions and, 57
explicit, 57
implicit, 54, 57
treatment affected by, 57
Bilevel positive airway pressure, 154b
Billing, ethics of, 82–83
Biological age, 128
Biological theories, of aging, 36–37, 37t
Bipolar disorder, 252
Black communities, systemic injustice against, 56
Bladder training, 112
Blindness, 169

Blood
	age-related changes to, 126b
	vasculature movement of, 147
Blood pressure, 127
Body functions, 42, 339
Body mass index (BMI), 195
Body structures
	assessment of, 226t
	description of, 42
Bone
	menopause-related loss of, 192
	remodeling of, 192–193
	trabecular, 192
	turnover rate for, 192
Bone density, 106
Bone health, 193
"Boomerang effect," 9
Borg CR10 Scale, 156b
Box and Block Test, 371
Braden Scale for Predicting Pressure Sore Risk, 180
Bradykinesia, 213, 221t
Brain
	age-related changes in, 212, 243
	magnetic resonance imaging of, 243
	stroke effects on, 216, 218f
	traumatic injury to, 220
Brain Injury Visual Assessment Battery for Adults, 172
Brain-derived neurotrophic factor, 253
Bridge employment, 326
Bristol Activities of Daily Living Scale, 271
British Pain Society, 498
Bronchitis, 129
Bronchodilators, 154b
Brown communities, systemic injustice against, 56
Burnout, caregiver, 89, 160, 361

C

C fibers, 181
Calcium-channel blockers, 152b
Canada
	healthcare system financing in, 446
	life expectancy in, 4
Canadian Model of Occupational Performance and Engagement (CMPO-E), 43, 373
Canadian Occupational Performance Measure (COPM), 13, 26, 133, 156b, 284, 316, 370–371, 376
Cancer
	aging and, 128b, 128–129
	caregiver care for, 362
	home-life intervention for, 492, 494, 494t
	lung, 153
	obesity as risk factor for, 128–129
Capillaries, 191
Cardiac cycle, 147f
Cardiac transplant, 152b
Cardiogenic shock, 152b
Cardiomyopathy, 151
Cardiopulmonary conditions
	acute respiratory distress syndrome, 153–154
	assessment of, 156b
	caregiver education about, 160
	chronic obstructive pulmonary disease, 129, 153
	client education about, 159
	diaphragmatic breathing for, 158
	dyspnea associated with, 158
	dyspnea-controlled postures for, 158
	energy conservation/work simplification for, 159–160
	interprofessional collaboration for, 161
	interstitial lung disease, 153
	lung cancer, 153
	nonsurgical interventions for, 154, 154b
	patient's response to activity/intervention for, monitoring of, 160–161
	practice frameworks for, 155–156
	psychosocial components associated with, 160
	pulmonary edema, 154
	pursed-lip breathing for, 158
	screening for, 156b
	surgical interventions for, 154, 154b
	treatment of, 156–161
Cardiopulmonary resuscitation (CPR), 84t
Cardiopulmonary system
	age-related changes, 148, 149t
	airways, 148
	alveolar capillary wall, 149
	chest wall, 149
	cycle of, 148f
	description of, 145–146
	intrinsic factors that affect, 149
	lung parenchyma, 148–149
	respiratory muscles, 149
Cardiovascular conditions
	assessment of, 156b
	cardiomyopathy, 151
	caregiver education about, 160
	client education about, 159
	congestive heart failure, 151
	coronary artery disease, 150–151
	diaphragmatic breathing for, 158
	dyspnea associated with, 158
	dyspnea-controlled postures for, 158
	energy conservation/work simplification for, 159–160
	functional impairment associated with, 152–153
	heart failure, 151
	hypertension. See Hypertension (HTN)
	interprofessional collaboration for, 161
	myocardial infarction, 151
	nonsurgical interventions for, 152, 152b
	patient's response to activity/intervention for, monitoring of, 160–161
	practice frameworks for, 155–156
	psychosocial components associated with, 160
	pursed-lip breathing for, 158
	surgical interventions for, 152, 152b
	treatment of, 156–161
Cardiovascular disease (CVD)
	aging and, 125–128
	depression and, 128
	description of, 267
	diabetes mellitus and, 126–127, 130
	hypertension and, 127, 127b
	mental health disorders and, 128
	noncommunicable disease deaths caused by, 123
	physical activity for prevention of, 134
Cardiovascular system
	age-related changes to, 126b, 134, 146–148, 148t
	anatomy of, 146, 147f
	cardiac cycle, 147f
	components of, 146, 147f
	description of, 145–146
	intrinsic factors that affect, 149
	smoking effects on, 126
	venous vasculature, 146
Care home, moving to, 30
Care of People with Dementia in their Environment (COPE), 249
Care partners
	problem-solving training for, 297
	training of, 288, 297
Caregiver Hospital Assessment Tool, 361
Caregiver-centered care, 361
Caregivers/caregiving. See also Family caregivers/caregiving
	burnout of, 89, 160, 361
	cancer care by, 362
	cardiopulmonary disease management by, 160
	cardiovascular disease management by, 160
	for chronic conditions, 362
	dementia care by, 248, 314
	depression in, 248
	education for, 160, 409
	in future, 511–512
	levels of prevention in, 359, 359f
	for life-limiting illness, 491
	robotics for assistance in, 511
	support of, 265, 377
Cartilage, 193, 193t
Case management, 444–445
Case managers, 332, 388t, 421, 444
Cataracts, 169
Cavities, 104–105
Cell senescence theory, 37, 37t
Centers for Disease and Control (CDC)
	aging in place as defined by, 8
	Stopping Elderly Accidents, Deaths and Injuries initiative, 113, 114f–115f
Centers for Medicaid and Medicare Services
	home care focus by, 508
	home health agencies and, 455, 458
	Hospitals Without Walls program, 508
	Outcome and Assessment Information Set, 458
Central auditory processing disorder, 175
Cerebellum, 211
Cerebral palsy (CP), 217t
Certified nurse assistants, 453
Certified therapeutic recreation specialists (CTRS), 318–319
Change
	in later life, 19
	stages of, 131
Charité Mobility Index, 375
Chedoke-McMaster Stroke Assessment (CMSA), 227
Chemosensory system
	age-related changes in, 176–177
	losses in, 177
Chest wall, 149
Chondroblasts, 194
Chronic Care Model (CCM), 405
Chronic conditions
	caregiving for, 362
	occupational therapy interventions for, 393
	prevalence of, 467
	primary care for, 362
	wellness affected by, 390

Chronic disease self-management, 411–412
Chronic Disease Self-Management Program (CDSMP), 136–137, 301–302, 393
Chronic inflammation, 128
Chronic obstructive pulmonary disease (COPD), 129, 153
Chronological age, 128, 441
Circadian rhythms, 135, 305
Cisgender, 68t
Cisgender females
  description of, 68
  sexual activity among, 70
  sexual response in, age-related changes in, 71t
Cisgender men
  sexual activity among, 70
  sexual dysfunction in, 70–71
  sexual response in, age-related changes in, 71t
Client-centered care, 317
Client-centered intervention planning, 330
Climate change, 505
Clinical ethicist, 92
Clinical note, 477
Clinical Test of Sensory Integration on Balance, 116
Clostriodiodes difficile colitis, 130
Coaching, health, 410, 410f
Cochlea, 174, 174f
Code of Ethics, 80, 82–83
Cognition
  aging and, 38–39, 238, 244
  assessment of, 156b, 249, 375–376, 409, 428, 472t
  dementia effects on, 247
  fall risks, 197
  functional, 38, 241–242
  home management affected by, 282
  screening of, 249, 428
  stimulation of, 252–253, 253t
Cognitive behavioral therapy, 136, 182, 196, 248
Cognitive capacity, 243
Cognitive conditions
  health management affected by, 296–297
  self-care abilities affected by, 267–268
Cognitive demand, 214b
Cognitive functioning
  in acute care setting, 428, 429f
  changes in, 238
  driving affected by, 341–342
  exercise benefits for, 253
  interprofessional collaboration for, 254–255
  in neuropathologies, 254
  neuropathologies that affect. *See* Neuropathologies
  optimizing of, 252–254
  physical activity benefits for, 253
  socialization benefits for, 253
  stroke effects on, 249
  summary of, 243–244
  theories of, 243
Cognitive health, 243
Cognitive impairment
  in acute care, 427–428
  description of, 271
  rehabilitation affected by, 442
Cognitive Orientation to Daily Occupational Performance (CO-OP), 250, 254, 299, 301, 303
Cognitive Performance Test, 271, 371

Cognitive processes
  age-related changes in, 239t
  attention, 238–239
  executive functioning, 240
  explicit processing, 241
  functional cognition, 241–242
  implicit processing, 241
  intellectual abilities, 240–241
  memory, 239
  wisdom, 241
Cognitive reserve, 252, 390–391
Cognitive restructuring, 136
Cognitive stage, of motor learning, 223
Cognitive stimulation, 245, 394
Cognitive theories of aging, 243
Cognitive-perceptual screening, for driving, 344
Cogwheel rigidity, 221t
Cohorts, 5, 6t
Cold therapy, for pain, 182
Collagen, 193, 193t
Coma Recovery Scale-Revised, 430
Communication
  acute care, 421–422
  dementia effects on, 247
Communities
  aging in, 30
  individuals and, intersectionality of, 53
  systemic injustice against, 56
  systems of power that affect, 56
Community Aging in Place—Advancing Better Living for Elders (CAPABLE), 317
Community level of environment, 50, 50t, 51f
Community mobility
  advocacy for, 349–350
  certification in, 343
  definition of, 338
  driving for. *See* Driving
  health conditions that affect, 341–342
  limitations to, 338
  options for, 338, 348–349
  overview of, 337–338
  paratransit options, 339f, 349
  participation facilitated by, 338f
  public transportation for, 339f, 349
Community-based institutions, 452
Community-based occupational therapists, 9
Community-based rehabilitation, 402
Community-based wellness services
  adult day centers, 385–386
  advocacy for, 396
  connecting older adults with, 387, 388t
  contexts of, 386–387
  description of, 384
  environmental factors, 386
  interprofessional partners for, 389
  PACE centers, 386
  senior centers, 384–385, 386b, 388t
  service barriers, 387
Comorbidities, 127, 281, 423–424, 442–443
Compassionate ageism, 54
Competence, 269
Comprehension, 20
Comprehensive geriatric assessment (CGA), 100, 108, 436, 443–444
Comprehensive outpatient rehabilitation facilities (CORFs), 439
Concentric strength, 189
Concepts, theories and, 35

Concrete value, 23
Conductive hearing loss, 173, 175
"Confined to home," 456b, 456–457
Confrontation testing, 172
Confusion Assessment Method for the Intensive Care Unit (CAM-ICU), 244
Congestive heart failure (CHF), 151. *See also* Heart failure (HF)
Congregate meal programs, 395–396
Connective tissue, 193
Constraint-induced movement therapy (CIMT), 220, 224
Construct validity, 372t
Content validity, 372t
Continuity Assessment Record and Evaluation (CARE), 371
Continuity theory, 41, 314, 327
Continuous positive airway pressure (CPAP), 154b
Contrast sensitivity, 167, 171–172, 341, 345
Co-occupation
  description of, 21
  examples of, 28
  occupational therapy intervention considering, 27–28
Coordinated movements, 215
Coordination
  age-related changes in, 214–215
  assessment of, 226t
  interventions for, 229
Cornea
  age-related changes in, 167–168
  anatomy of, 168f
Coronary artery bypass graft (CABG), 152b
Coronary artery disease (CAD), 150–151
Coronary heart disease
  obesity and, 126
  prevalence of, 150
Corticosteroids, 154b
Cougar Home Safety Assessment (CHSA), 285t
COVID-19 pandemic
  ageism during, 505
  elder abuse and neglect during, 85
  healthcare staffing affected by, 511
  leisure participation during, 315
  life expectancy affected by, 4
  living arrangements affected by, 504
  loneliness during, 69, 266
  negative social media messaging during, 10
  older adults during, 54, 81–82
  older workers affected by, 324
  physical activity during, 315
  retirement plans affected by, 324
  social isolation during, 69
  social network losses during, 65
  telehealth during, 403
C-reactive protein (CRP), 126
Creative occupations, 25, 27
Credit for Caring Act, 360
Criterion validity, 372t
Critical illness polyneuropathy myopathy (CIPNM), 424
Critical perspectives of aging, 41–42, 42t
Crystallized abilities, 38
Crystallized intelligence, 240
Cultural competency, 57
Cultural humility, 57–58, 372
Cultural perceptions, 57

Culture
  aging affected by, 10, 52–53
  definition of, 50–51
  driving and, 339
  environmental context of, 50, 50t
  ethnic group versus, 50
  individual choice affected by, 29
  personal health beliefs affected by, 55–56
  retirement affected by, 328
Current Procedural Terminology (CPT) codes, 363
Custodial care, 468
Cytokines, 128

D

Dance, 303
Day-care intervention, in hospice, 492, 493t
Day-care programs, 439–440
Death
  leading causes of, 5, 124t
  spiritual experiences and, 24
Decision making
  ethical, 90–93
  older adult's participation in, 422
Declarative memory, 39
Deconditioning, 425
Defibrillator, 152b
Dehydration
  assessment of, 108
  attention affected by, 390
  causes of, 107t
  definition of, 106
  interventions for, 109
Delirium, 244–245, 423, 425, 428
D.E.L.I.R.I.U.M. mnemonic, 244
Dementia
  Alzheimer disease as cause of, 246, 248t
  behavioral symptoms of, 247
  caregiving for, 248, 314
  cognitive symptoms of, 247, 296
  communication affected by, 247
  definition of, 245
  depression and, 296
  driving and, 341
  frontotemporal, 246–247
  institutionalized older adults with, 12
  instrumental activities of daily living completion affected by, 247
  irreversible, 246
  with Lewy bodies, 246
  in long-term care residents, 472, 476
  occupational therapy interventions for, 247–249
  prevalence of, 245–246, 296
  psychological symptoms of, 247
  rehabilitation affected by, 442
  reversible, 246
  risk factors for, 245
  self-care abilities affected by, 268
  vascular, 246
Dementia Carer Assessment of Support Needs Tool, 377
Dependency ratio, 10, 44
Depression
  antidepressants for, 251
  assessment of, 409, 472t
  cardiovascular disease and, 128
  in caregivers, 248

contributing factors, 251
  dementia and, 296
  Geriatric Depression Scale, 300t
  in long-term care residents, 472
  rehabilitation affected by, 442
  signs and symptoms of, 251
  type 2 diabetes mellitus and, 130
Dermis, 179
Descending tracts, 211
Descriptive assessments, 370–371
Developmental explanations, 38
Diabetes mellitus
  aging and, 129–130
  cardiovascular disease and, 126–127, 130
  driving performance and, 342
  peripheral artery disease risks, 199
  type 2, 129–130
Diabetic retinopathy (DR), 170–171
Diaphragmatic breathing, 158
Diastole, 147f
Diastolic heart failure, 151b
Dietary Approaches to Stop Hypertension (DASH), 132
Dietary habits, aging effects on, 107
Dietary patterns
  definition of, 132
  examples of, 133b
  metabolic syndrome managed with, 132–133, 133b
Dietitian, 93
Differential occupational patterns, 11
Diffusing capacity, 149
Digital ageism, 54
Digital divide, 331
Digital health literacy, 510
Digitally enabled care, 506
Disability
  causes of, 443
  late-life, in women, 11
  leisure participation affected by, 315
Disablement, 370
Disaster preparedness, 288
Discharge planning, 424, 437–438, 455
Discriminative assessments, 371
Disease, cultural influences on causes of, 55
Disengagement theory, 41
Distal determinant, 38t
Disuse atrophy, 190
Diuretics, 152b
Diverse social networks, 64
Divided attention, 238
DNA damage, 37
Do Live Well framework, 301–302
Do not resuscitate (DNR) order, 84t
Documentation
  acute care, 429–430
  home health care, 460–461
  long-term care services, 477
  palliative care, 495
  primary care, 412
  rehabilitation, 445
  wellness services, 396
Do-Live-Now framework, 392
Domestic migration, 9
Domiciliary care, 462
Dressing areas, 273
DriveAware, 345
Driverless cars, 511

DriveSafe, 345
Driving
  assessment of, 343–346, 409
  behind-the-wheel assessment for, 345–346
  cessation of, 346–348
  client factors that affect, 339–340
  cognitive functions and, 341–342, 346
  cognitive-perceptual screening for, 344
  cultural context of, 339
  diabetes mellitus and, 342
  driving performance and, 342
  environment considerations for, 339–340
  family involvement in decisions about, 348
  fatalities during, 341b
  field of view test for, 344
  fitness to drive assessment, 343, 345
  functional cognition and, 242
  health conditions that affect, 341–342, 342
  independence and, 339
  initiating decision to alter or stop, 347–348
  as instrumental activity of daily living, 338
  interprofessional team for, 342–343
  interventions to support, 346
  mobility alternatives to, 348–350
  motor vehicles crashes, 341b
  neuromusculoskeletal assessment for, 345
  as occupation, 338–340
  occupational therapy and, 342–343
  on-road assessments for, 345–346
  performance patterns associated with, 339
  performance skills for, 339
  technology application to, 340, 346
  vision screening for, 344–345
  visual function and, 341
Driving certification, 343
Driving history, 343–344
Driving performance, 341–342
Driving rehabilitation specialists, 343
Driving safety, 341–342
Driving simulator, 345–346
Drop-arm bedside commode, 426
Dry age-related macular degeneration, 170
Dual-process theory, 243
Durable power of attorney, 83t
Dynamic assessment, 376
Dynamic Loewenstein Occupational Therapy Assessment Geriatric Version (DLOTCA-G), 376
Dynamic stretching, 204
Dysarthria, 217
Dyslipidemia, 127
Dysphagia, 222t, 454
Dyspnea on exertion, 153
Dyspnea-controlled postures, 158

E

Ear, 174f
Early mobilization, 245
Eccentric strength, 190
Ecological model, of aging, 39, 40t
Ecological systems theory, 39–40, 40t
Economics, aging affected by, 11–12
Eden Alternative, 475
Education
  attitudes toward aging changed through, 10
  caregivers, 160, 409
  health, 393
eHEALS: the eHealth Literacy Scale, 300t
eHealth literacy, 296, 300t

Elastin, 193, 193t
Elder abuse and neglect
　abusers, 85
　ageism and, 88
　approaches for addressing, 88–89
　assessment instruments for, 87–88
　criminal justice approach to, 88–89
　definition of, 86t
　definitions, 86t
　family violence and, 88
　forms of, 86t, 86–88
　as geriatric syndrome, 88
　as human rights violation, 89
　laws regarding, 86
　multidisciplinary team management of, 89
　occupational therapist's role, 89
　prevalence of, 85
　as public health concern, 89
　reporting of, 86
　resources for, 89
　risk factors for, 85–88
　screening for, 87–88
　signs of, 86–88, 87f
　as social problem, 88
　statistics regarding, 85
　team management of, 89
Elder Justice Act, 86
Elder Maltreatment Screen and Follow-up Plan, 88
Elder speak, 54
Elderly Mobility Scale, 115, 375
Electronic magnification, 173t
Electronic medical record (EMR), 412
Emotional abuse, 86t
Emotional health, 301–302
Emotional support, 65
Emphysema, 129
Empowerment, 159
Endocrine theory, of aging, 36–37, 37t
End-of-life
　care during, 484, 488
　decision making at, 84
　ethical considerations at, 84, 84t, 90t
　family affected by, 490
　grief at, 490
　life-limiting diseases at, 484
　meaningful occupations at, 484f
　occupational therapy practitioners during, 85
Endurance, 156b
Energy conservation, 159–160, 286
Energy conservation/work simplification (ECWS), 159–160
Energy-balance behaviors, 136–137
EngAGED, 394
Enhanced activities of daily living (EADLs), 318
Enriched environments, 39
Environment
　aging affected by, 282
　assessment of, 272
　driving and, 339–340
　fall risks, 113
　leisure affected by, 314
　for low vision, 172
　medication management affected by, 103
　modifications of, for activities of daily living, 273, 273f
　rural. See Rural environments
　self-care affected by, 269, 272
　sleep affected by, 135–136, 304–305

Environmental press, 39, 282–283
Environmental systems
　community level of, 50, 50t, 51f
　cultural contexts, 50, 50t, 51f
　health outcomes of older adults affected by, 53–59
　immediate level of, 50, 50t, 51f, 55
　long-term stress in, 56–57
　physical activity affected by, 135
　proximal level of, 50, 50t, 51f
　societal level of, 50, 50t, 51f
Environmental theories, of aging, 39–40, 40t
Epidermis, 179
Epigenetics, 37, 37t
Epworth sleepiness scale, 301t
Ergonomics, 331
Erikson, Erik, 22
Error theories, of aging, 37
Ethical conflicts, 84
Ethical considerations
　advance care planning, 83
　advance directives, 83, 83t
　billing, 82–83
　at end-of-life, 84, 84t, 90t
　ethical issues, 90t
　ethical principles, 80, 89
　in functional performance evaluations, 372–373
　interprofessional practice, 91–93
　problem-solving framework, 91f
　productivity, 82–83
　resources for, 93b
　unique types of, 89–90
Ethical decision making, 90–93
Ethical dilemma, 80
Ethnic group, culture versus, 50
Eurobarometer, 81
European Association for Palliative Care (EAPC), 485, 485b, 498
Evaluation
　in acute care, 422–423
　meaningful occupations, 26
　in Model of Human Occupation, 132
Evaluative assessments, 371
Evaluative meanings, 23, 24t
Everyday Ageism Scale, 80
Exceptionalism, 53
Executive Function Performance Test (EFPT), 271, 285t, 300t, 376
Executive functioning, 240, 296
Executive processing, 282
Exercise. See also Physical activity
　adherence to, 202
　cognitive functioning affected by, 253
　fall prevention through, 303
　flexibility, 204
　guidelines for, 395t
　health benefits of, 395
　resistance, 203–204
　strength, 203–204, 204b
　stretching, 204
　wellness benefits of, 395
Existential meanings, 23–24, 24t
Expanded Chronic Care Model (ECCM), 405, 406f, 407t
Explicit biases, 57
Explicit processing, 241
Ex-PLISSIT communication, 73
Exploitation, 86t

Expressive aphasia, 232
Extended family, 66
Extrapyramidal system, 213
Eye
　age-related changes in, 167–168
　anatomy of, 168f

F

Facetime, 511
Falls
　activity modification to prevent, 117
　aging and, 112–117
　assessment of, 113–116, 114f–115f, 375
　balance assessments, 115
　common locations for, 113
　definition of, 112, 197
　delirium and, 425
　environmental hazards that cause, 113
　fear of, 297
　fractures caused by, 197–198
　in hospital, 425
　influencers of, 112–113
　injuries caused by, 197, 425
　in institutions, 113
　interventions for, 116–117, 303
　mechanical, 112
　medical conditions, 112–113
　multifactorial prevention programs for, 303
　nonmechanical, 112
　occupational therapy evaluations, 113, 115
　osteoarthritis as risk factor for, 197
　outcomes of, 113
　prevention of, 303, 425
　resources for, 101b
　risk factors for, 197, 297
　self-care considerations, 266
　sensory changes associated with, 113
　visual impairment as cause of, 427
Families of choice, 357
Family
　definition of, 65
　in driving decisions, 348
　extended, 66
　nuclear, 357
　structure of, 66, 357–358
Family and Medical Leave Act of 1993 (FMLA), 357, 360
Family caregivers/caregiving. See also Caregivers/caregiving
　cancer care by, 363
　care integration of, 361–362
　contextual characteristics of, 356
　continuous care by, 357t
　continuum of care for, 356
　definition of, 355
　demographics of, 356
　end-of-life care by, 357t
　episodic care by, 357t
　family structure differences and, 357–358
　filial obligation in, 357
　in future, 511–512
　gender differences, 356–357
　health promotion for, 362
　home care by, 357t
　interventions for, 362–363
　level of care, 356, 357t
　levels of prevention in, 359, 359f

for life-limiting illness, 491
long-term care by, 357t
occasional daily care by, 357t
palliative care by, 357t
policies to support, 359–361
prevalence of, 355–356, 358
public health issues, 358
recuperative care by, 357t
responsibilities of, 356–358
screening of, 361
trends affecting, 355–356
wellness promotion for, 362
women as, 356
Family constellations, 65–66
Family relationships, 65
Family-focused social networks, 64
Fast-twitch muscle fibers, 191, 212
Fatigue, 286, 298, 377
Fatigue Severity Scale, 377
Fear of falling, 297
Federally Qualified Health Centers (FQHCs), 402
Female sexual dysfunction (FSD), 70
Festinating gait, 222t
Fictive kin, 66
Fidelity, 80
Field of view test, 344
Filial obligation, 357
Finances, 11
Financial abuse, 86t, 88
Fine-motor coordination, 215
First responder retirement transition planning, 330–331
Fit, 39
Fitness programs, 395
Fitness to drive assessment, 343, 345
Five Wishes, 83
Five-personality trait theory, 406
Flavor enhancers, 109
Flexibility
  assessment of, 201
  exercises for, 204
Floaters, 167
Flow, 312
Fluid
  daily intake of, 245
  human requirements for, 106
  inadequate intake of, 107
Fluid intelligence, 38, 240
Focused attention, 238
Food(s)
  flavor enhancers for, 109
  functional, 106
Food insecurity, 133–134
Formal learning, 315
Foundational theories of aging, 39–40
401(k) plans, 10
Fractures, vertebral, 198
Frailty
  assessment of, 100, 409
  definition of, 99–100
  exercise programs for, 203
  features of, 442
  implications of, 100–101
  rehabilitation affected by, 442
  resources for, 101b
  risk enablement plan for, 100
Free radical theory, of aging, 37, 37t

Friends
  emotional support from, 65
  friend-focused social networks, 64
Frontotemporal dementia, 246–247
Fugl-Meyer Assessment of Sensorimotor Recovery After Stroke (FMA), 226–227
Function
  International Classification of Functioning, Disability, and Health definition of, 42–43
  neuromotor, 211, 215
  physical, 189f
  visual, 166t, 167–168, 341
Functional Autonomy Measurement Scale, 374
Functional Autonomy Measurement System, 377
Functional cognition, 38, 241–242
Functional foods, 106
Functional incidental training, 112
Functional incontinence, 110
Functional Independence Measure, 156b
Functional mobility
  assessment of, 374–375
  description of, 192, 346
Functional movements, 214–215
Functional performance, 370
Functional performance evaluation
  activities of daily living, 374
  assessments used in, 370–372
  caregiver support, 377
  cognition, 375–376
  descriptive purpose of, 370–371
  ethical considerations in, 372–373
  fatigue, 377
  importance of, 370
  instrumental activities of daily living, 374
  issues associated with, 376–377
  leisure, 376
  mobility, 374–375
  overview of, 369–370
  purpose of, 370–371
  sensory changes that affect, 376–377
  social participation, 376
  upper-extremity function, 375
Functional Reach Test (FRT), 115

G
Gait speed, 409
Gastrointestinal disorders, 130
Gender
  aging affected by, 11–12
  definition of, 68t
  life expectancy affected by, 11
  poverty and, 11
Gender diverse, 68t
Gender identity
  description of, 67–68
  sexual response by, 71t
  terminology associated with, 68t
Gender nonconforming, 68t
Generalized anxiety disorders, 251
Generation X, 6t, 329
Generation Y, 6t, 329
Generation Z, 6t
Generational characteristics, 5, 6t
Generational cohorts, 66
Genetic theories, of aging, 37
Genetics, 11
Geriatric Depression Scale, 300t

Geriatric Oral Health Assessment Index (GOHAI), 105
Geriatric rehabilitation, 438b
Geriatric syndromes, 423
Geriatrician, 441
Gerontologists, 36
Gerontology
  definition of, 36
  social, 36
Gerotechnology, 331
Glaucoma, 170, 282
Global Positioning System, 340f
Global Wellness Institute (GWI), 384
Glycoproteins, 193t
Goal setting, 136
"Grand-families," 512
Grandparent–grandchild relationship, 66
Grandparenting
  in Japan, 328
  as occupation, 27–28, 312
  as social relationship, 66
Great Depression, 5, 10
Great Recession, 10
Green House Model, 475
Grief, 442, 490–491
Grip strength, 375, 409
Guided imagery, 182
Guillain-Barré syndrome (GBS), 218t
Gustatory sense, 133

H
Habituation, 131–132
Happiness, 23
Health
  assessment tools for, 301t
  definition of, 294, 384
  determinants of, 3
  exercise benefits for, 395
  factors involved in, 293, 325
  self-assessments of, 294
  self-care effects on, 266
  social support benefits for, 282
  technology for monitoring of, 509–510
Health Belief Model (HBM), 131, 392
Health beliefs, cultural influences on, 55–56
Health coaching, 393, 410, 410f
Health conditions
  community mobility affected by, 341–342
  driving affected by, 341–342
  driving performance affected by, 342
  fall risks associated with, 297
  health management affected by, 296–298
  home management activities affected by, 280–282
  retirement affected by, 325
  self-care affected by, 267–269
  sleep and, 299
  work affected by, 325
Health education, 393
Health literacy
  description of, 7–8, 295–296, 302–303, 421
  digital, 510
  lack of, 510
Health management
  assessment of, 299, 300t–301t
  barriers to, 295
  cognitive changes and, 296–297
  definition of, 294

Index

elements of, 293
health care access and use, 295–296
health conditions that affect, 296–298
hearing loss effects on, 296
interventions for, 299, 301–305
mobility effects on, 297
occupations involved in, 294, 295t
overview of, 293–294
social determinants of health, 295
social support effects on, 297
socioeconomic status effects on, 297
symptom and condition management, 302
theoretical approaches to success in, 299
vision impairment effects on, 296
Health outcomes
  neighborhood influences on, 54–55
  social determinants of health effects on, 295
  structural ageism effects on, 53–54
Health promotion, 392–393
Health Resources and Services Administration (HRSA), 402
Health span, 505
Health status, 7
Healthcare
  access to
    barriers to, 404
    conceptual framework for, 404, 404f
    definition of, 404
    dimensions of, 404
    for older adults, 53–56, 93, 295–296
  ageism and, 81–82
  communication with, 300t, 302–303
  decision making, cultural influences on, 55
  funding issues in, 508–509
  interprofessional collaboration effects on, 507–508
  staff shortages in, 508–509
  technology in, 509–511
  transparency of services in, 404
  trends in, 506–509
Healthcare professions, 81
Healthy aging, 63, 384, 504
Healthy lifestyle behaviors, 132–138
Healthy People 2030, 7–8
Hearing
  age-related changes in, 166t
  anatomy of, 174f
  augmentation of, 245
  cognitive functioning and, 243
  measurement of, 173
Hearing aids, 176
Hearing loss
  activity limitations caused by, 268–269
  assistive listening devices for, 176, 177f
  central auditory processing disorder as cause of, 175
  communication strategies for, 176b
  conductive, 173, 175
  environmental modifications for, 176b
  health management affected by, 296
  prevalence of, 173
  sensorineural, 174
  social consequences of, 175–176
  speech perception affected by, 175
Hearing sensitivity, 175
Heart
  age-related changes, 126, 126b, 136, 148t
  anatomy of, 146, 147f

electrical behavior of, 136
mechanical behavior of, 136–137
Heart blocks, 136
Heart disease, 150
Heart failure (HF)
  description of, 151
  left-sided, 151b
  obesity and, 126
  right-sided, 151b
Heart rate
  age-related changes to, 126b
  maximum aerobic, 161
Heart transplant, 152b
Heat therapy, for pain, 182
Helicobacter pylori, 130
Heteronormativity, 72
Home
  acute care at, 508
  environmental modifications in, 287, 288t
  objects of meaning in, 29
  as place, 29
Home and Community Environment Instrument, 272
Home Environment Assessment Protocol (HEAP), 285t
Home Environment Lighting Assessment (HELA), 172
Home health. *See also* Home health services
  administrative staff in, 455
  advocacy in, 462–463
  assessment for, 457–459
  comprehensive assessment in, 458–459
  context of, 452–453
  definition of, 451
  documentation of, 460–461
  dressing in, 453
  initial evaluation for, 461
  initial visit, 458
  inpatient setting versus, 452
  international, 462
  interprofessional partners in, 453–455
  intervention in, 459–460, 463–464
  Medicare reimbursement for, 456–457, 462
  occupational therapy in, 453
  payment systems for, 461–462
  physical therapy in, 453–454
  problem areas encountered in, 460
  reassessments in, 461
  reimbursement for, 460–462
  skilled nursing in, 454
  social services in, 454–455
  speech therapy in, 454
Home health agencies
  administrative staff in, 455
  Centers for Medicaid and Medicare Services, 455, 458
  definition of, 455
  Medicare reimbursement to, 456–457, 462
  regulatory guidelines for, 455
Home health aides, 454–455
Home Health Compare, 458
Home health services
  assisted-living facilities, 452–453
  "confined to home" criterion for, 456b, 456–457
  definition of, 452
  outpatient services and, 462
  plan of care for, 457, 459

Home management
  activities associated with, 280, 281t
  assessment of, 284, 285t
  assistive technology for, 287
  care partner training for, 288
  cognitive changes and, 282
  definition of, 280
  disaster preparedness, 288
  energy conservation for, 286
  health conditions effect on, 280–282
  importance of, 281
  intervention for, 284–288
  physical changes that affect, 282
  task adaptation for, 286
  task-oriented approach to, 283
  task-specific skill training, 286–287
  theoretical approaches to, 282–283
Home safety
  assessments of, 284, 285t
  interventions for, 287
Homelessness, 9
Homeostatic hydration, 107
Home-Rx, 103, 300t
Hopkins Medication Schedule, 103
Hormone replacement therapy (HRT), 70
Hospice care
  day-care intervention in, 492, 493t
  description of, 84t, 453, 483–484
  history of, 484
  interprofessional partners in, 488–489
  occupational therapy in, 487–488
Hospital
  assistive technology in, 429
  cognitive impairment in, 427
  communication in, 421–422
  day hospital model, 440
  fall prevention in, 425
  multidisciplinary care in, 437
Hospital-associated deconditioning (HAD), 423
Hospitalization
  comorbidities of older adults, 423–424
  functional status decline caused by, 423
  rehabilitation after, 471
  spirituality concerns, 429
Huntington disease, 39
Hyaluronic acid, 193t
Hydration
  aging effects on, 105–109
  assessment of, 108–109
  homeostatic, 107
  influencers of, 106–107
  resources for, 101b
  wellness affected by, 390
Hypercholesterolemia, 129
Hyperglycemia, 126
Hyperinsulinemia, 128
Hyperlipidemia, 129
Hypertension (HTN)
  arterial, 126
  cardiovascular disease and, 127, 127b
  medication adherence and, 127
  organ damage caused by, 127
  pathogenesis of, 152
  risk factors for, 127b
  secondary, 127
  stroke risks and, 127
  treatment of, 152
Hypertensive crisis, 127

Hypertensive emergencies, 127
Hypertonia, 217
Hypertrophy, 126
Hypodermis, 179–180
Hypokinesia, 221t
Hypotonia, 217

I

ICU
  acute care in, 419
  early mobility in, 424
ICU-acquired weakness (ICUAW), 424
Identity
  components of, 51
  creativity and, 25
  gender. *See* Gender identity
  intersectionality of, 51
  meaning and, 24t, 24–25
  positionality of, 51
  transitions and, 25
  work effects on, 324
Immunologic theory, of aging, 37, 37t
Implicit Association Test, 57
Implicit biases, 54, 57
Implicit learning, 224
Implicit processing, 241
In Home Occupational Performance Evaluation (I-HOPE), 285t
Incontinence, urinary, 110–112
Incontinence Impact Questionnaire (IIQ), 111
Independent Living Scale, 285t
Independent Transportation Network (ITN America), 349
India, 12
Indigenous communities
  older adults in, 385
  systemic injustice against, 56
Indirect wellness care, 389
Individual Food Resource Profile (IFRP), 133
Individuals, community and, 53
Industrial revolution, 10
Informal learning, 315
Informational support, 65
In-Home Medication Management Performance Evaluation, 103
Inner ear, 174f
Inpatient rehabilitation units, 437–439
Institution(s)
  community-based, 452
  definition of, 452
  falls in, 113
  sleep routine in, 136
Institutionalization, 9, 12
Instrumental activities of daily living (IADLs)
  assessment of, 156b, 270, 284, 285t, 374, 409, 472t
  in cardiopulmonary conditions, 159
  in cardiovascular conditions, 159
  care partner training for, 288
  classification of, 264
  cognitive loss effects on performance of, 476
  cooking, 304
  dementia and, 247
  dementia effects on, 268
  difficulties in performing, prevalence of, 370
  driving as, 338
  in end-of-life care, 484
  functional cognition and, 241
  health conditions effect on, 280–282
  hearing loss effects on, 268–269
  home environmental modifications for, 287, 288t
  importance of, 281
  intervention for, 284–288, 460
  limitations of, prevalence of, 266–267
  musculoskeletal system functioning for, 188
  in palliative care, 487–488
  retraining, 159, 198
  stroke effects on, 267
  vision impairment effects on, 268
Instrumental meanings, 22–23, 24t
Instrumental support, 65
Integrated care, 420–421
Integrated care models, 444
Integrated Primary Care and Occupational Therapy for Aging and Chronic Disease Treatment to Preserve Independence and Functioning (IPROACTIF), 403
Integrative Medication Self-Management Intervention (IMedS), 137–138
Integumentary system, 179–180
Intellectual abilities, 240–241
Intensive Care Delirium Screening Checklist (ICDSC), 244
Intensive care unit. *See* ICU
Intergenerational service learning, 10
Internal consistency reliability, 372t
International Classification of Functioning, Disability, and Health (ICF)
  activity and participation, 42
  body functions, 42
  body structures, 42
  community mobility in, 338
  description of, 13
  disability in, 42
  domains of, 42f, 42–43
  framework of, 13f, 42, 42f, 146
  functioning as defined in, 42–43
  health care applicability of, 146
  looking after one's health, 294
  occupational therapist interventions based on, 146
  purpose of, 42, 373
International Consultation on Incontinence Questionnaire Short Form (ICIQ-SF), 111
International Council on Active Aging (ICAA), 384
International home health, 462
International migration, 9
Interprofessional collaboration
  cardiopulmonary conditions managed with, 161
  cardiovascular conditions managed with, 161
  cognitive functioning managed with, 254–255
  delirium managed with, 244–245
  healthcare delivery affected by, 507–508
  leisure managed with, 318–319
  metabolic syndrome managed with, 138
  neuromotor conditions managed with, 231–232
  patient transition affected by, 507
  retirement managed with, 331–332
  stroke managed with, 250
  work managed with, 331–332
Interprofessional Collaborative Relationship-Building Model, 441
Interprofessional integrated care, 420–421
Interprofessional practice, 91–93

Interprofessional team
  description of, 92–93, 342–343
  members of, 469
  occupational therapist in, 408
  in primary care, 408
Interrater reliability, 372t
Intersectionality
  with aging, 52–53
  definition of, 51
Intersex, 68t
Interstitial lung disease (ILD), 153
Interventions. *See* Occupational therapy interventions
In-the-canal (ITC) hearing aids, 176
In-the-ear (ITE) hearing aids, 176
Intra-aortic balloon pump (IABP), 152b
Intrusionary occupational therapy, 408
Ischemic stroke, 127
Isokinetic strength, 190, 203
Isolation
  driving cessation as cause of, 347
  leisure participation affected by, 315
  social, 69, 135, 390
Isometric strength, 189, 203
Isotonic strength, 203

J

Japan, 328
Jim Crow laws, 58
Job Accommodation Network, 330
Joint(s)
  age-related changes in, 193, 193t
  protection of, in acute care setting, 426–427
  range of motion of, 194, 201
  synovial, 194
Joint inflammation, 268
Joint replacement, 196
Justice, 80, 82

K

Katz Index of Daily Living, 271, 374
Kawa model, 44, 299
Kettle Test, 271
Kin ties, social support from, 65
Kitchen Picture Test (KPT), 285t
Kohlman Evaluation of Living Skills (KELS), 271, 285t, 374

L

Labrador Retriever personal robot, 511
Later life
  change in, 19
  characteristics of, 19
  disability in, 11
  Erikson's tasks for, 22
  learning in, 315
  occupational patterns in, 23
  physical activity in, 26
  well-being in, 26
Laws
  ageism and, 81, 81t
  elder abuse and neglect, 86
  federal, 81
  resources for, 93b
  state, 81
Lawton IADL Scale, 285t, 374, 409
LEA Low Contrast Flip Chart, 345

Lead pipe rigidity, 221t
Leading causes of death, 5, 124t
Learning
 formal, 315
 informal, 315
 lifelong, as leisure, 315–316
 nonformal, 315
Left ventricular assist device (LVAD), 152b
Left-sided heart failure, 151b
Legal blindness, 169
Leisure
 activities of, 311–312, 332
 aging and, 311
 assessment of, 316–317, 376, 472t
 benefits of, 312
 definition of, 311–312
 engagement and, 312, 314
 environment and, 314
 interprofessional collaboration for, 318–319
 lifelong learning as, 315–316
 in palliative care, 488
 participation in
  assistive technology to support, 318
  barriers to, 314
  disability effects on, 315
  interventions that support, 317–318
  isolation effects on, 315
 social justice and, 314–315
 social participation and, 312
 theoretical approaches, 313–314
 volunteerism and, 332–333
Leisure motivation, 312
Lens, 168
Levesque framework, 404
Lewin, Kurt, 39
Lewy bodies, dementia with, 246
LGBTQIA+ population
 aging concerns of, 67–69, 385
 families of choice for, 357
 older adults as, 67–69
 pronouns, 67
 sexuality among, 72
Life Adaptations Skills Training (LAST), 254
Life course approach, 327
Life course perspective of aging, 41, 42t
Life course theory, 314
Life crises, 21
Life expectancy
 in Canada, 4
 care challenges associated with, 44
 COVID-19 effects on, 4
 definition of, 4
 gender differences in, 11
 global increases in, 504
 increases in, 4, 504
 medical advances affecting, 4–5
 in premodern world, 4
 racial differences in, 5
 in United States, 4f
Life review, 27
Life satisfaction, 23
Life Satisfaction Index, 26
Life span
 definition of, 4
 future of, 505
Life span development theory, of aging, 22, 38, 38t
Life-limiting diseases, 484, 489
Lifelong learning, as leisure, 315–316

Lifelong Learning Institute (LLI) Network, 316
Life-span development, 327
Lifestyle
 interventions, 410
 noncommunicable diseases related to, 124t
 Western, 124
Lifestyle Redesign®, 27, 301–302, 317–318, 393–394, 410, 412
Lifestyle-based occupational therapy, 202b
Lil'Flo, 511
Limb amputation, 199–201
Living arrangements, 504–505
Living will, 83t
Lobectomy, 154b
Loewenstein Occupational Therapy Assessment Geriatric Version (LOTCA-G), 376
Loneliness, 7, 11, 20, 69, 266, 300t, 390
Long-term care facilities
 elder abuse in, 85
 sexuality in, 72
Long-Term Care (LTC) Ombudsman Program, 81
Long-term care services. *See also* Nursing home care
 advocacy for, 478–479
 assessment for, 469
 assessments in, 472t
 definition of, 467–468
 dementia, 472, 476
 depression, 472
 description of, 467
 dining experience, 475–476
 discharge planning in, 477
 documentation of, 477
 evaluation in, 472
 international reimbursement for, 478
 interprofessional partners in, 469–471
 Medicare reimbursement for, 477
 occupational therapy in
  description of, 469
  evaluation, 472
  interventions, 473t–474t, 473–476
  outcomes of, 476–477
  therapeutic environments, 475
  treatment plans, 473
 oral hygiene, 472
 payment systems for, 477–478
 rehabilitation after hospitalization, 471
 reimbursement for, 477–478
 restorative care, 471–472
 screening tools in, 472t
 settings for, 467
 state regulations regarding, 478
Looking after one's health, 294
Low vision
 description of, 169, 169b
 health management affected by, 296
 rehabilitation of, 172
Lower motor neuron, 211
Lubben Social Network Scale-6, 69
Lung(s)
 age-related changes, 149t
 parenchyma of, 148–149
 transplant of, 154b
Lung cancer, 153

M

Macula
 age-related degeneration of, 169–170
 anatomy of, 168

Magnifiers, 173t
Maintenance model, 440
Malnutrition
 causes of, 106, 107t
 description of, 105–106
 interventions for, 109
 micronutrient-related, 105
Manual muscle testing (MMT), 426
Mars Contrast Sensitivity Test, 172
Massage, 182
Mattering, 20
Maturists, 5, 6t
Maximum aerobic heart rate, 161
Meaning
 occupation and, 269
 in self-care, 269–270
Meaningful Activities Survey (EMAS), 26
Meaningful Activity and Life Meaning model (MALM), 26
Meaningful Activity Wants and Needs Assessment (MAWNA), 26
Meaningful occupations
 definition of, 20
 at end-of-life, 484f
 evaluation of, 26
 importance of, 367
 interventions to support, 26–28
 social engagement as, 22
Meaning/meaning in life
 assessment for, 26
 benefits of, 20
 comprehension and, 20
 definition of, 20
 evaluation of, 26, 29
 evaluative, 23, 24t
 existential, 23–24, 24t
 in home, 29
 identity and, 24t, 24–25
 instrumental, 22–23, 24t
 mattering and, 20
 occupation and, 20–21, 26
 occupational, 22–24
 in occupational therapy process, 25–29
 purpose and, 20
 religion and, 24
 search for, 19–21
 spirituality and, 24
 themes of, 21–24, 24t
Mechanical ventilation
 definition of, 154b
 at end-of-life, 84t
Media portrayals, of older adults, 10, 52–53
Medicaid
 billing of, 82
 history of, 80
Medical mismanagement, 90t
Medical Orders for Life-Sustaining Treatment (MOLST), 83t
Medicare
 beneficiaries of, 456–457
 billing of, 82
 comprehensive assessments, 458
 elder abuse policies of, 86
 history of, 80
 home health agencies and, 456–458, 462
 hospice benefits of, 360t
 Part A, 446, 455
 Part B, 446, 455

Part C, 455
Part D, 455
plan of care, 457, 459
Prospective Payment System, 478
reasonable and necessary therapy services, 457
rehabilitation funding by, 446, 477
wellness program studies by, 396
Medicare and Medicaid Act of 1965, 80
Medication(s)
 adherence to, 102–103, 127, 296
 aging body functions and structures that affect, 102–103
 effectiveness of, 102–103
 food flavor affected by, 133
 foods that affect, 103
 nonadherence to, 103
 pharmacodynamics of, 103
 pharmacokinetics of, 102
 sexuality affected by, 72
Medication management
 actions for, 137
 assessment of, 103, 300t
 assistive technology for, 103f
 description of, 102
 environmental considerations, 103
 Integrative Medication Self-Management Intervention, 137–138
 interventions for, 103–104, 303
 resources for, 101b
Mediterranean diet, 39
Meissner corpuscles, 179
Melbourne Low Vision ADL Index, 271
Memory
 declarative, 39
 description of, 239
 working, 239, 243, 296
Menopause, 192
Mental health
 cognitive behavioral therapy for, 136
 lifestyle behaviors that affect, 136
 occupational therapy interventions for, 253–254
 socioeconomic status and, 11
 state spending on, 437
 yoga benefits for, 303
Mental health conditions
 anxiety disorders, 251
 bipolar disorder, 252
 cardiovascular disease and, 128
 depression. *See* Depression
 prevalence of, 250
 schizophrenia, 251
 substance use disorders, 252
Mental illness, 250
Mental stimulation, 252–253, 253t
Mesenchymal stem cells (MSCs), 193
Metabolic conditions
 description of, 123
 noncommunicable diseases, 123–125
Metabolic equivalent (MET) levels, 157t, 157–158, 160–161
Metabolic syndrome (MetS)
 cancer associated with, 128
 cardiometabolic risk factors, 124
 chronic obstructive pulmonary disease and, 129
 gastrointestinal disorders associated with, 130
 interprofessional collaboration and referrals for, 138

 ischemic stroke risks, 127
 lung diseases associated with, 129
 Person-Environment-Occupation-Performance model application to, 132
 risk factors for, 126
 treatment of
  dietary patterns, 132–134, 133b
  medications, 137
  mental health, 136
  nutritious diet, 132–133
  physical activity, 134–135
  sedentary behavior minimization, 134–135
  sleep, 135–136
Micrographia, 221t
Micronutrient-related malnutrition, 105
Middle cerebral artery (MCA), 219t
Middle ear, 174f
Middle-old, 4, 9
Migration, 9
Mild cognitive impairment (MCI), 245, 346, 375
Millennials, 329
Mindfulness, 136
Mini-Balance Evaluation Systems Test, 226
Mini-Mental State Examination (MMSE), 156b, 172, 249, 375
Mitral valve replacement, 152b
Mixed incontinence, 110
MNA Short-Form, 108
Mobility
 early mobilization, 245
 functional, 192
 gait speed and, 409
 health management affected by, 297
Model of Human Occupation (MOHO), 25, 44, 131–132, 299, 330, 373–374
Model of Human Occupation Screening Tool (MOHOST), 13
Modified Ashworth Scale, 225
Modified Borg Scale, 156b, 161
Modified Food Guide Pyramid for 70+ Adults, 106
MOLST forms, 83t
Montessori method, 476
Montreal Cognitive Assessment (MoCA), 172, 245, 249, 344, 409
Moral distress, 90
Motivation
 adherence versus, 442
 goal-setting in, 442
 motor learning and, 223
 in rehabilitation, 442
Motivational interviewing (MI), 410–411
Motor control theories, 222
Motor learning
 client-centered approach to, 230
 definition of, 221–222
 intervention strategies for, 224
 motivation and, 223
 motor performance versus, 223
 three-stage model of, 223–224, 224t
Motor neuron diseases (MND), 217t
Motor performance, 223
Motor units, 212
Motor vehicles crashes, 341b
Multicontext Treatment Approach (MTA), 250
Multidimensional Fatigue Inventory, 377

Multi-Directional Reach Test, 227
Multidisciplinary care, 138
Multidisciplinary teams, 89
Multi-level leisure mechanisms framework (MLMF), 313, 313f
Multimorbidity, 188, 408–409
Multiple sclerosis, 217t, 228t, 229
Muscle
 atrophy of, 190
 fat accumulation in, 191
 skeletal, 191–192
 structure of, 190b, 190–192, 191f
Muscle fibers, 191
Muscle mass, 190–191
Muscle power
 age-related changes in, 189, 190b
 assessment of, 201–202
 definition of, 190
 functional mobility affected by, 192
Muscle strength
 age-related changes in, 189–190, 190b, 190f, 191f
 assessment of, 201–202, 225, 226t
 exercises for, 203–204
 functional mobility and, 192
 interventions for, 227–228
 isokinetic testing of, 201
 muscle mass and, 190
Muscle tone
 assessment of, 225, 226t
 interventions for, 227–228
Muscle wasting, 424
Musculoskeletal conditions
 amputation, 199–201
 driving performance affected by, 342
 falls, 197–199
 fractures, 197–198
 management of, 202–204
 osteoarthritis, 195–197
 osteoporosis, 197–199
Musculoskeletal system
 age-related changes in, 188–195, 203
 assessments, 201–205
 flexibility assessment, 201
 functioning of, 188
 overview of, 187–188
 range of motion assessment, 201
Myasthenia gravis, 217t
MyMobility Plan, 117
Myocardial infarction (MI), 151

N

Narrative ethics, 80
National Association for Home Care & Hospice (NAHC), 463
National Center for Transgender Equity, 67
National Center on Elder Abuse, 87
National Council on Aging, 85, 137
National Family Caregiver Support Program (NFCSP), 359–360, 360t
National Health Service (NHS), 462
National Institutes of Health (NIH) Institute on Aging, 86
National Sleep Foundation, 135
Native Americans, 5
Naturally occurring retirement communities (NORC), 9
Negative stereotypes of aging, 238, 505

Neglect, 86t. *See also* Elder abuse and neglect
Neighborhoods
  affluence of, 54–55
  definition of, 54
  health outcomes affected by, 54–55
  resource access in, 55
  socioeconomic level of, 54–55
Nervous system, 212b
Neurocognitive disorders
  description of, 267–268
  loneliness risks, 315
Neurodevelopmental theory, 222
Neurodevelopmental treatment (NDT), 221
Neurological assessment, 225b
Neuromotor conditions
  amyotrophic lateral sclerosis, 217t
  assessment of, 224–227, 226t
  cerebral palsy, 217t
  Guillain-Barré syndrome, 218t
  interprofessional collaboration for, 231–232
  interventions for, 227–230, 228t
  motor neuron diseases, 217t
  multiple sclerosis, 217t
  myasthenia gravis, 217t
  nurse collaboration for, 232
  Parkinson's disease. *See* Parkinson's disease
  physical therapy collaboration for, 232
  physician collaboration for, 232
  polymyositis, 218t
  social worker collaboration for, 232
  speech-language therapy collaboration for, 232
  spinal cord injury, 218t, 319
  stroke. *See* Stroke
  task-oriented approaches to, 222–224
  theories and practice frameworks for, 221–224
  traumatic brain injury, 220
Neuromotor function
  definition of, 211
  upper extremity, 215
Neuromotor system
  age-related changes in, 212–216
  balance, 213–214, 214b
  coordination, 214–215
  descending tracts of, 211
  overview of, 211–212
  proprioception, 213
Neuromuscular system, 211–212
Neuromusculoskeletal assessment, 345
Neuropathologies
  cognitive functioning in, 254
  delirium, 244–245
  dementia. *See* Dementia
  mild cognitive impairment, 245
Neuroplasticity theories, 39
Neuropsychologist, 92
Newest Vital Sign, 300t
NMDA receptors, 39
Nonbinary, 68t
Noncommunicable diseases (NCD), 123–125, 124t
Nondeclarative memory, 239
Nonformal learning, 315
Nonmaleficence, 80
Nonrapid eye movement (NREM) sleep, 298
Nonsmall cell lung cancer (NSCLC), 153
Non-ST elevation myocardial infarction (NSTEMI), 151
Nonstandardized assessments, 371

Nuclear family, 357
Nurse
  in acute care, 421
  in interprofessional team, 92
Nursing aides, 421
Nursing home care. *See also* Long-term care services
  care goals in, 475
  chronic disease in, 468
  COVID-19 pandemic effects on, 504–505
  custodial care, 468
  description of, 467–468
  Medicare reimbursement for, 477
  residents of, 468, 470
  risk factors for placement in, 468
  skilled care, 468
  state regulations regarding, 478
Nutrients, recommended, 106
Nutrition
  aging effects on, 105–108
  assessment of, 108, 301t
  environmental factors that affect, 108
  factors that affect, 133
  influencers of, 106–107
  interventions for, 109, 303–304
  resources for, 101b
  self-care effects on, 266
  wellness affected by, 390, 395–396

O

Obesity
  cancer risks, 128–129
  coronary heart disease and, 126
  lung dysfunction associated with, 129
  sarcopenic, 190
Objects, as symbolic, 29
Occupation(s)
  activity analysis for, 103
  becoming dimension of, 21
  being dimension of, 21
  belonging dimension of, 21
  creative, 25, 27
  cultural relevance of, 24
  dimensions of, 21
  doing dimension of, 21
  drive for, 25
  driving as, 338–340
  factors that interfere with, 21
  in health management, 294, 295t
  late-life, 24
  meaning and, 20–21, 26
  meaningfulness in, 269. *See also* Meaningful occupations
  metabolic equivalent levels of, 157t
  purpose for, 25
  religious, 24
  social participation as, 65
  spiritual, 24
  theory of, 25–26
Occupation Centered Intervention Assessment (OCIA), 508
Occupational adaptation theory, 44, 392
Occupational deprivation, 314
Occupational justice, 12
Occupational Justice Framework (OJF), 12
Occupational meaning, 22–24
Occupational performance, 370
Occupational performance assessment tools, 301t

Occupational performance evaluation
  assessments used in, 370–372
  ethical considerations in, 372–373
  importance of, 370
  overview of, 369–370
  social participation, 376
Occupational Performance Measure of Food Activities (OPMF), 133
Occupational profile, 26, 159, 469
Occupational Questionnaire, 316–317
Occupational therapists
  in acute care, 419–422, 424
  adaptability of, 406
  aging in place supported by, 8
  assumptions made by, 49
  consultant role of, 407
  Expanded Chronic Care Model and, 405
  function of, 3
  generalist role of, 407
  health literacy promotion by, 7–8
  in interprofessional team, 92, 408
  moral distress by, 90
  in patient-centered medical home, 407
  personality characteristics of, 406
  primary care role of, 406–408
  telehealth use by, 506–507
  visual impairment interventions, 173b
Occupational therapy
  in acute care, 419–422
  client outcomes of, 330
  as direct care, 388–389
  driving and, 342–343
  future implications for, 512
  in home health, 453
  in hospice care, 487–488
  intrusionary, 408
  Kawa model of, 44
  lifestyle-based, 202b
  in long-term care services, 469
  meaning supported during, 25–29
  in palliative care, 487–488
  rehabilitation and, 441
  service delivery types for, 402–403
Occupational Therapy Driver Off-Road Assessment battery, 373
Occupational therapy interventions
  in acute care setting, 431
  Cancer Home-Life Intervention, 492, 494, 494t
  chronic condition management, 393
  cognitive activities, 394
  communication in health care system, 302–303
  co-occupation and, 27–28
  dementia, 247–249
  falls, 116–117, 303
  health promotion, management, and maintenance focus of, 392–393
  in home health, 459–460
  in long-term care, 473t, 473–476
  medication management, 103–104, 303
  mental health, 253–254
  models that guide, 391–392
  nutrition management, 303–304
  oral health, 105
  personal device management, 304
  physical activity, 303
  postamputation, 200
  religious meanings, 28

resource-oriented intervention, 494–495, 495t–496t
sleep, 301–305
social activities, 394
spiritual meanings, 28
steps involved in, 473
stroke, 250
symptom and condition management, 302
Occupational Therapy Practice Framework (OTPF)
advocacy, 479
cardiopulmonary conditions, 155–156
description of, 13, 24, 26, 42–43, 90, 373, 469
interventions, 157b
leisure in, 332
sleep and rest, 135
Occupational value, 21
Occupation-based theories and models, 43–44
Occupation-Centered Intervention Assessment (OCIA), 474, 474f
Older adult(s)
ageism of, 52–53
in agrarian cultures, 5
categorization of, 4
cohort effects, 5
in COVID-19 pandemic, 54, 81–82
definition of, 323
demographic changes in, 504
domestic migration of, 9
geographic location effects on, 8
health care access for, 53–56, 93
historical roles of, 5
at home, 8
homelessness in, 9
identity of, 51
institutionalization of, 9, 12
international migration of, 9
justice for, 12
laws and policy that affect, 80–81
Levinson's stages for, 22
LGBTQIA+, 67–69
media portrayal of, 10, 52–53
multimorbidity in, 188, 408–409
in Native American groups, 5
physical environment effects on, 8–9
population growth of, 4, 80–81, 85
protective factors for, 11
recommended nutrients for, 106
in rural environments, 8, 349
in same-gendered relationships, 70
sleep in, 298–299
societal trends that affect, 504
sociocultural factors that affect, 9–10
stereotypes of, 10
in suburban environments, 8
transition stage for, 22
in urban environments, 7–8
Older Adult Disaster Preparation Booklet, 288
Older Adult Technology Services (OATS), 505b
Older Americans Act (OAA), 81, 359–360, 385, 396
Older men
loneliness in, 11
older women versus, 11
Older women. *See also* Women
bone density changes in, 106
older men versus, 11
social support among, 65
widowhood in, 67

Older workers
barriers to continued employment faced by, 327–328
benefits of using, 324
caregiving by, 325
culture and, 324–325
demographics of, 324–325
ergonomic for, 331
legislative issues for, 329–330
policy issues for, 329–330
reaction time of, 325
in workforce, factors that affect, 326b
Oldest-old, 4, 9
Olfactory sense, 133, 176–177
Opioids, for osteoarthritis, 196
OPTIMAL, 411
Optimal experiences, 20
Optimization, 38
Oral cancer, 104–105
Oral health
aging and, 104–105
assessment of, 105
diseases that affect, 104
interventions for, 105
resources for, 101b
Oral hygiene, 472
Organ of Corti, 174, 174f
Organizational health literacy, 295–296
Orthotics, 426
Osteoarthritis (OA), 195–197, 342
Osteoblasts, 192
Osteoclasts, 192
Osteoporosis, 197–199
Ottawa Charter for Health Promotion, 295, 393
Outcome and Assessment Information Set (OASIS), 458, 461
Outcome expectation, 202
Outer ear, 174f
Outpatient rehabilitation, 439
Outreach services, 402
Overactive bladder, 110
Overflow incontinence, 110
Oxidative stress, 126
Oxygen management training, 158
Oxygen saturation, 161

P
PACE centers, 386
Pacemaker, 152b
Pacinian corpuscles, 179
Pain
aging and, 180–181
assessment of, 181–182
cold therapy for, 182
definition of, 180
heat therapy for, 182
interventions for, 182, 346
medications for, 182
nonpharmacological treatments for, 182
perception of, 181, 181b
phantom limb, 200
treatment affected by, 181
Pain behaviors, 182
Pain management
in acute care, 425–426
at end-of-life, 84t
Pain rating scales, 182

Palliative care
activities of daily living in, 487–488
adaptive approaches for, 498
advocacy for, 498–499
definition of, 485b
description of, 84t, 483–484
documentation in, 495
duration of, 484
existential dimensions, 489
funding for, 495
grief in, 490–491
health policy in, 497
integrated care pathways in, 497
interprofessional partners in, 488–489
interventions in, 491–495, 495t–497t
occupational therapy in, 487–488
older adult needs in, 489–490
payment systems for, 495, 497–498
physical dimensions, 489
priorities for, 497–498
psychological dimensions, 489
resource-oriented intervention in, 494–495, 495t–496t
social dimensions, 489
World Health Organization guidelines for, 484–485
Palliative occupational therapy, 487
Palliative sedation, 84t
Paratransit, 339f, 349
Parenchyma, lung, 148–149
Parkinson's disease
dance participation benefits in, 303
description of, 39, 213
driving performance and, 342
eating challenges associated with, 133
interventions for, 228t, 231
management of, 220–221
motor manifestations of, 220, 221f, 221t–222t
resting tremor associated with, 220, 221t
rigidity associated with, 220, 221t
sexuality affected by, 71–72
social worker collaboration for, 232
visual impairments caused by, 171
Participation, 42
Participation restrictions, 42
Patient Driven Groupings Model (PDGM), 461–462
Patient Driven Payment Model (PDPM), 478
Patient navigation, 405
Patient-centered care, 408, 421
Patient-centered medical home (PCMH), 402, 407
Payment systems
for acute care, 430
for home health care, 461–462
for long-term care services, 477–478
for palliative care, 495, 497–498
for primary care, 412
for wellness services, 396
Peak bone mass (PBM), 192
Pelvic floor muscle training (PFMT), 111–112
Pensions, 10–11
Perceived control, 24
Perceived exertion, 150t, 161
Perception, 165
Performance Analysis of Driving Ability, 345
Performance Assessment of Self-Care Skills (PASS), 271, 285t, 300t
Performance capacity, 131–132

Performance skills, 339
Periodontal disease, 104–105
Peripheral artery disease (PAD), 199
Peripheral vision, 170
Personal activities of daily living (PADLs), 487–488
Personal device management, 304
Personal health beliefs, 55–56
Personal health literacy, 7–8, 295
Personal value, 269
Personality, aging and, 38, 38t
Personality trait explanations, 38
Person-centered care, 286, 470
Person-environment fit, 39
Person-Environment-Occupation (PEO) model
　dehydration causes, 107t
　description of, 40t, 43, 99
　hydration, 108
　malnutrition causes, 107t
　neuromuscular/neuromotor conditions, 225
　occupational profile, 103
　occupational therapy interventions, 134t
Person-Environment-Occupation-Performance (PEOP) model, 43, 132, 283, 283t, 299
Phantom limb pain, 200
Pharmacist
　in acute care, 421
　in interprofessional team, 92
Pharmacodynamics, 103
Pharmacokinetics, 102
Phased retirement, 326
Phonemic regression, 175
Physiatrist, 438–439
Physical abuse, 86t
Physical activity. *See also* Exercise
　age-related changes reduced through, 146
　assessment tools for, 301t
　cardiovascular disease risk reductions through, 134
　cognitive functioning affected by, 253
　during COVID-19 pandemic, 315
　guidelines for older adults, 198, 203
　interventions for, 303
　in later life, 26
　lifestyle-related noncommunicable diseases associated with lack of, 124t
　metabolic equivalent levels of, 157t, 157–158
　metabolic syndrome risk reductions through, 134
　physical health affected by, 504
　programs for, 395
　sarcopenia and, 134
　subjective scales of exertion responses, 150t
　in type 2 diabetes mellitus, 130
　wellness through, 390, 394–395
Physical Activity Scale for the Elderly, 376
Physical environment
　aging affected by, 8–9
　aging in place, 8–9
　place of residence, 8
　sleep affected by, 135
Physical function, 189f
Physical therapists
　description of, 331
　in home health, 453–454
　in interprofessional team, 92
Physical therapy
　in home health, 453–454
　Medicare payment for, 478
　in neuromotor rehabilitation, 232

Physical touch, 69–70
Physically dependent individuals, 188
Physically elite individuals, 188
Physically fit individuals, 188
Physically frail individuals, 188
Physically independent individuals, 188
Physician
　driving cessation and, 348b
　in interprofessional team, 92
Physician Orders for Life-Sustaining Treatment (POLST), 83t
Physiological age, 441–442
Pilates, 112
Pillbox Test, 103
Pill-rolling tremor, 221t
Pittsburgh Sleep Quality Index, 301t
Place
　aging in, 8–9, 29–30, 282
　home as, 29
Place integration, 40, 40t
Place of residence, 8
Pleurocentesis, 154b
PLISSIT communication, 73
Pneumonectomy, 154b
Pneumonia, 153
Pneumothorax, 153
Political economy of aging perspective, 41, 42t
POLST forms, 83t
Polymyositis, 218t
Population aging, 44
Population health, 44
Positionality, 51
Positive aging, 4, 12, 202, 264
Positive attitudes, 9, 12
Positive Education about Aging and Contact Experiences (PEACE) model, 10, 82
Positive psychology, 20
Posterior cerebral artery, 219t
Posterior inferior cerebral artery, 219t
Postural balance evaluation, 113
Postural control, 213, 214b. *See also* Balance
Postural instability, 216, 221t
Postural stability, 214
Postural sway, 227
Poverty
　gender differences in, 11
　Social Security effects on, 10
Practice Framework–OTPF 4th edition, 264
Predictive assessments, 371
Predictive validity, 372t
Premature ventricular contractions, 136
Presbycusis, 173, 175
Presbyopia, 167
Prescription reading glasses, 173t
Pressure, 179
Pressure ulcers, 426
Preventative Correction Proactive Model, 392
Primary care
　advocacy for, 412–413
　chronic conditions managed in, 362
　definition of, 402
　documentation in, 412
　Expanded Chronic Care Model for, 405, 406f, 407t
　functional assessment in, 409
　interprofessional partners in, 407–408
　models of, 402

　occupational therapists' role in, 406–408
　patient-centeredness in, 408–409
　payment systems in, 412
　rehabilitation professionals and services integrated into, 402–404
　reimbursement in, 412, 413t
　team-based care for, 408
　theoretical frameworks and approaches for, 403–406
Primary health care
　access to, 404
　definition of, 402
　occupational therapy approach, 405
Primary open-angle glaucoma (POAG), 170
Primary prevention, 359f
Problem-solving
　ethical, 91f
　interventions that promote, 136
Procedural memory, 239
Process of aging, 36
Productivity, ethics of, 82–83
Programmed longevity, 37, 37t
Programmed theories, of aging, 36–37
Progressive resistance training, 204b
PROMIS Global Health, 301t
Pronouns, 67
Proprioception, 213
Proprioceptive neuromuscular facilitation (PNF), 204, 221
Prospective memory, 239
Prospective Payment System (PPS), 478
Protein, 106
Proteoglycans, 193t
Proximal determinant, 38t
Proximal level of environment, 50, 50t, 51f
Psychological theories, of aging, 37–38, 38t
Psychological well-being, 266
Psychometric properties, 371, 372t
Psychosocial health, 488
Public policies
　description of, 10
　for family caregiver support, 359–360, 360t
　health care access affected by, 10
Public transportation, 339f, 349
Pulmonary conditions
　acute respiratory distress syndrome, 153–154
　assessment of, 156b
　chronic obstructive pulmonary disease, 129, 153
　interstitial lung disease, 153
　lung cancer, 153
　nonsurgical interventions for, 154, 154b
　practice frameworks for, 155–156
　pulmonary edema, 154
　screening for, 156b
　surgical interventions for, 154, 154b
　treatment of, 156–161
Pulmonary disease
　aging and, 129
　description of, 153
Pulmonary edema, 154
Pulmonary embolism, 154
Pulmonary fibrosis, 153
Pulmonary system
　age-related changes in, 129, 148
　functions of, 148
Pulmonary transplant, 154b
Pulse oximetry, 161

Purpose, 20
Pursed-lip breathing, 158

Q

Quality of life
  areas important to, 9
  assessment of, 472t
  co-occupation and, 21
  occupation and, 21
  promotion of, 202
  urinary incontinence effects on, 111
Quality of Life in Neurological Disorders (Neuro-QOL), 271

R

Race
  amputation and, 199
  health disparities, 56
  life expectancy based on, 5
Range of motion (ROM)
  in acute care settings, 426
  assessment of, 201, 225, 226t
  flexibility-specific interventions for increasing, 204b
  interventions for, 227–228
Rapid Clinical Test for Delirium Detection, 244
Rapid eye movement (REM) sleep, 298
Rapid Pace Walk, 345
Reactive control, 115
Reading glasses, 173t
Reasonable and necessary therapy services, 457
Receptive aphasia, 232
Reciprocity, 65
Recognize, Assist, Include, Support, and Engage (RAISE) Family Caregivers Act, 360
Refractive errors, 167
Rehabilitation
  advocacy for, 446–447
  in ambulatory care, 439
  in Australia, 446
  in Canada, 446
  case management in, 444–445
  cognitive impairment effects on, 442
  comorbidities that affect, 442–443
  comprehensive geriatric assessment in, 443–444
  in day-care programs, 439–440
  definition of, 435
  dementia effects on, 442
  depression effects on, 442
  documentation of, 445
  environmental factors that affect, 443
  frailty effects on, 442
  geriatric, 438b
  grief effects on, 442
  after hospitalization, 471
  inpatient, 437–439
  integrated care models in, 444
  interprofessional partners in, 441
  Medicare funding of, 446, 477
  motivation in, 442
  occupational therapy in, 441
  outpatient, 439
  overview of, 435–436
  payment systems for, 446
  personal factors that affect, 441–443
  pre-existing disability effects on, 442–443
  process of, 435f
  reimbursement for, 446, 477
  restorative, 438b
  service contexts for, 436–441
  skill training for, 272–273
  in skilled nursing facilities, 439
  social determinants of health and, 443
  telerehabilitation, 440
  in transitional care, 439
  in United States, 446
Rehabilitation aides, 421
Rehabilitation counselors, 331–332
Rehabilitation technicians, 421
Reimbursement
  for acute care, 430
  for home health care, 460–462
  for long-term care services, 477–478
  for primary care, 412, 413t
  for rehabilitation, 446
  for wellness services, 396
Relaxation, 136, 182
Reliability, 371, 372t
Religion
  meaning and, 24
  occupations, 24
  religious interventions, 28
Reminiscence, 27
Remodeling, of bone, 192–193
Residence, 8, 452
Resident-centered care, 470
Residual volume, 149
Resilience, 390
Resistance exercises, 203–204
Resource Utilization Groups (RUGs), 478
Resource-oriented intervention, 494–495, 495t–496t
Respiratory system, 129
Respiratory therapists, 421
Respite care, 360
Rest periods, 245, 301t
Resting tremor, 220, 221t
Restoration, 224
Restorative care, 471–472
Restorative rehabilitation, 438b
Restricted social networks, 64
Retirement
  adaptation to, 327
  adjustment to, 327
  aging and, 326
  assessments, 330
  assistive technologies for, 331
  Atchley's stages of, 327, 327b
  cultural perspectives on, 328
  cultural variations in, 328
  first responder retirement transition planning, 330–331
  generational perspectives on, 328
  global variations in, 328
  health conditions effect on, 325
  interprofessional collaboration for, 331–332
  interventions for, 330–331
  legislative issues regarding, 329–330
  models of, 326–328
  overview of, 323
  phased, 326
  policy issues regarding, 329–330
  satisfaction with, 327
  statistics regarding, 324
  theoretical approaches to, 327
  transition to, 326–328, 328f
  work-ending phase before, 326
Reverse mentoring, 10
Rheumatoid arthritis, 71, 268, 342
Right-sided heart failure, 151b
Rigidity, 220, 221t
Risky sexual behaviours, 72
Rivermead Behavioural Memory Test, 376
Road Scholar, 316
Robotics, 511
Roles, 25
Rural environments
  caregiving in, 511
  description of, 8
  health needs in, 504
  health outcomes affected by, 55
  social isolation in, 349

S

Saccades, 171
SAFER-Home V3, 285t
Safety
  home. *See* Home safety
  self-care effects on, 266
Safety Assessment of Function and Environment for Rehabilitation Health Outcome Measurement and Evaluation Version 3 (SAFER-HOME), 374
Same-gendered relationships, 70
Sarcoidosis, 153
Sarcopenia, 134, 190–191, 191f, 424
Sarcopenic obesity, 190
Satisfaction With Life Scale (SWLS), 26
Saunders, Cicely, 484
Schizophrenia, 251
Scotomas, 171
Secondary hypertension, 127
Secondary prevention, 359f
Section 188 of the Workforce Investment Act of 1988 (WIA), 81t
Section GG, 458
Sedentary behavior, 134–135
Selection, optimization, and compensation (SOC) model, 29
Selective attention, 238
Selective optimization with compensation theory, of aging, 38, 38t, 313
Self Determination Theory of Motivation (SDT), 269
Self-care
  arthritis effects on, 268
  assessments, 472t
  assistive devices for, 274
  cardiovascular disease effects on, 267
  cognitive impairment effects on, 271
  competence in, 269–270
  deficits in, 271
  definition of, 264
  dementia effects on, 268
  environment effects on, 269
  evaluation of, 271
  goal setting for, 272
  health conditions that affect, 267–269
  hearing loss effects on, 268–269
  joint inflammation effects on, 268

meaning in, 269–270
nutrition affected by, 266
overview of, 263
practical importance of, 266
psychological well-being affected by, 266
safety affected by, 266
self-identity through, 266
sensory problems that affect, 268–269
significance of, 265
smell sense effects on, 269
stroke effects on, 267
task modifications for, 274
touch sense effects on, 269
value in, 269–270
Self-efficacy, 24, 131, 202, 391
Self-identity, 266
Self-management
  of chronic disease, 411–412
  description of, 125, 159
  programs for, 302, 403
Self-reward value, 23
Semantic memory, 239
Senescence, 36
Senile miosis, 168
Senior centers, 384–385, 386b, 388t
Sensorineural hearing loss, 174
Sensory deficit theory, 243
Sensory function deficits, 271
Sensory memory, 239
Sensory problems
  health management affected by, 296
  self-care affected by, 268–269
  vision impairment. See Visual impairments
Sensory systems. See also Hearing; Smell sense; Taste sense; Vision
  age-related changes in, 166t, 376–377
  impairments in, 166
  interprofessional collaboration for, 182–183
  physiology of, 165–166
Serum plasma water osmolality, 108
Sex, 68t
Sex hormones, 71
Sexual abuse, 86t
Sexual dysfunction, 70–72
Sexuality
  age-related changes that affect, 70–72, 71t
  cognitive behavioral changes that affect, 72
  consent issues for, 72
  living environment considerations, 72
  in long term care facilities, 72
  medications that affect, 72
  metabolic changes that affect, 71
  musculoskeletal changes that affect, 71
  neuromotor changes that affect, 71–72
  Parkinson's disease and, 71–72
  rheumatoid arthritis effects on, 71
  well-being and, 70
Shivering, 180
Short-term memory, 239
Shoulder subluxation, 217, 219, 220f
Sierra Club, 332
Silent generation, 5, 6t
Simple reaction time (SRT), 214
Sit-and-reach test, 201
Sit-to-stand test, 202
Situational model of care, 40, 40f, 40t
Six-Minute Walk Test, 375

Skeletal muscle, 191–192
Skeletal system, 192–193
Skill acquisition, 223t
Skill training
  for activities of daily living, 272–273
  task-specific, 286–287
Skilled care, 468
Skilled nursing, 454, 457
Skilled nursing facilities (SNFs), 439, 446, 471
Skills2Care, 317
Skin
  age-related changes in, 179–180
  anatomy of, 179
"Skipped generation," 512
Sleep
  assessment of, 299, 301t
  chronic health conditions and, 299
  cognitive-behavioral interventions for, 304
  daily requirements, 298
  enhancement of, 245
  environmental modifications for, 304–305
  importance of, 298
  inadequate, 298
  interventions for, 299, 301–305
  metabolic syndrome risk reduction with, 135–136
  multicomponent interventions for, 305
  nonrapid eye movement, 298
  in older adults, 298–299
  in palliative care, 488
  parameters for, 135b
  poor-quality, daytime occupational performance affected by, 298–299
  rapid eye movement, 298
  recommendations for, 135
Sleep deprivation, 299
Sleep diary, 301t
Sleep education, 304
Sleep efficiency, 135b, 304
Sleep hygiene, 304
Sleep latency, 135b
Slow-twitch muscle fibers, 191
Smart homes, 510
Smart watches, 287
Smell sense
  age-related changes in, 166t
  losses in, 177
  self-care affected by declines in, 269
Smoking
  cardiovascular system affected by, 126
  chronic obstructive pulmonary disease risks, 129
Snellen acuity, 169
"Snowbirding," 9
Social breakdown/competence theory, 41
Social connections
  description of, 64
  maintaining of, 65
Social constructionist perspective, 41, 42t
Social constructivism, 41
Social determinants of health (SDOH)
  ageism effects on, 80–81
  definition of, 7, 295
  description of, 3, 7–8
  examples of, 295
  health outcomes affected by, 295
  health status affected by, 7
  negative, 7

rehabilitation affected by, 443
wellness promotion affected by, 390
Social engagement, 22
Social environments
  sleep affected by, 135
  technology in, 509–511
Social exchange theory, 41, 42t
Social gerontology, 36
Social health, 301–302
Social interaction, 22
Social isolation, 7, 69, 135, 347, 390
Social justice, 12, 314–315
Social networks
  characteristics of, 64–65
  composition of, 64–65
  description of, 64
  diverse, 64
  diversity of, 65
  family-focused, 64
  friend-focused, 64
  loss of, in COVID-19 pandemic, 65
  restricted, 64
Social participation, 65, 376
Social relationships
  description of, 64
  grandparenting, 66
  maintaining of, 65
  reciprocity for, 65
  spousal, 67
  widowhood and, 67
Social robotics, 511
Social Security, 10
Social Security Act (SSA), 80
Social Security Amendments Act, 80
Social support
  definition of, 65
  health affected by, 282
  health management affected by, 297
  immediate, 443
  types of, 282
Social worker
  in acute care, 421
  in home health, 454
  in interprofessional team, 92, 332
  in neuromotor rehabilitation, 232
  services offered by, 332
Socialization
  description of, 253
  programs for, 394t
Societal level of environment, 50, 50t, 51f
Society
  cultural perceptions of aging in, 52–53
  health care access in, 53–54
  living arrangements affected by, 504–505
  trends in, aging affected by, 504
Sociocultural factors, 9–10
Socioeconomic status (SES)
  cognitive function affected by, 11
  health management affected by, 297
  of neighborhood, 54–55
Socioemotional selectivity theory, of aging, 38, 38t, 313
Sociological theories, of aging, 41–44, 42t
Somatic mutation theory, 37, 37t
Somatosensory input, 165
Somesthesis, 179–180
SPEACS program, 429

Specialty Certificate in Driving and Community Mobility (SCDCM), 343
Speech discrimination, 175
Speech perception, 175
Speech therapy
 in home health, 454
 in neuromotor rehabilitation, 232
Speech-language pathologists, 421, 454, 470
Speed of processing theory, 243
Spinal cord injury (SCI), 218t, 319
Spiritual History Scale in Four Dimensions, 26
Spiritual interventions, 27–28
Spiritual occupations, 24
Spirituality, 24
Spirituality Index of Well-Being, 26
Splinting, 426–427
Spousal relationships, 67
Staff shortages, 508–509
Standardized assessments, 371, 372t
Start of care, 455, 458
Static stretching, 204
Statins, 152b
Staying-active programs, 395
ST-elevation myocardial infarction (STEMI), 151
Stereotypes
 ageism as, 52–54
 description of, 9–10
Sternotomy, 152b
Stigmatization, 56
Stopping Elderly Accidents, Deaths and Injuries (STEADI) initiative, 113, 114f–115f
Storytelling, 27
Strength and Vulnerability Integration (SAVI) model, 82
Strength exercises, 203–204, 204b
Stress incontinence, 110
Stress management, 156b
Stress Management Questionnaire, 156b
Stressful listening conditions, 175
Stretching exercises, 204
Stroke
 brain areas affected by, 216, 218f
 cognitive deficits caused by, 249
 cognitive functioning affected by, 249
 comorbidities in, 127
 constraint-induced movement therapy after, 220, 224
 definition of, 216
 description of, 217t
 hypertension as risk factor for, 127
 interprofessional collaboration for, 250
 interventions for, 228t
 ischemic, 127
 limb impairment contralateral to, 216
 motor relearning after, 224
 neuromotor impairments after, 216–217
 neuromotor manifestations of, 219–220
 occupational therapy interventions for, 250
 positioning for, 228, 229f
 rehabilitation for, 219–220, 250, 267
 risk factors for, 128b
 self-care abilities affected by, 267
 shoulder subluxation associated with, 217, 219, 220f
 signs and symptoms of, 219t
 upper extremity task training for, 231
 upper limb function assessments after, 227

Structural ageism, 53–54
Subjective usefulness, 23
Subjective well-being, 23
Substance use disorders (SUDs), 252
Suburban environments, 8
Suicide, 11
Superficial sensation, 166t
Supplemental oxygen (O_2) therapy, 154b
Supportive living environments, 135
Sustained attention, 238
Sweat glands, 180
Sweden, 4
Symbolic value, 23
Synovial joints, 194
Systems Engineering Initiative for Patient Safety (SEIPS) 3.0 model, 507
Systole, 147f
Systolic blood pressure, 126
Systolic heart failure, 151b

T

Tai chi chuan, 303, 395
Tailored Activity Program (TAP), 248–249
Task adaptation, 286
Task Force on Elder Abuse, 87–88
Task modifications, 274
Task performance, 230–231
Task-oriented approaches, 222–224, 283
Task-specific skill training, 286–287
Taste receptors, 177
Taste sense
 age-related changes in, 166t, 176–177
 losses in, 177
 self-care affected by declines in, 269
Teach-back method, 303
Team-based care, 408
TeamSTEPPS 2.0, 508
Technology
 activities of daily living monitoring using, 510
 assistive. See Assistive technology
 gerotechnology, 331
 in health monitoring, 509–510
 in healthcare, 509–511
 robotics, 511
 service delivery uses of, 403
 smart homes, 510
 in social environments, 509–511
 transportation, 511
 wearables, 509
 for work, 331
Teleconsultation, 440
Telehealth, 403, 440, 506–507
Telemonitoring, 440
Telerehabilitation, 440
Telescopes, 173t
Teletreatment, 440
Telomeres, 37
Temperature, 179–180
Tendons, 193, 193t
Tertiary prevention, 359f
Test-retest reliability, 372t
Texas Functional Living Scale, 285t
Theories of aging
 biological, 36–37
 cognition, 38t, 38–39
 contemporary, 40, 40t

critical perspectives of aging, 41–42, 42t
 definition of, 35
 endocrine, 36–37, 37t
 environmental, 39–40, 40t
 error, 37
 foundational, 39–40
 free radicals, 37, 37t
 genetic, 37
 immunologic, 37, 37t
 life course, 42t
 life course perspective, 41
 life span development, 22, 38, 38t
 occupation-based, 43–44
 overview of, 35–36
 personality, 38, 38t
 political economy of aging, 41, 42t
 programmed, 36–37
 psychological, 37–38
 selective optimization with compensation, 38, 38t
 social constructionist perspective, 41, 42t
 social exchange, 41, 42t
 socioemotional selectivity, 38, 38t
 sociological, 41–44, 42t
Theory
 concepts and, 35
 definition of, 35
 in gerontology, 34–35
Theory of occupational adaptation, 392
Therapeutic exercises programs, for osteoarthritis, 196
Thermoreceptors, 179–180
Thermoregulation, 179–180
Thoracostomy, 154b
Thoracotomy, 154b
Thorax, 149t
Three-Item Loneliness Scale, 69
Three-stage model of motor learning, 223–224, 224t
Timed Up & Go (TUG) test, 115, 303, 371, 375
Tinetti Balance and Gait Test, 115
Tinetti Performance Oriented Mobility Assessment, 375
Tinnitus, 175
Tooth decay, 104
Total joint replacement, 196
Total pain, 485
Touch, 69–70, 179–180
Touch sense, 269
Trabecular bone, 192
Traditionalists, 6t
Trail Making Test, 172, 344–345
Transdisciplinary care, 138
Transgender, 68t
Transgender females
 hormone replacement therapy in, 71
 sexual response in, age-related changes in, 71t
Transgender males
 hormone replacement therapy in, 71
 sexual activity among, 70
 sexual response in, age-related changes in, 71t
Transition stage, 22
Transitional care, 439, 507
Transitions, 507
Transportation
 in suburban environments, 8
 technology in, 511

Transtheoretical Model (TTM)
  description of, 131
  interventions based on, 136
  positive health-related behavior changes, 131
Trauma
  limb amputation caused by, 199
  traumatic brain injury (TBI), 220, 229
Tremors, 215, 221t
Type 2 diabetes mellitus, 129–130

U

UCLA three-item loneliness scale, 300t
Undernutrition, 105
United Nations Decade of Healthy Ageing (2021–2030), 12, 13b, 389, 395
United States
  life expectancy in, 4f
  older adult population in, 4
Universal design, 331
University of the Third age (U3A), 316
Upper extremity
  fractures of, 199
  function assessment of, 226t, 227, 375, 472t
  interventions for, 229
  movement of, 215
  task training, 231
Urban environments, 8
Urge incontinence, 110
Urinary incontinence, 110–112
Urinary management, 101b
Urinary tract infection (UTI), 109–110

V

VA MISSION Act, 359–360
Validity, 371, 372t
Value, 269
Value and Meaning in Occupations (ValMO), 23
Value-based payment, 412
Valve replacements, 152b
Vascular dementia, 246
Venous thromboembolism (VTE), 71
Venous vasculature, 146
Ventricular systole, 147f
Veracity, 80, 82
Vertebral basilar artery, 219t
Vertebral fractures, 198
Video-assisted thoracoscopic surgery (VATS), 154b
Virtual care, 506–507
Vision
  6/6, 169b
  20/20, 169b
  age-related changes in, 166t
  assessment of, 171–172, 245
  central, 170
  cognitive functioning and, 243
  loss of, 170–171
  low. See Low vision
  peripheral, 170
Visual disability questionnaires, 172
Visual function
  age-related changes in, 166t, 167–168
  driving affected by, 341
Visual impairments
  in acute care setting, 427
  description of, 169, 268
  driving affected by, 341
  falls caused by, 427
  health management affected by, 296
Visual system
  age-related changes in, 166t, 167–168
  age-related macular degeneration, 169–170
  assessment of, 171–172
  cataracts, 169
  diabetic retinopathy, 170–171
  driving performance affected by, 341
  glaucoma, 170
  interventions for, 172, 173b, 173t
  low vision, 169
  occupational therapist's role with, 173b
  Parkinson disease as cause of, 171
  treatment of, 171–172
Vitamin B6, 106
Vitamin B12, 106
Vitamin D, 106, 112
Vitamin E, 106
Volition, 131–132
Volunteering/volunteerism, 24–25, 332–333

W

Wake after sleep onset, 135b
Water, 106
Wearable technology, 509
Wedge resection, 154b
Weekly Calendar Planning Activity (WCPA), 371, 376
Well-being
  in aging in place, 337
  characteristics of, 63
  late-life activities that support, 26
  lifestyle-based occupational therapy intervention for, 202b
  psychological, 266
  sexuality and, 70
  social interaction and, 22
  subjective, 23
Well-being of Older People measure (WOOP), 300t
Wellness
  adaptation and, 390
  chronic conditions and, 390
  continuum of, 384f
  definition of, 384
  direct care, 388–389
  economic stability effects on, 390
  exercise benefits for, 395
  fitness programs for, 395
  goal of, 384
  health factors that affect, 390–391
  holistic models of, 390
  hydration effects on, 390
  indirect care, 389
  interventions for, 390–396
  nutrition and, 390, 395–396
  physical activity and, 390, 394–395
  program development for, 392
  psychosocial factors that affect, 390
  resilience and, 390
  self-efficacy and, 390
  social determinants of health that affect, 390
Wellness services
  advocacy for, 396
  community-based. See Community-based wellness services
  documentation of, 396
  payment systems for, 396
  reimbursement for, 396
Wellspring Program, 475
Wernicke-Korsakoff syndrome (WKS), 252
Westmead Home Safety Assessment (WeHSA), 285t
Wet age-related macular degeneration, 170
Widowhood, 67
Wolf Motor Function Test, 375
Women. See also Older women
  as family caregivers, 356
  financial difficulties for, 11
  late-life disability in, 11
  in poverty, 11
Work
  assessments, 330
  assistive technologies for, 331
  cultural perspectives on, 328
  cultural variations in, 328
  generational perspectives on, 328
  global variations in, 328
  health conditions effect on, 325
  interprofessional collaboration for, 331–332
  interventions for, 330–331
  overview of, 323
  self-identity affected by, 324
  technology for, 331
Work Environment and Impact Scale (WEIS), 330
Workbooks, 26
Work-ending phase, 326
Worker Role Interview (WRI), 330
Workforce Investment Act of 1988, Section 188 of, 81t
Working memory, 239, 243, 296
World Federation of Occupational Therapists (WFOT), 389, 391, 403
World Health Organization (WHO)
  Disability Assessment Schedule 2.0, 13, 271
  elder abuse statistics, 85
  health as defined by, 294, 384
  healthy aging as defined by, 504
  International Classification of Functioning, Disability, and Health. See International Classification of Functioning, Disability, and Health (ICF)
  interprofessional collaboration as defined by, 138
  Ottawa Charter for Health Promotion, 295
  palliative care guidelines, 484–485
  physical activity recommendations, 134
  poor nutritional status criteria, 105
  social determinants of health, 7
World War II, 5, 10

X

Xerosis, 179
Xerostomia, 104

Y

Yoga, 112, 303
Youngest-old, 4, 9

Z

Zoom, 511